facts and comparisons

nurses drug facts™

1997

AF886094

facts and comparisons

In Collaboration With

ANA

AMERICAN NURSES ASSOCIATION

Nurses Drug Facts™, 1997 Edition

ISBN 1-57439-000-7

ISBN 1-57439-002-3 (*Nurses Drug Facts* Reference Set)
ISBN 1-57439-001-5 (*Patient Drug Information*)

Printed in the United States of America

Published by
Facts and Comparisons
111 West Port Plaza, Suite 300
St. Louis, Missouri 63146-3098
314/878-2515
Toll free customer service 800/223-0554

Editor

David S. Tatro, PharmD
Drug Information Consultant
San Francisco, CA

Assistant Editors

Larry R. Borgsdorf, PharmD
Pharmacist Specialist
Ambulatory Care
Kaiser Permanente
Bakersfield, CA

Joseph T. Catalano, RN, CCRN, PhD
Professor of Nursing
East Central University
Ada, OK

Jennifer C. Lahl, RN, BSN
Children's Hospital Oakland
Nursing Administration
Oakland, CA

Julio R. Lopez, PharmD
Director of Drug Information
VA Medical Center
Martinez, CA

Kristina Frederick, RN, BSN, BA, MS
Emergency Department
Johns Hopkins Hospital
Baltimore, MD

Stephanie G. Metzger, MS, RNC, CPNP
Clinical Nurse Specialist
Nursing-Rehabilitation Coordinator
Children's Hospital
Richmond, VA

Marilyn Nelsen Pase, RN, MSN
Department of Nursing
New Mexico State University
Las Cruces, NM

Contributors

Jill E. Allen, PharmD, BCPS, Drug Information Consultant, Pin Oak Associates (UT)
Gloria Arthur, RN, MSN, Nursing Administration, Decatur General Hospital (AL)
Paul Badore, RPh, Drug Information Consultant (CT)
Sandra L. Beaird, PharmD, Drug Information Specialist, St. Louis College of Pharmacy (MO)
Renee Bellanger, PharmD, Department of Pharmacy, Methodist Women's and Children's Hospital (TX)
Juanita Bowsher, RNC, CS, PhD, Nursing Consultant (GA)
Lita A. Burns, RN, MSN, Allied Health, Central Wyoming College
Barbara Walsh Clark RN, MSN, BSN Completion Program, Midway College (KY)
Rebecca M. Coley, MS, PharmD, Assistant Director, National Center for Computer Education and Research in Healthcare, St. Louis College of Pharmacy (MO)
Joan W. Conklin, RNC, EdD, Presbyterian Division of Nursing, Bloomfield College (NJ)
Deborah Crawford, RN, BSN, CCRN, Nursing Resources, Hillcrest Center (OK)
Jolene M. Culbertson, MN, ARNP, CS, Nursing Instructor, Pacific Lutheran University (WA)
JoAnn Dever, RN, MSNEd, Health and Human Services (Chair), Indiana Vocational Technical College
Janet Duffy Dionne, RN, MS, Associate Professor, Nursing-Health and Human Services, Community College of Denver (CO)
Michael N. Dipirro, PharmD, Office of Mental Health, Western New York Regional Office
Carol Flom, BSN, MEd, MS, Mental Health Staff Nurse, Abbott Northwestern Hospital
Carolyn A. Gatschet, RN, MN, MS, Associate Professor of Nursing, Fort Hays State University (KS)
Diana Girdley, RN, MSN, School of Nursing, University of Wisconsin-Madison
John D. Grabenstein, BS, MS, EdM, FASHP, Major, Medical Service Corps, US Army (NC)
Sheila C. Grossman, RN, PhD, School of Nursing, Fairfield University (CT)
John W. Grunden, PharmD, Department of Pharmacy Services, University of Utah Hospital
Geneal E. Hall, RN, PhD, Department of Nursing, Jamestown College (ND)
Rebecca A. Hampton-Abelita, RN, MSN, Instructor, Miles Community College (MT)
Holly K. Hill, RN, Office of Managed Care, University of Utah Health Sciences Center
Mivic Hirose, RN, MS, Department of Nursing, San Francisco General Hospital Medical Center (CA)
Naomi B. Ingrim, PharmD, Specialist, Central Texas Poison Center
Tracy Kelly, RN, MSN, CPNP, Department of Pediatric Hematology-Oncology, Yale New Haven Hospital (CT)
Deborah L. Kern, RN, MSN, CCRN, Adjunct Assistant Professor, Montana State University

Jennifer Menchini Kirby, RN, MSN, Vice President of Nursing, Southern Maryland Hospital Center

Joan Klemballa, RN, PhD, School of Nursing & Health Sciences, The College of West Virginia

Barbara Konopka, RN, MSN, DNSc (CAND), CCRN, CEN, School of Nursing, Pennsylvania State University

Patricia Little, RN, MSN, Assistant Professor, University of Nevada

Jon E. Maesner, PharmD, Assistant Vice President, Clinical Pharmacy, Managed Pharmacy Division, CIGNA Healthcare (CT)

Jacqueline Mangnall, RN, MS, Nursing Department, Jamestown College (ND)

Grace Matthews, RN, BSN, Nurse Manager, University of Iowa Hospitals and Clinics

Kathleen S. Nance, PharmD, Consultant Pharmacist (LA)

Cindy Newman, RN, Medical-Surgical Department, University of Utah

Richard Oksas, PharmD, MPh, Medication Information Service (CA)

Cynthia A. Padula, PhD, RN, CS, College of Nursing, University of Rhode Island

Mary B. Pava, MSN, RN, Department of Nursing, Lincoln Memorial University (TN)

Pamela Pranke, RNC, MSN, Department of Nursing, Jamestown College (ND)

Jean Quiggle, RPh, BS Pharm, Compu-Dose Pharmacies (VA)

Teresa L. Rittenbach, RN, MS, CGNP, Assistant Professor of Nursing, Jamestown College (ND)

Maureen G. Roussel, RN, MSN, CCRN, CS, Cardiothoracic Clinical Nurse Specialist, Yale New Haven Hospital (CT)

Nichola Fay Rowden, MSN, RN, Department of Nursing, East Arkansas Community College

Alice F. Running, PhD, RN, MSN, CS, ANP, School of Nursing, University of Nevada - Reno

Victoria A. Sand, BSN, RN, Department of Nursing, Jamestown College (ND)

Alice Serey, RN, MSN, Associate Degree Nursing-Chair, Indian River Community College (FL)

Carol Shaw, RN, BSN, Instructor, Southeastern Community College (IA)

Donald S. Swanson, BA, BSN, RN, Psychiatric Nursing, University of Iowa Hospitals and Clinics

Burgunda V. Sweet, PharmD, Department of Pharmacy Services, University of Michigan Hospitals

Lisa Walworth, RPh, BS Pharm, Pharmacist II, Buffalo Psychiatric Center (NY)

Mary P. Watkins, PhD, RN, Department of Nursing, Delaware State University

Cora D. H. West, MSN, RN, Home Healthcare Consultant (IN)

Rosemarie C. Westberg, RN, MSN, CPN, Professor of Nursing, Northern Virginia Community College

Kaye M. Wothe, RN, BSN, CRNI, Staff Nurse, Coram Home Infusion (OR)

Rita M. Yeager, RN, MA, MSN, Professor, Chair Health Science, West Virginia Northern Community College

Doris I. Young, RN, MSN, MCCS, CPN, CSN, EdD, School of Nursing, Widener University (PA)

Reviewers

Special acknowledgement for additional efforts

Holly DelGiudice, RN, GYN Oncology, Yale New Haven Hospital (CT)

Deborah Eischens, RN, Department of Nursing, University of Iowa Hospital and Clinics

Mary K. McDonald, RN, BS, CCRN, Nurse Manager, Staff Development, Clinton Hospital (MA)

Donna Miller, RN, MA, CNRN, Assistant Director of Nursing, Mediplex Rehabilitation Hospital - Marlton (NJ)

Nancy O'Donnell, RN, BSN, MS, Department of Pediatrics, Medical College of Virginia

Lisa Shaver, RN, MS, Assistant Professor/Staff Nurse, Pediatrics, Medical College of Virginia Hospitals

LaDonna Weiler, RN, BSN, Nursing Consultant (PA)

General Reviewers

Gloria Arthur, RN, MSN, Nursing Administration, Decatur General Hospital (AL)

Danial Baker, PharmD, FASHP, FACP, Professor of Pharmacy Practice, Director Drug Information Center, Washington State University College of Pharmacy

Daniel Brown, PharmD, Director of Pharmacy Services, Merced Community Medical Center (CA)

Kelly Burch, PharmD, Consultant Pharmacist, The Manuscript Prescription (MO)

John M. Burke, PharmD, BCPS, Associate Professor of Pharmacy, St. Louis College of Pharmacy (MO)

Marianne Benoit, RN, Medical Nursing, Massachusetts General Hospital

Karen Borden, RN, BSN, GYN-Surgical-Oncology Department, Massachusetts General Hospital

Gina Briscoe, RN, Nursing Education, Decatur General Hospital (AL)

Carol Burns, MSN, CCRN, Pain Management Coordinator, Medical Center at Princeton (NJ)

Karen Sue Cassidy, RN, MSN, CCRN, CNS, Special Care Education Coordinator, Decatur General Hospital (AL)

Patricia Christensen, RN, MSN, Executive Director, The Nursing Spectrum (VA)

Sharon S. Cohen, RN, MSN, CEN, Trauma/Emergency Clinical Nurse Specialist, Broward General Medical Center (FL)

Shelby Sue Conner, RN, Staff Nurse, Surgery/Clinical Cancer Center, University of Iowa Hospital and Clinics

Susan Czarnecki, RN, MSN, Nursing Care Coordinator, Intermediate Surgical ICU, Thomas Jefferson University Hospital (PA)

Carlene Daley, RN, BSN, Nurse Clinician, Department of Nursing, University of Iowa Hospital and Clinics

Andrea DiNardo, RN, CCRN, Surgical Intensive Care Unit/Telemetry Unit, Cardiac Surgical Float Team, Massachusetts General Hospital

Nancy C. Edger, RN, BSN, MBA, Supervisor, Blood Bank, Thomas Jefferson University Hospital (PA)

Brian M. French, RN, MS, Staff Specialist, Quality, Research and Development, Massachusetts General Hospital

Diane French, MS, MBA, RN, CS, CDE, Medical Surgical Clinical Nurse Specialist, Robert Wood Johnson University Hospital (NJ)

Kathleen Gallo, RN, PhD, Administrative Director, Department of Emergency Medicine, North Shore University Hospital, (NY)

Joyce Generali, RPh, MS, Drug Information Service, University of Kansas Medical Center

Patricia C. Green, ADN, RN, Staff Nurse, University of Iowa Hospital and Clinics

Ann Smith Gregoire, RN, MSN, CRNP, CCRN, Tertiary Care Nurse Practitioner, The Mitton S. Hershey Medical Center (PA)

Ellen Hamburg, PharmD, BCPS, Associated Professor of Clinical Pharmacy, Arnold and Marie Schwartz College of Pharmacy and Health Sciences of Long Island University, and State University of New York Health Sciences Center at Brooklyn

Holly K. Hill, RN, Office of Managed Care, University of Utah Health Sciences Center

Mivic Hirose, RN, MS, Department of Nursing, San Francisco General Hospital (CA)

Gary Holt, PhD, School of Pharmacy, Northeast Louisianna University

Daniel A. Hussar, PhD, Philadelphia College of Pharmacy and Science (PA)

Janet Jaramilla, PharmD, BCPS, Louis A. Weiss Memorial Hospital, The University of Chicago Hospitals (IL)

Therese Johnson, RN, Staff Nurse, Department of Nursing, Multi-Speciality Services, University of Iowa Hospital and Clinics

Judy Karlsen, RN, Trauma Surgical Floor, San Francisco General Hospital (CA)

Tracy Kelly, RN, MSN, Department of Pediatric Hematology-Oncology, Yale New Haven Hospital (CT)

Diane M. Landers, RN, Infant Child Nurse Manager, Decatur General Hospital (AL)

Grace Matthews, RN, BSN, Nurse Manager, University of Iowa Hospital and Clinics

Renee C. Meade, RN, BSN, Staff Nurse, Surgical ICU, Critical Care Nursing SICU, University of Iowa Hospital and Clinics

Connie W. Menlove, RN, BSN, MSN, ONC, Nurse Manager, Orthopaedics, General Surgery and Gynecology, University of Utah

Lisa Mercugliano, RN, Staff Nurse, Clinical Research Specialist, Preferred Health Plans (CT)

Teri Jo Miller, BSN, RN, CEN, Staff Nurse, Emergency Department, Shawnee Mission Medical Center (KS)

JoAnne Morris, RN, BSN, CPAN, Staff Nurse, Post Anesthesia Care Unit, University of Utah Medical Center

Joan M. O'Brien, RN, MSN, ANP, Nurse Practitioner, Kentfield – Pacific Pain Treatment Center, Kentfield Rehabilitation Hospital (CA)

Julie C. Oki, PharmD, Assistant Professor of Medicine, University of Missouri – Kansas City

Carla Pies, RN, BSN, Staff Nurse II, University of Iowa Hospital and Clinics

Michael T. Reed, PharmD, Associate Professor of Clinical Pharmacy, Arnold and Marie Schwartz College of Pharmacy and Health Sciences of Long Island University, and The Mount Sinai Medical Center (NY)

Timothy Reilly, RN, Clinician, Acute Medicine, University Hospital At Stony Brook (NY)

Maureen G. Roussel, RN, MSN, CCRN, CS, Cardiothoracic Clinical Nurse Specialist, Yale New Haven Hospital (CT)

Maureen E. Savitsky, PharmD, Coordinator, Clinical and Drug Information Services, Geisinger Medical Center (PA)

Kevin Schnupp, PharmD, MBA, Vice President, Professional Services, Liberty Health Systems (MD)

Joan Stachnik, PharmD, BCPS, Drug Information Specialist, University of Illinois at Chicago

Carrie A. Sullivan, BSN, BS, Staff Nurse, University of Utah Health Sciences Center

Donald S. Swanson, BA, BSN, RN, Psychiatric Nursing, University of Iowa Hospital and Clinics

Carlos W. Tam, PharmD, Coordinator, Pharmacy Service, Department of Veterans Affairs Medical Center

Laurel R. Tenney, RN, Staff Nurse Leader, Medical Nursing, Massachusetts General Hospital

Nancy J. Usher, RN, MA, Geriatric/Medical Clinical Nurse Specialist, St. Anthony Hospital Central, Centura (CO)

Nancy Lawless White, RN, BSN, MSM, Admission Liaison, Shaughnessy-Kaplan Rehabilitation Hospital (MA)

Linda Young, RN, CCRN, Coronary Care Unit, Yale New Haven Hospital (CT)

Facts and Comparisons Staff

President	C. Sue Sewester
Publisher	Paul S. Heirendt
Director of Drug Information	Bernie R. Olin, PharmD
Business Development	Heidi L. Meredith
Editorial Development	Cathy H. Reilly
Print Products Mgr.	Noël A. Shamleffer
Assistant Editors	Angela J. Brantley Stephanie Hug Tim O'Brien Sara L. Schweain Brendan T. Sullivan

Table of Contents

Publisher's Preface

Nurses Drug Facts is a drug information reference designed for the practicing nurse.

This is an important distinction, since this premise guided many decisions in format, layout and content. The contributors to this book felt it necessary to emphasize the information that the busy nurse needs immediately in daily practice.

As any practicing nurse knows, drug therapy is an integral part of patient care. As one of the health care professionals most directly associated with the patient, the nurse is obligated to be knowledgeable about their medications. Drug administration must include knowledge of the proper medication, given at the proper time, in the proper fashion, monitored with proper vigilance, and often with proper instructions to the patient for self-medication. This is a daunting task; a nurse who graduated 10 years ago has seen approximately 250 new chemical entities enter the market and thousands of trade name/formulation changes.

The nurse needs a reliable and easy-to-use reference on drugs. *Nurses Drug Facts* comes to you from Facts and Comparisons, a leader in drug information publishing for 50 years. A large team of nurses and pharmacists, from many disciplines, have contributed to this publication and have developed an excellent drug information reference.

Nurses Drug Facts is designed in a very logical fashion. Each drug monograph, arranged alphabetically, has two sections; Drug Information and Nursing Considerations. These sections are well land marked with consistent icons for rapid location of needed information. Both sections are designed to give you the information you need quickly, so that you can get back to your patients. An extensive color guide is included, arranged by color flow, to rapidly identify that unknown tablet or capsule.

The nurse also knows the importance of administering reliable and useful information to the patient, along with the "bottle of pills". *Nurses Drug Facts* has a companion book, *Patient Drug Information*. This book provides brief drug information and detailed patient instructions on a single page, to be copied and given to the patient. The page numbers are cross referenced in the *Nurses Drug Facts* drug monograph, for easy reference.

The publisher of *Nurses Drug Facts*, Facts and Comparisons, has a longstanding reputation for quality clinical drug information. The principles that have guided us for 50 years are applied to every publication: current, accurate, unbiased, concise and standardized format. Drug information is collected and analyzed daily from thousands of sources.

I am very excited about this publication and I feel confident that you will find it a valuable addition to your practice. However, it will be incomplete until we hear from you. Please feel free to contact us with any comment, question or criticisms of *Nurses Drug Facts, as well as any suggestions for future editions.*

C. Sue Sewester
President and Publisher, Facts and Comparisons

Foreword

Every citizen needs health care and every patient deserves a nurse. Despite sweeping changes in health care delivery, the explosion of health and medical knowledge, and new challenges for nurses, one constant remains: The patient's need for expert nursing care and our unmatched ability to provide it. Our patients and their families rely on us as never before to interpret complex medical diagnoses, to explain the risks and benefits of a treatment or procedure, and to discuss when and how to take medications. Nurses have always excelled at patient teaching, and, because we so often serve as the consumer's primary contact point with the health care system, we are uniquely positioned to inform and educate.

Because patients turn to nurses first, the American Nurses Association has partnered with Facts and Comparisons to publish Nurses Drug Facts. The alliance between ANA, nursing's oldest and largest professional association, and Facts and Comparisons, a publisher with a 50-year history of providing unbiased drug information, is a natural fit. The result is *Nurses Drug Facts* - a ready reference for the practicing nurse with quick access to information on prescription and over-the-counter medications. And because our patients rely on us for education, *Nurses Drug Facts* is designed with a companion patient counseling guide with single page information sheets to photocopy for patients and their families.

In the dynamic health care environment, every nurse needs timely, comprehensive information in a format that promotes patient education. The American Nurses Association will continue to offer nurses professional information of the highest quality to support and enhance our practice. Every patient deserves a well-informed nurse.

Beverly Malone, PhD, RN, FAAN
President, American Nurses Association

Introduction

Nurses Drug Facts was developed with the practicing nurse in mind. The book is designed to provide vital drug information in a format that is both easy to understand and readily accessible. *Nurses Drug Facts* contains more than 600 full drug monographs, plus abbreviated monographs for combination drugs, orphan drugs, investigational agents, and AIDS drugs in development. Each monograph covers pharmacology considerations and nursing considerations. Most monographs are also cross-referenced to the *Patient Drug Information* companion product. The companion serves as a patient counseling tool, summarizing important drug information in lay language. The *Patient Drug Information* monographs are designed to be photocopied and given to the patient and/or family.

Monographs are organized alphabetically by generic drug name. Consistent sections and unique icons are used to create a visual roadmap to help navigate the information. The standard format used throughout the book makes the information clear and easy to find. The following outlines what you'll find in each category.

Monograph Organization

Pharmacology considerations: The top half of each monograph contains detailed drug information. The following sections are included:

1. **Drug Name:** Generic drug name and common synonyms are listed in each monograph header. A slash between drug names indicates a combination product.
2. **Phonetic Pronunciation:** A guide is provided for generic drug names. Pronunciations for commonly used terms, such as acid, have not been given. The pronunciations are based on the USAN Council officially designated pronunciations. The syllable in capital letters receives the emphasis.
3. **Trade Name:** U.S. trade names are listed for each drug in italics. If none are available the statement "available as generic only" appears. Common Canadian trade names are provided whenever possible following the list of U.S. names. A maple leaf appears at the beginning of the Canadian list. If a trade name is available both in the U.S. and Canada it appears under the U.S. list only.
4. **Class:** Facts and Comparisons' drug classification is used. A semicolon separates two equal therapeutic classes (eg, Cardiovascular; Antineoplastic) when a drug is indicated for very different uses (eg, corticosteroids for cancer or for poison ivy). A slash is used to separate a class and a subclass (eg, Antibiotic/Cephalosporin).
5. **Action:** A brief, simple description of the drug's action is provided.
6. **Indications:** All approved indications are included. For some antibiotics a general statement regarding susceptible microorganisms is listed instead of listing the entire microbial spectrum, which could be quite lengthy. Common unlabeled uses and orphan drug uses are included when appropriate.

7 **Contraindications:** All known contraindications are included. Hypersensitivity to a given drug is always a contraindication and, therefore, this fact is assumed and has not been repeated for every monograph. "Standard Considerations" appears when there are no specific contraindications other than hypersensitivity.

8 **Route/Dosage:** Route of administration and the pertinent dosages are provided. Standard abbreviations are used when possible (see Standard Abbreviations, page xix). Route and dosage are organized by age group, route and specific condition when appropriate.

9 **Interactions:** Potential drug interactions are listed alphabetically followed by any incompatibilities. "None well documented" appears when there is no specific information.

10 **Lab Test Interferences:** Potential lab test interferences are listed alphabetically. "None well documented" appears when there is no specific information.

11 **Adverse Reactions:** Common (1% or greater incidence) or life-threatening reactions are included. Adverse reactions are classified according to abbreviated body system (see Standard Abbreviations, page xix).

12 **Precautions:** Information regarding pregnancy (including FDA category), lactation, children, elderly, and special risk patients is included. For pregnancy Category X drugs, any applicable information regarding birth control use is also included.

114 BUSPIRONE HCL

1 **Buspirone HCl**

2 (byoo-SPY-rone HIGH-droe-KLOR-ide)

3 *BuSpar*

4 **Class:** Antianxiety

5 **Action** Mechanism unknown; does not exert anticonvulsant or muscle relaxant effects.

6 **Indications** Treatment of anxiety disorders; short-term relief of anxiety symptoms. **Unlabeled use:** Reduction of symptoms of PMS.

7 **Contraindications** Severe liver and kidney impairment.

8 **Route/Dosage** ADULTS: Initial dose: PO 5 mg tid; may increase by 5 mg/day q 2-3 days prn (maximum 60 mg/day in divided doses).

Interactions 9
Haloperidol: May elevate haloperidol serum levels. *MAO inhibitors:* May elevate BP. *Trazodone:* May elevate serum concentrations of ALT.

Lab Test Interferences 10
None well documented.

Adverse Reactions 11
CV: Chest pain; cerebrovascular accident; CHF; MI. *CNS:* Dizziness; headache; nervousness; lightheadedness; insomnia; excitement; dream disturbances. *GI:* Nausea. *HEMA:* Eosinophilia; leukopenia; thrombocytopenia.

Precautions 12
Pregnancy: Category B. *Lactation:* Undetermined. Nursing should be avoided. *Children* < *18 yr:* Safety and efficacy not established.

Nursing Considerations: The bottom half of each monograph contains information specific to nursing care. The following sections are included:

13 **Administration/Storage:** Information includes timing of administration, methods of administration, whether or not to crush, chew or swallow certain dose forms, reconstitution/dilution specifics, general storage guidelines, safe handling and disposal. Storage temperature ranges are given and generally are as follows:

Controlled Room Temperature	=	20° to 25°C (68° to 77°F)
Refrigeration	=	2° to 8°C (36° to 46°F)
Freezing	=	–20° to –10°C (–4° to 14°F)

14 **Assessment/Interventions:** Information includes actions to take before/during/after drug administration, assessing for allergy, history, preconditions, dietary and social habits.

15 **Overdosage:** Information not available for all drugs. Specific signs and symptoms that might signal an overdose are included when appropriate.

16 **Patient/Family Education:** Information to share with patient and/or family is listed, including how/when to take medication, side effects to watch for, actions to take to counteract/minimize side effects, cautions on hazardous activities, and general safety precautions. All monographs are cross-referenced to the *Patient Drug Information* companion. The companion product supplies one page drug summaries for photocopying and giving to the patient and/or family.

NURSING CONSIDERATIONS

13 **Administration/Storage**

- Administer with food, which may decrease rate of absorption and increase bioavailability of drug.
- Store in a dry place at room temperature.

14 **Assessment/Interventions**

- Obtain patient history, including drug history and any known allergies. Assess for drug abuse potential and suicidal tendencies.
- If patient is currently taking benzodiazepines or other sedative-hypnotic drugs, dosages of these drugs should be tapered gradually until discontinued because buspirone hydrochloride will not block withdrawal symptoms.
- If patient is currently taking digoxin, assess for cardiac arrhythmias or signs of escalating symptoms of CHF.
- If patient has history of drug misuse or abuse, monitor for behaviors such as drug tolerance or drug seeking.

OVERDOSAGE: SIGNS & SYMPTOMS 15

Nausea, vomiting, dizziness, drowsiness, miosis, gastric distress

Patient/Family Education 16

- Advise patient that optimal therapeutic results usually do not occur until after 3-4 wk of treatment. However, some improvement may be noted within 7-10 days.
- Caution patient to avoid intake of alcoholic beverages and other CNS depressants.
- Instruct patient to report any of these symptoms to physician: dizziness, drowsiness, insomnia, nervousness, headache, nausea, fatigue or abnormal movements.
- Advise patient that drug may cause drowsiness and dizziness and to use caution while driving or performing other tasks requiring mental alertness.

See Patient Guide, p. 78.

The following information is not stated because it is assumed that, for every drug, the nurse will take these patient education actions:

1. Discuss name, action, and side effects of drug.
2. Instruct patient to take medication exactly as prescribed. Tell patient not to adjust dosage, skip dose, or discontinue medication without notifying the prescriber.
3. Advise patient that if a dose is missed, contact prescriber.
4. Instruct patient to complete full course of medication as prescribed unless otherwise directed by prescriber.
5. Instruct patient to keep medication out of reach of children.
6. Give patient written information if appropriate.

New Drugs

Recently approved drugs are included on the screened pages following the alphabetical listings. These drugs were approved by the FDA late in the production of *Nurses Drug Facts*. In order to include them they were added out of the alphabetical sequence of the other monographs. These complete and comprehensive monographs follow the same monograph organization outlined above.

Combination Drugs

Combination drugs not included in the general monograph section are summarized in table format. Generic name, trade name, strength and average adult dose are listed.

Investigational Agents

Drugs that are in late clinical trials (Phase III or later) or in earlier trials but considered news worthy.

Orphan Drugs

Drug or biological products for the diagnosis, treatment or prevention of rare diseases or conditions. A rare disease is one which affects <200,000 persons in the U.S. or one which affects >200,000 persons but for which there is no reasonable expectation that the cost of developing the drug and making it available will be recovered from sales of that drug in the U.S.

AIDS Drugs in Development

Investigational agents specific to AIDS that are in any phase of clinical trials, usually Phase II or later.

Appendices

The appendices include a variety of reference material designed to offer a quick guide to often needed information. They include the FDA Pregnancy Categories, General Management of Acute Overdosage, Management of Hypersensitivity Reactions, Calculations, International System of Units, Normal Laboratory Values, Drug Names That Look Alike and Sound Alike, and Oral Dosage Forms That Should Not Be Crushed Or Chewed.

Color Locator

A four-color drug identification guide follows Appendix H. More than 900 prescription drugs are represented. Each photograph includes designated schedule, trade name, strength and identification imprint (if available). The photographs are organized by color and are indexed according to their Color Locator page (eg, CL-22).

Using the Index

The index includes both generic and trade drug names followed by the number of their monograph page and Color Locator page, if it exists. Trade drug names appear in italics. The Color Locator pages are preceded by a CL (eg, CL-22).

Standard Abbreviations

ABGs	arterial blood gases
AIDS	acquired immunodeficiency syndrome
ALT	alanine aminotransferase (previously SGPT)
APTT	activated partial thromboplastin time
ARDS	adult respiratory distress syndrome
AST	aspartate aminotransferase (previously SGOT)
AV	atrioventricular
bid	twice daily
bpm	beats per minute
BP	blood pressure
BSA	body surface area
BUN	blood urea nitrogen
°C	degrees Celsius
Cal	Calorie (kilocalorie)
CBC	complete blood count
cc	cubic centimeter
CDC	Centers for DiseaseControl and Prevention
CHF	congestive heart failure
CN	cranial nerve
CNS	central nervous system
COPD	chronic obstructive pulmonary disease
CPK	creatine phosphokinase
CSF	cerebrospinal fluid
CT	computed tomography
cu	cubic
Cu	copper
CV	cardiovascular
CVP	central venous pressure
D5W	5% Dextrose in Water
D10W	10% Dextrose in Water
DERM	dermatologic
DIC	disseminated intravascular coagulation
dl	deciliter (100 ml)
DNA	deoxyribonucleic acid
ECG	electrocardiogram
EDTA	ethylenediamine tetraacetic acid
EEG	electroencephalogram
EENT	eye, ear, nose, throat
ELISA	enzyme-linked immunosorbent assay
EMIT	enzyme-multiplied immunoassay test
°F	degrees Fahrenheit
FDA	Food and DrugAdministration
G-6-PD	glucose-6-phosphate dehydrogenase
GABA	gamma-aminobutyric acid
GI	gastrointestinal
gtt	drops
GU	genitourinary
Hct	hematocrit
HDL	high-density lipoprotein
HEMA	hematologic
HEPA	hepatic
Hgb	hemoglobin
HIV	human immunodeficiency virus
hr	hour
I&O	intake and output
IM	intramuscular
IND	investigational new drug
IOP	intraocular pressure
IU	international units
IV	intravenous
kg	kilogram
L	liter
LDH	lactate dehydrogenase
LDL	low-density lipoprotein
LOC	level of consciousness
m	meter
m^2	square meter
MAO	monoamine oxidase
mcg	microgram
mEq	milliequivalent
META	metabolic
mg	milligram
MI	myocardial infarction
min	minute
ml	milliliter
mm	millimeter
mm^3	cubic millimeter
mm Hg	millimeters of mercury
mo	month
mOsm	milliosmole
MRI	magnetic resonance imaging
npo	nothing by mouth
NSAID	nonsteroidal anti-inflammatory drug
ng	nanogram
NK	natural killer (cells)
otc	over-the-counter (nonprescription)
oz	ounce
PABA	para-aminobenzoic acid
PAC	premature atrial contraction
pH	negative log of hydrogen ion concentration
PMS	premenstrual syndrome
pCO_2	carbon dioxide pressure (tension)
pO_2	oxygen pressure (tension)
PO	by mouth
ppm	parts per million
prn	as needed
PR	per rectum
pt	pint
PT	prothrombin time
PTT	partial thromboplastin time
PVC	premature ventricular contraction
q	every
qd	every day
q hr	every hour
qid	four times daily

qod	every other day
q 2 hr	every 2 hours
qt	quart
RBC	red blood cell count
RDA	Recommended Dietary Allowance
RDS	respiratory distress syndrome
RNA	ribonucleic acid
SC	subcutaneous
sec	second
SIADH	syndrome of inappropriate secretion of antidiuretic hormone
SL	sublingual
SLE	systemic lupus erythematosus
SPF	sun protection factor
STD	sexually transmitted disease
tid	three times daily
Tbsp	tablespoon
TPN	total parenteral nutrition
TSH	thyroid-stimulating hormone
tsp	teaspoon
U	unit
UTI	urinary tract infection
VHDL	very high density lipoprotein
VLDL	very low density lipoprotein
WBC	white blood cell count
WHO	World Health Organization
wk	week
yr	year

Abciximab

(ab-SICK-sih-mab)
ReoPro
Class: Antiplatelet

Action Binds to glycoprotein IIb/IIIa receptors on surface of platelets thereby preventing platelet aggregation.

Indications Adjunct to percutaneous transluminal coronary angioplasty (PTCA) to prevent ischemic complications in patients at high risk of abrupt closure of the treated vessel. Intended for use with aspirin and heparin.

Contraindications Active internal bleeding; recent (6 weeks) GI/GU bleeding, major surgery or trauma; history of CVA in the past 2 years or CVA with significant residual neurological deficit; use of oral anticoagulants within 7 days unless prothrombin time < 1.2 times control; thrombocytopenia; severe uncontrolled hypertension; vasculitis; intracranial neoplasm, aneurysm or arteriovenous malformation; or the recent or current use of IV dextran.

Route/Dosage
ADULTS: **IV** 0.25 mg/kg bolus 10-60 minutes before PTCA followed by continuous infusion at 10 µg/min for 12 hours.

Interactions None well documented.

Lab Test Interferences
None well documented.

Adverse Reactions
HEMA: Bleeding; thrombocytopenia; anemia; leukocytosis. *CV:* Hypotension; bradycardia; atrial fibrillation; pulmonary edema; AV block; supraventricular tachycardia. *GI:* Nausea, vomiting. *CNS:* Hypesthesia; confusion; dizziness. *EENT:* Abnormal vision. *RESP:* Pleural effusion; pneumonia. *MISC:* Pain; peripheral edema.

Precautions
Pregnancy: Category C. *Lactation:* Undetermined. *Children:* Safety and efficacy not established. *Readministration:* Abciximab may cause antibody development. Readministration may be associated with allergic reactions. *Bleeding:* Since risk of bleeding is increased, use cautiously, if at all, with thrombolytics, oral anticoagulants, non-steroidal anti-inflammatory drugs (NSAIDs), dipyridamole and ticlopidine. Institute bleeding precautions. *Thrombocytopenia:* Monitor platelet counts.

NURSING CONSIDERATIONS

Administration/Storage
- Use only NS or D_5W for IV infusion. Add no other medication for the infusion.
- Do not use drug if vial contains visibly opaque particles.
- Withdraw medication through a 0.2 or 2.2 micron filter.
- Administer drug through a separate IV line with filter.
- Store vials at 2° to 8°C (36° to 46°F). Do not freeze. Do not shake. Discard any unused portion.

Assessment/Interventions
- Obtain patient history.
- If symptoms of sensitivity occur any time during therapy, discontinue drug and initiate symptomatic and supportive therapy. Have epinephrine, dopamine, theophylline, antihistamines and corticosteroids available.
- If serious bleeding occurs that is not controlled with pressure, stop infusion of abciximab and heparin.
- Avoid non-compressible sites when obtaining IV access.
- Discontinue heparin at least 4 hours prior to removal of arterial sheath. Following removal, apply pressure for

at least 30 minutes, then apply a pressure dressing.
- Maintain the patient on bedrest for 6 to 8 hours.
- Frequently check insertion site and distal pulses while sheath is in place and 6 hours after removal. Measure any hematoma and monitor for enlargement.
- Avoid other invasive procedures during therapy.
- Prior to administration, check platelet count, PTT and APTT. Monitor during and after treatment.

Patient/Family Education
- Advise patient to report any bleeding or bruising to healthcare provider immediately.

No patient monograph available.

Acarbose

(A-car-bose)
Precose
Class: Antidiabetic

Action Inhibits intestinal enzymes that digest carbohydrate, thereby reducing carbohydrate digestion after meals. This lowers postprandial glucose elevation in diabetics.

Indications Patients with NIDDM who have failed dietary therapy. May be used alone or in combination with sulfonylureas.

Contraindications Diabetic ketoacidosis; cirrhosis; inflammatory bowel disease; colonic ulceration; intestinal disorders of digestion or absorption; partial or predisposition to intestinal obstruction; conditions that may deteriorate as a result of increased intestinal gas production.

Route/Dosage
ADULTS: PO 25 mg tid with the start of each meal. Increase by 25 mg/dose at 4-8 week intervals according to response up to a maximum based on blood glucose response (maximum: 150/day if < 60 kg; 300 mg/day if > 60 kg).

Interactions
Intestinal absorbents (eg, charcoal); digestive enzymes: May lower the efficacy of acarbose. *Drugs that produce hyperglycemia (eg, corticosteroids, diuretics, thyroid preparations):* May lead to loss of glucose control.

Lab Test Interferences
None well documented.

Adverse Reactions
GI: Abdominal pain; diarrhea; flatulence. *HEPA:* Elevated serum transaminases rarely associated with jaundice.

Precautions
Pregnancy: Category B. Insulin is recommended to maintain blood glucose levels during pregnancy. *Lactation:* Undetermined. *Children:* Safety and efficacy not established. *Hypoglycemia:* Acarbose does not produce hypoglycemia; however, hypoglycemia may develop if used together with sulfonylureas. *Loss of blood glucose control:* Certain medical conditions (eg, surgery, fever, infection or trauma) and drugs (eg diuretics, corticosteroids, oral contraceptives, etc) affect glucose control. In these situations, it may be necessary to adjust dose of acarbose and other antidiabetic drugs. *Renal impairment:* Acarbose not recommended.

NURSING CONSIDERATIONS

Administration/Storage
- The medication should be taken at the start (ie, first bite) of each meal.
- Store below 25°C (77°F), in a tightly closed container, protected from moisture.

Assessment/Interventions ◆ Renal function should be assessed prior to starting medication.
◆ Therapy is monitored by periodic blood glucose tests.
◆ Check serum transaminases every 3 months during the first year of treatment.
◆ Assess for hypoglycemia if this medication is combined with a sulfonylurea.
◆ If hypoglycemia develops, use oral or parenteral glucose to increase blood glucose instead of sucrose (table sugar), since metabolism of sucrose is inhibited by acarbose.

OVERDOSAGE: SIGNS & SYMPTOMS

Increased flatulence, diarrhea and abdominal discomfort may occur

Patient/Family Education ◆ Advise patient to take the drug with first bite of each meal. May be taken during the meal if not taken with the first bite. Do not take after meal is completed.
◆ Encourage patient to participate in regular physical activity and follow diabetic meal plan.
◆ Counsel patient on regular monitoring of blood glucose.
◆ Advise women of childbearing age that this medication should not be used during pregnancy. Insulin is preferred agent to control blood glucose.
◆ Advise patient/family that "cane sugar" (sucrose) should not be used to treat hypoglycemia reactions. Glucose or glucagon are necessary to increase blood sugar.
◆ Advise patient to inform healthcare provider if gas, diarrhea or abdominal discomfort occurs.

See Patient Guide, p. 1.

Acebutolol HCl

(ass-cee-BYOO-toe-lahl HIGH-droe-KLOR-ide)

Sectral, *Monitan*, *Rhotral*

Class: Beta-adrenergic blocker

Action Blocks beta-receptors, primarily affecting heart (slows rate), vascular musculature (decreases BP) and lungs (reduces function).

Indications Management of hypertension and premature ventricular contractions.

Contraindications Hypersensitivity to beta-blockers; persistently severe bradycardia; greater than first-degree heart block; CHF, unless secondary to tachyarrhythmia treatable with beta-blockers; overt cardiac failure; sinus bradycardia; cardiogenic shock.

Route/Dosage

Hypertension

ADULTS: **PO** 400 mg qd initially in single or divided doses; usual response range is 200-1200 mg/day. ELDERLY PATIENTS: May require lower maintenance doses. Dosage should not exceed 800 mg qd.

Ventricular Arrhythmia

ADULTS: **PO** 400 mg (200 mg bid); may be titrated up to 1200 mg qd.

Interactions *Clonidine:* May enhance or reverse acebutolol's antihypertensive effect; potentially life-threatening situations may occur, especially on withdrawal. *NSAIDs:* Some agents may impair antihypertensive effect. *Prazosin:* May cause increase in orthostatic hypotension. *Verapamil:* Effects of both drugs may be increased.

Lab Test Interferences Antinuclear antibodies may develop; usually reversible on discontinuation. Acebutolol may interfere with glucose or insulin tolerance tests. May cause changes in serum lipids.

Adverse Reactions *CV:* Hypotension; bradycardia; CHF; cold extremities; heart block. *RESP:* Bronchospasm; dyspnea; wheezing. *CNS:*Insomnia; fatigue; dizziness;

depression; lethargy; drowsiness; forgetfulness. *EENT:* Dry eyes; blurred vision; tinnitus; slurred speech; sore throat. *GI:* Nausea; vomiting; diarrhea; dry mouth. *GU:* Impotence; painful, difficult or frequent urination. *HEMA:* Agranulocytosis; thrombocytopenia purpura. *DERM:* Rash; hives; fever; alopecia. *OTHER:* Weight changes; facial swelling; muscle weakness.

Precautions

Pregnancy: Category B. *Lactation:* Excreted in breast milk. *Abrupt withdrawal:* Associated with adverse effects; gradually decrease dose over 1-2 wk. *Anaphylaxis:* Serious reactions may occur; aggressive therapy may be required. *CHF:* Administer cautiously in patients taking digitalis and diuretics for CHF. *Diabetes:* Acebutolol may mask signs of hypoglycemia (eg, tachycardia, BP changes). May potentiate insulin-induced hypoglycemia. *Nonallergic bronchospasm (eg, chronic bronchitis, emphysema):* In general, do not give beta-blockers to patients with bronchospastic disease. *Peripheral vascular disease:* Acebutolol may precipitate or aggravate symptoms of arterial insufficiency. *Renal/hepatic function impairment:* Reduction in daily dose is advised. *Thyrotoxicosis:* Acebutolol may mask clinical signs of developing or continuing hyperthyroidism (eg, tachycardia). Abrupt withdrawal may exacerbate symptoms of hyperthyroidism, including thyroid storm.

NURSING CONSIDERATIONS

Administration/Storage

- Before giving initial dose, take patient's pulse. If pulse is < 60 bpm, do not administer medication; notify physician.
- During initial phase of therapy, continue taking patient's pulse before administering each dose. After initial phase, take pulse before first dose of day and measure BP twice weekly.
- Store at room temperature.

Assessment/Interventions

- Obtain patient history, including drug history and any known allergies.
- Monitor serum lipid levels and thyroid function.
- Assess for signs of CHF (shortness of breath, edema, decreased output) or respiratory involvement (dyspnea, cough); if present, withhold drug and notify physician.

Patient/Family Education

- Teach patient to take pulse every day and record. If < 60 bpm, tell not to take medication and to notify physician.
- Instruct diabetic patients to monitor blood sugar level every 6 hr. Drug may mask symptoms of hypoglycemia.
- Caution patient not to stop taking drug suddenly since doing so may exacerbate angina and increase possibility of MI.
- Explain that drug may cause dizziness. Advise patient to avoid sudden position changes to prevent orthostatic hypotension.
- Advise patient that drug may cause drowsiness and to use caution while driving or performing other tasks requiring mental alertness.
- Instruct patient not to take any otc medications without consulting physician.

See Patient Guide, p. 2.

Acetaminophen (*N*-Acetyl-*p*-Aminophenol; APAP)

(ass-cet-ah-MEE-noe-fen)

Acephen, Apacet, Arthritis Pain Formula Aspirin Free, Banesin, Children's Feverall, Dapa, Datril Extra-Strength, Dolanex, Genapap Extra Strength, Genebs, Halenol, Liquiprin, Meda Cap, Myapap, Oraphen-PD, Panadol, Panex, Phenaphen, Snaplets-FR, Tapanol Extra Strength, Tempra, Tylenol, ♣ *Abenol, Atasol, Atasol Forte, Children's Acetaminophen Elixir Drops, Children's Acetaminophen Oral Solution, Tantaphen, 222 AF Regular Strength, 222 AF Extra Strength*

Class: Analgesic/antipyretic

Action Inhibits prostaglandins in CNS but lacks anti-inflammatory effects in periphery; reduces fever through direct action on hypothalmic heat-regulating center.

Indications Relief of mild to moderate pain; treatment of fever. **Unlabeled uses:** Pain and fever prophylaxis after vaccination.

Contraindications Standard considerations.

Route/Dosage

Oral

ADULTS: **PO** 325-650 mg prn q 4-6 hr or 1 g 3-4 times/day. Do not exceed 4 g/day. CHILDREN: **PO** 10-15 mg/kg/dose prn q 4-6 hr; do not exceed 5 doses/24 hr.

Suppositories

ADULTS: **PR** 650 mg q 4-6 hr; do not exceed 6 suppositories/24 hr. CHILDREN: 3-6 YR: **PR** 120 mg q 4-6 hr; do not exceed 720 mg/24 hr. CHILDREN: 6-12 YR: **PR** 325 mg q 4-6 hr; do not exceed 2.6 g/24 hr.

Interactions

Ethanol: Chronic excessive use may increase risk of hepatotoxicity. *Hydantoins, sulfinpyrazone:* May decrease therapeutic effect of APAP; concomitant long-term use may increase risk of hepatoxicity.

Lab Test Interferences

With Chemstrip bG, Dextrostix, Visidex II home blood glucose measurement systems, drug may cause > 20% decrease in mean glucose.

Adverse Reactions

HEMA: Hemolytic anemia; neutropenia; leukopenia; pancytopenia; thrombocytopenia. *HEPA:* Jaundice. *OTHER:* Hypoglycemia; allergic skin eruptions or fever.

Precautions

Pregnancy: Category B. *Lactation:* Excreted in breast milk. *Hepatic impairment:* Chronic alcoholics should not exceed 2 g/day. *Persistent pain or fever:* May indicate serious illness. Physician should be consulted.

NURSING CONSIDERATIONS

Administration/Storage

- Administer with water 30 min before or 2 hr after meals.
- Store tablets and capsules at room temperature in tightly closed container. Refrigerate suppositories. Refrigeration of elixir improves palatability.

Assessment/Interventions

- Obtain patient history, including drug history and any known allergies.
- Assess for pain and fever before and 1-2 hr after administration.
- Assess serum glucose and liver enzyme levels before long-term therapy.

OVERDOSAGE: SIGNS & SYMPTOMS

Nausea, vomiting, abdominal pain, diarrhea, anorexia, malaise, diaphoresis, confusion, low BP, cardiac arrhythmias, jaundice, acute renal failure, liver failure

Patient/Family Education

- Instruct family to consult physician for use in children < 3 yr and not to continue taking drug more than 5 days unless advised by physician.
- Instruct adult patients not to continue taking drug more than 10 days for pain or 3 days for fever.
- Instruct patient/family to contact physician if pain or fever (> 103°F) persists more than 3 days.
- Advise diabetic patients to use sugar-free form of drug.

See Patient Guide, p. 3.

Acetaminophen with Codeine Phosphate

(ass-cet-ah-MEE-noe-fen with KOE-deen FOSS-fate)

Tylenol with Codeine, Margesic, Phenaphen with Codeine, ♣ *Empracet, Triatec 30*

Class: Narcotic analgesic combination

Action Inhibits synthesis of prostaglandins; binds to opiate receptors in CNS and peripherally blocks pain impulse generation; produces antipyresis by direct action on hypothalamic heat-regulating center; causes cough suppression by direct central action in medulla; may produce generalized CNS depression; does not have significant anti- inflammatory or antiplatelet effects.

Indications Relief of mild to moderate pain; analgesic-antipyretic therapy in presence of aspirin allergy, hemostatic disturbances, bleeding diatheses, upper GI disease and gouty arthritis.

Contraindications Hypersensitivity to codeine phosphate or similar compounds.

Route/Dosage

Tylenol No. 2 equals 15 mg codeine, 300 mg acetaminophen. Tylenol No. 3 equals 30 mg codeine, 300 mg acetaminophen. Tylenol No. 4 equals 60 mg codeine, 300 mg acetaminophen. Maximum adult dose: Codeine equals 360 mg/day; acetaminophen equals 4 g/day.

Tablets

ADULTS: **PO** Usually 1-2 tablets q 4 hr (varies according to product). CHILDREN < 12 YR: **PO** 0.5-1 mg codeine/kg/dose q 4-6 hr; 10-15 mg acetaminophen/kg/dose q 4 hr to maximum of 2.6 g/24 hr.

Elixir

CHILDREN > 12 YR: **PO** 15 ml q 4 hr prn. CHILDREN 7-12 YR: **PO** 10 ml tid-qid prn. CHILDREN 3-6 YR: **PO** 5 ml tid-qid prn.

Interactions

Carbamazepine, hydantoins, sulfinpyrazone: May result in increased risk of hepatotoxicity. *Cimetidine:* Effects of codeine may be enhanced, increasing toxicity. *CNS depressants (barbiturates, ethyl alcohol, other narcotics):* May result in additive CNS depressant effects and toxicity. *Tricyclic antidepressants, phenothiazines:* May cause additive CNS depressant effects and toxicity.

Lab Test Interferences

With Chemstrip bG, Dextrostix and Visidex II home blood glucose systems, drug may cause false decrease in mean glucose values. False-positive results may occur in urinary 5-hydroxyindoleacetic acid test.

Adverse Reactions

CV: Flushing. *RESP:* Dyspnea; respiratory depression; decreased cough reflex. *CNS:* Lightheadedness; dizziness; sedation; euphoria; insomnia; disorientation; uncoordination. *GI:* Nausea; vomiting; dry mouth; constipation; abdominal pain. *DERM:* Pruritus. *OTHER:* Histamine release.

Precautions

Pregnancy: Category C. *Lactation:* Excreted in breast milk. *Sulfite sen-*

sitivity: Caution is needed with sulfite-sensitive patients; some commercial preparations contain sodium bisulfite.

Hepatic impairment: Acetaminophen intake must be limited to ≤ 2 g/day.

NURSING CONSIDERATIONS

Administration/Storage

- Give with food or milk if GI distress occurs.
- Store in airtight, light-resistant container at room temperature.

Assessment/Interventions

- Obtain patient history, including drug history and any known allergies. Note pulmonary or hepatic disease, alcoholism, head injury, Addison's disease, hypothyroidism or previous addiction to narcotic drugs.
- Assess baseline level of pain before administration.
- Take vital signs before administration. Withhold dose if respiratory rate is < 12 breaths/min (< 20 in children) and notify physician.
- Consider related factors that may lower pain threshold, such as anxiety, fear, boredom or environmental stressors.
- Assess cough for productiveness and effectiveness; auscultate for rales.
- Administer scheduled dose before pain becomes severe.
- Use adjunctive pain relief measures: massage, emotional support and diversion.
- If visual acuity is decreased by pupil constriction, keep room well lit during waking hours.
- Assess therapeutic effectiveness 1 hr after administration of dose based on patient's report of relief. Do not rely on objective signs.
- Reassess respiratory rate, depth and rhythm after each dose. Notify physician if rate is < 10 breaths/min or breathing is shallow.
- Assess for dizziness, sedation, euphoria or confusion.
- Monitor for urinary retention or constipation.
- Monitor special risk patients carefully: elderly; debilitated; those with increased intracranial pressure; pulmonary disease or conditions involving hypoxia or hypercapnia; history of drug dependence.
- Record degree and duration of pain relief. Notify physician if therapy is ineffective.
- Record any adverse or unusual reactions.
- If drowsiness or sedation occurs, institute safety precautions.
- Provide diet high in fiber; increase fluids to 2-3 L unless contraindicated.
- If constipation occurs, notify physician.
- Encourage patient to void q 3-4 hr.

OVERDOSAGE: SIGNS & SYMPTOMS

Blood dyscrasias, respiratory depression, hepatic damage (may occur up to several days after overdose)

Patient/Family Education

- Caution patient that drug dependency or tolerance may result from long-term use.
- Instruct patient not to discontinue medication abruptly after long-term regular use.
- Caution patient to avoid intake of alcohol and other CNS depressants without consulting physician.
- Advise patient that drug may cause drowsiness and to use caution while driving or performing other tasks requiring mental alertness.
- Instruct patient to notify physician if these signs/symptoms occur: persistence or recurrence of pain before next scheduled dose; difficulty breathing; blurred vision; increased drowsiness; severe nausea; vomiting; urinary retention or yellowing of skin, sclera or gums.
- Warn patient that orthostatic hypotension may occur; instruct patient to

change positions slowly and to sit or lie down if symptoms occur.

- Explain that diaphoresis is a common side effect and does not indicate a problem.
- Warn patient that constipation may occur. Advise patient to increase dietary fiber and fluids unless contraindicated.
- Caution patient against taking otc medications that contain acetaminophen.

See Patient Guide, p. 4.

Acetazolamide

(uh-seet-uh-ZOLE-uh-mide)

Diamox, Diamox Sequels, Ak-Zol, Dazamide, ♣ *APO-Acetazolamide*

Class: Anticonvulsant/carbonic anhydrase inhibitor

Action Inhibits carbonic anhydrase enzyme, reducing rate of aqueous humor formation and thus lowering IOP; produces diuretic effect; retards neuronal conduction in brain.

Indications Adjunctive treatment of chronic simple (open-angle) glaucoma and secondary glaucoma; preoperative treatment of acute congestive (closed-angle) glaucoma; prevention or lessening of symptoms associated with acute mountain sickness; adjunctive treatment of (1) edema caused by CHF or drug-induced edema and (2) centrencephalic epilepsies (eg, petit mal, generalized seizures).

Contraindications Hypersensitivity to other sulfonamides; depressed sodium or potassium serum levels; marked kidney and liver disease or dysfunction; suprarenal gland failure; hyperchloremic acidosis; adrenocortical insufficiency; severe pulmonary obstruction with increased risk of acidosis; cirrhosis; long-term use in chronic noncongestive angle-closure glaucoma. Sustained release dosage form is not recommended for use as anticonvulsant or for treatment of edema caused by CHF or drug-induced edema.

Route/Dosage

Epilepsy

ADULTS & CHILDREN: **PO** 8-30 mg/kg/day in divided doses; optimum range 375-1000 mg daily. When drug is given in combination with other anticonvulsants, initial dosage is 250 mg once daily.

Chronic Simple (Open-Angle) Glaucoma

ADULTS: **PO** 250 mg-1 g/day, usually in divided doses for amounts > 250 mg.

Secondary Glaucoma/Preoperative Treatment of Closed-Angle Glaucoma

ADULTS: SHORT-TERM CARE: **PO** 250 mg q 4 hr or 250 mg bid. ACUTE CARE: **PO** Initially 500 mg; then 125-250 mg q 4 hr. IV therapy may be used for rapid relief of increased IOP. Direct IV administration is preferred because IM route is painful. CHILDREN: ACUTE CARE: **IM/IV** 5-10 mg/kg/dose q 6 hr. LONG-TERM CARE: **PO** 10-15 mg/kg/day in divided doses q 6-8 hr.

Diuresis in CHF

ADULTS: Initially **PO** 250-375 mg (5-10 mg/day) q AM; then give on alternate days or for 2 days alternating with 1 day of rest.

Drug-Induced Edema

ADULTS: **PO** 250-376 mg qd for 1-2 days. CHILDREN: **PO/IV** 5 mg/kg q AM. Most effective if given every other day or for 2 days alternating with 1 day of rest.

Acute Mountain Sickness

ADULTS: **PO** 500-1000 mg/day in divided doses.

Interactions

Diflunisal: May cause significant decrease in IOP. *Primidone:* Primidone concentrations may be decreased. *Quinidine:* Quinidine serum levels may be increased. *Salicylates:* May cause acetazolamide accumulation and toxicity, including CNS depression and metabolic acidosis.

Lab Test Interferences

False-positive urinary protein results may occur because of alkalinization of urine.

Adverse Reactions

CNS: Drowsiness; confusion; sensory disturbances, including paresthesia and loss of appetite; convulsions. *EENT:* Transient myopia; photosensitivity; hearing disturbances; sore throat. *GI:* Nausea; vomiting; diarrhea; melena. *GU:* Polyuria; hematuria; glycosuria. *HEMA:* Blood dyscrasias, including agranulocytosis and aplastic anemia; unusual bleeding or bruising. *HEPA:* Hepatic insufficiency. *DERM:* Skin rash; urticaria. *OTHER:* Flaccid paralysis; fever; flank or loin pain; severe adverse reactions associated with sulfonamides, including Stevens-Johnson syndrome and toxic epidermal necrolysis.

Precautions

Pregnancy: Category C. *Lactation:* Undetermined. *Dose increases:* Increasing dose does not augment diuresis but may increase drowsiness and paresthesias. *Pulmonary conditions:* Use in pulmonary obstruction and emphysema may aggravate or precipitate acidosis.

NURSING CONSIDERATIONS

Administration/Storage

- Administer with food. Tablets can be crushed and mixed with sweet foods to mask bitter taste.
- Do not crush sustained release capsules; open and sprinkle contents on food.
- To prevent dehydration, give patient 2000-3000 ml/day of fluids, unless contraindicated.
- Store in a cool, dry location at room temperature.

Assessment/Interventions

- Obtain patient history, including drug history and any known allergies.
- Assess baseline CBC and platelet count before initiating therapy. Monitor at regular intervals.
- If medication is being used as diuretic, monitor weight and I&O throughout therapy.
- Monitor electrolyte levels throughout therapy.
- Take appropriate seizure precautions.
- Observe for signs of sulfonamide allergy and toxicity (fever, rash, fluid retention).
- Check for signs of hypokalemia (eg, low serum potassium levels, muscle weakness, cardiac arrhythmia) and metabolic acidosis (eg, confusion, drowsiness, lethargy, headache, abdominal pain, cardiac arrhythmia, Kussmaul respirations).
- In patients with glaucoma, monitor IOP frequently.
- Notify physician immediately if patient develops increased difficulty in breathing or signs of toxicity (drowsiness, anorexia, nausea, vomiting, dizziness, paresthesia, ataxia, tremor, tinnitus).
- Notify physician if these signs occur: sore throat, fever, unusual bleeding or bruising, tingling or tremors in hands or feet, loin pain or skin rash.

Patient/Family Education

- Advise patient to take medication with food to decrease gastric irritation and upset.
- Instruct seizure patients not to stop taking medication suddenly because doing so can cause seizures.
- Caution patient to avoid sudden or rapid position changes to prevent orthostatic hypotension.
- Advise patient to eat foods high in potassium and to avoid black licorice.
- Caution patient about possible temporary difficulty with far vision.
- Advise patient that drug may cause drowsiness and to use caution while driving or performing other tasks requiring mental alertness.
- Encourage patient to carry medical

ID card or wear Medi-Alert bracelet if taking drug for control of seizures.
- Instruct patient not to take any otc medications without consulting physician.

See Patient Guide, p. 5.

Acetohexamide

(uh-seet-toe-HEX-uh-mide)

Dymelor, *Dimelor*

Class: Antidiabetic/sulfonylurea

Action Decreases blood glucose by stimulating release of insulin from pancreas.

Indications Adjunctive therapy, used with dietary modification, in patients with non-insulin-dependent diabetes mellitus (type II) for lowering blood glucose level.

Contraindications Hypersensitivity to sulfonylureas; diabetes complicated by ketoacidosis; sole therapy of insulin-dependent (type I) diabetes mellitus; diabetes complicated by pregnancy.

Route/Dosage
ADULTS: **PO** 250 mg-1.5 g/day. In patients receiving ≤ 1 g daily, condition can be controlled with once-daily dosage; 1.5 g/day is given bid (maximum 1.5 g/day).

Interactions
Androgens, chloramphenicol, clofibrate, fenfluramine, H_2 *antagonists,* MAO *inhibitors, phenylbutazone, probenecid, salicylates, sulfonamides:* Hypoglycemic effect may be increased. *Diazoxide, rifampin, thiazide diuretics:* Hypoglycemic effect of acetohexamide may be decreased.

Lab Test Interferences
Elevated liver function. Mild to moderate elevations in BUN and creatinine.

Adverse Reactions
CV: Possible increased risk of cardiovascular mortality as compared with treatment with diet alone. *CNS:* Dizziness; vertigo. *EENT:* Tinnitus. *GI:* Nausea; epigastric fullness; heartburn; cholestatic jaundice (rare, discontinue drug if this occurs). *GU:* Mild diuresis. *HEMA:* Leukopenia; thrombocytopenia; aplastic anemia; agranulocytosis; hemolytic anemia; pancytopenia. *HEPA:* Hepatic porphyria. *DERM:* Allergic skin reactions; eczema; pruritus; erythema; urticaria; morbilliform or maculopapular eruptions, lichenoid reactions; photosensitivity. *META:* Hypoglycemia. *OTHER:* Disulfiram-like reaction; weakness; paresthesia, fatigue; malaise.

Precautions
Pregnancy: Category C. Insulin is recommended to maintain blood glucose levels during pregnancy. Prolonged severe neonatal hypoglycemia can occur if sulfonylureas are administered at time of delivery. *Lactation:* Undetermined. *Children:* Safety and efficacy not established. *Elderly or debilitated patients:* Particularly susceptible to hypoglycemic effects of drug. *Disulfiram-like syndrome:* Alcohol may cause facial flushing and breathlessness. *Hepatic and renal impairment:* Cautious use is necessary. *Hypoglycemia:* May be difficult to recognize in elderly patients or in patients receiving beta-blockers. *Loss of blood glucose control:* Stress (eg, fever or surgery) or secondary drug failure may precipitate loss of blood glucose control.

NURSING CONSIDERATIONS

Administration/Storage
- Administer at same time each day, with food if desired.
- Do not give > 1.5 g/day.
- For amounts > 1 g, administer in divided doses before morning and evening meals.

- Store tablets in tightly closed container at room temperature.

Assessment/Interventions

- Obtain patient history, including drug history and any known allergies.
- Assess condition of patient's feet, and routinely perform foot care.
- Note baseline liver function, BUN and creatinine. Monitor for elevated levels.
- Assess current blood glucose levels. Observe patient for signs of hyperglycemia (frequent urination, thirst, weakness, weight loss, ketoacidosis) and hypoglycemia (tingling of lips and tongue, nausea, diminished cerebral function [e.g., lethargy, confusion], tachycardia, sweating, convulsions, coma). Have oral glucose or carbohydrates and IV glucose available.
- Monitor liver and renal function regularly.
- Monitor effectiveness of diabetes control through individualized treatment plan, including diet, daily blood glucose levels, medication and exercise.

OVERDOSAGE: SIGNS & SYMPTOMS

Hypoglycemia, mild hypoglycemia without loss of consciousness and no neurologic findings, severe hypoglycemic reactions

Patient/Family Education

- Advise patient that drug may be taken with food if nausea occurs.
- Review symptoms of hypoglycemia and hyperglycemia.
- Emphasize importance of wearing Medi-Alert bracelet at all times.
- Instruct patient to call physician if any of these symptoms occur: nausea, vomiting, heartburn, diarrhea, fever, sore throat, rash, itching, weakness, unusual bruising, bleeding.
- Caution patient about possible effects of alcohol intake: flushing, weakness, dizziness, tingling sensation, headache.
- Caution patient to avoid exposure to sunlight and to use sunscreen or wear protective clothing to avoid photosensitivity reaction.
- Advise patient not to take any otc medications without consulting physician.

See Patient Guide, p. 6.

Acetylcysteine
(N-Acetylcysteine)

(ASS-cee-till-SIS-teen)

Acetylcysteine, Mucomyst, Mucomyst-10, Mucosil-10, Mucosil-20

Class: Respiratory inhalant/mucolytic

Action Decreases thickness of mucous secretions in lung.

Indications Reduction of viscosity of bronchopulmonary mucous secretions in patients with chronic or acute lung diseases, pulmonary complications associated with cystic fibrosis, surgery, anesthesia, atelectasis caused by mucous obstruction; diagnostic bronchial studies; prevention or lessening of liver damage after potentially toxic quantity of acetaminophen. **Unlabeled uses:** Ophthalmic preparation for dry eye; enema for bowel obstruction. **Orphan drug use:** IV form for acetaminophen overdose.

Contraindications Standard considerations.

Route/Dosage

ADULTS: **Nebulization (face mask, mouthpiece, tracheostomy)** 1-10 ml (usually 2-5 ml) of 20% solution or 2-20 ml (usually 6-10 ml) of 10% solution q 2-6 hr (usually tid or qid); **(nebulization tent)** large volumes (up to 300 ml) during treatment period. **Instillation** 1-2 ml of 10 to 20% solution as often as every hour. DIAGNOSTIC BRONCHOGRAMS: 2-3 administrations of 1-2 ml of 20% solution or 2-4 ml of 10% solution q 1-4 hr by instillation before procedure. ACETAMINOPHEN OVERDOSE: After appropriate overdose procedures (eg, lavage or induction of emesis), 140 mg/kg as oral loading dose (diluted with soft drink). Then 70 mg/kg orally 4 hr after loading dose and repeated at 4 hr intervals for total of 17 doses, unless acetaminophen assay indicates otherwise.

Interactions None well documented. INCOMPATIBILITIES: Do not mix with tetracycline, chlortetracycline, oxytetracycline, erythromycin lactobionate, amphotericin B, ampicillin sodium, iodized oil, chymotrypsin, trypsin or hydrogen peroxide.

Lab Test Interferences None well documented.

Adverse Reactions *CV:* Tachycardia; hypotension; hypertension; chest tightness. *RESP:* Bronchospasm; bronchial irritation. *CNS:* Drowsiness. *EENT:* Rhinorrhea. *GI:* Nausea; vomiting; stomatitis. *DERM:* Rash; pruritis; angioedema. *OTHER:* Fever; clamminess.

Precautions *Pregnancy:* Category B. *Lactation:* Undetermined. *Bronchial secretions:* Increased secretion volume may occur. When cough is inadequate, open airway may need to be maintained by mechanical suction. *Asthmatic bronchospasm:* If bronchospasm progresses, medication must be discontinued immediately. *Antidotal use:* If allergic reaction, encephalopathy or severe, persistent vomiting occurs, discontinuation of drug may be necessary.

NURSING CONSIDERATIONS

Administration/Storage

Mucolytic

- Use Sodium Chloride for Injection or Inhalation or Sterile Water for Injection or Inhalation to prepare 20% solution.
- Do not dilute 10% solution unless instructed by physician.
- Do not use nebulization equipment that contains iron, copper or rubber because of potential for corrosion. Use glass, plastic, aluminum, anodized aluminum, chromed metal, or stainless steel equipment.
- Refrigerate unused or undiluted solution and use within 96 hr.

Acetaminophen Overdosage

- Administer orally immediately if 24 hr or less after ingestion of acetaminophen.
- Dilute 20% solution 1:3 with soft drink or juice to mask odor.
- Cover glass with aluminum foil and push straw through cover to help patient ingest without smelling medication and vomiting.
- Use fresh dilution within 1 hr.
- Undiluted opened vials will last for 96 hr under refrigeration.

Assessment/Interventions

- Obtain patient history, including drug history and any known allergies.
- Assess airway patency, baseline lung sounds and effectiveness of cough.
- Assess for urticaria, rashes, hemoptysis or stomatitis.
- Review baseline liver enzyme levels and monitor throughout therapy.
- If rapid onset of bronchospasm occurs, discontinue medication immediately and notify physician.
- If patient vomits loading dose or maintenance dose within 1 hr of administration, repeat dose.
- If patient's cough is inadequate, maintain open airway by mechanical suction or clear airway by endotrachial aspiration.
- Notify physician of these signs/symptoms: chest tightness, tachycardia or severe and persistent vomiting.

Patient/Family Education

- Explain that medication has disagreeable odor.

- Advise patient of likelihood for significant increase in respiratory secretions and need to cough.
- Caution patient to notify physician of rash, urticaria, wheezing, chest tightness, severe vomiting, hemoptysis, fever or severe malaise.
- Provide follow-up counseling as needed for acetaminophen overdose.

See Patient Guide, p. 7.

Acyclovir

(A-SIKE-low-vihr)

Zovirax, ♣ *Zovirax 200, Zovirax 400 Wellstat Pac*

Class: Anti-infective/antiviral

Action Inhibits viral DNA replication by interfering with viral DNA polymerase.

Indications
Parenteral form: Treatment of initial or recurrent mucosal and cutaneous herpes simplex viruses (HSV) and varicella zoster (shingles) infections in immunocompromised patients; treatment of herpes simplex encephalitis in infants > 6 mo; treatment of severe clinical episodes of genital herpes. *Oral form:* Treatment of initial and recurrent episodes of genital herpes in certain patients; acute treatment of shingles and chickenpox; suppressive therapy for frequent recurrence of genital herpes. *Topical form:* Treatment of initial episodes of herpes genitalis and some mucotaneous HSV infections in immunocompromised patients. **Unlabeled uses:** Treatment of cytomegalovirus and HSV infection after bone marrow or renal transplant; treatment of infectious mononucleosis, varicella pneumonia, chickenpox and other HSV infections.

Contraindications Standard considerations.

Route/Dosage
Parenteral
For IV infusion only; rapid or bolus IV must be avoided. ADULTS: **IV** 15-30 mg/kg/day in 3 divided doses given q 8 hr over 1 hr. CHILDREN: **IV** 250-500 mg/m^2 q 8 hr.

Oral
Initial genital herpes: ADULTS: **PO** 200 mg q 4 hr 5 times/day for 10 days. **Suppressive therapy for recurrent genital herpes:** ADULTS: **PO** 400 mg bid or 200 mg q 8 hr. **Intermittent therapy for recurrent genital herpes:** ADULTS: **PO** 200 mg q 4 hr 5 times/day for 5 days at earliest sign or symptom of recurrence. **Herpes zoster:** ADULTS: **PO** 800 mg q 4 hr 5 times/day for 7-10 days. **Chickenpox:** ADULTS & CHILDREN: **PO** 20 mg/kg/dose (maximum 800 mg/dose) qid for 5 days.

Topical
ADULTS & CHILDREN: Apply to lesions q 3 hr 6 times/day.

Interactions
Zidovudine: Increased propensity for lethargy. INCOMPATIBILITIES: Precipitation may occur with bacteriostatic water. Do not add acyclovir to biologic or colloidal fluids.

Lab Test Interferences
None well documented.

Adverse Reactions
CV: Phlebitis at injection site. *CNS:* Encephalopathic changes; lethargy; obtundation; tremor; confusion; hallucinations; headache; agitation; seizures; coma. *GI:* Nausea; vomiting. *HEPA:* Transient elevations of serum creatinine, BUN, transaminases. *DERM:* Inflammation at injection site; itching; rash; hives. *OTHER:* Asthenia; paresthesia. *Topical form:* Burning or stinging; pruritis. Topical use may cause same adverse reactions as systemic use.

Precautions
Pregnancy: Category C. *Lactation:* Excreted in breast milk. *Children:* Safety and efficacy in children < 2 yr not established. *Encephalopathic changes:* Patients with underlying neurologic abnormalities or severe hypoxia may have

increased risk of neurotoxic effects. *Cutaneous use:* Care must be taken to avoid getting drug in eyes. *Renal impairment:* Dosage adjustment may be needed. With parenteral use, acyclovir may precipitate as crystals in renal tubules. *Genital herpes:* Sexual intercourse must be avoided when lesions are present. Use of acyclovir does not prevent transmission.

NURSING CONSIDERATIONS

Administration/Storage

Topical

- Use finger cot or rubber glove when applying topical ointment to prevent spread of infection.
- Cover entire lesion with ointment 6 times/day for 7 days. A ½-inch ribbon of ointment covers approximately 4 sq inches.

Parenteral

- Administer at room temperature. Be certain any precipitate in refrigerated solution dissolves at room temperature.
- Administer after hemodialysis.
- Avoid rapid or bolus IV administration.
- Establish infusion rate to administer over at least 1 hr.
- Use reconstituted solution within 12 hr.

Oral/Suspension/Capsules

- Shake suspension before using.
- Store capsules at room temperature.

Assessment/Interventions

- Obtain patient history, including drug history and any known allergies.
- Monitor IV site for redness, swelling or heat.
- Rotate IV sites frequently.
- Monitor vital signs frequently during infusion.
- Monitor serum BUN and creatinine.
- Assess for nausea and vomiting.
- Monitor I&O.
- Notify physician if lesion does not improve or recurs.

OVERDOSAGE: SIGNS & SYMPTOMS

Increased BUN and serum creatinine, renal failure

Patient/Family Education

- Advise patient to avoid sexual intercourse while genital herpes lesions are present.
- Tell patient that acyclovir is a treatment, not a cure.
- Instruct patient to notify physician if there is no reduction in severity or frequency of lesions.
- Advise patient that ointment is for external use only.
- Teach patient to apply ointment with finger cot or glove and to completely cover lesion every 3 hr 6 times/day.
- Advise patient that transient burning, stinging, itching or rash may occur and to notify physician if these symptoms are pronounced or persistent.
- Caution patient to start treatment as soon as symptoms occur.
- Tell patient not to use medication on or near eyes.
- Advise patient to notify physician if nausea, vomiting, diarrhea, headache, numbness, tingling or general body discomfort occurs with oral dosing.

See Patient Guide, p. 8.

Adenosine

(ah-DEN-oh-seen)

Adenocard

Class: Antiarrhythmic

Action Slows conduction through atrioventricular (AV) node; can interrupt reentry pathways through AV node and restore normal sinus rhythm.

Indications Conversion to sinus rhythm of paroxysmal supraventricular tachycardia (PSVT), including that associated with Wolff-Parkinson-White syndrome. **Unlabeled use:** Noninvasive assessment of patients with suspected coronary artery disease in conjunction with thallium tomography. **Orphan drug use:** Used with BCNU for treatment of brain tumors.

Contraindications Second- or third-degree AV block or sick sinus syndrome (except in patients with functioning artificial pacemaker); atrial flutter; atrial fibrillation; ventricular tachycardia.

Route/Dosage

ADULTS: Initial dose: **IV** 6 mg as rapid IV bolus (over 1-2 sec). REPEAT ADMINISTRATION: If first dose does not eliminate PSVT within 1-2 min, give 12 mg as rapid IV bolus; 12 mg dose may be repeated a second time if necessary. Doses > 12 mg are not recommended.

Interactions

Caffeine, theophylline: Antagonize effects of adenosine; larger doses of adenosine may be needed. *Carbamazepine:* May produce higher degrees of heart block. *Dipyridamole:* Potentiates effects of adenosine; smaller doses may be adequate.

Lab Test Interferences

None well documented.

Adverse Reactions

CV: Facial flushing; headache; chest pain; hypotension. *RESP:* Dyspnea; shortness of breath; chest pressure. *CNS:* Lightheadedness, dizziness, tingling in arms; numbness. *GI:* Nausea.

Precautions

Pregnancy: Category C. *Lactation:* Undetermined. *Arrhythmias:* At time of conversion to normal sinus rhythm, new arrhythmias may appear on ECG; these are usually self-limiting. *Asthma:* Adenosine may cause bronchoconstriction. *Heart block:* Drug may produce short-lasting heart block. Patients in whom high-level heart block (eg, third-degree) develops after one dose should not receive repeat doses.

NURSING CONSIDERATIONS

Administration/Storage

- Administer by rapid IV bolus only.
- Administer either directly into vein or, if given into IV line, in most proximal IV line and follow with rapid saline solution flush.
- Do not administer if solution is cloudy or if sediment is present.
- Discard unused portion.
- Store at room temperature.
- Do not refrigerate because crystallization may occur. If crystallization has occurred, dissolve crystals by warming to room temperature.

Assessment/Interventions

- Obtain patient history, including drug history and any known allergies or asthma.
- Monitor BP and cardiac rhythm during and after administration.
- Monitor for transient asystole, which may develop during administration.

Patient/Family Education

- Inform patient to report these symptoms to physician: facial flushing, headache, shortness of breath, chest pressure, lightheadedness, dizziness, tingling in arms, numbness or nausea.

No patient monograph available.

Albumin Human (Normal Serum Albumin)

(al-BYOO-MIN human)

Albuminar-5, -25; Albutein 5%, 25%; Buminate 5%, 25%; Plasbumin-5, -25

Class: Plasma protein fraction

Action Maintains plasma colloid osmotic pressure and serves as carrier of intermediate metabolites in transport and exchange of tissue products.

Indications Symptomatic relief and supportive treatment in management of shock, burns, hypoprothrombinemia, adult respiratory distress syndrome, cardiopulmonary bypass, acute liver failure, acute nephrosis, sequestration of protein-rich fluids, erythrocyte resuspension, hypotension or shock during renal dialysis, hyperbilirubinemia and erythroblastosis fetalis.

Contraindications Severe anemia; cardiac failure; renal insufficiency; presence of normal or increased intravascular volume; chronic nephrosis; hypoprothrombinemic states associated with chronic cirrhosis; malabsorption; protein-losing enteropathies, pancreatic insufficiency; undernutrition.

Route/Dosage

Burns

Initial treatment usually consists of large amounts of crystalloid infusions (eg, normal saline, lactated Ringer's) with lesser amounts of 5% albumin to maintain adequate plasma volume. After first 24 hr, ratio of alblumin and crystalloid should maintain plasma albumin level of approximately 2.5 g ± 0.5 g/100 ml or total plasma protein level of about 5.2 g/100 ml. This is best achieved with albumin 25% solution.

NORMAL SERUM ALBUMIN, 5%

Shock

Give as rapidly as necessary to improve patient's condition and restore normal blood volume. ADULTS: Initial dose: **IV** 500 ml of 5% albumin given as rapidly as tolerated. If response in 30 min is inadequate, give additional 500 ml. In patients with slightly low or normal blood volume, rate is 2-4 ml/min. CHILDREN: **IV** Rate of administration is ¼ to ½ adult rate. NEONATES & INFANTS: **IV** 10-20 ml/kg 5% albumin based on clinical response, BP and assessment of anemia.

Hypoproteinemia

To replace protein loss, 5% albumin may be given.

ALBUMIN HUMAN, 25%

Shock

ADULTS & CHILDREN: Initial dose: **IV** Determined by patient's condition and response to treatment. Therapy is guided by degree of venous or pulmonary congestion or Hct measurements.

Hypoproteinemia

ADULTS: **IV** 50-75 g/day at rate not exceeding 2 ml/min. CHILDREN: **IV** 25 g/day at rate not exceeding 2 ml/min.

Acute Nephrosis

ADULTS: **IV** 100 ml 25% albumin in combination with loop diuretic repeated daily for 7-10 days.

Renal Dialysis

ADULTS: **IV** Approximately 100 ml 25% albumin.

Hyperbilirubinemia and Erythroblastosis Fetalis

NEONATES & INFANTS: **IV** 1 g/kg 1-2 hr before transfusion.

Interactions None well documented.

Lab Test Interferences None well documented.

Adverse Reactions

CV: Hypotension after rapid infusion (> 10 ml/min) or intra-arterial administration to patients undergoing cardiopulmonary bypass; rapid administration may cause vascular overload, dyspnea or pulmonary edema. *OTHER:* Allergic or pyogenic reactions (characterized by fever and chills).

Precautions
Pregnancy: Category C. *Lactation:* Undetermined. *Special risk patients:* Circulatory overload may develop in patients with CHF, renal insufficiency or stabilized chronic anemia. *Concomitant blood administration:* Relative anemia can be avoided by supplementing or replacing large quantities of albumin with whole blood. *Hepatic or renal impairment:* Caution is needed because of added protein load.

NURSING CONSIDERATIONS

Administration/Storage
- Administer by IV infusion only, using accompanying administration set and large-gauge needle or catheter.
- Give medication as supplied; do not dilute.
- Administer slowly to prevent too-rapid expansion of blood volume. *Exception:* May be administered rapidly if there is severe loss of plasma volume.
- Do not administer if solution is cloudy or sediment is present.
- Store at room temperature. Do not freeze.

Assessment/Interventions
- Obtain patient history, including drug history and any known allergies. Note severe anemia, hepatic or renal impairment.
- Assess baseline Hct before infusion.
- Take pulse and BP before and during infusion.
- Monitor liver and kidney function, Hct, electrolytes, plasma albumin and total serum protein before and during therapy.
- Assess for signs of fluid overload before and during infusion.
- If venous or pulmonary congestion worsens or if hypotension occurs, slow or discontinue infusion and notify physician.
- Monitor I&O.
- Monitor for dehydration. Patient may require additional fluids.
- If patient has sustained injury or has had surgery, observe for new bleeding points as BP increases.
- Monitor for allergic or pyogenic reactions characterized by fever and chills. If these symptoms occur, discontinue treatment and notify physician.
- Do not infuse if intravascular volume is normal or increased or if patient has potential for fluid volume overload.

Patient/Family Education
- Explain rationale for infusion of drug and need for frequent monitoring.
- Instruct patient to report these symptoms to physician: fever, chills, headache or back pain.

No patient monograph available.

Albuterol

(al-BYOO-ter-ahl)

Proventil, Proventil Repetabs, Ventolin, Ventolin Rotacaps

Class: Bronchodilator/sympathomimetic

Action Produces bronchodilation by relaxing bronchial smooth muscle through beta-2 receptor stimulation.

Indications Prevention and treatment of reversible bronchospasm associated with asthma and other obstructive pulmonary diseases. **Unlabeled use:** Adjunctive treatment of hyperkalemia in patients undergoing dialysis.

Contraindications Cardiac tachyarrhythmias.

Route/Dosage
Inhalation Aerosol
ADULTS & CHILDREN ≥ 4 YR: 1-2 in-

halations q 4-6 hr. PREVENTION OF EXERCISE-INDUCED BRONCHOSPASM: 2 inhalations 15 min before exercise.

Inhalation Solution

ADULTS & CHILDREN ≥ 12 YR: 2.5 mg/dose 3-4 times/day by nebulization.

Inhalation Capsules

ADULTS & CHILDREN ≥ 4 YR: 1-2 capsules q 4-6 hr using Rotahaler inhalation device.

Oral

ADULTS & CHILDREN ≥ 12 YR: PO 2-4 mg/dose 3-4 times/day. Do not exceed 32 mg/day. CHILDREN 6-12 YR: PO 2 mg/dose 3-4 times/day. Do not exceed 24 mg/day. CHILDREN 2-6 YR: PO 0.1-0.2 mg/kg/dose 3 times/day. Do not exceed 12 mg/day.

Interactions

Digoxin: Albuterol may decrease serum digoxin levels.

Lab Test Interferences

None well documented.

Adverse Reactions

CV: Palpitations; tachycardia; elevated BP. *RESP:* Cough, bronchospasm. *CNS:* Tremor; dizziness; hyperactivity; nervousness; headache; insomnia. *EENT:* Dry mouth; throat irritation. *GI:* Nausea; vomiting; heartburn; diarrhea. *GU:* Urinary retention.

Precautions

Pregnancy: Category C. *Lactation:* Unknown. *Labor and delivery:* May inhibit uterine contractions. *Cardiovascular effects:* Toxic symptoms may occur in patients with cardiovascular disorders. *CNS effects:* CNS stimulation may occur; use cautiously in patients with history of seizures or hyperthyroidism. *Diabetes:* Dosage adjustment of insulin or oral hypoglycemic agent may be required. *Excessive use:* Paradoxical bronchospasm and cardiac arrest have been associated with excessive inhalant use. *Hypokalemia:* Decreases in potassium levels have occurred. *Tolerance:* If previously effective dose fails to provide relief, therapy may need to be reassessed.

NURSING CONSIDERATIONS

Administration/Storage

- Do not crush tablets.
- Administer oral preparations with meals to minimize GI upset.
- Use before other inhalation therapy and before postural drainage.
- Allow 1-2 min between metered-dose inhalations and 5 min before administering other inhalant medications. Permit patient to rinse mouth after each completed inhalation dose.
- Store at room temperature. Refrigeration of syrup improves palatability.

Assessment/Interventions

- Obtain patient history, including drug history and any known allergies.
- Check pulse, BP, respirations and lung sounds before and after administration.
- Review baseline and any follow-up ECG. If patient takes digoxin, check baseline and any follow-up serum digoxin levels.
- If patient is diabetic, check baseline and follow-up blood sugar levels.
- If bronchospasm occurs, withhold drug and report to physician.
- During pregnancy, monitor fetal heart rate and report tachycardia (> 140 bpm).

> **OVERDOSAGE: SIGNS & SYMPTOMS**
>
> Tremor, palpitations, tachycardia, elevated BP, seizures

Patient/Family Education

- Tell patient not to chew or crush capsules.
- Teach patient correct method for using metered-dose inhaler. Have patient demonstrate proper technique, including timing between inhalations.

- Instruct patient in home monitoring of pulse and BP.
- Advise patient to maintain fluid intake of 2000 ml/day and to rinse mouth after each complete dose.
- Instruct patient not to use otc inhalers without consulting physician.
- Instruct patient to contact physician if symptoms are not relieved by normal dose.
- Tell patient to report adverse reactions or side effects.

See Patient Guide, p. 9.

Aldesleukin (Interleukin-2; IL-2)

(al-dess-LOO-kin)
Proleukin
Class: Antineoplastic

Action Produces immunologic effects, including (1) activation of cellular immunity with profound lymphocytosis, eosinophilia and thrombocytopenia; (2) production of cytokines, including tumor necrosis factor, interleukin-1 and interferon gamma and (3) inhibition of tumor growth.

Indications Treatment of metastatic renal cell carcinoma. **Unlabeled uses:** Treatment of Kaposi's sarcoma (in combination with zidovudine), metastatic melanoma (with low-dose cyclophosphamide), colorectal cancer, non-Hodgkin's lymphoma.

Contraindications Abnormal thallium stress test results; abnormal pulmonary function test results; organ allografts; retreatment in patients who experienced toxicity in previous aldesleukin therapy.

Route/Dosage
Metastatic Renal Cell Carcinoma
ADULTS: **IV** 600,000 IU/kg (0.037 mg/kg) by 15 min infusion q 8 hr for total of 14 doses over 5 days. After 9-day rest, repeat for another 14 doses. RETREATMENT: In patients with tumor shrinkage, allow minimum rest period of 7 wk from date of last hospital discharge.

Interactions
Cardiotoxic agents (eg, doxorubicin), hepatotoxic agents (eg, methotrexate), myelotoxic agents (eg, cytotoxic chemotherapy), nephrotoxic agents (eg, aminoglycosides): Aldesleukin may increase organ toxicity when given with these agents. *Psychotropic agents*: Aldesleukin may interfere with actions of these medications.

Lab Test Interferences
None well documented.

Adverse Reactions
CV: Hypotension; sinus tachycardia; arrhythmias; bradycardia; premature ventricular contractions; premature atrial contractions; myocardial ischemia or infarction; cardiac arrest; CHF; stroke; gangrene; myocarditis; endocarditis; pericardial effusion; thrombosis; edema. *RESP*: Pulmonary congestion; dyspnea; pulmonary edema; respiratory failure; tachypnea; pleural effusion; wheezing; apnea; pneumothorax. *CNS*: Mental status changes; dizziness; sensory dysfunction; special sensory disorder of vision, speech, taste; syncope; motor dysfunction; coma; seizures. *EENT*: Conjunctivitis; permanent or transient blindness. *GI*: Nausea; vomiting; stomatitis; anorexia; GI bleeding; bowel necrosis; dyspepsia; constipation; intestinal perforation; pancreatitis. *GU*: Oliguria; anuria; proteinuria; hematuria; dysuria; renal impairment requiring dialysis; increased BUN, serum creatinine. *HEMA*: Anemia; thrombocytopenia; leukopenia; coagulation disorders; leukocytosis; eosinophilia; hypocalcemia; hypomagnesemia; hypophosphatemia; hypokalemia; hyperkalemia; hyperuricemia; hyponatremia. *HEPA*: Jaundice; ascites; hepatomegaly; elevated bilirubin, transaminase, alkaline phosphatase. *DERM*: Pruritus, erythema; rash; dry skin; exfo-

liative dermatitis; purpura; petechiae; urticaria; alopecia; injection site reactions. *META:* Acidosis; alkalosis; hyperglycemia; hypoglycemia; hypoproteinemia; hypoalbuminemia. *OTHER:* Fever; chills; pain; fatigue; weakness; malaise; infection; weight gain or loss; malignant hyperthermia.

Precautions

Pregnancy: Category C. *Lactation:* Undetermined. *Children:* Safety and efficacy in children < 18 yr not established. *Bacterial infections:* Aldesleukin is associated with impaired neutrophil function and increased risk of disseminated infection. *Capillary leak syndrome (CLS):* Results from extravasation of plasma proteins and fluid into extravascular space and loss of vascular tone. CLS may begin immediately after treatment is begun. *CNS metastases:* Aldesleukin may exacerbate disease symptoms in patients with clinically unrecognized or untreated CNS metastases. *Mental status changes:* May indicate sepsis. *Renal or hepatic impairment:* Occurs often during treatment.

NURSING CONSIDERATIONS

Administration/Storage

- Reconstitute each vial containing 22 million IU with 1.2 ml of Sterile Water for Injection. Discard unused portion.
- Do not shake contents of vial during reconstitution. Use gentle swirling motion to avoid excess foaming.
- Dilute reconstituted aldesleukin in 50 ml of 5% Dextrose Injection. Use plastic container for dilution.
- Infuse over 15 min. Do not use in-line filters during administration.
- Refrigerate vial and administer within 48 hr of reconstitution. Bring to room temperature before infusion. Do not freeze.

Assessment/Interventions

- Obtain patient history, including drug history and any known allergies.
- Take vital signs and record weight daily during therapy.
- Monitor hematologic status, including CBC, platelets and blood chemistries.
- Monitor serum electrolytes and renal, hepatic and pulmonary function.
- Notify physician of signs of these conditions: *CLS*—hypotension, hypoperfusion, edema, effusion; *cardiac/pulmonary dysfunction*—arrhythmias, ECG changes, chest pain, shortness of breath; *renal dysfunction*—decreased urine output, elevated BUN, elevated creatinine; *anemia, hypovolemia* or *thrombocytopenia*—shortness of breath, fatigue, headache, bruising, unusual bleeding; *infection/sepsis*—fever, chills, tachycardia; *mental status changes*—irritability, agitation, confusion, seizures, lethargy.

Patient/Family Education

- Instruct patient to report any difficulty in breathing, chest pain, palpitations, abnormal bleeding, decreased urine output or edema.

No patient monograph available.

Alendronate Sodium

(al-LEN-droe-nate SO-dee-uhm)

Fosamax

Class: Hormone/Bisphosphonates

Action Inhibits bone resorption and increases bone density.

Indications Treatment of osteoporosis in postmenopausal women; Paget's disease.

Contraindications Hypocalcemia.

Route/Dosage

Osteoporosis

ADULTS: PO 10 mg QD.

Paget's Disease

ADULTS: PO 40 mg QD for 6 months. Retreatment may be considered for patients who relapse after a 6-month observation period.

Interactions

Food: Absorption of alendronate is decreased by food. *Ranitidine:* Increased alendronate absorption; clinical importance unknown. *Calcium supplements, antacids:* Decreased alendronate absorption. *Aspirin:* Risk of upper GI adverse effects is increased by concomitant use of aspirin and alendronate doses over 10 mg/day.

Lab Test Interferences

None well documented.

Adverse Reactions

CNS: Headache. *GI:* Abdominal pain; constipation; diarrhea; flatulence; esophageal ulcer; dysphagia. *OTHER:* Musculoskeletal pain.

Precautions

Pregnancy: Category C. *Lactation:* Undetermined. *Children:* Safety and efficacy not established. *Renal:* Not recommended for patients with creatinine clearance < 35 ml/min. *GI Disorders:* Not recommended for patients with upper GI problems. *Hypocalcemia:* Correct before starting alendronate. *Nutrition:* Maintain adequate calcium and vitamin D intake during alendronate therapy. *Concomitant estrogen replacement therapy:* Not recommended. *Absorption:* Food, beverages other than water, and medication inhibit absorption. Must be taken first thing in the morning with a full glass of water at least 30 minutes before any food, beverages or medications. Must remain sitting or standing for 30 minutes after taking.

NURSING CONSIDERATIONS

Administration/Storage

- Divide the dose if GI upset occurs.
- Avoid high calcium food, vitamins with mineral supplements, and antacids high in metals within 2 hours of dosing.
- Take 30 minutes before the first meal, medication or drink of the day. Take with 6-8 oz of plain water only.
- Store at room temperature in well closed container.

Assessment/Interventions

- Obtain patient history.
- Assess for hypersensitivity reaction.
- Assess for severe renal insufficiency prior to administration.

OVERDOSAGE: SIGNS & SYMPTOMS

Hypocalcemia, hypophosphatemia, upper GI adverse effects expected

Patient/Family Education

- Instruct the patient to take the medication with plain water 30 minutes before the first food or drink of the day.
- Take medication with a full glass of water. Do not lie down for 30 minutes following administration.
- Do not suck or chew on the tablet; swallow whole.
- Patient should take supplemental calcium (1,500 mg) and vitamin D (400 PO daily) if dietary intake is not adequate.
- Patient should be encouraged to perform weight-bearing exercises and modify behaviors that promote osteoporosis (eg, avoid alcohol and cigarette smoking).
- Patient should read package insert before starting therapy.

See Patient Guide, p. 10.

Alfentanil HCl

(al-FEN-tuh-NILL HIGH-droe-KLOR-ide)

Alfenta

Class: Narcotic agonist analgesic

Action Binds opioid receptors in CNS.

Indications Induction of analgesia and anesthesia in specific situations.

Contraindications Hypersensitivity to narcotics; diarrhea caused by poisoning until toxic agent is identified; acute bronchial asthma; upper airway obstruction.

Route/Dosage

Obese Patients

Calculate dosage on basis of lean body weight.

Incremental Injection

ADULTS: Initial dose: **IV** 8-50 mcg/kg; maintenance: 3-15 mcg/kg or 0.5-1 mcg/kg/min.

Anesthetic Induction

ADULTS: Initial dose: **IV** 130-245 mcg/kg; maintenance: **IV** 0.5-1.5 mcg/kg/min (or use general anesthetic).

Continuous Infusion

ADULTS: Initial dose: **IV** 50-75 mcg/kg; maintenance: 0.5-3 mcg/kg/min.

Interactions *CNS depressants:* May increase CNS and cardiovascular effects of alfentanil. *Erythromycin:* May increase levels of alfentanil, causing prolonged anesthesia.

Lab Test Interferences Amylase or lipase concentration test results may be unreliable for 24 hr after administration of alfentanil.

Adverse Reactions *CV:* Hypotension; hypertension; tachycardia; bradycardia; asystole hypercarbia; arrhythmia. *RESP:* Respiratory depression; bronchospasm; apnea. *CNS:* Sedation; dizziness. *EENT:* Blurred vision. *GI:* Nausea; vomiting. *OTHER:* Muscular rigidity.

Precautions *Pregnancy:* Category C. *Lactation:* Undetermined. *Labor:* Narcotics cross placenta and can affect neonate. *Children:* Hypotension has occurred in neonates receiving alfentanil. Not recommended for children < 12 yr. *Elderly:* Decreased dosage may be necessary. *Cardiac effects:* Drug may cause bradycardia and hypotension; may aggravate arrhythmias. *CNS depression:* Patient may be sensitive to depressive effects of alfentanil. *Head injury:* Alfentanil may increase intracranial pressure. *Respiratory effects:* Alfentanil may decrease respiratory drive and cause apnea. *Seizures:* Alfentanil may cause or aggravate seizure disorder.

NURSING CONSIDERATIONS

Administration/Storage

- Drug is to be administered only by those qualified to give IV anesthetics.
- For accurate administration of small volumes, use tuberculin syringe or equivalent.
- Slow IV administration (90 sec-3 min) reduces incidence of adverse reactions.
- Infusion should be discontinued 10-15 min before surgery is complete.

Assessment/Interventions

- Obtain patient history, including drug history and any known allergies.
- Monitor vital signs frequently during and after administration.
- Monitor serum amylase or lipase concentrations for elevations.
- Assist patient with ambulation.

OVERDOSAGE: SIGNS & SYMPTOMS

Respiratory depression, CNS depression, circulatory collapse (usually after rapid IV administration)

Patient/Family Education

- Instruct preoperative patient about possible side effects.
- Advise postoperative patient to rise from bed slowly and to call for assistance in ambulation.
- Instruct patient to avoid intake of alcoholic beverages or other CNS depressants for 24 hr after outpatient surgery.

No patient monograph available.

Allopurinol

(AL-oh-PURE-ee-nahl)

Zyloprim, ♣ *APO-Allopurinol; Purinol-100, -200, -300*

Class: Analgesic/gout

Action Inhibits xanthine oxidase, enzyme responsible for conversion of hypoxanthine to xanthine and then to uric acid.

Indications Treatment of primary or secondary gout, hyperurecemia resulting from chemotherapy for malignancies, recurrent calcium oxalate renal calculi. **Unlabeled uses:** Prevention of fluorouracil-induced stomatitis and fluorouracil-induced granulocyte suppression.

Contraindications Standard considerations.

Route/Dosage

Control of Gout/Hyperuricemia

ADULTS: **PO** 100-800 mg/day. For amounts > 300 mg, give divided doses.

Secondary Hyperurecemia Associated with Malignancies

CHILDREN 6-10 YR: **PO** 300 mg/day. CHILDREN < 6 YR: **PO** 150 mg/day.

Prevention of Uric Acid Nephropathy in Vigorous Chemotherapy of Neoplastic Disease

ADULTS: **PO** 600-800 mg/day for 2-3 days.

Reduction of Risk of Acute Gouty Attacks

ADULTS: Initial oral dose of 100 mg/day is increased by 100 mg at weekly intervals until adequate response is achieved or maximum recommended dose (800 mg/day) is reached.

Interactions

Aluminum salts, uricosuric agents: May lessen effectiveness of allopurinol. *Ampicillin:* May increase incidence of ampicillin-induced skin rash. *Cyclophosphamide:* May enhance bone marrow suppression. *Theophyllines:* Theophylline clearance may be decreased, leading to toxicity. *Thiopurines (eg, azathioprine, mercaptopurine):* Toxicity of these drugs may be increased.

Lab Test Interferences

None well documented.

Adverse Reactions

CNS: Headache; peripheral neuropathy; neuritis; paresthesias; drowsiness. *EENT:* Epistaxis; taste disturbance; myopathy. *GI:* Nausea; vomiting; diarrhea; abdominal pain; gastritis; dyspepsia; granulomatous changes. *GU:* Renal failure; uremia. *HEMA:* Leukopenia; leukocytosis; eosinophilia; thrombocytopenia; bone marrow depression. *HEPA:* Elevated liver enzymes; reversible hepatomegaly; cholestatic jaundice; hepatitis; hepatic necrosis. *DERM:* Skin rash; ecchymosis; alopecia; allergic vasculitis. Allergic reactions may be severe and sometimes fatal. *OTHER:* Arthralgia; acute gouty attacks; fever; myopathy; necrotizing angiitis.

Precautions

Pregnancy: Category C. *Lactation:* Excreted in breast milk. *Children:* Allopurinol is rarely indicated for use in children, except for hyperuricemia resulting from malignancy or with certain rare inborn errors of purine metabolism. *Acute gouty attacks:* May occur during initial stages of therapy. *Bone marrow depression:* Reported in patients given allopurinol. *Hypersensitivity:* Discontinue drug at first appearance of skin rash or other signs of allergic reaction. Rash may be followed by more severe hypersensitivity reactions and, rarely, death. *Renal function impairment:* Reduced dose is given in patients with this condition. Drug may exacerbate renal failure in certain patients.

NURSING CONSIDERATIONS

Administration/Storage

- Administer immediately after meals. For patients who have difficulty swallowing, crush tablets and mix with food.
- Store in tightly closed container in cool location.

Assessment/Interventions

- Obtain patient history, including drug history and any known allergies.
- Assess for renal toxicity and failure.
- Increase fluid intake to 2000-3000 ml/day (unless contraindicated) to prevent calculi formation.
- Obtain baseline CBC. Monitor frequently.
- For treatment of gout, obtain baseline uric acid level. Monitor every 1-2 wk for dosage adjustment; then monitor every few months.
- Monitor liver and kidney function, including BUN, serum creatinine and creatinine clearance, especially during early therapy.
- Monitor for decrease in joint swelling and pain.
- If urine output is decreased, dosage may need to be decreased. Consult physician.

Patient/Family Education

- Encourage patient to focus on weight loss or control.
- Tell patient to avoid purine-rich foods (eg, organ meats).
- Caution patient to avoid excessive intake of alcohol.
- Explain that gouty attacks may not end for 2-6 wk after beginning of therapy.
- Instruct patient to stop taking medication and notify physician if rash or flu-like symptoms develop.
- Advise patient that drug may cause drowsiness and to use caution while driving or performing other tasks requiring mental alertness.
- Instruct patient not to take otc medications without consulting physician.

See Patient Guide, p. 11.

Alprazolam

(al-PRAY-zoe-lam)

Xanax, ♣ *APO-Alpraz, Novo-Alprazol, Nu-Alpraz*

Class: Antianxiety/benzodiazepine

Action Potentiates action of GABA (gamma-aminobutyric acid), an inhibitory neurotransmitter, resulting in increased neuronal inhibition and CNS depression, especially in limbic system and reticular formation.

Indications Management of anxiety, anxiety associated with depression, panic disorder with or without agoraphobia. **Unlabeled uses:** Treatment of irritable bowel syndrome, depression, PMS, agoraphobia with social phobia.

Contraindications Hypersensitivity to other benzodiazepines; psychoses; acute narrow-angle glaucoma.

Route/Dosage

Anxiety Disorder

ADULTS: PO 0.25-0.5 mg tid; maximum 4 mg/day in divided doses.

Elderly/Debilitated Patients

ADULTS: PO 0.25 mg bid-tid; may increase dose gradually.

Panic Disorder

Initial dose: PO 0.5 mg tid; if needed, increase by maximum 1 mg/day q 3-4 day. May require > 4 mg/day.

Interactions

Alcohol and other CNS depressants: Produce additive CNS depressant effects. *Cimetidine, oral contraceptives, disulfiram:* May increase effects of alprazolam, producing excessive sedation and impaired psychomotor function. *Digoxin:* Serum digoxin concentrations may increase. *Omeprazole:* May increase serum levels of alprazolam and enhance alprazolam's effects. *Theophyllines:* May antagonize sedative effects of alprazolam.

Lab Test Interferences

None well documented.

Adverse Reactions

CV: Hypotension. *CNS:* Drowsiness; confusion; ataxia; dizziness; fatigue; apathy; memory impairment; disorientation; anterograde amnesia; restlessness; headache; slurred speech; aphonia; stupor; coma; euphoria; irritability; vivid dreams; psychomotor retardation; paradoxical reactions (eg, anger, hostility, mania, insomnia, muscle spasms). *EENT:* Visual or auditory disturbances; depressed hearing. *GI:* Constipation; diarrhea; dry mouth; coated tongue; nausea; anorexia; vomiting. *HEMA:* Blood dyscrasias, including agranulocytosis; anemia; thrombocytopenia; leukopenia; neutropenia; decreased hematocrit levels. *HEPA:* Hepatic dysfunction, including hepatitis and jaundice. *DERM:* Rash. *OTHER:* Elevated LDH, ALT, AST and alkaline phosphatase.

Precautions

Pregnancy: Category D. *Lactation:* Excreted in breast milk. *Children:* Safety and efficacy in children < 18 yr not established. *Dependence:* Prolonged use can lead to physical and psychological dependence. Withdrawal syndrome has occurred within 4-6 wk of treatment, especially if abruptly discontinued. Cautious use and tapering of dosage are necessary. *Psychiatric disorders:* Not intended for patients with primary depressive disorder, psychoses or disorders in which anxiety is not prominent. *Renal or hepatic impairment:* Caution is needed to avoid accumulation of drug. *Suicide:* Use with caution in patients with suicidal tendencies; do not allow patient access to large quantities of drug.

NURSING CONSIDERATIONS

Administration/Storage

- May be given with food if GI upset occurs.
- If patient has difficulty swallowing, crush tablets.
- Store in light-resistant container at room temperature.

Assessment/Interventions

- Obtain patient history, including drug history and any known allergies. Note hypersensitivity to other benzodiazepines and presence of narrow-angle glaucoma.
- Assess patient's mental status and extent of anxiety before initiation of therapy.
- Assess for signs of withdrawal syndrome: confusion, abnormal perception of movement, depersonalization, muscle twitching, psychosis, paranoid delusions, seizures.
- Notify physician if signs/symptoms of these conditions occur: *digoxin toxicity*—anorexia, nausea, vomiting, diarrhea, visual disturbances, arrhythmias; *hepatic dysfunction*—fatigue, jaundice, abdominal pain, elevated liver enzyme levels; *paradoxical reactions*—anger, hostility, episodes of

mania and hypomania; or *cardiovascular reactions*—tachycardia, arrhythmias, hypotension.

Patient/Family Education

- Advise patient against reducing or suddenly discontinuing this medication, which may cause withdrawal symptoms (sweating, vomiting, muscle cramps, tremors, seizures).
- Caution patient to avoid sudden position changes to prevent orthostatic hypotension.
- Instruct patient to avoid intake of alcoholic beverages or other CNS depressants.
- Caution patient that prolonged use of this medication can lead to dependence.
- Advise patient that drug may cause drowsiness and to use caution while driving or performing other tasks requiring mental alertness.

See Patient Guide, p. 12.

Alprostadil (PGE$_1$; Prostaglandin E$_1$)

(al-PRAHST-uh-dill)

Caverject, Prostin VR Pediatric

Class: Prostaglandin/patent ductus arteriosus, agent for impotence

Action Relaxes smooth muscle of ductus arteriosus. Produces vasodilation, inhibits platelet aggregation and stimulates intestinal and uterine smooth muscle. Induces erection by relaxation of trabecular smooth muscle and by dilation of cavernosal arteries.

Indications Palliative therapy to maintain patency of ductus arteriosus temporarily, until surgery can be performed, in neonates who have congenital heart defects (eg, pulmonary stenosis, tricuspid atresia) and who depend on patent ductus for survival. Treatment of erectile dysfunction due to nerogenic, vasculogenic, psychogenic, or mixed etiology.

Contraindications Standard considerations. *Caverject:* Conditions that might predispose patients to priapism (eg, sickle cell anemia or trait, multiple myeloma leukemia); patients with anatomical deformation of the penis (eg, angulation, cavernosal fibrosis, Peyronie's disease); patients with penile implants; use in women, children or newborns; use in men for whom sexual activity is inadvisable or contraindicated.

Route/Dosage

NEONATES: **IV** 0.01-0.4 mcg/kg/min. Drug is infused for shortest time and at lowest effective dose.

Impotence

Erectile dysfunction of vasculogenic, psychogenic, or mixed etiology—Initiate dose titration at 2.5 mcg. If there is a partial response, the dose may be increased by 2.5 mcg to a dose of 5 mcg and then in increments of 5 to 10 mcg, depending on erectile response, until the dose that produces an erection suitable for intercourse and not exceeding a duration of 1 hour is reached. If there is no response to the initial 2.5 mcg dose, the second dose may be increased to 7.5 mcg, followed by increments of 5 to 10 mcg. If there is no response, then the next higher dose may be given within 1 hour. If there is a response, then there should be a 1-day interval before the next dose is given.

Erectile dysfunction of pure neurogenic etiology (spinal cord injury)—Initiate dosage titration at 1.25 mcg. The dose may be increased by 1.25 mcg to a dose of 2.5 mcg, followed by an increment of 2.5 mcg to a dose of 5 mcg, and then in 5 mcg increments until the dose that produces an erection suitable for intercourse and not exceeding a duration of 1 hour is reached. If there is no response, then the next higher dose may be given within 1 hour. If there is a response, then there should be at least a 1-day interval before the next dose is given. *Maintenance therapy*—The first interjections of alprostadil must be done at the physician's office by medically trained personnel. Self-injection therapy by the patient can be started only after the patient is properly instructed and well-trained in the self-injection technique. The physician should make a careful assessment of the patient's skills and competence with the procedure.

Interactions None well documented.

Lab Test Interferences
None well documented.

Adverse Reactions
CV: Flushing; bradycardia; hypotension; tachycardia; cardiac arrest; edema. Other rare, but serious cardiovascular effects include CHF; hyperemia; second-degree heart block; shock; spasm of right ventricle infundibulum; supraventricular tachycardia; ventricular fibrillation. *RESP:* Apnea. *CNS:* Fever; seizures; cerebral bleeding. *GI:* Diarrhea. *HEMA:* DIC; bleeding. *OTHER:* Cortical proliferation of long bones; sepsis. *Caverject only:* Penile pain; prolonged erection; penile fibrosis; injection site hematoma; penis disorder; injection site ecchymosis.

Precautions
Hemostatic effects: Use cautiously in neonates with bleeding tendencies because alprostadil inhibits platelet aggregation. *Respiratory status:* Apnea has occurred in some neonates treated with alprostadil. *Priapism* (erection lasting > 6 hours): Prolonged erection has been known to occur following intracavernosal administration of vasoactive substances, including alprostadil. To minimize the chances of priapism, titrate slowing to the lowest effective dose. If priapism is not treated immediately, penile tissue damage and permanent loss of potency may result. *Penile fibrosis:* Discontinue treatment in patients who develop penile angulation, cavernosal fibrosis, or Peyronie's disease.

NURSING CONSIDERATIONS

Administration/Storage
Prostin VR Pediatric

- Drug is to be given only by trained personnel in PICU via continuous IV infusion into large vein or through umbilical artery catheter.
- Dilute medication with normal saline or D5W only.
- Use volumetric IV pump to regulate delivery.
- Monitor infant closely during administration.
- Discard preparation after 24 hr and mix new solution.

Caverject

- Bacteriostatic water for injection or sterile water, both preserved with benzyl alcohol 0.945% w/v, must be used as the diluent for reconstitution.
- After reconstitution, immediately use the solution and do not store or freeze.
- Do not shake the contents of the reconstituted vial.
- Discard vials with precipitates or discoloration.
- The intracavernosal injection must be done under sterile conditions. The site of injection is usually along the dorso-lateral aspect of the proximal third of the penis. Avoid visible veins. The side of the penis that is injected and the site of injection must be alternated; the injection site must be cleansed with an alcohol swab.

Assessment/Interventions

- Obtain patient history, including drug history and any known allergies.
- Assess infant's cardiac status before administration.
- Do not administer if infant is in respiratory distress.
- Obtain baseline CBC, ABGs, PT, PTT and pulmonary function tests.

- Monitor arterial pressure intermittently. If pressure decreases significantly, notify physician immediately. Infusion rate will need to be decreased.
- Monitor respiratory status throughout treatment. Have ventilatory equipment at bedside.
- Monitor BP during administration.
- Notify physician and decrease or stop infusion if infant develops: (1) increased respiratory distress; (2) bleeding, bruising or hematoma formation; (3) sudden changes in cardiac status (eg, decreased BP, bradycardia, cardiac arrest, cyanosis). Decrease or stop infusion until physician gives new orders.
- *Caverject only:* Exercise careful follow-up of the patient while in the self-injection program. This is especially true for the initial self-injections, since adjustments in the dose of alprostadil may be needed. While on self-injection treatment, it is recommended that the patient visit the prescribing physician's office every 3 months. At that time, assess the efficacy and safety of the therapy and adjust the dosage.

OVERDOSAGE: SIGNS & SYMPTOMS

Apnea, bradycardia, pyrexia, hypotension, flushing

Patient/Family Education

Prostin VR Pediatric

- Explain to parents about infant's congenital heart disease and purpose and expected outcome of treatment.
- Keep parents/family informed of course of treatment; alert them to usual side effects (eg, flushing of skin).
- Promote parent-infant bonding by encouraging parent involvement in infant's care.
- Encourage parents to express their emotions. Show compassion and understanding and help them to cope.

Caverject

- Thoroughly instruct and train the patient in the self-injection technique before he begins intracavernosal treatment at home. Establish the desired dose in the physician's office.
- Inform the patient that the established dose should not be changed without consulting the physician or healthcare provider.
- The patient may expect an erection to occur within 5 to 20 minute. A standard treatment goal is to produce an erection lasting no longer than 1 hour.
- Instruct the patient that alprostadil generally should be used no more than 3 times per week, with at least 24 hours between each use.
- Instruct the patient to seek immediate medical attention if an erection persists for more than 6 hours.
- Patient should report any penile pain that was not previously present or that increased in intensity, as well as the occurrence of nodules or hard tissue in the penis to his physician as soon as possible.
- Advise patient that the use of intracavernosal alprostadil offers no protection from the transmission of sexually transmitted diseases. Counsel individuals who use alprostadil about the protective measures necessary to guard against the spread of STDs, including HIV.
- The injection of alprostadil can induce a small amount of bleeding at the site of injection. In patients infected with blood-borne diseases, this could increase the risk of transmission of blood-borne diseases between partners.

Caverject—See Patient Guide, p. 13.

Prostin VR Pediatric—No patient monograph available.

Alteplase, Recombinant

(AL-tuh-PLACE)

Activase, ♣ *Activase rt-PA*, *Lysatec rt-PA*

Class: Tissue plasminogen activator

Action Aids in dissolution of blood clots.

Indications Lysis of thrombi in management of acute MI or acute massive pulmonary embolism. **Unlabeled use:** Treatment of unstable angina pectoris.

Contraindications Active internal bleeding; history of cerebrovascular accident; recent (within 2 mo) intracranial or intraspinal surgery or trauma; intracranial neoplasm; arteriovenous malformation or aneurysm; bleeding diathesis; severe uncontrolled hypertension.

Route/Dosage

ADULTS: **IV** 100 mg over 3 hr, given as 60 mg first hr, with 6-10 mg bolus over next 1-2 min; then 20 mg/hr over next 2 hr. Dosage not to exceed 150 mg because of increased risk of intracranial bleeding.

Acute MI

Patients < 65 kg may receive 1.25 mg/kg over 3 hr, as described above.

Interactions

Aspirin, dipyridamole or heparin: May increase risk of bleeding. INCOMPATIBILITIES: Do not add other medications to infusion solution.

Lab Test Interferences

Results of tests for coagulation or fibrinolytic activity may be unreliable because of degradation of fibrinogen in blood.

Adverse Reactions

CV: Hypotension. *HEMA:* Bleeding, both superficial (eg, venous cutdowns, arterial punctures, sites of surgical intervention) and internal (eg, GI tract, GU tract, pericardial, retroperitoneal or intracranial sites). *OTHER:* Mild hypersensitivity (eg, urticaria), fever.

Precautions

Pregnancy: Category C. *Lactation:* Undetermined. *Bleeding:* Most frequent and serious adverse effect.

NURSING CONSIDERATIONS

Administration/Storage

- Reconstitute immediately before use. Use large-bore (18-gauge) needle for reconstitution.
- Do not use if vacuum has been broken.
- Reconstitute only with accompanying Sterile Water for Injection. Do not use Bacteriostatic Water for Injection.
- Administer by IV infusion only.
- Do not administer if solution is discolored or if sediment is present.
- Store lyophilized alteplase at room temperature or refrigerate. May be used for IV administration within 8 hr when stored at room temperature.

Assessment/Interventions

- Obtain patient history, including drug history and any known allergies. Note cerebrovascular disease, hypertension or recent internal bleeding.
- Obtain drug history, noting use of aspirin, dipyridamole or heparin because these drugs may increase risk of bleeding.
- Ensure that coagulation studies have been performed before administration. These tests provide baseline values against which to monitor patient's response to therapy.
- Take pulse and BP before administration and monitor frequently during infusion.
- Observe for internal or external bleeding before and during infusion.
- Carefully monitor potential bleeding

sites (eg, catheter insertion sites, arterial puncture sites) because fibrin will be lysed during therapy, resulting in new or increased bleeding.

- Avoid IM injections and nonessential handling of patient during treatment.
- Minimize number of arterial and venous punctures.
- If arterial punctures are necessary, use site accessible to manual compression. Use manual pressure for at least 30 min, apply pressure dressing and check site frequently for evidence of bleeding.
- If serious bleeding occurs, stop infusion and any concomitant heparin and notify physician.
- Observe for indications of hypersensitivity (eg, urticaria, fever). Nausea, vomiting, hypotension and fever are frequent sequelae of MI and may or may not be attributable to therapy.
- If anaphylactic reaction occurs, stop infusion, notify physician and initiate appropriate therapy.

Patient/Family Education

- Explain drug action and need for frequent monitoring, including blood tests and vital signs.
- Instruct patient to report any new bleeding sites or increased bleeding, dizziness, headache, numbness or tingling.
- Tell patient to report urticaria or fever.
- Instruct patient to avoid getting out of bed without assistance during treatment.

No patient monograph available.

Altretamine (Hexamethylmelamine)

(ahl-TRETT-uh-meen)

Hexalen

Class: Antineoplastic

Action Produces cytotoxicity, which may be caused by interaction with cellular macromolecules, including DNA.

Indications Treatment of recurrent or persistent ovarian cancer after other therapies.

Contraindications Preexisting bone marrow depression; severe neurologic toxicity.

Route/Dosage
Dosage calculation based on BSA. ADULTS: **PO** 260 mg/m^2/day in 4 divided doses for 14 or 21 consecutive days in 28-day cycle.

Interactions
MAO inhibitors: May cause severe orthostatic hypotension, especially in elderly patients.

Lab Test Interferences
None well documented.

Adverse Reactions
CNS: Peripheral sensory neuropathy; mood disorders; disorders of consciousness; ataxia; dizziness; vertigo; anorexia; fatigue; seizures. *GI:* Nausea; vomiting; increased alkaline phosphatase. *GU:* Increased serum creatinine and BUN levels. *HEMA:* Leukopenia; thrombocytopenia; anemia.

Precautions
Pregnancy: Category D. *Lactation:* Undetermined. *Children:* Safety and efficacy not established. *Carcinogenesis, mutagenesis and fertility impairment:* Similar drugs are carcinogenic. *Hematologic:* Altretamine causes mild to moderate myelosuppression. *Neurotoxicity:* Altretamine causes mild to moderate neurotoxicity (eg, peripheral neuropathy, ataxia, mood disorders). More common with higher doses; usually reversible. *Special risk patients:* Patients with GI intolerance, neurotoxicity or low blood counts should receive decreased doses.

NURSING CONSIDERATIONS

Administration/Storage

- Administer orally.
- Store in dry environment.

Assessment/Interventions

- Obtain patient history, including drug history and any known allergies.
- Assess patient's neurologic status.
- Monitor CBC (with differential) and serum creatinine and BUNs.
- Notify physician if decreased LOC or seizures occur.
- Monitor for signs of bleeding, infection or anemia. Report signs of infection to physician.
- Observe for nausea and vomiting. Notify physician if GI symptoms are severe.

Patient/Family Education

- Advise patient to notify physician if seizures, severe nausea or vomiting occurs.
- Caution patient to call physician if hematuria, melena stools or unusual sleeping patterns are noted.

See Patient Guide, p. 14.

Aluminum Salts

(uh-LOO-min-uhm salts)

Aluminum Carbonate
Basaljel

Aluminum Hydroxide
AlternaGEL Liquid, Alu-Cap, Alu-Tab, Amphojel, Dialume, Rolaids

Aluminum Phosphate
Phosphaljel

Dihydroxyaluminum Sodium Carbonate
Rolaids Antacid

Class: Antacid

Action Neutralizes gastric acid, thus increasing pH of stomach and duodenal bulb. Increases lower esophageal sphincter tone and inhibits smooth muscle contraction and gastric emptying. Aluminum carbonate and aluminum hydroxide bind with phosphate ions in intestine to form insoluble aluminum phosphate, which is excreted in feces.

Indications *Aluminum carbonate, aluminum hydroxide, dihydroxyaluminum sodium carbonate:* Symptomatic relief of GI upset associated with hyperacidity, including heartburn, gastroesophageal reflux, acid indigestion and sour stomach; peptic ulcer; gastritis. *Aluminum carbonate:* Management of hyperphosphatemia or adjunctive therapy (with low-phosphate diet) to prevent formation of phosphate urinary stones. *Aluminum phosphate:* Reduction of fecal excretion of phosphates.

Contraindications Standard considerations.

Route/Dosage

Aluminum Carbonate Gel, Basic

ADULTS: ANTACID: **PO** 2 capsules, 2 tablets or 10 ml suspension (in water or fruit juice) as often as q 2 hr, up to 12 times daily. HYPERPHOSPHATEMIA: **PO** 2 capsules, 2 tablets or 12 ml suspension (in water or fruit juice) tid or qid with meals.

Aluminum Hydroxide Gel

ADULTS: **PO** 500-1800 mg 3-6 times/day between meals and at bedtime. CHILDREN (HYPERPHOSPHATEMIA): **PO** 50-150 mg/kg/24 hr in divided doses q 4-6 hr; titrated to maintain normal serum phosphorus.

Aluminum Phosphate Gel

ADULTS: **PO** 15-30 ml undiluted q 2 hr between meals and at bedtime.

Dihydroxyaluminum Sodium Carbonate

ADULTS: **PO** 1-2 chewable tablets prn.

Interactions *Iron:* Absorption of iron salts may be decreased. *Ketoconazole:* Effects of ketoconazole may be reduced. *Penicillamine:* Pharmacologic effect of penicillamine may be decreased. *Salicylates:* Serum levels of salicylates may be reduced. *Sodium polystyrene sulfonate:* Concomitant use may cause metabolic alkalosis in patients with renal failure. *Tetracyclines:* Drug may decrease pharmacologic effect of tetracyclines.

Lab Test Interferences

None well documented.

Adverse Reactions

CNS: Neurotoxicity; encephalopathy. *GI:* Constipation; intestinal obstruction. *META:* Hypophosphatemia. *OTHER:* Osteomalacia; bone pain; muscular weakness; malaise; decreased fluoride absorption; aluminum accumulation in serum, bone and CNS.

Precautions

Pregnancy: Consult physician. *Lactation:* Consult physician. *GI hemorrhage:* Use aluminum hydroxide with care in patients who have undergone recent massive upper GI hemorrhage. *Renal impairment:* Use cautiously. *Sodium content:* May be significant. Use low-sodium product in patients with hypertension or CHF or in those following low-sodium diets.

NURSING CONSIDERATIONS

Administration/Storage

- Administer other medications 1-2 hr before or after antacid.

Aluminum Hydroxide Gel

- Administer between meals and at bedtime.

Aluminum Phosphate Gel

- Give undiluted gel q 2 hr between meals and at bedtime.

Aluminum Carbonate Gel, Basic

- Dilute suspension in water or juice. Shake well.

Dihydroxyaluminum Sodium Carbonate

- Have patient chew tablet thoroughly and then drink full glass of water.

Assessment/Interventions

- Obtain patient history, including drug history and any known allergies.
- Increase fluid intake to 2-3 L/day unless contraindicated.
- Monitor serum electrolytes, calcium and phosphate.
- Monitor I&O. Strain urine if monitoring for renal calculi.
- Monitor bowel sounds. Assess for constipation.
- Observe for black tarry stools, "coffee grounds" emesis or bright red blood in emesis.
- Monitor patients with hypertension or CHF or those on sodium restricted diet throughout therapy.

Patient/Family Education

- Remind patient to shake liquid well before pouring.
- Instruct patient to chew chewable tablets thoroughly before swallowing and to follow with glass of water.
- Instruct patient not to take antacids within 1-2 hr of other drugs because antacids may interfere with absorption of other medications.
- Inform patient (especially if elderly) that aluminum-containing products may cause constipation and that laxatives or stool softeners may be needed.
- Instruct patient to increase fluid intake to 2-3 L/day, unless contraindicated, and to increase bulk in diet.
- Advise patients with hypertension or CHF or those following restricted low-sodium diet to use low-sodium preparation.
- Advise patients with ulcers to adhere strictly to prescribed dosage schedule.
- Caution patient not to use maximum dosage for more than 2 wk unless under physician's supervision.
- Advise patient to inform physician if no improvement is noted with antacid.
- Instruct patient to report these symptoms to physician: black tarry stools, "coffee grounds" emesis or bright red blood in emesis.

See Patient Guide, p. 15.

Amantadine HCl

(uh-MAN-tuh-deen HIGH-droe-KLOR-ide)

Symadine, Symmetrel, ♣ *Endantadine*

Class: Antiparkinson/antiviral

Action Exact mechanism is unknown; thought to facilitate dopamine release from intact dopaminergic terminals, increasing dopamine concentration at dopaminergic terminals. Exhibits antiviral activity against influenza A virus by inhibiting entry of virus into host cell.

Indications Symptomatic treatment of several forms of Parkinson's disease or syndrome and drug-induced extrapyramidal reactions; prevention and treatment of influenza A viral respiratory illness, especially in high-risk patients.

Contraindications Standard considerations.

Route/Dosage

Parkinson's Disease

ADULTS: PO 100 mg bid when used as single agent. Initial dose: PO 100 mg/day if patient is debilitated or receiving high doses of other antiparkinson drugs. If necessary, dose may be titrated to maximum of 400 mg/day.

Drug-Induced Extrapyramidal Reactions

ADULTS: PO 100 mg bid; up to 300 mg/day may be given in divided doses.

Influenza A Viral Infection (Symptomatic Treatment)

ADULTS: PO 200 mg/day as single dose or 100 mg bid. ELDERLY AND PATIENTS WITH PRIOR SEIZURE DISORDERS: PO 100 mg qd. CHILDREN 9-12 YR: PO 100 mg bid. CHILDREN 1-9 YR: PO 4.4-8.8 mg/kg/day; not to exceed 150 mg/day.

Influenza A Viral Infection (Prophylaxis)

Same dosages as for symptomatic treatment. However, start in anticipation of contact or as soon as possible after exposure. Continue drug administration for at least 10 days after known exposure. When influenza A virus vaccine is unavailable or contraindicated, administer amantadine for up to 90 days. In conjunction with the vaccine, administer amantadine for 2-3 wk after vaccination.

Interactions None well documented.

Lab Test Interferences
None well documented.

Adverse Reactions
CNS: Lightheadedness; dizziness; insomnia; depression; anxiety; irritability; hallucinations; confusion; ataxia; headache. *GI:* Nausea; anorexia; constipation; dry mouth. *EENT:* Visual disturbances. *OTHER:* Livedo reticularis; peripheral edema; orthostatic hypotension.

Precautions
Pregnancy: Category C. *Lactation:* Excreted in breast milk. *Neonates & infants:* Safety and efficacy not established. *Elderly patients:* Decreased dosage is necessary. *CHF:* CHF has developed in patients taking amantadine. *Renal impairment:* Reduced dose is required in renal impairment. *Seizures:* Reduced dose is necessary in patients with prior seizure disorders, including epilepsy.

NURSING CONSIDERATIONS

Administration/Storage

- Administer after meals or with food.
- Do not administer at bedtime because drug may cause insomnia.
- Store in tightly closed container in cool location.

Assessment/Interventions

- Obtain patient history, including drug history and any known allergies. Note cardiac or renal disease.
- Assess for psychotic or abnormal behavior during therapy.
- Assess for suppression of parkinsonian symptoms during therapy.
- Monitor cardiac, GI and GU functioning throughout therapy.
- In patients with prior seizure disorders, observe patient carefully. Notify physician immediately if seizures occur.
- Notify physician if orthostatic hypertension develops.

Patient/Family Education

- Explain that full effectiveness of medication may not occur for several days after initiation of drug therapy.
- When medication is used for Parkinson's disease, explain that doses will be tapered gradually before stopping.
- Advise patient that during first week of therapy, blurred vision, redness and mottling of skin are common but these signs and symptoms will subside later.
- Instruct patient to take sips of water frequently, suck on ice chips or sugarless hard candy, or chew sugarless gum if dry mouth occurs.
- Instruct patient to avoid sudden position changes to prevent orthostatic hypotension.
- Advise patient that drug may cause drowsiness and to use caution while driving or performing other tasks requiring mental alertness.
- Warn patient to avoid alcoholic beverages.
- Instruct patient not to take otc medications without consulting physician.

See Patient Guide, p. 16.

Amifostine

(am-ih-FOSS-teen)
Ethyol
Class: Cytoprotective

Action Converted to an active free thiol metabolite that binds toxic cisplatin metabolites and also scavenges free radicals, protecting normal tissues from cisplatin toxicity. It does not appear to reduce the effectiveness of cisplatin.

Indications Reduction of cumulative renal toxicity in patients given repeated administration of cisplatin for advanced ovarian cancer.

Contraindications Hypersensitivity to aminothiol compounds or mannitol.

Route/Dosage
ADULTS: **IV Infusion** 910 mg/m^2 once daily over 15 minutes starting within 30 minutes before chemotherapy.

Interactions
Antihypertensives: May potentiate blood pressure lowering effect.

Lab Test Interferences
None well documented.

Adverse Reactions
CV: Transient hypotension. *CNS:* Somnolence; dizziness. *GI:* Nausea; vomiting. *OTHER:* Flushing; chills; feeling of warmth or coldness; hiccups; sneezing; hypocalcemia, allergic reactions (rash, rigors).

Precautions
Pregnancy: Category C. *Lactation:* Undetermined. *Children:* Safety and efficacy not established. *Elderly:* Safety has not been established in elderly patients with pre-existing cardiovascular or cerebrovascular conditions. *Chemotherapy antagonism:* Amifostine should not be given to patients with neoplasms that are potentially curable. *Hypotension:* Do not give to patients who are hypotensive, dehydrated or who cannot discontinue antihypertensive therapy 24 hours before administra-

tion. Infusion of amifostine for longer than 15 minutes increases the likelihood of hypotension. BP needs to be monitored every 5 minutes during the infusion. *Nausea and vomiting:* Antiemetic medication should be administered prior to and in conjunction with amifostine.

NURSING CONSIDERATIONS

Administration/Storage

- For IV administration only.
- Medication must be reconstituted with 9.5 ml of 0.9% normal saline for IV infusion.
- Begin administration of amifostine within 30 minutes prior to start of chemotherapy.
- Infuse over 15 minutes. Longer administration times are associated with a higher incidence of side effects. Infusion times less than 15 minutes have not been studied.
- Administer antiemetic medications or dexamethasone before and during administration.
- Solutions that contain particulate matter, are discolored or cloudy should not be used.
- Diluted solution may be stored in PVC containers for 5 hours at room temperature, and up to 24 hours under refrigeration.
- Lypholized powder (for reconstitution) should be stored in refrigerator.

Assessment/Interventions

- Obtain patient history.
- Obtain baseline blood pressure and note any hypotension.
- Ensure adequate hydration of patient before infusing.
- Keep patient in supine position during infusion.
- Monitor blood pressure every 5 minutes during infusion.
- If blood pressure drops, stop infusion and treat hypotension with fluid infusion and postural management.
- If blood pressure returns to normal within 5 minutes and patient is asymptomatic, restart infusion and finish full dose of medication.

OVERDOSAGE: SIGNS & SYMPTOMS
Hypotension

Patient/Family Education

- Explain why medication is being given and its desired effects.
- Warn patient of possible side effects, especially hypotension.
- Because medication is only administered with chemotherapy medications, include usual teaching concerning avoidance of infections.
- If the full dose of amifostine cannot be administered because of hypotension, subsequent doses should be reduced (740 mg/m^2).

See Patient Guide, p. 17.

Amikacin Sulfate

(am-ih-KAE-sin SULL-fate)
Amikin
Class: Antibiotic/aminoglycoside

Action Inhibits production of bacterial protein, causing bacterial cell death.

Indications Treatment of infections caused by susceptible strains of microorganisms, especially gram-negative bacteria.

Contraindications Generally not indicated for long-term therapy because of ototoxicity and nephrotoxicity.

Route/Dosage
ADULTS, CHILDREN & INFANTS: **IV/IM** 15 mg/kg (ideal body weight)/day in 2 or 3 divided doses. Treatment in heavier patients should not exceed 1.5 g/day. UNCOMPLICATED UTIS: **IV/IM** 250 mg bid. NEONATES: **IV/IM** Loading dose of 10

mg/kg is recommended followed by 7.5 mg/kg q 12 hr. Lower doses may be needed in first 2 wk of life.

Interactions

Drugs with nephrotoxic potential (eg, cephalosporins, enflurane, methoxyflurane and vancomycin): May increase risk of nephrotoxicity. *Loop diuretics (eg, furosemide)*: May increase risk of auditory toxicity. *Neuromuscular blocking agents (eg, tubocurarine)*: Amikacin may enhance effects of these agents. INCOMPATIBILITIES: Do not mix with beta-lactam antibiotics (eg, carbenicillin, ticarcillin).

Lab Test Interferences

None well documented.

Adverse Reactions

EENT: Hearing loss; deafness; loss of balance. *GU*: Oliguria; proteinuria; increased serum creatinine; urinary casts; red and white blood cells in urine; azotemia. *OTHER*: Decreased serum magnesium.

Precautions

Pregnancy: Category D. *Lactation*: Undetermined. *Children*: Cautious use is necessary in premature infants and neonates because of renal immaturity. *Nephrotoxicity/ototoxicity*: If patient has signs and symptoms of nephrotoxicity or ototoxicity, discontinuation or dosage adjustment is needed. *Renal impairment*: Dosage adjustment is needed in patients with this condition.

NURSING CONSIDERATIONS

Administration/Storage

- Dilute with normal saline or D5W according to instructions.
- Administer by IV or IM route only.
- Use volumetric IV pump to regulate delivery.
- Avoid overrapid administration, which may result in respiratory depression and arrest; give over 30-60 min.
- Do not mix with or administer within 1 hr of other IV medications because of potential for incompatibility or inactivation.
- Discard diluted solution after 24 hr.
- When giving by IM route, use deep, slow injection; rotate sites to prevent tissue irritation or breakdown.

Assessment/Interventions

- Obtain patient history, including drug history and any known allergies. Note hypersensitivity to aminoglycosides.
- Assess renal and auditory function before administration and monitor periodically during therapy to detect nephrotoxicity or ototoxicity.
- Blood should be sent for culture and sensitivity before beginning therapy.
- Monitor patient for signs and symptoms of yeast infections during therapy.
- Monitor I&O during therapy; maintain good hydration.
- Assess patient for signs of infection to determine effectiveness of therapy.
- Notify physician and stop infusion if patient has signs of oliguria or shows signs of renal failure (edema, shortness of breath, pruritus), ototoxicity or anaphylactic reaction.

Patient/Family Education

- Encourage patient to increase fluid intake to 2000-3000 ml/day, unless contraindicated.
- Warn patient that diarrhea and abdominal bloating are common side effects of antibiotics.
- Inform patient that improvement should be seen in 3-5 days.
- Instruct patient to report these signs to physician: hypersensitivity, tinnitus, vertigo or hearing loss.
- Teach patient signs of renal failure and instruct to notify physician immediately if these signs occur.

No patient monograph available.

Amiloride HCl

(uh-MILL-oh-ride HIGH-droe-KLOR-ide)

Midamor

Class: Potassium-sparing diuretic

Action Interferes with sodium reabsorption at distal tubule, resulting in increased excretion of water and sodium and decreased excretion of potassium.

Indications Treatment of CHF or hypertension (in combination with thiazide or loop diuretics) and diuretic-induced hypokalemia. **Unlabeled use:** Reduction of lithium-induced polyuria. **Aerosol form:** Slowed reduction of pulmonary function in patients with cystic fibrosis.

Contraindications Serum potassium > 5.5 mEq/L; potassium supplementation; impaired renal function: spironolactone or triamterene therapy.

Route/Dosage

ADULTS: **PO** 5-10 mg daily. LITHIUM-INDUCED POLYURIA: **PO** 10-20 mg daily. CYSTIC FIBROSIS: Dissolve in 0.3% saline and deliver by nebulizer.

Interactions

Angiotensin-converting enzyme inhibitors: May result in severely elevated serum potassium levels. *Potassium preparations:* May severely increase serum potassium levels, possibly resulting in cardiac arrhythmias or cardiac arrest. Do not administer to patients taking potassium preparations.

Lab Test Interferences

None well documented.

Adverse Reactions

CV: Angina pectoris; orthostatic hypotension; arrhythmia. *RESP:* Cough; dyspnea. *CNS:* Headache; dizziness; encephalopathy; paresthesia; tremors; vertigo; nervousness; mental confusion; insomnia; decreased libido; depression. *EENT:* Visual disturbances; tinnitus; nasal congestion. *GI:* Nausea; anorexia; diarrhea; vomiting; abdominal pain; gas pain; appetite changes; constipation; GI bleeding; abdominal fullness; thirst; dry mouth; heartburn; flatulence. *GU:* Impotence; polyuria; dysuria; urinary frequency. *HEMA:* Aplastic anemia; neutropenia. *HEPA:* Jaundice. *DERM:* Skin rash; itching; pruritus. *META:* Increased serum potassium levels. *OTHER:* Musculoskeletal (weakness; fatigue; muscle cramps; joint/back/chest pain; neck or shoulder ache).

Precautions

Pregnancy: Category B. *Lactation:* Undetermined. *Children:* Safety and efficacy not established. *Diabetes mellitus:* Hyperkalemia may occur. *Electrolyte imbalances and BUN increase:* Hyperkalemia, hyponatremia, hypochloremia and increases in BUN may occur. *Hepatic impairment:* With severe liver disease, hepatic encephalopathy (tremors, confusion, coma, jaundice) may occur. *Renal impairment:* Use cautiously in patients with this condition.

NURSING CONSIDERATIONS

Administration/Storage

- Administer medication with food, preferably in AM.
- Store in tightly closed container in cool location.

Assessment/Interventions

- Obtain patient history, including drug history and any known allergies. Note BP and renal disease or history of potassium supplement use.
- Monitor potassium, BUN and creatinine levels.
- If sudden elevation in serum potassium level (> 5.5 mEq/L) occurs, withhold dose and notify physician.
- Monitor fluid and electrolyte balance

during therapy (I&O, daily weight, edema).

- If drug is given in combination with another antihypertensive, monitor BP throughout administration.
- If hypokalemia is suspected, obtain periodic ECG during therapy.
- If ECG changes occur (peaked T waves, abnormal S or P waves), withhold dose and notify physician.
- Monitor for signs of hyperkalemia (fatigue, muscle weakness, cardiac irregularities).
- Monitor for signs of hyponatremia.
- Monitor renal function.

Patient/Family Education

- Explain that dietary considerations are very important while taking this medication. Advise patient to avoid the following: eating excessive amounts of potassium-rich foods (bananas, citrus fruits, raisins, nuts), using salt substitutes, taking medications high in potassium and eating foods high in sodium (tomatoes, pickled foods, canned foods, luncheon meats).
- Teach patient to monitor BP daily.
- Instruct patient to take medication as directed, even if feeling well.
- Encourage patient to avoid sudden changes in position to prevent orthostatic hypotension.
- Advise patient that drug may cause dizziness and blurred vision and to use caution while driving or performing other tasks requiring mental alertness.
- Inform patient that this medication causes increased urine output.
- Teach patient signs and symptoms of hyperkalemia and hyponatremia.
- Caution patient to notify any physician or dentist seen about taking this medication and notify physician of cramps or chronic fatigue and weakness, which are serious side effects.

See Patient Guide, p. 18.

Aminocaproic Acid

(uh-mee-no-kuh-PRO-ik acid)

Amicar

Class: Hemostatic

Action Inhibits fibrinolysis to stop bleeding.

Indications Treatment of excessive bleeding from systemic hyperfibrinolysis and urinary fibrinolysis. **Unlabeled uses:** Prevention of recurrence of subarachnoid hemorrhage; management of amegakaryocytic thrombocytopenia; abortion or prevention of attacks of hereditary angioneurotic edema.

Contraindications Active intravascular clotting; DIC; administration to newborns.

Route/Dosage

Adults: **IV/PO** 4-5 g in first hour; then 1-1.25 g/hr for 8 hr or until bleeding is controlled. Dosage > 30 g/24 hr is not recommended.

Interactions

Oral contraceptives or estrogens: May lead to increase in clotting factors, producing state of hypercoagulation.

Lab Test Interferences

Serum potassium level may be elevated, especially in impaired renal function.

Adverse Reactions

CV: Hypotension. *CNS:* Dizziness; headache; delirium; auditory, visual and kinesthetic hallucinations; weakness; convulsions. *EENT:* Conjunctival suffusion; tinnitus; nasal congestion. *GI:* Nausea; diarrhea; abdominal cramps. *GU:* Reversible acute renal failure; intrarenal obstruction. *HEMA:* Thrombophlebitis. *DERM:* Skin rash. *OTHER:* Malaise; myopathy (characterized by weakness, fatigue, elevated levels of serum enzymes such as creatinine phosphokinase); rhabdomyolysis.

Precautions

Pregnancy: Category C. *Lactation:* Undetermined. *Upper urinary tract bleeding:* Not used in treatment of hematuria of upper UT origin unless possible benefits outweigh risks.

NURSING CONSIDERATIONS

Administration/Storage

IV Infusion

- Dilute as 1 g/50 ml diluent. Compatible diluents include Sterile Water for Injection, normal saline, D5W and Ringer's solution.
- Use infusion pump for IV administration. Closely monitor rate of infusion because this drug is not intended for rapid IV injection or in undiluted form.
- Infuse dose over 30 min-1 hr.

Oral Administration

- Give with full glass of water.
- Encourage fluid intake between doses.
- Store in tightly closed container at room temperature.

Assessment/Interventions

- Obtain patient history, including drug history and any known allergies.
- Determine baseline BP and pulse before starting IV infusion.
- Assess patient's respiratory and neurologic status.
- Note presence of menstrual bleeding.
- Monitor serum potassium levels, clotting factors and platelet counts.
- Monitor vital signs, especially BP and pulse, and respiratory and neurologic status throughout therapy.
- Monitor I&O. Note any increase or decrease in urinary output.
- Observe for signs of internal bleeding (eg, petechiae, gingival oozing, hematuria, epistaxis or ecchymosis).
- Have vitamin K or protamine sulfate available for emergency use.

Patient/Family Education

- Caution patient to avoid sudden position changes to prevent orthostatic hypotension.
- Advise patient to use soft toothbrush or sponge for dental care.
- Instruct patient to report these symptoms to physician: gingival bleeding, epistaxis, hematuria, skin changes such as ecchymosis and petechiae, difficulty in urination, reddish-brown urine, chest or leg pain, or breathing difficulty.

See Patient Guide, p. 19.

Aminophylline (Theophylline Ethylenediamine)

(am-in-AHF-ih-lin)

Phyllocontin, Truphylline, ♣ *Phyllocontin-350*

Class: Bronchodilator/xanthine derivative

Action Relaxes bronchial smooth muscle and pulmonary blood vessels; stimulates central respiratory drive; increases diaphragmatic contractility.

Indications Prevention or treatment of reversible bronchospasm associated with asthma or COPD. **Unlabeled uses:** Treatment of apnea and bradycardia of prematurity.

Contraindications Hypersensitivity to xanthines (eg, caffeine, theobromine) or ethylenediamine; peptic ulcer; seizure disorders not treated with medication. Aminophylline suppositories are contraindicated in presence of irritation or infection of rectum or lower colon.

Route/Dosage

Dosage is calculated on basis of lean body weight.

ORAL/RECTAL

Dose is determined by percentage of theophylline content in aminophylline salt. Aminophylline is 79% theophylline.

Loading Dose

ADULTS & CHILDREN: **PO/PR** 5 mg/kg.

Maintenance Dose

HEALTHY NONSMOKERS: **PO/PR** 3 mg/kg q 8 hr. ELDERLY & PATIENTS WITH COR PULMONALE: 2 mg/kg q 8 hr. PATIENTS WITH CHF: 1-2 mg/kg q 12 hr. CHILDREN 9-16 YR & YOUNG ADULT SMOKERS: 3 mg/kg q 6 hr. CHILDREN 1-9 YR: 4 mg/kg q 6 hr.

PARENTERAL

Loading Dose

ADULTS & CHILDREN NOT RECEIVING THEOPHYLLINE: **IV** 6 mg/kg. ADULTS & CHILDREN RECEIVING THEOPHYLLINE: **IV** 0.6-3.1 mg/kg.

Maintenance Dose

HEALTHY NONSMOKERS: **IV** 0.5-0.7 mg/kg/hr. ELDERLY & PATIENTS WITH COR PULMONALE: **IV** 0.3-0.6 mg/kg/hr. PATIENTS WITH CHF: **IV** 0.1-0.5 mg/kg/hr. CHILDREN 9-16 YR & YOUNG ADULT SMOKERS: **IV** 0.8-1 mg/kg/hr. CHILDREN 1-9 YR: **IV** 1-1.2 mg/kg/hr. NEONATES-INFANTS < 6 MO: Not recommended. Weigh benefits against risks. INFANTS 26-52 WK: Divide into q 6 hr dosing. INFANTS UP TO 26 WK: Divide into q 8 hr dosing. INFANTS 6-52 WK: [(0.2 x Age in Weeks) + 5] = 24 hr dosage (mg). PREMATURE INFANTS > 24 DAYS POSTNATAL: **IV** 1.5 mg/kg q 12 hr. PREMATURE INFANTS < 24 DAYS POSTNATAL: **IV** 1 mg/kg q 12 hr.

Interactions

Allopurinol, nonselective beta-blockers, calcium channel blockers, cimetidine, oral contraceptives, corticosteroids, disulfiram, ephedrine, influenza virus vaccine, interferon, macrolide antibiotics, mexiletine, quinolone antibiotics, thyroid hormones: May increase aminophylline levels. *Aminoglutethimide, barbiturates, hydantoins, ketoconazole, rifampin, smoking (tobacco and marijuana), sulfinpyrazone, sympathomimetics:* May decrease aminophylline levels. *Benzodiazepines, propofol:* Aminophylline may antagonize sedative effects. *Beta-agonists:* Effects of both drugs may be antagonized. *Carbamazepine, isoniazid, loop diuretics:* May increase or decrease aminophylline levels. *Food:* Sustained-released medications are taken on empty stomach to avoid rapid drug release. Low-protein, high-carbohydrate diet may increase aminophylline levels. Charcoal-broiled foods or high-protein, low-carbohydrate diet may decrease aminophylline levels. *Halothane:* May cause catecholamine-induced arrhythmias. *Ketamine:* May result in seizures. *Lithium:* Aminophylline may reduce lithium levels. *Nondepolarizing muscle relaxants:* May antagonize neuromuscular blockade. INCOMPATIBILITIES: Do not mix with anileridine hydrochloride, ascorbic acid, chlorpromazine, codeine phosphate, dimenhydrinate, dobutamine hydroide, epinephrine, erythromycin gluceptate, hydralazine, insulin, levorphanol tartrate, meperidine, methadone, methicillin, morphine sulfate, norepinephrine bitartrate, oxytetracycline, penicillin G potassium, phenobarbital, phenytoin, prochlorperazine, promazine, promethazine, tetracycline, vancomycin, verapamil, vitamin B complex with vitamin C.

Lab Test Interferences

None well documented.

Adverse Reactions

CV: Palpitations; tachycardia; hypotension; arrhythmias. *RESP:* Tachypnea; respiratory arrest. *CNS:* Irritability; headache; insomnia; muscle twitching; seizures. *GI:* Nausea; vomiting; anorexia, diarrhea; gastroesophageal reflux; epigastric pain. *GU:* Proteinuria; diuresis. *OTHER:* Fever; flushing; hyperglycemia; inappropriate antidiuretic hormone secretion; sensitivity reactions (exfoliative dermatitis and urticaria).

Precautions

Pregnancy: Category C. *Lacta-*

tion: Excreted in breast milk. *Children:* Safety and efficacy not established in children < 1 yr. *Cardiac effects:* Aminophylline may cause or worsen preexisting arrhythmias. *GI effects:* Aminophylline may cause or worsen preexisting ulcers or gastroesophageal reflux. *Status asthmaticus:* In this medical emergency parenteral medication and close monitoring in intensive care unit are recommended. *Toxicity:* Patients with liver impairment or cardiac failure and those > 55 yr are at greatest risk.

NURSING CONSIDERATIONS

Administration/Storage

- Store at room temperature.

Tablets and Liquid

- Give on empty stomach (½-1 hr before meals or 2 hr after meals).
- Do not crush or chew extended release forms; capsules may be opened and contents mixed with soft food. Scored tablets can be cut in half and then swallowed.

IV Infusion

- Do not administer if solution is discolored or if crystals are present.
- Rapid infusion may cause cardiac arrest.
- Give undiluted drug at rate of 25 mg/min.
- Dilute in dextrose or saline solutions or Lactated Ringer's. Administer diluted drug at rate of 25 mg/min (maximum). Once mixed, solution must be refrigerated and used within 24 hr.
- Use of infusion pump is recommended for precise administration.
- Do not mix aminophylline solution in syringe with other drugs. Separate IV infusion is recommended because of IV incompatibilities.

Suppositories

- Do not use rectal route when irritation or infection is present.
- May have special storage requirements.

IM Injection

- IM route is usually not used because this method produces intense prolonged pain.

Assessment/Interventions

- Obtain patient history, including drug history and any known allergies. Note sensitivity to xanthines (caffeine or chocolate), peptic ulcer, seizure disorders, liver disease and current medication regimen.
- Take vital signs before and after administration.
- Note baseline ECG.
- Assess lung sounds.
- Measure and record I&O.
- Position patient with head of bed elevated or place in position of comfort to reduce dyspnea.
- Encourage fluid intake to liquefy bronchial secretions.
- Reduce patient's intake of cola, coffee and chocolate and use of cigarettes.
- Report carbohydrate or protein restrictions in patient's diet because theophylline dosage may need to be adjusted.
- Monitor vital signs and cardiac status. If significant tachycardia or ventricular arrhythmias occur, withhold drug and report to physician.
- In patients receiving theophylline products, monitor serum theophylline levels for toxicity. If levels are above therapeutic range (10-20 mcg/ml), report to physician.
- In patients receiving erythromycin, beta-blockers (eg, atenolol, metoprolol, nadolol, propanolol), cimetidine or allopurinol, monitor for toxicity.
- In patients receiving phenobarbital, rifampin, carbamazepine or lithium, monitor effectiveness of aminophylline; dosage may not be sufficient.

Patient/Family Education

- Advise patient not to smoke. If patient changes smoking habits or stops smoking, dosage adjustment may be necesssary.

- Instruct patient to report these symptoms to physician: unusual worsening of symptoms, nausea, vomiting, excessive nervousness, insomnia or irregular heartbeat.
- For patients taking theophylline, emphasize that serum theophylline levels should be tested every 6-12 mo.
- Advise elderly patients to take safety precautions (rise slowly, use handrails, request assistance in ambulation) if dizziness occurs.
- Instruct patient to avoid foods or beverages containing caffeine and to limit intake of charcoal-broiled foods.
- Advise patient not to take otc cough, cold or breathing medications without consulting physician.

See Patient Guide, p. 20.

Aminosalicylate Sodium (Para-Aminosalicylate Sodium; PAS)

(uh-MEE-no-suh-LIS-ih-late SO-dee-uhm)

Sodium P.A.S.

Class: Anti-infective/antitubercular

Action Competitively antagonizes metabolism of para-aminobenzoic acid, resulting in bacteriostatic activity against *Mycobacterium tuberculosis*.

Indications Treatment of tuberculosis (in combination with other antituberculous drugs) caused by susceptible strains of tubercle bacilli.

Contraindications Severe hypersensitivity to aminosalicylate sodium and its congeners.

Route/Dosage

ADULTS: **PO** 14-16 g/day in 2-3 divided doses. CHILDREN: **PO** 275-420 mg/kg/day in 3-4 divided doses.

Interactions

Digoxin: May reduce oral absorption and serum levels of digoxin. *Rifampin:* May decrease absorption of rifampin. *Vitamin B_{12}:* May decrease GI absorption of oral vitamin B_{12}.

Lab Test Interferences

None well documented.

Adverse Reactions

GI: Nausea; vomiting; diarrhea; abdominal pain. *META:* Goiter with or without myxedema. *OTHER:* Hypersensitivity (eg, fever, skin eruptions, infectious mononucleosis–like syndrome, leukopenia, agranulocytosis, thrombocytopenia, hemolytic anemia, jaundice, hepatitis, encephalopathy, Loffler's syndrome, vasculitis).

Precautions

Pregnancy: Category C. *Lactation:* Excreted in breast milk. *CHF:* Use with caution because of high sodium content (55 mg of sodium per 500 mg tablet). *Crystalluria:* Maintain urine at neutral or alkaline pH to avoid crystalluria. *Gastric ulcer:* Use with caution. *Hepatic or renal function impairment:* Use with caution. *Hypersensitivity:* Stop medication if hypersensitivity symptoms develop. Restart cautiously.

NURSING CONSIDERATIONS

Administration/Storage

- Administer with food or meals. Product may cause GI upset.
- Do not leave medication in extreme heat or direct sunlight. Moisture, extreme heat or direct sunlight may reduce effectiveness of product.
- Do not use products that are brown or purple in color.

Assessment/Interventions

- Obtain patient history, including drug history and any known allergies.
- Review results of renal and hepatic function studies and assess patient for undesirable side effects and adverse reactions. Notify physician of any untoward response.

- Check patient record for notation of prescription for parenteral administration of vitamin B_{12} when aminosalicylate sodium will be given for more than a few weeks or if patient is malnourished.
- Do not discontinue without consulting physician.
- Monitor urine pH and report any change toward acidity or crystal formation.
- If patient is taking digoxin, monitor for signs of reduced serum levels of digoxin and notify physician of any associated signs, symptoms or lab data.

Patient/Family Education

- Instruct patient to take medication with meals or immediately after meals to minimize GI symptoms and to maintain adequate fluid intake.
- Explain to patients taking digoxin that dose may be increased while taking aminosalicylate sodium.
- Instruct patient to report these symptoms to physician: fever, sore throat, unusual bleeding or bruising or skin rash.
- Teach patient importance of maintaining urine at neutral or alkaline pH and demonstrate method for testing urine pH.
- Instruct patient not to take otc medications without consulting physician.

See Patient Guide, p. 21.

Amiodarone

(A-MEE-oh-duh-rone)

Cordarone

Class: Antiarrhythmic

Action Prolongs action potential duration and refractory period in myocardial cells; acts as noncompetitive inhibitor of alpha- and beta-adrenergic receptors.

Indications Treatment of life-threatening recurrent ventricular arrhythmias (ie, ventricular fibrillation and hemodynamically unstable ventricular tachycardia) that do not respond to other antiarrhythmic agents. **Unlabeled uses:** Treatment of refractory sustained or paroxysmal atrial fibrillation, paroxysmal supraventricular tachycardia (PSVT) and symptomatic atrial flutter. In low doses, may produce benefits in left ventricular ejection fraction, exercise tolerance and ventricular arrhythmias in patients with CHF.

Contraindications Severe sinus-node dysfunction, causing marked sinus bradycardia; second- or third-degree atrioventricular (AV) block; when bradycardia produces syncope, unless used with pacemaker.

Route/Dosage

Life-Threatening Recurrent Ventricular Arrhythmias

Loading dose: **PO** 800-1600 mg/day for 1-3 wk. Reduce doses of other antiarrhythmic agents gradually. When adequate arrhythmia control is achieved, reduce dose to 600-800 mg/day for 1 mo. Usual maintenance dose: **PO** 400 mg/day.

Paroxysmal Atrial Fibrillation, PSVT, Symptomatic Atrial Flutter

PO 600-800 mg/day for 7-10 days, then 200-400 mg/day.

Arrhythmias in Patients with CHF

PO 200 mg/day.

Interactions

Anticoagulants: Effect of anticoagulant may be increased. Use of product may require 30%-50% decrease in anticoagulant dose. *Digoxin:* Serum digoxin levels may be increased. *Flecainide:* Serum levels of flecainide may be increased. *Hydantoins (eg, phenytoin):* Serum concentrations of hydantoins may be increased with potential for symptoms of hydantoin toxicity; also, amiodarone levels may be decreased. *Procainamide:* Serum levels of procainamide may be increased. *Quinidine:* Serum quinidine levels may increase, creating potential for fatal cardiac arrhythmias.

Lab Test Interferences

May alter results of thyroid and liver function tests.

Adverse Reactions

CV: Exacerbation of arrhythmias; CHF; bradycardia; sinoatrial node dysfunction; heart block; sinus arrest; flushing. *RESP:* Pulmonary inflammation or fibrosis; progressive dyspnea, pulmonary toxicosis and death. *CNS:* Fatigue; malaise; tremor/abnormal involuntary movements; lack of coordination; abnormal gait/ataxia; dizziness; paresthesias; decreased libido; insomnia; headache; sleep disturbances; abnormal sense of smell. *EENT:* Visual disturbances; reversible asymptomatic corneal microdeposits; photophobia; abnormal taste. *GI:* Nausea; vomiting; constipation; anorexia; abdominal pain; abnormal salivation. *HEMA:* Coagulation abnormalities. *HEPA:* Nonspecific hepatic disorders. *DERM:* Photosensitivity; solar dermatitis; blue discoloration of skin. *OTHER:* Edema; hyperthyroidism or hypothyroidism.

Precautions

Pregnancy: Category D. *Lactation:* Excreted in breast milk. *Children:* Safety and efficacy not established.

NURSING CONSIDERATIONS

Administration/Storage

- Administer with meals.
- Store at room temperature and protect from light.

Assessment/Interventions

- Obtain patient history, including drug history and any known allergies.
- Review baseline clotting factor studies and serum levels of digoxin, flecainide, quinidine, procainamide and theophylline, as available, and continue to monitor these parameters during treatment.
- Review thyroid and liver function test results and note any changes after initiation of therapy.
- Consult chest x-ray, and review findings from any pulmonary function tests performed prior to and after initiation of therapy.
- Repeat history and physical examination every 3-6 mos and consult chest radiographs as available.
- Assess for changes in pulmonary status, and notify physician of any trends that could be associated with pulmonary toxicity such as dyspnea, fatigue, cough or pleuritic pain. Document and report any fever to physician.
- Assess for symptoms of hyperthyroidism or hypothyroidism.
- Assess baseline pulse and BP and monitor during treatment. Report symptomatic bradycardia (fatigue, light-headedness or syncope).
- Assess for CNS side effects (eg, muscle weakness) and report to physician.
- Monitor cardiac rhythm continuously during initiation of treatment and regularly during maintenance therapy. Notify physician of exacerbation of presenting arrhythmia, bradycardia, heart block or sinus arrest.

Patient/Family Education

- Instruct patient to report any cough or shortness of breath.
- Show patient how to take pulse. Explain that heart rate < 60 bpm should be reported to physician.
- Caution patient to avoid exposure to sunlight and to use sunscreen or wear protective clothing to avoid photosensitivity reaction. Sun exposed skin may appear blue-gray. Also, explain that discomfort of photophobia may be decreased by wearing sunglasses.
- Explain that eating small, frequent meals or dividing daily dose and taking 2 or 3 doses with meals may help if patient experiences GI upset.
- Instruct patient to report these symptoms to physician: halos around lights; any vision problems; GI distress; loss of appetite; tremors;

twitches; fatigue; unsteady walking; dizziness; numbness and tingling in hands or feet; insomnia; headache; slowing of heartbeat; irregular heart rhythm; difficulty breathing; coughing; sensitivity to sunlight, including blue-gray patches on skin; dermatitis; bruising; hair loss; flushing; abnormal sense of taste or smell; fluid retention; loss of sex drive.

See Patient Guide, p. 22.

Amitriptyline HCl

(am-ee-TRIP-tih-leen HIGH-droe-KLOR-ide)

Elavil, Endep, Enovil, ♣ *APO-Amitriptylene*

Class: Tricyclic antidepressant

Action Inhibits presynaptic reuptake of norepinephrine and serotonin in CNS.

Indications Palliative treatment of depression. **Unlabeled uses:** Management of chronic pain associated with migraine, tension headache, diabetic neuropathy, peripheral neuropathy, cancer or arthritis; treatment of panic and eating disorders.

Contraindications Hypersensitivity to any tricyclic antidepressant; use during acute recovery phase of MI; concomitant use with monoamine oxidase (MAO) inhibitors, except under close medical supervision.

Route/Dosage

ADULTS: Titrate dosage over 2 wk-1 mo. Give maintenance dose 6 mo-1 yr. Do not interrupt therapy abruptly; reduce over 2 wk period. OUTPATIENTS: **PO** 75-150 mg/day in divided doses; give in evening or at bedtime because of sedative effects. HOSPITALIZED PATIENTS: **PO** 100-300 mg/day. ADOLESCENT & ELDERLY PATIENTS: **PO** 10 mg tid and 20 mg at bedtime. MAINTENANCE: **PO** 40-100 mg/day. PARENTERAL FORM: Do *not* use IV route. **IM** 20-30 mg qid. Change to oral dosing as soon as possible.

Interactions

Barbiturates, charcoal: May cause decreased blood levels of amitriptyline. *Cimetidine, fluoxetine:* May cause increased blood levels of amitriptyline. *Clonidine:* Use with product may result in hypertensive crisis. *CNS depressants:* Depressant effects may be additive. *MAOIs:* May cause hyperpyretic crises, severe convulsions and death when given with amitriptyline.

Lab Test Interferences

None well documented.

Adverse Reactions

CV: Orthostatic hypotension; hypertension; tachycardia; palpitations; arrhythmias; ECG changes. *RESP:* Pharyngitis; rhinitis; sinusitis; cough. *CNS:* Confusion; hallucinations; disturbed concentration; decreased memory; delusions; nervousness; restlessness; agitation; panic; insomnia; nightmares; mania; exacerbation of psychosis; drowsiness; dizziness; weakness; emotional lability; numbness; tremors; extrapyramidal symptoms (pseudoparkinsonism, movement disorders, akathesia); seizures. *EENT:* Conjunctivitis; blurred vision; increased IOP; mydriasis; tinnitus; nasal congestion; peculiar taste in mouth. *GI:* Nausea; vomiting; anorexia; GI distress; diarrhea; flatulence; dry mouth; constipation. *GU:* Impotence; sexual dysfunction; menstrual irregularities; dysmenorrhea; nocturia; urinary frequency; UTI; vaginitis; cystitis; urinary retention and hesitancy. *HEMA:* Bone marrow depression, including agranulocytosis; eosinophilia; purpura; thrombocytopenia; leukopenia. *HEPA:* Jaundice. *DERM:* Rash; pruritus; photosensitivity reaction; dry skin; acne; itching. *META:* Elevation or depression of blood sugar levels. *OTHER:* Breast enlargement.

Precautions

Pregnancy: Category C. *Lactation:* Excreted in breast milk. *Children:* Not recommended for children < 12 yr. *Changing from MAO inhibitor to amitriptyline:* Waiting period of 7-10 days is necessary to prevent hypertensive crisis. *Special risk patients:* Caution is needed with history of seizures; urinary retention; urethral or ureteral spasm; angle-closure glaucoma or increased IOP; cardiovascular disorders; hyperthyroidism and patients receiving thyroid medication; hepatic or renal impairment; schizophrenia; paranoia.

NURSING CONSIDERATIONS

Administration/Storage

- Use IM route only if patient is unable to take oral form.
- Give drug with or immediately after food or fluid and in late afternoon or at bedtime because of sedative effect. Tablets may be crushed.
- Store at room temperature and protect from light.

Assessment/Interventions

- Obtain patient history, including drug history and any known allergies.
- Take vital signs and monitor during initial therapy.
- Assess patient's mental status, affect, energy level, sleeping and eating habits and suicidal tendencies.
- Record I&O, noting bowel elimination pattern.
- Encourage high intake of fiber and fluid, and offer laxatives or stool softeners as necessary.
- Restrict amount of medication available to patient. Check patient's mouth after administration to detect possible hoarding of medication or noncompliance with therapy.
- Provide frequent oral hygiene.
- Assist patient to rise slowly. Supervise ambulation and institute measures to prevent falling.
- Monitor ECG, WBC with differential, serum glucose level and cardiac, renal and hepatic function regularly.
- Document patient's mental status and vital signs every shift until reponse to therapy is evaluated.
- Monitor closely for oversedation, especially if patient is taking antihistamines, narcotic analgesics or sedatives/hypnotics.
- If systolic BP increases or decreases 10-20 mm Hg from baseline or if pulse rate or rhythm shows significant change, withhold drug and notify physician.

OVERDOSAGE: SIGNS & SYMPTOMS

Confusion, agitation, hallucinations, seizures, status epilepticus, clonus, choreoathetosis, hyperactive reflexes, positive Babinski's sign, coma, cardiac arrhythmias, renal failure, flushing, dry mouth, dilated pupils, hyperpyrexia

Patient/Family Education

- Caution patient not to stop taking medication abruptly without consulting physician.
- Reinforce importance of follow-up visits to physician for monitoring drug's effectiveness and side effects.
- Explain that drug effects may not be evident for 2-3 wk but that side effects are usually noted early.
- Tell patient that side effects are reduced if drug is taken at bedtime.
- Advise patient that weight gain often results from increased appetite caused by drug.
- Inform patient that urine may turn blue-green.
- Emphasize the need for regular dental care because oral dryness can increase risk for dental caries.
- Instruct patient to report these symptoms to physician: blurred vision, increased heart rate, impaired coordination, difficult urination, excessive sedation or seizures.

- Instruct patient to take sips of water frequently, suck on ice chips or sugarless hard candy, or chew sugarless gum if dry mouth occurs.
- Caution patient to avoid sudden position changes to prevent orthostatic hypotension.
- Instruct patient to avoid intake of alcohol beverages or other CNS depressants.
- Advise patient that drug may cause drowsiness and to use caution while driving or performing other tasks requiring mental alertness.
- Caution patient to avoid exposure to sunlight and to use sunscreen or wear protective clothing to avoid photosensitivity reaction.
- Instruct patient not to take otc medications without consulting physician.

See Patient Guide, p. 23.

Amlodipine

(am-LOW-dih-PEEN)

Norvasc

Class: Calcium channel blocker

Action Inhibits movement of calcium ions across cell membrane in systemic and coronary vascular smooth muscle.

Indications Hypertension; chronic stable angina; vasospastic (Prinzmetal's or variant) angina.

Contraindications Sick sinus syndrome; second- or third-degree atrioventricular (AV) block, except with a functioning pacemaker.

Route/Dosage

ADULTS: PO 5-10 mg qd. ELDERLY: PO Initially 2.5 mg qd.

Hepatic Impairment

PO Initially 2.5 mg qd.

Interactions

Beta-blockers: May cause increased adverse cardiac effects as a result of myocardial depression. *Fentanyl:* Severe hypotension or increased fluid volume requirements have occurred with similar drug.

Lab Test Interferences

None well documented.

Adverse Reactions

CV: Palpitations; peripheral edema; syncope; tachycardia; bradycardia; arrhythmias; ventricular asystoles. *RESP:* Shortness of breath; dyspnea; wheezing. *CNS:* Headache; dizziness; lightheadedness; fatigue; lethargy; somnolence. *GI:* Nausea; abdominal discomfort; cramps; dyspepsia. *DERM:* Dermatitis; rash; pruritus; urticaria. *OTHER:* Flushing; sexual difficulties; muscle cramps, pain or inflammation.

Precautions

Pregnancy: Category C. *Lactation:* Undetermined. *Children:* Safety and efficacy not established. *CHF:* Cautious use is required with this condition. *Hepatic impairment:* Cautious use is required.

NURSING CONSIDERATIONS

Administration/Storage

- Administer medication in AM.
- If patient has difficulty swallowing, crush tablets.
- Store in tightly closed container in cool location.

Assessment/Interventions

- Obtain patient history, including drug history and any known allergies. Note any diabetes, liver disease, cardiac disease or sensitivity to calcium channel blockers.
- Monitor BP and pulse before administration.
- Review baseline ECG.
- Assess for signs of withdrawal syndrome. Abrupt withdrawal may cause increased frequency and duration of

angina. Gradual tapering of dose is necessary.
- Assess patient for signs of CHF during therapy.
- If chest pain occurs, assess for location, intensity, duration and radiation. Nitroglycerin preparations may be administered in conjunction with this medication.
- If drug is used with other calcium channel blockers or beta-blockers, observe for intensification of side effects.
- Withhold medication and notify physician if any of these signs and symptoms occur: sudden severe dyspnea; edema of hands and feet; changes in ECG (widened QRS, prolonged QT segments); pulse falls below 50 bpm.
- If the patient experiences chest pain not relieved by medication, continue medication and notify physician.

OVERDOSAGE: SIGNS & SYMPTOMS

Nausea, weakness, dizziness, drowsiness, confusion, slurred speech, hypotension, bradycardia, second- or third-degree AV block

Patient/Family Education
- Teach patient how to monitor pulse before taking medication. Tell patient not to take medication if pulse if < 50 bpm and to call physician.
- Explain to patient how to monitor BP daily.
- Instruct patient not to stop taking this medication suddenly because doing so can cause chest pain and MI.
- Teach patient importance of good oral hygiene and frequent visits to dentist while taking medication.
- Inform patient that frequent follow-up appointments with physician are important to adjust medication dosage.
- Caution patient to avoid sudden position changes to prevent orthostatic hypotension.
- Instruct patient to avoid intake of alcoholic beverages or other CNS depressants.
- Advise patient that drug may cause drowsiness and to use caution while driving or performing other tasks requiring mental alertness.
- Instruct patient not to take otc medications without consulting physician.

See Patient Guide, p. 24.

Amobarbital Sodium

(am-oh-BAR-bih-tahl SO-dee-uhm)

Amytal Sodium

Class: Sedative and hypnotic/barbiturate

Action Depresses sensory cortex; decreases motor activity; alters cerebellar function and produces drowsiness, sedation and hypnosis.

Indications Relief of anxiety; short-term therapy for insomnia; induction of preanesthetic sedation.

Contraindications Hypersensitivity to barbiturates; history of addiction to sedative-hypnotic drugs; history of porphyria; severe liver impairment; respiratory disease with dyspnea; patients with nephritis.

Route/Dosage

Insomnia

ADULTS: **PO/IM/IV** 65-200 mg at bedtime.

Sedation

ADULTS: **PO/IM/IV** 30-50 mg bid or tid. CHILDREN: **PO/IM** 2-6 mg/kg/dose.

Interactions

Alcohol, CNS depressants: Depressant effects of these drugs may be enhanced. *Anticoagulants, beta-blockers, calcium-channel blockers (eg, Verapamil) theophyllines:* Activity of these drugs may be reduced. *Anticonvulsants:* Serum concentrations of carbamazepine, valproic acid and succinimides may be reduced. Valproic acid may increase barbiturate serum levels. *Corticosteroids:* Effectiveness may be reduced. *Estrogens, estrogen-containing oral contraceptives:* Effectiveness may be reduced.

Lab Test Interferences

Decreased serum bilirubin; false-positive phentolamine test results.

Adverse Reactions

CV: Bradycardia; hypotension; syncope. *RESP:* Hypoventilation; apnea; laryngospasm; bronchospasm. *CNS:* Drowsiness; agitation; confusion; headache; hyperkinesia; ataxia; CNS depression; paradoxical excitement; nightmares; psychiatric disturbances; hallucinations; insomnia; dizziness. *GI:* Nausea; vomiting; constipation. *HEMA:* Blood dyscrasias (agranulocytosis, thrombocytopenia). *HEPA:* Liver damage. *OTHER:* Hypersensitivity reactions (angioedema, rashes, exfoliative dermatitis); fever; injection site reactions (local pain, thrombophlebitis).

Precautions

Pregnancy: Category D. *Lactation:* Excreted in breast milk. *Children:* Safety and efficacy not established in children < 6 yr. *Elderly:* Dosage should be reduced. *Drug dependence:* Tolerance or psychologic and physical dependence may occur with continued use. *Renal or hepatic impairment:* Use with caution; dosage should be reduced.

NURSING CONSIDERATIONS

Administration/Storage

- May be given in oral, IM (deep) or IV form. Do not administer SC.
- Reconstitute solution with Sterile Water for Injection, rotating vial to mix. Do not shake vial. Solution should clear within 5 min.
- Do not dilute with Lactated Ringer's solution.
- Do not administer if solution is discolored or if precipitate is present.
- After reconstitution, solution should be injected within 30 min.
- Do not exceed IV infusion rate of 1 ml/min or 100 mg/min. Overrapid administration may result in respiratory depression, apnea and hypertension.
- To avoid tissue irritation, no more than 5 ml should be injected IM into any one site.
- Store at room temperature. Do not freeze.

Assessment/Interventions

- Obtain patient history, including drug history and any known allergies.
- Ensure that serum bilirubin level has been determined before beginning long-term therapy, especially in patients with hepatic disease.
- Monitor vital signs before and during IV infusion.
- Assess sleep patterns and mental status before beginning therapy and monitor periodically during therapy.
- Observe IV site during and after infusion. Extravasation or inadvertent intra-arterial injection may cause tissue necrosis, arterial spasm, thrombosis or gangrene.
- Monitor children and elderly patients for adverse reactions, including marked excitement, confusion, restlessness or depression.
- If hypersensitivity reaction develops, withhold dose and notify physician.
- When administering by IV infusion, keep resuscitation equipment at bedside.
- If signs of extravasation or phlebitis appear at injection site, discontinue IV infusion and notify physician.
- Implement safety measures to prevent falls, especially with elderly patients.
- Restrict amount of drug available to patient during early therapy.

OVERDOSAGE: SIGNS & SYMPTOMS

Respiratory depression, CNS depression progressing to Cheyne-Stokes respiration, oliguria, tachycardia, hypotension, hypothermia, coma, shock, cessation of electrical activity in brain (extreme overdose)

Patient/Family Education

- Advise patient not to increase dosage or stop therapy without advice of physician.
- Instruct patient to avoid alcohol, nicotine and caffeine products.
- Advise patient that drug may cause drowsiness and to use caution while driving or performing other tasks requiring mental alertness.
- Inform patient to report these symptoms to physician: excessive sleepiness, fatigue, nausea or vomiting.

See Patient Guide, p. 25.

Amobarbital/Secobarbital

(am-oh-BAR-bih-tahl/see-koe-BAR-bih-tahl)

Tuinal 100 mg Pulvules, Tuinal 200 mg Pulvules

Class: Sedative and hypnotic/barbiturate

Action Depresses sensory cortex, decreases motor activity, alters cerebellar function and produces drowsiness, sedation and hypnosis.

Indications Treatment of short-term insomnia; induction of preanesthetic sedation.

Contraindications Hypersensitivity to barbiturates; history of addiction to sedative-hypnotic drugs; history of porphyria; severe liver impairment; respiratory disease with dyspnea; nephrosis.

Route/Dosage

ADULTS: **PO** 1 capsule (50 mg/50 mg or 100 mg/100 mg) at bedtime or 1 hr before surgery.

Interactions

Alcohol, CNS depressants: Depressant effects of these drugs may be enhanced. *Anticoagulants, beta-blockers, calcium channel blockers (eg, Verapamil), theophyllines:* Activity of these drugs may be reduced. *Anticonvulsants:* Serum concentrations of carbamazepine, valproic acid and succinimides may be reduced. Valproic acid may increase barbiturate serum levels. *Corticosteroids:* Effectiveness may be reduced. *Estrogens, estrogen-containing oral contraceptives:* Effectiveness may be reduced.

Lab Test Interferences

Decreased serum bilirubin; false-positive phentolamine test results.

Adverse Reactions

CV: Bradycardia; hypotension; syncope. *RESP:* Hypoventilation; apnea; laryngospasm; bronchospasm. *CNS:* Drowsiness; agitation; confusion; headache; hyperkinesia; ataxia; CNS depression; paradoxical excitement; nightmares; psychiatric disturbances; hallucinations; insomnia; dizziness. *GI:* Nausea; vomiting; constipation. *HEMA:* Blood dyscrasias (agranulocytosis, thrombocytopenia). *HEPA:* Liver damage. *OTHER:* Hypersensitivity reactions (angioedema, rashes, exfoliative dermatitis); fever; injection site reactions (local pain, thrombophlebitis).

Precautions

Pregnancy: Category D. *Lactation:* Excreted in breast milk. *Children:* Safety and efficacy not established. *Elderly:* Dosage should be reduced. *Drug dependence:* Tolerance or psychologic and physical dependence may occur with continued use. *Renal or hepatic impairment:* Use with caution; dosage should be reduced.

Administration/Storage
◆ Administer at bedtime or 1-2 hr prior to procedure.
◆ May be crushed and given mixed with food or fluid.
◆ Store at room temperature in tightly closed container.

Assessment/Interventions
◆ Obtain patient history, including drug history and any allergies. Note history of drug abuse.
◆ Assess patient's sleep patterns and mental status before beginning therapy and monitor periodically during long-term therapy.
◆ Assess vital signs prior to initial dose.
◆ Ensure that hepatic function tests have been performed and hematology test results and serum folate and vitamin D levels have been determined before beginning long-term therapy.
◆ Darken room, provide quiet environment and offer caffeine-free warm beverage to promote sleep at bedtime.
◆ If signs of respiratory depression or overdosage develop, withhold dose and notify physician.
◆ Report unexpected responses (particularly in elderly) such as marked excitement, confusion, restlessness or depression.
◆ Implement safety measures to prevent falls, especially in elderly patients.

OVERDOSAGE: SIGNS & SYMPTOMS

Respiratory depression, CNS depression progressing to Cheyne-Stokes respiration, oliguria, tachycardia, hypotension, hypothermia, coma, shock, cessation of electrical activity in brain (extreme overdose)

Patient/Family Education
◆ Instruct patient to avoid intake of alcohol or other CNS depressants (eg, sedatives or tranquilizers).
◆ Caution patient to avoid nicotine and caffeine.
◆ Advise patient that drug may cause drowsiness and to avoid driving or performing other activities requiring mental alertness or coordination.
◆ Instruct patient to keep medication in daily-dose system or in locked cabinet to avoid accidental overdosage.
◆ Teach patient appropriate exercise and stress-reduction techniques to promote rest.

See Patient Guide, p. 26.

Amoxapine

(am-OX-uh-peen)
Asendin
Class: Tricyclic antidepressant

Action Inhibits reuptake of norepinephrine and serotonin in CNS.

Indications Relief of symptoms of depression.

Contraindications Hypersensitivity to tricyclic antidepressants; not recommended for use during acute recovery phase of MI. Drug should not be used concomitantly with MAO inhibitors except under close medical supervision.

Route/Dosage
ADULTS: **PO** 200-300 mg/day; may be given in single daily dose at bedtime once effective dosage is established. Divided doses are given for amounts > 300 mg/day. Hospitalized patients refractory to antidepressant therapy and with no history of seizures may be cautiously titrated to 600 mg/day in divided doses. ELDERLY PATIENTS: **PO** Initially 25 mg bid or tid. If well tolerated, may be increased to 50 mg bid or tid. Some patients may need up to 300 mg/day.

Interactions
Barbiturates, charcoal: May decrease amoxapine blood levels. *Cimetidine, fluoxetine:* May increase amoxapine blood levels. *Clonidine:* May result

in hypertensive crisis. *CNS depressants:* Depressant effects may be additive. *MAO inhibitors:* May cause serious and possibly fatal hypertensive crisis.

Lab Test Interferences None well documented.

Adverse Reactions Effects can generally be minimized by starting with low doses and increasing gradually. *CV:* Orthostatic hypotension; hypertension; tachycardia; palpitations; arrythmias; ECG changes. *RESP:* Pharyngitis; rhinitis; sinusitis, cough. *CNS:* Confusion; hallucinations; delusions; nervousness; restlessness; disturbed concentration; decreased memory; agitation; panic; insomnia; nightmares; mania; exacerbation of psychosis; drowsiness; dizziness; weakness; emotional liability; seizures. *EENT:* Conjunctivitis; blurred vision; increased intraocular pressure; mydriasis; tinnitus; nasal congestion; peculiar taste in mouth. *GI:* Nausea; vomiting; anorexia; GI distress; diarrhea; flatulence; dry mouth; constipation. *GU:* Impotence; sexual dysfunction; nocturia; urinary frequency, retention or hesitancy; urinary tract infection; vaginitis; cystitis. *HEMA:* Bone marrow depression including agranulocytosis; eosinophilia; purpura; thrombocytopenia; leukopenia. *HEPA:* Hepatitis; jaundice. *DERM:* Rash; pruritus; photosensitivity reaction; dry skin; acne; itching. *META:* Elevation or depression of blood glucose levels. *OTHER:* Numbness; tremors; menstrual irregularities, dysmenorrhea; breast enlargement in males and females; extrapyramidal symptoms (pseudoparkinsonism, movement disorders, akathesia); tardive dyskinesia.

Precautions
Pregnancy: Category C. *Lactation:* Excreted in breast milk. *Children:* Not recommended in children < 16 yr. *Neuroleptic malignant syndrome (NMS):* Potentially fatal condition that has been reported with amoxapine. Signs and symptoms include hyperpyrexia, muscle rigidity, altered mental status, irregular pulse, irregular blood pressure, tachycardia and diaphoresis. Notify physician. Amoxapine and nonessential drugs should be discontinued. *Patients switching from MAOI to amoxapine:* Wait 7-10 days to prevent hypertensive crisis. *Special risk patients:* Use with caution in patients with history of seizures, urinary retention, urethral or ureteral spasm, angle-closure glaucoma or increased intraocular pressure, cardiovascular disorders, hyperthyroid patients or those patients receiving thyroid medication, hepatic or renal impairment, schizophrenic or paranoid patients.

NURSING CONSIDERATIONS

Administration/Storage

- Administer by oral route only.
- Administer with or immediately after meals to reduce GI irritation.
- May be crushed and given mixed with food or fluid.
- Dosage is titrated during first week(s). Once effective dosage is determined, may be given as single bedtime dose.
- Store at room temperature in tightly closed container.

Assessment/Interventions

- Obtain patient history, including drug history and any allergies. Note glaucoma, pre-existing cardiovascular disease, history of prostatic hypertrophy and seizures.
- Restrict amount of drug available to patient during early therapy.
- Implement suicide precautions.
- Assist patient to ambulate and change positions to prevent orthostatic hypotension.
- Offer frequent liquids or oral hygiene.
- Assess mental status, affect and suicidal tendencies.
- Obtain baseline BP and monitor daily.
- Ensure that baseline hepatic, renal, and pancreatic function tests have

been performed before therapy and monitor results during long-term therapy.

- Review baseline ECG and monitor CBC and differential counts during long-term therapy.
- Monitor for sedation and initial antidepressant effect during first 4-7 days of therapy.
- Monitor I&O and evaluate bowel elimination.
- In diabetic patient, monitor blood glucose levels periodically during therapy.

Patient/Family Education

- Explain that full effectiveness of drug may not occur for up to 2-3 wk after initiation of drug therapy and that dosage will be tapered slowly before stopping.
- Advise patient that changes in smoking habits can alter drug effectiveness.
- Instruct patient to monitor food intake: weight gain can occur because of increased appetite and craving for sweets.
- Emphasize importance of regular dental care, because oral dryness can increase risk for dental caries.
- Instruct patient to report these symptoms to physician: persistent dry mouth, constipation, urinary retention or muscle rigidity.
- Instruct patient to take sips of water frequently, suck on ice chips or sugarless hard candy or chew sugarless gum if dry mouth occurs. Suggest patient increase fluids and fiber in diet to alleviate constipation.
- Instruct patient to avoid intake of alcohol or other CNS depressants.
- Caution patient to avoid exposure to sunlight and to use sunscreen or wear protective clothing to avoid photosensitivity reaction.
- Instruct patient not to take otc medications without consulting physician.

See Patient Guide, p. 27.

Amoxicillin

(a-MOX-ih-sil-in)

Amoxil, Amoxil Pediatric, Biomox, Polymox, Trimox, Wymox, ♣ *APO-Amoxi, Nu-Amoxi*

Class: Antibiotic/penicillin

Action Inhibits bacterial cell wall mucopeptide synthesis.

Indications Treatment of infections due to susceptible strains of certain microorganisms.

Contraindications Hypersensitivity to penicillins, cephalosporins or imipenem. Not used to treat severe pneumonia, empyema, bacteremia, pericarditis, meningitis and purulent or septic arthritis during acute stage.

Route/Dosage

ADULTS: **PO** 250-500 mg q 8 hr. CHILDREN: **PO** 20-40 mg/kg/day in divided doses given q 8 hr.

Gonococcal Infections

ADULTS: **PO** 3 g plus 1 g probenecid followed by doxycycline.

Bacterial Endocarditis Prophylaxis

ADULTS: **IM/IV** 3 g 1 hr before invasive procedure, then **PO/IM/IV** 1.5 g 6 hr after initial dose. CHILDREN: **IM/IV** 50 mg/kg 1 hr before invasive procedure, then **PO/IM/IV** 25 mg/kg 6 hr after initial dose.

Unlabeled Use

CHLAMYDIA TRACHOMATIS IN PREGNANCY: **PO** 500 mg tid for 7 days.

Interactions

Contraceptives, oral: May reduce efficacy of oral contraceptives. *Tetracyclines:* May impair bactericidal effects of amoxicillin.

Lab Test Interferences

May cause false-positive urine glucose test results with Benedict's Solution, Fehling's Solution, or Clinitest tablets (enzyme-based tests, eg,

Clinistix, Tes-Tape, are recommended); false-positive direct Coombs' test result in certain patient groups; false-positive protein reactions with sulfosalicylic acid and boiling test, acetic acid test, biuret reaction and nitric acid test (bromphenol blue test, Multi-Stix, is recommended).

Adverse Reactions

CNS: Dizziness; fatigue; insomnia; reversible hyperactivity. *EENT:* Itchy eyes; glossitis; stomatitis; sore or dry mouth or tongue; black "hairy" tongue; abnormal taste sensation; laryngospasm; laryngeal edema. *GI:* Gastritis; anorexia; nausea; vomiting; abdominal pain or cramps; epigastric distress; diarrhea or bloody diarrhea; rectal bleeding; flatulence; enterocolitis; pseudomembranous colitis. *GU:* Interstitial nephritis (eg, oliguria, proteinuria, hematuria, hyaline casts, pyuria); nephropathy; vaginitis. *HEMA:* Anemia; hemolytic anemia; thrombocytopenia; thrombocytopenic purpura; eosinophilia; leukopenia; granulocytopenia; neutropenia; bone marrow depression; agranulocytosis; reduced hemoglobin or hematocrit; prolonged bleeding and prothrombin time; increased or decreased lymphocyte count; increased monocytes, basophils, platelets. *HEPA:* Transient hepatitis; cholestatic jaundice. *DERM:* Urticaria; maculopapular to exfoliative dermatitis; vesicular eruptions; erythema multiforme; skin rashes. *META:* Elevated serum alkaline phosphatase and hypernatremia; reduced serum potassium, albumin, total proteins and uric acid. *OTHER:* Hyperthermia.

Precautions

Pregnancy: Category B. *Lactation:* Excreted in breast milk. *Hypersensitivity:* Reactions range from mild to life threatening. Use cautiously in cephalosporin-sensitive patients because of possible cross-allergenicity. *Streptococcal infections:* Minimum of 10 days required for effective treatment. *Superinfection:* May result in overgrowth of nonsusceptible bacterial or fungal organisms.

NURSING CONSIDERATIONS

Administration/Storage

- Use liquid preparations for patients with swallowing difficulties. Shake liquid preparations well before using.
- Time doses for equal distribution throughout day to achieve optimal blood levels.
- Be certain chewable tablets are crushed or chewed before swallowing. Supply water after each dose.
- Refrigerate liquid preparations as indicated after reconstitution. Discard after 14 days. Use tight lid to avoid evaporation of moisture.

Assessment/Interventions

- Obtain patient history, including drug history and any known allergies.
- Review results of culture and sensitivity testing as available.
- Monitor patient closely for several hours after administering first dose even when there is no history of allergy. Notify physician of any signs of potential hypersensitivity or anaphylactic reaction.
- Monitor renal and GI function. Notify physician of severe gastrointestinal distress.

OVERDOSAGE: SIGNS & SYMPTOMS

Hyperexcitability, convulsions

Patient/Family Education

- Instruct patient to time doses evenly over a 24-hour period.
- Inform patient that the medication works best on empty stomach but may be taken with food if there is GI upset.
- Instruct patient to increase fluid intake to 2000-3000 ml/day unless contraindicated.
- Advise patient to discard oral liquid preparations that are more than 14 days old.

- If therapy is changed because of allergic reaction, explain significance of penicillin allergy and inform patient of potential sensitivity to cephalosporins.
- Instruct patient to report these symptoms to physician: rash, difficulty breathing.

See Patient Guide, p. 28.

Amoxicillin/Potassium Clavulanate

(a-MOX-ih-sil-in/poe-TASS-ee-uhm CLAV-you-lon-ate)

Augmentin, ♣ *Clavulin*

Class: Antibiotic/penicillin

Action Amoxicillin inhibits bacterial cell wall mucopeptide synthesis. Clavulanate inhibits plasmid- and chromosomal-mediated beta-lactamase enzymes commonly found in microorganisms resistant to penicillin.

Indications Treatment of lower respiratory infections, otitis media, sinusitis, skin and skin-structure infections and urinary tract infections caused by susceptible beta-lactamase–producing microorganisms. **Unlabeled uses:** Treatment of chancroid *(Haemophilus ducreyi)*; treatment of disseminated gonococcal infections.

Contraindications Hypersensitivity to penicillins, cephalosporins or imipenem. Not used to treat severe pneumonia, empyema, bacteremia, pericarditis, meningitis and purulent or septic arthritis during acute stage.

Route/Dosage

ADULTS: **PO** 250-500 mg q 8 hr. CHILDREN < 40 KG: **PO** 20-40 mg/kg/day in divided doses given q 8 hr. CHILDREN > 40 KG: Usual adult dose.

Chancroid (Haemophilus Ducreyi)

ADULTS: **PO** 500 mg tid for 7 days.

Disseminated Gonococcal Infections

ADULTS: **PO** (after appropriate parenteral therapy) 500 mg tid.

Interactions

Contraceptives, oral: May reduce efficacy of oral contraceptives. *Tetracyclines:* May impair bactericidal effects of amoxicillin/clavulanate.

Lab Test Interferences

May cause false-positive urine glucose test results with Benedict's Solution, Fehling's Solution, or Clinitest tablets (enzyme-based tests, eg, Clinistix, Tes-Tape, are recommended); false-positive direct Coombs' test in certain patient groups; positive direct antiglobulin tests; false-positive protein reactions with sulfosalicylic acid and boiling test, acetic acid test, biuret reaction and nitric acid test (the bromphenol blue test, Multi-Stix, is recommended).

Adverse Reactions

CNS: Dizziness; fatigue; insomnia; reversible hyperactivity. *EENT:* Itchy eyes; stomatitis; glossitis; sore or dry mouth or tongue; black "hairy" tongue; abnormal taste sensation; laryngospasm; laryngeal edema. *GI:* Gastritis; anorexia; nausea; vomiting; abdominal pain or cramps; epigastric distress; diarrhea or bloody diarrhea; rectal bleeding; flatulence; enterocolitis; pseudomembranous colitis. *GU:* Interstitial nephritis (eg, oliguria, proteinuria, hematuria, hyaline casts, pyuria); nephropathy; vaginitis. *HEMA:* Anemia; hemolytic anemia; thrombocytopenia; thrombocytopenic purpura; eosinophilia; leukopenia; granulocytopenia; neutropenia; bone marrow depression; agranulocytosis; reduced hemoglobin or hematocrit; prolonged bleeding and prothrombin time; increased or decreased lymphocyte count; increased monocytes, basophils, platelets. *HEPA:* Transient hepatitis; cholestatic jaundice. *DERM:* Urticaria; maculopapular to exfoliative dermatitis; vesicular eruptions; erythema multiforme; skin rashes. *META:*

Elevated serum alkaline phosphatase and hypernatremia; reduced serum potassium, albumin, total proteins and uric acid. *OTHER:* Hyperthermia.

Precautions

Pregnancy: Category B. *Lactation:* Excreted in breast milk. *Hypersensitivity:* Reactions range from mild to life threatening. Use cautiously in cephalosporin-sensitive patients because of possible cross-allergenicity. *Streptococcal infections:* Minimum treatment is 10 days. *Superinfection:* May result in overgrowth of nonsusceptible bacterial or fungal organisms.

NURSING CONSIDERATIONS

Administration/Storage

- Use liquid preparations for patients with swallowing difficulties. Shake liquid preparations well before using.
- Time doses for even distribution throughout day to achieve optimal blood levels.
- Be certain chewable tablets are crushed or chewed before swallowing. Supply water with each dose.
- Refrigerate liquid preparations as indicated after reconstitution. Keep lid tight to avoid evaporation of moisture, and discard after 14 days.

Assessment/Interventions

- Obtain patient history, including drug history and any known allergies.
- Review results of culture and sensitivity testing as available.
- Monitor patient closely for several hours after administering first dose even if there is no history of allergy, and notify physician of any signs or symptoms of hypersensitivity or anaphylactic reaction.
- Monitor renal and GI function and assess blood studies during therapy. Notify physician of severe GI distress.

OVERDOSAGE: SIGNS & SYMPTOMS

Hyperexcitability, convulsions

Patient/Family Education

- Instruct patient to time doses for even distribution over 24 hr.
- Inform patient that medication works best on empty stomach but may be taken with food if there is GI upset.
- Inform patient to increase fluid intake to 2000-3000 ml/day unless contraindicated.
- Advise patient to discard oral liquid preparations that are more than 14 days old.
- If therapy is changed because of allergic reaction, explain significance of penicillin allergy and inform of potential for sensitivity to cephalosporins.
- Instruct patient to report these symptoms to physician: rash, difficulty breathing.

See Patient Guide, p. 29.

Amphetamine (Racemic Amphetamine Sulfate)

(am-FET-uh-meen)

Available as generic only

Class: CNS stimulant/amphetamine

Action Activates noradrenergic neurons, causing CNS and respiratory stimulation; stimulates satiety center in brain, causing appetite suppression.

Indications Narcolepsy; attention deficit disorder with hyperactivity; short-term (ie, few weeks) exogenous obesity adjunct used only when alternative therapy has been ineffective.

Contraindications Advanced arteriosclerosis; symptomatic cardiovascular disease; moderate to severe hypertension; hyperthyroidism; hypersensitivity to sympathomimetic amines;

glaucoma; agitated states; history of drug abuse. Drug should not be used concomitantly with or within 14 days of MAO inhibitor use.

Route/Dosage

Narcolepsy

ADULTS & CHILDREN > 12 YR: **PO** 10 mg/day; may be increased weekly by 10 mg to maximum of 60 mg/day in divided doses. CHILDREN 6-12 YR: **PO** 5 mg/day; may be increased weekly by 5 mg to maximum of 60 mg/day in divided doses.

Attention Deficit Disorder

CHILDREN ≥ 6 YR: **PO** 5 mg/day; may be increased weekly by 5 mg to maximum of 40 mg/day in divided doses. Usual range: 0.1-0.5 mg/kg/dose q AM. CHILDREN 3-5 YR: **PO** 2.5 mg/day; may be increased weekly by 2.5 mg. Usual range: 0.1-0.5 mg/kg/dose in morning.

Exogenous Obesity

ADULTS & CHILDREN > 12 YR: **PO** 5-10 mg 30-60 min before meals, up to 30 mg/day.

Interactions

Guanethidine: Effectiveness may be decreased. *MAO inhibitors, furazolidone:* May cause hypertensive crisis and intracranial hemorrhage. *Tricyclic antidepressants:* May decrease amphetamine effect. *Urinary acidifiers (ammonium chloride, ascorbic acid):* May decrease amphetamine effect. *Urinary alkalinizers (acetazolamide, sodium bicarbonate):* May increase amphetamine effect.

Lab Test Interferences

Plasma and urine steroid levels may be altered.

Adverse Reactions

CV: Palpitations; tachycardia; hypertension; arrhythmias. *CNS:* Hyperactivity; dizziness; restlessness; tremors; insomnia; euphoria; headache. *EENT:* Dry mouth; unpleasant taste. *GI:* Diarrhea; constipation; anorexia. *GU:* Impotence. *DERM:* Urticaria.

Precautions

Pregnancy: Category C. *Lactation:* Excreted in breast milk. *Children:* Should not be used as anorectic agent in children < 12 yr. Not recommended for attention deficit disorder in children < 3 yr. *Drug dependence:* Has high potential for dependence and abuse. *Tolerance:* May occur; recommended dose should not be exceeded.

NURSING CONSIDERATIONS

Administration/Storage

- Administer drug as supplied; do not crush or have patient chew sustained-release or long-acting tablets.
- Administer in AM or at least 6 hr before bedtime to avoid insomnia.
- Store at room temperature.

Assessment/Interventions

- Obtain patient history, including drug history and any allergies (particularly aspirin). Note cardiovascular disease, hypertension, history of drug abuse.
- Obtain blood pressure initially and monitor periodically during therapy.
- Ensure that serum thyroxine (T_4), plasma corticosteroid and urinary steroid levels have been obtained before beginning therapy.
- Review ECG for arrhythmias before beginning therapy.
- Assess mental status. Depressed patients are more likely to misuse drug to induce euphoria and mood elevation.
- Implement safety precautions to prevent falls.
- If hypertensive crisis occurs, administer phentolamine.
- Monitor patient drug use pattern closely. Physical and psychologic dependency can occur quickly with these agents.
- Observe for early signs of overdosage: restlessness, irritability, fever, hyperpnea, confusion.
- Closely monitor growth rate of chil-

dren during therapy. Effect of drug on growth rate is unknown.
- Observe for dizziness and dry mucous membranes.

OVERDOSAGE: SIGNS & SYMPTOMS

Restlessness, tremor, hyperreflexia, confusion, hallucinations, panic, fatigue, depression, convulsions, coma, arrhythmias, hypertension, hypotension, circulatory collapse, nausea, vomiting, diarrhea, abdominal cramps

Patient/Family Education
- Caution patient to take medication exactly as ordered and not to increase dosage unless advised by physician.
- Advise patient to avoid caffeine, which increases drug effect.
- Instruct patient to report these symptoms to physician: insomnia, skin discolorations, GI disturbances.
- Instruct patient to take sips of water frequently, suck on ice chips or sugarless hard candy or chew sugarless gum if dry mouth occurs.
- Advise patient that drug may cause drowsiness and to use caution while driving or performing tasks requiring mental alertness.

See Patient Guide, p. 30.

Amphotericin B

(am-foe-TER-ih-sin B)

Fungizone, Fungizone Intravenous
Class: Anti-infective/antifungal

Action Alters fungal cell membrane permeability.

Indications Treatment of progressive, potentially fatal infections caused by certain fungal species. *Topical preparations:* Treatment of fungal infections caused by *Candida* species.

Contraindications Standard considerations.

Route/Dosage
ADULTS: Test dose: **IV** 1 mg given by slow infusion over 6 hr in concentration of 0.1 mg/ml to determine patient tolerance. Initial dose: **IV** 0.25 mg/kg by slow infusion over 6 hr. Dose is increased gradually up to 1 mg/kg (1.5 mg/kg for qod therapy). Maximum daily dose: 1.5 mg/kg/day. Total doses of > 5 g are associated with greater renal toxicity.

Sporotrichosis
ADULTS: **IM** usual dose: 20 mg per injection. Up to 9 mo of therapy may be required.

Topical
2-4 times/day for 1-4 wk.

Fungal Meningitis
ADULTS: **Intrathecal/intraventricular** 0.1-0.5 mg q 48-72 hr.

Candidal Cystitis
ADULTS: 5-15 mg/dl may be instilled periodically or continuously by bladder irrigation for 5-10 days.

Interactions
Corticosteroids: Increased potential for hypokalemia. *Cyclosporine:* May increase nephrotoxic effects. *Nephrotoxic agents (eg, aminoglycosides):* Possible synergistic nephrotoxicity. INCOMPATIBILITIES: Do not mix with other IV medications.

Lab Test Interferences
None well documented.

Adverse Reactions
CV: Arrhythmias; ventricular fibrillation; cardiac arrest. *CNS:* Headache; convulsions; peripheral neuropathy. *EENT:* Hearing loss. *GI:* Anorexia; nausea; vomiting; dyspepsia; diarrhea; cramping; epigastric pain; hemorrhagic gastroenteritis. *GU:* Hypokalemia; azotemia; hyposthenuria; nephrocalcinosis; renal tubular acidosis; anuria; oliguria; permanent renal damage. *HEMA:* Normochromic, normocytic anemia; thrombocytopenia; leukopenia; agranulocytosis; eosinophilia; leukocytosis. *DERM:* Topical preparations may

cause local irritation (eg, erythema, pruritis or burning sensation) or dryness. *OTHER:* Fever (sometimes with shaking chills); malaise; generalized pain, including muscle and joint pains; venous pain at injection site with phlebitis and thrombophlebitis; weight loss; anaphylactoid reactions.

Precautions

Pregnancy: Category B. *Lactation:* Undetermined. *Children:* Safety and efficacy not established. *Nephrotoxicity:* Drug is toxic and should be used with caution under close supervision. Renal damage is most important toxic effect. Despite its dangerous side effects, amphotericin B frequently is only effective treatment for potentially fatal fungal diseases. *Topical use:* Avoid contact with eyes. *Pulmonary reactions:* Acute dyspnea, hypoxemia and interstitial infiltrates can occur in neutropenic patients receiving amphotericin B and leukocyte transfusions.

NURSING CONSIDERATIONS

Administration/Storage

- IV infusion should be administered only in acute care setting under close supervision. Test dose is usually given before administering first therapeutic dose.
- Follow manufacturer's instructions for reconstitution and administration. Use Sterile Water for Injection without a bacteriostatic agent. Do not reconstitute with saline. Preservatives, bacteriostatic agents and saline may cause precipitation.
- Use solutions prepared for IV infusion promptly after reconstitution.
- Use aseptic technique while handling medication.
- Wear gloves while applying topical ointments.
- Use volumetric IV pump to regulate delivery over recommended 6 hr period. (Shorter infusion times have also been used.)
- Use IV filter (1 µm or greater) during administration.
- Agitate hanging solution to mix every 30-60 min.
- Do not mix with other IV medications.
- Do not administer if solution is discolored or if precipitate is present.
- Medication is stable for 24 hr at room temperature or 7 days if kept refrigerated.
- Store in dark area. Protect from light during administration.

Assessment/Interventions

- Obtain patient history, including drug history and any allergies.
- Ensure that fungal culture (blood or urine, as appropriate) of organism has been obtained before beginning therapy.
- Monitor pulse and BP every 15 min during test dose.
- Monitor IV injection site closely during administration for signs of infiltration.
- Monitor laboratory values, including liver function tests, CBC, renal function tests, and magnesium levels during therapy.
- Monitor I&O during therapy.
- Monitor temperature 4 hr after administration; may be elevated.
- Assess for symptoms of hypokalemia, especially disorientation and weakness.
- If patient experiences infusion-related symptoms (chills, fever, hypotension, joint pain), nonsteroidal anti-inflammatory drug, corticosteroid, or other antipyretic may be given before administering drug. Administration of heparin, rapid infusion, removal of needle after infusion, rotation of infusion sites and administration through large central vein or distal vein may lessen incidence of thrombophlebitis.
- If severe side effects or signs of anaphylactic reaction occur, stop infusion and notify physician.

Patient/Family Education

- Explain need for prolonged therapy and for close monitoring during course of therapy.
- Encourage patient to increase fluid intake to 2000-3000 ml/day if allowed.
- Inform patient to report any discomfort at injection site immediately.
- Instruct patient to report symptoms of chills, malaise or fever.
- Warn patient that contact with topical preparation can cause discoloration of fabrics. However, this is easily removed by washing with soap and water or applying common stain removers.

See Patient Guide, pp. 31-32.

Ampicillin

(am-pih-SILL-in)

D-Amp, Omnipen, Omnipen-N, Polycillin, Polycillin-N, Polycillin Pediatric, Polycillin-PRB (with probenecid), Principen, Probampacin (with probenecid), Totacillin, Totacillin-N, ♣ *Ampicin, APO-Ampi, Novo Ampicillin, Nu-Ampi, Penbritin*

Class: Antibiotic/penicillin

Action Inhibits bacterial cell wall mucopeptide synthesis.

Indications Treatment of respiratory tract and soft tissue infections, bacterial meningitis, septicemia and gonococcal infections caused by susceptible microorganisms; prophylaxis in rape victims and for bacterial endocarditis. **Unlabeled use:** Prophylaxis in cesarean section in certain high risk patients.

Contraindications Hypersensitivity to penicillins, cephalosporins or imipenem. Oral form not used to treat severe pneumonia, empyema, bacteremia, pericarditis, meningitis and purulent or septic arthritis during acute stage.

Route/Dosage

ADULTS: **PO/IV/IM** 1-12 g/day in divided doses q 4-6 hr. **PO** 1-2 g/day in divided doses q 6 hr. CHILDREN: **PO/IV/IM** 50-200 mg/kg/day in divided doses q 4-6 hr. INFANTS > 7 DAYS & > 2000 G: **IV/IM** 100 mg/kg/day in divided doses q 6 hr. INFANTS > 7 DAYS & < 2000 G: **IV/IM** 75 mg/kg/day in divided doses q 8 hr. INFANTS < 7 DAYS & > 2000 G: **IV/IM** 75 mg/kg/day in divided doses q 8 hr. INFANTS < 7 DAYS & < 2000 G: **IV/IM** 50 mg/kg/day in divided doses q 12 hr.

Respiratory Tract and Soft Tissue Infections

ADULTS ≥ 40 KG: **IV** 250-500 mg q 6 hr. ADULTS < 40 KG: **IV** 25-50 mg/kg/day in divided doses q 6-8 hr. CHILDREN ≥ 40 KG: **IV** 250-500 mg q 6 hr. CHILDREN < 40 KG: **IV** 25-50 mg/kg/day in divided doses q 6-8 hr. CHILDREN ≥ 20 KG: **PO** 250 mg q 6 hr. CHILDREN < 20 KG: **PO** 50 mg/kg/day in divided doses q 6-8 hr.

Bacterial Meningitis

ADULTS: **PO/IV/IM** 8-14 g/day in divided doses q 3-4 hr. CHILDREN: **IV/IM** 100-200 mg/kg/day in divided doses q 3-4 hr.

Septicemia

ADULTS: **IV/IM** 150-200 mg/kg/day q 3-4 hr. CHILDREN: **IV/IM** 150-200 mg/kg/day q 3-4 hr.

Gonococcal Infections

ADULTS & CHILDREN ≥ 45 KG: **IV** 1 g q 6 hr.

Rape Victim Infection Prophylaxis

ADULTS & CHILDREN ≥ 45 KG: **PO** 3.5 g with 1 g probenecid.

Bacterial Endocarditis Prophylaxis

ADULTS: **IM/IV** 1-2 g 30 min before invasive procedure and 8 hr after initial dose. CHILDREN: **IM/IV** 50 mg/kg 30 min before invasive procedure and 8 hr after initial dose.

Cesarean Section Prophylaxis
ADULTS: IV Single dose immediately after cord clamping.

Interactions
Allopurinol: Increases potential for ampicillin-induced skin rash. *Atenolol:* Antihypertensive and antianginal effects may be impaired. *Contraceptives, oral:* May reduce efficacy of oral contraceptives. *Tetracyclines:* May impair bactericidal effects of ampicillin. INCOMPATIBILITIES: Do not mix with aminoglycosides (eg, gentamicin).

Lab Test Interferences
May cause false-positive urine glucose test results with Benedict's Solution, Fehling's Solution, or Clinitest tablets (enzyme-based tests, eg, Clinistix, Tes-tape, are recommended); false-positive direct Coombs' test result in certain patient groups; false-positive protein reactions with sulfosalicylic acid and boiling test, acetic acid test, biuret reaction and nitric acid test (the bromphenol blue test, Multistix, is recommended).

Adverse Reactions
CV: Thrombophlebitis at injection site. *CNS:* Dizziness; fatigue; insomnia; reversible hyperactivity; neurotoxicity (lethargy, neuromuscular irritability, hallucinations, convulsions, seizures). *EENT:* Itchy eyes; laryngospasm; laryngeal edema. *GI:* Diarrhea; pseudomembranous colitis. *GU:* Interstitial nephritis (eg, oliguria, proteinuria, hematuria, hyaline casts, pyuria); nephropathy; increased BUN and creatinine; vaginitis. *HEMA:* Decreased Hgb, Hct, RBC, WBC, neutrophils, lymphocytes, platelets; increased lymphocytes, monocytes, basophils, eosinophils and platelets. *DERM:* Urticaria; maculopapular to exfoliative dermatitis; vesicular eruptions; erythema multiforme; skin rashes. *META:* Elevated serum alkaline phosphatase, glutamic oxaloacetic transaminase, ALT, AST, and LDH; reduced serum albumin and total proteins. *OTHER:* Pain at injection site; hyperthermia.

Precautions
Pregnancy: Category B. *Lactation:* Excreted in breast milk. *Hypersensitivity:* Reactions range from mild to life-threatening. Use cautiously in cephalosporin-sensitive patients because of possible cross-allergenicity. *Superinfection:* May result in overgrowth of nonsusceptible bacterial or fungal organisms. *Renal impairment:* Use cautiously with altered dosing interval.

NURSING CONSIDERATIONS

Administration/Storage

- Use liquid preparations for patients with swallowing difficulties. Follow manufacturer's instructions for reconstitution, and handle liquids carefully to prevent contact dermatitis.
- Time doses at equal intervals to achieve optimal blood levels.
- To achieve maximum benefit, administer 1 hour before or 2 hours after a meal.
- Monitor renal function.
- Shake liquid preparations well before using.
- Administer IM and IV solutions within 1 hr of reconstitution.
- Allow foaming to subside before administering IV preparations. Do not administer if discolored or cloudy. Use volumetric IV pump to regulate delivery over 10-15 min period. Do not mix with other IV medications.
- Be certain chewable tablets are crushed or chewed before swallowing. Supply water following dose.
- Refrigerate liquid preparations after reconstitution, and discard after 14 days. Discard after 7 days if not refrigerated.
- Store tablets and capsules in dry, tightly closed container.

Assessment/Interventions

- Obtain patient history, includ-

ing drug history and any known allergies.

- Review results of culture and sensitivity testing, as available.
- Monitor patient's condition closely for several hours after administering the first dose even when there is no history of allergy. Notify physician of any signs or symptoms of hypersensitivity or anaphylactic reaction.
- Monitor renal and GI function during therapy, and notify physician of severe GI distress.
- Evaluate skin daily for presence of classic ampicillin rash, usually maculopapular, pruritic and generalized.
- Monitor for bleeding in patients receiving anticoagulant therapy.

OVERDOSAGE: SIGNS & SYMPTOMS

Hyperexcitability, convulsive seizures

Patient/Family Education

- Instruct patient to time the doses evenly over a 24-hour period.
- Inform patient that medication works best on an empty stomach, but may be taken with food if there is GI upset.
- Tell patient to increase fluid intake to 2000-3000 ml/day, unless contraindicated.
- Advise patient to refrigerate oral liquid preparations and to discard unrefrigerated preparations that are more than 7 days old.
- Inform patient to notify physician immediately if rash develops or if patient has difficulty breathing.
- Warn diabetic patient that product may cause false-positive glucose urine test results, and identify alternative tests.
- If therapy is changed because of allergic reaction, explain the significance of penicillin allergy and inform of potential sensitivity to cephalosporins.

See Patient Guide, p. 33.

Ampicillin Sodium/ Sulbactam Sodium

(am-pih-SILL-in SO-dee-uhm/sull-BAK-tam SO-dee-uhm)

Unasyn

Class: Antibiotic/penicillin

Action Ampicillin inhibits bacterial cell wall mucopeptide synthesis. Sulbactam inhibits plasmid-medicated beta-lactamase enzymes commonly found in microorganisms resistant to ampicillin.

Indications Treatment of infections of skin and skin structure, intra-abdominal and gynecologic infections caused by susceptible microorganisms, and mixed infections caused by ampicillin-susceptible organisms and beta-lactamase–producing organisms.

Contraindications Hypersensitivity to penicillins, cephalosporins or imipenem.

Route/Dosage

ADULTS: **IV/IM** 1.5-3 g q 6 hr not to exceed 4 g/day sulbactam (1.5 g of product contains 0.5 g sulbactam).

Interactions

Allopurinol: Increases potential for ampicillin-induced skin rash. *Contraceptives, oral:* May reduce efficacy of oral contraceptives. *Tetracyclines:* May impair bactericidal effects of ampicillin/sulbactam. INCOMPATIBILITIES: Do not mix with aminoglycosides (eg, gentamicin).

Lab Test Interferences

May cause false-positive urine glucose test results with Benedict's Solution, Fehling's Solution, or Clinitest tablets (enzyme-based tests, eg, Clinistix, Tes-tape, are recommended); false-positive direct Coombs' test result in certain patient groups; false-positive protein reactions with sulfosalicylic acid and boiling test, acetic acid test, biuret reaction and nitric acid test (the bromphenol blue test, Multistix, is recommended).

Adverse Reactions

CV: Thrombophlebitis at injection site. *CNS:* Dizziness; fatigue; insomnia; reversible hyperactivity. *EENT:* Itchy eyes; laryngospasm; laryngeal edema. *GI:* Diarrhea; pseudomembranous colitis. *GU:* Interstitial nephritis (eg, oliguria, proteinuria, hematuria, hyaline casts, pyuria); nephropathy; increased BUN and creatinine; vaginitis. *HEMA:* Decreased Hgb, Hct, RBC, WBC, neutrophils, lymphocytes, platelets; increased lymphocytes, monocytes, basophils, eosinophils and platelets. *DERM:* Urticaria; maculopapular to exfoliative dermatitis; vesicular eruptions; erythema multiforme; skin rashes. *META:* Elevated serum alkaline phosphatase, glutamic oxaloacetic transaminase, ALT, AST, and LDH; reduced serum albumin and total proteins. *OTHER:* Pain at injection site; hyperthermia.

Precautions

Pregnancy: Category B. *Lactation:* Excreted in breast milk. *Children:* Safety and efficacy not established. *Hypersensitivity:* Reactions range from mild to life-threatening. Use cautiously in cephalosporin-sensitive patients because of possible cross-allergenicity. *Superinfection:* May result in overgrowth of nonsusceptible bacterial or fungal organisms. *Renal impairment:* Use cautiously with altered dosing interval.

NURSING CONSIDERATIONS

Administration/Storage

- Do not mix in same IV solution with aminoglycosides.
- Administer IM and IV solutions within 1 hr of reconstitution.
- Allow foaming to subside before administering IV preparations. Do not administer if discolored or cloudy. Use volumetric IV pump to regulate delivery over 10-15 min period.
- Do not infuse with other IV medications.
- Do not administer other antibiotics within 1 hr.
- Monitor renal function.
- Rotate IM injection sites.
- Keep refrigerated after reconstitution. Medication is stable for 2 hr at room temperature, 72 hr if refrigerated.

Assessment/Interventions

- Obtain patient history, including drug history and any known allergies.
- Review results of culture and sensitivity testing as available.
- Monitor I&O during therapy.
- Monitor patient's condition closely for several hours after administration even if there is no history of known penicillin allergy. Notify physician of any signs and symptoms of hypersensitivity or anaphylactic reaction.

OVERDOSAGE: SIGNS & SYMPTOMS

Hyperexcitability, convulsive seizures

Patient/Family Education

- Explain rationale for hospitalization during course of therapy.
- Inform patient of potential side effects, and encourage a report of any problems.
- Encourage patient to increase fluid intake to 2000-3000 ml/day, unless contraindicated.
- Inform diabetic patients that this medication may cause false-positive glucose urine test results and identify types that will be more reliable.
- If therapy is changed because of allergic reaction, explain significance of penicillin allergy, and inform of potential sensitivity to cephalosporins.

See Patient Guide, p. 34.

Amrinone Lactate

(AM-rih-nohn LAK-tate)

Inocor

Class: Cardiovascular/positive inotropic

Action Positive inotropic agent with vasodilator activity.

Indications Short-term management of CHF in patients whose condition can be closely monitored and who have not responded adequately to digitalis, diuretics or vasodilators.

Contraindications Hypersensitivity to bisulfites.

Route/Dosage

ADULTS: **IV** Initial dose: 0.75 mg/kg bolus slowly over 2-3 min. Maintenance: 5-10 mcg/kg/min; additional 0.75 mg/kg bolus may be given 30 min after initiating therapy, not to exceed total daily dose of 10 mg/kg.

Interactions None well documented. INCOMPATIBILITIES: *Dextrose-containing solutions:* Chemical interaction occurs slowly over 24 hr when mixed directly. *Furosemide:* Do not inject furosemide into IV line containing amrinone; immediate precipitate forms.

Lab Test Interferences

None well documented.

Adverse Reactions

CV: Arrhythmia; hypotension. *GI:* Nausea; vomiting. *HEMA:* Thrombocytopenia.

Precautions

Pregnancy: Category C. *Lactation:* Undetermined. *Children:* Safety and efficacy not established. *Arrhythmias:* Supraventricular and ventricular arrhythmias have occurred. *Fluid balance:* Vigorous diuretic therapy may cause inadequate response to amrinone therapy; liberalization of fluids may be needed. CVP monitoring has been advocated. *Hepatotoxicity:* Dose may be reduced or drug may be discontinued if there are alterations in liver enzymes; if alterations occur with clinical symptoms, drug is discontinued. *Post MI:* Not recommended during acute phase. *Severe aortic or pulmonic valvular disease:* Not recommended. *Sulfite sensitivity:* May cause allergic-type reaction in susceptible patients. *Thrombocytopenia:* More common in patients on prolonged therapy.

NURSING CONSIDERATIONS

Administration/Storage

IV Infusion

- Administer as supplied or dilute in normal saline or ½ normal saline to a concentration of 1-3 mg/ml.
- Do not dilute in dextrose-containing solutions, although product may be injected into running dextrose infusion through Y-connector or directly into tubing. Do not infuse product and furosemide through same line.
- Administer maintenance infusion 5 to 10 µg/kg/min, preferably with infusion pump; adjust rate according to patient response.
- Use diluted solutions within 24 hr.
- Protect ampules from light.

Assessment/Interventions

- Obtain patient history, including drug history and any known allergies. Determine presence or history of asthma.
- Review baseline ECG and assess ongoing cardiac monitoring. Notify physician of any arrhythmias.
- Assess cardiac rate and rhythm throughout therapy.
- Assess vital signs, especially blood pressure and pulse, before and during therapy. Notify physician of excessive hypotension and slow or stop infusion.
- Monitor I&O, including changes (increase or decrease) in output.
- Monitor laboratory values for altera-

tions in liver enzymes, renal functions, platelets, and serum electrolytes. Notify physician of any changes.

- Monitor for nausea and vomiting and for signs of hepatotoxicity.

OVERDOSAGE: SIGNS & SYMPTOMS
Arrhythmias; excessive hypotension

Patient/Family Education

- Instruct patient to avoid sudden position changes to prevent orthostatic hypotension.
- Advise patient to notify physician of shortness of breath and increased chest pain.

No patient monograph available.

Amyl Nitrite

(A-mill NYE-trite)

Amyl Nitrite Aspirols, Amyl Nitrite Vaporole

Class: Antianginal

Action Relaxes smooth muscle of venous and arterial vasculature.

Indications Relief of angina pectoris.

Contraindications Hypersensitivity to nitrates; pregnancy; severe anemia; closed-angle glaucoma; orthostatic hypotension; head trauma; cerebral hemorrhage.

Route/Dosage

ADULT: INHALATION: 0.3 ml prn. 1-6 inhalations from 1 capsule are usually sufficient. May be repeated in 3-5 min.

Interactions

Alcohol: Severe hypotension and cardiovascular collapse may occur. *Aspirin:* Increased nitrate concentration and actions may occur. *Calcium channel blockers:* Symptomatic orthostatic hypotension may occur. *Heparin:* Effects of heparin may be decreased.

Lab Test Interferences

May cause false report of reduced serum cholesterol with Zlatkis-Zak color reaction.

Adverse Reactions

CV: Tachycardia; palpitations; hypotension; syncope; arrhythmias; edema. *RESP:* Bronchitis; pneumonia. *CNS:* Headache; apprehension; weakness; vertigo; dizziness; agitation; insomnia. *EENT:* Blurred vision. *GI:* Nausea; vomiting; diarrhea; dyspepsia. *GU:* Dysuria; impotence. *HEMA:* Methemoglobinemia; hemolytic anemia. *DERM:* Cutaneous vasodilation with flushing. *OTHER:* Arthralgia; perspiration; pallor; cold sweat.

Precautions

Pregnancy: Category X. *Lactation:* Contraindicated. *Children:* Safety and efficacy not established. *Angina:* May aggravate angina caused by hypertrophic cardiomyopathy. *Drug abuse:* May be abused for sexual stimulation or for effects of lightheadedness, dizziness and euphoria. *Glaucoma:* May increase intraocular pressure. *Orthostatic hypotension:* May occur even with small doses; alcohol accentuates this reaction. *Withdrawal:* Dose is gradually reduced to prevent withdrawal reaction.

NURSING CONSIDERATIONS

Administration/Storage

- Help patient into sitting or reclining position.
- Crush capsule, wave under patient's nose and instruct to breathe deeply; 1 to 6 inhalations are usually sufficient. May repeat in 3-5 min.
- Keep capsules in original container and keep container tightly closed.

Assessment/Interventions

- Obtain patient history, including drug history and any known allergies.

- Assess current status of cardiac, renal and hepatic function.
- Assess vital signs, especially BP and pulse. Also assess for signs of tolerance to or abuse of the product.
- Evaluate relief of symptoms and monitor for any adverse effects such as GI symptoms, headache, tachycardia, postural hypotension, skin flushing, rash or possible arrhythmia.
- Note any changes in serum cholesterol levels.

OVERDOSAGE: SIGNS & SYMPTOMS
Severe headache, severe hypotension, flushing, tachycardia, vertigo, confusion, syncope, nausea, slow breathing or dyspnea, cyanosis, metabolic acidosis, convulsions, coma, death

Patient/Family Education

- Caution patient that this medication must not be taken during pregnancy or when pregnancy is possible. Advise patient to use reliable form of birth control while taking this drug.
- Advise use of acetaminophen for relief of headache.
- Show patient how to crush capsule. Remind patient not to remove cloth-like covering.
- Show patient how to keep record of usage, including frequency, dosage and level of pain relief.
- Explain potential for abuse.
- Instruct patient to report these symptoms to physician: blurred vision, dry mouth or persistent headache occurs or symptoms are not relieved.
- Caution patient to avoid sudden position changes to prevent orthostatic hypotension.
- Instruct patient to avoid intake of alcoholic beverages or other CNS depressants and aspirin.

See Patient Guide, p. 35.

Anastrozole

(an-ASS-troe-zole)

Arimidex

Class: Antineoplastic/antiestrogen

Action Blocks the formation of estradiol, a hormone that stimulates the growth of certain breast neoplasms.

Indications Advanced breast cancer in postmenopausal women with estrogen receptor-positive tumors who progress despite tamoxifen therapy.

Contraindications Standard considerations.

Route/Dosage
ADULTS: PO 1 mg QD.

Interactions None well documented.

Lab Test Interferences
None well documented.

Adverse Reactions
GI: Diarrhea; nausea; vomiting; constipation; abdominal pain; anorexia. *ENT:* Dry mouth; pharyngitis. *RESP:* Dyspnea; increased cough; bronchitis; rhinitis. *CNS:* Dizziness; headache; somnolence; confusion; anxiety; insomnia; paresthesia; depression. *GU:* Pelvic pain; vaginal hemorrhage; vaginal dryness. *DERM:* Rash; pruritus. *META:* Increased alkaline phosphotase. *CV:* Hypertension; thrombophlebitis. *HEPA:* Increased liver function tests. *HEMA:* Anemia; leukopenia. *OTHER:* Asthenia; hot flushes; sweating; pain; chest pain; weight gain; edema; fever.

Precautions
Pregnancy: Category D. *Lactation:* Undetermined. *Children:* Safety and efficacy not established. *Hepatic impairment:* Monitor patient for side effects. Dosage adjustment does not appear to be necessary with mild-to-moderate liver impairment.

NURSING CONSIDERATIONS

Administration/Storage

- Administer without regard to food or meals. Give with food if GI upset occurs.
- Store at room temperature.

Assessment/Interventions

- Before starting treatment, pregnancy should be excluded.
- Obtain patient history.
- Report any side effects to physician.

Patient/Family Education

- Instruct patient to inform healthcare provider if pregnancy occurs while receiving this medication.
- Try to take about the same time each day.
- Take without regard to meals. Take with food if GI upset occurs.

See Patient Guide, p. 36.

Anistreplase

(uh-NISS-truh-place)

Eminase

Class: Thrombolytic enzyme

Action Aids in dissolution of blood clots.

Indications Lysis of obstructing coronary thrombi for management of acute MI.

Contraindications Hypersensitivity to streptokinase; active internal bleeding; history of cerebrovascular accident; recent (within 2 mon) intracranial or intraspinal surgery or trauma; intracranial neoplasm; arteriovenous malformation or aneurysm; known bleeding diathesis; uncontrolled hypertension.

Route/Dosage

ADULTS: **IV** 30 U over 2-5 min into IV line or vein.

Interactions

Anticoagulants (eg, heparin, warfarin) and antiplatelet agents (eg, aspirin, dipyridamole): May increase risk of bleeding. INCOMPATIBILITIES: Do not add to any infusion fluids. Do not add other medications to vial or syringe containing anistreplase.

Lab Test Interferences

Can cause decreases in plasminogen and fibrinogen levels and increases in thrombin time, activated partial thromboplastin time and prothrombin time, making results of coagulation tests unreliable.

Adverse Reactions

CV: Arrhythmia and conduction disorders; hypotension. *HEMA:* Bleeding at puncture site, non–puncture-site hematoma; hematuria; hemoptysis; GI hemorrhage; intracranial bleeding; mouth and gum hemorrhage; epistaxis; ocular hemorrhage; nonspecific hemorrhage.

Precautions

Pregnancy: Category C. *Lactation:* Undetermined. *Children:* Safety and efficacy not established. *Hypersensitivity:* Rarely anaphylactic and anaphylactoid reactions (with bronchospasm or angioedema) may occur. *Readministration:* Because of formation of antistreptokinase antibody, anistreplase may not be effective if administered > 5 days-6 mon after prior anistreplase or streptokinase therapy or after streptococcal infection.

NURSING CONSIDERATIONS

Administration/Storage

- Reconstitute powder with 5 ml of Sterile Water for Injection. Do not shake vial during reconstitution; try to minimize foaming. Do not further dilute reconstituted anistreplase.
- Administer 30 U of anistreplase by IV injection over 2-5 min.

- Store lyophilized anistreplase under refrigeration.
- Discard any reconstituted anistreplase not administered within 30 min of reconstitution.

Assessment/Interventions

- Obtain patient history, including drug history and any known allergies.
- Identify factors that may contribute to bleeding risk, including baseline coagulation and fibrinolytic activity test results.
- Determine if and when previous fibrinolytic therapy was administered.
- Have epinephrine and emergency treatment provisions available during administration of anistreplase.
- Avoid nonessential handling of patient during anistreplase therapy.
- If arterial puncture is necessary after administration of anistreplase, it is preferable to use upper extremity vessel that is accessible to manual compression. Apply pressure dressing; check puncture site frequently for evidence of bleeding. Control minor bleeding with manual pressure.
- Remember that allergic-type reactions may occur in milder forms up to 1-2 wk after therapy.
- Evaluate data from cardiac monitoring and report any arrhythmias.
- Monitor diligently for signs or symptoms of internal or surface bleeding. Remember that lab values for coagulation tests and measurements of fibrinolytic activity after anistreplase therapy may be unreliable.
- Monitor vital signs, especially BP and pulse, because severe hypotension may occur.

Patient/Family Education

- Explain to patient the need for bedrest and minimal handling of patient.
- Instruct patient to report these symptoms to physician: bruising, bleeding and hypersensitivity reactions (eg, urticaria, flushing, itching, rashes).
- Caution patient to avoid sudden position changes to prevent orthostatic hypotension.

No patient monograph available.

Ascorbic Acid (Vitamin C)

(ASS-kor-bik acid)

Ascorbicap, Cebid Timecelles, Cecon, Cetane, Cevalin, Cevi-Bid, Ce-Vi-Sol, Dull-C, Flavorcee, N'ice Vitamin C Drops, Vita-C, ♣ *APO-C, Redoxon, Revitalose-C-1000, TimeTec Timed Release Vitamin C, Timedose Vitamin C*

Class: Vitamin

Action Essential vitamin believed important for synthesis of cellular components, catecholamines, steroids and carnitine.

Indications Prevention and treatment of scurvy. **Unlabeled uses:** Treatment of idiopathic methemoglobinemia; combination therapy with methenamine to increase acidity of urine. Although not proven scientifically, prevention of common colds and treatment of cancer, asthma, atherosclerosis, burns and other wounds.

Contraindications Standard considerations.

Route/Dosage

ADULTS: **PO** Recommended daily allowance 60 mg; average protective dose 70-150 mg/day. INFANTS: **PO** Average protective dose 30 mg; usual curative dose 100-300 mg/day. PREMATURE INFANTS: **PO/IV/IM** May require 75-100 mg/day.

Parenteral

Used in acute deficiency or when oral absorption is uncertain. Rapid IV administration should be avoided. SCURVY: **IV/IM/SC** 75-150 mg/day; up to 6 g/day has been administered without toxicity. ENHANCED WOUND HEALING: **PO** 300-500 mg/day for 7-10 days has been given.

Interactions None well documented.

Lab Test Interferences
Amine-dependent tests for occult blood in stool: May cause false-negative results. *Urine glucose determinations:* May cause false-negative determinations.

Adverse Reactions
CNS: Faintness or dizziness may occur with rapid IV administration. *GI:* Diarrhea; nausea; vomiting. *GU:* Excessive doses over long period of time may cause precipitation of cystine, oxalate or urate crystals in kidney. *OTHER:* Injection site irritation may occur with IM or SC administration.

Precautions
Pregnancy: Category C. *Lactation:* Excreted in breast milk. *Excessive doses:* Diabetics, patients prone to renal calculi, patients on sodium restricted diets and those taking anticoagulants should not take excessive doses (> 5 g/day) over extended periods of time. *Sulfite sensitivity:* Some products contain sulfites, which may precipitate a reaction in sensitive individuals. *Tartrazine sensitivity:* Some products contain tartrazine, which can precipitate breathing difficulties in sensitive individuals.

NURSING CONSIDERATIONS

Administration/Storage

- Check expiration date on container for oral tablets; product is relatively unstable after exposure to air and light.
- Cover IV bag to protect from light if being administered IV.
- Refrigerate when possible, although storage at room temperature is acceptable.
- Discard IV solution after 24 hours.

Assessment/Interventions

- Obtain patient history, including drug history and any known allergies.
- Evaluate patient for signs of vitamin C deficiency before and during therapy.
- Monitor pH of urine if patient is being treated for renal stones.
- If patient experiences dizziness or syncope, stop administration and notify physician.
- Rotate injection or infusion sites to reduce irritation.

Patient/Family Education

- Explain that taking product with foods high in iron will enhance absorption of iron.
- Explain to any patient scheduled for glucose studies that product should not be taken for at least 48-72 hours before test.

See Patient Guide, p. 37.

Asparaginase

(ass-PAR-uh-jin-aze)

Elspar, ♣ *Kidrolase*

Class: Antineoplastic

Action Inhibits cell reproduction by depriving tumor cells of required amino acid.

Indications Used in combination with other chemotherapeutic agents to induce remission in acute lymphocytic leukemia. Not used for maintenance therapy. **Unlabeled uses:** Other leukemia types; lymphosarcoma.

Contraindications Active pancreatitis or history of pancreatitis.

Route/Dosage
ADULTS: **IV/IM** INDUCTION WITH OTHER CHEMOTHERAPEUTIC AGENTS: 1000 IU/kg/day for 10 consecutive days; varies per protocol. ADULTS & CHILDREN: **IV** INDUCTION AS SOLE AGENT: 200 IU/kg/day for 28 days. IN-

TRADERMAL SKIN TEST: **Intradermal** 2 IU (double dilution needed). Observe for positive reaction, erythema or wheal formation for 1 hour.

Interactions

Methotrexate: Product may diminish or abolish effect of methotrexate on malignant cells and is not used with or after asparaginase therapy while asparaginase levels are below normal. *Vincristine and prednisone:* Concurrent administration may increase toxicity.

Lab Test Interferences

Drug may interfere with interpretation of thyroid function test results.

Adverse Reactions

CNS: Depression; somnolence; fatigue; coma; confusion; agitation; hallucinations; parkinson-like syndrome with tremor and progressive increase in muscle tone; headache; irritability. *GI:* Nausea, vomiting, anorexia, abdominal cramps; pancreatitis and acute hemorrhagic pancreatitis. *GU:* Prerenal azotemia. Rarely, acute renal shut-down and fatal renal insufficiency. *HEMA:* Bone marrow depression; bleeding; hypoprothrombinemia; low levels of clotting factors; intracranial hemorrhage; fatal bleeding. *HEPA:* Reversible elevations of AST, ALT, alkaline phosphatase and bilirubin; depression of serum albumin, cholesterol and plasma fibrinogen; serum lipid fluctuations. *META:* Hyperglycemia with glucosuria and polyuria. Syndrome resembles hyperosmolar, nonketotic hyperglycemia.

Precautions

Pregnancy: Category C. *Lactation:* Undetermined. *Hepatotoxicity:* Occurs in most patients; may increase preexisting liver impairment; may affect other drugs metabolized by liver. *Hypersensitivity:* Reactions are frequent; anaphylaxis and death have been reported. Patients who have been exposed previously to asparaginase are at high risk.

NURSING CONSIDERATIONS

Administration/Storage

- Have readily available resuscitation equipment and drugs for treatment of hypersensitivity reaction (eg, diphenhydramine, epinephrine, corticosteroids).
- Filter reconstituted solution through a 5-micron filter to remove any particulate matter.
- Administer within 8 hours of reconstitution. Do not administer if solution is cloudy.
- Store under refrigeration.

Assessment/Interventions

- Obtain patient history, including drug history and any known allergies.
- Assess results of intradermal skin test and notify physician of positive reaction.
- Review results of baseline liver function tests, CBC, blood sugar, PT, PTT, creatinine and BUN and monitor blood sugar and other test results frequently.
- Notify physician of significant bleeding, decrease in level of consciousness, hematemesis, chills or fever or of signs or symptoms of allergic or anaphylactic reaction.

Patient/Family Education

- Advise patient of predictability of adverse reactions.
- Advise patient to report any unusual symptoms to nursing staff or physician.

No patient monograph available.

Aspirin (Acetylsalicylic Acid; ASA)

(ASS-pihr-in)

Ascriptin A/D, Aspergum, Genuine Bayer, Bayer Children's, Bufferin, Cama Arthritis Pain Reliever, Easprin, Ecotrin, Empirin, Genprin, ½ Halfprin, Magnaprin, ZORprin, ♣ *APO-Asa, Asaphen, Entrophen, Entrophen Extra Strength, Entrophen 10, Entrophen 15 Maximum Strength, Novasen, PMS-ASA*

Class: Analgesic/salicylate

Action Inhibits prostaglandin synthesis, resulting in analgesia, anti-inflammatory activity and platelet aggregation inhibition; reduces fever by acting on the brain's heat-regulating center to promote vasodilation and sweating.

Indications Treatment of mild to moderate pain; fever; various inflammatory conditions; reduction of risk of death or MI in patients with previous infarction or unstable angina pectoris or recurrent transient ischemic attacks or stroke in men who have had transient brain ischemia caused by platelet emboli. **Unlabeled uses:** Prevention of cataract formation; prevention of toxemia of pregnancy; improvement of inadequate uteroplacental blood flow in pregnancy.

Contraindications Hypersensitivity to salicylates or NSAIDs; hemophilia, bleeding ulcers or hemorrhagic states.

Route/Dosage

Analgesic/Antipyretic

ADULTS: **PO** 325-650 mg q 4 hr prn; 500 mg q 3 hr prn; 1000 mg q 6 hr prn. CHILDREN (2-12 YR): **PO** 10-15 mg/kg/dose q 4 hr prn (up to 80 mg/kg/day).

Arthritis and Other Rheumatic Conditions

ADULTS: **PO** 3.2-6 g/day in divided doses.

Juvenile Rheumatoid Arthritis

CHILDREN: **PO** 60-110 mg/kg/day in divided doses q 6-8 hr.

Acute Rheumatic Fever

ADULTS: **PO** 5-8 g/day, initially, for up to 2 wk. Subsequent doses are based on patient response. CHILDREN: **PO** 75-100 mg/kg/day.

Transient Ischemic Attacks in Men

ADULTS: **PO** 1300 mg/day in 2-4 doses.

Myocardial Infarction Prophylaxis

ADULTS: **PO** 160-325 mg/day.

Kawasaki Disease

CHILDREN: **PO** 80-180 mg/kg/day during acute febrile period; 10 mg/kg/day after fever resolves.

Interactions

Alcohol: May increase risk of GI ulceration and prolong bleeding time. *Antacids, urinary alkalinizers, and corticosteroids:* May decrease aspirin levels. *Anticoagulants, oral and heparin:* May increase risk of bleeding. *Carbonic anhydrase inhibitors (eg, acetohexamide), methotrexate, valproic acid:* May increase levels of these drugs. *Probenecid, sulfinpyrazone:* May decrease uricosuric effect. *Sulfonylureas, insulin:* Aspirin (> 2 g/day) may potentiate glucose lowering.

Lab Test Interferences

May increase levels of serum uric acid, cause false-positive readings of urine glucose by copper reduction method (Clinitest) and false-negative readings by glucose oxidase method (Clinistix); may interfere with urine tests of 5-hydroxyindoleacetic acid, ketone, phenolsulfonphthalein, vanillylmandelic acid.

Adverse Reactions

EENT: Dizziness; tinnitus. *GI:* Nausea; dyspepsia; heartburn; bleeding. *HEMA:* Increased bleeding times; anemia; decreased iron concentration. *OTHER:* Hypersensitivity reactions may include urticaria, hives, rashes, angioedema and anaphylactic shock.

Precautions
Pregnancy: Category D. *Lactation:* Excreted in breast milk. *Children:* Reye's syndrome has been associated with aspirin administration to children (including teenagers) with acute febrile illness. Do not use without consulting physician. *GI disorders:* Can cause gastric irritation and bleeding. *Hepatic impairment:* May cause hepatotoxicity in patients with impaired liver function. *Hypersensitivity:* Reaction may include bronchospasm and generalized urticaria or angioedema; patients with asthma or nasal polyps have greatest risk. *Renal impairment:* May decrease renal function or aggravate kidney diseases. *Surgical patients:* Aspirin may increase risk of postoperative bleeding. If possible, avoid use 1 week before surgery.

NURSING CONSIDERATIONS

Administration/Storage

- Administer after meals, with food or with antacid to minimize gastric irritation.
- Do not crush or have patient chew enteric-coated or timed-release caplets.
- Store oral forms at room temperature in tightly closed container. Store suppositories in a cool location or refrigerate. Do not freeze.

Assessment/Interventions

- Obtain patient history, including drug history and any known allergies, particularly to tartrazine (yellow dye #5). Note asthma, hay fever and nasal polyps.
- Ensure that bleeding time and prothrombin time have been evaluated before beginning large dose long-term therapy.
- Monitor hemoglobin or guaiac (hemoccult) stool periodically during therapy.
- Monitor during long-term therapy for tinnitus, GI disturbances, bleeding from gums, black tarry stools or prolonged fever lasting more than 3 days.
- If signs of bleeding, black tarry stools or tinnitus occur, withhold medication and notify physician.
- Observe for rash, urticaria, dyspnea or anaphylactic reaction. If these occur, notify physician immediately.

OVERDOSAGE: SIGNS & SYMPTOMS

Nausea, vomiting, tinnitus, dizziness, respiratory alkalosis, metabolic acidosis, hemorrhage, convulsions

Patient/Family Education

- Instruct patient to take drug with food or after meals and with full glass of water. Explain that antacids should be avoided within 1-2 hr after ingestion of enteric-coated tablets.
- Tell patient to discard any aspirin that has a vinegar-like odor.
- Instruct patient to report ringing in ears or unusual bleeding, bruising or persistent GI pain.
- Advise patient on long-term therapy to inform physician or dentist before seeking surgery or dental care.
- Tell patient on sodium-restricted diet to limit use of effervescent or buffered aspirin preparations.
- Caution parents to avoid giving aspirin to children or teenagers with flu-like symptoms or chickenpox without first consulting physician.
- Instruct patient to avoid intake of alcoholic beverages or other CNS depressants.

See Patient Guide, p. 38.

Astemizole

(ASS-TEM-ih-zole)
Hismanal
Class: Antihistamine

Action Competitively antagonizes histamine at H_1 receptor sites.

Indications Symptomatic relief of allergic rhinitis and chronic idiopathic urticaria. **Unlabeled uses:** Symptomatic relief of vasomotor rhinitis; allergic conjunctivitis; allergic and nonallergic pruritus; mild, uncomplicated urticaria and angioedema.

Contraindications Hypersensitivity to antihistamines; significant hepatic dysfunction; concomitant erythromycin, ketoconazole or itraconazole therapy.

Route/Dosage
ADULTS & CHILDREN > 12 YR: **PO** 10 mg/day. Do not exceed recommended dose.

Interactions
Drug/food: Absorption is reduced by 60% when taken with food. *Fluconazole, itraconazole, ketoconazole, miconazole, macrolide antibiotics (eg, erythromycin):* May increase astemizole plasma levels, leading to serious cardiovascular effects.

Lab Test Interferences
May diminish or prevent positive reactions to skin testing procedures.

Adverse Reactions
CV: Angioedema; rarely death, cardiac arrest, torsade de pointes and other ventricular arrhythmias have occurred in patients with significant hepatic dysfunction or concomitant administration of azole antifungals or macrolide antibiotics (See Contraindications) or in overdosage. *RESP:* Bronchospasm. *CNS:* Headache; nervousness; dizziness. Drug appears to have little to no sedative effects. *EENT:* Conjunctivitis; pharyngitis. *GI:* Nausea; diarrhea; abdominal pain. *HEMA:* Epistaxis. *DERM:* Rash, pruritus. *META:* Increased appetite; weight gain. *OTHER:* Arthralgia; edema; myalgia. Drug appears to have little to no anticholinergic effects.

Precautions
Pregnancy: Category C. *Lactation:* Unknown. *Children:* Safety not established in children < 12 yr. *Elderly patients:* Use not recommended.

NURSING CONSIDERATIONS

Administration/Storage
- Administer medication on empty stomach, 1 hr before or 2 hr after meals.
- Store in tightly closed container in cool location. Avoid exposure to light.

Assessment/Interventions
- Obtain patient history, including drug history and any allergy, especially to antihistamines. Note cardiac disease.
- Assess allergic symptoms for which medication is being ordered.
- Obtain baseline BP, respirations and pulse before beginning therapy.
- Monitor closely for signs of hypersensitivity if patient has history of allergic reactions to other antihistamines.
- If patient develops palpitations or syncope, stop medication and notify physician immediately.

OVERDOSAGE: SIGNS & SYMPTOMS
Serious ventricular arrhythmias, including torsade de pointes

Patient/Family Education
- Warn patient not to increase dose to try to obtain quicker relief of symptoms.
- If patient is to have allergy skin testing, advise to avoid taking medication for 4 days before test.
- Advise female patients of childbearing age to avoid becoming pregnant during therapy and for 4 mo after discontinuing drug.
- Caution patient to avoid sudden position changes to prevent orthostatic hypotension.
- Instruct patient to avoid intake of alcoholic beverages or other CNS depressants.

- Advise patient not to take otc medications without notifying physician.

See Patient Guide, p. 39.

Atenolol

(ah-TEN-oh-lahl)

Tenormin, ♣ *APO-Atenol, Novo-Atenol, Nu-Atenol*

Class: Beta-adrenergic blocker

Action Blocks beta receptors, primarily affecting heart (slows rate), vascular system (decreases BP) and, to lesser extent, lungs (reduces function).

Indications Treatment of hypertension (used alone or in combination with other drugs), angina pectoris resulting from coronary atherosclerosis, acute MI. **Unlabeled uses:** Migraine prophylaxis, alcohol withdrawal syndrome, ventricular arrhythmias, supraventricular arrhythmias or tachycardias, esophageal varices rebleeding, anxiety.

Contraindications Hypersensitivity to beta-blockers; sinus bradycardia; greater than first-degree heart block; CHF unless secondary to tachyarrhythmia treatable with beta-blockers; overt cardiac failure; cardiogenic shock.

Route/Dosage

Hypertension

ADULTS: **PO** 50-100 mg/day.

Angina Pectoris

May require up to 200 mg/day.

Acute MI

IV 5 mg over 5 min; second **IV** dose 10 min later. Follow with **PO** 50-100 mg/day.

Interactions

Ampicillin: May impair antihypertensive and antianginal effects. *Clonidine:* May add to or reverse antihypertensive effects; potentially life-threatening situations may occur, especially on withdrawal. *NSAIDs:* Some agents may impair antihypertensive effect. *Prazosin:* May increase orthostatic hypotension. *Verapamil:* Effects of both drugs may be increased.

Lab Test Interferences

None well documented.

Adverse Reactions

CV: Hypotension; bradycardia; CHF; cold extremities; second- or third-degree heart block. *RESP:* Bronchospasm; dyspnea; wheezing. *CNS:* Insomnia; fatigue; dizziness; depression; lethargy; drowsiness; forgetfulness; slurred speech. *EENT:* Dry eyes; blurred vision; tinnitus; dry mouth; sore throat. *GI:* Nausea; vomiting; diarrhea. *GU:* Impotence; painful, difficult or frequent urination. *HEMA:* Agranulocytosis; thrombocytopenic purpura. *HEPA:* Elevated liver enzymes and bilirubin. *DERM:* Rash; hives; fever; alopecia. *OTHER:* Weight changes; facial swelling; muscle weakness; hyperglycemia; hypoglycemia; antinuclear antibodies; hyperlipidemia.

Precautions

Pregnancy: Category C. *Lactation:* Excreted in breast milk. *Children:* Safety not established. *Anaphylaxis:* Deaths have occurred; aggressive therapy may be required. *CHF:* Should be administered cautiously in patients with CHF controlled by digitalis and diuretics. *Diabetes mellitus:* May mask symptoms of hypoglycemia (eg, tachycardia, BP changes). *Elderly:* Dosage reduction may be necessary. *Nonallergic bronchospastic diseases (eg, chronic bronchitis, emphysema):* In general, do not give beta-blockers to patients with bronchospastic diseases. *Peripheral vascular disease:* May precipitate or aggravate symptoms of arterial insufficiency. *Thyrotoxicosis:* May mask clinical signs (eg, tachycardia) of developing or continuing hyperthyroidism. Abrupt withdrawal may exacerbate symptoms of hyperthyroidism, including thyroid storm.

Renal/hepatic impairment: Dose should be reduced.

NURSING CONSIDERATIONS

Administration/Storage

- May be administered with or without food.
- If patient has difficulty swallowing, tablet may be crushed and mixed with fluid.
- Store in a tightly closed container in a cool location.

Assessment/Interventions

- Obtain patient history, including drug history and any allergies. Note diabetes; respiratory, liver or cardiac disease or sensitivity to other beta-blockers.
- Review baseline ECG.
- Assess BP and pulse before administration. If pulse is below 60 bpm, withhold medication and notify physician.
- Monitor I&O and daily weight during therapy for signs of fluid retention.
- If sudden severe dyspnea or edema of hands and feet develops, withhold medication and notify physician.
- If chest pain occurs, assess for location, intensity, duration and radiation. Nitroglycerin preparations may be administered in conjunction with this medication if ordered.
- If patient experiences chest pain not relieved by medication, continue medication and notify physician.
- If there are changes in the ECG (long PR interval, low- or high-grade heart blocks, ventricular ectopic beats), withhold dose and notify physician.

OVERDOSAGE: SIGNS & SYMPTOMS

Bradycardia, hypotension, CHF, cardiogenic shock, hypertension, cardiac arrhythmias, seizures, respiratory depression, coma, pulmonary edema, bronchospasm, hypoglycemia

Patient/Family Education

- Explain that full effectiveness of drug may not occur for up to 1-2 wk after initiation of therapy and that dosage will be tapered slowly before stopping. Warn that sudden discontinuation can cause chest pain or heart attack.
- Teach patient how to take pulse and instruct to check before taking drug. Warn patient not to take drug if pulse is < 60 bpm, and to call physician.
- When medication is being used for treatment of hypertension, teach patient how to take BP and advise to take daily.
- Advise patient that medication may cause increased sensitivity to cold.
- Inform diabetic patient to monitor blood glucose level carefully. It may be necessary to alter insulin dose while taking drug.
- Inform patient that frequent follow-up appointments with physician are important to adjust medication dosage.
- Instruct patient to report these symptoms to physician: difficulty breathing; swelling of feet, legs, hands, etc.; irregular heart beat; altered mood or depression.
- Caution patient to avoid sudden position changes to prevent orthostatic hypotension.
- Advise patient that drug may cause drowsiness and to use caution while driving or performing other tasks requiring mental alertness.
- Caution patient not to take otc medications without consulting physician.

See Patient Guide, p. 40.

Atenolol/Chlorthalidone

(ah-TEN-oh-lahl/klor-THAL-ih-dohn)

Tenoretic-50, Tenoretic-100

Class: Antihypertensive

Action Atenolol is beta-adrenergic blocking agent that slows heart rate, reduces cardiac output and lowers BP. Chlorthalidone is diuretic agent that reduces body water by increasing urine output.

Indications Treatment of hypertension.

Contraindications Hypersensitivity to sulfonamide-derived drugs, sinus bradycardia, heart block greater than first degree, cardiogenic shock, overt cardiac failure, anuria. Not for initial therapy of hypertension.

Route/Dosage

ADULTS: **PO** 50 mg atenolol/25 mg chlorthalidone or 100 mg atenolol/25 mg chlorthalidone once daily.

Interactions

Clonidine: Beta blockers may exacerbate rebound hypertension associated with clonidine withdrawal. Atenolol/chlorthalidone should be tapered and withdrawn several days before gradual withdrawal of clonidine. *Digitalis glycosides:* Diuretic-induced hypokalemia may potentiate digitalis toxicity. *Lithium:* May increase therapeutic and toxic effects of lithium; avoid concomitant use. *Nondepolarizing muscle relaxants:* May increase effects of these agents. *Norepinephrine:* May decrease arterial responsiveness to norepinephrine. *Other antihypertensive agents:* May increase antihypertensive effects. *Sulfonylureas:* May decrease hypoglycemic effects.

Lab Test Interferences

May increase serum protein-bound iodine levels without signs of thyroid disturbances.

Adverse Reactions

CV: Bradycardia; orthostatic hypotension; cold extremities; leg pain; CHF; slow atrioventricular (AV) conduction; intensification of AV block. *RESP:* Bronchospasm; wheezing; dyspnea. *CNS:* Fatigue; dizziness; vertigo; light-headedness; lethargy; drowsiness; depression; dreaming. *GI:* Diarrhea; nausea. *GU:* Peyronie's disease; impotence; diminished libido. *HEMA:* Thrombocytopenia; agranulocytosis. *HEPA:* Elevated liver enzymes; jaundice; pancreatitis. *DERM:* Rash. *META:* Hyperuricemia; hyponatremia; hypochloremic alkalosis; hypokalemia. *OTHER:* Development of lupus syndrome with antinuclear antibodies.

Precautions

Pregnancy: Category D. *Lactation:* Atenolol is excreted in breast milk and may produce clinically significant effects in infants. *Children:* Safety and efficacy not established. *Anaphylaxis:* Deaths have occurred with anaphylactic reactions to beta-blockers; aggressive therapy may be required. *Cardiac failure:* Use with caution in patients with history of heart failure. *Diabetes mellitus:* May mask symptoms of hypoglycemia (eg, tachycardia, BP changes). May potentiate insulin-induced hypoglycemia. *Elderly:* Dose may need to be reduced. *Hypertension:* Fixed-dose combinations of drugs are not intended for initial therapy of hypertension but are used for convenience once patient has been stabilized. *Nonallergic bronchospastic diseases (eg, chronic bronchitis, emphysema):* In general, do not give beta-blockers to patients with bronchospastic diseases. *Peripheral vascular disease:* May precipitate or aggravate symptoms of arterial insufficiency. *Renal and hepatic impairment:* Use with caution in patients with renal or hepatic disease; dose may need to be reduced. *Thyrotoxicosis:* May mask clinical signs (eg, tachycardia), of developing or continuing hyperthyroidism. Abrupt withdrawal may exacerbate symptoms of hyperthyroidism, including thyroid storm.

NURSING CONSIDERATIONS

Administration/Storage

- Give in morning with food or milk.
- If patient has difficulty swallowing, tablet may be crushed and mixed with fluid.
- Store at room temperature in tightly closed, light-resistant container.

Assessment/Interventions

- Obtain patient history, including drug history and any known allergies. Note asthma, diabetes and respiratory, liver or cardiac disease.
- Ensure that baseline creatinine clearance levels have been obtained in patients with impaired renal function and monitor periodically during therapy, along with serum electrolytes.
- Assess BP and apical pulse before administering. If systolic BP is < 90 mm Hg or pulse is < 60 bpm, withhold drug and notify physician.
- Monitor I&O and daily weight during therapy for signs of fluid retention.
- Monitor for fluid overload (eg, jugular venous distension, dyspnea, rales, peripheral edema). Notify physician if these signs occur.
- Withhold medication and notify physician if the following symptoms occur: hypotension, bradycardia or dyspnea, difficulty breathing on exertion or lying down, night cough, edema of hands and feet.

Patient/Family Education

- Explain that dosage will be tapered slowly before stopping. Warn that sudden discontinuation may cause adverse effects (eg, exacerbation of angina, precipitation of MI).
- Teach patient proper technique for taking pulse and BP and instruct to check before taking medication.
- Advise patient not to take medication in evening to avoid prolonged diuretic effects.
- Instruct diabetic patient to monitor blood glucose level carefully.
- Counsel patient that impotence or decrease in libido is common side effect and advise to contact physician if either symptom occurs.
- Caution patient to avoid sudden position changes to prevent orthostatic hypotension.
- Advise patient that drug may cause drowsiness and to use caution while driving or performing other tasks requiring mental alertness until individual effects can be determined.
- Instruct patient not to take otc medications without consulting physician.

See Patient Guide, p. 41.

Atovaquone

(uh-TOE-vuh-KWONE)

Mepron

Class: Anti-infective/antiprotozoal

Action Inhibits mitochondrial electron transport in metabolic enzymes of microorganisms. This may cause inhibition of nucleic acid and adenosine triphosphate synthesis.

Indications Treatment of mild to moderate *Pneumocystis carinii* pneumonia (PCP) in patients who are intolerant of trimethoprim-sulfamethoxazole.

Contraindications Standard considerations.

Route/Dosage

ADULTS: **PO** 750 mg with food tid for 21 days.

Interactions

Food: Food, particularly fats, increases absorption threefold. *Highly protein-bound drugs:* Atovaquone is highly protein bound; interactions may occur because of competition for binding sites.

Lab Test Interferences None well documented.

Adverse Reactions *RESP*: Cough. *CNS*: Headache; insomnia; dizziness; anxiety. *EENT*: Sinusitis; rhinitis; altered taste. *GI*: Nausea; diarrhea; vomiting; abdominal pain; constipation; oral monilia; anorexia; dyspepsia. *GU*: Elevated creatinine; elevated BUN. *HEMA*: Anemia; neutropenia. *HEPA*: Elevated liver enzymes. *DERM*: Rash; pruritus. *OTHER*: Fever; sweating; weakness; decreased sodium concentration; elevated amylase.

Precautions *Pregnancy*: Category C. *Lactation*: Undetermined. *Children*: Safety and efficacy not established. *Elderly*: Atovaquone has not been systematically evaluated in patients > 65 yr. *Severe PCP*: Treatment of severe episodes of PCP has not been evaluated. Efficacy in patients not responding to trimethoprim-sulfamethoxazole has not been established. Atovaquone has not been evaluated for prophylaxis of PCP.

NURSING CONSIDERATIONS

Administration/Storage

- Most effective if administered with food, particularly proteins and fats.
- Do not freeze.

Assessment/Interventions

- Obtain patient history, including drug history and any known allergies, particularly to antifungal medications. Note existing GI disorders, because these may limit absorption of orally administered drug.
- Monitor patient closely for several hours after administering the first dose even if there is no history of allergy.
- Monitor renal and GI function during therapy.
- Observe for signs of superinfection during therapy (yeast infections, black "hairy" tongue, itching in groin area).
- Monitor for effectiveness during therapy (decreased temperature, decreased lung congestion).
- If signs and symptoms of hypersensitivity occur (rash, shortness of breath), withhold medication and notify physician.
- If no improvement in infection occurs within 5 days, notify physician.
- If severe gastrointestinal side effects occur, notify physician.

Patient/Family Education

- Inform the patient that medication is most effective when taken with food (particularly fatty foods) and to notify physician if unable to eat.
- Inform patient that slight rash may develop while taking medication.
- Teach patient to recognize signs of oral fungal infections.

See Patient Guide, p. 42.

Atropine

(AT-troe-peen)

Atropine-1, Atropine Care, Atropine Injectable, Atropine Sulfate S.O.P., Atropisol, Isopto Atropine, ♣ *Dioptic's Atropine, R.O.-Atropine*

Class: Anticholinergic; antispasmodic

Action Inhibits action of acetylcholine or other cholinergic stimuli at postganglionic cholinergic receptors, including smooth muscles, secretory glands and CNS sites.

Indications Administration prior to anesthesia to reduce or prevent secretions of respiratory tract; to control rhinorrhea; treatment of parkinsonism; restoration of cardiac rate and arterial pressure in some situations; treatment of peptic ulcers; management of hypersecretion, irritation or inflammation of stomach, intestines or pancreas; treatment of diarrhea; relief of infant colic; management of spasms of bile tract; treatment of hypertonicity of small intestine and uterus; management of hypermotility of colon; prevention of spasm of pylorus, biliary tree, ureters, and bronchi; treatment of frequent urination and bedwetting; therapy for certain bradycardias and heart blocks; treatment of closed head injury with acetylcholine release; reduction of laughing and crying associated with brain lesions; treatment of alcohol withdrawal symptoms; relief of motion sickness. Antidote for cardiovascular collapse in certain overdoses or poisonings. Ophthalmic preparation: Production of cycloplegia and mydriasis. Short-term treatment and prevention of bronchospasm associated with chronic bronchial asthma, bronchitis and COPD.

STOP **Contraindications** Hypersensitivity to anticholinergics; narrow-angle glaucoma; adhesions between iris and lens; prostatic hypertrophy; obstructive uropathy; myocardial ischemia; unstable cardiac status caused by hemorrhage; tachycardia; myasthenia gravis; pyloric or intestinal obstruction; asthma; hyperthyroidism; renal disease; hepatic disease; toxic megacolon; intestinal atony or paralytic ileus.

Route/Dosage

ADULTS: **PO** 0.4-0.6 mg q 4-6 hr. CHILDREN: **PO** Use lowest effective dose beginning at 0.01 mg/kg q 4-6 hr not to exceed 0.4 mg q 4-6 hr.

Surgery

ADULTS: **SC/IM/IV** 0.4-0.6 mg q 4-6 hr. CHILDREN: **SC/IM/IV** 0.01 mg/kg to maximum of 0.4 mg q 4-6 hr. INFANTS < 5 KG: **SC/IM/IV** 0.04 mg/kg. INFANTS > 5 KG: **SC/IM/IV** 0.03 mg/kg.

Bradyarrhythmias

ADULTS: **SC/IM/IV** 0.4-2 mg q 1-2 hr prn. CHILDREN: **SC/IV/IM** 0.01-0.03 mg/kg, q 1-2 hr prn.

Antidote

Insecticide poisoning. ADULTS: Parenteral: At least 2-3 mg, repeated until signs of poisoning subside or signs of intoxication appear. CHILDREN: 0.02-0.05 mg/kg/dose q 10-20 min until signs of atropic effect are observed, then q 1-4 hr for at least 24 hr.

Ophthalmic

Uveitis

ADULT: 1-2 drops 0.5%-1% solution qid or ointment tid. CHILDREN: 1-2 drops 0.5% solution tid.

Refraction

ADULT: 1-2 drops of 1% solution 1 hour before refraction examination. CHILDREN: 1-2 drops 0.5% solution bid 1-3 days before refraction examination.

Interactions

Haloperidol: Worsened schizophrenic symptoms; decreased serum haloperidol concentrations. *Phenothiazines:* Decreased antipsychotic effects and increased anticholinergic effects may occur. *Other anticholinergic agents:* Additive anticholinergic effects.

Lab Test Interferences

None well documented.

Adverse Reactions

CV: Palpitations; bradycardia; tachycardia; orthostatic hypotension. *RESP:* Bronchospasm. *CNS:* Headache; nervousness; drowsiness; weakness; dizziness; confusion; insomnia; fever; excitability; restlessness; tremor. *EENT:* Nasal congestion; altered taste. *GI:* Xerostomia; nausea; vomiting; dysphagia; heartburn; constipation; bloated feeling; paralytic ileus. *GU:* Urinary hesitancy and retention; impotence. *DERM:* Allergic reactions; urticaria; rash; flushing. *OTHER:* Suppression of lactation; decreased sweating.

Precautions

Pregnancy: Category C. *Lactation:* If possible, do not use. *Infants:* Use cautiously. *Special risk patients:* Use cautiously in elderly patients and in patients with Down's syndrome, brain damage or spastic paralysis. *Anticholinergic psychosis:* Has occurred in sensitive patients. *Diarrhea:* May be an early symptom of incomplete intestinal obstruction. *Gastric ulcer:* May delay gastric emptying time and complicate therapy. *Glaucoma:* Determine intraocular IOP and depth of angle of anterior chamber before and during ophthalmic use to avoid glaucoma attacks. *Heat prostration:* May occur at high ambient temperature.

NURSING CONSIDERATIONS

Administration/Storage

Oral

- Administer 30 min before meals and at bedtime for GI disorders.
- Store in airtight, light-resistant container at room temperature.

Intramuscular/Subcutaneous

- Draw solution carefully into syringe. Accidental eye exposure results in blurred vision.
- Administer 30-60 min before surgery if used for preanesthesia.
- Give after patient has voided.

Intravenous

- Do not add to IV solutions.

Ophthalmic

- Compress inner canthus gently for 1-3 min after installation.
- Wash hands after administration to avoid accidental eye exposure.

Assessment/Interventions

- Obtain patient history, including drug history and any known allergies.
- Identify baseline signs and symptoms, and monitor patient according to indications for use: increased heart rate when used for bradycardia (notify physician of paradoxical bradycardia); decreased secretions for preanesthesia; decreased GI motility or decreased abdominal pain in GI disorders; pupil dilation in eye disorders; decreased tremor, rigidity and drooling in Parkinson's disease.
- Monitor elderly patient for agitation or drowsiness.
- Monitor vital signs. Remember that pulse rate is particularly sensitive to atropine.
- Assess for urinary retention, particularly in elderly male patients and in those with pre-existing prostatic hypertrophy and other obstructive/retentive disorders.
- Dim room lighting to comfort level or provide sunglasses if necessary.
- Keep room cool and provide adequate hydration to prevent hyperpyrexia.
- Institute safety precautions if visual or CNS disturbances occur.
- Provide frequent oral hygiene, skin care and lubricating eye drops if dry mouth/skin/eyes occur.
- Notify physician immediately if eye pain, diarrhea or significant tachycardia or bradycardia occurs.

OVERDOSAGE: SIGNS & SYMPTOMS

Dry mouth, thirst, vomiting, nausea, abdominal distention, CNS stimulation, delirium, drowsiness, restlessness, stupor, fever, seizures, hallucinations, convulsions, coma, circulatory failure, tachycardia, weak pulse, hypertension, hypotension, respiratory depression, palpitations, urinary urgency, blurred vision, dilated pupils, photophobia, rash, dry and hot skin

Patient/Family Education

- Warn patient that temporary mild stinging and blurred vision may occur with ophthalmic preparations.
- Instruct patient to withhold ophthalmic preparations if eye pain, redness, or rapid, irregular pulse occurs and to notify physician immediately.
- Instruct patient in and observe return demonstration of patient's technique for installation of ophthalmic preparations.
- Instruct patient to take oral dose 30 min before meals and at bedtime.
- Caution patient to avoid hazardous activities until vision clears.

- Advise patients that eyes may be more sensitive to light and to wear sunglasses, as needed.
- Tell patients to increase dietary fiber and fluids, unless contraindicated, to reduce constipation.
- Explain importance of frequent oral hygiene and regular dental care when mouth is dry. Explain that chewing sugarless gum or sucking on ice chips or hard candy may relieve dry mouth.
- Caution patient to avoid vigorous exercise in warm environment and to avoid hot baths or saunas.
- Advise male patients that if impotence occurs, it may be a result of drug therapy and to notify physician.
- Tell patient to notify physician immediately if these symptoms occur: rapid, irregular pulse; headaches; hot, dry skin; difficulty swallowing; urinary retention; constipation; difficulty breathing; loss of coordination; restlessness; tremors; disorientation; hallucinations.
- If patient is taking drug for symptoms of Parkinson's disease, warn patient that drug should not be discontinued abruptly, because withdrawal-like symptoms may occur.

See Patient Guide, pp. 43-44.

Atropine Sulfate/ Scopolamine Hydrobromide/ Hyoscyamine Sulfate/ Phenobarbital

(AT-troe-peen SULL-fate/skoe-POLE-uh-meen HIGH-droe-BROE-mide/high-oh-SIGH-uh-meen SULL-fate/fee-no-BAR-bih-tahl)

Donnatal

Class: Anticholinergic; antispasmodic

Action Promotes peripheral anticholinergic/antispasmodic action (decreases GI motility); provides mild sedation.

Indications Possibly effective for treatment of irritable bowel syndrome and acute enterocolitis. Also may be useful as adjunctive therapy for duodenal ulcer.

Contraindications Glaucoma; obstructive uropathy; obstructive disease of the gastrointestinal tract; paralytic ileus; intestinal atony in elderly or debilitated patient; severe ulcerative colitis; toxic megacolon complicating ulcerative colitis; hepatic or renal disease; tachycardia; myocardial ischemia; unstable cardiovascular status in acute hemorrhage; myasthenia gravis; acute intermittent porphyrinuria.

Route/Dosage
ADULTS: **PO** 1 to 2 tablets or capsules tid to qid; 1 extended-release tablet q 12 hr; 5 to 10 ml elixir tid to qid according to condition and severity of symptoms. CHILDREN: **PO** 0.5 to 5.0 ml elixir: q 4 hr to q 6 hr, according to body weight.

Interactions
Anticoagulants: Anticoagulant effects may be decreased. *Anticholinergic agents:* Additive anticholingeric effects. *Haloperidol:* Worsened schizophrenic symptoms; decreased haloperidol concentrations. *Phenothiazines:* Decreased antipsychotic effects and increased anticholinergic effects may occur.

Lab Test Interferences
None well documented.

Adverse Reactions
CV: Palpitations; bradycardia; tachycardia; flushing. *CNS:* Headache; nervousness; drowsiness; weakness; dizziness; confusion; insomnia; fever (especially in children); mental confusion or excitement (especially in the elderly, even with small doses); CNS stimulation (restlessness, tremor), psychosis. *EENT:* Blurred vision; mydriasis; photophobia; cycloplegia; increased IOP; dilated pupils; nasal congestion; altered taste perception. *GI:* Xerostomia; nausea; vomiting; dysphagia; heartburn;

constipation; bloated feeling; paralytic ileus. *GU:* Urinary hesitancy and retention; impotence. *DERM:* Urticaria and other dermal manifestations of allergic reaction. *OTHER:* Severe allergic reactions, including anaphylaxis; suppression of lactation; decreased sweating.

Precautions

Pregnancy: Category C. *Lactation:* If possible, do not use. *Elderly patients:* May react with agitation, drowsiness and other untoward manifestations even with small doses. *Special risk patients:* Used with caution in patients with neuropathy, hepatic or renal disease, hyperthyroidism, coronary artery disease, CHF, arrhythmias, hypertension or tachycardia. May complicate gastric ulcer treatment. *Diarrhea:* May be symptom of incomplete intestinal obstruction, especially in patients with ileostomy or colostomy and, therefore, may serve as contraindication. *Heat prostration:* Can occur in presence of high ambient temperature due to interference with normal sweating. *Potentially hazardous tasks:* May produce drowsiness, dizziness or blurred vision. *Addiction potential:* May be habit forming; when possible, not given to addiction-prone individual.

NURSING CONSIDERATIONS

Administration/Storage

- Available for oral use only.
- Store in a cool, dry place.

Assessment/Interventions

- Obtain patient history, including drug history and any known allergies.
- Monitor vital signs and LOC. Note any signs of hyperactivity or sedation.
- Monitor I&O and bowel sounds. Notify physician of abdominal distention.
- In patient with chronic lung disease, monitor lung sounds and effectiveness of cough.

OVERDOSAGE: SIGNS & SYMPTOMS

Dry mouth, thirst, vomiting, nausea, abdominal distention, CNS stimulation, delirium, drowsiness, restlessness, stupor, fever, seizures, hallucinations, convulsions, coma, "flat" EEG, circulatory failure, tachycardia, weak pulse, hypertension, hypotension, respiratory depression, palpitations, arrhythmias, urinary urgency, blurred vision, dilated pupils, photophobia, rash, dry and hot skin

Patient/Family Education

- Caution patient to have adequate oral intake.
- Advise patient to include fiber in diet to prevent constipation.
- Caution patient to limit exposure to high ambient temperatures.
- Advise patient that dilated pupils may be experienced.
- Warn patient that product may cause excitability or sedation. Remind patient not to drive or operate heavy machinery if sedation occurs.
- Advise patient to notify physician if confusion, disorientation, ataxia, nausea, vomiting, diarrhea, abdominal distention or elevated body temperature occurs. With ophthalmic preparations, also tell the patient to notify the doctor if eye pain is experienced.

See Patient Guide, p. 45.

Auranofin

(or-RAIN-oh-fin)
Ridaura
Class: Analgesic/antirheumatic agent/ gold compound

Action Gold compounds relieve symptoms of arthritis but do not cure this disease; decrease rheumatoid factor concentrations and immunoglobulins.

Indications Relief of symptoms of active adult rheumatoid arthritis poorly controlled with other therapies. **Unlabeled uses:** Treatment of pemphigus and psoriatic arthritis.

Contraindications Standard considerations.

Route/Dosage
ADULTS: PO 6 mg/day or 3 mg bid. If no response by 6 months, dose may be increased to 3 mg tid. Parenteral route may be used when control cannot be achieved by oral form. CHILDREN: Auranofin is not recommended for children; safety and efficacy have not been established. If prescribed, however, the following doses have been recommended: *Initial*—0.1 mg/kg/day; *maintenance*—0.15 mg/kg/day; *maximum*—0.2 mg/kg/day.

Interactions None well documented.

Lab Test Interferences
None well documented.

Adverse Reactions Reactions can occur months after therapy is discontinued. *CNS:* Confusion; hallucinations; seizures. *RESP:* Interstitial pneumonitis; pulmonary fibrosis. *EENT:* Mucositis that may be preceded by metallic taste; conjunctivitis; corneal gold deposition; metallic taste; inflammation of the upper respiratory tract; pharyngitis. *GI:* Diarrhea; abdominal pain; anorexia; dyspepsia; flatulence; GI bleeding; enterocolitis; gastritis; colitis; tracheitis. *GU:* Nephrotic syndrome and glomerulitis with proteinuria and hematuria. *HEMA:* Anemia; thrombocytopenia; leukopenia; aplastic anemia. *HEPA:* Elevated liver enzymes; jaundice; hepatitis. *DERM:* Dermatitis; pruritus; grey-blue pigmentation on sun-exposed skin; exfoliative dermatitis; angioedema. *OTHER:* Vaginitis; glossitis.

Precautions
Pregnancy: Category C. *Lactation:* Excreted in breast milk. *Children:* Safety and efficacy not established. *Elderly:* Tolerance decreases with age. *Special risk patients:* Use with caution in patients with diabetes mellitus, CHF, history of blood dyscrasias, allergy or hypersensitivity to other gold products, skin rash, previous kidney or liver disease, marked hypertension, compromised circulation or inflammatory bowel disease.

NURSING CONSIDERATIONS

Administration/Storage
- Administer with food or fluid.
- Protect product from light and moisture.

Assessment/Interventions
- Obtain patient history, including drug history and any known allergies.
- Observe patient for early symptoms of toxicity such as a metallic taste in the mouth, pruritus or rash.
- Review laboratory values for indications of gold toxicity such as decreased hemoglobin, < 4000 WBC/mm^3, platelets < 100,000-150,000/cu mm, proteinuria, and elevated liver enzymes.
- If given parenterally, stay with patient for 15 minutes after injection and monitor for signs of adverse reaction: anaphylactic shock; syncope; bradycardia; thickening of tongue;

dysphagia; dyspnea; and angioneurotic edema. Notify physician of any problems.

- Observe for diarrhea and loose stools, a common adverse reaction that usually can be managed by a reduction in dosage.

OVERDOSAGE: SIGNS & SYMPTOMS

Renal damage (eg, hematuria, proteinuria), hematologic reactions (eg, thrombocytopenia), nausea, vomiting, diarrhea, fever, skin disorders

Patient/Family Education

- Instruct patient to immediately report any adverse effects of therapy including dermatitis and pruritus, weakness, fatigue, hematuria, sore mouth, indigestion, diarrhea, metallic taste in mouth or unusual bruising.
- Caution patient to minimize exposure to the sun and other sources of ultraviolet light. Explain the need to wear sunscreen and protective clothing outdoors.
- Advise patient to keep appointments with health care providers for continued assessment and monitoring of renal, hepatic and hematologic functions.
- Review oral hygiene, including use of soft toothbrush, daily flossing and avoidance of strong, commercial mouthwashes. If mild stomatitis develops, an isotonic NaCl and sodium bicarbonate solution can be used.
- Alert female patients to the potential risks of using gold therapy during pregnancy.

See Patient Guide, p. 46.

Azathioprine

(AZE-uh-THIGH-oh-preen)

Imuran

Class: Immunosuppressive

Action Suppresses cell-mediated hypersensitivities; alters antibody production and may reduce inflammation.

Indications Adjunct for prevention of rejection in renal homotransplantation; treatment in adults for severe, active, erosive rheumatoid arthritis not responsive to conventional management. **Unlabeled uses:** Treatment of chronic ulcerative colitis, Crohn's disease, myasthenia gravis and Behçet's syndrome.

Contraindications Pregnancy in patients with rheumatoid arthritis.

Route/Dosage

Renal Transplantation

ADULTS & CHILDREN: **IV/PO** Initiate with 3 to 5 mg/kg/day as single daily dose. Maintenance levels are 1-3 mg/kg/day.

Rheumatoid Arthritis

ADULTS: **PO** Initial dose is 1 mg/kg given as single dose or twice daily. Dose is increased by 0.5 mg/kg/day at 6-8 wk, then every 4 wk if there are no serious toxicities and if initial response is unsatisfactory. Maximum dose is 2.5 mg/kg/day. **IV** Reserved for patients unable to tolerate oral medications.

Interactions

Allopurinol: Decreases metabolism of azathioprine. Dose of azathioprine is reduced to approximately one third to one fourth usual dose when used concomitantly. *Non-depolarizing muscle relaxants (eg, tubocurarine, pancuronium):* Azathioprine may resist or reverse neuromuscular blockade.

Lab Test Interferences

None well documented.

Adverse Reactions

GI: Nausea; vomiting. *HEMA:* Leukopenia; thrombocytopenia; macrocytic anemia; bleeding; selective erythrocyte aplasia. *DERM:* Rash. *OTHER:* Serious infections; neoplasias.

Precautions

Pregnancy: Category D. *Lactation:* Excreted in breast milk. *Children:* Safety and efficacy not established. *Carcinogenesis/mutagenesis:* Chronic immunosuppression with azathioprine increases risk of neoplasia. Patients with rheumatoid arthritis previously treated with alkylating agents (eg, cyclophosphamide, chlorambucil, melphalan) may have prohibitive risk of neoplasia. *GI toxicity:* Hypersensitivity reaction with severe nausea and vomiting may occur. Frequency of gastric disturbances can be reduced by giving in divided doses or after meals. *Hematologic effects:* Severe hematologic toxicities may occur; blood counts should be monitored. *Hepatoxicity:* Occurs primarily in allograft recipients. Rare but life-threatening hepatic veno-occlusive disease has occurred in transplant patients; liver function tests should be monitored. *Superinfection:* Serious fungal, viral, bacterial and protozoal infections may develop in patients on long-term immunosuppression.

NURSING CONSIDERATIONS

Administration/Storage

- Do not vigorously shake solution when reconstituting IV preparations.
- Divide daily dosage to reduce GI upset.
- Administer with food or immediately after meals.
- Store in a tightly closed container in a cool location.
- Discard reconstituted IV preparations after 24 hr. Follow any procedures required for proper disposal of immunosuppressant/antimetabolite.

Assessment/Interventions

- Obtain patient history, including drug history and any known allergies.
- Review baseline CBC, renal studies and liver studies.
- Assess for signs of infection before administration.
- Monitor I&O and daily weight during therapy.
- Monitor patient for signs of superinfection during therapy.
- Notify physician if patient displays sudden, severe dyspnea, bleeding from the gums or mucous membranes or blood in urine or stools.

OVERDOSAGE: SIGNS & SYMPTOMS

Bone marrow hypoplasia, bleeding, infection, death

Patient/Family Education

- Instruct patient that if once-daily dose is forgotten to skip the dose, but if two daily doses are missed call physician. Next dose may be doubled.
- Explain importance of precautions regarding contact with individuals who have active infections and individuals who have recently received oral polio vaccine.
- Identify signs of transplant rejection (localized redness, tenderness and swelling in the area of the transplant, and decreased transplant organ function) and remind patient that this or similar medication will be required indefinitely to prevent transplant rejection.
- Explain that frequent follow-up appointments with physician are important to adjust medication dosage.
- Instruct patient to report these symptoms to physician: unusual bleeding, decreased urine output or abdominal pain.
- Caution patient not to take otc medications without consulting physician.

See Patient Guide, p. 47.

Azithromycin

(UHZ-ith-row-MY-sin)

Zithromax

Class: Antibiotic/macrolide

Action Interferes with microbial protein synthesis.

Indications

Adults: Treatment of infections of the respiratory tract, skin and skin structure, and sexually transmitted diseases caused by susceptible organisms. *Children:* Treatment of acute otitis media caused by susceptible organisms; treatment of pharyngitis/tonsillitis caused by *Streptococcus pyogenes* in patients who cannot use first-line therapy.

Contraindications Hypersensitivity to azithromycin, erythromycin or to any macrolide antibiotic.

Route/Dosage

Acute Otitis Media

CHILDREN: **PO** 10 mg/kg as a single dose on the first day, not to exceed 500 mg/day. Then give 5 mg/kg for 4 more days, not to exceed 250 mg/day.

Bacterial Infections

ADULTS: **PO** 500 mg as single dose on first day, then 250 mg/day for 4 more days.

Pharyngitis/Tonsillitis

CHILDREN: **PO** 12 mg/kg/day for 5 days, not to exceed 500 mg/day.

Sexually Transmitted Diseases

ADULTS: **PO** Single 1 g dose.

Interactions

Tacrolimus: Increased tacrolimus plasma levels with increased risk of toxicity.

Lab Test Interferences

None well documented

Adverse Reactions

CV: Palpitations; chest pain. *CNS:* Dizziness; headache; vertigo; somnolence; fatique. *GI:* Diarrhea; nausea; vomiting; abdominal pain; dyspepsia; flatulence; melena. *GU:* Vaginitis; monilia, nephritis. *HEPA:* Cholestatic jaundice. *DERM:* Rash; photosensitivity. *OTHER:* Angioedema; anaphylaxis.

Precautions

Pregnancy: Category B. *Lactation:* Undetermined. *Cardiac effects:* Serious cardiovascular events have occurred with other macrolide antibiotics, especially when given concomitantly with certain antihistamines (eg, terfenadine, astemizole). *Gonorrhea/syphilis:* Ineffective for treatment of these infections. *Hepatic/renal impairment:* Use cautiously. *Pneumonia:* Only effective for mild community-acquired pneumonia. *Pseudomembranous colitis:* May be factor in patients who develop diarrhea.

NURSING CONSIDERATIONS

Administration/Storage

- Administer 1 hour before or 2 hours after meal.
- Time doses evenly throughout day for optimal blood levels.
- Do not give antacids for at least 2 hours after administration of product.
- Do not crush capsules.
- Give patient 6 to 8 ounces of water or noncitrus juice with medication.
- Store in tightly closed container at room temperature.

Assessment/Interventions

- Obtain patient history, including drug history and any known allergies.
- Review C&S report as available.
- Monitor renal, liver and GI function during therapy. Notify physician of any gastrointestinal side effects.
- Observe for signs of superinfection during therapy (yeast infections, black hairy tongue, itching in groin area).
- Monitor for bleeding in patients re-

ceiving concomitant oral anticoagulant therapy.

- Notify physician if signs and symptoms of anaphylaxis occur.

Patient/Family Education

- Instruct patient to time doses for even distribution over a 24-hour period.
- Inform patient that the medication works best on empty stomach, but may be taken with food if there is GI upset.
- Instruct patient to take medication with full glass of water or noncitrus juice.
- Encourage patient to increase fluid intake to 2000-3000 ml/day, if not contraindicated.
- Instruct patient to notify physician if rash develops or difficult breathing occurs.
- Explain that antacids should be avoided while this medication is being taken.

See Patient Guide, p. 48.

Aztreonam

(AZZ-TREE-oh-nam)

Azactam

Class: Antibiotic/monobactam

Action Inhibits bacterial cell wall synthesis.

Indications Treatment of infections of urinary tract, lower respiratory tract, skin and skin structure, intra-abdominal infections, gynecologic infections, surgical infections and septicemia caused by susceptible microorganisms. **Unlabeled use:** Treatment of acute, uncomplicated gonorrhea in patients with penicillin-resistant gonococci.

Contraindications Standard considerations.

Route/Dosage

Urinary Tract Infection

ADULTS: **IM/IV** 500 mg or 1 g q 8-12 hr.

Systemic Infections

ADULTS: **IM/IV** 1-2 g q 6-12 hr. CHILDREN: **IM/IV** 30-50 mg/kg q 4-8 hr.

Acute Uncomplicated Gonorrhea

IM 1 g. Maximum recommended dosage is 8 g/day.

Interactions

Beta-lactamase–inducing antibiotics (eg, cefoxitin, imipenem): May antagonize activity of aztreonam and should not be used concurrently. INCOMPATIBILITIES: *Nafcillin sodium, cephradine, metronidazole:* Incompatible in admixture.

Lab Test Interferences

None well documented.

Adverse Reactions

RESP: Dyspnea. *CNS:* Seizures. *GI:* Diarrhea; nausea; vomiting; pseudomembranous colitis. *DERM:* Rash. *OTHER:* Phlebitis/thrombophlebitis after IV administration; pain/swelling at IM injection site.

Precautions

Pregnancy: Category B. *Lactation:* Excreted in breast milk. *Children:* Safety and efficacy not established. *Hypersensitivity:* Reactions range from mild to life-threatening. Administer cautiously to penicillin- or cephalosporin-sensitive patients because of possible cross-reactivity. *Renal impairment:* Reduced dose required. *Superinfection:* May result in overgrowth of nonsusceptible bacterial or fungal organisms.

NURSING CONSIDERATIONS

Administration/Storage

- Follow manufacturer's instructions for reconstitution.
- Shake reconstituted solutions vigorously immediately after mixing. Reconstituted solutions stable at room

temperature for 48 hours; stable under refrigeration for 7 days. Discard unused solutions.

- Avoid administering concurrently with other IV medications.
- Administer by deep IM injection in large muscle masses due to localized tissue irritation.

Assessment/Interventions

- Obtain patient history, including drug history and any known allergies.
- Review culture and sensitivity of organism as available.
- Monitor patient closely for several hours after initial dose even without a history of allergy.
- Closely monitor renal and GI function during therapy.
- In patients with hepatic impairment, monitor for signs of hepatitis and jaundice.
- Observe for signs of superinfection during therapy (yeast infections, black hairy tongue, itching in groin area).
- Monitor IV site continuously during administration.
- Notify physician if signs and symptoms of hypersensitivity occur (rash, shortness of breath), and stop medication.
- Notify physician if severe gastrointestinal side effects occur.
- Call physician and stop infusion if infusion site becomes red, streaked, warm or painful.
- Notify physician of any signs of unusual bleeding.

Patient/Family Education

- Encourage patient to increase fluid intake to 2000-3000 ml per day, if allowed.
- Inform patient to notify physician if rash or difficulty breathing is experienced.
- If therapy is discontinued because of allergic reaction, explain significance of penicillin allergy and of potential problems with cephalosporins.
- Caution patient against skipping doses or stopping treatment early, which could result in recurrence of symptoms and potential resistance of the organism to this product.

No patient monograph available.

Baclofen

(BACK-low-fen)

Lioresal, ♣ *Alpha-Baclofen*

Class: Skeletal muscle relaxant/ centrally acting

Action May inhibit transmission of reflexes at spinal level, possibly by action (hyperpolarization) at primary afferent fiber terminals resulting in relief of muscle spasticity; has CNS depressant properties.

Indications

Oral: Treatment of reversible spasticity resulting from multiple sclerosis. *Intrathecal:* Treatment of severe spasticity of spinal cord origin in patients who are unresponsive to or cannot tolerate oral baclofen therapy. Used intrathecally in single bolus test doses; chronic use requires implantable pump.

Unlabeled uses: *Oral:* Therapy for trigeminal neuralgia (tic douloureux); tardive dyskinesia. *Intrathecal:* Cerebral palsy spasticity in children.

Contraindications Treatment of spasms from rheumatic disorders, stroke, cerebral palsy and Parkinson's disease; use of intrathecal form via IV, IM, SC or epidural routes.

Route/Dosage

ADULTS: Initial dose: **PO** 5 mg tid; may be increased by 5 mg/dose q 3 days prn to maximum of 80 mg/day (20 mg qid). **Intrathecal** Refer to manufacturer's manual for implantable pump.

Screening

1 ml of 50 mcg/ml dilution is administered into the intrathecal space by barbotage over 1 min and patient is observed for 4-8 hr; may be repeated 24

hr later with 75 mcg/1.5 ml and 48 hr later with 100 mcg/2 ml. Patients not responding to 100 mcg bolus should not be given implantable pump.

Postimplant Dose Titration Period
Double amount of effective screening dose is given over 24 hr and increased by 10%-30% q 24 hr until desired effect is achieved. However, if effect of screening dose lasts more than 12 hr, starting dose should be screening dose administered over 24 hr. *Maintenance:* **Intrathecal** Dose is increased by 10%-40% or decreased by 10%-20% based on response; usual dose: 300-800 µg/day. Sudden requirement for substantial dose escalation typically indicates catheter complication; reservoir refilling must be performed by specially trained personnel. **Intrathecal** Because of possible life threatening side effects, this route must be used in a medically supervised and adequately equipped environment. Physician must be trained and educated in chronic intrathecal infusion therapy.

Interactions

CNS depressants: May cause increased sedative effects. *Morphine (epidural):* May cause hypotension and dyspnea.

Lab Test Interferences

May cause false elevation of AST, alkaline phosphatase or blood glucose.

Adverse Reactions

CV: Hypotension; palpitations; chest pain. *RESP:* Dyspnea. *CNS:* Drowsiness; weakness in lower extremities; dizziness; seizures; headache; numbness; euphoria; depression; confusion; lethargy; insomnia. *EENT:* Tinnitus; blurred vision; taste disorder; nasal congestion. *GI:* Nausea; vomiting; dry mouth; constipation; diarrhea; abdominal pain; anorexia. *GU:* Urinary frequency; enuresis; dysuria; impotence. *DERM:* Pruritus; rash. *OTHER:* Hypotonia; slurred speech; muscle pain; ankle edema; excessive perspiration; weight gain.

Precautions

Pregnancy: Category C. *Lactation:* Excreted in breast milk. *Children:* Safety of oral baclofen in children < 12 yr and of intrathecal baclofen in children < 18 yr has not been established. *Intrathecal use:* Only specially trained personnel should administer drug intrathecally because of potentially life-threatening CNS depression, cardiovascular collapse or respiratory failure. *Fatalities:* Fatalities occurred in premarketing trials of intrathecal baclofen; role of baclofen in these deaths is unknown. *Epilepsy and psychotic disorders:* Use with caution because of potential exacerbations. *Infection:* Patients should be infection-free before screening trial with baclofen injection. *Renal impairment:* Should be administered with caution. Dosage reduction may be necessary. *Stroke:* Drug has not significantly benefited patients with stroke; these patients also have poor drug tolerance.

NURSING CONSIDERATIONS

Administration/Storage

- Administer with milk or food to avoid GI upset.
- Dilute intrathecal medication per manufacturer's instructions.
- Have resuscitation equipment available during trial drug period if intrathecal administration is being considered. Patient must have positive response to trial of intrathecal medication before use of implantable pump.
- Store at room temperature in tightly closed container.

Assessment/Interventions

- Obtain patient history, including drug history and any known allergies. Note any signs of infection.
- Assess muscle spasticity and monitor throughout course of therapy.
- Monitor renal function prior to administration.

OVERDOSAGE: SIGNS & SYMPTOMS

Oral: Vomiting, muscular hypotonia, muscle twitching, drowsiness, accommodation disorders, coma, respiratory depression, seizures. *Intrathecal:* Drowsiness, lightheadedness, dizziness, somnolence, respiratory depression, seizures

Patient/Family Education

- Instruct patient to take drug exactly as prescribed. If dose is missed it should be taken within 1 hr. Warn patient not to double up on doses.
- Explain that full effectiveness of drug may not occur until several weeks after initiation of drug therapy.
- Warn patient not to discontinue medication abruptly. Explain that hallucinations or seizures may occur.
- Instruct patient to avoid intake of alcoholic beverages or other CNS depressants.
- Teach patient to avoid sudden position changes to prevent orthostatic hypotension.
- Caution diabetic patient that false elevation of blood glucose may occur. Instruct patient to monitor blood glucose carefully.
- Instruct patient to report these symptoms to physician: dizziness, nausea, hypotension, urinary frequency, retention, painful urination, headache, seizures and weakness.
- Advise patient that drug may cause drowsiness and to use caution while driving or performing other tasks requiring mental alertness.

See Patient Guide, p. 49.

Beclomethasone Dipropionate

(BEK-low-METH-uh-zone die-PRO-pee-oh-NATE)

Beclovent, Beconase, Beconase AQ, Vancenase, Vancenase AQ, Vanceril, ♣ *Beclodisk, Becloforte Inhaler, Beclomethasone Diproprionate Inhalation, Beclomethasone Dipropionate Nasal Aerosol, Beclovent Rotacaps, Propaderm*

Class: Corticosteroid

Action Has potent anti-inflammatory effect on respiratory tract and in nasal passages.

Indications *Oral inhalation:* Chronic corticosteroid treatment of bronchial asthma and related bronchospastic states. *Intranasal:* Treatment of seasonal or perennial rhinitis not responsive to conventional therapy with antihistamines or decongestants; prevention of recurrence of nasal polyps after surgery; therapy for nonallergic (vasomotor) rhinitis.

Contraindications Primary treatment of status asthmaticus or acute episodes of asthma; systemic fungal infections; positive sputum cultures of *Candida albicans* or *Aspergillus niger*. Intranasal: Untreated localized infections of nasal mucosa.

Route/Dosage

Bronchial Asthma

ADULTS: **PO inhalation** 2 inhalations (84 mcg) tid-qid or 4 inhalations (168 mcg) bid. Do not exceed 20 inhalations daily. CHILDREN (6-12 YR): **PO inhalation** 1-2 inhalations tid-qid or 2-4 inhalations bid. Do not exceed 10 inhalations daily.

Rhinitis

ADULTS & CHILDREN > 12 YR: **Nasal inhalation** 1 inhalation (42 µg) in each nostril bid-qid. CHILDREN (6-12 YR): 1 inhalation in each nostril bid.

Interactions None well documented.

Lab Test Interferences None well documented.

Adverse Reactions *RESP:* Coughing; wheezing; pulmonary infiltrates. *CNS:* Headache, lightheadedness. *EENT:* Nasal bleeding; sneezing; throat and nasal irritation, burning or stinging; hoarseness or dysphonia; nasal, laryngeal or pharyngeal fungal infection. *GI:* Dry mouth. *META:* Suppression of hypothalamic-pituitary-adrenal (HPA) function. *OTHER:* Hypersensitivity reaction with rash, urticaria, angioedema and bronchospasm; facial edema.

Precautions

Pregnancy: Category C. *Lactation:* Undetermined. *Children:* Safety and efficacy in children < 6 yr not established. *Acute asthma:* Not indicated for relief of bronchospasm. *Fungal infections:* Antifungal treatment or discontinuance of corticosteroid therapy may be necessary. *Hypersensitivity:* Immediate and delayed hypersensitivity reactions have occurred. *Systemic effects:* Use cautiously in patients taking daily or alternate-day prednisone; may increase likelihood of hypothalamic-pituitary-adrenal suppression. Exceeding recommended dose may cause systemic effects.

NURSING CONSIDERATIONS

Administration/Storage

- May be administered singly or with concomitant systemic steroids.
- Shake inhaler well before administration.
- Before oral inhalation administration, give patient drink of water to moisten throat. Place inhaler mouthpiece 2 fingerbreaths away from patient's mouth. Tilt patient's head back slightly. Instruct patient to take slow, deep breath while inhaler is being activated and to hold breath for 5-10 sec and then breathe slowly. A spacing device (eg, Aerochanger) may be used to enhance delivery of medication. Have patient rinse mouth with water after inhalations are complete.
- Before nasal inhalation, instruct patient to blow nose gently to clear nasal passages. A topical decongestant may be used 15 min before administration to ensure adequate tissue penetration. Nasal lavage with saline also may help remove secretions.
- Insert nozzle into patient's nostril. Use your finger to keep other nostril closed. Instruct patient to inhale while you activate medication. Repeat with other nostril.
- If patient is also receiving bronchodilators by inhalation, administer bronchodilator before beclomethasone to enhance penetration of latter drug into bronchial tree.
- Store at room temperature; do not refrigerate.
- Do not store or use near open flame or discard in incinerator.

Assessment/Interventions

- Obtain patient history, including drug history and any known allergies, particularly to other corticosteroids.
- If change is made from systemic (oral) to inhaled or intranasal corticosteroids, observe patient carefully for signs of steroid withdrawal (nausea, fatigue, dizziness, hypotension, depression, joint and muscle pain). Notify physician if these signs occur. Deaths caused by adrenal insufficiency have occurred during and after transfer to aerosol corticosteroids.
- Have epinephrine 1:1000 available for immediate or delayed hypersensitivity reaction.

OVERDOSAGE: SIGNS & SYMPTOMS

Hypercorticism, adrenal suppression

Patient/Family Education

- Review proper administration technique. Have patient demonstrate technique.
- Explain that effects of drug are not immediate. Benefit requires daily use as instructed and usually occurs after several days. Caution patient not to continue intranasal therapy beyond 3 wk if there is no improvement.

- Instruct patient not to exceed prescribed dose.
- Advise patient that dosage will be tapered slowly before stopping.
- Remind patient to wash inhaler daily with warm water and dry thoroughly.
- Tell patient to store inhaler at room temperature, away from excessive heat or cold; do not refrigerate.
- Instruct patient to use with caution if sores develop or injuries occur in nasal passages. Drug may prevent or slow proper healing.
- Warn patient not to use for acute severe asthma attack requiring rapid relief.
- Instruct patient to carry Medi-Alert card if he or she experiences acute severe asthma attacks requiring rapid systemic relief.
- Advise patient to report these symptoms to physician: sore throat or mouth, cough, dry mouth, rash, facial swelling or difficult breathing with oral inhalation therapy; sneezing, nasal irritation or nosebleed with intranasal therapy.
- Inform patient to report any fungal infection of the nose or throat to physician.
- If patient is being converted from oral steroids to inhaler/nasal steroids, review signs and symptoms of adrenal insufficiency, which may occur days or weeks after conversion is complete.
- Warn patient not to take otc medications without consulting physician.

See Patient Guide, pp. 50-51.

Benazepril HCl

(BEN-AZE-uh-prill HIGH-droe-KLOR-ide)

Lotensin

Class: Antihypertensive/ACE inhibitor

Action Competitively inhibits angiotensin I–converting enzyme, resulting in the prevention of angiotensin I conversion to angiotensin II, a potent vasoconstrictor that stimulates aldosterone secretion. Results in decrease in sodium and fluid retention, decrease in blood pressure and increase in diuresis.

Indications Treatment of hypertension.

Contraindications Hypersensitivity to ACE inhibitors.

Route/Dosage
ADULTS: Initial dose: **PO** 10 mg qd. In patients taking diuretics that cannot be discontinued, initial dose of 5 mg should be given. Maintenance: **PO** 20-40 mg/day as single dose or in 2 divided doses; doses up to 80 mg have been used.

Interactions
Allopurinol: Greater risk of hypersensitivity possible with coadministration. *Antacids:* May decrease bioavailability of benazepril; separate administration by 1-2 hr. *Capsaicin:* Cough may be exacerbated. *Digoxin:* Increased digoxin levels. *Diuretics:* May cause symptomatic hypotension after initial dose of benazepril. *Indomethacin:* May reduce effects of benazepril, especially in low-renin or volume-dependent hypertensive patients. *Lithium:* May increase lithium levels and symptoms of lithium toxicity. *Phenothiazines:* May increase effects of benazepril. *Potassium preparations, potassium-sparing diuretics:* May increase serum potassium levels.

Lab Test Interferences
None well documented.

Adverse Reactions
CV: Hypotension; ECG changes. *RESP:* Chronic dry cough. *CNS:* Headache; dizziness; fatigue; hypertonia. *GI:* Nausea. *HEPA:* Elevated liver enzymes, elevated serum bilirubin. *DERM:* Hypersensitivity reaction (dermatitis, pruritus or rash with or without fever).

META: Hyperkalemia; hyponatremia; elevated uric acid; elevated blood glucose. *OTHER:* Arthralgia; myalgia; angioedema; leukopenia; eosinophilia; proteinuria.

Precautions

Pregnancy: Category D (second and third trimester); Category C (first trimester). ACE inhibitors can cause injury or death to fetus if used during second or third trimester. When pregnancy is detected, discontinue ACE inhibitors as soon as possible. *Lactation:* Excreted in breast milk; avoid use in nursing mothers if possible. *Children:* Safety and efficacy not established. *Angioedema:* Use with extreme caution in patients with hereditary angioedema. Angioedema associated with laryngeal edema may be fatal. *Hypotension/first-dose effect:* Significant decreases in blood pressure may occur after first dose, especially in severely salt- or volume-depleted patients (eg, those undergoing dialysis or vigorous diuretic therapy), or those with heart failure. Risk is minimized by discontinuing use of diuretics, increasing salt intake approximately 1 wk before initiating benazepril or decreasing benazepril dose. *Neutropenia/agranulocytosis:* Has occurred with other ACE inhibitors. *Renal impairment:* Dosage should be reduced.

NURSING CONSIDERATIONS

Administration/Storage

- May be administered with or without food.
- Store in tightly closed container in a cool location.

Assessment/Interventions

- Obtain patient history, including drug history and any known allergies. Note liver disease, CHF, concurrent use of diuretics or dialysis.
- Ensure that kidney function tests and baseline electrolytes have been obtained prior to administration and monitor during therapy.
- Review baseline ECG.
- Assess BP and pulse before administration. If systolic BP is < 90 mm Hg, withhold medication and notify physician.
- Monitor for hyperkalemia in patients with impaired renal function, diabetes mellitus, and patients receiving potassium supplementation or potassium-sparing diuretics.
- Monitor closely for at least 2 hr after initial dose and during first 2 wk of therapy. If patient experiences sudden marked decrease in BP, withhold medication and notify physician.
- If sudden severe dyspnea, swelling of lips or eyes, or edema of hands and feet develops, withhold medication and notify physician.

OVERDOSAGE: SIGNS & SYMPTOMS

Hypotension

Patient/Family Education

- Instruct patient not to discontinue medication suddenly. Loss of BP control can result.
- Explain that exercise, salt restriction and weight loss will enhance efficacy of medication and may allow for lowering of dosage.
- Tell patient that missed doses should be taken as soon as remembered but not to double up on doses.
- Explain that frequent follow-up appointments with physician are very important to adjust medication dosage.
- Teach patient how to monitor BP and instruct to check before taking drug. Warn patient not to take drug if systolic BP is < 90 mm Hg and to call physician.
- Advise patient to avoid intake of caffeine, salt substitutes and foods high in potassium or sodium.
- Instruct patient to avoid sudden position changes to prevent orthostatic hypotension.

- Tell patient that medication causes dizziness and to avoid driving.
- Instruct patient to notify physician if chronic dry cough or other persistent symptoms occur.
- Explain that drug may cause impaired taste perception. Tell patient to notify physician if this symptom occurs.
- Tell patient not to take otc medications without notifying physician.

See Patient Guide, p. 52.

Benzphetamine HCl

(benz-FET-uh-meen HIGH-droe-KLOR-ide)

Didrex

Class: CNS stimulant/anorexiant

Action Stimulates satiety center in brain, causing appetite suppression.

Indications Short-term (8-12 wk) adjunct to diet plan to reduce weight.

Contraindications Hypersensitivity to sympathomimetic amines; pregnancy; advanced arteriosclerosis; symptomatic cardiovascular disease; moderate to severe hypertension; hyperthyroidism; glaucoma; agitated states; history of drug abuse; during or within 14 days of MAO inhibitor use; coadministration with other CNS stimulants.

Route/Dosage

ADULTS: PO 25-50 mg 1-3 times/day.

Interactions

Guanethidine: May decrease hypotensive effect. *MAO inhibitors, furazolidone:* May cause hypertensive crisis and intracranial hemorrhage.

Lab Test Interferences

None well documented.

Adverse Reactions

CV: Palpitations; tachycardia; arrhythmias; hypertension; hypotension; chest pain. *CNS:* Hypersensitivity; dizziness; insomnia; euphoria; tremor; headache; restlessness; overstimulation; nervousness; anxiety; agitation. *EENT:* Mydriasis; blurred vision; unpleasant taste. *GI:* Dry mouth; nausea; diarrhea; constipation; stomach pain. *GU:* Dysuria; urinary frequency; impotence; menstrual disturbances. *HEMA:* Bone marrow depression; agranulocytosis; leukopenia. *DERM:* Urticaria; rash; erythema; hair loss. *OTHER:* Excessive sweating; flushing; myalgia; gynecomastia.

Precautions

Pregnancy: Category X. *Lactation:* Undetermined. *Children:* Not recommended for children < 12 yr. *Drug dependence:* Has high potential for dependence and abuse. Tolerance may occur. *Tartrazine sensitivity:* Some products contain tartrazine, which may cause allergic-type reactions in susceptible individuals.

NURSING CONSIDERATIONS

Administration/Storage

- Administer midmorning or midafternoon. Anorexiant effects occur within 1-2 hr and last up to 4 hr.
- Administer last dose several hours before bedtime.
- Store at room temperature in tightly closed, light-resistant container.

Assessment/Interventions

- Obtain patient history, including drug history and any known allergies. Note cardiovascular disease, hypertension, glaucoma, history of drug or alcohol abuse.
- Monitor renal function.
- Take vital signs and auscultate heart and lungs before administration.
- Assess mental status. Depressed patients are more likely to misuse

drug to induce euphoria and mood elevation.

- If hypertension, dysrhythmias, marked agitation, restlessness, depression, or other adverse effects occur, withhold medication and notify physician.
- For best results medication should be administered concurrently with a program to improve eating habits, increase motivation, and improve self-image.

OVERDOSAGE: SIGNS & SYMPTOMS

Restlessness, tremor, rapid respirations, tachypnea, dizziness, confusion, mood changes, panic states, dysrhythmias, palpitations, and hypertension or hypotension

Patient/Family Education

- Caution patient that this medication must not be taken during pregnancy or when pregnancy is possible. Advise patient to use reliable form of birth control while taking this drug.
- Remind patient to take medication on empty stomach (1 hr before meal or 2 hr after meal).
- Instruct patient to avoid taking medication within 6 hr of bedtime because it may cause insomnia.
- Explain that anorexiant effects are temporary and tolerance to medication and dependence can occur.
- Instruct patient to notify physician immediately if any of these symptoms occur: chest pain, palpitations, nervousness, or dizziness.
- Warn patient not to drive or perform tasks that require mental alertness if dizziness or blurred vision occur. Notify physician of these disturbances.
- Tell patient to report excessive dryness of mouth, constipation, or prolonged insomnia because dosage may need to be adjusted.
- Inform patient that weight reduction requires strict adherence to dietary restrictions.

See Patient Guide, p. 53.

Benztropine Mesylate

(BENZ-troe-peen MEH-sih-LATE)

Cogentin, ♣ *Apo-Benztropine, PMS Benztropine*

Class: Antiparkinson/anticholinergic

Action Thought to act by competitively antagonizing acetylcholine receptors in corpus striatum to restore neuromuscular balance.

Indications Treatment of all forms of parkinsonism; control of extrapyramidal disorders (except tardive dyskinesia) due to neuroleptic drugs.

Contraindications Angle-closure glaucoma; myasthenia gravis; pyloric or duodenal obstruction; stenosing peptic ulcer; prostatic hypertrophy or bladder neck obstructions; megacolon; tardive dyskinesia; children < 3 yr old.

Route/Dosage

Parkinsonism

ADULTS: PO 1-2 mg/day; range: 0.5-6 mg. Individualize dosage. IDIOPATHIC PARKINSONISM: ADULTS: PO Initially 0.5-1 mg at bedtime; 4-6 mg/day may be required. POSTENCEPHALITIC PARKINSONISM: ADULTS: PO 2 mg/day in 1 or more doses; some patients may require initial dose of 0.5 mg.

Drug-Induced Extrapyramidal Disorders

ADULTS: 1-4 mg qd or bid.

Acute Dystonic Reactions

ADULTS: PO/IM/IV Initial dose: IM/IV 1-2 mg; then PO 1-2 mg bid.

Interactions

Amantadine: May increase anticholinergic effects. *Digoxin:* May increase digoxin serum levels, especially with slow-dissolution oral digoxin tablets. *Haloperidol:* May worsen schizophrenic symptoms; may decrease haloperidol serum levels; tardive dyskinesia may develop. *Phenothiazines:* May decrease action of phenothiazines. May increase incidence of anticholinergic effects.

Lab Test Interferences

None well documented.

Adverse Reactions

CV: Tachycardia; bradycardia. *CNS:* Toxic psychosis including confusion, disorientation, memory impairment, visual hallucinations; exacerbation of pre-existing psychosis; nervousness; depression; finger numbness. *EENT:* Blurred vision; dilated pupils; narrow-angle glaucoma. *GI:* Paralytic ileus; constipation; nausea; vomiting; dry mouth. *GU:* Urinary retention; dysuria. *DERM:* Skin rash. *OTHER:* Heat stroke; hyperthermia; fever; weakness; inability to move particular muscle groups.

Precautions

Pregnancy: Category C. *Lactation:* Undetermined. *Children:* Safety and efficacy not established. *Elderly patients:* Patients > 60 yr may have increased side effects; dosage reduction and observation may be needed. *Special risk patients:* Use with caution in patients with glaucoma, prostatic hypertrophy, epilepsy, cardiac arrhythmias, hypertension, hypotension, tendency toward urinary retention, liver or kidney disorders, obstructive disease of GI or GU tract, tachycardia or those who are taking other drugs with anticholinergic activity. *Heat illness:* Fatal hyperthermia has occurred. Use with caution during hot weather. *Ophthalmic:* Narrow-angle glaucoma may occur. *Tardive dyskinesia:* May aggravate tardive dyskinesia.

NURSING CONSIDERATIONS

Administration/Storage

- When given PO, administer with food to prevent GI irritation.
- If patient has difficulty swallowing, tablet may be crushed.
- May be given IM or IV in acute dystonic reaction. However, because onset and efficacy are equivalent for IM and IV route, IV administration is usually unnecessary.
- Store in a dry place in tightly closed, light-resistant container.

Assessment/Interventions

- Obtain patient history, including drug history and any allergies. Note glaucoma, urinary retention, prostatic hypertrophy or constipation.
- Monitor vital signs and I&O for anticholinergic side effects (hypotension and urinary retention).
- Monitor patient for reduction of rigidity and decrease in tremors during therapy.
- Monitor frequency of bowel movements. Patient may need stool softener.

OVERDOSAGE: SIGNS & SYMPTOMS

Circulatory collapse, cardiac arrest, respiratory depression, CNS depression or stimulation, shock, coma, stupor, seizures, convulsions, ataxia, anxiety, incoherence, hyperactivity, smelly breath, decreased bowel sounds, dilated and sluggish pupils

Patient/Family Education

- Explain that full effectiveness of drug may not occur for 2-3 days after initiation of drug therapy. Explain that doses will be tapered gradually before stopping.
- Advise patient that increasing fluid intake will help decrease dry mouth and constipation.
- Instruct patient to take sips of water frequently, suck on ice chips or sugarless hard candy, or chew sugarless gum if dry mouth occurs.
- Warn patient to pay particular attention to dental hygiene because of problems associated with decreased salivation.

- Tell patient that stool softeners may be used if constipation occurs.
- Warn patient to drink plenty of fluids and take precautions against hyperthemia in hot weather.
- Tell patient that vision may be blurry during the first 2-3 wk of treatment.
- Advise patient that wearing sunglasses outdoors will help to minimize photophobia.
- Instruct patient that drug may cause drowsiness and to use caution while driving or performing other tasks requiring mental alertness.
- Advise patient to avoid intake of alcoholic beverages or other CNS depressants.
- Instruct patient to obtain periodic eye examinations during long-term treatment to monitor for glaucoma.

See Patient Guide, p. 54.

Beractant

(ber-ACT-ant)

Survanta

Class: Lung surfactant

Action Replaces deficient endogenous pulmonary surfactant and restores surface activity of lung.

Indications Prevention and treatment ("rescue") of neonatal respiratory distress syndrome (RDS) in premature infants.

Contraindications Standard considerations.

Route/Dosage

NEONATES & INFANTS: **Intratracheal** PREVENTION: 25 mg/kg/instillation for 4 instillations (total dose of 100 mg/kg is administered in 4 quarter doses); dose is started within 15 min. of birth. RESCUE: 25 mg/kg/instillation for 4 instillations (total dose 100 mg/kg). May be repeated for continued or progressive RDS.

Interactions None well documented.

Lab Test Interferences
None well documented.

Adverse Reactions
CNS: Intracranial hemorrhage.

Precautions Drug should be administered only by trained personnel in a closely supervised setting. *Nosocomial sepsis:* Occurred in controlled clinical trials.

NURSING CONSIDERATIONS

Administration/Storage

- Warm medication by allowing it to stand at room temperature for 20 min or in hand for 8 min. Do not use artificial warming methods.
- If settling has occurred, swirl gently; do not shake.
- If preventive dose is planned, begin preparation before infant's birth.
- Before administering, assure proper placement and patency of endotracheal (ET) tube. If suctioning is required, allow patient to stabilize before administering.
- Instill through small (5 Fr) catheter inserted into ET tube with tip above carina. Do not instill into main stem bronchus. Attach catheter to syringe. Fill with medication and discard any excess through catheter to ensure that total dose to be given remains in syringe. After each quarter dose remove catheter and mechanically ventilate patient for 30 sec. Continue procedure until total dose is achieved. Administer each quarter dose with infant in different position.
- Store unopened vials under refrigeration and protect from light.
- Warmed unopened vials (< 8 hr) can be returned to refrigerator for future use. Drug should not be warmed and refrigerated more than once. Discard any open vials.

Assessment/Interventions

- If possible, review mother's patient history.
- Take baseline vital signs and monitor during and after medication administration.
- Avoid suctioning patient for 1 hr after administration unless airway is obstructed.
- Have emergency equipment available for cardiac or respiratory complications.
- Monitor lung sounds for any changes (eg, rales or moist sounds).
- Observe for signs of nosocomial infection/sepsis.
- Continually monitor oxygen and carbon dioxide measurements. If oxygen saturation decreases or bradycardia develops, discontinue administration until patient is stabilized.

OVERDOSAGE: SIGNS & SYMPTOMS

Acute airway obstruction (based on animal studies)

Patient/Family Education

- Advise family of infant's condition and offer frequent updates.
- Encourage active family participation in care whenever possible.
- Provide emotional support; offer hospital services and support groups.

No patient monograph available.

Betamethasone

(BAY-tuh-METH-uh-zone)

Celestone, ✤ *Betnesol*

Betamethasone Sodium Phosphate

Celestone Phosphate, Selestoject, Cel-U-Jec, ✤ *Celestone Repetabs*

Betamethasone Sodium Phosphate and Betamethasone Acetate

Celestone Soluspan

Betamethasone Valerate

Betatrex, Beta-Val, Valisone, Betatrex, Beta-Val, ✤ *Betacort Scalp Lotion, Betaderm, Betaderm Scalp Lotion, Betnovate, Celestoderm-V, Rholosone, Rholosone Scalp Lotion*

Betamethasone Dipropionate

Alphatrex, Diprosone, Maxivate, Teladar, ✤ *Rhoprosone, Rhoprolene, Taro-Sone*

Betamethasone Benzoate

Uticort, ✤ *Beben*

Augmented Betamethasone Dipropionate

Diprolene, Diprolene AF

Class: Adrenal cortical steroid/glucocorticoid

Action Synthetic, long-acting glucocorticoid that depresses formation, release and activity of endogenous mediators of inflammation including prostaglandins, kinins, histamine, liposomal enzymes and complement system. Also modifies body's immune response.

Indications Systemic treatment of primary or secondary adrenal cortex insufficiency, rheumatic disorders, collagen diseases, dermatologic diseases, allergic states, allergic and inflammatory ophthalmic processes, respiratory diseases, hematologic disorders, neoplastic diseases, edematous states (resulting from nephrotic syndrome), GI diseases, multiple sclerosis, tuberculous meningitis and trichinosis with neurologic or myocardial involvement. *Topical:* Relief of inflammatory and pruritic manifestations of corticosteroid-responsive dermatoses.

Contraindications Systemic fungal infections; IM use in idiopathic thrombocytopenic purpura; administration of live virus vaccines when patient is receiving immunosuppressive doses. *Topical:* Do not use as monotherapy in primary bacterial infections. Do not use on face, groin or axilla or for ophthalmic treatments.

Route/Dosage

Betamethasone

PO 0.6-7.2 mg/day.

Betamethasone Sodium Phosphate
IV/IM or into joint or soft tissue 0.5-9 mg/day.

Betamethasone Sodium Phosphate and Betamethasone Acetate
Intrabursal, intra-articular, intradermal or intralesional: 0.5-9 mg/day.

Topical (Betamethasone Dipropionate, Betamethasone Valerate, Betamethasone Benzoate)
Sparingly to affected areas 2-4 times/day.

Interactions

Anticholinesterases: May antagonize anticholinesterase effects in myasthenia gravis. *Anticoagulants, oral:* May alter anticoagulant dose requirements. *Barbiturates:* May decrease pharmacologic effect of betamethasone. *Hydantoins:* May increase clearance and decrease therapeutic efficacy of betamethasone. *Nondepolarizing muscle relaxants (eg, tubocurarine).* May potentiate or counteract neuromuscular blocking action. *Rifampin:* May increase clearance and decrease therapeutic efficacy of betamethasone. *Salicylates:* May reduce serum levels and efficacy of salicylates. *Troleandomycin:* May increase effects of betamethasone.

Lab Test Interferences

Increased urine glucose and serum cholesterol; decreased serum levels of potassium, T_3 and T_4; decreased uptake of I^{131}; false-negative nitroblue-tetrazolium test.

Adverse Reactions

CV: Thromboembolism or fat embolism; thrombophlebitis; necrotizing angiitis; cardiac arrhythmias or ECG changes; syncopal episodes; hypertension; myocardial rupture; CHF. *CNS:* Convulsions; increased intracranial pressure with papilledema (pseudotumor cerebri); vertigo; headache; neuritis/paresthesias; psychosis; fatigue; insomnia. *EENT:* Posterior subcapsular cataracts; increased IOP, glaucoma; exophthalmos. *GI:* Pancreatitis; abdominal distension; ulcerative esophagitis; nausea; vomiting; increased appetite and weight gain; peptic ulcer with perforation and hemorrhage; small and large bowel perforation. *GU:* Increased or decreased motility and number of spermatozoa. *HEMA:* Leukocytosis. *DERM:* Impaired wound healing; thin fragile skin; petechiae and ecchymoses; erythema; lupus erythematosus–like lesions; suppression of skin test reactions; subcutaneous fat atrophy; purpura; striae; hirsutism; acneiform eruptions; allergic dermatitis; urticaria; angioneurotic edema; perineal irritation; hyperpigmentation or hypopigmentation. Topical application may cause burning; itching; irritation; erythema; dryness; folliculitis; hypertrichosis; pruritus; perioral dermatitis; allergic contact dermatitis; numbness of fingers; stinging and cracking/tightening of skin; maceration of skin; secondary infections; skin atrophy; striae; miliaria; telangiectasia. *META:* Sodium and fluid retention; hypokalemia; hypokalemic alkalosis; metabolic alkalosis; hypocalcemia; hypothalamic-pituitary-adrenal (HPA) axis suppression; endocrine abnormalities (menstrual irregularities; cushingoid state; growth suppression in children secondary to adrenocortical and pituitary unresponsiveness; increased sweating; decreased carbohydrate tolerance; hyperglycemia; glycosuria; increased insulin or sulfonylurea requirements in diabetics; manifestations of latent diabetes mellitus; negative nitrogen balance caused by protein catabolism; hirsutism). *OTHER:* Musculoskeletal (weakness, myopathy, tendon rupture, osteoporosis, aseptic necrosis of femoral and humeral heads, spontaneous fractures including vertebral compression fractures and pathologic fracture of long bones); hypersensitivity, including anaphylactic reactions; aggravation or masking of infections; malaise. Topical use may produce same adverse reactions seen with systemic use.

Precautions

Pregnancy: Systemic use: Safety

not established. Topical use: Category C. *Lactation:* Excreted in breast milk. *Children:* Growth and development of infants and children on prolonged therapy must be monitored, even with topical treatment. *Adrenal suppression:* Prolonged therapy may lead to HPA suppression. *Cardiovascular:* Use with caution in patients with recent myocardial infarction. *Elderly:* May require lower doses. Consider benefits relative to risks. *Fluid and electrolyte balance:* Can cause elevated blood pressure, salt and water retention and increased potassium and calcium excretion. Dietary salt restriction and potassium supplementation may be necessary. *Hepatitis:* May be harmful in chronic active hepatitis positive for hepatitis B surface antigen. *Hypersensitivity:* Anaphylactoid reactions have occurred rarely. *Infections:* May mask signs of infection. May decrease host-defense mechanisms. *Ocular effects:* Use cautiously in ocular herpes simplex because of possible corneal perforation. *Peptic ulcer:* May contribute to peptic ulceration, especially in large doses. *Stress:* Increased dosage of rapidly acting corticosteroid may be needed before, during and after stressful situations. *Sulfites:* Some products contain sulfites, which may cause allergic-type reactions in susceptible individuals. *Withdrawal:* Abrupt discontinuation may result in adrenal insufficiency. Use is discontinued gradually, while supplementation is increased during times of stress.

NURSING CONSIDERATIONS

Administration/Storage

- Administer before 9 AM for minimal suppression of adrenal cortex activity.
- Give with meals or snacks.
- For large doses administer antacids between meals.

Assessment/Interventions

- Obtain patient history, including drug history and any known allergies.
- Review baseline lab results before therapy, including liver and renal function studies.
- Monitor BP, body weight, 2-hr postprandial blood glucose (at regular intervals) and electrolytes. Note potassium and calcium levels and any radiographic findings.
- Assess for signs of infection before initiation of therapy, because product may mask signs of infection and exacerbate systemic fungal infections.
- Report to physician any weight increase, edema, elevated BP or low potassium, GI bleeding, nausea or vomiting.

OVERDOSAGE: SIGNS & SYMPTOMS

Acute overdosage: Fever, myalgia, arthralgia, malaise, anorexia, nausea, skin desquamation, orthostatic hypotension, dizziness, fainting, dyspnea, hypoglycemia
Chronic overdosage: Cushingoid changes, moonface, central obesity, striae, hirsutism, acne, eccymoses, hypertension, osteoporosis, myopathy, sexual dysfunction, diabetes, hyperlipidemia, peptic ulcer, infarction, electrolyte and fluid imbalance

Patient/Family Education

- Tell patient to take with meals or snacks to avoid nausea.
- Explain that medication should be taken before 9 AM for best results.
- When multiple doses are to be taken, show patient how to space them evenly throughout day.
- If patient has diabetes, discuss importance of closely monitoring blood glucose for possible increase in insulin dosage.
- If patient is receiving long-term therapy, tell patient to carry identification containing notification of steroid therapy.

- Tell patient not to stop taking medication suddenly.
- Instruct patient to report these symptoms to physician: unusual weight gain or weight loss, swelling of lower extremities, muscle weakness, black tarry stools or vomiting blood, puffing face, prolonged sore throat, fever or cold, anorexia, nausea, vomiting, diarrhea, weakness, dizziness.

Topical Use

- Demonstrate proper technique for cleaning affected area before applying medication and for applying sparingly as a thin film.
- Tell patient to avoid contact with eyes and to avoid tight-fitting clothing on treated area.
- Explain that alcohol-containing preparations should not be applied to area, because of drying/irritation.
- Caution patient to discontinue medication and notify physician if affected area worsens or develops irritation, redness, burning, swelling or stinging.

See Patient Guide, p. 55.

Betamethasone/ Clotrimazole

(BAY-tuh-METH-uh-zone/kloe-TRIM-uh-zole)

Lotrisone

Class: Topical/corticosteroid/antifungal

Action Clotrimazole increases cell membrane permeability in susceptible fungi. Betamethasone has anti-inflammatory, antipruritic and vasoconstrictive actions.

Indications Topical treatment of tinea pedis, tinea cruris and tinea corporis caused by *Trichophyton rubrum*, *T. mentagrophytes*, *Epidermophyton floccosum*, *Microsporum canis*.

Contraindications Hypersensitivity to other corticosteroids or imidazoles.

Route/Dosage

Topical 1 application bid (2 wk for tinea cruris and tinea corporis; 4 wk for tinea pedis).

Interactions None well documented.

Lab Test Interferences

None well documented.

Adverse Reactions

CNS: Paresthesias. *DERM:* Maculopapular rash; erythema; stinging; blistering; peeling; pruritus; urticaria; burning; itching; dryness; acne; decreased pigmentation; striae; skin atrophy. *OTHER:* Edema; secondary infection; adrenal suppression with long-term use over large areas of skin.

Precautions

Pregnancy: Category C. *Lactation:* Undetermined. *Children:* Safety and efficacy not established. *Adrenal suppression:* Patients who receive large doses over large surface areas may experience hypothalamic-pituitary adrenal axis suppression. *Ophthalmic use:* Do not use for eye infections.

NURSING CONSIDERATIONS

Administration/Storage

- Wear gloves. Apply medication sparingly and rub in lightly. Notify physician if signs of hypersensitivity or irritation are noted.
- Avoid contact with eyes, mouth and nose.
- Do not cover treated area with dressings or use tight-fitting diapers, plastic pants or underwear over treated area.
- Store cream at room temperature.

Assessment/Interventions

- Obtain patient history, including drug history and any known allergies.
- Monitor treated sites for irritation or signs of secondary infection and

report any adverse reactions to physician.

Patient/Family Education

- Remind patient that medication is for external application only and to avoid contact with eyes, nose and mouth.
- Demonstrate application technique, cautioning patient to apply sparingly and to rub in lightly.
- Tell patient to notify physician if there is no improvement after 1 week for tinea cruris or tinea corporis or after 2 weeks for tinea pedis.
- Caution patient against using dressings, tight-fitting diapers or plastic pants over treated area.
- Tell patients with tinea corporis (ringworm) to wash clothes separately from those of other family.
- Remind patient to wash hands before and after each application of product.
- Advise patient to complete prescribed treatment, even if infection clears, to prevent relapse.
- Instruct patient to report these symptoms to physician: burning, itching, rash, swelling, redness or blistering in treated area.

See Patient Guide, p. 56.

Betaxolol HCl

(BAY-TAX-oh-lahl HIGH-droe-KLOR-ide)

Betoptic, Betoptic S

Class: Beta-adrenergic blocker

Action Blocks beta receptors, primarily affecting cardiovascular system (decreases heart rate, cardiac contractility and BP) and lungs (promotes bronchospasm). Ophthalmic use reduces intraocular pressure, probably by reducing aqueous production.

Indications Hypertension. *Ophthalmic preparation:* Ocular hypertension and chronic open-angle glaucoma.

Contraindications Hypersensitivity to beta-blockers; sinus bradycardia; greater than first-degree heart block; CHF unless secondary to tachyarrhythmia treatable with beta-blockers; overt cardiac failure; cardiogenic shock.

Route/Dosage

Hypertension

ADULTS: **PO** 10-20 mg/day. ELDERLY: **PO** Initial dose should be reduced to 5 mg/day.

Glaucoma

ADULTS: **Ophthalmic** 1 drop bid in affected eye(s).

Interactions

Clonidine: May enhance or reverse antihypertensive effect; potentially life-threatening situations may occur, especially on withdrawal. *NSAIDs:* Some agents may impair antihypertensive effect. *Prazosin:* May increase postural hypotension. *Verapamil:* May increase effects of both drugs.

Lab Test Interferences

None well documented.

Adverse Reactions

CV: Hypotension; bradycardia; CHF; cold extremities; second- or third-degree heart block; arrhythmias; syncope. *RESP:* Bronchospasm; dyspnea; wheezing. *CNS:* Insomnia; fatigue; dizziness; depression; lethargy; drowsiness; forgetfulness; headache. *EENT:* Dry eyes; blurred vision; tinnitus; slurred speech; dry mouth; sore throat. Ophthalmic use may cause eye discomfort or stinging; tearing; keratitis; blepharoptosis; visual disturbances; diplopia; ptosis. *GI:* Nausea; vomiting; diarrhea; constipation. *GU:* Impotence; painful, difficult or frequent urination. *HEMA:* Agranulocytosis; thrombocytopenic purpura. *HEPA:* Elevated liver function tests. *DERM:* Rash; hives; alopecia. *META:* Acidosis; diabetes; hypercholesterolemia; hyperlipidemia; increased LDH; hypokalemia. *OTHER:* Weight changes; fever; facial swelling;

muscle weakness. Ophthalmic betaxolol may produce the same adverse drug reactions seen with systemic use; antinuclear antibodies may develop.

Precautions

Pregnancy: Category C. *Lactation:* Undetermined. *Children:* Safety and efficacy not established. *Anaphylaxis:* Deaths have occurred with anaphylactic reactions to beta-blockers; aggressive therapy may be required. *Angle-closure glaucoma:* To effectively reduce elevated intraoccular pressure in angle-closure glaucoma, use with miotic agent. *Cessation of therapy:* Withdrawal should be done gradually, over approximately 2 wk. Patients should be observed carefully and be allowed minimal physical activity. *CHF:* Should be administered cautiously in patients whose CHF is controlled by digitalis and diuretics. *Diabetes mellitus:* May mask symptoms of hypoglycemia (eg, tachycardia, BP changes). May potentiate insulin-induced hypoglycemia. *Elderly:* Dosage reduction may be necessary. *Nonallergic bronchospastic disease (eg, chronic bronchitis, emphysema):* In general, beta-blockers are not given to patients with bronchospastic diseases. *Peripheral vascular disease:* May precipitate or aggravate symptoms of arterial insufficiency. *Renal/hepatic impairment:* Use with caution. *Systemic absorption:* Ophthalmic betaxolol may produce same adverse reactions seen with systemic use, because of absorption. *Thyrotoxicosis:* May mask clinical signs (eg, tachycardia) of developing or continuing hyperthyroidism. Abrupt withdrawal may exacerbate symptoms of hyperthyroidism, including thyroid storm.

NURSING CONSIDERATIONS

Administration/Storage

- For ophthalmic solution, pull out lower eyelid to make pocket, administer drop without touching eye, release lower lid, close eye and apply gentle pressure on inner canthus to avoid systemic absorption.
- Store ophthalmic form at room temperature. Do not freeze.
- Store oral form in cool location.

Assessment/Interventions

- Obtain patient history, including drug history and any known allergies. Note CHF, diabetes mellitus or hyperthyroidism.
- Ensure that baseline serum lipid and glucose levels have been obtained before initiating treatment with systemic medication.
- Monitor BP and pulse frequently when starting oral medication or when dosage is changed.
- In diabetic patient, monitor blood glucose and diabetic medication closely.
- Carefully monitor patients with CHF or chronic obstructive pulmonary disease who are taking oral form of medication.

OVERDOSAGE: SIGNS & SYMPTOMS

Bradycardia, CHF, hypotension, bronchospasm, hypoglycemia

Patient/Family Education

- Explain that full effectiveness of drug may not occur for up to 1-2 wk after initiation of therapy and that dosage will be tapered slowly before stopping to prevent adverse effects (eg, hypotension, tachycardia, anxiety, angina, MI).
- Teach patient how to monitor pulse before taking oral medication, and advise to contact physician if pulse remains < 50 bpm.
- Inform diabetic patient to monitor blood glucose level closely.
- Advise patient that ophthalmic solution may cause initial burning or stinging when first instilled in eye.
- Warn patient that medication may need to be gradually discontinued before surgery or dental work. Instruct

patient to discuss with physician or other health care provider.

- Explain that measurements of intraocular pressure will need to be performed on a regular basis to assess the therapeutic effect of the ophthalmic medication.
- Instruct patient to report these symptoms to physician: dizziness, decreased pulse, shortness of breath, confusion, rash or any unusual bleeding.
- Instruct patient not to take otc medications (including diet aids, cold or nasal preparations [alpha-adrenergic stimulants]) without consulting physician.
- Advise patient that drug may cause drowsiness and to use caution while driving or performing other tasks requiring mental alertness.

See Patient Guide, pp. 57-58.

Bethanechol Chloride

(beth-AN-ih-kole KLOR-ide)

Urecholine, Duvoid, Myotonachol, ♣ *PMS-Bethanechol Chloride*

Class: Urinary tract product/cholinergic stimulant

Action Stimulates parasympathetic nervous system, increasing tone to muscles of urinary bladder, stimulates gastric motility and tone and may restore rhythmic peristalsis.

Indications Treatment of acute postoperative and postpartum nonobstructive urinary retention and neurogenic atony of the urinary bladder with retention. **Unlabeled uses:** Diagnosis and treatment of reflux esophagitis.

Contraindications Hyperthyroidism; peptic ulcer; latent or active asthma; pronounced bradycardia; atrioventricular conduction defects; vasomotor instability; coronary artery disease; epilepsy; parkinsonism; coronary occlusion; hypotension; hypertension; bladder neck obstruction; spastic GI disturbances; acute inflammatory lesions of the GI tract; peritonitis; marked vagotonia. Not used when strength or integrity of GI or bladder wall is in question or in presence of mechanical obstruction, when increased muscular activity of GI tract or urinary tract may prove harmful (eg, after recent urinary bladder surgery, GI resection and anastomosis or possible GI obstruction).

Route/Dosage

ADULTS: **PO** 10-50 mg tid-qid on empty stomach. **SC** 2.5-5 mg at 15-30 min intervals for maximum of 4 doses; then minimum effective dose may be repeated tid-qid prn.

Unlabeled Uses

ADULTS & CHILDREN: DIAGNOSIS OF REFLUX ESOPHAGITIS: **SC** two 50 mcg/kg doses given 15 min apart. TREATMENT OF REFLUX ESOPHAGITIS: **SC** 25 mg qid. INFANTS & CHILDREN: **PO** 3 mg/m^2/dose tid has been used for gastroesophageal reflux.

Interactions

Cholinergic agents: Possible toxicity because of additive effects. *Ganglionic blocking compounds:* Severe hypotension, usually preceded by severe abdominal symptoms. *Quinidine or procainamide:* Antagonism of anticholinergic effects of bethanechol.

Lab Test Interferences

None well documented.

Adverse Reactions

CV: Fall in blood pressure with reflex tachycardia; vasomotor response. *RESP:* Bronchial constriction; asthmatic attacks. *CNS:* Headache. *EENT:* Lacrimation; miosis. *GI:* Abdominal cramps or discomfort; colicky pain; nausea; belching; diarrhea; rumbling and gurgling of stomach; salivation. *GU:* Urinary urgency. *DERM:* Flushing with feeling of warmth; sensation of heat about face; sweating. *OTHER:* Malaise.

Precautions
Pregnancy: Category C. *Lactation:* Undetermined. *Children:* Safety and efficacy not established. *Reflux infection:* May occur if bethanechol administration fails to relax urinary sphincter and urine is forced back into renal pelvis. *Tartrazine sensitivity:* Some products contain tartrazine, which may cause allergic-type reactions (eg, bronchial asthma) in susceptible individuals.

NURSING CONSIDERATIONS

Administration/Storage
- Give oral form on empty stomach.
- Use only SC route for parenteral administration. Violent symptoms of cholinergic overstimulation (hypotension, circulatory collapse, cardiac arrest) may occur with IM or IV administration.
- Do not administer with quinidine or procainamide.

Assessment/Interventions
- Obtain patient history, including drug history and any known allergies.
- Note any history of GI or urinary tract surgery or obstructions.
- Establish baseline blood pressure and pulse and monitor blood pressure, pulse and voiding patterns. Notify physician if urinary retention persists.
- Report symptoms of asthma or bronchial constriction.

OVERDOSAGE: SIGNS & SYMPTOMS
Abdominal discomfort, salivation, flushing of skin, sweating, nausea, vomiting, low blood pressure, shock, cardiac arrest

Patient/Family Education
- Caution patient about potential side effects such as increased salivation, sweating, flushing or stomach discomfort.
- Instruct patient to take medication on empty stomach.
- Show patient how to monitor I&O and tell patient to report abdominal distention or urinary retention to physician.
- Instruct patient to report these symptoms to physician: abdominal pain or discomfort, diarrhea, visual disturbances, dizziness or any other disturbing response to medication.

See Patient Guide, p. 59.

Biperiden

(by-PURR-ih-den)
Akineton
Class: Antiparkinson/anticholinergic

Action Thought to act by competitively antagonizing acetylcholine receptors in corpus striatum to restore neuromuscular balance.

Indications Treatment of all forms of parkinsonism; control of extrapyramidal disorders secondary to neuroleptic drug therapy.

Contraindications Narrow-angle glaucoma; bowel obstruction; megacolon.

Route/Dosage
Parkinsonism
ADULTS: **PO** 2 mg tid-qid to maximum of 16 mg/day. Dosage must be individualized.

Drug-Induced Extrapyramidal Disorders
ADULTS: **PO** 2 mg qd-tid. **IM/IV** 2 mg repeated q 30 min until symptoms resolve, but not more than 4 consecutive doses (or 8 mg) per day.

Interactions
Amantadine: May increase anticholinergic side effects. *Digoxin:* May increase digoxin serum levels, especially with slow-dissolution oral digoxin tablets. *Haloperidol:* May worsen schizo-

phrenic symptoms; may decrease haloperidol serum levels; tardive dyskinesia may develop. *Phenothiazines:* May decrease action of phenothiazines. May increase incidence of anticholinergic side effects.

Lab Test Interferences

None well documented.

Adverse Reactions

CV: Mild transient orthostatic hypotension; bradycardia; tachycardia. *EENT:* Blurred vision; narrow-angle glaucoma; pupillary dilation. *CNS:* Drowsiness; euphoria; disorientation; agitation; memory loss; disturbed behavior. *GI:* Dry mouth; constipation; GI irritation. *GU:* Urinary retention. *DERM:* Skin rash. *OTHER:* Hyperthermia; heat stroke.

Precautions

Pregnancy: Category C. *Lactation:* Undetermined. *Children:* Safety and efficacy not established. *Elderly:* Patients > 60 yr may have increased side effects; dosage reduction and observation may be needed. *Heat illness:* Fatal hyperthermia has occurred. Use with caution during hot weather. *Ophthalmic:* Narrow-angle glaucoma may occur. *Special risk patients:* Use with caution in patients with glaucoma, prostatic hypertrophy, epilepsy, cardiac arrhythmias, hypertension, hypotension, tendency toward urinary retention, liver or kidney disorders, obstructive disease of GI or GU tract, tachycardia or those who are taking other drugs with anticholinergic activity.

NURSING CONSIDERATIONS

Administration/Storage

- When given PO, administer with or after meals to prevent GI irritation.
- If patient has difficulty swallowing, tablet may be crushed.
- May be given IM or IV in acute dystonic reactions. When given IV, have patient remain recumbent during administration and for 15 min afterward.
- Store in dry place in tightly closed light-resistant container.

Assessment/Interventions

- Take patient history, including drug history and any known allergies. Note glaucoma, urinary retention, prostatic hypertrophy or constipation.
- Monitor vital signs and I&O routinely for anticholinergic side effects (hypotension and urinary retention).
- Monitor patient for reduction of rigidity and decrease in tremors during therapy.
- Monitor frequency and consistency of bowel movement. Patient may need stool softeners or laxatives.

OVERDOSAGE: SIGNS & SYMPTOMS

Characterized by adverse reactions. Also: Circulatory collapse, cardiac arrest, respiratory depression or arrest, CNS depression preceded or followed by stimulation, intensification of mental symptoms or toxic psychosis in mentally ill patients treated with neuroleptic drugs (eg, phenothiazines), shock, coma, stupor, seizures, convulsions, ataxia, anxiety, incoherence, hyperactivity, combativeness, anhidrosis, hyperpyrexia, fever, hot/dry/flushed skin, dry mucous membranes, dysphagia, foul-smelling breath, decreased bowel sounds, dilated and sluggish pupils

Patient/Family Education

- Explain that doses will be tapered gradually before stopping to avoid withdrawal reaction.
- Advise patient that increasing fluid intake will help decrease dry mouth and constipation.
- Instruct patient to pay particular attention to dental hygiene because of problems associated with decreased salivation (eg, increased risk of caries).
- Tell patient that stool softeners may

be used if constipation occurs. Small doses of milk of magnesia may be helpful.

- Warn patient to drink plenty of fluids and take precautions against hyperthermia in hot weather.
- Instruct patient to obtain periodic eye exams during long-term treatment to monitor for glaucoma.
- Advise patient that wearing sunglasses outdoors will help to minimize photophobia.
- Tell patient that vision may be blurry during first 2-3 wk of treatment.
- Instruct patient to take sips of water frequently, suck on ice chips or sugarless hard candy or chew sugarless gum if dry mouth occurs.
- Caution patient to avoid sudden position changes to prevent orthostatic hypotension.
- Instruct patient to avoid intake of alcoholic beverages or other CNS depressants.
- Advise patient that drug may cause drowsiness and to use caution while driving or performing other tasks requiring mental alertness.

See Patient Guide, p. 60.

Bisacodyl

(BISS-uh-koe-dill)

Biscolax, Dulcagen, Dulcolax, Fleet, Bisacodyl Uniserts, ♣ *APO-Bisacodyl, PMS-Bisacodyl*

Class: Laxative

Action Acts as cathartic stimulant.

Indications Short-term treatment of constipation; evacuation of colon for rectal and bowel evaluations; preparation for delivery or surgery.

Contraindications Nausea, vomiting or other symptoms of appendicitis; acute surgical abdomen; fecal impaction; intestinal obstruction; undiagnosed abdominal pain; ulcerative lesions of colon; rectal fissures; ulcerative hemorrhoids.

Route/Dosage

Oral

ADULTS: **PO** 10-15 mg. PREPARATION OF LOWER GI TRACT: Up to 30 mg. CHILDREN > 6 YR: **PO** 5-10 mg (0.3 mg/kg).

Suppository

ADULTS: **PR** 10 mg. CHILDREN > 2 YR: **PR** 10 mg. CHILDREN < 2 YR: **PR** 5 mg.

Interactions

Milk or antacids: May cause enteric coating of tablets to dissolve, resulting in gastric lining irritation or gastric indigestion.

Lab Test Interferences

None well documented.

Adverse Reactions

CV: Palpitations. *CNS:* Dizziness, fainting. *GI:* Excessive bowel activity (griping, diarrhea, nausea, vomiting); perianal irritation; bloating; flatulence; abdominal cramping; proctitis and inflammation. *OTHER:* Sweating, weakness. Suppositories may cause proctitis and inflammation with long-term use.

Precautions

Pregnancy: Category B. *Lactation:* Undetermined. *Children:* Tablet form not recommended for children < 6 yr. *Abuse/Dependency:* Long-term use may lead to laxative dependency. Long-term abuse results in cathartic colon (poorly functioning colon). *Rectal bleeding or failure to produce bowel movement:* May indicate serious condition that may require further medical attention.

NURSING CONSIDERATIONS

Administration/Storage

- Administer tablet at bedtime or before breakfast.
- Do not administer within 1 hr of patient ingesting antacids, milk or cimetidine.
- Have patient take tablets whole with full glass of water. Tablets should not be crushed or chewed.
- Insert suppository at time bowel movement is desired or 1-2 hr before scheduled procedure. Onset of action is 6-8 hr for tablets and 15-60 min for suppositories.
- Moisten suppository with lukewarm water, insert high into rectum and instruct patient to retain suppository in rectum for as long as possible until urge to defecate is felt.
- Store tablets and suppositories in tightly closed containers in cool location.

Assessment/Interventions

- Obtain patient history, including drug history and any known allergies.
- Assess living and dietary habits, including bulk or fiber intake, exercise, fluid intake and use of laxatives.
- Assess for presence of bowel sounds and usual pattern of bowel function.
- Assess for abdominal distention, excessive bowel activity, abdominal cramping, weakness, fluid and electrolyte imbalance, perianal irritation.
- Monitor color, consistency and amount of stool produced.
- Notify physician of unrelieved constipation, rectal bleeding and signs and symptoms of electrolyte imbalance (muscle cramps or pain, weakness, dizziness).

Patient/Family Education

- Inform patient not to take bisacodyl when constipation is accompanied by abdominal pain, fever, nausea or vomiting.
- Advise patient to use laxative only for short-term therapy; do not use > 1 wk.
- Caution patient that prolonged, frequent, or excessive use of drug may result in dependence and/or electrolyte imbalance.
- Encourage patient to incorporate high-fiber foods in diet, increase fluid intake (at least 6-8 glasses daily) and increase or maintain exercise level.
- Instruct patient to report these symptoms to physician: unrelieved constipation, rectal bleeding, muscle cramps, pain, weakness or dizziness.

See Patient Guide, p. 61.

Bismuth Subsalicylate

(BISS-muth sub-suh-LIS-ih-late)

Bismatrol, Bismatrol Extra Strength, Pepto-Bismol Maximum Strength, Pepto-Bismol, Pink Bismuth

Class: Antidiarrheal

Action Produces antisecretory and antimicrobial effects; may have anti-inflammatory effect.

Indications Treatment of indigestion without causing constipation, nausea, abdominal cramps; diarrheal control, including traveler's diarrhea. **Unlabeled uses:** Treatment of recurrent ulcers, chronic infantile diarrhea, gastroenteritis associated with Norwalk virus; prevention of traveler's diarrhea.

Contraindications Viral illness such as chickenpox or influenza in patients < 18 yr.

Route/Dosage
ADULTS: **PO** 2 tablets (262 mg each) or 30 ml suspension q 30-60 min prn (maximum 8 doses/day). CHILDREN 9-12 YR: **PO** 1 tablet or 15 ml suspension q 30-60 min prn (maximum 8 doses/day). CHILDREN 6-9 YR: **PO** ⅔ tablet or 10 ml suspension q 30-60 min prn (maximum 8 doses/day). CHILDREN 3-6 YR: **PO** ⅓ tablet or 5 ml suspension q

30-60 min prn (maximum 8 doses/day). CHILDREN < 3 YR: Consult physician.

Interactions

Aspirin or other salicylates: May cause salicylate toxicity. *Corticosteroids:* May decrease effectiveness. *Insulin:* Drug may increase glucose-lowering effect of insulin. *Methotrexate:* Drug may increase effects and toxicity of methotrexate. *Spironolactone:* Drug may interfere with diuretic effect. *Sulfinpyrazone:* Drug may interfere with uricosuric effect. *Tetracyclines:* Bismuth subsalicylate may reduce GI absorption of tetracyclines and diminish their effectiveness. *Valproic acid:* Drug may increase free fraction of valproic acid, leading to toxicity.

Lab Test Interferences

Radiologic examination: Bismuth subsalicylate is radiopaque and may interfere with radiologic examination of GI tract.

Adverse Reactions

EENT: Tinnitus; discoloration of tongue. *GI:* Discoloration of stools; impaction.

Precautions

Pregnancy: Category C. *Lactation:* Excreted in breast milk. *Children:* May cause impaction. *Debilitated patients:* May cause impaction.

NURSING CONSIDERATIONS

Administration/Storage

- Tablets may be crushed, chewed or allowed to dissolve in mouth. Do not allow patient to swallow whole.
- Before administering, shake suspension well.
- Store at room temperature.
- Protect from light.

Assessment/Interventions

- Obtain patient history, including drug history and any known allergies.
- Assess patient for risk of Reye's syndrome.
- Determine if patient is taking otc medications for colds, fever and pain; many contain salicylates, which may produce additive toxicity.
- Observe for discoloration of stool produced by drug (may mask GI bleeding).
- Discontinue use when symptoms subside.

OVERDOSAGE: SIGNS & SYMPTOMS

Ringing in ears, respiratory alkalosis, nausea, vomiting, hypokalemia, neurologic abnormalities (eg, disorientation, seizures), dehydration, hyperthermia, unusual bleeding or bruising

Patient/Family Education

- Counsel patient to maintain adequate fluid intake (2-3 L/day) to prevent dehydration.
- Instruct patient to notify physician if diarrhea is accompanied by high fever or continues > 2 days or if abdominal pain occurs.
- Advise patient not to use medication if concurrent viral illness is present.
- Instruct patient to consult with physician before taking drug if concurrently taking other salicylates, anticoagulants or medications for diabetes or gout.
- Instruct patient to inform physician regarding bismuth subsalicylate administration before any scheduled radiologic studies or stool examinations.
- Inform patient of possibility of salicylate toxicity and associated symptoms, and instruct patient to notify physician if these symptoms occur.
- Explain that stools may become black or gray and tongue may darken.

See Patient Guide, p. 62.

Bisoprolol Fumarate

(bih-SO-pro-lahl FYU-mah-rate)
Zebeta
Class: Beta-adrenergic blocker

Action Blocks beta receptors, primarily affecting cardiovascular system (decreases heart rate, cardiac contractility and BP) and lungs (promotes bronchospasm).

Indications Hypertension. **Unlabeled uses:** Angina pectoris; supraventricular tachycardias; premature ventricular contractions.

Contraindications Hypersensitivity to beta-blockers; sinus bradycardia; greater than first-degree heart block; CHF unless secondary to tachyarrhythmia treatable with beta-blockers; overt cardiac failure; cardiogenic shock.

Route/Dosage
Hypertension
ADULTS: **PO** 5-20 mg qd. Dosage should be individualized; some patients may be given starting dose of 2.5 mg/day.

Interactions
Clonidine: May enhance or reverse antihypertensive effect; potentially life-threatening situations may occur, especially on withdrawal. *NSAIDs:* Some agents may impair antihypertensive effect. *Prazosin:* May increase orthostatic hypotension. *Verapamil:* May potentiate effects of both drugs.

Lab Test Interferences
None well documented.

Adverse Reactions
CV: Hypotension; bradycardia; CHF; cold extremities; second- or third-degree heart block. *RESP:* Bronchospasm; dyspnea; wheezing. *CNS:* Insomnia; fatigue; dizziness; depression; lethargy; drowsiness; forgetfulness; anxiety; headache; slurred speech. *EENT:* Dry eyes; blurred vision; tinnitus; sore throat. *GI:* Nausea; vomiting; diarrhea; constipation; abdominal pain; dry mouth. *GU:* Impotence; painful, difficult or frequent urination; increased creatinine and BUN. *HEMA:* Agranulocytosis; thrombocytopenic purpura. HEPA: Elevated liver function test results. *DERM:* Rash; hives; alopecia. *META:* Hyperglycemia; hypoglycemia. *OTHER:* Weight changes; fever; facial swelling; muscle weakness; increased serum uric acid, potassium and phosphorus; elevated serum lipids; possible development of antinuclear antibodies.

Precautions
Pregnancy: Category C. *Lactation:* Undetermined. *Children:* Safety and efficacy not established. *Anaphylaxis:* Deaths have occurred; aggressive therapy may be required. *CHF:* Should be administered cautiously in patients whose CHF is controlled by digitalis and diuretics. *Diabetes mellitus:* May mask symptoms of hypoglycemia (eg, tachycardia, BP changes). May potentiate insulin-induced hypoglycemia. *Nonallergic bronchospastic disease (eg, chronic bronchitis, emphysema):* In general, beta-blockers are not given to patients with bronchospastic diseases. *Peripheral vascular disease:* May precipitate or aggravate symptoms of arterial insufficiency. *Renal/hepatic impairment:* Daily dose should be reduced. *Thyrotoxicosis:* May mask clinical signs (eg, tachycardia) of developing or continuing hyperthyroidism. Abrupt withdrawal may exacerbate symptoms of hyperthyroidism, including thyroid storm.

NURSING CONSIDERATIONS

Administration/Storage
- May be given without regard to meals.

Assessment/Interventions
- Obtain patient history, including drug history and any known aller-

gies. Note CHF, diabetes mellitus or hypertension.

- Assess for withdrawal syndrome. Beta-blocker withdrawal syndrome (hypertension, tachycardia, anxiety, angina, MI) may occur 1-2 wk after sudden discontinuation. Gradually withdraw therapy over 1-2 wk if possible.
- Ensure that baseline AST, ALT, uric acid, creatinine, BUN, serum potassium, glucose and phosphorus levels have been obtained before starting treatment with this medication.
- Monitor BP and pulse prior to each dosage.
- In diabetic patient monitor blood glucose level and diabetic medications closely.
- Carefully monitor patients with CHF, COPD or asthma and report changes in cardiac or respiratory status to physician.

> **OVERDOSAGE: SIGNS & SYMPTOMS**
> Bradycardia, CHF, hypotension, bronchospasm, hypoglycemia

Patient/Family Education

- Explain that drug will be tapered slowly before stopping to prevent rebound symptoms and adverse effects.
- Teach patients how to monitor pulse before taking oral medication and advise to contact physician if pulse is < 50 bpm.
- Inform diabetic patient to monitor blood glucose level closely.
- Instruct patient to report these symptoms to physician: dizziness, decreased pulse, shortness of breath, confusion, rash or any unusual bleeding.
- Advise patient that drug may cause drowsiness and to use caution while driving or performing other tasks requiring mental alertness.
- Instruct patient not to take otc medications (including diet aids, cold or nasal preparations [alpha-adrenergic stimulants]) without consulting physician.

See Patient Guide, p. 63.

Bitolterol Mesylate

(by-TOLE-ter-ole MEH-sih-LATE)

Tornalate

Class: Bronchodilator/sympathomimetic

Action Relaxes bronchial smooth muscle through beta-2 receptor stimulation.

Indications Prevention and treatment of reversible bronchospasm associated with asthma or other obstructive pulmonary diseases.

Contraindications Standard considerations.

Route/Dosage

ADULTS & CHILDREN > 12 YR: ORAL INHALATION: ACUTE BRONCHOSPASM: 2-3 inhalations at interval of 2-3 min, followed by third inhalation if necessary. PREVENTION OF BRONCHOSPASM: 2 inhalations q 8 hr, not to exceed 3 inhalations q 6 hr or 2 inhalations q 4 hr.

Interactions None well documented.

Lab Test Interferences May cause decreased potassium level.

Adverse Reactions

CV: Palpitations; tachycardia; irregular pulse; hypertension. *RESP:* Cough; increased chest discomfort; rhinitis; bronchospasm. *CNS:* Tremor; lightheadedness; dizziness; nervousness; headache; tiredness. *EENT:* Throat and mouth irritation. *GI:* GI distress; nausea.

Precautions

Pregnancy: Category C. *Lactation:* Undetermined. *Children:* Safety and efficacy in children < 12 yr not established. *Cardiovascular disorders:* Toxic symptoms may occur. *CNS effects:* Drug may cause CNS stimulation; cautious use is needed in patients with history of seizures or hyperthyroidism. *Diabetes mellitus:* Dosage adjustment of insulin or oral hypoglycemic agent may be required. *Elderly:* Lower doses may be required. *Excessive use:* Paradoxical bronchospasm and cardiac arrest have been associated with excessive inhalant use. *Labor and delivery:* May inhibit uterine contractions and delay preterm labor. *Tolerance:* May occur.

NURSING CONSIDERATIONS

Administration/Storage

- To administer, instruct patient to tilt head back and put inhaler mouthpiece between lips or 2 inches from open mouth. Tell patient to inhale slowly, press down on canister, hold breath at least 10 sec or as long as comfortable, remove mouthpiece, then exhale slowly.
- Use spacing device (eg, Aerochanger) to enhance drug delivery.
- Pressurized inhalation should be administered during second half of inspiration to achieve better distribution of medication, because airways are opened wider at this time. If second inhalation is necessary, wait at least 1 full min between inhalations.
- Store metered-dose inhaler in pressurized container at room temperature; do not freeze. Keep away from extreme heat. Do not store or use near open flame or discard in incinerator.

Assessment/Interventions

- Obtain patient history, including drug history and any known allergies.
- Review baseline ECG for cardiac dysrhythmias associated with tachycardia.
- Take heart rate before administration of drug. If tachycardia, cardiac arrhythmia, or chest pain is present, hold medication and notify physician immediately.
- Have epinephrine 1:1000 available for immediate or delayed hypersensitivity reaction.
- Obtain baseline blood values and monitor during therapy. Notify physician of abnormal results.

OVERDOSAGE: SIGNS & SYMPTOMS

Exaggerated side effects, such as tremors, tachycardia, seizures, hypokalemia, anginal pain and hypertension

Patient/Family Education

- Ask patient to demonstrate correct use of inhaler. It may be necessary to repeat instructions and demonstrations more than once. Consider use of spacing device.
- Explain that tolerance may occur with prolonged use, but temporary cessation of drug usually restores its original effectiveness. Instruct patient to notify physician if medication is ineffective.
- Warn patient to avoid excessive use, which can lead to side effects or loss of effectiveness.
- Instruct patient to rinse mouth with water or commercial mouthwash after use to remove residue and reduce irritation.
- Tell patient to store inhaler at room temperature, away from excessive heat or cold.
- Warn patient receiving concurrent corticosteroid therapy not to stop or reduce medication without consulting physician even if patient feels better.
- Instruct patient to wash inhaler daily with warm water and to dry thoroughly.
- Caution patient to avoid getting aerosol spray in eyes.
- Instruct patient to report these symptoms to physician: palpitations, chest pain, muscle tremors, dizziness, increased nervousness, headache, flush-

ing, breathing problems or difficult urination.

- Instruct patient not to take otc medications without consulting physician.

See Patient Guide, p. 64.

Bleomycin Sulfate

(BLEE-oh-MY-sin SULL-fate)

Blenoxane

Class: Antineoplastic

Action Appears to inhibit DNA and, to lesser extent, RNA synthesis, blocking cell division.

Indications Palliative treatment of lymphomas, squamous cell carcinomas and testicular carcinomas. **Unlabeled uses:** Sclerosis of malignant pleural effusions.

Contraindications Idiosyncratic reaction to bleomycin.

Route/Dosage
ADULTS: Initial dose **IV/IM/SC** 0.25-0.5 units/kg (10-20 units/m^2) 1 or 2 times/wk. MAINTENANCE THERAPY, HODGKIN'S DISEASE: **IV/IM** 1 unit/day or 5 units/wk. LYMPHOMA PATIENTS: **IV/IM/SC** Give test dose of < 2 units for first 2 doses because of increased risk of anaphylactoid reactions. Avoid cumulative dose > 400 units because of increased risk of pulmonary toxicity.

Interactions
Digoxin: Drug may decrease digoxin serum levels. Digitoxin and digoxin capsules do not appear to be affected. *Other antineoplastic agents:* Pulmonary toxicity may occur at lower doses. *Phenytoin:* Drug may decrease phenytoin serum levels.

Lab Test Interferences
None well documented.

Adverse Reactions
CV: Vascular toxicity (eg, MI, stroke, thrombotic microangiopathy, cerebral arteritis); peripheral vasoconstriction; hypotension. *RESP:* Pneumonitis; pulmonary fibrosis. *EENT:* Mucositis. *GI:* Nausea; vomiting; stomatitis; anorexia. *DERM:* Erythema; rash; striae; vesiculation; hyperpigmentation; skin tenderness; hyperkeratosis; nail changes; alopecia; pruritus. *OTHER:* Fever; chills; weight loss (may persist long after bleomycin administration); idiosyncratic reaction consisting of hypotension, mental confusion, fever, chills, wheezing; pain or necrosis at tumor site; phlebitis at IV site.

Precautions
Pregnancy: Safety not established. *Lactation:* Undetermined. *Idiosyncratic reactions:* Have occurred in patients with lymphoma; similar to anaphylaxis. Reactions, which usually occur after first or second dose, may be immediate or delayed for several hours. *Pulmonary complications:* Interstitial pneumonitis and fatal pulmonary fibrosis have occurred; greater risk with high doses and in elderly. Earliest symptom is dyspnea. *Renal or hepatic toxicity:* Has occurred, beginning as deterioration in renal or liver function tests.

NURSING CONSIDERATIONS

Administration/Storage

- Administer according to manufacturer's guidelines under continual supervision of health care professional certified in cancer chemotherapy. Small initial test dose is given to assess for hypersensitivity.
- Can be given alone or with other chemotherapeutic agents in combination therapy.
- When giving by IM route, use deep, slow injection. Rotate sites to prevent tissue irritation.
- Prepare solution under laminar airflow hood. Wear gloves, gown and mask while reconstituting or prepar-

ing medication. Discard used supplies in appropriately marked containers.

- After reconstitution, drug is stable for 24 hr at room temperature.
- Refrigerate unopened vials.

Assessment/Interventions

- Obtain patient history, including drug history and any known allergies.
- Monitor CBC for signs of increased thrombocytopenia and leukopenia prior to administration of agent.
- Compare hemoglobin and hematocrit to baseline values. If hemoglobin falls below 8 g/dl, withhold medication and contact physician. Anticipate possible blood transfusion.
- Monitor urinary output and renal function during therapy. Because high percentage of drug is excreted via kidneys in active form, patients with impaired renal function require decreased dosage.
- Auscultate lungs for crackles (rales) and observe for dyspnea and other signs of respiratory difficulty.
- Avoid oxygen levels above an FIO_2 of 25%, because lung damage can occur at levels usually considered safe. Concomitant use with radiation increases risk of pulmonary toxicity.
- Observe for signs of skin toxicity, including sensitivity, hyperpigmentation, rashes, and thickening of the skin, especially during the second or third week of treatment.
- Observe for anaphylactic and idiosyncratic reactions (hypotension, confusion, fever, chills, dyspnea, wheezing). Symptomatic treatment includes antihistamines, steroids, epinephrine, volume expanders and pressor agents.
- Monitor patient closely for febrile reactions. These are common when drug is given via IV route, less common when given via intrapleural or intraperitoneal routes. Reactions usually occur 1-3 hr after administration. If symptoms of pulmonary toxicity (rales, dyspnea, tachypnea), spiking temperatures (to 104°F) or shaking rigors (chills) occur, notify physician immediately.

Patient/Family Education

- Explain that temporary hair loss and/or changes in hair texture or color may occur. Discuss possible coping strategies and use of scarves or wigs.
- Instruct patient to check mucous membranes for signs of inflammation and ulceration. Discuss importance of oral hygiene in prevention of stomatitis.
- If stomatitis occurs, instruct patient to rinse mouth often with water. Teeth should be brushed with soft brush, sponge or cotton-tipped applicators. Tell patient to use mouthwash such as isotonic solution of sodium chloride and sodium bicarbonate and to avoid strong commercial mouthwashes.
- Instruct patient to notify physician if eating problems or persistent mouth pain occur. Topical or systemic analgesics such as viscous lidocaine mouthwashes may be ordered.
- Encourage patient not to smoke, because this may worsen pulmonary toxicity.
- Explain that routine laboratory tests will be scheduled to evaluate drug's effectiveness and to monitor for adverse reactions.
- Instruct patient to report these symptoms to physician: respiratory problems, erythema, rash, hyperpigmentation, nail changes, alopecia, pruritus or stomatitis.
- Caution patient not to take otc medications or have medical treatments such as vaccinations without consulting physician.

No patient monograph available.

Bretylium Tosylate

(breh-TILL-ee-uhm TAH-sill-ate)
Bretylol
Class: Antiarrhythmic

Action Causes a chemical sympathectomy–like state by inhibiting norepinephrine release and depressing adrenergic nerve terminal excitability; produces a positive inotropic effect on the myocardium.

Indications Prophylaxis and treatment of ventricular fibrillation; treatment of life-threatening ventricular arrhythmia that has failed to respond to first-line antiarrhythmic agents. **Unlabeled use:** Second-line therapy (following lidocaine) for the treatment of ventricular arrythmia during advanced cardiac life support in CPR.

Contraindications Standard considerations.

Route/Dosage

Life-Threatening Ventricular Arrythmias

ADULTS: Initial dose: **IV** 5-10 mg/kg (undiluted) by rapid IV injection; if arrhythmia persists, adjust dosage as necessary. Maintenance (for continuous suppression): Infuse diluted solution at 1-2 mg/min. Alternately, infuse diluted solution at 5-10 mg/kg over > 8 min q 6 hr. CHILDREN: **IV** 5 mg/kg/dose followed by 10 mg/kg at 10-30 min intervals (maximum total dose 30 mg/kg). Maintenance: 5-10 mg/kg/dose q 6 hr.

Other Ventricular Arrythmias

ADULTS: **IV** 5-10 mg/kg (diluted) over 8 min; if arrhythmia persists, give subsequent doses q 1-2 hr. Maintenance: Administer same dose q 6 hr or infuse 1-2 mg/min. **IM** 5-10 mg/kg (undiluted); if arrhythmia persists, give subsequent doses at 1-2 hr intervals. Maintain same dosage q 6-8 hr. CHILDREN: 5-10 mg/kg/dose q 6 hr.

Interactions

Antihypertensives: May cause severe hypotension. *Catecholamines:* Enhance pressor effects of catecholamines. *Digoxin:* May aggravate arrhythmias caused by digitalis toxicity.

Lab Test Interferences

None well documented.

Adverse Reactions

CV: Orthostatic hypotension; bradycardia; increased premature ventricular contractions and other arrythmias; transient hypertension; angina; sensation of substernal pressure. *CNS:* Dizziness; lightheadedness; syncope; vertigo. *GI:* Nausea and vomiting after rapid IV injection.

Precautions

Pregnancy: Category C. *Lactation:* Undetermined. *Children:* Safety and efficacy not established. *Renal impairment:* Increase dosage interval. *Fixed cardiac output:* Because severe hypotension may occur, avoid use in patients with fixed cardiac output (eg, severe aortic stenosis, pulmonary hypertension). Orthostatic hypotension is common (50%); keep patient supine until tolerance develops or medication is withdrawn.

NURSING CONSIDERATIONS

Administration/Storage

- Use for short-term therapy only.
- For maintenance administration, dilute each dose in at least 50 ml of 5% Dextrose in Water or 0.9% Sodium Chloride for Injection. Larger amounts can be diluted in any amount of solution (1 g in 250 ml = 4 mg/ml; 1 g in 500 ml = 2 mg/ml; 1 g in 1000 ml = 1 mg/ml).
- Use slow injection (over 10 min) to prevent nausea and vomiting.
- Rotate IM injection sites frequently to prevent atrophy and necrosis of

muscle tissue. Do not give > 5 ml in any one site.

- Store at room temperature. Protect from freezing.

Assessment/Interventions

- Obtain patient history, including drug history and any known allergies.
- Anticipate nausea and vomiting to occur after rapid IV administration.
- Monitor patient's vital signs frequently, including cardiac rhythm. Transient increase in arrhythmias and hypertension may occur within 1 hr after initial administration. Especially note slow or irregular pulse or significant hypotension. If BP is < 75 mm Hg, notify physician.
- Monitor I&O if nausea or vomiting develops, if patient has renal impairment or demonstrates decreased cardiac output.
- Take safety precautions if dizziness, lightheadedness, vertigo or syncope occurs.
- Keep bed in low position and supervise ambulation.
- Keep the patient in supine position until tolerance to orthostatic hypotension develops.
- If systolic BP is < 75 mm Hg, notify physician.
- Observe for increased anginal pain.

OVERDOSAGE: SIGNS & SYMPTOMS

Hypertension followed by refractory hypotension

Patient/Family Education

- Instruct patient to make position changes slowly and to request assistance with ambulation.
- Advise male patients to sit on toilet while urinating.

No patient monograph available.

Bromocriptine Mesylate

(BROE-moe-KRIP-teen MEH-sih-LATE)

Parlodel

Class: Antiparkinson

Action Stimulates dopamine receptors in the corpus striatum, relieving parkinsonian symptoms. Inhibits prolactin, which is responsible for lactation, and lowers elevated blood levels of growth hormone in acromegaly.

Indications Treatment of hyperprolactinemia-associated disorders (amenorrhea with or without galactorrhea, infertility, hypogonadism) in patients with prolactin-secreting adenomas; therapy for female infertility associated with hyperprolactinemia; treatment of acromegaly; therapy for Parkinson's disease (idiopathic or postencephalitic). **Unlabeled uses:** Treatment of hyperprolactinemia associated with pituitary adenomas; therapy for neuroleptic malignant syndrome; treatment of cocaine addiction.

Contraindications Sensitivity to ergot alkaloids; severe ischemic heart disease or peripheral vascular disease; pregnancy.

Route/Dosage

Hyperprolactinemia-Associated Disorders

Initial dose: **PO** 1.25-2.5 mg/day; 2.5 mg may be added as tolerated every 3-7 days until optimum response. (Dosage range: 2.5-15 mg/day).

Acromegaly

Initial dose: **PO** 1.25-2.5 mg for 3 days at bedtime; may be increased by 1.25-2.5 mg as tolerated every 3-7 days until optimum response occurs. Dosage range: 20-30 mg/day, not to exceed 100 mg/day.

Parkinson's Disease

Initial dose: **PO** 1.25 mg bid titrated individually. Dosage range: 10-40 mg/day, not to exceed 100 mg/day.

Interactions

Dopamine antagonists (eg, phenothiazines, butyrophenones, metoclopramide): May reduce bromocriptine efficacy. *Erythromycin:* May increase bromocriptine serum levels.

Lab Test Interferences

None well documented.

Adverse Reactions

CV: Hypotension (including orthostatic); syncope; hypertension; stroke, digital vasospasm. *RESP:* Shortness of breath; pulmonary infiltrates; pleural effusion; pleural thickening. *CNS:* Headache; dizziness; fatigue; lightheadedness; fainting; drowsiness; psychosis; seizures; abnormal involuntary movements; hallucinations; confusion; ataxia; insomnia; depression; vertigo; "on-off" phenomenon. *EENT:* Visual disturbances, nasal congestion. *GI:* Nausea; vomiting; abdominal cramps; constipation; diarrhea; anorexia; indigestion/dyspepsia; GI bleeding. *OTHER:* Exacerbation of Raynaud's syndrome; asthenia.

Precautions

Pregnancy: Pregnancy category undetermined. *Lactation:* Contraindicated in nursing women. *Children:* Safety and efficacy in children < 15 yr not established. *Pituitary tumors:* Evaluate pituitary before treatment to determine if tumor is present. *Symptomatic hypotension:* Do not administer to postpartum patients until blood pressure normalizes. Use caution in patients with pre-eclampsia and in those who have received other drugs that may alter blood pressure. *Acromegaly:* Cold-sensitive digital vasospasms and severe GI bleeding from peptic ulcers have been reported in patients with acromegaly; institute appropriate treatment. Possible tumor expansion has occurred; monitor patient's condition and discontinue treatment if necessary. *Parkinson's disease:* Safe use > 2 yr has not been established. Periodic evaluation of hepatic, hematopoietic, CV and renal functions is necessary.

NURSING CONSIDERATIONS

Administration/Storage

- Give with milk or meals to reduce gastric distress. Initial dose is usually given at bedtime because of adverse CNS reactions (dizziness, fainting).
- Tablet may be crushed if patient has difficulty swallowing.
- If dose must be delayed for > 4 hr, omit dose. Do not give double dose.
- Response to bromocriptine varies with individuals. Titrate dose to balance risks/benefits.
- Store at room temperature in tightly closed container.

Assessment/Interventions

- Obtain patient history, including drug history and any known allergies.
- Monitor BP prior to and during drug therapy. Severe hypotension may occur. Have patient remain supine for several hours after initial dose.
- Observe for lessening of symptoms of Parkinson's disease (rigidity, akinesia, tremors, pill rolling, shuffling gait, mask facies) prior to and during drug therapy.
- Assess breasts for decrease in engorgement.
- Assess for exacerbation of Raynaud's syndrome (muscle cramps in hands or feet, cold feet).
- Ensure safety and assess for risk of falls if dizziness occurs.

Patient/Family Education

- Tell patient not to skip doses or take double doses.
- Caution patient not to discontinue drug suddenly, to avoid rapid recurrence of original symptoms. Explain that dosage will be tapered slowly before stopping use of drug.
- Advise women of childbearing age to use nonhormonal methods of birth control during therapy.

- Instruct patient to inform physician immediately if pregnancy is suspected.
- When used for infertility, instruct patient to obtain daily basal body temperatures to determine when ovulation occurs.
- Advise patients who are taking drug to suppress lactation that breast engorgement may occur as therapy is discontinued.
- Inform patient that side effects are common, especially during initial phase of therapy.
- Instruct patient to notify physician if increasing dyspnea or nasal congestion occurs.
- Caution patient to avoid sudden position changes to prevent orthostatic hypotension.
- Advise patient to avoid intake of alcoholic beverages.
- Advise patient that drug may cause drowsiness and to use caution while driving or performing other tasks requiring mental alertness.

See Patient Guide, p. 65.

Brompheniramine Maleate

(brome-fen-AIR-uh-meen MAL-ee-ate)

Bromphen, Codimal-A, Cophene-B, Dehist, Dimetane, Dimetane Extentabs, Diamine T.D., Histaject, Nasahist B

Class: Antihistamine/alkylamine

Action Competitively antagonizes histamine at H1 receptor sites.

Indications Symptomatic relief of perennial and seasonal allergic rhinitis, treatment of vasomotor rhinitis, allergic conjunctivitis; temporary relief of runny nose and sneezing caused by common cold; treatment of allergic and nonallergic pruritic symptoms; temporary relief of mild, uncomplicated urticaria and angioedema; amelioration of allergic reactions to blood or plasma; adjunctive therapy in anaphylactic reactions.

Contraindications Newborn and premature infants; nursing mothers; narrow-angle glaucoma; stenosing peptic ulcer; symptomatic prostatic hypertrophy; asthmatic attack; bladder neck obstruction; pyloroduodenal obstruction; MAOI therapy.

Route/Dosage

Oral

ADULTS & CHILDREN (12 YR & OLDER): **PO** 4 mg q 4-6 hr, or 8-12 mg of sustained release form q 8-12 hr (maximum 24 mg/day). CHILDREN 6-12 YR: **PO** 2 mg q 4-6 hr (maximum 12 mg/day). Administer sustained release preparations only at direction of physician. CHILDREN < 6 YR: Use only as directed by physician.

Parenteral

ADULTS: **SC/IM/IV** 10 mg (range 5-20 mg) (maximum 40 mg/day). Twice daily administration is usually sufficient (maximum 40 mg/day). CHILDREN < 12 YR: **SC** 0.5 mg/kg/day or 15 mg/m^2/day in 3 or 4 divided doses.

Interactions

Alcohol, CNS depressants: May cause additive CNS depressant effects. MAO *inhibitors:* Anticholinergic effects of brompheniramine may increase.

Lab Test Interferences

In skin testing procedures, antihistamines may prevent or diminish an otherwise positive reaction to dermal reactivity indicators.

Adverse Reactions

CV: Orthostatic hypotension; palpitations; bradycardia; tachycardia; reflex tachycardia; extrasystoles; faintness. *RESP:* Thickening of bronchial secretions; chest tightness; wheezing; nasal stuffiness; sore throat; respiratory depression. *CNS:* Drowsiness (often transient); sedation; dizziness; syncope; disturbed coordination. *GI:* Epigastric distress; nausea; vomiting; diarrhea; dry mouth, nose and throat; constipation; change in bowel habits. *HEMA:* Agranulocytosis. *META:* Increased appetite; weight gain. *OTHER:* Photosensitivity.

Precautions

Pregnancy: Category C. *Lactation:* Contraindicated in nursing mothers. *Children:* Antihistamines may diminish mental alertness; in young child, they may produce paradoxical excitation. *Elderly:* Greater likelihood of dizziness, excessive sedation, syncope, toxic confusional states and hypotension in patients > 60 years. Dosage reduction may be required. *Special-risk patients:* Use with caution in patients with predisposition to urinary retention, history of bronchial asthma, increased intraocular pressure, hyperthyroidism, cardiovascular disease or hypertension. Avoid use in patients with history of sleep apnea. *Hepatic function impairment:* Use with caution in patients with cirrhosis or other liver disease. *Respiratory disease:* Generally not recommended to treat lower respiratory tract symptoms including asthma.

NURSING CONSIDERATIONS

Administration/Storage

- Give tablets with food or milk to reduce GI irritation. Tablets can be crushed and mixed with small amounts of food.
- Administer sustained release preparations as supplied. Do not allow patient to crush, break or chew.
- Use IM or SC preparations without dilution.
- Give via slow IV infusion (over 60 min), preferably with patient in recumbent position.

Assessment/Interventions

- Obtain patient history, including drug history and any known allergies.
- Note history of respiratory problems, hypertension, cardiac arrhythmias, glaucoma, urinary retention, ulcers or GI obstruction.
- Monitor vital signs closely after establishing a baseline and report irregularities to physician.
- Monitor intake and output routinely to determine whether patient has urinary retention.
- Maintain patient's oral hygiene and hydration to decrease mouth dryness.
- Closely monitor elderly (> age 60) because of possible intensified effects of medication.

OVERDOSAGE: SIGNS & SYMPTOMS

Large overdose: Hallucinations, convulsions, death

Patient/Family Education

- Caution against use if asthmatic symptoms (eg, wheezing) are present.
- Warn against taking drugs that cause CNS depression such as alcohol, sedatives, or analgesics except as directed by physician.
- Tell patient to notify physician if heart palpitations are noticed.
- Instruct patient to report any GI pain or evidence of blood in stool to physician.
- Caution patient to avoid taking during pregnancy or while breastfeeding unless instructed by physician.
- Instruct patient to stand slowly from sitting or prone position to avoid dizziness.
- Advise patient that drug may cause drowsiness and to use caution when driving, operating heavy equipment or performing other tasks requiring mental alertness.
- Instruct patient to take sips of water frequently or to suck on ice chips, sugarless hard candy or chewing gum if dry mouth occurs.

- Advise patient that skin tests performed while taking this drug may yield inaccurate results.

See Patient Guide, p. 66.

Budesonide

(byoo-DESS-oh-nide)
Rhinocort
Class: Corticosteroid

Action Exerts potent anti-inflammatory effect on nasal passages.

Indications Management of symptoms of seasonal and perennial allergic rhinitis in adults and children; management of nonallergic perennial rhinitis in adults.

Contraindications Untreated localized infections involving the nasal mucosa; hypersensitivity to the drug or drug compound of the product.

Route/Dosage
ADULTS & CHILDREN ≥ 6 YR: **Intranasal** *Initially:* 2 sprays in each nostril in the morning and evening or 4 sprays in each nostril in the morning. *Maintenance:* Smallest amount necessary to control symptoms. Maximum: 4 sprays/nostril daily.

Interactions
None well documented.

Lab Test Interferences
None well documented.

Adverse Reactions
RESP: Increased cough. *EENT:* Nasal irritation/bleeding; burning; stinging; sneezing; pharyngitis. *GI:* Dry mouth; indigestion.

Precautions
Pregnancy: Category C. *Lactation:* Undetermined. *Children:* Not recommended for children < 6 yr. *Fungal infections:* Antifungal treatment or discontinuation of corticosteroid therapy may be necessary. *Hypersensitivity:* Immediate hypersensitivity reactions have occurred. *Systemic effects:* Use cautiously in patients taking daily or alternate day steroid therapy; may increase likelihood of hypothalamic-pituitary-adrenal suppression. Exceeding recommended dose may cause systemic effects.

NURSING CONSIDERATIONS

Administration/Storage

- Shake well before using.
- Before nasal inhalation, instruct patient to blow gently to clear nasal passages. A topical decongestant may be used 15 minutes before administration to ensure adequate penetration. Nasal lavage with saline also may help remove secretions.
- Insert nozzle into patient nostril. Use your finger to keep other nostril closed. Instruct patient to inhale while you activate medication. Repeat with other nostril.
- Must be used within 6 months after opening the aluminum pouch.
- Store at room temperature in a low humidity environment with the valve downward. Cold temperatures reduce effectiveness.
- Do not puncture or incinerate container. Storing container above 120°F (50°C) may cause canister to burst.

Assessment/Interventions

- Obtain patient history.
- If change is made from systemic (oral) to inhaled or intranasal corticosteroids, observe patient carefully for signs of steroid withdrawal (nausea, fatigue, dizziness, hypotension, depression, joint and muscle pain). Notify physician if these signs occur. Deaths caused by adrenal insufficiency have occurred during and after transfer to aerosol corticosteroids.

- Have epinephrine 1:1000 available for immediate or delayed hypersensitivity reaction.

OVERDOSAGE: SIGNS & SYMPTOMS

Hypercorticism, adrenal suppression

Patient/Family Education

- Review administration technique. Have patient demonstrate technique.
- Before nasal inhalation, instruct patient to blow gently to clear nasal passages. A topical decongestant may be used 15 minutes before administration to ensure adequate penetration.
- Open and lock nasal adaptor into place.
- Hold inhaler upright. Shake well.
- Insert inhaler into one nostril, close other nostril by pressing on nose with finger.
- Begin to inhale through nostril; breathe and actuate dose by pressing on the canister.
- Repeat procedure for other nostril.
- Teach patient to clean plastic parts by removing from aerosol canister, and soaking in warm – not hot – water with a mild detergent. Allow parts to dry before replacing.
- Stress importance of using the medication as prescribed. Instruct patient not to exceed prescribed dose.
- Warn patient to call the healthcare provider if signs of nasal, oral or pharyngeal infections develop.
- If patient is being converted from oral to nasal steroids, review signs and symptoms of adrenal insufficiency, which may occur days or weeks after conversion is complete.
- Instruct patient to use caution if sores develop or injuries occur in nasal passages. Drug may prevent or slow proper healing.
- Inform patient to report any fungal infections of the nose or throat to healthcare provider.
- Explain that effects of drug are not immediate. Benefit requires daily use as instructed and usually occurs after several days. Caution patient not to continue therapy after 3 weeks if there is no improvement.
- Advise patient to contact healthcare provider if symptoms do not improve, if condition worsens, or if sneezing or nasal irritation occurs.
- Advise patient not to take over-the-counter medications without consulting a healthcare provider.

See Patient Guide, p. 67.

Bumetanide

(BYOO-MET-uh-nide)

Bumex

Class: Loop diuretic

Action Inhibits reabsorption of sodium and chloride in proximal tubules and loop of Henle.

Indications Treatment of edema associated with CHF, hepatic cirrhosis and renal disease. **Unlabeled use:** Relief of adult nocturia.

Contraindications Hypersensitivity to other loop diuretics or to sulfonylureas; anuria; hepatic coma or states of severe electrolyte depletion until condition is improved or corrected.

Route/Dosage

ADULTS: **PO** 0.5-2 mg/day as single dose. If inadequate response, give second or third dose at 4-5 hr intervals up to maximum of 10 mg/day. **IM/IV** 0.5-1 mg/day over 1-2 min. May repeat at 2-3 hr intervals, up to maximum of 10 mg/day. Reserve parenteral route for situations in which GI absorption is impaired or when oral administration is not practical; replace with oral therapy as soon as possible.

Interactions

Aminoglycosides: Increased auditory toxicity. *Cisplatin:* Additive ototoxicity. *Digitalis glycosides:* Electrolyte disturbances may predispose to digitalis-induced arrhythmias. *Lithium:* Increased plasma lithium levels and toxicity. *NSAIDs:* Decreased effects of bumetanide. *Salicylates:* Impaired diuretic response in patients with cirrhosis and ascites. *Thiazide diuretics:* Synergistic effects that may result in profound diuresis and serious electrolyte abnormalities.

Lab Test Interferences

None well documented.

Adverse Reactions

CV: Hypotension; ECG changes; chest pain. *RESP:* Hyperventilation. *CNS:* Asterixis; encephalopathy with preexisting liver disease; vertigo; headache; dizziness. *EENT:* Impaired hearing; ear discomfort; tinnitus; deafness. *GI:* Upset stomach; dry mouth; nausea; vomiting; diarrhea; pain. *GU:* Premature ejaculation; difficulty maintaining erection; renal failure. *HEMA:* Thrombocytopenia; deviations in Hgb, Hct, prothrombin time and WBC, platelets and differential counts. *DERM:* Hives; pruritus; itching; nipple tenderness; rash; photosensitivity. *META:* Glucosuria and proteinuria; hyperuricemia; gout; hypochloremia; hypokalemia; azotemia; hyponatremia; increased serum creatinine; hyperglycemia; variations in phosphorus, CO_2 content, bicarbonate, and calcium; increases in LDL, total cholesterol and triglycerides; decreases in HDL cholesterol. *OTHER:* Musculoskeletal weakness; arthritic pain; pain; muscle cramps; fatigue; dehydration; sweating.

Precautions

Pregnancy: Category C. *Lactation:* Undetermined. *Children:* Safety and efficacy not established in children < 18 yr. *Dehydration:* Excessive diuresis may cause dehydration and decreased blood volume with circulatory collapse and possible vascular thrombosis and embolism, especially in elderly patients. *Hepatic cirrhosis and ascites:* Sudden alterations of electrolyte balance may precipitate hepatic encephalopathy and coma. *Ototoxicity:* Associated with rapid injection, very large doses or concurrent use of other ototoxic drugs. *Renal impairment:* In severe chronic renal insufficiency, patients may benefit from continuous infusion (12 mg over 12 hr) rather than from intermittent bolus therapy. Renal function should be monitored and drug stopped if renal function decreases further. *Systemic lupus erythematosus:* May be exacerbated or activated.

NURSING CONSIDERATIONS

Administration/Storage

- Give with food or milk to reduce GI upset.
- Administer by parenteral route only in patients with impaired GI absorption or when oral route is not practical.
- Drug is most effective when given on alternate days or for 3-4 days with rest intervals of 1-2 days.
- If given by IV infusion, use solution within 24 hr of preparation.
- Store at room temperature in tightly closed container.

Assessment/Interventions

- Obtain patient history, including drug history and any known allergies. Note systemic lupus erythematosus or renal impairment.
- Ensure that baseline electrolytes have been obtained prior to administration. Do not administer to electrolyte-depleted patients.
- Check that baseline creatine, BUN, calcium, uric acid and CBC have been obtained before beginning therapy and monitor throughout therapy.
- Monitor BP and pulse rate frequently.
- Monitor I&O and daily weight during therapy.
- Observe for ototoxicity, especially in patients receiving drug via IV infusion and in those taking other ototoxic drugs.

- Ensure that patient maintains adequate hydration to prevent dehydration.
- Have epinephrine 1:1000 available if hypersensitivity reaction occurs.
- If tinnitus, hearing impairment or fullness in ears is reported, notify physician.

OVERDOSAGE: SIGNS & SYMPTOMS

Profound water loss, volume and electrolyte depletion (characterized by weakness, dizziness, mental confusion, anorexia, lethargy, vomiting, cramps), dehydration, reduction in blood volume, circulatory collapse with possible thrombosis and embolism

Patient/Family Education

- Instruct patient to take as single dose early in day. Drug can be taken with food or milk to reduce GI upset.
- Advise patient to drink adequate fluids to prevent dehydration unless fluid restrictions apply.
- Caution patient to get out of bed slowly on arising and to avoid sudden position changes to prevent orthostatic hypotension.
- If patient is not taking a potassium supplement, advise to increase potassium-rich foods in daily diet.
- Instruct patient to report these symptoms to physician: signs of bleeding, weakness, cramps, nausea or dizziness.
- Caution patient to avoid exposure to sunlight and to use sunscreen or wear protective clothing to avoid photosensitivity reaction.
- Advise diabetic patients to monitor blood glucose carefully because drug may cause loss of glycemic control.

See Patient Guide, p. 68.

Bupropion HCl

(byoo-PRO-pee-ahn HIGH-droe-KLOR-ide)

Wellbutrin

Class: Antidepressant

Action Exact mechanism of antidepressant activity unknown; does not inhibit monoamine oxidase.

Indications Treatment of depression.

Contraindications Seizure disorder; current or prior diagnosis of bulimia or anorexia nervosa; concurrent treatment with or within 14 days of discontinuation of MAO inhibitors.

Route/Dosage

ADULTS: **PO** 100 mg bid initially; may increase to 100 mg tid after 3 days. Maximum daily dose 450 mg; maximum single dose 150 mg.

Interactions

MAO *inhibitors*, *selegiline*: May increase risk of acute bupropion toxicity. MAO inhibitors should be discontinued at least 14 days before starting bupropion.

Lab Test Interferences

None well documented.

Adverse Reactions

CV: Edema; chest pain; ECG abnormalities (eg, premature beats, nonspecific ST-T segment changes); MI. *RESP*: Bronchitis; shortness of breath or dyspnea; pulmonary embolism. *CNS*: Agitation; anxiety; insomnia; hallucinations; suicidal ideation; seizures; headache/migraine; tremor. *EENT*: Dilated pupils; visual disturbances. *GI*: Dry mouth; stomatitis; nausea; vomiting; decreased appetite; thirst disturbance; colitis; GI bleeding; constipation. *GU*: Nocturia; decreased sexual function or impotence; painful erection; painful or retarded ejaculation; urinary tract infection. *HEMA*: Anemia; lymphadenopathy; pancytopenia. *HEPA*: Liver damage. *DERM*: Rash; dry skin. *META*: Gynecomastia. *OTHER*: Flulike symptoms; increased sweating;

weight loss; decreased electrolytes (especially potassium).

Precautions

Pregnancy: Category B. *Lactation:* Undetermined. *Children:* Safety and efficacy not established. *Heart disease:* Use with caution in patients with history of MI or unstable heart disease. *Psychosis or mania:* May precipitate mania in bipolar patients or activate latent psychosis in other patients. *Seizures:* May occur; dose-related risk. Use with caution in patients with history of head trauma or CNS tumor and in patients taking other drugs known to increase risk of seizures. *Suicide:* Patients at risk should not receive excessive quantities of drug.

NURSING CONSIDERATIONS

Administration/Storage

- Help patient to avoid insomnia from medication by avoiding bedtime doses.
- Store in dry place away from heat, light and moisture.

Assessment/Interventions

- Obtain patient history, including drug history and any known allergies.
- Consider potential for abuse or suicide.
- Assess for conditions affecting elimination, including liver disease, CHF, age, or renal function, which may affect accumulation of active secondary metabolites.
- Review laboratory reports to assist in ongoing evaluations of hepatic and renal function.
- Carefully monitor patients at risk of seizure.
- Institute suicide precautions if indicated. (Risk of suicide can be present until significant remission of depression occurs.)
- Observe for hoarding of drug.
- Monitor patient for signs of increased restlessness, agitation, anxiety, insomnia, or anorexia, and report to physician any related findings.
- Watch for signs of psychotic problems including hallucinations, delusions and paranoia, and report to physician any related findings.
- Monitor cardiovascular status for signs of chest pain, arrhythmia and symptoms of MI.

OVERDOSAGE: SIGNS & SYMPTOMS

Seizures, hallucinations, loss of consciousness, tachycardia, cardiac arrest

Patient/Family Education

- Instruct patient to take medication in 3-4 equally divided doses a day to minimize risk of seizures.
- Caution patient not to consume alcohol while taking this drug because of risk of seizure.
- Inform patient and family of adverse effects of product and instruct them to notify physician of potential problems. Explain that symptoms of psychosis, anorexia, or seizure should be reported immediately.
- Advise patient that drug may adversely affect their performance and to avoid or use caution while driving, operating machinery or performing other tasks requiring mental alertness.

See Patient Guide, p. 69.

Buspirone HCl

(byoo-SPY-rone HIGH-droe-KLOR-ide)

BuSpar

Class: Antianxiety

Action Mechanism unknown; does not exert anticonvulsant or muscle relaxant effects.

Indications Treatment of anxiety disorders; short-term relief of anxiety symptoms. **Unlabeled use:** Reduction of symptoms of PMS.

Contraindications Severe liver and kidney impairment.

Route/Dosage
ADULTS: Initial dose: **PO** 5 mg tid; may increase by 5 mg/day q 2-3 days prn (maximum 60 mg/day in divided doses).

Interactions
Haloperidol: May elevate haloperidol serum levels. MAO *inhibitors:* May elevate BP. *Trazodone:* May elevate serum concentrations of ALT.

Lab Test Interferences
None well documented.

Adverse Reactions
CV: Chest pain; cerebrovascular accident; CHF; MI. *CNS:* Dizziness; headache; nervousness; lightheadedness; insomnia; excitement; dream disturbances. *GI:* Nausea. *HEMA:* Eosinophilia; leukopenia; thrombocytopenia.

Precautions
Pregnancy: Category B. *Lactation:* Undetermined. Nursing should be avoided. *Children < 18 yr:* Safety and efficacy not established.

NURSING CONSIDERATIONS

Administration/Storage

- Administer with food, which may decrease rate of absorption and increase bioavailability of drug.
- Store in a dry place at room temperature.

Assessment/Interventions

- Obtain patient history, including drug history and any known allergies. Assess for drug abuse potential and suicidal tendencies.
- If patient is currently taking benzodiazepines or other sedative-hypnotic drugs, dosages of these drugs should be tapered gradually until discontinued because buspirone hydrochloride will not block withdrawal symptoms.
- If patient is currently taking digoxin, assess for cardiac arrhythmias or signs of escalating symptoms of CHF.
- If patient has history of drug misuse or abuse, monitor for behaviors such as drug tolerance or drug seeking.
- If patient displays suicidal tendencies, institute suicide precautions immediately and inform physician.

OVERDOSAGE: SIGNS & SYMPTOMS

Nausea, vomiting, dizziness, drowsiness, miosis, gastric distress

Patient/Family Education

- Advise patient that optimal therapeutic results usually do not occur until after 3-4 wk of treatment. However, some improvement may be noted within 7-10 days.
- Caution patient to avoid intake of alcoholic beverages and other CNS depressants.
- Instruct patient to report any of these symptoms to physician: dizziness, drowsiness, insomnia, nervousness, headache, nausea, fatigue or abnormal movements.
- Advise patient that drug may cause drowsiness and dizziness and to use caution while driving or performing other tasks requiring mental alertness.
- Instruct patient not to take otc medications without consulting physician.

See Patient Guide, p. 70.

Busulfan

(byoo-SULL-fan)

Myleran

Class: Antineoplastic/alkylator

Action Acts predominantly against granulocytic cells and WBCs; thought to interact with cellular thiol groups.

Indications Palliative treatment of chronic myelogenous leukemia (myeloid, myelocytic, granulocytic). **Unlabeled uses:** Treatment of myelofibrosis; therapy for polycythemia vera; treatment of thrombocytosis.

Contraindications Disease demonstrating prior resistance to drug (total dose). Not effective in chronic lymphocytic leukemia, acute leukemia, or in "blastic crisis" of chronic myelogenous leukemia.

Route/Dosage
ADULTS: Remission induction: **PO** 4-8 mg/day. Maintenance: 1-3 mg/day; dosage is based on total leukocyte count. CHILDREN: **PO** Approximately 60 μg/kg.

Interactions
Myelosuppressive drugs: Additive myelosuppression may occur. *Thioguanine:* Combined, long-term use may cause esophageal varices and abnormal liver function test results.

Lab Test Interferences
None well documented.

Adverse Reactions
RESP: Bronchopulmonary dysplasia with interstitial pulmonary fibrosis. *EENT:* Cataracts. *GI:* Dry mouth. *HEMA:* Severe bone marrow hypoplasia or failure; pancytopenia; anemia; leukopenia; thrombocytopenia. *HEPA:* Cholestatic jaundice. *DERM:* Hyperpigmentation; urticaria; erythema multiforme; erythema nodosum; alopecia; porphyria cutanea tarda; skin dryness and fragility. *META:* Syndrome resembling adrenal insufficiency (eg, weakness, severe fatigue, anorexia, weight loss, nausea, vomiting and melanoderma); hyperuricemia; hyperuricosuria. *OTHER:* Gynecomastia; myasthenia gravis.

Precautions
Pregnancy: Category D. *Lactation:* Undetermined. *Carcinogenesis/mutagenesis:* May be carcinogenic and mutagenic in human beings. *Cellular dysplasia:* May cause cellular dysplasia in many organs including lungs, lymph nodes, pancreas, thyroid, adrenal glands, liver and bone marrow. *Fertility impairment:* May cause ovarian suppression, with menopausal symptoms in premenopausal females. Sterility, azospermia and testicular atrophy have been reported in males.

NURSING CONSIDERATIONS

Administration/Storage
- Give medication at the same time each day.
- Administer on empty stomach to reduce nausea and vomiting.
- Store at room temperature in tightly closed container.

Assessment/Interventions
- Obtain patient history, including drug history and any known allergies.
- Ensure that baseline BUN, serum creatinine, uric acid and liver function tests have been obtained and monitor during course of therapy.
- Assess gums, urine and stools for signs of bleeding. Observe for frequent bruising, petechiae and emesis.
- Observe for signs of infection, fever, cough and sore throat. Notify physician if these occur.
- Check for signs of gout (joint pain and swelling).
- Monitor I&O and daily weight. Notify physician of significant or steady change in weight.
- Verify CBC and differential count

weekly. Notify physician if WBC falls below 15,000 mm (drug is normally withdrawn at this point) or if sudden drop occurs.

- Protect patient from infection. Do not allow visitors who have recently had symptoms of cold, flu or elevated temperature.
- Avoid IM injections.
- Minimize number of arterial and venous punctures. Maintain pressure on venipuncture sites for at least 10 min.
- Encourage patient to increase fluid intake to 2 L/day, unless contraindicated.
- If signs of infection occur, notify physician.

OVERDOSAGE: SIGNS & SYMPTOMS

Bone marrow suppression, CNS stimulation, convulsions

Patient/Family Education

- Instruct patient to take drug on empty stomach and at same time each day.
- Inform patient that the following side effects are common but should be reported to physician only if pronounced: darkening of skin, fatigue, anorexia, nausea, vomiting, diarrhea, hair loss.
- Discuss use of scarves or wigs and coping strategies related to hair loss.
- Advise patient to use soft toothbrush and electric razor to minimize risk of tissue injury and bleeding.
- Caution patient to avoid crowds and individuals with infections.
- Warn patient to avoid contact with anyone who has recently received oral polio vaccine. Explain that patient should receive vaccinations only with consent of physician.
- Instruct patient to report these symptoms to physician: cold or flu symptoms; infection; difficulty breathing; persistent cough; unusual bleeding or bruising; abdominal, flank or joint pain.
- Warn patient to avoid use of aspirin and alcoholic beverages, which may precipitate GI bleeding.
- Advise patient that frequent blood tests are necessary to monitor response to therapy and toxicity.

See Patient Guide, p. 71.

Butalbital/ Acetaminophen/Caffeine

(BYOO-TAL-bih-tuhl/uh-seet-uh-MIN-oh-fen/kaff-EEN)

Amaphen, Anoquan, Arcet, Butace, Endolor, Esgic, Esgic-Plus, Femcet, Fioricet, Medigesic, Repan, Tencet, Triad, Two-Dyne

Class: Nonnarcotic analgesic

Action Butalbital has generalized depressant effect on CNS and, in very high doses, has peripheral effects. Acetaminophen has analgesic and antipyretic effects; its analgesic effects may be mediated through inhibition of prostaglandin synthetase enzyme complex. Caffeine is thought to produce constriction of cerebral blood vessels.

Indications Relief of symptom complex of tension (or muscle contraction) headache.

Contraindications Hypersensitivity to acetaminophen, caffeine or barbiturates; porphyria.

Route/Dosage

ADULTS: PO 1-2 tablets or capsules q 4 hr; maximum is 6 tablets or capsules/day.

Interactions

Beta-blockers (eg, propranolol), corticosteroids, doxycycline, estrogens (including oral contraceptives), felodipine, griseofulvin, nifedipine, phenylbutazone, quinidine, theophylline, warfarin: Effects of these drugs may be decreased. *Carbamazepine, sulfinpyrazone:* May increase risk of hepatotoxicity. MAO *inhibitors:* May increase CNS effects. *Other CNS depressants (ethanol, narcotics, general anesthetics, tranquilizers, sedative-hypnotics)*: Increased drowsiness, dizziness and other CNS depressive effects may occur. *Tricyclic antidepressants*: Antidepressant effect may decrease.

Lab Test Interferences

With Chemstrip bG and Dextrostix home blood glucose systems, may cause false decrease in mean glucose values; may give false-positive urinary 5-hydroxyindoleacetic acid test result.

Adverse Reactions

CNS: Drowsiness; dizziness; lightheadedness; confusion. *GI*: Nausea; vomiting; flatulence. *DERM*: Rash.

Precautions

Pregnancy: Category C. *Lactation*: Undetermined. *Children*: Safety and efficacy in children < 12 yr not established. *Drug dependency*: Prolonged use may produce drug tolerance and dependency (psychologic and physical).

NURSING CONSIDERATIONS

Administration/Storage

- Give with food or water.
- Store in airtight, light-resistant container at room temperature.

Assessment/Interventions

- Obtain patient history, including drug history and any known allergies.
- Assess pain before administration to establish baseline.
- Assess vital signs before administration.
- Assess related factors that may precipitate or worsen pain such as anxiety, fear or stress.
- Administer scheduled dose before pain is severe.
- Utilize adjunct pain relief measures, such as massage, positioning and maintaining quiet environment to enhance effectiveness.
- Assess therapeutic effectiveness 1 hr after dose based on patient report of relief. Do not rely on objective signs.
- Reassess vital signs.
- Assess for dizziness, sedation or euphoria.
- Record degree and duration of pain relief. Notify physician if product is ineffective.
- Institute safety precautions if drowsiness or sedation occurs.

OVERDOSAGE: SIGNS & SYMPTOMS

Blood dyscrasias, respiratory depression, hepatic damage, drowsiness, confusion, coma, hypotension, tachycardia, hypovolemic shock, nausea, vomiting, insomnia, restlessness, tremor

Patient/Family Education

- Caution patient that dependency/tolerance may result from regular long-term use.
- Tell patient to take drug with full glass of water.
- Instruct patient not to discontinue drug abruptly after long-term regular use.
- Caution patient to avoid intake of alcoholic beverages and other CNS depressants without physician approval.
- Advise patient to avoid any hazardous activity (driving or smoking) if dizziness, drowsiness or a decrease in mental acuity occurs.
- Warn patient that orthostatic hypotension may occur. Instruct patient to change positions slowly and to sit or lie down if symptoms occur.
- Instruct patient not to take otc or other medications unless directed by physician.
- Inform patient to report these symptoms to physician: persistent or recurrent pain before next scheduled dose, difficulty breathing, increased drowsi-

ness, vomiting or yellowing of skin or gums.

See Patient Guide, p. 72.

Butalbital/ Acetaminophen/Caffeine/ Codeine Phosphate

(BYOO-TAL-bih-tuhl/uh-seet-uh-MIN-oh-fen/kaff-EEN/KOE-deen FOSS-fate)

Amaphen with Codeine #3; Fioricet with Codeine

Class: Narcotic analgesic

Action Butalbital has generalized depressant effect on CNS and, in very high doses, has peripheral effects. Acetaminophen has analgesic and antipyretic effects; its analgesic effects may be mediated through inhibition of prostaglandin synthetase enzyme complex. Caffeine is thought to produce constriction of cerebral blood vessels. Codeine binds to opiate receptors in the CNS, causing inhibition of ascending pain pathways and altering perception of and response to pain.

Indications Relief of symptom complex of tension (or muscle contraction) headache.

Contraindications Hypersensitivity to acetaminophen, caffeine, opiates or barbiturates; porphyria.

Route/Dosage

ADULTS & CHILDREN ≥ 12 YR: **PO** 1-2 tablets or capsules q 4 hr; maximum is 6 tablets or capsules/day.

Interactions

Beta-blockers (eg, propranolol), corticosteroids, doxycycline, estrogens (including oral contraceptives), felodipine, griseofulvin, nifedipine, phenylbutazone, quinidine, theophylline, warfarin: Effects of these drugs may be decreased. *Carbamazepine, sulfinpyrazone:* May increase risk of hepatotoxicity. *MAO inhibitors:* May increase CNS effects. *Other CNS depressants (ethanol, narcotics, general anesthetics, tranquilizers, sedative-hypnotics):* Increased drowsiness, dizziness and other CNS depressive effects may occur. *Tricyclic antidepressants:* Antidepressant effects may decrease.

Lab Test Interferences

With Chemstrip bG and Dextrostix home blood glucose systems, may cause false decrease in mean glucose values; may increase serum amylase; may give false-positive urinary 5-hydroxyindoleacetic acid test results.

Adverse Reactions

CV: Tachycardia. *RESP:* Shortness of breath. *CNS:* Drowsiness; dizziness; lightheadedness; confusion; intoxicated feeling. *GI:* Nausea; vomiting; flatulence; constipation. *DERM:* Rash.

Precautions

Pregnancy: Category C. *Labor:* Delivery may be prolonged and neonate may experience respiratory depression or withdrawal. *Lactation:* Undetermined. *Children:* Safety and efficacy in children < 12 years not established. *Head injury:* Respiratory depressant effects may be enhanced and CSF pressure may be increased. *Drug dependency:* Prolonged use may produce drug tolerance and dependency (psychologic and physical).

NURSING CONSIDERATIONS

Administration/Storage

- Give with food or water.
- Store in airtight, light-resistant container at room temperature.

Assessment/Interventions

- Obtain patient history, including drug history and any known allergies.
- Assess pain prior to administration to establish baseline.
- Assess related factors that may precipitate or worsen pain such as anxiety, fear or stress.

- Take vital signs prior to administration. Withhold dose if respiratory rate < 12 bpm (< 20 bpm in children) and notify physician.
- Assess cough for productiveness and effectiveness. Auscultate for rales.
- Administer scheduled dose before pain is severe.
- Utilize adjunct pain relief measures (massage, positioning, maintaining quiet environment and emotional support) to enhance effectiveness.
- Assess therapeutic effectiveness 1 hr after dose based on patient report of relief. Do not rely on objective signs.
- Record degree and duration of pain relief. Notify physician if product is ineffective.
- Reassess vital signs; notify physician if there is significant change.
- Assess for dizziness, sedation or euphoria.
- Assess for urinary retention or constipation.
- Institute safety precautions if drowsiness or sedation occurs.
- Provide high-fiber diet with 2-3 L of fluids unless contraindicated.
- If constipation occurs, arrange for a stool softener or bulk laxative.
- Encourage patient to void q 3-4 hr.

OVERDOSAGE: SIGNS & SYMPTOMS

Blood dyscrasias, respiratory depression, hepatic damage, drowsiness, confusion, coma, hypotension, hypovolemic shock, nausea, tremor, vomiting, tachycardia, insomnia, restlessness

Patient/Family Education

- Caution patient that dependency/tolerance may result from long-term use.
- Remind patient to take medication with full glass of water.
- Instruct patient not to discontinue drug abruptly after long-term regular use.
- Caution patient to avoid intake of alcoholic beverages and other CNS depressants without physician approval.
- Caution patient to avoid any hazardous activity (driving or operating heavy machinery) if dizziness, drowsiness or a decrease in mental acuity occurs.
- Warn patient that orthostatic hypotension may occur. Instruct patient to change positions slowly and to sit or lie down if symptoms occur.
- Instruct patient not to take otc or other medications without consulting physician.
- Warn patient that constipation could occur. Advise patient to increase dietary fiber and fluids unless contraindicated.
- Instruct patient to report these symptoms to physician: persistent or recurrent pain occurs before next scheduled dose, difficulty breathing, blurred vision, increased drowsiness, vomiting, constipation, urinary retention or yellowing of skin or gums.

See Patient Guide, p. 73.

Butalbital/Aspirin/Caffeine

(BYOO-TAL-bih-tuhl/ASS-pihr-in/kaff-EEN)

Fiorinal, Fiorgen PF, Fortabs, Idenal, Isollyl Improved, Lanorinal

Class: Nonnarcotic analgesic

Action Butalbital has generalized depressant effect on CNS and, in very high doses, has peripheral effects. Aspirin has analgesic, antipyretic, anti-inflammatory and antirheumatic effects; its analgesic and anti-inflammatory effects may be mediated through inhibition of prostaglandin synthetase enzyme complex. Aspirin also irreversibly inhibits platelet aggregation. Caffeine is thought to produce constriction of cerebral blood vessels.

Indications Relief of symptom complex of tension (or muscle contraction) headache.

Contraindications Hypersensitivity to salicylates, aspirin, caffeine, or barbiturates; porphyria; bleeding disorders; syndrome of nasal polyps, angioedema and bronchospastic reactivity to aspirin or other NSAIDs; peptic ulcer.

Route/Dosage
ADULTS & CHILDREN ≥ 12 YR: PO 1-2 tablets or capsules q 4 hr; maximum is 6 tablets or capsules/day.

Interactions
Beta-blockers (eg, propranolol), doxycycline, estrogens (including oral contraceptives), felodipine, griseofulvin, nifedipine, phenylbutazone, quinidine, theophylline: Effects of these drugs may be increased. *Corticosteroids:* May enhance renal clearance of aspirin; sudden discontinuation of corticosteroids may result in symptoms of salicylism; effects of corticosteroids may be decreased. *Insulin, oral antidiabetic agents:* Hypoglycemic effects may be increased. *MAO inhibitors:* May increase CNS effects. *Methotrexate, 6-mercaptopurine:* Bone marrow toxicity may occur. *NSAIDs:* Increased GI ulceration or bleeding may occur. *Other CNS depressants (ethanol, narcotics, general anesthetics, tranquilizers, sedative-hypnotics):* Increased drowsiness, dizziness and other CNS depressive effects may occur. *Sulfinpyrazone, probenecid:* Uricosuric effects may be decreased. *Tricyclic antidepressants:* Antidepressant levels/effect may decrease. *Warfarin:* Anticoagulant effects may be increased or decreased.

Lab Test Interferences
Blood tests: serum amylase; fasting blood glucose; cholesterol; protein; serum hepatic aminotransferase (ALT); uric acid; prothrombin time. *Urine tests:* glucose, 5-hydroxyindoleacetic acid; Gerhardt ketone, vanillylmandelic acid; uric acid; diacetic acid; spectrophotometric detection of barbiturates.

Adverse Reactions
CV: Tachycardia. *CNS:* Drowsiness; dizziness; lightheadedness; confusion; mental depression; unusual excitement; nervousness. *GI:* Nausea; vomiting; flatulence; heart-burn; abdominal pains; constipation. *DERM:* Rash.

Precautions
Pregnancy: Category C. *Lactation:* Undetermined. *Children:* Safety and efficacy in children < 12 years not established. *Drug dependency:* Prolonged use may produce drug dependency (psychologic and physical) and tolerance. *Peptic ulcer, coagulation abnormalities and preoperative states:* Use with extreme caution because of increased bleeding time. *Renal or hepatic impairment:* Use with caution due to decreased elimination. *Reye's syndrome:* May occur in children due to aspirin component; should not be used for chickenpox or flu symptoms.

NURSING CONSIDERATIONS

Administration/Storage
- Give with food or water.
- Discard if strong vinegarlike odor is present.
- Store in airtight, light-resistant container at room temperature.

Assessment/Interventions
- Obtain patient history, including drug history and any known allergies.
- Assess pain prior to administration to establish baseline.
- Take vital signs prior to administration.
- Assess related factors that may precipitate or worsen pain such as anxiety, fear or stress.
- Administer scheduled dose before pain is severe.
- Record degree and duration of pain relief. Notify physician if product is ineffective.

- Assess therapeutic effectiveness 1 hr after dose based on patient report of relief. Do not rely on objective signs.
- Reassess vital signs.
- Assess for dizziness, sedation or euphoria.
- Institute safety precautions if drowsiness or sedation occurs.
- Use adjunct pain relief measures (massage, positioning, maintaining quiet environment and emotional support) to enhance effectiveness.

OVERDOSAGE: SIGNS & SYMPTOMS

Hyperthermia, tachycardia, respiratory depression, bleeding, drowsiness, confusion, coma, hypotension, hypovolemic shock, nausea, vomiting, tremor, tinnitus, fluid and electrolyte abnormalities, insomnia, restlessness

Patient/Family Education

- Caution patient that dependency/tolerance may result from long-term use.
- Tell patient to take with food or full glass of water.
- Instruct patient not to discontinue abruptly after long-term regular use.
- Caution patient to avoid intake of alcoholic beverages and other CNS depressants without physician approval.
- Warn patient to avoid any hazardous activity (driving or smoking) if dizziness, drowsiness or decrease in mental acuity occurs.
- Instruct patient to avoid sudden position changes to avoid orthostatic hypotension.
- Advise patient to notify physician if any surgical procedures are required. Aspirin therapy should be discontinued 5 days prior to surgery to reduce potential for bleeding problems.
- Instruct patient not to take otc medications without consulting physician.
- Advise patient to report these symptoms to physician: persistent or recurrent pain before next scheduled dose, difficulty breathing, buzzing in ears, increased drowsiness, vomiting, abdominal pain, tarry stools, unusual bruising or bleeding.

See Patient Guide, p. 74.

Butalbital/Aspirin/Caffeine/Codeine Phosphate

(BYOO-TAL-bih-tuhl/ASS-pihr-in/Kaff-EEN/KOE-deen FOSS-fate)

Fiorinal with Codeine; ♣ *Fiorinal-C*

Class: Narcotic analgesic

Action Butalbital has generalized depressant effect on CNS and, in very high doses, has peripheral effects. Aspirin has analgesic, antipyretic, anti-inflammatory and antirheumatic effects; its analgesic and anti-inflammatory effects may be mediated through inhibition of prostaglandin synthetase enzyme complex. Aspirin also irreversibly inhibits platelet aggregation. Caffeine is thought to produce constriction of cerebral blood vessels. Codeine binds to opiate receptors in CNS, causing inhibition of ascending pain pathways and altering perception of and response to pain.

Indications Relief of symptom complex of tension (or muscle contraction) headache.

Contraindications Hypersensitivity to salicylates, aspirin, caffeine, opiates or barbiturates; porphyria; bleeding disorders; syndrome of nasal polyps, angioedema and bronchospastic reactivity to aspirin or other NSAIDs; peptic ulcer.

Route/Dosage

ADULTS & CHILDREN ≥ 12 YR: **PO** 1-2 tablets or capsules q 4 hr; maximum is 6 tablets or capsules/day.

Interactions

Beta-blockers (eg, propranolol), doxycycline, estrogens (including oral contraceptives), felodipine, griseofulvin, nifedipine, phenylbutazone, quinidine, theophylline: Effects of these drugs may be decreased. *Corticosteroids:* May enhance renal clearance of aspirin; sudden discontinuation of corticosteroids may result in symptoms of salicylism; effects of corticosteroid may be decreased. *Insulin, oral antidiabetic agents:* Hypoglycemic effects may be increased. *MAO inhibitors:* May increase CNS effects. *Methotrexate, 6-mercaptopurine:* Bone marrow toxicity may occur. *NSAIDs:* Increased GI ulceration may occur. *Other CNS depressants (ethanol, narcotics, general anesthetics, tranquilizers, sedative-hypnotics):* Increased drowsiness, dizziness and other CNS depressive effects may occur. *Probenecid, sulfinpyrazone:* Uricosuric effects may be decreased. *Tricyclic antidepressants:* Antidepressant effects may decrease. *Warfarin:* Anticoagulant effects may be increased or decreased.

Lab Test Interferences

Blood tests: serum amylase; fasting blood glucose; cholesterol; protein; serum hepatic aminotransferase (ALT); uric acid; prothrombin time. *Urine tests:* glucose; 5-hydroxyindoleacetic acid; Gerhardt ketone, vanillylmandelic acid; uric acid; diacetic acid; spectrophotometric detection of barbiturates. Codeine component may increase serum amylase or lipase levels.

Adverse Reactions

CV: Tachycardia. *CNS:* Drowsiness; dizziness; lightheadedness; confusion; mental depression; unusual excitement; nervousness. *GI:* Nausea; vomiting; flatulence; heartburn; abdominal pain; constipation. *DERM:* Rash; pruritus.

Precautions

Pregnancy: Category C. *Lactation:* Undetermined. *Children:* Safety and efficacy in children < 12 yr not established. *Drug dependency:* Prolonged use may produce drug tolerance and dependency (psychologic and physical). *Head injury:* Respiratory depressant effects may be enhanced and CSF pressure may be increased. *Peptic ulcer, coagulation abnormalities and preoperative states:* Use extreme caution because of increased bleeding time. *Renal or hepatic impairment:* Use caution because of decreased elimination. *Reye's syndrome:* May occur in children due to aspirin component; should not be used for chickenpox or flu symptoms.

NURSING CONSIDERATIONS

Administration/Storage

- Give with food or water.
- Discard if strong vinegarlike odor is present.
- Store in airtight, light-resistant container at room temperature.

Assessment/Interventions

- Obtain patient history, including drug history and any known allergies.
- Assess pain before administration to establish baseline.
- Assess vital signs before administration. Withhold dose if respiratory rate < 12 bpm (< 20 bpm in children) and notify physician.
- Assess related factors that may precipitate or worsen pain such as anxiety, fear or stress.
- Assess cough for productiveness and effectiveness. Auscultate for rales.
- Administer scheduled dose before pain is severe.
- Assess therapeutic effectiveness 1 hr after dose based on patient report of relief. Do not rely on objective signs.
- Record degree and duration of pain relief. Notify physician if product is ineffective.
- Reassess vital signs. Notify physician of any significant change.
- Assess for dizziness, sedation or euphoria. Institute safety precautions as needed.

- Assess for urinary retention or constipation.
- Use adjunct pain relief measures (massage, positioning, maintaining quiet environment and emotional support) to enhance effectiveness.
- Provide high-fiber diet with 2-3 L of fluid unless contraindicated.
- If constipation occurs, arrange for a stool softener or bulk laxative.
- Encourage patient to void q 3-4 hr.

OVERDOSAGE: SIGNS & SYMPTOMS

Hyperthermia, tachycardia, respiratory depression, bleeding, drowsiness, confusion, coma, hypotension, hypovolemic shock, nausea, vomiting, tremor, fluid and electrolyte abnormalities, insomnia, restlessness

Patient/Family Education

- Caution patient that dependency/tolerance may result from long-term use.
- Tell patient to take with food or full glass of water.
- Instruct patient not to discontinue abruptly after long-term regular use.
- Caution patient to avoid intake of alcoholic beverages and other CNS depressants.
- Warn patient to avoid any hazardous activity (driving or operating heavy machinery) if dizziness, drowsiness or a decrease in mental acuity occurs.
- Instruct patient to avoid sudden position changes to prevent orthostatic hypotension.
- Tell patient to notify physician if any surgical procedures are required. Aspirin therapy should be discontinued 5 days before surgery to reduce potential for bleeding problems.
- Instruct patient not to take otc medications without consulting physician.
- Advise patient to report these symptoms to physician: persistent or recurring pain before next scheduled dose, difficulty breathing, blurred vision, buzzing in ears, increased drowsiness, vomiting, abdominal pain, tarry stools, unusual bruising or bleeding.

See Patient Guide, p. 75.

Butoconazole Nitrate

(BYOO-toe-KOE-nuh-zole NYE-trate)

Femstat

Class: Topical/antifungal

Action Increases cell membrane permeability in susceptible fungi.

Indications Local treatment of vulvovaginal candidiasis (moniliasis).

Contraindications Hypersensitivity to imidazoles.

Route/Dosage

NONPREGNANT FEMALES: Intravaginal: 1 applicator (approx. 5 g) at bedtime for 3 days; may continue up to 6 days if needed. PREGNANT FEMALES: Intravaginal: Use only during second or third trimester, 1 applicator (approx. 5 g) at bedtime for 6 days.

Interactions None well documented.

Lab Test Interferences

None well documented.

Adverse Reactions

GU: Vulvar/vaginal burning; urinary frequency.

Precautions

Pregnancy: Category C. *Lactation:* Undetermined. *Children:* Safety and efficacy not established. *Intractable candidiasis:* May be symptom of unrecognized diabetes or reinfection; patient should be evaluated carefully. *Irritation or sensitization:* If this occurs, use is discontinued.

NURSING CONSIDERATIONS

Administration/Storage

- Open applicator immediately before administration to prevent contamination.
- Use care not to contaminate applicator during use.
- With patient in supine position, (at bedtime or while in bed) insert medication high in vagina.
- Complete full course of therapy even during menstrual period.
- Store at room temperature. Avoid heat above 40°C (104°F). Do not freeze.

Assessment/Interventions

- Obtain patient history, including drug history and any known allergies.
- Observe for vulvar or vaginal burning or urinary frequency. Notify physician of any signs of tissue changes at site of application.
- If patient has diabetes, monitor blood sugar and provide necessary interventions to control condition.

Patient/Family Education

- Teach patient correct application technique.
- Instruct patient to use sanitary napkin to prevent staining clothing.
- Caution patient to refrain from sexual intercourse or advise partner to use condom to prevent reinfection.
- Explain importance of informing sexual partner of possible infection and of seeking appropriate medical treatment.
- Caution patient against using tampons during treatment.
- Tell patient to notify physician if any of these symptoms occur after initiation of therapy: headache; body aches; local irritation, burning or rash; vaginal swelling or discharge; sensitivity to light.

See Patient Guide, p. 76.

Butorphanol Tartrate

(byoo-TORE-fan-ahl TAR-trate)

Stadol, Stadol NS

Class: Narcotic agonist-antagonist analgesic

Action Potent analgesic that stimulates and inhibits opiate receptors in CNS. Antagonist effects decrease (but do not eliminate) abuse potential and may cause withdrawal symptoms in patients with opiate dependence.

Indications Parenteral/nasal: management of pain, including postoperative and migraine. Parenteral: Preoperative or preanesthetic medication (to supplement balanced anesthesia); relief of pain during labor.

Contraindications Standard considerations.

Route/Dosage

Pain

ADULTS: **IV** 0.5-2 mg q 3-4 hr prn. **IM** 1-4 mg q 3-4 hr prn. Single doses not > 4 mg. **Nasal** 1 mg (1 spray in one nostril). If no relief in 30-90 min, may repeat as 1 mg dose. For severe pain initial dose of 2 mg can be used if patient can remain lying down. Do not repeat for 3-4 hr. ELDERLY: **IV/IM** ½ normal dose at twice normal interval. Titrate subsequent doses to response. **Nasal** Initial dose: 1 mg. Wait 90-120 min before giving second 1 mg dose.

Preoperative/Preanesthetic

ADULTS: Usual dose: **IM** 2 mg 60-90 min before surgery.

Labor

ADULTS: **IV/IM** 1-2 mg in early labor at term; repeat after 4 hr.

Kidney or Liver Impairment

ADULTS: **IM/IV** Increase dosing interval to q 6-8 hr initially. Titrate subsequent doses to response.

Interactions

Barbiturate anesthetics: Increased CNS and respiratory depression. *CNS depressants (eg, tranquilizers, sedatives, alcohol):* Additive CNS depression.

Lab Test Interferences

None well documented.

Adverse Reactions

CV: Vasodilation; palpitations. *RESP:* Respiratory depression; dyspnea (nasal use). *CNS:* Sedation; floating sensation; dizziness; confusion; headache; lethargy; insomnia. *EENT:* Nasal use: Tinnitus; ear pain; nasal and sinus congestion; epistaxis; nasal irritation; upper respiratory infections; unpleasant taste. *GI:* Nausea; vomiting; anorexia; constipation; dry mouth. *DERM:* Sweating; clammy skin.

Precautions

Pregnancy: Category C. *Lactation:* Excreted in breast milk. *Children:* Not recommended for children < 18 yr. *Cardiovascular disease:* Drug increases cardiac workload. Severe hypertension has occurred. *Drug dependence:* Although potential for physical dependence is low, abuse may occur. Tolerance and psychological and physical dependence may occur with long-term use. Use in patients physically dependent on opiate agonists may precipitate withdrawal symptoms. *Elderly:* More sensitive to effects; reduce dose. *Head injury or increased intracranial pressure:* Use with caution; drug can increase cerebrospinal fluid pressure.

NURSING CONSIDERATIONS

Administration/Storage

- When giving by IM route, use deep, slow injection.
- When giving by direct IV infusion, drug may be given undiluted. Administer over 3-5 min.
- Store at room temperature, away from light.

Assessment/Interventions

- Obtain patient history, including drug history and any known allergies. Note history of drug abuse; neurologic, cardiovascular, renal or liver disease.
- Take vital signs and auscultate heart and lungs before administration. Do not administer if respiratory rate is < 12/min.
- Institute fall precautions and assist with ambulation after administration.
- Monitor BP frequently to check for widening pulse pressure. If hypertension develops, withhold medication and call physician.
- Shallow respirations (< 10/min) may indicate impending respiratory arrest and need for respiratory assistance or stimulation.
- If drug is used during labor, observe fetal heart rate for signs of distress and newborn for signs of respiratory depression.

OVERDOSAGE: SIGNS & SYMPTOMS

Hyperventilation, cardiovascular insufficiency, coma

Patient/Family Education

- Demonstrate proper use of nasal spray for patients receiving drug via this route.
- Advise elderly patients to take safety precautions (rise slowly, use handrails, request assistance with ambulation) if dizziness occurs.
- Explain that physical dependency can result from extended use.
- Instruct patient to avoid intake of alcoholic beverages or other CNS depressants.
- Advise patient that drug may cause drowsiness and to use caution while driving or performing other tasks requiring mental alertness.
- Instruct patient not to take otc medications without consulting physician.

See Patient Guide, p. 77.

Calcitonin–Human

(kal-sih-TOE-nin–human)
Cibacalcin
Class: Hormone

Action Decreases rate of bone turnover, presumably by regulating bone metabolism (blocking bone resorption). In conjunction with parathyroid hormone endogenous calcitonin regulates serum calcium.

Indications Treatment of moderate to severe Paget's disease.

Contraindications Standard considerations.

Route/Dosage
ADULTS: Initial dose: **SC** 0.5 mg/day. Improvement may occur with 0.5 mg given 2-3 times/wk or 0.25 mg/day. Severe cases may require up to 1 mg/day (0.5 mg bid).

Interactions None well documented.

Lab Test Interferences
None well documented.

Adverse Reactions
CV: Chest pressure. *RESP:* Shortness of breath. *CNS:* Headache; dizziness; paresthesia. *EENT:* Eye pain; nasal congestion; metallic taste; salty taste. *GI:* Nausea with or without vomiting (decreases with continued administration); anorexia; diarrhea; epigastric discomfort; abdominal pain. *GU:* Increased urinary frequency; nocturia. *DERM:* Flushing of face or hands; pruritus of ear lobes; edema of feet; skin rashes. *META:* Mild tetanic symptoms (rare). *OTHER:* Feverish sensation; chills; weakness; tender palms and soles.

Precautions
Pregnancy: Category C. *Lactation:* Undetermined. *Children:* Safety and efficacy not established. *Allergy:* Systemic allergic reactions may occur. *Antibody formation:* Risk is less than with calcitonin-salmon. *Hypocalcemic tetany:* May occur with calcitonin, although no cases have been reported. *Osteogenic sarcoma:* Known to increase in Paget's disease.

NURSING CONSIDERATIONS

Administration/Storage
- Administer by SC injection only.
- Rotate injection sites to prevent skin irritation.
- Administer at bedtime to reduce nausea and flushing.
- Use within 6 hr of reconstitution.
- Store at room temperature and protect from light.

Assessment/Interventions
- Obtain patient history, including drug history and any known allergies.
- Intradermal testing should be considered before first full therapeutic dose is given, to determine hypersensitivity.
- During early therapy have parenteral calcium available in case of hypocalcemia or tetany.
- Assess for bone pain and weakness during therapy.
- Have epinephrine (1:1000), antihistamines and resuscitation equipment available in case anaphylaxis occurs.
- Use padded siderails and keep bed in low position if twitching or paresthesia occurs.
- Institute safety precautions to prevent falls.
- Monitor serum calcium levels weekly during initial therapy.
- Periodically monitor BUN, serum creatinine, parathyroid hormone levels and electrolytes.
- Monitor serum alkaline phosphatase and urinary hydroxyproline excretion

before and during early phase of long-term therapy.
- Notify physician immediately if signs of hypersensitivity reaction occur.
- Assess patient for signs of hypocalcemia: tachycardia, paresthesia, muscle cramps, laryngospasm, twitching, colic, Chvostek's or Trousseau's sign. Notify physician if any of these signs occur.

OVERDOSAGE: SIGNS & SYMPTOMS
Nausea, vomiting

Patient/Family Education
- Teach patient aseptic injection technique.
- Remind patient to follow low-calcium diet if ordered and to avoid high-calcium foods such as bok choy, broccoli, canned salmon and sardines, clams, cream soups, milk and dairy products, blackstrap molasses, oysters, spinach, tofu.
- Instruct patient to rotate injection sites.
- Explain comfort measures to be used for injection sites.
- Emphasize importance of maintaining adequate intake of vitamin D by incorporating fish liver, fish oil, fortified breads, milk and cereals in diet.
- Explain that nausea is common side effect, usually occurring 30 min after injection, and will lessen during course of therapy. Remind patient that taking dose at bedtime will reduce nausea and flushing.
- Tell patient that other side effects include anorexia, vomiting, diarrhea and flushing of face, ears, hands and feet.
- Remind patient that follow-up office visits and lab tests are necessary.
- Instruct patient not to take otc medications without consulting physician.

See Patient Guide, p. 78.

Calcitonin–Salmon

(kal-sih-TOE-nin–salmon)
Calcimar, Miacalcin
Class: Hormone

Action Decreases rate of bone turnover, presumably by regulating bone metabolism (blocking bone resorption). In conjunction with parathyroid hormone endogenous calcitonin regulates serum calcium.

Indications Treatment of moderate to severe Paget's disease, postmenopausal osteoporosis, hypercalcemia. **Orphan drug use:** Nasal spray for treatment of symptomatic Paget's disease.

Contraindications Standard considerations.

Route/Dosage

Paget's Disease
ADULTS: Initial dose: **SC/IM** 100 IU/day; maintenance: **SC/IM** 50 IU/day or qod is usually sufficient.

Postmenopausal Osteoporosis
ADULTS: **SC/IM** 100 IU/day with supplemental calcium and adequate vitamin D intake. **Intranasal** 200 IU per day, alternating nostrils.

Hypercalcemia
ADULTS: Starting dose: **SC/IM** 4 IU/kg q 12 hr. Titrate gradually on basis of response to maximum dose of 8 IU/kg q 6 hr.

Interactions None well documented.

Lab Test Interferences
None well documented.

Adverse Reactions
EENT: Eye pain; salty taste. *GI:* Nausea with or without vomiting (decreases with continued administration); anorexia; diarrhea; epigastric discomfort; abdominal pain. *GU:* Nocturia. *DERM:* Injection site inflammation; flushing of face or hands; pruritus of ear lobes; edema of feet; skin rashes. *OTHER:* Feverish sensation.

Precautions

Pregnancy: Category C. *Lactation:* Undetermined. *Children:* Safety and efficacy not established. *Allergy:* Systemic allergic reactions, including anaphylaxis, may occur. *Antibody formation:* Circulating antibodies to calcitonin–salmon may occur after 2-18 mo of treatment. Treatment may or may not remain effective. *Hypocalcemic tetany:* May occur with calcitonin, although no cases have been reported. *Osteogenic sarcoma:* Known to increase in Paget's disease.

NURSING CONSIDERATIONS

Administration/Storage

- Administer by SC or IM injection. For doses > 2 ml, use IM site.
- Rotate injection sites to prevent skin irritation.
- Give medication at bedtime to reduce nausea and flushing.
- Keep medication under refrigeration.

Assessment/Interventions

- Obtain patient history, including drug history and any known allergies. Inquire about possible allergy to fish protein.
- Intradermal testing should be considered before first full therapeutic dose is given, to determine hypersensitivity.
- Have epinephrine (1:1000), antihistamines and resuscitation equipment available in case anaphylaxis occurs.
- Use padded siderails and keep bed in low position if twitching or paresthesia occurs.
- Institute safety precautions to prevent falls.
- During early therapy have parenteral calcium available in case hypocalcemia occurs.
- Monitor serum calcium levels weekly during initial therapy.
- Periodically monitor BUN, serum creatinine, alkaline phosphatase, urinary hydroxyproline excretion (every 24 hr), parathyroid hormone levels and electrolytes.
- Observe for signs of anaphylaxis, especially early in treatment. Notify physician immediately if any of these signs occur.
- Assess patient for signs of hypocalcemia: tachycardia, paresthesia, muscle cramps, laryngospasm, twitching, colic, Chvostek's or Trousseau's sign. Notify physician if any of these signs occur.

OVERDOSAGE: SIGNS & SYMPTOMS

Nausea, vomiting

Patient/Family Education

- Teach patient aseptic injection technique.
- Instruct patient to rotate injection sites.
- Explain comfort measures to be used for injection sites.
- Emphasize importance of maintaining adequate intake of vitamin D.
- Explain that nausea is a common side effect, usually occurring 30 min after injection, and will lessen during course of therapy.
- Tell patient that other side effects include anorexia, vomiting, diarrhea and flushing of face, ears, hands and feet.
- If patient is taking medication for osteoporosis, explain need for maintaining proper levels of total calcium (1.5 g/day) and vitamin D.
- Remind patient that follow-up office visits and lab tests are necessary.
- Caution patient to follow low-calcium diet if ordered and to avoid high-calcium foods such as bok choy, broccoli, canned salmon/sardines, clams, cream soups, milk and dairy products, blackstrap molasses, oysters, spinach, tofu.
- Instruct patient not to take otc medications without consulting physician.

See Patient Guide, p. 79.

Calcium

(KAL-see-uhm)

Calcium Carbonate

Alka-Mints, Amitone, Cal Carb-HD, Cal-Plus, Calci-Chew, Calci-Mix, Calciday-667, Calcium 600, Caltrate 600, Caltrate Jr., Chooz, Dicarbosil, Equilet, Florical, Gencalc 600, Mallamint, Nephro-Calci, Os-Cal 500, Oysco 500, Oyst-Cal 500, Oystercal 500, Rolaids Calcium Rich, Tums, Tums E-X Extra Strength

Calcium Citrate

Citracal

Calcium Glubionate

Neo-Calglucon

Calcium Chloride, Calcium Gluceptate, Calcium Gluconate and Calcium Lactate

Available as generic only

Calcium Carbonate

♣ *Calcite 500, Calsan*

Class: Mineral/antacid

Action Essential for development of bones, teeth, nerves and muscles and for normal cardiac contractility and blood coagulation.

Indications Treatment of calcium deficiency, dyspepsia, hypocalcemia, hyperphosphatemia, magnesium intoxication. **Unlabeled uses:** Treatment of black widow spider bites, calcium channel blocker toxicity, osteoporosis, rhabdomyolysis, tetany, PMS.

Contraindications Presence of renal calculi; hypercalcemia; hypophosphatemia; ventricular fibrillation; taking of digitalis.

Route/Dosage

Calcium Carbonate

ADULTS: **PO** 0.5-1 g tid with meals.

Calcium Chloride

ADULTS: **IV** 0.5-1 g as recommended. Administer slowly (0.5-2 ml/min). Do not give by IM injection.

Calcium Citrate

ADULTS: **PO** 0.9-1.9 g tid-qid.

Calcium Glubionate

ADULTS AND CHILDREN (≥ 4 YR): **PO** 15 ml tid-qid before meals. CHILDREN (< 4 YR): **PO** 10 ml tid before meals. INFANTS: 5 ml 5 times daily.

Calcium Gluceptate

ADULTS **IM** 0.44-1.1 g; **IV** 1.1-4.4 g at rate of 36 mg/min. CHILDREN: **IM/IV** 0.44-1.1 g.

Calcium Gluconate

ADULTS: **PO** 8.8-16.5 g/day in divided doses; **IV** 2.3-14 mEq as recommended. CHILDREN: **PO** 0.5-0.7 g/kg/body weight; **IV** 0.5-0.7 mEq/kg/body weight.

Calcium Lactate

ADULTS: **PO** 1.5-3 g tid with meals. CHILDREN: 0.34-0.5 g/kg/body weight daily in divided doses.

Interactions *Calcium channel blockers:* Antihypertensive effect may be decreased. *Iron salts:* Absorption of iron may be reduced. *Quinolones:* Effectiveness of norfloxacin may be decreased. Ciprofloxacin and oflaxacin do not appear to be affected. *Salicylates:* Salicylate serum levels may decrease when these agents are given with calcium-containing antacids. *Tetracyclines:* Oral calcium may decrease absorption and effects of tetracyclines. *Thiazide diuretics:* May predispose patient to milk-alkali syndrome. INCOMPATIBILITIES: IV solutions are incompatible with aminophylline, amphotericin B, tetracyclines, ascorbic acid, carbonates, citrates, phosphates, sulfates, tartrates, 10% IV fat emulsions.

Lab Test Interferences Because calcium competes with magnesium for absorption, decreased magnesium levels may occur.

Adverse Reactions CV: Arrhythmias and cardiac dysfunction may result from rapid IV injection; vasodilation; bradycardia. *GI:* Constipation; rebound hyperacidity; flatulence; GI irritation; metallic taste. *GU:* Nephrolithiasis. *HEMA:*

Calcium chloride injectable: Possible thrombosis. *DERM:* Calcium chloride and calcium gluconate injectable (IM or SC): necrosis; sloughing; abscess. *OTHER:* Muscle weakness, lethargy; coma with hypercalcemia.

Precautions

Pregnancy: Category C. *Lactation:* Undetermined. *Calcium acetate (PhosLo):* Do not give other calcium supplements in combination with calcium acetate. Hypercalcemia may develop in patients with end-stage renal failure when calcium is given with meals. *Extravasation:* Calcium chloride and calcium gluconate can cause severe necrosis, sloughing and abscesses with IM or SC administration. *IV:* Do not give by rapid injection.

NURSING CONSIDERATIONS

Administration/Storage

Milligram doses of calcium chloride, calcium gluconate and calcium gluceptate are not equal. Doses are noted as milligrams or milliequivalents of elemental calcium.

Oral

- Administer oral calcium supplement with meals to enhance absorption.
- Ensure that patient chews chewable tablets thoroughly and then drinks full glass of water.
- Sprinkle powdered calcium salts on food.

Intravenous

- Administer IV calcium by slow injection and in small amounts to avoid causing arrhythmias.
- Administer IV calcium cautiously to prevent irritation of vein.

Intramuscular

- Do not administer calcium chloride or calcium gluconate by IM injection.
- Use IM route only when IV route is impossible. Use a large muscle (eg, gluteal) to avoid irritation. Rotate injection sites.

Assessment/Interventions

- Obtain patient history, including drug history and any known allergies. Note any history of ventricular fibrillation, cardiac disease, renal disease or respiratory acidosis.
- Notify physician if signs of hypercalcemia develop: fatigue and CNS depression.
- Discontinue IV infusion if extravasation occurs. Apply warm, moist compresses to affected area.
- If patient is taking calcium channel blockers, monitor for decreased response to those medications.
- During IV administration, monitor ECG, BP and flow rate because IV injection may be accompanied by sudden drop in BP; advise patient to stay in bed for at least 15-30 min after administration.
- Monitor serum calcium levels. Report any abnormal test results to physician.
- Monitor patient's ECG for cardiac changes.
- Assess patient for symptoms of hypocalcemia: excitability of nerves, numbness and tingling of fingers, lips and toes.
- Assess for tissue damage at injection sites.

OVERDOSAGE: SIGNS & SYMPTOMS

Nausea, vomiting, weakness, lethargy, coma, sudden death

Patient/Family Education

- Teach patient and family to recognize and report signs of hypercalcemia: drowsiness, confusion, muscle weakness, headache, constipation.
- Advise patient that calcium may cause constipation and to notify physician if it occurs. Teach methods to prevent this effect.
- Unless patient is taking calcium carbonate, encourage patient to eat foods high in vitamin D (fortified milk, breads, cereals) to enhance calcium absorption. Eating foods high in

vitamin D while taking calcium carbonate can lead to milk-alkali syndrome.

- Instruct patient to eat foods high in calcium such as milk, leafy vegetables and sardines.
- Instruct patient to take calcium tablets with, or soon after, meals to enhance absorption.
- Stress importance of follow-up blood monitoring and examinations to determine effectiveness of drug and to assess for side effects.
- Instruct patient not to use maximum dosage of antacid for > 2 wk, except under medical supervision.

See Patient Guide, pp. 80-81.

Capsaicin

(kap-SAY-uh-sin)

Zostrix, Zostrix-HP

Class: Topical/analgesic

Action May deplete and prevent reaccumulation of substance P, principal transmitter of pain impulses, from periphery to CNS.

Indications Temporary relief of pain from rheumatoid arthritis and osteoarthritis; relief of neuralgias (eg, pain after shingles, diabetic neuropathy). **Unlabeled uses:** Temporary relief of pain of psoriasis, vitiligo, intractable pruritus, postmastectomy and postamputation neuroma (phantom limb syndrome), vulvar vestibulitis, apocrine chromidrosis, reflex sympathetic dystrophy.

Contraindications Standard considerations.

Route/Dosage

ADULTS & CHILDREN ≥ 2 YR: Apply to affected area no more than 3-4 times/day. Wash hands immediately after application.

Interactions None well documented.

Lab Test Interferences

None well documented.

Adverse Reactions

RESP: Cough; respiratory irritation. *DERM:* Burning; stinging; erythema.

Precautions

Pregnancy: Safety undetermined. *Lactation:* Undetermined. Capsaicin is for external use only.

NURSING CONSIDERATIONS

Administration/Storage

- Wear gloves during application and avoid contact with eyes and broken or irritated skin.
- If bandage is needed, apply loosely to application area.
- Store at room temperature.

Assessment/Interventions

- Obtain patient history, including drug history and any known allergies.
- Note that transient burning may occur during initial course of therapy but will decrease in a few days. Burning is more common when medication is applied more than 3 times/day.
- Assess location and intensity of pain periodically throughout therapy.

Patient/Family Education

- Remind patient that this medication is for external use only.
- Teach patient correct method of application: wear gloves, avoid contact with eyes and broken or irritated skin and wash hands immediately after application.
- Caution patient to use care when handling contact lens after application.
- Advise patient to keep bandage placed loosely over application area.
- Emphasize that following prescribed regimen reduces transient burning associated with infrequent administration. Remind patient not to apply medication more than 3 times/day.

- Instruct patient to discontinue treatment and notify physician if pain persists 14-28 days or returns a few days after initiation of therapy or if signs of infection occur.
- Counsel patient to notify physician if persistent cough accompanies therapy.

See Patient Guide, p. 82.

Captopril

(KAP-toe-prill)

Capoten, ♣ *APO-Capto, Novo-Captopril, Nu-Capto, Syn-Captopril*
Class: Antihypertensive/ACE inhibitor

Action Competitively inhibits angiotensin I–converting enzyme, preventing conversion of angiotensin I to angiotension II, a potent vasoconstrictor that also stimulates aldosterone secretion. Results in decreased BP, potassium retention and reduced sodium reabsorption.

Indications Treatment of hypertension, CHF in patients unresponsive to or uncontrolled by conventional therapy, left ventricular dysfunction after MI, diabetic nephropathy. **Unlabeled uses:** Treatment of hypertensive crisis, neonatal and childhood hypertension; rheumatoid arthritis; diagnosis of anatomic renal artery stenosis and primary aldosteronism; treatment of hypertension related to scleroderma renal crisis and Takayasu's disease, idiopathic edema, Bartter's and Raynaud's syndrome, asymptomatic left ventricular dysfunction after MI.

Contraindications Hypersensitivity to ACE inhibitors.

Route/Dosage

Hypertension

ADULTS: Initial dose: **PO** 25 mg bid-tid; then gradually increase q 1-2 wk if satisfactory effect is not achieved. Usual dose: 25-150 mg bid-tid. Maximum daily dose: 450 mg.

Severe Hypertension

CHILDREN: **PO** 0.01-0.5 mg/kg/day.

Heart Failure

ADULTS: Initial dose: **PO** 6.25-12.5 mg tid; then titrate to usual daily dosage within next several days.

Left Ventricular Dysfunction after MI

ADULTS: **PO** 6.25 mg 3 days after MI; then 12.5 mg tid and 25 mg tid for next several days. Target dose: 50 mg tid over next several weeks.

Diabetic Nephropathy

ADULTS: **PO** 25 mg tid.

Interactions

Allopurinol: Greater risk of hypersensitivity with coadministration. *Antacids:* May decrease bioavailability of captopril. *Capsaicin:* Cough may be exacerbated. *Digoxin:* Increased digoxin levels. *Food:* Reduces bioavailability of captopril. *Indomethacin:* Hypotensive effects may be reduced, especially in low-renin or volume-dependent hypertensive patients. *Lithium:* Increased lithium levels and symptoms of lithium toxicity may occur. *Phenothiazines:* May increase effect of captopril. *Potassium preparations, potassium-sparing diuretics:* May increase serum potassium levels. *Probenecid:* Increased captopril blood levels and decreased total clearance.

Lab Test Interferences

False-positive urine acetone test may occur.

Adverse Reactions

CV: Chest pain; palpitations; tachycardia; orthostatic hypotension. *RESP:* Chronic dry cough: dyspnea; eosinophilic pneumonitis. *CNS:* Headache; sleep disturbances; paresthesias; dizziness; fatigue; malaise. *EENT:* Rhinitis. *GI:* Nausea; abdominal pain; vomiting; gastric irritation; aphthous ulcers; peptic ulcer; jaundice; cholestasis; diarrhea; dysgeusia; anorexia; constipation; dry mouth. *GU:* Oliguria; proteinuria. *HEPA:* Elevated liver enzymes and serum bilirubin. *HEMA:* Neutropenia; agranulocytosis; thrombocytopenia; pancytopenia. *DERM:* Rash; pruritus; alopecia. *META:* Hyperkalemia; hyponatremia; elevated uric acid and blood glucose. *OTHER:* Gynecomastia; myasthenia.

Precautions

Pregnancy: Category D (second and third trimester); category C (first trimester). ACE inhibitors can cause injury or death to fetus if used during second or third trimester. When pregnancy is detected, discontinue ACE inhibitors as soon as possible. *Lactation:* Excreted in breast milk. *Children:* Safety and efficacy not established. *Angioedema:* Use with extreme caution in patients with hereditary angioedema. *Hypotension/first-dose effect:* Significant decreases in BP may occur after first dose, especially in patients with severe salt or volume depletion or those with CHF. *Neutropenia and agranulocytosis:* Risk appears greater with renal dysfunction, CHF. *Proteinuria:* May occur, especially in patients with prior renal disease or those receiving high doses of drug (> 150 mg/day); generally resolves within 6 mo. *Renal impairment:* Reduce dosage. In renal insufficiency stable elevations in BUN and serum creatinine may occur because of inadequate renal perfusion.

NURSING CONSIDERATIONS

Administration/Storage

- Administer either 1 hr before or 2 hr after meals because food reduces absorption of drug.
- If tablets are used to prepare a solution, store in glass bottles. Syrup is stable 7 days refrigerated or at room temperature. Solution with distilled water is stable 7 days at room temperature or 14 days refrigerated. Solution with distilled water plus sodium ascorbate is stable 14 days at room temperature or 56 days refrigerated.
- If patient is taking antacids, separate administration of captopril and antacid by 1-2 hr.
- Store at room temperature and protect from light.

Assessment/Interventions

- Obtain patient history, including drug history and any known allergies. Note any cardiac disease or concurrent dialysis therapy.
- Determine whether patient is taking antihypertensives, diuretics (especially potassium-sparing), salt substitutes or potassium replacement drugs.
- Monitor BP closely for at least 2 hr after initial dose and during first 2 wk of therapy. Observe for sudden exaggerated hypotensive response.
- Monitor BP and pulse throughout therapy.
- Monitor blood studies, electrolytes and renal and liver function throughout therapy.
- Assess urine for protein during first 6 mo of therapy and periodically thereafter.
- If patient is undergoing diuretic therapy, monitor weight and assess for resolution of fluid overload.
- Report increased serum potassium and decreased sodium ions to physician.
- If signs of hyperkalemia or hyponatremia occur, report to physician.

OVERDOSAGE: SIGNS & SYMPTOMS

Hypotension

Patient/Family Education

- Teach patient or family member how to monitor and record BP daily (or as indicated).
- Instruct patient to weigh self daily at consistent time and to notify physician of 5 lb weight fluctuation.
- If patient is overweight, advise to enroll in medically supervised weight management program.
- Counsel patient to adhere to low-

sodium diet and to check with physician before using any salt substitute.

- Caution patient to avoid smoking and alcohol intake.
- Emphasize importance of daily physical exercise routine.
- Advise patient to be alert for symptoms of hypotension, especially in early therapy. Stress importance of avoiding rapid posture changes and dangling feet before getting out of bed.
- Explain effect of captopril on water retention and lowering BP. Tell patient to expect increased urine output.
- Explain that if patient becomes dehydrated (eg, from flu or excessive sweating), hypotensive effect of drug may be increased and dizziness may be noted. Advise patient to contact physician if this occurs.
- Tell patient that chronic cough is common side effect and to notify physician if this effect occurs.
- Instruct patient to report these symptoms to physician: vomiting, diarrhea; swelling of eyes, face, lips, tongue or throat; difficulty breathing, speaking or swallowing.
- Emphasize importance of complying with dosage schedule. Caution patient not to discontinue taking drug and not to take otc medications without consulting physician.

See Patient Guide, p. 83.

Carbamazepine

(KAR-bam-AZE-uh-peen)

Epitol, Tegretol ♣ *APO-Carbamazepine, Novocarbamaz, Tegretol CR*

Class: Anticonvulsant

Action Mechanism appears to act by reducing polysynaptic responses and blocks post-tetanic potentiation.

Indications Treatment of epilepsy (partial seizures with complex symptoms, generalized tonic-clonic seizures [grand mal], mixed seizure patterns or other partial or generalized seizures), in patients refractory to or intolerant of other agents. Treatment of pain of trigeminal neuralgia. **Unlabeled uses:** Management of neurogenic diabetes insipidus; treatment of certain psychiatric disorders; management of alcohol, cocaine and benzodiazepine withdrawal; relief of restless legs syndrome. Nonhereditary chorea in children.

Contraindications Hypersensitivity to tricyclic antidepressants; history of bone marrow depression; active liver disease. Discontinue MAO inhibitors at least 14 days before administration of carbamazepine.

Route/Dosage

Epilepsy

ADULTS: Initial dose: **PO** 200 mg bid (tablets) or 100 mg qid (suspension). Increase weekly by up to 200 mg/day in 3-4 divided doses to reach minimum effective dose (maximum 1200 mg/day). CHILDREN > 15 YR: Initial dose: **PO** 200 mg bid (tablets) or 100 mg qid (suspension). Increase weekly by up to 200 mg/day in 3-4 divided doses to reach minimum effective dose (maximum 1200 mg/day). CHILDREN 12-15 YR: Initial dose: **PO** 200 mg bid (tablets) or 100 mg qid (suspension). Increase weekly by up to 200 mg/day in 3-4 divided doses to reach minimum effective dose (maximum 1000 mg/day). ADULTS & CHILDREN > 12 YR: Maintenance: 800-1200 mg/day. CHILDREN 6-12 YR: Initial dose: **PO** 100 mg bid (tablets) or 50 mg qid (suspension). Increase weekly by 100 mg/day in 3-4 divided doses to reach minimum effective dose (maximum 1000 mg/day). (Alternative regimen: 20-30 mg/kg/day in divided doses tid or qid). Maintenance: 400-800 mg/day in 3-4 divided doses.

Trigeminal Neuralgia

ADULTS: Initial dose: **PO** 100 mg bid (tablets) or 50 mg qid (suspension). May increase by up to 200 mg/day in 3-4 divided doses (tablets: 100 mg increments q 12 hr; suspension: 50 mg qid) prn (maximum 1200 mg/day). Maintenance: 200-1200 mg/day. Use minimum effective dose or discontinue drug once every 3 mo.

Interactions

Anticoagulants: May decrease anticoagulant effects. *Barbiturates:* May result in decreased carbamazepine serum concentrations, possibly leading to decreased effectiveness. *Charcoal, activated:* May reduce absorption of carbamazepine. *Cimetidine:* May result in carbamazepine toxicity. *Contraceptives, oral:* Causes breakthrough bleeding and reduces effectiveness of contraceptives. *Diltiazem, verapamil, danazol, propoxyphene, macrolide antibiotics (except azithromycin):* May increase carbamazepine levels and may result in toxicity. *Doxycycline hyclate:* May decrease doxycycline hyclate levels. *Felbamate:* May decrease concentrations of felbamate or carbamazepine. *Felodipine:* May decrease effects of felodipine. *Haloperidol:* May decrease effects of haloperidol. *Hydantoins (eg, phenytoin):* May decrease carbamazepine levels; may alter hydantoin levels. *Isoniazid:* May result in toxicity of isoniazid, carbamazepine or both. *Lithium:* May cause adverse CNS effects regardless of drug levels. *Nondepolarizing muscle relaxants:* May make these agents less effective. *Primidone:* Decreased carbamazepine levels. Primidone's active metabolite (phenobarbital) may be increased. *SSRIs (fluoxetine, fluvoxamine):* Increased carbamazepine levels with possible toxicity. *Theophylline:* May reduce effects of theophylline and carbamazepine. Theophylline levels may be increased or decreased. *Tricyclic antidepressants:* May increase carbamazepine levels; may decrease tricyclic antidepressant levels. *Valproic acid:* May decrease valproic acid levels; may alter carbamazepine levels.

Lab Test Interferences

None well documented.

Adverse Reactions

CV: AV block; CHF; hypertension; hypotension; syncope; edema; thrombophlebitis; aggravation of coronary artery disease; arrhythmias. *RESP:* Pulmonary hypersensitivity (eg, fever, dyspnea, pneumonitis or pneumonia). *CNS:* Dizziness; drowsiness; unsteadiness; confusion; headache; hyperacusis; fatigue; speech disturbances; abnormal involuntary movements; peripheral neuritis and paresthesias; depression with agitation; talkativeness; behavior changes (children); paralysis. *EENT:* Blurred vision; visual hallucinations; diplopia; nystagmus; punctate cortical lens opacities; conjunctivitis; tinnitus; dryness and irritation of the mouth and throat. *GI:* Nausea; vomiting; gastric distress; abdominal pain; diarrhea; constipation; anorexia. *GU:* Urinary frequency or retention; oliguria with hypertension; renal failure; azotemia; impotence; albuminuria; glycosuria; elevated BUN; urinary microscopic deposits. *HEMA:* Aplastic anemia; leukopenia; agranulocytosis; eosinophilia; leukocytosis; thrombocytopenia; pancytopenia; bone marrow depression. *HEPA:* Abnormal liver function tests; jaundice; hepatitis. *DERM:* Pruritic and erythematous rashes; exfoliative dermatitis; erythema muetiforme and nodosum; purpura; aggravation of disseminated lupus erythematosus; toxic epidermal necrolysis; urticaria; photosensitivity; pigment changes; alopecia; diaphoresis; Stevens-Johnson syndrome. *META:* Hyponatremia; hypothyroidism. *OTHER:* Aching joints and muscles; leg cramps; adenopathy; lymphadenopathy; fever; chills; SIADH.

Precautions

Pregnancy: Category C. *Lactation:* Excreted in breast milk. *Children:* Safety and efficacy in children < 6 yr not established. *Elderly:* May make elderly more prone to CNS side effects; may cause confusion, agitation or activation of latent psychosis. *Special-risk patients:* Use with caution in patient with prior adverse hematologic reactions to any drug; glaucoma; cardiac, hepatic or renal disease; and mixed seizure disorders, including absence seizures.

NURSING CONSIDERATIONS

Administration/Storage

- Discontinue MAO inhibitors for minimum 2 wk before administering carbamazepine.
- Give with food to reduce GI irritation. Tablets can be crushed and mixed with food.
- Carbamazepine suspension may produce higher peak level than equivalent tablet dose. Adjust dose accordingly when switching from one form of drug to other.
- Shake suspension thoroughly before administration.
- To minimize loss via nasogastric tube due to adherence to polyvinylchloride tubing, dilute suspension with equal volume of diluent and flush tube after administration.
- Store in cool, dry environment.

Assessment/Interventions

- Obtain patient history, including drug history and any known allergies.
- Note hypersensitivity to tricyclic antidepressants.
- Determine if MAO inhibitors have been taken within last 2 wk.
- Perform pretreatment baseline hematologic studies (CBC, platelets, reticulocyte, serum iron), liver function tests, eye examination, urinalysis and BUN, and continue to monitor monthly for first 2 mo and then yearly throughout treatment.
- Monitor drug levels if noncompliance or toxicity is suspected.
- If signs of bone marrow suppression occur (infections, sore throat, bruising, unusual bleeding), notify physician immediately.
- If signs of liver dysfunction occur (jaundice, dark urine, light-colored stools), withhold drug and notify physician immediately.
- If signs of renal dysfunction occur (decreased urine output, elevated BUN, elevated creatinine), notify physician immediately.

OVERDOSAGE: SIGNS & SYMPTOMS

Irregular breathing, respiratory depression, tachycardia, hypotension, hypertension, shock, coma, LOC, convulsions, muscle twitching, tremor, ataxia, drowsiness, dizziness, nystagmus, nausea, vomiting, anuria, urinary retention, abnormal EEG

Patient/Family Education

- Instruct patient to carry/wear identification indicating use of this drug.
- Advise patient that drowsiness, dizziness, and ataxia are common reactions during first few days of therapy.
- Inform patient with epilepsy that abrupt withdrawal from this drug may precipitate seizures.
- Advise patient to use nonhormonal form of contraception.
- If drowsiness, sedation or blurred vision occurs, institute safety precautions.
- Instruct patient to report these symptoms to physician: nosebleeds, mouth ulcers, sore throat, petechiae, unusual bleeding, fever, jaundice, dark urine or light-colored stools.
- Caution patient to avoid exposure to sunlight and to use sunscreen or wear protective clothing to avoid photosensitivity reaction.

See Patient Guide, p. 84-85.

Carbenicillin Indanyl Sodium

(car-BEN-ih-SILL-in IN-duh-nil SO-dee-uhm)

Geocillin ♣ *Geopen Oral, Pyopen*
Class: Antibiotic/penicillin

Action Inhibits mucopeptide synthesis in bacterial cell wall.

Indications Treatment of acute and chronic infections of the upper and lower urinary tract, prostatitis and asymptomatic bacteriuria caused by susceptible microorganisms.

Contraindications Hypersensitivity to penicillins, cephalosporins or imipenem. Do not treat severe pneumonia, empyema, bacteremia, pericarditis, meningitis and purulent or septic arthritis with oral carbenicillin during acute stage.

Route/Dosage
ADULTS: **PO** 382-764 mg qid.

Interactions
Contraceptives, oral: May reduce efficacy of oral contraceptives. Use nonhormonal form of contraception during carbenicillin therapy. *Tetracyclines:* May impair bactericidal effects of carbenicillin.

Lab Test Interferences
Antiglobulin (Coombs') test: Drug may cause false-positive results. *Urine glucose test:* Drug may cause false-positive results with copper sulfate tests (Benedict's test, Fehling's test or Clinitest tablets); enzyme-based tests (eg, Clinistix, Tes-tape) are not affected. *Urine protein determinations:* May cause false-positive reactions with sulfosalicylic acid and boiling test, acetic acid test, biuret reaction and nitric acid test; bromphenol blue test (Multi-Stix) is not affected.

Adverse Reactions
CNS: Dizziness; fatigue; insomnia; reversible hyperactivity. *EENT:* Itchy eyes; furry tongue; black "hairy" tongue; abnormal taste sensation; laryngeal edema; laryngospasm. *GI:* Gastritis; nausea; vomiting; abdominal pain or cramps; diarrhea or bloody diarrhea; flatulence; pseudomembranous colitis. *GU:* Interstitial nephritis (eg, oliguria, proteinuria, hematuria, hyaline casts, pyuria); nephropathy; increased BUN and creatinine. *HEMA:* Anemia; hemolytic anemia; thrombocytopenia; thrombocytopenic purpura; eosinophilia; leukopenia; granulocytopenia; neutropenia; bone marrow depression; agranulocytosis; reduced hemoglobin or hematocrit; prolonged bleeding and prothrombin time; increased or decreased lymphocyte count; increased monocytes, basophils, platelets. *HEPA:* Transient hepatitis and cholestatic jaundice. *DERM:* Urticaria; vesicular eruptions; erythema multiforme; skin rash. *META:* Elevated serum alkaline phosphatase and hypernatremia; reduced serum potassium, albumin, total proteins and uric acid. *OTHER:* Hypersensitivity reactions (urticaria, angioneurotic edema, laryngospasm, bronchospasm, hypotension, vascular collapse, death, maculopapular to exfoliative dermatitis, vesicular eruptions, erythema multiforme, serum sickness, laryngeal edema, skin rash, prostration); vaginitis; hyperthermia; fever.

Precautions
Pregnancy: Category B. *Lactation:* Excreted in breast milk. *Children:* Safety and efficacy in infants and children < 12 yr not established. *Cystic fibrosis:* Associated with higher incidence of side effects with drug (eg, rash, fever). *Renal impairment:* Use drug cautiously; dosage adjustment may be required.

NURSING CONSIDERATIONS

Administration/Storage

- Administer on empty stomach 1 hr before meals or 2 hr after meals.
- Give with full glass of water.

Assessment/Interventions

- Obtain patient history, including drug history and any known allergies, especially to drugs in penicillin family or related drugs (eg, cephalosporins).
- Obtain specimens for culture and sensitivity before beginning therapy.
- Keep epinephrine, antihistamine, and resuscitation equipment close by in event of anaphylactic reaction.
- Monitor renal function throughout therapy.
- If rash, itching, hives, shortness of breath, wheezing or other signs of allergic reaction and anaphylaxis occur, withhold drug and notify physician.
- If dizziness, black tongue, sore throat, nausea, diarrhea, vomiting, fever, swollen joints or any unusual bruising occurs, withhold drug and notify physician.

Patient/Family Education

- If allergy to carbenicillin is demonstrated, inform patient that this allergy extends to all penicillins, cephalosporins and imipenem.
- Advise patient to take medication with full glass of water, *not* with food, fruit juice or carbonated beverages because doing so may inactivate drug.
- Caution patient to stop taking drug and notify physician if difficulty breathing, rash or other allergic response occurs.
- Advise patient to take medication at even intervals if possible.
- Instruct patient to report these symptoms to physician: decreased urinary output, nausea, vomiting, unpleasant aftertaste and smell, dry mouth, "furry" tongue, unexplained bruising or nosebleeds, foul-smelling diarrhea/stool or vaginal discharge.

See Patient Guide, p. 86.

Carbidopa

(CAR-bih-doe-puh)

Lodosyn

Class: Antiparkinson

Action Inhibits peripheral decarboxylation of levodopa, making more levodopa available for transport to brain.

Indications Has no effect as single agent. For use with levodopa in treatment of idiopathic Parkinson's disease, postencephalitic parkinsonism and symptomatic parkinsonism associated with carbon monoxide or manganese poisoning. **Unlabeled uses:** Reduction of breakdown of L-5-hydroxytryptophan for treatment of postanoxic intention myoclonus.

Contraindications Hypersensitivity to carbidopa or levodopa.

Route/Dosage

ADULTS: **PO** in 1:10 ratio to levodopa (eg, 10 mg carbidopa/100 mg levodopa) tid-qid. With regimen of 10 mg carbidopa/100 mg levodopa, additional 12.5-25 mg carbidopa may be administered qd or qod with first dose if needed. With regimen of 25 mg carbidopa/250 mg levodopa, 12.5-25 mg carbidopa may be added by ½-1 tablet qd or qod to maximum of 8 tablets/day (2 tablets qid) for optimal therapeutic response (maximum 200 mg/day). INITIATING COMBINATION THERAPY: Do not give carbidopa and levodopa together until at least 8 hr after last dose of levodopa was taken alone. Lower levodopa dose to 20%-25% of previous daily dose and administer both drugs at same time.

Interactions None well documented. (See *Levodopa.*)

Lab Test Interferences

May cause false-positive test result for urinary ketones when test tape is used to determine ketonuria. False-negative test results may occur with glucose-oxidase methods of testing for urinary glucose.

Adverse Reactions

Only adverse reactions seen with carbidopa have been associated with combined use of carbidopa and levodopa.

Precautions

Pregnancy: Undetermined. *Lactation:* Undetermined. Do not administer to nursing mothers. *Children:* Safety and efficacy not established for children < 18 yr. *Dyskinesias:* Dyskinesias caused by levodopa may occur sooner or at lower doses of levodopa when levodopa and carbidopa are given concomitantly than when levodopa is administered alone. *Elderly patients:* May require lower doses of carbidopa/levodopa. *Neuroleptic malignant-like syndrome:* Muscular rigidity, fever, mental changes and increased serum creatinine phosphokinase may occur when dose of levodopa is reduced abruptly or discontinued.

NURSING CONSIDERATIONS

Administration/Storage

- Do not administer carbidopa and levodopa together until at least 8 hr after last dose of levodopa was taken alone.
- Administer carbidopa at same time as levodopa.
- Administer with food to reduce GI upset.
- Instruct patient not to crush or chew sustained-release tablets.
- Store in light-resistant container at room temperature.

Assessment/Interventions

- Obtain patient history, including drug history and any known allergies.
- Monitor vital signs during period of dose adjustment.
- Monitor glucose closely in diabetic patients. Report any abnormal results to physician.
- If patient experiences any CNS effects (uncontrollable movements of the face, eyelids, mouth, tongue, neck, arms, hands or legs; mood or mental changes) notify physician.

OVERDOSAGE: SIGNS & SYMPTOMS

Blepharospasm

Patient/Family Education

- Remind patient to take medication with food to prevent GI upset.
- Advise patient that onset of effect of first morning dose may be delayed by up to 1 hr.
- Inform patient it may take several wk to few mo to experience benefit from this drug.
- Caution patient that this drug may interfere with results of urine tests for glucose/ketones.
- Advise patient that harmless darkening of urine and sweat may occur.
- Caution patient to avoid sudden position changes to prevent orthostatic hypotension.
- Advise patient that this drug may cause drowsiness and to use caution while driving or performing tasks requiring mental alertness.
- Instruct patient not to take otc medications without consulting physician.

No patient monograph available.

Carboplatin

(car-boe-PLATT-in)

Paraplatin, ♣ *Carboplatin injection*, *Paraplatin-AQ*

Class: Antineoplastic/alkylating

Action Produces DNA cross-links. Apparently cell-cycle non-specific.

Indications Alone or in combination therapy with cyclophosphamide in initial treatment of advanced ovarian carcinoma; secondary palliative treatment of ovarian carcinoma after prior chemotherapy. **Unlabeled uses:** Treatment of small cell lung cancer, advanced or recurrent squamous cell carcinoma of head and neck, advanced endometrial cancer, relapsing and refractory acute leukemia, seminoma of testicular cancer.

Contraindications History of severe allergy to cisplatin or other platinum compounds or mannitol; severe bone marrow depression; significant bleeding.

Route/Dosage

ADULTS: *As single agent:* **IV** 360 mg/m^2 as single dose on day 1 q 4 wk. *As part of combination therapy with cyclophosphamide:* **IV** 300 mg/m^2 plus cyclophosphamide IV 600 mg/m^2 as single dose on day 1 q 4 wk for 6 cycles.

Interactions

Phenytoin: Reduced effectiveness of phenytoin. INCOMPATIBILITIES: *Aluminum:* Aluminum-containing needles or IV administration sets may reduce potency of carboplatin and cause platinum precipitation.

Lab Test Interferences

None well documented.

Adverse Reactions

CNS: Peripheral neuropathies; mild paresthesias. *EENT:* Visual disturbances; ototoxicity. *GI:* Nausea; vomiting. *GU:* Nephrotoxicity with abnormal renal function tests (eg, BUN, serum creatinine). *HEMA:* Bone marrow suppression (dose-limiting toxicity); thrombocytopenia; neutropenia; granulocytopenia; leukopenia. *HEPA:* High doses result in severe abnormal test results in alkaline phosphatase, AST and total bilirubin. *META:* Decreased serum electrolytes. *OTHER:* Pain; asthenia; alopecia; sensory disturbances including taste; hypersensitivity (eg, rash, urticaria, erythema, pruritus, bronchospasm).

Precautions

Pregnancy: Category D. *Lactation:* Undetermined. Consider discontinuing nursing. *Bone marrow suppression:* This condition is dose-limiting toxicity. Can result in infection or hemorrhagic complications including death. *Carcinogenesis/mutagenesis:* Drug is mutagenic; similar drugs have carcinogenic potential. *Emesis:* Antiemetic premedication may reduce intensity; also, using slow 24 hr infusion or dividing total dose over 5 consecutive daily pulse doses may reduce emetogenic potential. *Nephrotoxicity:* Patients with renal function impairment may need dosage adjustment. *Peripheral neurotoxicity:* Reported in 4% of patients. More likely to occur in patients > 65 yr (10%) or those previously given cisplatin (10%). Prolonged treatment may cause cumulative neurotoxicity.

NURSING CONSIDERATIONS

Administration/Storage

- Wear disposable gloves, mask and gown when preparing solutions. Wash immediately with soap and water if drug accidentally comes into contact with skin or mucosa.
- Reconstitute contents of each vial with Sterile Water for Injection, D5W or Sodium Chloride for Injection for concentration of 10 mg/ml.
- Solution can be diluted further with

D5W or Sodium Chloride for Injection to 0.5 mg/ml.

- Use within 8 hr of reconstitution.
- Pretreatment or posttreatment hydration or forced diuresis is not needed.
- Administer as infusion lasting 15 min.
- Store unopened vials at room temperature.
- Protect from light.

Assessment/Interventions

- Obtain patient history, including drug history and any known allergies.
- Note concurrent use of any ototoxic or nephrotoxic drugs.
- Assess for previous allergic reaction to cisplatin or platinum compounds.
- Assess results of CBC and renal function tests before initiation of therapy.
- Administer antiemetic medication 30-60 min before initiating therapy to control nausea and vomiting.
- Continue antiemetic administration as necessary throughout treatment.
- If signs of anaphylaxis (facial edema, wheezing, tachycardia, hypotension) occur, withhold drug and notify physician. These reactions may occur within minutes of administration. Epinephrine and resuscitation equipment should be available.
- Assess patency of IV site frequently during therapy.
- Blood counts should be performed weekly and doses then adjusted on basis of results.
- Do not repeat intermittent course of single agent or combination therapy until neutrophil and platelet counts are acceptable. Median nadir in circulating platelets and leukocytes occurs at day 21.
- Assess for fever, chills, sore throat and other signs of infection.
- Monitor BUN and serum creatinine to assess potential nephrotoxicity.

OVERDOSAGE: SIGNS & SYMPTOMS

Bone marrow suppression, hepatic toxicity

Patient/Family Education

- Instruct patient to report pain at IV site immediately.
- Caution patient to avoid crowds and anyone with known infection.
- Instruct patient to report signs of thrombocytopenia, leukopenia and anemia to physician: bruising, unexplained bleeding, petechiae, fever, sore throat, any signs of infection, fatigue, shortness of breath, faintness.
- Advise patient to immediately report signs of neurotoxicity to physician: tingling, numbness, tremors of extremities.
- Instruct patient to immediately report any signs of nephrotoxicity to physician: decreased urine output, weight gain, edema, anorexia, nausea and vomiting.

No patient monograph available.

Carisoprodol

(car-eye-so-PRO-dole)

Soma

Class: Skeletal muscle relaxant/centrally acting.

Action Produces skeletal muscle relaxation, probably as result of its sedative properties.

Indications Adjunctive treatment of acute, painful musculoskeletal conditions (eg, muscle strain).

Contraindications Acute intermittent porphyria; hypersensitivity to related compounds such as meprobamate; suspected porphyria.

Route/Dosage

ADULT: PO 350 mg tid or qid.

Interactions

Alcohol and other CNS depressants: May cause additive CNS depression.

Lab Test Interferences

None well documented.

Adverse Reactions

CV: Tachycardia; orthostatic hypotension; facial flushing. *CNS:* Dizziness; drowsiness; vertigo; ataxia; tremor; agitation; irritability; headache; depressive reactions; syncope; insomnia. *GI:* Nausea; vomiting; hiccoughs; epigastric distress. *OTHER:* Allergic or idiosyncratic reactions within first to fourth doses, including skin rash, erythema multiforme, pruritus, eosinophilia and fixed drug eruption; severe reactions include asthma, fever, weakness, dizziness, angioneurotic edema, hypotension and anaphylactoid shock.

Precautions

Pregnancy: Undetermined. *Lactation:* Excreted in breast milk. *Children:* Not recommended in children < 12 yr. *Dependency:* Use with caution in addiction-prone patients. *Renal or hepatic impairment:* Use with extreme caution. *Tartrazine sensitivity:* Some products contain tartrazine, which may cause allergic reactions (including bronchial asthma) in susceptible individuals. Such patients often also have aspirin hypersensitivity.

NURSING CONSIDERATIONS

Administration/Storage

- Give with food or milk if GI upset occurs.
- Administer last dose at bedtime.
- Store in tightly closed container in cool, dry place.

Assessment/Interventions

- Obtain patient history, including drug history and any known allergies. Note history of porphyria and hypersensitivity or allergy to meprobamate or carisoprodol.
- Obtain baseline liver function tests, serum BUN and creatinine.
- Note history of drug dependence.
- Monitor for signs of idiosyncratic response: disorientation, agitation, vision disturbances, impaired verbal communication, extreme weakness, transient quadriplegia, dizziness, ataxia and euphoria. These reactions may appear within minutes or hours of first dose. Symptoms usually subside over several hours. If such reactions occur, withhold drug and notify physician.
- Monitor liver function tests, BUN and creatinine.
- Notify physician if patient experiences hiccough, hives or shortness of breath.

OVERDOSAGE: SIGNS & SYMPTOMS

Stupor, coma, shock, respiratory depression

Patient/Family Education

- Instruct patient to take last daily dose at bedtime.
- Tell patient to take medication with meals if GI upset occurs.
- Instruct patient to report these symptoms to physician: palpitations, tremors, hiccough or ataxia.
- Advise patient to avoid intake of alcoholic beverages or other CNS depressants.
- Caution patient that drug may cause drowsiness and to use caution while driving or performing other tasks requiring mental alertness.

See Patient Guide, p. 87.

Carmustine (BCNU)

(CAR-muss-teen)

BiCNU

Class: Antineoplastic/alkylating

Action Alkylates DNA and RNA and inhibits several enzymes.

Indications Palliative therapy alone or in combination chemotherapy in treatment of certain brain tumors, multiple myeloma (in combination with prednisone) and as secondary therapy in combination with other drugs in treatment of relapsing or nonresponsive Hodgkin's disease and non-Hodgkin's lymphoma.

Contraindications Standard considerations.

Route/Dosage
ADULTS: IV 150-200 mg/m² as single dose q 6 wk or as divided daily injections (ie, 75-100 mg/m²) over 2 days.

Interactions
Cimetidine: May enhance myelosuppressive toxicity of carmustine. *Combination chemotherapy (including carmustine):* May lower blood levels of digoxin and phenytoin.

Lab Test Interferences
None well documented.

Adverse Reactions
RESP: Pulmonary infiltrates or fibrosis; pulmonary toxicity. *EENT:* Ocular nerve fiber–layer infarcts; retinal hemorrhage; neuroretinitis. *GI:* Nausea; vomiting. *GU:* Decreased kidney size; progressive azotemia; renal failure. *HEMA:* Delayed myelosuppression; thrombocytopenia and leukopenia; anemia. *HEPA:* Reversible liver toxicity with elevated transaminase, alkaline phosphatase and bilirubin levels. *OTHER:* Localized burning at injection site; localized thrombosis; skin flushing; suffusion of conjunctiva.

Precautions
Pregnancy: Category D. *Lactation:* Undetermined. *Children:* Safety and efficacy not established. *Bone marrow suppression:* Dosage adjustment is required when drug is given in combination with other myelosuppressive drugs or if bone marrow reserve is depleted. *Carcinogenesis:* Nitrosourea therapy has carcinogenic potential in humans. *Ocular toxicity:* Carmustine given by intraarterial intracarotid investigational route may cause ocular toxicity.

NURSING CONSIDERATIONS

Administration/Storage

- Exercise caution when handling drug by protecting skin and using gloves while preparing solution. If solution contacts skin, wash immediately with soap and water.
- Give prophylactic antiemetics to patient before administration to reduce nausea and vomiting.
- Administer solution by slow IV drip over 1-2 hr to reduce discomfort at injection site. Shorter infusion time may result in pain and burning at injection site.
- Avoid starting infusion in dorsum of hand, wrist or antecubital veins, to prevent damage to underlying tendons and nerves.
- Check flow rate and blood return frequently. Observe IV site for redness, burning or pain. Check patency of IV line and restart if necessary.
- Do not give repeat dose until blood count returns to acceptable levels (ie, adequate number of neutrophils on peripheral blood smear, platelets > 100,000/mm³, leukocytes > 4000/mm³).
- Do not repeat dose before 6 wk because of delayed and cumulative toxicity.
- After initial dose adjust to lower dose if nadir of leukocytes was < 3000/mm³ or if nadir of platelets was < 75,000/mm³.
- After reconstitution carmustine is stable for 8 hr at room temperature and 24 hr under refrigeration.
- Store carmustine only in glass containers and refrigerate.

Assessment/Interventions

- Obtain patient history, including drug history and any known allergies.
- Review baseline vital signs, pulmonary function studies, CBC and renal

and liver function tests. Monitor as ordered by physician.

- Determine if patient is taking digoxin, phenytoin or cimetidine; notify physician if patient is taking any of these drugs because of possible interactions.
- Determine if patient has history of lung disease.
- Ensure that IV line is patent before administration to prevent collection of medication in tissue and resultant tissue damage.
- Conduct pulmonary, liver and renal function tests.
- Administer prophylactic antiemetics to reduce nausea and vomiting.
- Monitor blood counts weekly for at least 6 wk after dose.
- If bleeding or signs of infection, renal failure, thrombocytopenia, leukopenia, visual disturbances or pulmonary dysfunction occur, notify physician.

Patient/Family Education

- Caution patient that facial flushing may occur for up to 3 hr after administration of drug.
- Discuss with patient possibility of hair loss and appropriate coping strategies.
- Instruct patient to maintain good oral hygiene and inspect mouth for sores or irritation.
- Advise patient to report any signs of hepatic toxicity (dark urine, jaundice, pruritus, light-colored stools) or renal impairment (dysuria, oliguria, hematuria, swelling of legs and feet).
- Caution patient not to take aspirin or aspirin products for nosebleeds.
- Instruct patient to report these symptoms to physician: any signs of infection, bleeding, respiratory difficulties or nausea and vomiting.
- Instruct patient not to take otc medications without consulting physician.

See Patient Guide, p. 88.

Carteolol HCl

(CAR-tee-oh-lahl HIGH-droe-KLOR-ide)

Ocupress

Class: Beta-adrenergic blocker

Action Blocks beta-receptors, primarily affecting cardiovascular system (decreases heart rate, cardiac contractility and BP) and lungs (promotes bronchospasm). Ophthalmic use reduces IOP, probably by decreasing aqueous production.

Indications Management of hypertension. *Ophthalmic preparation* for control of intraocular hypertension and chronic open-angle glaucoma. **Unlabeled use:** Treatment of angina.

Contraindications Hypersensitivity to beta-blockers; persistently severe bradycardia; > first-degree atrioventricular block; CHF unless secondary to tachyarrhythmia treatable with beta-blockers; overt cardiac failure; sinus bradycardia; cardiogenic shock; bronchial asthma or brochospasm, including severe COPD.

Route/Dosage

ADULTS: **PO** 2.5-10 mg qd. OPHTHALMIC USE: 1 gtt bid in affected eye(s).

Interactions

Clonidine: May enhance or reverse antihypertensive effect; may cause potentially life-threatening increases in BP, especially on simultaneous discontinuation of both drugs. *Epinephrine:* May cause initial hypertensive episode followed by bradycardia. *Ergot alkaloids:* May cause peripheral ischemia with cold extremities. Peripheral gangrene possible. *NSAIDs:* May impair antihypertensive effect. *Prazosin:* May increase orthostatic hypotension. *Systemic beta-blocker:* When administered concomitantly with ophthalmic carteolol hydrochloride solution, may cause additive effects and toxicity. *Theophyllines:* May reduce elimination of theophylline. May cause pharmacologic antagonism, reducing effects of one or both drugs. *Verapamil:* May increase effects of both drugs.

Lab Test Interferences

None well documented.

Adverse Reactions

CV: Hypotension; bradycardia; CHF; cold extremities; first, second- or third-degree atrioventricular block; arrhythmias; syncope. *RESP:* Bronchospasm; shortness of breath; wheezing. *CNS:* Insomnia; fatigue; dizziness; depression; lethargy; drowsiness; forgetfulness; headache. *EENT:* Dry eyes; blurred vision; tinnitus; slurred speech; dry mouth; sore throat. With ophthalmic use: eye discomfort or stinging; tearing; keratitis; drooping eyelids; visual disturbances; diplopia; ptosis. *GI:* Nausea; vomiting; diarrhea; constipation. *GU:* Impotence; painful, difficult or frequent urination. *HEMA:* Agranulocytosis; thrombocytopenic purpura. *DERM:* Rash; hives; alopecia. *META:* Hyperglycemia; hypoglycemia; unstable diabetes mellitus; hypercholesterolemia; hyperlipidemia; increased LDH. *OTHER:* Weight changes; fever; facial swelling; cramps; muscle weakness. Antinuclear antibodies may develop.

Precautions

Pregnancy: Category C. *Lactation:* Excreted in breast milk. *Children:* Safety and efficacy not established. *Cessation of therapy:* Should be done gradually, over approximately 2 wk, with careful observation of patient and limited physical activity. *CHF:* Should be administered cautiously in patients with CHF treated with digitalis and diuretics. *Diabetes mellitus:* Drug may mask signs and symptoms of hypoglycemia (eg, tachycardia, blood pressure changes). May potentiate insulin-induced hypoglycemia. *Peripheral vascular disease:* Drug may precipitate or aggravate symptoms of arterial insufficiency. *Renal and hepatic impairment:* Requires dosage adjustment. *Thyrotoxicosis:* May mask clinical signs of developing or continuing hyperthyroidism (eg, tachycardia). Abrupt withdrawal may exacerbate symptoms of hyperthyroidism, including thyroid storm.

NURSING CONSIDERATIONS

Administration/Storage

- For ophthalmic solution, pull out lower lid to create pocket, administer drop without touching eye, release lower lid, close eye and apply gentle pressure on inner canthus of eye to avoid systemic absorption.
- Store at room temperature.

Assessment/Interventions

- Obtain patient history, including drug history and any known allergies. Note history of CHF, asthma, diabetes, hypertension or sensitivity to sulfite preservatives, which may be present in ophthalmic solution.
- Determine baseline serum lipids and glucose before initiating treatment with systemic medication.
- Perform measurements of IOP on regular basis to assess therapeutic effect of ophthalmic medication.
- At end of drug regimen, taper dosage slowly under physician supervision to prevent rebound symptoms and adverse effects.
- In patients with diabetes monitor blood glucose and diabetic medications closely. Changes in diabetic medications may be required.
- Monitor BP and pulse frequently when starting oral medication or when dosage is changed.
- Note that ophthalmic solution may produce same adverse reactions as oral form because of absorption.
- Be aware that systemic medication may mask signs of hyperthyroidism.
- If signs of anaphylactic reaction are noted, withhold drug and notify physician.
- Notify physician at first sign or symp-

tom of CHF or unexplained respiratory problem.

- Observe patient for signs of withdrawal syndrome: hypertension, tachycardia, anxiety, angina, MI.

OVERDOSAGE: SIGNS & SYMPTOMS

Bradycardia, cardiac failure, hypotension, bronchospasm, hypoglycemia

Patient/Family Education

- Instruct patient in proper method of instilling eye drops.
- Teach patient how to monitor pulse before taking oral medication and to notify physician if pulse remains below 50 bpm after taking drug and fatigue and dizziness occur.
- Instruct patient to inform physician of any scheduled surgery or dental work; dosage may need to be gradually tapered (and ophthalmic solution discontinued) before surgery or treatment.
- Caution patient not to discontinue medication without consulting physician.
- Instruct diabetic patient to monitor blood glucose closely because carteolol hydrochloride may mask signs of hypoglycemia.
- Inform patient that ophthalmic solution may cause burning or stinging when first instilled in eye.
- Instruct patient to report these symptoms to physician: CHF, dizziness, decreased pulse, confusion, shortness of breath, rash or any unusual bleeding.
- Advise patient that drug may cause drowsiness and to use caution while driving or performing other tasks requiring mental alertness.
- Instruct patient not to take otc medications without consulting physician.

See Patient Guide, pp. 89-90.

Castor Oil

(KASS-ter Oil)

Emulsoil, Purge, Fleet Flavored Castor Oil
Class: Laxative

Action Acts as GI stimulant to induce bowel movement.

Indications Short-term treatment of constipation; evacuation of bowel for colon and rectal examinations and surgery.

Contraindications Nausea, vomiting or other symptoms of appendicitis; acute surgical abdomen; fecal impaction; intestinal obstruction; undiagnosed abdominal pain; pregnancy.

Route/Dosage
Dosing varies by product, concentration, and formulation (liquid or emulsion); see specific product information. ADULTS: **PO** 15-60 ml as single dose. CHILDREN: **PO** 5-15 ml as single dose. INFANTS: **PO** 1.25-7.5 ml as single dose.

Interactions None well documented.

Lab Test Interferences
None well documented.

Adverse Reactions
CV: Palpitations. *CNS:* Dizziness; fainting. *GI:* Excessive bowel activity (griping, diarrhea, nausea, vomiting); perianal irritation; bloating; flatulence; abdominal cramping. *OTHER:* Sweating; weakness, electrolyte imbalance.

Precautions
Pregnancy: Do not use during pregnancy; may induce preterm labor. *Lactation:* Undetermined. *Abuse/Dependency:* Chronic use of stimulant laxatives may lead to laxative dependency, which may result in fluid and electrolyte imbalances, steatorrhea, osteomalacia, and vitamin and mineral deficiencies. Cathartic colon (poorly functioning co-

lon) results from chronic abuse of stimulant cathartics. Pathologic presentation may resemble ulcerative colitis. *Fluid and electrolyte imbalance*: Excessive laxative use may lead to significant fluid and electrolyte imbalance. *Rectal bleeding or failure to induce bowel movement*: May indicate serious condition that may require further medical attention.

NURSING CONSIDERATIONS

Administration/Storage

- Administer with full glass of water, juice or carbonated beverage. This medication is most effective when given on empty stomach.
- Medication should not be given at bedtime. Effects usually occur within 2-6 hr.
- Castor oil should be used for only short period of time (ie, < 1 wk). Its cathartic effect is too strong to warrent use for common constipation.
- Store at room temperature.

Assessment/Interventions

- Obtain complete history, including drug history and any known allergies. Note GI symptoms of cramping and constipation.
- Assess frequency and duration of patient use of laxative.
- Check for chronic use of laxatives and monitor electrolyte levels.
- Notify physician if persistent diarrhea or constipation occurs.

Patient/Family Education

- Instruct patient that proper dietary fiber, adequate fluid intake and regular exercise are vital to normal bowel function.
- Caution patient that laxatives are for temporary use (< 1 wk) only.
- Instruct patient to notify physician if persistent diarrhea, abdominal cramping, signs of electrolyte imbalance (muscle cramping, weakness, dizziness), rectal bleeding or unrelieved constipation occurs.

See Patient Guide, p. 91.

Cefaclor

(SEFF-uh-klor)

Ceclor

Class: Antibiotic/cephalosporin

Action Inhibits mucopeptide synthesis in bacterial cell wall.

Indications Treatment of infections of respiratory tract, urinary tract, skin and skin structures; treatment of otitis media due to susceptible strains of specific microorganisms.

Contraindications Hypersensitivity to cephalosporins.

Route/Dosage

ADULTS: **PO** 250-500 mg q 8 hr. CHILDREN: **PO** 20-40 mg/kg/day in divided doses q 8 hr (for otitis media and pharyngitis: q 12 hr). (Maximum 1 g/day).

Interactions

Probenecid: Inhibition of renal excretion of cefaclor.

Lab Test Interferences

May cause false-positive urine glucose test results with Benedict's solution, Fehling's solution, or Clinitest tablets but not with enzyme-based tests (eg, Clinistix, Tes-tape); false-positive test results for proteinuria with acid and denaturization-precipitation tests; false-positive direct Coombs' test results in certain patients (eg, those with azotemia); false elevations in urinary 17-ketosteroid values.

Adverse Reactions

GI: Nausea; vomiting; diarrhea; anorexia; abdominal pain or cramps; flatulence; colitis, including pseudomembranous colitis. *GU:* Pyuria; renal dysfunction; dysuria; reversible interstitial nephritis; hematuria; toxic nephropathy. *HEMA:* Eosinophilia; neutropenia; lymphocytosis; leukocytosis; thrombocytopenia; decreased platelet function; anemia; aplastic anemia; hemorrhage. *HEPA:* Hepatic dysfunction, abnormal liver function test results. *OTHER:* Hypersensitivity, including Stevens-Johnson syndrome, erythema multiforme and toxic epidermal necrolysis; serum sickness–like reactions (eg, skin rash, polyarthritis, arthralgia, fever); candidal overgrowth.

Precautions

Pregnancy: Category B. *Lactation:* Excreted in breast milk. *Children:* In infants, consider benefits relative to risks. Safety and efficacy in children < 1 mo not established. *Hypersensitivity:* Reactions range from mild to life-threatening. Administer drug with caution to penicillin-sensitive patients due to possible cross-reactivity. *Pseudomembranous colitis:* Should be considered in patients in whom diarrhea develops. *Renal impairment:* Use drug with caution in patients with renal impairment. Dosage adjustment based on renal function may be required. *Superinfection:* May result in bacterial or fungal overgrowth of nonsusceptible microorganisms.

NURSING CONSIDERATIONS

Administration/Storage

- Administer with food or milk if GI upset occurs.
- After reconstitution, oral suspension must be refrigerated and will remain stable for up to 14 days. Do not freeze. Shake well before use. Do not administer if solution is cloudy or precipitate is present.

Assessment/Interventions

- Obtain patient history, including drug history and any known allergies. Note renal impairment and allergy to cephalosporins or penicillins.
- Obtain specimens for culture and sensitivity before beginning therapy and periodically during treatment.
- Monitor renal function carefully during treatment.
- Monitor for signs of infection, especially fever, and for positive response to antibiotic therapy.
- Assess for signs and symptoms of anaphylaxis (shortness of breath, wheezing, laryngeal spasm). Have resuscitation equipment available.
- Assess for symptoms of superinfection, such as vaginitis or stomatitis.
- Assess for severe diarrhea with blood or pus, which may be symptom of pseudomembranous colitis. Symptoms may occur after antibiotic treatment.

OVERDOSAGE: SIGNS & SYMPTOMS

Seizures

Patient/Family Education

- Instruct patient to complete full course of therapy.
- Instruct patient to check body temperature daily. If fever persists for more than a few days or if high fever (> 102°F) or shaking chills are noted, physician should be notified immediately.
- Advise patient to maintain normal fluid intake while using this medication.
- Advise diabetic patient to use enzyme-based tests (eg, Clinistix, Tes-tape) for monitoring urine glucose because drug may give false results with other tests.
- Instruct patient to report these symptoms to physician: nausea, vomiting, diarrhea, skin rash, hives, muscle or joint pain.
- Advise patient to report signs of superinfection: black "furry" tongue, white patches in mouth, foul-smelling stools, vaginal itching or discharge.
- Warn patient that diarrhea that contains blood or pus may be a sign of serious disorders. Tell patient to seek medical care and not to treat at home.
- Instruct patient to seek emergency

care immediately if wheezing or difficulty in breathing occurs.

See Patient Guide, p. 92.

Cefadroxil

(SEFF-uh-DROX-ill)

Duricef, Ultracef

Class: Antibiotic/cephalosporin

Action Inhibits mucopeptide synthesis in bacterial cell wall.

Indications Treatment of infections of urinary tract, skin and skin structures; treatment of pharyngitis and tonsillitis due to susceptible strains of specific microorganisms.

Contraindications Hypersensitivity to cephalosporins.

Route/Dosage

ADULTS: **PO** 1-2 g/day in single dose or two divided doses. CHILDREN: **PO** 30 mg/kg/day in single dose or two divided doses.

Interactions

Probenecid: Inhibition of renal excretion of cefadroxil.

Lab Test Interferences

May cause false-positive urine glucose test results with Benedict's solution, Fehling's solution, or Clinitest tablets but not with enzyme-based tests (eg, Clinistix, Tes-tape); false-positive test results for proteinuria with acid and denaturization-precipitation tests; false-positive direct Coombs' test results in certain patients (eg, those with azotemia); false elevations in urinary 17-ketosteroid values.

Adverse Reactions

GI: Nausea; vomiting; diarrhea; anorexia; abdominal pain or cramps; flatulence; colitis, including pseudomembranous colitis. *GU:* Pyuria; renal dysfunction; dysuria; reversible interstitial nephritis; hematuria; toxic nephropathy. *HEMA:* Eosinophilia; neutropenia; lymphocytosis; leukocytosis; thrombocytopenia; decreased platelet function; anemia; aplastic anemia; hemorrhage. *HEPA:* Hepatic dysfunction, abnormal liver function test results. *OTHER:* Hypersensitivity, including Stevens-Johnson syndrome, erythema multiforme and toxic epidermal necrolysis; serum sickness–like reactions (eg, skin rash, polyarthritis, arthralgia, fever); candidal overgrowth.

Precautions

Pregnancy: Category B. *Lactation:* Excreted in breast milk. *Children:* In infants, consider benefits relative to risks. Drug may accumulate in neonates. *Hypersensitivity:* Reactions range from mild to life-threatening. Administer drug with caution to penicillin-sensitive patients due to possible cross-reactivity. *Pseudomembranous colitis:* Should be considered in patients in whom diarrhea develops. *Renal impairment:* Use drug with caution in patients with renal impairment. Dosage adjustment based on renal function may be required. *Superinfection:* May result in bacterial or fungal overgrowth of nonsusceptible microorganisms.

NURSING CONSIDERATIONS

Administration/Storage

- Administer with food or milk if GI upset occurs.
- Oral suspension must be refrigerated and will remain stable for up to 14 days. Do not freeze. Shake well before use.

Assessment/Interventions

- Obtain patient history, including drug history and any known allergies. Note renal impairment and allergy to cephalosporins or penicillins.
- Obtain specimens for culture and sensitivity before beginning therapy and periodically during treatment.

- Monitor renal function carefully during treatment.
- Monitor for signs of infection, especially fever, and for positive response to antibiotic therapy.
- Assess for signs and symptoms of anaphylaxis (shortness of breath, wheezing, laryngeal spasm). Have resuscitation equipment available.
- Assess for symptoms of superinfection, such as vaginitis or stomatitis.
- Assess for severe diarrhea with blood or pus, which may be symptom of pseudomembranous colitis. Symptoms may occur after antibiotic treatment.

OVERDOSAGE: SIGNS & SYMPTOMS
Seizures

Patient/Family Education

- Instruct patient to complete full course of therapy.
- Instruct patient to check body temperature daily. If fever persists more than a few days or if high fever (> 102°F) or shaking chills are noted, physician should be notified immediately.
- Advise patient to maintain normal fluid intake while using this medication.
- Advise diabetic patient to use enzyme-based tests (eg, Clinistix, Tes-tape) for monitoring urine glucose because drug may give false results with other tests.
- Instruct patient to report these symptoms to physician: nausea, vomiting, diarrhea, skin rash, hives, muscle or joint pain.
- Instruct patient to report signs of superinfection: black "furry" tongue, white patches in mouth, foul-smelling stools, vaginal itching or discharge.
- Warn patient that diarrhea that contains blood or pus may be a sign of serious disorders. Tell patient to seek medical care and not to treat at home.
- Instruct patient to seek emergency care immediately if wheezing or difficulty in breathing occurs.

See Patient Guide, p. 93.

Cefamandole Nafate

(SEFF-uh-MAN-dahl NA-fate)
Mandol
Class: Antibiotic/cephalosporin

Action Inhibits mucopeptide synthesis in bacterial cell wall.

Indications Treatment of infections of lower respiratory tract, urinary tract, skin and skin structures, bone and joint; treatment of mixed infections; treatment of septicemia and peritonitis due to susceptible strains of specific microorganisms; perioperative prophylaxis.

Contraindications Hypersensitivity to cephalosporins.

Route/Dosage
ADULTS: **IV/IM** 500 mg- 1 g q 4-8 hr (life-threatening infections or infections due to less susceptible organisms: up to 2 g q 4 hr) (maximum 12 g/day). CHILDREN > 1 MO: **IV/IM** 50-150 mg/kg/day in equally divided doses q 4-8 hr (maximum 12 g/day). PERIOPERATIVE PROPHYLAXIS: ADULTS: **IV/IM** 1-2 g ½-1 hr prior to surgical procedure followed by 1-2 g q 6 hr for 24-48 hr. CHILDREN ≥ 3 MO: **IV/IM** 50-100 mg/kg/day in equally divided doses q 6 hr for 24-48 hr.

Interactions
Alcohol: May cause acute alcohol intolerance (disulfiram-like reaction); reaction may occur up to 3 days after last dose of cefamandole nafate. *Aminoglycosides:* May increase risk of nephrotoxicity. *Anticoagulants, oral:* May increase anticoagulant effect; may cause bleeding complications. *Probenecid:* Inhibition of renal excretion of cefamandole. INCOMPATIBILITIES: Aminoglycosides: Do not add aminoglycosides to cefa-

mandole solutions because inactivation of both drugs may result; administer at separate sites if concurrent therapy is indicated.

Lab Test Interferences
May cause false-positive urine glucose test results with Benedict's solution, Fehling's solution, or Clinitest tablets but not with enzyme-based tests (eg, Clinistix, Tes-tape); false-positive test result for proteinuria with acid and denaturization-precipitation tests; false-positive direct Coombs' test result in certain patients (eg, those with azotemia); false elevations in urinary 17-ketosteroid values.

Adverse Reactions
GI: Nausea; vomiting; diarrhea; anorexia; abdominal pain or cramps; flatulence; colitis, including pseudomembranous colitis. *GU:* Pyuria; renal dysfunction; dysuria; reversible interstitial nephritis; hematuria; toxic nephropathy. *HEMA:* Eosinophilia; neutropenia; lymphocytosis; leukocytosis; thrombocytopenia; decreased platelet function; anemia; aplastic anemia; hemorrhage. *HEPA:* Hepatic dysfunction and cholestatic jaundice; abnormal liver function tests. *OTHER:* Hypersensitivity, including Stevens-Johnson syndrome, erythema multiforme, toxic epidermal necrolysis; candidal overgrowth; serum sickness–like reactions (eg, skin rash, polyarthritis; arthralgia, fever); phlebitis, thrombophlebitis and pain at injection site.

Precautions
Pregnancy: Category B. *Lactation:* Excreted in breast milk. *Children:* Safety and efficacy in children < 1 mo not established. *Coagulation abnormalities:* Cefamandole nafate may interfere with hemostasis. There is increased risk of bleeding abnormalities associated with hepatic and renal dysfunction, thrombocytopenia and concomitant use of anticoagulants or other drugs that affect hemostasis (eg aspirin). *Pseudomembranous colitis:* Should be considered in patients in whom diarrhea develops. *Renal impairment:* Use drug with caution. Dosage adjustment based on renal function may be required. *Superinfection:* Drug may cause bacterial or fungal overgrowth of nonsusceptible microorganisms.

NURSING CONSIDERATIONS

Administration/Storage

- For IM administration, dilute in ratio of 1 g/3 ml of Sterile Water for Injection, Bacteriostatic Water for Injection, 0.9% Sodium Chloride for Injection or Bacteriostatic Sodium Chloride. Shake well until dissolved.
- For IV administration, reconstitute in ratio of 1 g/10 ml of Sterile Water for Injection, D5W or 0.9% Sodium Chloride for Injection.
- Administer intravenously or inject deep into large muscle mass to minimize pain.
- Store open vials at room temperature.
- May store drug at room temperature for 24 hr after reconstitution. Do not administer if solution is cloudy or precipitate is present.
- May refrigerate reconstituted drug for 96 hr.
- When drug is administered for perioperative prophylaxis, administration is usually discontinued 24-48 hr after surgical procedure but can be continued for up to 3-5 days postoperatively following complicated surgical procedures.

Assessment/Interventions

- Obtain patient history, including drug history and any known allergies. Note allergy to cephalosporins and penicillins.
- Obtain specimens for culture and sensitivity before beginning therapy.
- Monitor renal function.
- Monitor for coagulation abnormalities. Elevated prothombin time or abnormal platelet count may occur. If

bleeding occurs and PT is prolonged, vitamin K may be indicated.

- Monitor for signs of infection, especially fever, and for positive response to antibiotic therapy.
- Assess for signs and symptoms of anaphylaxis (shortness of breath, wheezing, laryngeal spasm). Have resuscitation equipment available.
- Assess for signs of superinfection, such as vaginitis or stomatitis.
- Assess for diarrhea with blood or pus, which may be symptom of pseudomembranous colitis. Symptoms may occur after antibiotic treatment.
- Monitor IV site for infiltration, infection, and thrombophlebitis.

OVERDOSAGE: SIGNS & SYMPTOMS
Seizures

Patient/Family Education

- Instruct patient to check body temperature daily. If fever persists for more than a few days or if high fever (> 102°F) or shaking chills are noted, physician should be notified immediately.
- Advise patient to maintain normal fluid intake while using this medication.
- Advise patient not to drink alcoholic beverages or take alcohol-containing medications while taking this medication and for several days after discontinuing it.
- Instruct patient to report any increase in ecchymoses, petechiae, nose bleeds.
- Advise patient to report signs of superinfection: black "furry" tongue, white patches in mouth, foul-smelling stools, vaginal itching or discharge.
- Instruct patient in good personal hygiene (especially mouth and perineal area care).
- Instruct patient to eat/drink 4 oz of yogurt or buttermilk a day as a prophylaxis against intestinal superinfection.
- Advise diabetic patient to use enzyme-based tests (eg. Clinistix, Tes-tape) for monitoring urine glucose because drug may give false results with other tests.
- Instruct patient to report these symptoms to physician: nausea, vomiting, diarrhea, skin rash, hives, sore throat, bruising, bleeding, muscle or joint pain.
- Warn patient that diarrhea that contains blood or pus may be a sign of serious disorders. Tell patient to seek medical care and not to treat at home.
- Instruct patient to seek emergency care if wheezing or difficulty breathing occurs.

See Patient Guide, p. 94.

Cefazolin Sodium

(seff-UH-zoe-lin SO-dee-uhm)

Ancef, Kefzol, Zolicef

Class: Antibiotic/cephalosporin

Action Inhibits mucopeptide synthesis in bacterial cell wall.

Indications Treatment of infections of respiratory tract, genitourinary tract, skin and skin structures, biliary tract, bone and joint; perioperative prophylaxis; treatment of septicemia and endocarditis due to susceptible strains of specific microorganisms.

Contraindications Hypersensitivity to cephalosporins.

Route/Dosage

ADULTS: **IV/IM** 250 mg - 1.5 g q 6-12 hr (severe infections: up to 12 g/day). CHILDREN > 1 MO: **IV/IM** 25-50 mg/kg/day in 3-4 equal divided doses q 6-8 hr (severe infections: up to 100 mg/kg/day). PERIOPERATIVE PROPHYLAXIS: ADULTS: **IV/IM** 1 g ½-1 hr prior to surgery; 0.5-1 g at appropriate intervals (≥ 2 hr) during surgery; 0.5-1 g q 6-8 hr for 24 hr (up to 5 days) after surgery. CHILDREN > 1 MO: **IV/IM** 25-50 mg/kg/day divided into 3-4 equal doses; (maximum 100 mg/kg/day).

Interactions

Aminoglycosides: May increase risk of nephrotoxicity. *Probenecid:* Inhibition of renal excretion of cefazolin. INCOMPATIBILITIES: Aminoglycosides: Do not add aminoglycosides to cefazolin solutions because inactivation of both drugs may result; administer at separate sites if concurrent therapy is indicated.

Lab Test Interferences

May cause false-positive urine glucose test results with Benedict's solution, Fehling's solution, or Clinitest tablets but not with enzyme-based tests (eg, Clinistix, Tes-tape); false-positive test results for proteinuria with acid and denaturization-precipitation tests; false-positive direct Coombs' test result in certain patients (eg, those with azotemia); false elevations in urinary 17-ketosteroid values.

Adverse Reactions

GI: Nausea; vomiting; diarrhea; anorexia; abdominal pain or cramps; colitis, including pseudomembranous colitis. *GU:* Renal dysfunction; anal pruritus. *HEPA:* Hepatic dysfunction; abnormal liver function test results. *HEMA:* Eosinophilia; neutropenia; lymphocytosis; leukocytosis; thrombocytopenia; theombocythemia; decreased platelet function; anemia; aplastic anemia; hemorrhage. *OTHER:* Hypersensitivity, including Stevens-Johnson syndrome, erythema multiforme, toxic epidermal necrolysis; candidal overgrowth; serum sickness–like reactions (eg, skin rash, polyarthritis, arthralgia, fever); phlebitis, thrombophlebitis and pain at injection site.

Precautions

Pregnancy: Category B. *Lactation:* Excreted in breast milk. *Children:* Safety and efficacy in children < 1 mo not established. *Pseudomembranous colitis:* Should be considered in patients in whom diarrhea develops. *Renal impairment:* Use drug with caution. Dosage adjustment based on renal function may be needed. *Superinfection:* Drug may cause bacterial or fungal overgrowth of nonsusceptible microorganisms.

NURSING CONSIDERATIONS

Administration/Storage

- For IM administration, dilute in ratio of 1 g/3 ml of Sterile Water for Injection, Bacteriostatic Water for Injection, 0.9% Sodium Chloride for Injection or Bacteriostatic Sodium Chloride. Shake well until dissolved. Inject deep into large muscle mass to minimize pain.
- For IV administration, reconstitute in ratio of 1 g/10 ml of Sterile Water for Injection, D5W or 0.9% Sodium Chloride for Injection. Solution can be frozen in original container for up to 12 wk. Thaw premixed frozen solution at room temperature. May store at room temperature for 48 hr after thawing or may refrigerate for 10 days. Do not refreeze. Do not administer if solution is cloudy or precipitate is present.
- Store unopened vials at room temperature.
- May store drug at room temperature for 24 hr after reconstitution.
- May refrigerate reconstituted drug for 96 hr.
- Reconstituted solution should be light yellow to amber. Do not administer if solution is cloudy or precipitate is present.
- When drug is administered for perioperative prophylaxis, administration is usually discontinued 24 hr postoperatively but can be continued for up to 3-5 days following complicated surgical procedures.

Assessment/Interventions

- Obtain patient history, includ-

ing drug history and any known allergies. Note allergy to cephalosporins and penicillins.

- Obtain specimens for culture and sensitivity before beginning therapy and periodically during treatment.
- Monitor for signs of infection, especially fever, and for positive response to antibiotic therapy.
- Assess for signs and symptoms of anaphylaxis (shortness of breath, wheezing, laryngeal spasm). Have resuscitation equipment available.
- Assess for signs of superinfection, such as vaginitis or stomatitis.
- Assess for diarrhea with blood or pus, which may be symptom of pseudomembranous colitis. Symptoms may occur after antibiotic treatment.
- Monitor IV site for infiltration, infection, and thrombophlebitis.
- Monitor for coagulation abnormalities. Elevated prothrombin time or abnormal platelet count may occur. If bleeding occurs and PT is prolonged, vitamin K may be indicated.

OVERDOSAGE: SIGNS & SYMPTOMS
Seizures

Patient/Family Education

- Instruct patient to check body temperature daily. If fever persists for more than a few days or if high fever (> 102°F) or shaking chills are noted, physician should be notified immediately.
- Advise patient to maintain normal fluid intake while using this medication.
- Advise patient to report signs of superinfection: black "furry" tongue, white patches in mouth, foul-smelling stools, vaginal itching or discharge.
- Instruct patient in good personal hygiene (especially mouth and perineal care).
- Advise patient to report any increase in ecchymoses, petechiae, nose bleeds.
- Instruct patient to eat/drink 4 oz of yogurt or buttermilk a day as a prophylaxis against intestinal superinfection.
- Advise diabetic patient to use enzyme-based tests (eg, Clinistix, Tes-tape) for monitoring urine glucose because drug may give false results with other tests.
- Instruct patient to report these symptoms to physician: nausea, vomiting, diarrhea, skin rash, hives, sore throat, bruising, bleeding, muscle or joint pain.
- Warn patient that diarrhea that contains blood or pus may be a sign of serious disorders. Tell patient to seek medical care and not to treat at home.
- Instruct patient to seek emergency care if wheezing or difficulty in breathing occurs.

See Patient Guide, p. 95.

Cefixime

(SEFF-IKS-eem)
Suprax
Class: Antibiotic/cephalosporin

Action Inhibits mucopeptide synthesis in bacterial cell wall.

Indications Treatment of uncomplicated urinary tract infections, otitis media, pharyngitis and tonsillitis, acute bronchitis, exacerbation of chronic bronchitis, and uncomplicated gonorrhea due to susceptible strains of specific microorganisms.

Contraindications Hypersensitivity to cephalosporins.

Route/Dosage

Infection

ADULTS & CHILDREN > 12 YR OR > 50 KG: PO 400 mg/day as single dose or two divided doses q 12 hr. CHILDREN 6 MO-12 YR: PO 8 mg/kg/day as single dose or two divided doses q 12 hr.

Uncomplicated Gonorrhea
ADULTS: PO 400 mg or 800 mg as single dose.

Interactions

Probenecid: Inhibition of renal excretion of cefixime.

Lab Test Interferences

May cause false-positive urine glucose test results with Benedict's solution, Fehling's solution, or Clinitest tablets but not with enzyme-based tests (eg, Clinistix, Tes-tape); false-positive test results for proteinuria with acid and denaturization-precipitation tests; false-positive direct Coombs' test result in certain patients (eg, those with azotemia); false elevations in urinary 17-ketosteroid values.

Adverse Reactions

GI: Nausea; vomiting; diarrhea; anorexia; abdominal pain or cramps; flatulence; colitis, including pseudomembranous colitis. *GU:* Pyuria; dysuria; renal dysfunction; reversible interstitial nephritis; hematuria; toxic nephropathy. *HEMA:* Eosinophilia; neutropenia; lymphocytosis; leukocytosis; thrombocytopenia; decreased platelet function; anemia; aplastic anemia; hemorrhage. *HEPA:* Hepatic dysfunction; abnormal liver function test results. *OTHER:* Hypersensitivity, including Stevens-Johnson syndrome, erythema multiforme and toxic epidermal necrolysis; serum sickness–like reactions (eg, skin rash, polyarthritis, arthralgia, fever); candidal overgrowth.

Precautions

Pregnancy: Category B. *Lactation:* Excreted in breast milk. *Children:* In infants, consider benefits relative to risks. Safety and efficacy in children < 6 mo not established. *Hypersensitivity:* Reactions range from mild to life-threatening. Administer drug with caution to penicillin-sensitive patients due to possible cross-reactivity. *Pseudomembranous colitis:* Should be considered possibility in patients in whom diarrhea develops. *Renal impairment:* Use drug with caution in patients with renal impairment. Dosage adjustment based on renal function may be required. *Superinfection:* May result in bacterial or fungal overgrowth of nonsusceptible microorganisms.

NURSING CONSIDERATIONS

Administration/Storage

- Administer with food or milk if GI upset occurs.
- Suspension should be used in treatment of otitis media because it results in higher peak blood concentrations.
- At room temperature oral suspension will remain stable for up to 14 days. Do not freeze. Shake well before use.

Assessment/Interventions

- Obtain patient history, including drug history and any known allergies. Note renal impairment and allergy to cephalosporins and penicillins.
- Obtain specimens for culture and sensitivity before beginning therapy and periodically during treatment.
- Monitor renal function carefully during treatment.
- Monitor for signs of infection, especially fever, and for positive response to antibiotic therapy.
- Assess for signs and symptoms of anaphylaxis (shortness of breath, wheezing, laryngeal spasm). Have resuscitation equipment available.
- Assess for symptoms of superinfection, such as vaginitis or stomatitis.
- Assess for severe diarrhea with blood or pus, which may be symptom of pseudomembranous colitis. Symptoms may occur after antibiotic treatment.

OVERDOSAGE: SIGNS & SYMPTOMS
Seizures

Patient/Family Education

- Instruct patient to complete full course of therapy.

- Remind patient to check body temperature daily. If fever persists more than a few days or if high fever (> 102°F) or shaking chills are noted, physician should be notified immediately.
- Advise patient to maintain normal fluid intake while using this medication.
- Advise diabetic patient to use enzyme-based test (eg, Clinistix, Tes-tape) for monitoring urine glucose because drug may give false results with other tests.
- Instruct patient to report these symptoms to physician: nausea, vomiting, diarrhea, skin rash, hives, muscle or joint pain.
- Instruct patient to report signs of superinfection: black "furry" tongue, white patches in mouth, foul-smelling stools, vaginal itching or discharge.
- Warn patient that diarrhea that contains blood or pus may be a sign of serious disorders. Tell patient to seek medical care and not to treat at home.
- Instruct patient to seek emergency care immediately if wheezing or difficulty in breathing occurs.

See Patient Guide, p. 96.

Cefmetazole

(seff-MET-uh-zole)

Zefazone

Class: Antibiotic/cephalosporin

Action Inhibits mucopeptide synthesis in bacterial cell wall.

Indications Treatment of infections of urinary tract, lower respiratory tract, skin and skin structure; treatment of intra-abdominal infections due to susceptible microorganisms; perioperative prophylaxis.

Contraindications Hypersensitivity to cephalosporins.

Route/Dosage

ADULTS: **IV** 2 g q 6-12 hr.

Perioperative Prophylaxis

ADULTS: **IV** 1-2 g at specified times prior to surgery.

Abdominal Hysterectomy/ Cholecystectomy (High-Risk)

ADULTS: **IV** 1 g 30-90 min before surgery and repeated 8 hr and 16 hr later.

Cesarean Section

ADULTS: **IV** 2 g after clamping cord or 1 g after clamping cord and repeated 8 hr and 16 hr later.

Colorectal Surgery/Vaginal Hysterectomy

ADULTS: **IV** 2 g 30-90 min before surgery or 1-2 g 30-90 min before surgery and repeated 8 hr and 16 hr later.

Interactions

Alcohol: May cause acute alcohol intolerance (disulfiram-like reaction); reaction may occur several days after last dose of cefmetazole. *Aminoglycosides:* May increase risk of nephrotoxicity. *Anticoagulants, oral:* May increase anticoagulant effects; may cause bleeding complications. *Probenecid:* Inhibition of renal excretion of cefmetazole. INCOMPATIBILITIES: Aminoglycosides: Do not add aminoglycosides to cefmetazole solutions because inactivation of both drugs may result; administer at separate sites if concurrent therapy is indicated.

Lab Test Interferences

May cause false-positive urine glucose test results with Benedict's solution, Fehling's solution, or Clinitest tablets but not with enzyme-based tests (eg, Clinistix, Tes-tape); false-positive test results for proteinuria with acid and denaturization-precipitation tests; false-positive direct Coombs' test results in certain patients (eg, those with azotemia); false elevations in urinary 17-ketosteroid values.

Adverse Reactions

CV: Hypotension; shock. *RESP:* Shortness of breath; pleural effusion.

CNS: Headache; hot flashes. *GI:* Nausea; vomiting; diarrhea; abdominal pain or cramps; flatulence; colitis, including pseudomembranous colitis. *GU:* Renal dysfunction; increased BUN; increased creatinine. *HEMA:* Eosinophilia; neutropenia; lymphocytosis; leukocytosis; thrombocytopenia; decreased platelet function; anemia; aplastic anemia; hemorrhage. *HEPA:* Hepatic dysfunction; abnormal liver function test results. *OTHER:* Hypersensitivity, including Stevens-Johnson syndrome, erythema multiforme, toxic epidermal necrolysis; candidal overgrowth; serum sickness–like reactions (eg, skin rash, polyarthritis, arthralgia, fever); phlebitis, thrombophlebitis and pain at injection site.

Precautions

Pregnancy: Category B. *Lactation:* Excreted in breast milk. *Children:* Safety and efficacy not established. *Pseudomembranous colitis:* Should be considered in patients in whom diarrhea develops. *Renal impairment:* Use drug with caution. Dosage adjustment based on renal function may be required. *Superinfection:* Drug may cause bacterial or fungal overgrowth of nonsusceptible microorganisms.

NURSING CONSIDERATIONS

Administration/Storage

- Administer intravenously.
- Reconstitute in ratio of 1 g/10 ml of Sterile Water for Injection, D5W or 0.9% Sodium Chloride for Injection.
- May store drug at room temperature for 24 hr after reconstitution. Reconstituted drug is stable for 7 days if refrigerated and for 6 wk if frozen. Do not use if solution is cloudy or precipitate is present.

Assessment/Interventions

- Obtain patient history, including drug history and any known allergies. Note allergy to cephalosporins or penicillins.
- Obtain specimens for culture and sensitivity before beginning therapy and during treatment.
- Monitor renal function during therapy.
- Monitor IV site during infusion.
- Monitor for signs of infection, especially fever, and for positive response to antibiotic therapy.
- Assess for signs and symptoms of anaphylaxis (shortness of breath, wheezing, laryngeal spasm). Have resuscitation equipment available.
- Assess for signs of superinfection, such as vaginitis or stomatitis.
- Assess for diarrhea with blood or pus, which may be symptom of pseudomembranous colitis. Symptoms may occur after antibiotic treatment.
- Monitor IV site for infiltration, infection, and thrombophlebitis.

OVERDOSAGE: SIGNS & SYMPTOMS

Seizures

Patient/Family Education

- Instruct patient to check body temperature daily. If fever persists for more than a few days or if high fever (> 102°F) or shaking chills are noted, physician should be notified immediately.
- Advise patient to maintain normal fluid intake while using this medication.
- Advise diabetic patient to use enzyme-based tests (eg, Clinistix, Testape) for monitoring urine glucose because drug may give false results with other tests.
- Instruct patient to report these symptoms to physician: nausea, vomiting, diarrhea, skin rash, hives, sore throat, bruising, bleeding, muscle or joint pain.
- Instruct patient to report signs of superinfection: black "furry" tongue, white patches in mouth, foul-smelling stools, vaginal itching or discharge.
- Warn patient that diarrhea that con-

tains blood or pus may be a sign of serious disorders. Tell patient to seek medical care and not to treat at home.

- Instruct patient to seek emergency care if wheezing or difficulty in breathing occurs.
- Advise patient not to drink alcoholic beverages or to take alcohol-containing medications while receiving cefmetazole and for several days after discontinuing drug.

See Patient Guide, p. 97.

Cefonicid Sodium

(seh-FAHN-ih-SID SO-dee-uhm)

Monocid

Class: Antibiotic/cephalosporin

Action Inhibits mucopeptide synthesis in bacterial cell wall.

Indications Treatment of infections of lower respiratory tract, urinary tract, skin and skin structures, bone and joint; treatment of septicemia due to susceptible microorganisms; preoperative prophylaxis.

Contraindications Hypersensitivity to cephalosporins.

Route/Dosage

Infections

ADULTS: **IV/IM** 1-2 g/24 hr.

Preoperative Prophylaxis

ADULTS: **IV/IM** 1 g 1 hr prior to surgical procedure; daily doses may be repeated for 2 additional days; may be given to patients undergoing prosthetic arthroplasty or open heart surgery.

Interactions

Aminoglycosides: May increase risk of nephrotoxicity. *Probenecid:* Inhibition of renal excretion of cefonicid.

Lab Test Interferences

May cause false-positive urine glucose test result with Benedict's solution, Fehling's solution, or Clinitest tablets but not with enzyme-based tests (eg, Clinistix, Tes-tape); false-positive test result for proteinuria with acid and denaturization-precipitation tests; false-positive direct Coombs' test result in certain patients (eg, those with azotemia); false elevations in urinary 17-ketosteroid values.

Adverse Reactions

GI: Diarrhea; pseudomembranous colitis. *GU:* Renal dysfunction; pyuria; dysuria; reversible interstitial nephritis; hematuria; toxic nephropathy. *HEMA:* Eosinophilia; neutropenia; lymphocytosis; leukocytosis; thrombocytopenia; decreased platelet function; anemia; aplastic anemia; hemorrhage. *HEPA:* Hepatic dysfunction; abnormal liver function test results. *OTHER:* Hypersensitivity, including Stevens-Johnson syndrome, erythema multiforme, toxic epidermal necrolysis; candidal overgrowth; serum sickness–like reactions (eg, skin rashes, polyarthritis; arthralgia, fever); phlebitis, thrombophlebitis and pain at injection site.

Precautions

Pregnancy: Category B. *Lactation:* Excreted in breast milk. *Children:* Safety and efficacy in children not established. *Hypersensitivity:* Reactions range from mild to life-threatening. Administer drug with caution to penicillin-sensitive patients due to possible cross-reactivity. *Pseudomembranous colitis:* Should be considered in patients in whom diarrhea develops. *Renal impairment:* Use drug with caution. Dosage adjustment based on renal function may be required. *Superinfection:* May result in bacterial or fungal overgrowth of nonsusceptible microorganisms.

NURSING CONSIDERATIONS

Administration/Storage

- For IM administration, inject deeply within body of large muscle (eg, gluteus muscle). When giving 2 g IM doses once daily, divide dose in ½ and give in different large muscle masses.

- For direct bolus injection, administer reconstituted solution slowly over 3-5 min.
- For IV infusion, administer reconstituted solution over 20-30 min.
- After reconstitution or dilution, solution is stable for 24 hr at room temperature or 72 hr if refrigerated. Do not administer if solution is cloudy or precipitate is present.

Assessment/Interventions

- Obtain patient history, including drug history and any known allergies. Note allergy to cephalosporins and penicillins.
- Obtain specimen for culture and sensitivity before beginning therapy and periodically during treatment.
- Monitor for signs of infection, especially fever, and for positive response to antibiotic therapy.
- Assess for signs and symptoms of anaphylaxis (shortness of breath, wheezing, laryngeal spasm). Have resuscitation equipment available.
- Assess for signs of superinfection, such as vaginitis or stomatitis.
- Assess for diarrhea with blood or pus, which may be symptom of pseudomembranous colitis. Symptoms may occur after antibiotic treatment.
- Monitor IV site for infiltration, infection, and thrombophlebitis.

OVERDOSAGE: SIGNS & SYMPTOMS

Seizures

Patient/Family Education

- Instruct patient to check body temperature daily. If fever persists for more than a few days or if high fever (> 102°F) or shaking chills are noted, physician should be notified immediately.
- Advise patient to maintain normal fluid intake while using this medication.
- Advise patient not to drink alcoholic beverages or take alcohol-containing medications while taking this medication and for several days after discontinuing it.
- Inform diabetic patient to use enzyme-based tests (eg, Clinistix, Testape) for monitoring urine glucose because drug may give false results with other tests.
- Instruct patient to report these symptoms to physician: nausea, vomiting, diarrhea, skin rash, hives, sore throat, bruising, bleeding, muscle or joint pain.
- Instruct patient to report signs of superinfection: black "furry" tongue, white patches in mouth, foul-smelling stools, vaginal itching or discharge.
- Warn patient that diarrhea that contains blood or pus may be a sign of serious disorders. Tell patient to seek medical care and not to treat at home.
- Instruct patient to seek emergency care if wheezing or difficulty in breathing occurs.

See Patient Guide, p. 98.

Cefoperazone Sodium

(SEFF-oh-PURR-uh-zone SO-dee-uhm)

Cefobid

Class: Antibiotic/cephalosporin

Action Inhibits mucopeptide synthesis in bacterial cell wall.

Indications Treatment of infections of respiratory tract, skin and skin structures, treatment of pelvic inflammatory disease; treatment of septicemia and peritonitis due to susceptible microorganisms.

Contraindications Hypersensitivity to cephalosporins.

Route/Dosage

ADULTS: **IV/IM** 2-4 g/day in equally divided doses q 12 hr (severe infections: 6-12 g/day in equally divided doses [1.5-4 g/dose] q 6, 8 or 12 hr).

Interactions

Alcohol: May cause acute alcohol intolerance (disulfiram-like reaction); reaction may occur up to 3 days after last dose of cefoperazone. *Aminoglycosides:* May increase risk of nephrotoxicity. *Anticoagulants, oral:* May increase anticoagulant effect; bleeding complications may occur. INCOMPATIBILITIES: Aminoglycosides: Do not add aminoglycosides to cefoperazone solutions because inactivation of both drugs may result; administer at separate sites if concurrent therapy is indicated.

Lab Test Interferences

May cause false-positive urine glucose test results with Benedict's solution, Fehling's solution, or Clinitest tablets but not with enzyme-based tests (eg, Clinistix, Tes-tape); false-positive test result for proteinuria with acid and denaturization-precipitation tests; false-positive direct Coombs' test result in certain patients (eg, those with azotemia); false elevations in urinary 17-ketosteroid values.

Adverse Reactions

GI: Nausea, vomiting, diarrhea; pseudomembranous colitis. *GU:* Renal dysfunction; elevation in serum creatinine. *HEMA:* Eosinophilia; neutropenia; lymphocytosis; leukocytosis; thrombocytopenia; decreased platelet function; anemia; aplastic anemia; hemorrhage. *HEPA:* Hepatitis; abnormal liver function test results. *OTHER:* Hypersensitivity, including Stevens-Johnson syndrome, erythema multiforme, toxic epidermal necrolysis; candidal overgrowth; serum sickness–like reactions (eg, skin rashes, polyarthritis; arthralgia, fever); phlebitis, thrombophlebitis and pain at injection site.

Precautions

Pregnancy: Category B. *Lactation:* Small quantities may be excreted in breast milk. *Children:* Safety and efficacy in children not established. *Coagulation abnormalities:* Cefoperazone may interfere with hemostasis. Bleeding abnormalities are greater risk in presence of hepatic and renal dysfunction, thrombocytopenia, concomitant use of anticoagulants or other drugs that affect hemostasis (eg, aspirin) and in elderly, malnourished or debilitated patients. *Hepatic impairment:* Since cefoperazone is extensively excreted in bile, serum concentrations may be elevated; monitor levels at doses > 4 g. *Hypersensitivity:* Reactions range from mild to life-threatening. Administer drug with caution to penicillin-sensitive patients due to possible cross-reactivity. *Pseudomembranous colitis:* Should be considered in patients in whom diarrhea develops. *Superinfection:* May result in bacterial or fungal overgrowth of nonsusceptible microorganisms.

NURSING CONSIDERATIONS

Administration/Storage

- If drug is administered intramuscularly with concentration > 250 mg/ml, give with 0.5% lidocaine or any other suitable diluent.
- For IV infusion, dilute reconstituted drug in 50-100 ml 0.9% sodium chloride or D5W and infuse over 30 min.
- For IM administration, inject deeply within body of large muscle (eg, gluteus muscle).
- May freeze medication. Thaw at room temperature and discard unused portions. Do not refreeze.
- Before reconstitution, protect from light and store at cool temperature.
- Solutions are stable for 24 hr at room temperature and 5 days if refrigerated. Do not administer if solution is cloudy or precipitate is present.

Assessment/Interventions

- Obtain patient history, including drug history and any known allergies. Note allergy to cephalosporins and penicillins.

- Obtain specimens for culture and sensitivity before beginning therapy and periodically during treatment.
- Monitor renal function carefully during treatment.
- Monitor for signs of infection, especially fever, and for positive response to antibiotic therapy.
- Assess for signs and symptoms of anaphylaxis (shortness of breath, wheezing, laryngeal spasm). Have resuscitation equipment available.
- Assess for signs of superinfection, such as vaginitis or stomatitis.
- Assess for diarrhea with blood or pus, which may be symptom of pseudomembranous colitis. Symptoms may occur after antibiotic treatment.
- Monitor IV site for infiltration, infection, and thrombophlebitis.
- Monitor for coagulation abnormalities. Elevated prothrombin time or abnormal platelet count may occur. If bleeding occurs and PT is prolonged, vitamin K may be indicated.

OVERDOSAGE: SIGNS & SYMPTOMS
Seizures

Patient/Family Education

- Instruct patient to check body temperature daily. If fever persists for more than a few days or if high fever (> 102°F) or shaking chills are noted, physician should be notified immediately.
- Advise patient to maintain normal fluid intake while using this medication.
- Advise diabetic patient to use enzyme-based tests (eg, Clinistix, Testape) for monitoring urine glucose because drug may give false results with other tests.
- Instruct patient to report these symptoms to physician: nausea, vomiting, diarrhea, skin rash, hives, sort throat, bruising, bleeding, muscle or joint pain.
- Warn patient that diarrhea that contains blood or pus may be a sign of serious disorders. Tell patient to seek medical care and not to treat at home.
- Instruct patient to seek emergency care if wheezing or difficulty in breathing occurs.
- Advise patient to report signs of superinfection: black "furry" tongue, white patches in mouth, foul-smelling stools, vaginal itching or discharge.
- Instruct patient not to drink alcoholic beverages or to take alcohol-containing medications while taking this medication and for several days after discontinuing it.

See Patient Guide, p. 99.

Cefotaxime Sodium

(seff-oh-TAX-eem SO-dee-uhm)
Claforan
Class: Antibiotic/cephalosporin

Action Inhibits mucopeptide synthesis in bacterial cell wall.

Indications Treatment of infections of lower respiratory tract, urinary tract, skin and skin structures, bone and joints; treatment of bacteremia/septicemia, CNS infections, intra-abdominal infections and gynecological infections due to susceptible strains of specific microorganisms; perioperative prophylaxis.

Contraindications Hypersensitivity to cephalosporins.

Route/Dosage
Infection
ADULTS: **IV/IM** Up to 12 g/day in divided doses (from q 4 hr for septicemia to q 12 hr for uncomplicated infection) usually for 7-10 days. IV route is preferable for severe infections. CHILDREN 1 MO-12 YR: **IV/IM** 50-200 mg/kg/day in 4-6 divided doses. INFANTS 1-4 WK: **IV** 50 mg/kg q 8 hr. NEONATES < 1 WK: **IV** 50 mg/kg q 12 hr.

Gonorrhea

ADULTS: **IM** 1 g as single dose.

Perioperative Prophylaxis

ADULTS: **IV/IM** 1 g 30-90 min prior to surgery.

Cesarean Section

ADULTS: **IV** 1 g as soon as umbilical cord is clamped; second and third dose IV/IM at 6- and 12-hr intervals after first dose.

Interactions

Aminoglycosides: Increased risk of nephrotoxicity. INCOMPATIBILITIES: Do not add aminoglycosides to cefotaxime solutions because inactivation of both drugs may result; administer at separate sites if concurrent therapy is indicated.

Lab Test Interferences

May cause false-positive urine glucose test results with Benedict's solution, Fehling's solution or Clinitest tablets but not with enzyme-based tests (eg, Clinistix, Tes-tape); false-positive test results for proteinuria with acid and denaturization-precipitation tests; false-positive direct Coombs' test results in certain patients (eg, those with azotemia); false elevations in urinary 17-ketosteroid values.

Adverse Reactions

CNS: Headache; dizziness; fatigue; paresthesia; confusion; nervousness; sleeplessness. *GI:* Nausea; vomiting; diarrhea; anorexia; abdominal pain or cramps; flatulence; colitis, including pseudomembranous colitis. *GU:* Pyuria; renal dysfunction; transient elevations in BUN and creatinine; dysuria; reversible interstitial nephritis; hematuria; toxic nephropathy. *HEMA:* Eosinophilia; neutropenia; lymphocytosis; leukocytosis; thrombocytopenia; decreased platelet function; anemia; aplastic anemia; hemorrhage. *HEPA:* Hepatic dysfunction; abnormal liver function test results. *OTHER:* Hypersensitivity, including Stevens-Johnson syndrome, erythema multiforme, pruritus, fever, toxic epidermal necrolysis; candidal overgrowth; serum sickness–like reactions (eg, skin rashes, polyarthritis, arthralgia, fever); phlebitis, thrombophlebitis and pain at injection site.

Precautions

Pregnancy: Category B. *Lactation:* Excreted in breast milk. *Children:* Cephalosporins may accumulate in neonates. *Hypersensitivity:* Reactions range from mild to life-threatening. Administer drug with caution to penicillin-sensitive patients due to possible cross-reactivity. *Pseudomembranous colitis:* Should be considered in patients in whom diarrhea develops. *Renal and hepatic impairment:* Use drug with caution in patients with renal and hepatic impairment. Dosage adjustment based on renal and hepatic function may be required. *Superinfection:* May result in bacterial or fungal overgrowth of nonsusceptible microorganisms.

NURSING CONSIDERATIONS

Administration/Storage

- Reconstituted solution should be light yellow to amber. Do not administer if solution is cloudy or precipitate is present.
- When giving by IM route, inject deeply into large muscle (eg, upper outer quadrant of gluteus muscle or lateral thigh). Massage well.
- Divide IM 2 g dose and administer in two separate sites.
- When giving by IV route, administer slowly over 3-5 min. Reconstituted drug may be diluted in 50-100 ml D5W or 0.9% sodium chloride injection and infused over 20-30 min. Change IV sites q 48-72 hr.
- For perioperative surgical prophylaxis, administer cefotaxime 30-90 min before surgical incision.
- Store sterile powder at room temperature and protect from light.
- Reconstituted solutions are stable at room temperature for 24 hr.

Assessment/Interventions

- Obtain patient history, including drug history and any known allergies. Note allergy to cephalosporins or penicillins.
- Obtain specimens for culture and sensitivity before beginning therapy and periodically during treatment. Repeat cultures are indicated if resistance is suspected.
- Monitor renal function carefully during treatment.
- Monitor for signs of infection, especially fever, and for positive response to antibiotic therapy.
- Assess for signs and symptoms of anaphylaxis (shortness of breath, wheezing, laryngeal spasm). Have resuscitation equipment available.
- Assess for signs of superinfection, such as vaginitis or stomatitis.
- Assess for severe diarrhea with blood or pus, which may be symptom of pseudomembranous colitis. Symptoms may occur after antibiotic treatment.
- Monitor IV site for infiltration, infection, and thrombophlebitis.

OVERDOSAGE: SIGNS & SYMPTOMS

Seizures, acute renal failure, acidosis, hypernatremia

Patient/Family Education

- Instruct patient to check body temperature daily. If fever persists for more than a few days or if high fever (> 102°F) or shaking chills are noted, physician should be notified immediately.
- Advise patient to maintain normal fluid intake while using this medication.
- Advise diabetic patient to use enzyme-based tests (eg, Clinistix, Tes-tape) for monitoring urine glucose because drug may give false results with other tests.
- Instruct patient to report these symptoms to physician: nausea, vomiting, diarrhea, skin rash, hives, sore throat, bruising, bleeding, muscle or joint pain.
- Warn patient that diarrhea that contains blood or pus may be a sign of serious disorders. Tell patient to seek medical care and not to treat at home.
- Instruct patient to seek emergency care if wheezing or difficulty in breathing occurs.
- Instruct patient to report signs of superinfection: black "furry" tongue, white patches in mouth, foul-smelling stools, vaginal itching or discharge.

See Patient Guide, p. 100.

Cefotetan Disodium

(SEFF-oh-tee-tan die-SO-dee-uhm)

Cefotan

Class: Antibiotic/cephalosporin

Action Inhibits mucopeptide synthesis in bacterial cell wall.

Indications Treatment of infections of urinary tract, lower respiratory tract, skin and skin structures, bone and joint; treatment of gynecological infections; treatment of intra-abdominal infections due to susceptible strains of specific microorganisms; perioperative prophylaxis.

Contraindications Hypersensitivity to cephalosporins.

Route/Dosage

Infection

ADULTS: **IV/IM** 1-2 g q 12 hr (life-threatening infections: up to 3 g q 12 hr) for 7-10 days.

Perioperative Prophylaxis

ADULTS: **IV** 1-2 g 30-60 min prior to surgery. In cesarean section, give dose as soon as umbilical cord is clamped.

Interactions

Alcohol: Acute alcohol intolerance (disulfiram-like reaction) may occur up to 3 days after last dose of cefotetan. *Aminoglycosides:* Increased risk of nephrotoxicity. *Anticoagulants, oral:* Increased anticoagulant effect; bleeding complications may occur. INCOMPATIBILITIES: Aminoglycosides: Do not add aminoglycosides to cefotetan solutions because inactivation of both drugs may result; administer at separate sites if concurrent therapy is indicated.

Lab Test Interferences

May cause false-positive urine glucose test results with Benedict's solution, Fehling's solution, or Clinitest tablets but not with enzyme-based tests (eg, Clinistix, Tes-tape); false-positive test result for proteinuria with acid and denaturization-precipitation tests; false-positive direct Coombs' test results in certain patients (eg, those with azotemia); false elevations in urinary 17-ketosteroid values. High concentrations may interfere with creatinine concentrations measured by the Jaffe reaction, producing false results; serum samples should not be analyzed for creatinine if obtained within 2 hr of drug administration.

Adverse Reactions

GI: Nausea; vomiting; diarrhea; anorexia; abdominal pain or cramps; flatulence; colitis, including pseudomembranous colitis. *GU:* Pyuria; renal dysfunction; dysuria; reversible interstitial nephritis; hematuria; toxic nephropathy. *HEMA:* Eosinophilia; neutropenia; lymphocytosis; leukocytosis; thrombocytopenia; decreased platelet function; anemia; aplastic anemia; hemorrhage. *HEPA:* Hepatic dysfunction; abnormal liver function test results. *OTHER:* Hypersensitivity, including Stevens-Johnson syndrome, erythema multiforme, toxic epidermal necrolysis; candidal overgrowth; serum sickness–like reactions (eg, skin rashes, polyarthritis; arthralgia, fever); phlebitis, thrombophlebitis and pain at injection site.

Precautions

Pregnancy: Category B. *Lactation:* Excreted in breast milk. *Children:* Safety and efficacy in children not established. *Hypersensitivity:* Reactions range from mild to life-threatening. Administer drug with caution to penicillin-sensitive patients due to possible cross-reactivity. *Pseudomembranous colitis:* Should be considered in patients who develop diarrhea. *Renal impairment:* Use drug with caution in patients with renal impairment. Dosage adjustment based on renal function may be required. *Superinfection:* May result in bacterial or fungal overgrowth of nonsusceptible microorganisms.

NURSING CONSIDERATIONS

Administration/Storage

- Reconstituted solution may be light yellow to amber. Do not administer if solution is cloudy or precipitate is present.
- For IM injection, drug may be reconstituted with 0.5% or 1% lidocaine without epinephrine to minimize pain on injection.
- When giving by IM route, inject deeply into large muscle (eg, upper outer quadrant of gluteus muscle or lateral thigh). Massage well.
- When giving by IV route, administer slowly over 3-5 min. Reconstituted drug may be diluted in 50-100 ml of D5W or 0.9% sodium chloride and infused over 20-30 min. Change IV sites q 48-72 hr.
- For perioperative prophylaxis, administer cefotetan 50-120 min before surgical incision.
- Store sterile powder at room temperature and protect from light.

Assessment/Interventions

- Obtain patient history, including drug history and any known allergies. Note allergy to cephalosporins or penicillins.
- Obtain specimens for culture and sensitivity before beginning therapy and periodically during treatment.

- Monitor renal function carefully during treatment.
- Monitor for coagulation abnormalities. Elevate prothrombin time or abnormal platelet count may occur. If bleeding occurs and PT is prolonged, vitamin K may be indicated.
- Monitor for signs of infection, especially fever, and for positive response to antibiotic therapy.
- Assess for signs and symptoms of anaphylaxis (shortness of breath, wheezing, laryngeal spasm). Have resuscitation equipment available.
- Assess for signs of superinfection, such as vaginitis or stomatitis.
- Assess for diarrhea with blood or pus, which may be symptom of pseudomembranous colitis. Symptoms may occur after antibiotic treatment.
- Monitor IV site for infiltration, infection and thrombophlebitis.

OVERDOSAGE: SIGNS & SYMPTOMS

Seizures

Patient/Family Education

- Instruct patient to check body temperature daily. If fever persists for more than a few days or if high fever (> 102°F) or shaking chills are noted, physician should be notified immediately.
- Advise patient to maintain normal fluid intake while using this medication.
- Advise patient not to drink alcoholic beverages or take alcohol-containing medications while taking cefamandole nafate and for several days after discontinuing drug.
- Advise diabetic patient to use enzyme-based tests (eg, Clinistix, Testape) for monitoring urine glucose because drug may give false results with other tests.
- Instruct patient to report these symptoms to physician: nausea, vomiting, diarrhea, skin rash, hives, sore throat, bruising, bleeding, muscle or joint pain.
- Warn patient that diarrhea that contains blood or pus may be a sign of serious disorders. Tell patient to seek medical care and not to treat at home.
- Instruct patient to seek emergency care if wheezing or difficulty in breathing occurs.
- Instruct patient to report signs of superinfection: black "furry" tongue, white patches in mouth, foul-smelling stools, vaginal itching or discharge.

See Patient Guide, p. 101.

Cefoxitin Sodium

(seff-OX-ih-tin SO-dee-uhm)

Mefoxin

Class: Antibiotic/cephalosporin

Action Inhibits mucopeptide synthesis in bacterial cell wall.

Indications Treatment of infections of lower respiratory tract, urinary tract, skin and skin structures, bone and joint; treatment of intra-abdominal infections, gynecological infections and septicemia due to susceptible microorganisms; perioperative prophylaxis.

Contraindications Hypersensitivity to cephalosporins.

Route/Dosage

Infection

ADULTS: **IV/IM** 1-2 g q 6-8 hr. CHILDREN ≥ 3 MO: **IV/IM** 80-160 mg/kg/day in divided doses q 4-6 hr (maximum 12 g/day).

Surgical Prophylaxis

ADULTS: **IV/IM** 2 g just prior to surgery then 2 g q 6 hr for 24 hr. CHILDREN ≥ 3 MO: **IV/IM** 30-40 mg/kg just prior to surgery then 30-40 mg/kg q 6 hr for 24 hr.

Interactions

Aminoglycosides: May increase

risk of nephrotoxicity. *Probenecid:* Inhibition of renal excretion of cefoxitin. INCOMPATIBILITIES: Do not add aminoglycosides to cefoxitin solutions because inactivation of both drugs may result; administer at separate sites if concurrent therapy is indicated.

Lab Test Interferences

May cause false-positive urine glucose test results with Benedict's solution, Fehling's solution, or Clinitest tablets but not with enzyme-based tests (eg, Clinistix, Tes-tape); false-positive test result for proteinuria with acid and denaturization-precipitation tests; false-positive direct Coombs' test result in certain patients (eg, those with azotemia); false elevations in urinary 17-ketosteroid values. High concentrations may interfere with creatinine concentrations measured by the Jaffe reaction, producing false results; serum samples should not be analyzed for creatinine if obtained within 2 hr of drug administration.

Adverse Reactions

CV: Hypotension. *GI:* Nausea; vomiting; diarrhea; colitis, including pseudomembranous colitis. *GU:* Renal dysfunction; elevated renal function tests; pyuria; dysuria; reversible interstitial nephritis; hematuria; toxic nephropathy. *HEMA:* Eosinophilia; neutropenia; lymphocytosis; leukocytosis; thrombocytopenia; decreased platelet function; anemia; hemolytic anemia; aplastic anemia; hemorrhage. *HEPA:* Hepatic dysfunction; jaundice; abnormal liver function test results. *OTHER:* Hypersensitivity, including Stevens-Johnson syndrome, erythema multiforme, toxic epidermal necrolysis; candidal overgrowth; serum sickness–like reactions (eg, skin rashes, polyarthritis; arthralgia, fever); phlebitis, thrombophlebitis and pain at injection site.

Precautions

Pregnancy: Category B. *Lactation:* Excreted in breast milk. *Children:* In children ≥ 3 mo, high doses of cefoxitin have been associated with increased incidence of eosinophilia and elevated AST. *Hypersensitivity:* Reactions range from mild to life-threatening. Administer drug with caution to penicillin-sensitive patients due to possible cross-reactivity. *Pseudomembranous colitis:* Should be considered in patients in whom diarrhea develops. *Renal impairment:* Use drug with caution. Dosage adjustment based on renal function may be required. *Superinfection:* May result in bacterial or fungal overgrowth of nonsusceptible microorganisms.

NURSING CONSIDERATIONS

Administration/Storage

- For IM administration reconstitute each gram with 2 ml of Sterile Water for Injection or 2 ml of 0.5% lidocaine without epinephrine to minimize discomfort. Inject deeply into large muscle (eg, gluteus or lateral thigh).
- For IV use, reconstitute each gram with 10 ml of Sterile Water for Injection. Administer slowly over 3-5 min. Reconstituted drug may be diluted in 50-100 ml of 0.9% Sodium Chloride or D5W and infused over 30 min.
- Change IV sites every 48-72 hr.
- Solutions are stable for 24 hr at room temperature and for 1 wk if refrigerated.
- May freeze medication. Thaw at room temperature. After thawing, discard unused portion. Do not refreeze. Do not administer if solution is cloudy or precipitate is present.

Assessment/Interventions

- Obtain patient history, including drug history and any known allergies. Note allergy to cephalosporins and penicillins.
- Obtain specimens for culture and sensitivity before beginning therapy and periodically during treatment.

- Monitor renal function carefully during treatment.
- Monitor for signs of infection, especially fever, and for positive response to antibiotic therapy.
- Monitor for coagulation abnormalities. Elevated prothrombin time or abnormal platelet count may occur. If bleeding occurs and PT is prolonged, vitamin K may be indicated.
- Assess for signs and symptoms of anaphylaxis (shortness of breath, wheezing, laryngeal spasm). Have resuscitation equipment available.
- Assess for signs of superinfection, such as vaginitis or stomatitis.
- Assess for diarrhea with blood or pus, which may be symptom of pseudomembranous colitis. Symptoms may occur after antibiotic treatment.
- Monitor IV site for vein irritation, infiltration, infection and thrombophlebitis.

OVERDOSAGE: SIGNS & SYMPTOMS

Seizures

Patient/Family Education

- Instruct patient to check body temperature daily. If fever persists for more than a few days or if high fever (> 102°F) or shaking chills are noted, physician should be notified immediately.
- Advise patient to maintain normal fluid intake while using this medication.
- Advise diabetic patient to use enzyme-based tests (eg, Clinistix, Tes-tape) for monitoring urine glucose because drug may give false results with other tests.
- Warn patient to report these symptoms to physician: nausea, vomiting, diarrhea, skin rash, hives, sore throat, bruising, bleeding, muscle or joint pain.
- Instruct patient to report signs of superinfection: black "furry" tongue, white patches in mouth, foul-smelling stools, vaginal itching or discharge.
- Warn patient that diarrhea that contains blood or pus may be a sign of serious disorders. Tell patient to seek medical care and not to treat at home.
- Instruct patient to seek emergency care if he or she experiences wheezing or difficulty breathing.

See Patient Guide, p. 102.

Cefpodoxime Proxetil

(SEF-pode-OX-eem PROX-uh-til)

Vantin

Class: Antibiotic/cephalosporin

Action Inhibits mucopeptide synthesis in bacterial cell wall.

Indications Treatment of infections of respiratory tract, urinary tract, skin and skin structures; treatment of sexually transmitted diseases due to susceptible strains of specific microorganisms.

Contraindications Hypersensitivity to cephalosporins.

Route/Dosage

ADULTS: PO 100-400 mg q 12 hr. CHILDREN 6 MO-12 YR: PO 10 mg/kg/day in divided doses q 12 hr (maximum 200 mg/dose).

Interactions

Probenecid: Inhibition of renal excretion of cefpodoxime.

Lab Test Interferences

May cause false-positive urine glucose test results with Benedict's solution, Fehling's solution, or Clinitest tablets but not with enzyme-based tests (eg, Clinistix, Tes-tape); false-positive test results for proteinuria with acid and denaturization-precipitation tests; false-positive direct Coombs' test result in certain patients (eg, those with azotemia); false elevations in urinary 17-ketosteroid values.

Adverse Reactions

GI: Nausea; vomiting; diarrhea;

anorexia; abdominal pain or cramps; flatulence; colitis, including pseudomembranous colitis. *GU:* Pyuria; renal dysfunction; dysuria; reversible interstitial nephritis; hematuria; toxic nephropathy. *HEMA:* Eosinophilia; neutropenia; lymphocytosis; leukocytosis; thrombocytopenia; decreased platelet function; anemia; aplastic anemia; hemorrhage. *HEPA:* Hepatic dysfunction; abnormal liver function test results. *OTHER:* Hypersensitivity, including Stevens-Johnson syndrome, erythema multiforme, toxic epidermal necrolysis; serum sickness–like reactions (eg, skin rashes, polyarthritis, arthralgia, fever); candidal overgrowth.

Precautions

Pregnancy: Category B. *Lactation:* Excreted in breast milk. *Children:* Consider benefits relative to risks. Safety and efficacy in children < 6 mo not established. *Hypersensitivity:* Reactions range from mild to life-threatening. Administer drug with caution to penicillin-sensitive patients due to possible cross-reactivity. *Pseudomembranous colitis:* Should be considered in patients in whom diarrhea develops. *Renal impairment:* Use drug with caution in patients with renal impairment. Dosage adjustment based on renal function may be required. *Superinfection:* May result in bacterial or fungal overgrowth of nonsusceptible microorganisms.

NURSING CONSIDERATIONS

Administration/Storage

- Administer with food to enhance absorption.
- Oral suspension must be refrigerated and will remain stable for up to 14 days. Do not freeze. Shake well before use.

Assessment/Interventions

- Obtain patient history, including drug history and any known allergies. Note renal impairment and allergy to cephalosporins or penicillins.
- Obtain specimens for culture and sensitivity before beginning therapy and periodically during treatment.
- Monitor renal function carefully during treatment.
- Monitor for signs of infection, especially fever, and for positive response to antibiotic therapy.
- Assess for signs and symptoms of anaphylaxis (shortness of breath, wheezing, laryngeal spasm). Have resuscitation equipment available.
- Assess patient for symptoms of superinfection, vaginitis or stomatitis.
- Assess for diarrhea with blood or pus, which may be symptom of pseudomembranous colitis. Symptoms may occur after antibiotic treatment.

OVERDOSAGE: SIGNS & SYMPTOMS

Seizures

Patient/Family Education

- Instruct patient to complete full course of therapy.
- Advise patient to take with food to enhance absorption.
- Remind patient to check body temperature daily. If fever persists for more than a few days or if high fever (> 102°F) or shaking chills are noted, physician should be notified immediately.
- Advise patient to maintain normal fluid intake while using this medication.
- Advise diabetic patient to use enzyme-based tests (eg, Clinistix, Testape) for monitoring urine glucose because drug may give false results with other tests.
- Instruct patient to report these symptoms to physician: nausea, vomiting, diarrhea, skin rash, hives, muscle or joint pain.
- Instruct patient to report signs of superinfection: black "furry" tongue, white patches in mouth, foul-smelling stools, vaginal itching or discharge.

- Warn patient that diarrhea that contains blood or pus may be a sign of serious disorders. Tell patient to seek medical care and not to treat at home.
- Instruct patient to seek emergency care immediately if wheezing or difficulty breathing occurs.

See Patient Guide, p. 103.

Cefprozil

(SEFF-pro-zill)

Cefzil

Class: Antibiotic/cephalosporin

Action Inhibits mucopeptide synthesis in bacterial cell wall.

Indications Treatment of infections of skin and skin structures, bronchitis, pharyngitis, tonsillitis and otitis media due to susceptible strains of specific microorganisms.

Contraindications Hypersensitivity to cephalosporins.

Route/Dosage

ADULTS: **PO** 250-500 mg q 12-24 hr. CHILDREN 6 MO-12 YR: **PO** 7.5-15 mg/kg q 12 hr.

Interactions

Probenecid: Inhibition of renal excretion of cefprozil.

Lab Test Interferences

May cause false-positive urine glucose test results with Benedict's solution, Fehling's solution, or Clinitest tablets but not with enzyme-based tests (eg, Clinistix, Tes-tape); false-positive test results for proteinuria with acid and denaturization-precipitation tests; false-positive direct Coombs' test result in certain patients (eg, those with azotemia); false elevations in urinary 17-ketosteroid values.

Adverse Reactions

CNS: Headache, dizziness; fatigue; paresthesia; confusion; nervousness; sleeplessness; insomnia. *GI:* Nausea; vomiting; diarrhea; abdominal pain or cramps; flatulence; colitis, including pseudomembranous colitis. *GU:* Genital pruritus; vaginitis; renal dysfunction. *HEMA:* Eosinophilia; neutropenia; lymphocytosis; leukocytosis; thrombocytopenia; decreased platelet function; anemia; aplastic anemia; hemorrhage. *HEPA:* Hepatic dysfunction; cholestatic jaundice; abnormal liver function test results. *OTHER:* Hypersensitivity, including Stevens-Johnson syndrome, erythema multiforme, toxic epidermal necrolysis; candidal overgrowth; serum sickness–like reactions (eg, skin rashes, polyarthritis; arthralgia, fever).

Precautions

Pregnancy: Category B. *Lactation:* Excreted in breast milk. *Children:* Safety and efficacy in children < 6 mo not established. *Hypersensitivity:* Reactions range from mild to life-threatening. Administer drug with caution to penicillin-sensitive patients due to possible cross-reactivity. *Pseudomembranous colitis:* Should be considered in patients in whom diarrhea develops. *Renal impairment:* Use drug with caution in patients with renal impairment. Dosage adjustment based on renal function may be required. *Superinfection:* May result in bacterial or fungal overgrowth of nonsusceptible microorganisms.

NURSING CONSIDERATIONS

Administration/Storage

- May be given without regard to meals. Administer with food or milk if GI upset occurs. Food slows but does not decrease absorption.
- Administer after hemodialysis because drug is partially removed by dialysis.
- After reconstitution, oral suspension must be refrigerated. Solution may be stored for up to 14 days in refrigerator. Do not freeze. Shake well before use.

- Store tablets at room temperature.

Assessment/Interventions

- Obtain patient history, including drug history and any known allergies. Note renal or hepatic impairment and allergy to cephalosporins or penicillins.
- Obtain specimens for culture and sensitivity before beginning therapy and periodically during treatment.
- Monitor renal function carefully during treatment.
- Monitor for signs of infection, especially fever, and for positive response to antibiotic therapy.
- Assess for signs and symptoms of anaphylaxis (shortness of breath, wheezing, laryngeal spasm). Have resuscitation equipment available.
- Assess for signs of superinfection, such as vaginitis or stomatitis.
- Assess for severe diarrhea with blood or pus, which may be symptom of pseudomembranous colitis. Symptoms may occur after antibiotic treatment.

OVERDOSAGE: SIGNS & SYMPTOMS

Seizures

Patient/Family Education

- Instruct patient to complete full course of therapy.
- Remind patient to check body temperature daily. If fever persists for more than a few days or if high fever (> 102°F) or shaking chills are noted, physician should be notified immediately.
- Advise patient to maintain normal fluid intake while using this medication.
- Remind diabetic patient to use enzyme-based tests (eg, Clinistix, Tes-tape) for monitoring urine glucose because drug may give false results with other tests.
- Advise patient to report these symptoms to physician: nausea, vomiting, diarrhea, skin rash, hives, muscle or joint pain.
- Instruct patient to report signs of superinfection: black "furry" tongue, white patches in mouth, foul-smelling stools, vaginal itching or discharge.
- Warn patient that diarrhea that contains blood or pus may be a sign of serious disorders. Tell patient to seek medical care and not to treat at home.
- Instruct patient to seek emergency care immediately if he or she experiences wheezing or difficulty breathing.
- Caution patient to avoid alcohol intake while taking medication.

See Patient Guide, p. 104.

Ceftazidime

(seff-TAZE-ih-deem)

Ceptaz, Fortaz, Tazicef, Tazidine

Class: Antibiotic/cephalosporin

Action Inhibits mucopeptide synthesis in bacterial cell wall.

Indications Treatment of infections of lower respiratory tract, skin and skin structures, urinary tract, bone and joint; treatment of gynecological infections; treatment of intra-abdominal infections; treatment of septicemia and meningitis due to susceptible strains of specific microorganisms.

Contraindications Hypersensitivity to cephalosporins.

Route/Dosage

ADULTS: **IV/IM** 250 mg-2 g q 8-12 hr. CHILDREN 1 MO-12 YR: **IV** 30-50 mg/kg q 8 hr (maximum: 6 g/day). NEONATES < 4 WK: **IV** 30 mg/kg q 12 hr.

Interactions

Aminoglycosides: Increased risk of nephrotoxicity. INCOMPATIBILITIES: Aminoglycosides: Do not add aminoglycosides to ceftazidime solutions because inactivation of both drugs may result; administer at separate sites if concurrent therapy is indicated. Sodium bicarbonate: Do not dilute ceftazidine with sodium bicarbonate.

Lab Test Interferences

May cause false-positive urine glucose test results with Benedict's solution, Fehling's solution, or Clinitest tablets but not with enzyme-based tests (eg, Clinistix, Tes-tape); false-positive test results for proteinuria with acid and denaturization-precipitation tests; false-positive direct Coombs' test result in certain patients (eg, those with azotemia); false elevations in urinary 17-ketosteroid values.

Adverse Reactions

GI: Nausea; vomiting; diarrhea; anorexia; abdominal pain or cramps; flatulence; colitis, including pseudomembranous colitis. *GU:* Pyuria; renal dysfunction; dysuria; reversible interstitial nephritis; hematuria; toxic nephropathy. *HEMA:* Eosinophilia; neutropenia; lymphocytosis; leukocytosis; thrombocytopenia; thrombocytosis; decreased platelet function; anemia; aplastic anemia; hemorrhage. *HEPA:* Hepatic dysfunction; cholestatic jaundice; abnormal liver function test results. *OTHER:* Hypersensitivity, including Stevens-Johnson syndrome, erythema multiforme, toxic epidermal necrolysis; candidal overgrowth; serum sickness–like reactions (eg, skin rashes, polyarthritis, arthralgia, fever); phlebitis; thrombophlebitis and pain at injection site.

Precautions

Pregnancy: Category B. *Lactation:* Excreted in breast milk. *Hypersensitivity:* Reactions range from mild to life-threatening. Administer drug with caution to penicillin-sensitive patients due to possible cross-reactivity. *Pseudomembranous colitis:* Should be considered in patients in whom diarrhea develops. *Renal impairment:* Use drug with caution in patients with renal impairment. Dosage adjustment based on renal function may be required. *Superinfection:* May result in bacterial or fungal overgrowth of nonsusceptible microorganisms.

NURSING CONSIDERATIONS

Administration/Storage

- Administer by parenteral route (IV or IM) only.
- Follow manufacturer's instructions for reconstitution and dilution.
- Reconstituted solution should be light yellow to amber; darkened solution or powder does not indicate altered potency. Do not administer if solution is cloudy or precipitate is present.
- When giving by IM route, add 3 ml diluent to 1-g vial to yield 280 mg/ml. Inject deeply into large muscle (eg, upper outer quadrant of gluteus muscle or lateral thigh); massage well.
- When giving by IV route, add 10 ml Sterile Water for Injection to 1-g vial to yield 280 mg/ml. Administer slowly over 3-5 min. Change IV sites q 48-72 hr.
- For intermittent infusions, reconstituted solution can be further diluted with 50-100 ml of D5W or 0.9% sodium chloride and infused over 30 min.
- Store sterile powder at room temperature and protect from light.
- When reconstituted with Sterile Water for Injection, solution is stable for 7 days if refrigerated and for 18-24 hr when stored at room temperature. If frozen immediately after reconstitution, solution is stable for 3 mo. Completely thaw frozen preparation at room temperature before use. After thawing, solution may be stored for 18-24 hr at room temperature or 4 days in refrigerator. Do not refreeze.

Assessment/Interventions

- Obtain patient history, including drug history and any known allergies. Note renal impairment and allergy to cephalosporins or penicillins.

- Obtain specimens for culture and sensitivity before beginning therapy and periodically during treatment.
- Monitor renal function carefully during treatment.
- Monitor for signs of infection, especially fever, and for positive response to antibiotic therapy.
- Assess for signs and symptoms of anaphylaxis (shortness of breath, wheezing, laryngeal spasm). Have resuscitation equipment available.
- Assess for signs of superinfection, such as vaginitis or stomatitis.
- Assess for diarrhea with blood or pus, which may be symptom of pseudomembranous colitis. Symptoms may occur after antibiotic treatment.
- Monitor IV site for infiltration, infection, thrombophlebitis and bleeding.

OVERDOSAGE: SIGNS & SYMPTOMS

Neuromuscular excitability, asterixis, seizures, encephalopathy

Patient/Family Education

- Remind patient to check body temperature daily. If fever persists for more than a few days or if high fever (> 102°F) or shaking chills are noted, physician should be notified immediately.
- Advise patient to maintain normal fluid intake while using this medication.
- Remind diabetic patient to use enzyme-based tests (eg, Clinistix, Testape) for monitoring urine glucose because drug may give false results with other tests.
- Advise patient to report these symptoms to physician: nausea, vomiting, diarrhea, skin rash, hives, sore throat, bruising, bleeding, muscle or joint pain.
- Instruct patient to report signs of superinfection: black "furry" tongue, white patches in mouth, foul-smelling stools, vaginal itching or discharge.
- Warn patient that diarrhea that contains blood or pus may be a sign of serious disorders. Tell patient to seek medical care and not to treat at home.
- Instruct patient to seek emergency care immediately if wheezing or difficulty breathing occurs.
- Advise patient not to drink alcoholic beverages or to take alcohol-containing medications while taking this medication and for several days after discontinuing it.

See Patient Guide, p. 105.

Ceftibuten

(seff-TIE-byoo-ten)

Cedax

Class: Antibiotic/cephalosporin

Action Inhibits mucopeptide synthesis in bacterial cell wall.

Indications Treatment of pharyngitis/tonsillitis caused by *S. pyogenes*, otitis media caused by *M. Catarrhalis*, *H. influenzae* (including beta-lactamase-producing strains) or *S. pyogenes*, and acute bacterial exacerbation of chronic bronchitis caused by *S. pneumoniae* (penicillin-susceptible strains), *H. influenzae* (including beta-lactamase-producing strains) or *M. catarrhalis* (including beta-lactamase-producing strains).

Contraindications Hypersensitivity to cephalosporins.

Route/Dosage

ADULTS & CHILDREN ≥ 12 YR: PO 400 mg QD for 10 days. CHILDREN < 12 YR: PO 9 mg/kg QD (maximum 400 mg) for 10 days. Give suspension 2 hours before or 1 hour after a meal.

Interactions None well documented.

Lab Test Interferences

May cause false-positive urine glucose test results with Benedict's solution, Fehling's solution or Clinitest tablets, but not with enzyme-based tests (eg, Clinistix, Test-tape); false-positive test results for proteinuria with acid and denaturization-precipitation tests; false-positive direct Coombs' test results in certain patients (eg, those with azotemia); false elevations in urinary 17-ketosteroid values.

Adverse Reactions

GI: Nausea; vomiting; diarrhea; anorexia; abdominal pain or cramps; flatulence; colitis. *GU:* Pyuria; dysuria; renal dysfunction; reversible interstitial nephritis; hematuria; toxic nephropathy. *HEMA:* Eosinophilia; neutropenia; lymphocytosis; leukocytosis; thrombocytopenia; decreased platelet function; anemia; aplastic anemia; hemorrhage. *HEPA:* Hepatic dysfunction; abnormal liver function test results. *OTHER:* Hypersensitivity, including Stevens-Johnson syndrome, erythema multiforme and toxic epidermal necrolysis; serum sickness-like reactions (eg, skin rash, polyarthritis, arthralgia, fever); candidal overgrowth.

Precautions

Pregnancy: Category B. *Lactation:* Undetermined. *Children:* In infants consider benefits relative to risks. Safety and efficacy in children < 6 MO not established. *Hypersensitivity:* Reactions range from mild to life-threatening. Administer drug with caution to penicillin-sensitive patients due to possible cross-sensitivity. *Pseudomembranous colitis:* Should be considered possibility in patients in whom diarrhea develops. *Renal impairment:* Use drug with caution in patients with renal impairment. Dosage adjustment based on renal function may be required. *Superinfection:* May result in bacterial or fungal overgrowth on non-susceptible microorganisms. *Hemodialysis patients:* A single 400 mg capsule or 9 mg/kg (maximum 400 mg) dose may be administered at the end of each hemodialysis session.

NURSING CONSIDERATIONS

Administration/Storage

- Administer oral suspension 2 hours before or 1 hour after meal.
- After mixing, the suspension may be kept for 14 days stored in refrigerator. Keep tightly closed. Shake well before use. Capsules may be stored at room temperature.

Assessment/Interventions

- Assess for hypersensitivity reaction or previous penicillin allergy.
- Assess renal function prior to starting therapy.
- Obtain specimens for culture and sensitivity before beginning therapy and periodically during treatment.
- Monitor for signs of infection, especially fever, and for positive response to antibiotic therapy.
- Assess for signs and symptoms of anaphylaxis. Have resuscitation equipment available.
- Assess for signs of superinfection, such as vaginitis or stomatitis.
- Assess for severe diarrhea with blood or pus, which may be symptom of pseudomembranous colitis. Symptoms may occur after antibiotic treatment is discontinued.

OVERDOSAGE: SIGNS & SYMPTOMS

Seizures

Patient/Family Education

- Inform diabetic patients that oral suspension contains 1 gm sucrose/teaspoon of suspension.
- Instruct patient to complete full course of therapy.
- Have patient take drug with food or milk to avoid GI upset.
- Notify healthcare provider if patient has penicillin allergy or cephalosporin allergy.
- Notify healthcare provider of nausea, vomiting or diarrhea, especially if severe or contains blood, mucus or pus.
- Remind diabetic patient to use an enzyme-based test for urine glucose or

may otherwise obtain a false-positive result.

- Remind patient to check body temperature daily. If fever persists for more than a few days or if high fever (> 102°F) or shaking chills are noted, physician should be notified.
- Instruct patient to report signs of superinfection: black "furry" tongue, white patches in mouth, foul-smelling stools, vaginal itching or discharge.
- Instruct patient to seek emergency care if he or she experiences wheezing or difficulty breathing.

See Patient Guide, p. 106.

Ceftizoxime Sodium

(SEFF-tih-ZOX-eem SO-dee-uhm)

Cefizox

Class: Antibiotic/cephalosporin

Action Inhibits mucopeptide synthesis in bacterial cell wall.

Indications Treatment of infections of lower respiratory tract, urinary tract, skin and skin structures, bone and joint; treatment of intra-abdominal infections, pelvic inflammatory disease, gonorrhea, septicemia and meningitis due to susceptible microorganisms.

Contraindications Hypersensitivity to cephalosporins.

Route/Dosage
ADULTS: **IV/IM** 1-2 g q 8-12 hr (life-threatening infections: **IV** up to 2 g q 4 hr or 3-4 g q 8 hr). CHILDREN > 6 MO: **IV/IM** 50 mg/kg q 6-8 hr up to 200 mg/kg/day (maximum 12 g/day).

Interactions
Aminoglycosides: Increased risk of nephrotoxicity. *Probenecid:* Inhibition of renal excretion of ceftizoxime. INCOMPATIBILITIES: Aminoglycosides: Do not add aminoglycosides to ceftizoxime solutions because inactivation of both drugs may result; administer at separate sites if concurrent therapy is indicated.

Lab Test Interferences
May cause false-positive urine glucose test results with Benedict's solution, Fehling's solution, or Clinitest tablets but not with enzyme-based tests (eg, Clinistix, Tes-tape); false-positive test results for proteinuria with acid and denaturization-precipitation tests; false-positive direct Coombs' test results in certain patients (eg, those with azotemia); false elevations in urinary 17-ketosteroid values.

Adverse Reactions
GI: Nausea; vomiting; diarrhea; anorexia; abdominal pain or cramps; flatulence; colitis, including pseudomembranous colitis. *GU:* Pyuria; renal dysfunction; dysuria; reversible interstitial nephritis; hematuria; toxic nephropathy. *HEMA:* Eosinophilia; neutropenia; lymphocytosis; leukocytosis; thrombocytopenia; decreased platelet function; anemia; aplastic anemia; hemorrhage. *HEPA:* Hepatic dysfunction; abnormal liver function test results. *OTHER:* Hypersensitivity, including Stevens-Johnson syndrome, erythema multiforme, toxic epidermal necrolysis; candidal overgrowth; serum sickness–like reactions (eg, skin rashes, polyarthritis, arthralgia, fever); phlebitis; thrombophlebitis and pain at injection site.

Precautions
Pregnancy: Category B. *Lactation:* Excreted in breast milk. *Children:* Safety and efficacy in infants < 6 mo not established. In infants, consider benefits relative to risks. *Hypersensitivity:* Reactions range from mild to life-threatening. Administer drug with caution to penicillin-sensitive patients due to possible cross-reactivity. *Pseudomembranous colitis:* Should be considered in patients who develop diarrhea. *Renal impairment:* Use drug with caution in patients with baseline renal impair-

ment. Dosage adjustment based on renal function may be required. *Superinfection:* May result in bacterial or fungal overgrowth of nonsusceptible microorganisms.

NURSING CONSIDERATIONS

Administration/Storage

- IV route may be preferable for life-threatening infections.
- Administer after hemodialysis, because drug is partially removed by dialysis.
- When giving by IM route, inject deeply into large muscle (eg, upper outer quadrant of gluteus muscle or lateral thigh); massage well. For amounts > 2 g, divide dose and administer in different muscle masses.
- Reconstituted solution should be light yellow to amber. Do not administer if solution is cloudy or precipitate is present.
- When giving by IV route, administer slowly over 3-5 min using direct (bolus) injection. Change IV sites q 48-72 hr.
- When drug is administered by intermittent IV infusion, reconstituted solution can be further diluted with 50-100 ml of 0.9% Sodium Chloride or D5W and infused over 30 min.
- Completely thaw frozen preparations at room temperature before use. Do not introduce additives. After thawing, solution is stable for 24 hr at room temperature or for 10 days if refrigerated. Do not refreeze.
- Store sterile powder at room temperature and protect from light.
- Reconstituted solution is stable for 96 hr if refrigerated and 24 hr when stored at room temperature.

Assessment/Interventions

- Obtain patient history, including drug history and any known allergies. Note renal impairment and allergy to cephalosporins or penicillins.
- Obtain specimens for culture and sensitivity before beginning therapy and periodically during treatment.
- Monitor renal function carefully during treatment.
- Monitor for signs of infection, especially fever, and for positive response to antibiotic therapy.
- Assess for signs and symptoms of anaphylaxis (shortness of breath, wheezing, laryngeal spasm). Have resuscitation equipment available.
- Assess for signs of superinfection, such as vaginitis or stomatitis.
- Assess for severe diarrhea with blood or pus, which may be symptom of pseudomembranous colitis. Symptoms may occur after antibiotic treatment.
- Monitor IV site for infiltration, infection, thrombophlebitis and bleeding.

OVERDOSAGE: SIGNS & SYMPTOMS

Seizures

Patient/Family Education

- Remind patient to check body temperature daily. If fever persists for more than a few days or if high fever (> 102°F) or shaking chills are noted, physician should be notified immediately.
- Advise patient to maintain normal fluid intake while using this medication.
- Instruct diabetic patient to use enzyme-based tests (eg, Clinistix, Tes-tape) for monitoring urine glucose because drug may give false results with other tests.
- Advise patient to report these symptoms to physician: nausea, vomiting, diarrhea, sore throat, bruising, bleeding, hives, bone or joint pain.
- Instruct patient to report signs of superinfection: black "furry" tongue, white patches in mouth, foul-smelling stools, vaginal itching or discharge.
- Warn patient that diarrhea that contains blood or pus may be a sign of

serious disorders. Tell patient to seek medical care and not to treat at home.
- Instruct patient to seek emergency care immediately if wheezing or difficulty in breathing occurs.
- Advise patient to avoid ingesting alcohol.

See Patient Guide, p. 107.

Ceftriaxone Sodium

(SEFF-TRY-AXE-own SO-dee-uhm)

Rocephin

Class: Antibiotic/cephalosporin

Action Inhibits mucopeptide synthesis in bacterial cell wall.

Indications Treatment of infections of lower respiratory tract, skin and skin structures, bone and joint, urinary tract; treatment of pelvic inflammatory disease, intra-abdominal infections, gonorrhea, meningitis and septicemia due to susceptible microorganisms; preoperative prophylaxis. **Unlabeled use:** Treatment of Lyme disease in patients refractory to penicillin G.

Contraindications Hypersensitivity to cephalosporins.

Route/Dosage

Infection

ADULTS: **IV/IM** 1-2 g/day or in equally divided doses q 12 hr (maximum 4 g/day). CHILDREN: **IV/IM** 50-75 mg/kg/day in equally divided doses q 12 hr (maximum 2 g/day).

Uncomplicated Gonococcal Infections

ADULTS: **IM** 250 mg as single dose.

Surgical Prophylaxis

ADULTS: **IV/IM** 1 g as single dose ½-2 hr before surgery.

Pediatric Meningitis

CHILDREN: **IV/IM** 75 mg/kg as loading dose then 100 mg/kg/day in divided doses q 12 hr (maximum 4 g/day).

Interactions

Aminoglycosides: Increased risk of nephrotoxicity. INCOMPATIBILITIES: Other antimicrobial drugs.

Lab Test Interferences

May cause false-positive urine glucose test result with Benedict's solution, Fehling's solution, or Clinitest tablets but not with enzyme-based tests (eg, Clinistix, Tes-tape); false-positive test results for proteinuria with acid and denaturization-precipitation tests; false-positive direct Coombs' test results in certain patients (eg, those with azotemia); false elevations in urinary 17-ketosteroid values.

Adverse Reactions

GI: Nausea; vomiting; diarrhea; colitis, including pseudomembranous colitis. *GU:* Renal dysfunction; pyuria; dysuria; reversible interstitial nephritis; hematuria; toxic nephropathy, urinary casts. *HEMA:* Eosinophilia; neutropenia; lymphocytosis; leukocytosis; thrombocytopenia; decreased platelet function; anemia; aplastic anemia; hemorrhage. *HEPA:* Hepatic dysfunction; jaundice; abnormal liver function test results. *OTHER:* Hypersensitivity, including Stevens-Johnson syndrome, erythema multiforme, toxic epidermal necrolysis; candidal overgrowth; serum sickness–like reactions (eg, skin rashes, polyarthritis; arthralgia, fever); phlebitis, thrombophlebitis and pain at injection site.

Precautions

Pregnancy: Category B. *Lactation:* Excreted in breast milk. *Children:* Cephalosporins may accumulate in neonates. *Hypersensitivity:* Reactions range from mild to life-threatening. Administer drug with caution to penicillin-sensitive patients due to possible cross-reactivity. *Pseudomembranous colitis:* Should be considered in patients in whom diarrhea develops. *Superinfection:* May result in bacterial or fungal overgrowth of nonsusceptible microorganisms.

NURSING CONSIDERATIONS

Administration/Storage

- Reconstituted solution should be light yellow to amber. Do not administer if solution is cloudy or precipitate is present.
- When giving by IM route, inject deeply into large muscle (eg, upper outer quadrant of gluteus muscle or lateral thigh); massage well.
- When giving by IV route, administer slowly over 3-5 min. Change IV sites q 48-72 hr.
- Reconstituted drug should not be mixed with other antibiotics.
- For piggyback infusion, reconstituted solution may be diluted with D5W or 0.9% Sodium Chloride infused over 30-60 min.
- For preoperative surgical prophylaxis, administer ceftriaxone 50-120 min before surgical incision.
- When reconstituted with 250 ml of diluent, use within 24 hr when stored at room temperature and within 3 days if refrigerated.
- When reconstituted with 100 ml of Sterile Water for Injection, 0.9% Sodium Chloride or 5% Dextrose, use within 3 days when stored at room temperature and within 10 days if refrigerated.
- Completely thaw frozen preparations at room temperature before use; do not refreeze.
- Store sterile powder at room temperature and protect from heat or light.

Assessment/Interventions

- Obtain patient history, including drug history and any known allergies. Note allergy to cephalosporins or penicillins.
- Obtain specimens for culture and sensitivity before beginning therapy and periodically during treatment.
- Monitor renal function carefully during treatment.
- Monitor for signs of infection, especially fever, and for positive response to antibiotic therapy.
- Assess for signs and symptoms of anaphylaxis (shortness of breath, wheezing, laryngeal spasm). Have resuscitation equipment available.
- Assess for signs of superinfection, such as vaginitis or stomatitis.
- Assess for diarrhea with blood or pus, which may be symptom of pseudomembranous colitis. Symptoms may occur after antibiotic treatment.
- Monitor for coagulation abnormalities. Elevated prothrombin time or abnormal platelet count may occur. If bleeding occurs and PT is prolonged, vitamin K may be indicated.
- Monitor IV site for infiltration, infection, thrombophlebitis and bleeding.

OVERDOSAGE: SIGNS & SYMPTOMS

Seizures

Patient/Family Education

- Remind patient to check body temperature daily. If fever persists for more than a few days or if high fever (> 102°F) or shaking chills are noted, physician should be notified immediately.
- Advise patient to maintain normal fluid intake while using this medication.
- Instruct diabetic patient to use enzyme-based tests (eg, Clinistix, Tes-tape) for monitoring urine glucose because drug may give false results with other tests.
- Instruct patient to report these symptoms to physician: nausea, vomiting, diarrhea, skin rash, hives, sore throat, bruising, bleeding, muscle or joint pain.
- Advise patient to report signs of superinfection: black "furry" tongue, white patches in mouth, foul-smelling stools, vaginal itching or discharge.
- Warn patient that diarrhea that contains blood or pus may be a sign of serious disorders. Tell patient to seek medical care and not to treat at home.
- Instruct patient to seek emergency care immediately if wheezing or difficulty in breathing occurs.

See Patient Guide, p. 108.

Cefuroxime

(SEFF-yur-OX-eem)
Ceftin, Kefurox, Zinacef
Class: Antibiotic/cephalosporin

Action Inhibits mucopeptide synthesis in bacterial cell wall.

Indications
Oral form: Treatment of infections of lower respiratory tract, urinary tract, skin and skin structures; treatment of uncomplicated gonorrhea, otitis media, pharyngitis and tonsillitis due to susceptible strains of specific microorganisms. *Parenteral form:* Treatment of infections of lower respiratory tract, urinary tract, skin and skin structures, bone and joint; preoperative prophylaxis; treatment of septicemia, gonorrhea and meningitis due to susceptible strains of specific microorganisms.

Contraindications Hypersensitivity to cephalosporins.

Route/Dosage
Infection
ADULTS & CHILDREN ≥ 12 YR: **PO** 125-500 mg bid. **IV/IM** 750 mg-1.5 g q 8 hr. CHILDREN < 12 YR: **PO** 125-250 mg bid. INFANTS & CHILDREN (> 3 MO): **IV/IM** 50-150 mg/kg/day (not to exceed adult dose) in equally divided doses q 6-8 hr.

Bacterial Meningitis
ADULTS & CHILDREN ≥ 12 YR: **IV/IM** Up to 3 g q 8 hr. INFANTS & CHILDREN 3 MO-12 YR: **IV/IM** 200-240 mg/kg/day in divided doses q 6-8 hr.

Uncomplicated Gonorrhea
ADULTS & CHILDREN ≥ 12 YR: **PO** 1 g as single dose. **IM** 1.5 g as single dose.

Preoperative Prophylaxis
ADULTS: **IV/IM** 1.5 g ½-1 hr before surgery then 750 mg q 8 hr for duration of surgery.

Interactions
Aminoglycosides: Increased risk of nephrotoxicity with parenteral cefuroxime. *Probenecid:* Inhibition of renal excretion of cefuroxime. INCOMPATIBILITIES: Aminoglycosides: Do not add aminoglycosides to cefuroxime solutions because inactivation of both drugs may result; administer at separate sites if concurrent therapy is indicated.

Lab Test Interferences
May cause false-positive urine glucose test results with Benedict's solution, Fehling's solution, or Clinitest tablets but not with enzyme-based tests (eg, Clinistix, Tes-tape); false-positive test results for proteinuria with acid and denaturization-precipitation tests; false-positive direct Coombs' test results in certain patients (eg, those with azotemia); false elevations in urinary 17-ketosteroid values; false-negative reaction in ferricyanide test for blood glucose.

Adverse Reactions
GI: Nausea; vomiting; diarrhea; anorexia; abdominal pain or cramps; flatulence; colitis, including pseudomembranous colitis. *GU:* Pyuria; renal dysfunction; dysuria; reversible interstitial nephritis; hematuria; toxic nephropathy. *HEMA:* Eosinophilia; neutropenia; lymphocytosis; leukocytosis; thrombocytopenia; decreased platelet function; anemia; aplastic anemia; hemorrhage. *HEPA:* Hepatic dysfunction; abnormal liver function test results. *OTHER:* Hypersensitivity, including Stevens-Johnson syndrome, erythema multiforme, toxic epidermal necrolysis; candidal overgrowth; serum sickness–like reactions (eg, skin rashes, polyarthritis, arthralgia, fever); phlebitis, thrombophlebitis and pain at injection site.

Precautions
Pregnancy: Category B. *Lactation:* Excreted in breast milk. *Children:* Safety and efficacy in children < 3 mo not established. *Hypersensitivity:* Reac-

tions range from mild to life-threatening. Administer drug with caution to penicillin-sensitive patients due to possible cross-reactivity. *Pseudomembranous colitis:* Should be considered in patients in whom diarrhea develops. *Renal impairment:* Use drug with caution in patients with renal impairment. Dosage adjustment based on renal function may be required. *Superinfection:* May result in bacterial or fungal overgrowth of nonsusceptible microorganisms.

NURSING CONSIDERATIONS

Administration/Storage

- Sodium salt is for parenteral administration. Axetil salt is for oral administration.
- Administer oral form with food to enhance absorption.
- May crush and mix with food or beverages; however, crushed tablets have strong, persistent bitter taste. Consider alternative therapy if children cannot swallow whole tablets.
- Reconstituted solution should be light yellow to amber. Do not administer if solution is cloudy or precipitate is present.
- When giving by IM route, shake IM suspension gently before administration. Aspirate to prevent injection into blood vessel. Inject deeply into large muscle (eg, upper outer quadrant of gluteus muscle or lateral thigh); massage well. Rotate injection sites.
- When giving by IV route, use direct intermittent infusion. Administer slowly over 3-5 min. Change IV sites q 48-72 hr.
- For intermittent IV infusion with Y-type administration set, administer over 30 min. and temporarily stop other solutions at Y-site.
- For continuous infusion, reconstituted solution may be further diluted with D5W or 0.9% Sodium Chloride.
- Reconstituted solution is stable for 24 hr at room temperature. When refrigerated, solution in vials is stable for 48 hr; IV solution is stable for 7 days when refrigerated.
- Completely thaw frozen solution at room temperature before use; do not refreeze.
- Do not add supplementary medication to premixed solution.
- Store sterile powder at room temperature and protect from light.
- Store tablets at room temperature.

Assessment/Interventions

- Obtain patient history, including drug history and any known allergies. Note renal impairment and allergy to cephalosporins or penicillins.
- Obtain specimens for culture and sensitivity before beginning therapy and periodically during treatment.
- Monitor renal function carefully during treatment.
- Monitor for signs of infection, especially fever, and for positive response to antibiotic therapy.
- Assess for signs and symptoms of anaphylaxis (shortness of breath, wheezing, laryngeal spasm). Have resuscitation equipment available.
- Assess for signs of superinfection, such as vaginitis or stomatitis.
- Assess for diarrhea with blood or pus, which may be symptom of pseudomembranous colitis. Symptoms may occur after antibiotic treatment.
- Monitor IV site for infiltration, infection and thrombophlebitis.

OVERDOSAGE: SIGNS & SYMPTOMS

Seizures

Patient/Family Education

- Instruct patient to complete full course of therapy.
- Advise patient to take with meals to enhance absorption. If tablet must be crushed, mix with food or beverage.
- Advise parent to contact physician if child is unable to tolerate crushed tablet with food or beverage.
- Remind patient to check body temperature daily. If fever persists for

more than a few days or if high fever (> 102°F) or shaking chills are noted, physician should be notified immediately.
- Advise patient to maintain normal fluid intake while using this medication.
- Advise diabetic patient to use enzyme-based tests (eg, Clinistix, Tes-tape) for monitoring urine glucose because drug may give false results with other tests.
- Instruct patient to report these symptoms to physician: nausea, vomiting, diarrhea, skin rash, sore throat, bruising, hives, muscle or joint pain.
- Instruct patient to report signs of superinfection: black "furry" tongue, white patches in mouth, foul-smelling stools, vaginal itching or discharge.
- Warn patient that diarrhea that contains blood or pus may be a sign of serious disorders. Tell patient to seek medical care and not to treat at home.
- Instruct patient to seek emergency care immediately if wheezing or difficulty breathing occurs.

See Patient Guide, pp. 109-110.

Cephalexin

(seh-fuh-LEX-in)

Biocef, Keflex, Keftab, ♣ *APO-Cephalex, Novolexin, Nu-Cephalex*

Class: Antibiotic/cephalosporin

Action Inhibits mucopeptide synthesis in bacterial cell wall.

Indications Treatment of infections of respiratory tract, urinary tract, skin and skin structures and bone; treatment of otitis media due to susceptible strains of specific microorganisms.

Contraindications Hypersensitivity to cephalosporins.

Route/Dosage

ADULTS: **PO** 1-4 g/day in divided doses (maximum 4 g/day). CHILDREN: **PO** (cephalexin monohydrate only) 25-100 mg/kg/day in divided doses.

Interactions

Probenecid: Inhibition of renal excretion of cephalexin.

Lab Test Interferences

May cause false-positive urine glucose test results with Benedict's solution, Fehling's solution, or Clinitest tablets but not with enzyme-based tests (eg, Clinistix, Tes-tape); false-positive test results for proteinuria with acid and denaturization-precipitation tests; false-positive direct Coombs' test results in certain patients (eg, those with azotemia); false elevations in urinary 17-ketosteroid values.

Adverse Reactions

GI: Nausea; vomiting; diarrhea; anorexia; abdominal pain or cramps; flatulence; colitis, including pseudomembranous colitis. *GU:* Pyuria; renal dysfunction; dysuria; reversible interstitial nephritis; hematuria; toxic nephropathy. *HEMA:* Eosinophilia; neutropenia; lymphocytosis; leukocytosis; thrombocytopenia; decreased platelet function; anemia; aplastic anemia; hemorrhage. *HEPA:* Hepatic dysfunction; abnormal liver function test results. *OTHER:* Hypersensitivity, including Stevens-Johnson syndrome, erythema multiforme, toxic epidermal necrolysis; candidal overgrowth; serum sickness–like reactions (eg, skin rash, polyarthritis, arthralgia, fever).

Precautions

Pregnancy: Category B. *Lactation:* Excreted in breast milk. *Children:* Safety and efficacy of cephalexin HCl monohydrate (Keftab) in children not established. Cephalosporins may accumulate in neonates. *Hypersensitivity:* Reactions range from mild to life-threatening. Administer drug with caution to penicillin-sensitive patients due to possible cross-reactivity. *Pseudomem-*

branous colitis: Should be considered in patients in whom diarrhea develops. *Renal impairment:* Use drug with caution in patients with renal impairment. Dosage adjustment based on renal function may be required. *Superinfection:* May result in bacterial or fungal overgrowth of nonsusceptible microorganisms.

NURSING CONSIDERATIONS

Administration/Storage

- Administer with food or milk if GI upset occurs. Food slows but does not decrease absorption.
- Shake oral suspension well before administering. Space doses evenly around clock.
- Oral suspension is stable up to 14 days after reconstitution when refrigerated.
- Store capsules and tablets at room temperature.

Assessment/Interventions

- Obtain patient history, including drug history and any known allergies. Note renal impairment and allergy to cephalosporins or penicillins.
- Obtain specimens for culture and sensitivity before beginning therapy and periodically during treatment.
- Monitor renal function carefully during treatment.
- Monitor for signs of infection, especially fever, and positive response to antibiotic therapy.
- Assess for signs and symptoms of anaphylaxis (shortness of breath, wheezing, laryngeal spasm). Have resuscitation equipment available.
- Assess for signs of superinfection, such as vaginitis or stomatitis.
- Assess for diarrhea with blood or pus, which may be symptom of pseudomembranous colitis. Symptoms may occur after antibiotic treatment.

OVERDOSAGE: SIGNS & SYMPTOMS

Seizures

Patient/Family Education

- Instruct patient to complete full course of therapy.
- Advise patient to take with food or milk if GI distress occurs.
- Remind patient to check body temperature daily. If fever persists for more than a few days or if high fever (> 102°F) or shaking chills are noted, physician should be notified immediately.
- Advise patient to maintain normal fluid intake while using this medication.
- Advise diabetic patient to use enzyme-based tests (eg, Clinistix, Testape) for monitoring urine glucose because drug may give false results with other tests.
- Instruct patient to report these symptoms to physician: nausea, vomiting, diarrhea, skin rash, hives, muscle or joint pain.
- Instruct patient to report signs of superinfection: black "furry" tongue, white patches in mouth, foul-smelling stools, vaginal itching or discharge.
- Warn patient that diarrhea that contains blood or pus may be a sign of serious disorders. Tell patient to seek medical care and not to treat at home.
- Instruct patient to seek emergency care immediately if wheezing or difficulty breathing occurs.

See Patient Guide, p. 111.

Cephalothin Sodium

(seff-AY-low-thin SO-dee-uhm)
Keflin
Class: Antibiotic/cephalosporin

Action Inhibits mucopeptide synthesis in bacterial cell wall.

Indications Treatment of infections of respiratory tract, urinary tract, skin and soft tissue, bone and joint; treatment of GI infections, meningitis and septicemia due to susceptible strains of specific microorganisms; perioperative prophylaxis.

Contraindications Hypersensitivity to cephalosporins.

Route/Dosage

Infection

ADULTS: **IV/IM** 500 mg-2 g q 4-6 hr. INFANTS & CHILDREN: **IV/IM** 80-160 mg/kg/day in divided doses.

Perioperative Prophylaxis

ADULTS: **IV** 1-2 g ½-1 hr before surgery then 1-2 g q 6 hr for 24 hr. CHILDREN: **IV** 20-30 mg/kg ½-1 hr before surgery then q 6 hr for 24 hr.

Interactions

Aminoglycosides: Increased risk of nephrotoxicity. *Probenecid:* Inhibition of renal excretion of cephalothin. INCOMPATIBILITIES: Aminoglycosides, bleomycin, calcium salts, diphenhydramine, erythromycin, penicillin, ranitidine. Syringe: metoclopramide.

Lab Test Interferences

May cause false-positive urine glucose test results with Benedict's solution, Fehling's solution, or Clinitest tablets but not with enzyme-based tests (eg, Clinistix, Tes-tape); false-positive test results for proteinuria with acid and denaturization-precipitation tests; false-positive direct Coombs' test results in certain patients (eg, those with azotemia); false elevations in urinary 17-ketosteroid values. High concentrations of cephalothin may interfere with creatinine concentrations measured by the Jaffe reaction, producing false results.

Adverse Reactions

GI: Nausea; vomiting; diarrhea; anorexia; abdominal pain or cramps; flatulence; colitis, including pseudomembranous colitis. *GU:* Pyuria; renal dysfunction; dysuria; reversible interstitial nephritis; hematuria; toxic nephropathy. *HEMA:* Eosinophilia; neutropenia; lymphocytosis; leukocytosis; thrombocytopenia; decreased platelet function; anemia; aplastic anemia; hemorrhage. *HEPA:* Hepatic dysfunction; abnormal liver function test results. *OTHER:* Hypersensitivity, including Stevens-Johnson syndrome, erythema multiforme, toxic epidermal necrolysis; candidal overgrowth; serum sickness–like reactions (eg, skin rashes, polyarthritis, arthralgia, fever); phlebitis, thrombophlebitis and pain at injection site.

Precautions

Pregnancy: Category B. *Lactation:* Excreted in breast milk. *Children:* In infants, consider benefits relative to risks. Cephalosporins may accumulate in neonates. *Hypersensitivity:* Reactions range from mild to life-threatening. Administer drug with caution to penicillin-sensitive patients due to possible cross-reactivity. *Pseudomembranous colitis:* Should be considered in patients in whom diarrhea develops. *Renal impairment:* Use drug with caution in patients with renal impairment. Dosage adjustment based on renal function may be required. *Superinfection:* May result in bacterial or fungal overgrowth of nonsusceptible microorganisms.

NURSING CONSIDERATIONS

Administration/Storage

- Reconstituted solution should be light yellow to amber; darkened solution does not indicate altered potency. Do not administer if solution is cloudy or precipitate is present.
- When giving by IM route, inject deeply into large muscle (eg, upper outer quadrant of gluteus muscle or lateral thigh); massage well. Rotate injection sites.
- When giving by IV route, administer slowly by direct infusion over 3-5 min or by intermittent infusion. Change IV site q 48-72 hr.
- For intermittent IV infusion, slowly

inject solution of 1 g in 10 ml of diluent directly into vein over 3-5 min or give through IV tubing.
- Administer solution for IM and intermittent IV infusion within 12 hr after reconstitution. For prolonged IV infusion, replace freshly prepared solution q 24 hr.
- Reconstituted solution retains potency for 96 hr when refrigerated.

Assessment/Interventions
- Obtain patient history, including drug history and any known allergies. Note renal impairment and allergy to cephalosporins or penicillins.
- Obtain specimens for culture and sensitivity before beginning therapy and periodically during treatment.
- Monitor renal function carefully during treatment.
- Monitor for signs of infection, especially fever, and for positive response to antibiotic therapy.
- Assess for signs and symptoms of anaphylaxis (shortness of breath, wheezing, laryngeal spasm). Have resuscitation equipment available.
- Assess for signs of superinfection, such as vaginitis or stomatitis.
- Assess for diarrhea with blood or pus, which may be symptom of pseudomembranous colitis. Symptoms may occur after antibiotic treatment.
- Monitor IV site for signs of infiltration, infection and thrombophlebitis.

OVERDOSAGE: SIGNS & SYMPTOMS
Seizures

Patient/Family Education
- Remind patient to check body temperature daily. If fever persists for more than a few days or if high fever (> 102°F) or shaking chills are noted, physician should be notified immediately.
- Advise patient to maintain normal fluid intake while using this medication.
- Instruct patient to report signs of superinfection: black "furry" tongue, white patches in mouth, foul-smelling stools, vaginal itching or discharge.

See Patient Guide, p. 112.

Cephapirin Sodium

(SEFF-uh-PIE-rin SO-dee-uhm)

Cefadyl

Class: Antibiotic/cephalosporin

Action Inhibits mucopeptide synthesis in bacterial cell wall.

Indications Treatment of infections of respiratory tract, urinary tract, skin and skin structures; treatment of endocarditis, osteomyelitis, septicemia due to susceptible strains of specific microorganisms; perioperative prophylaxis.

Contraindications Hypersensitivity to cephalosporins.

Route/Dosage

Infection

ADULTS: **IV/IM** 500 mg-2 g q 4-6 hr. (serious or life-threatening infections: up to 12 g/day). CHILDREN > 3 MO: **IV/IM** 40-80 mg/kg/day in 4 equally divided doses.

Perioperative Prophylaxis

ADULTS: **IV/IM** 1-2 g ½-1 hr before surgery then 1-2 g q 6 hr for 24 hr.

Interactions

Aminoglycosides: Increased risk of nephrotoxicity. *Probenecid:* Inhibition of renal excretion of cephapirin.

Lab Test Interferences

May cause false-positive urine glucose test results with Benedict's solution, Fehling's solution, or Clinitest tablets but not with enzyme-based tests (eg, Clinistix, Tes-tape); false-positive test results for proteinuria with acid and denaturization-precipitation tests; false-positive direct Coombs' test result in certain patients (eg, those with azotemia); false elevations in urinary 17-ketosteroid values.

Adverse Reactions

GI: Nausea; vomiting; diarrhea; anorexia; abdominal pain or cramps; flatulence; colitis, including pseudomembranous colitis. *GU:* Pyuria; renal dysfunction; dysuria; reversible interstitial nephritis; hematuria; toxic nephropathy. *HEMA:* Eosinophilia; neutropenia; lymphocytosis; leukocytosis; thrombocytopenia; decreased platelet function; anemia; aplastic anemia; hemorrhage. *HEPA:* Hepatic dysfunction; abnormal liver function test results. *OTHER:* Hypersensitivity, including Stevens-Johnson syndrome, erythema multiforme, toxic epidermal necrolysis; candidal overgrowth; serum sickness–like reactions (eg, skin rashes, polyarthritis, arthralgia, fever); phlebitis, thrombophlebitis and pain at injection site.

Precautions

Pregnancy: Category B. *Lactation:* Excreted in breast milk. *Children:* In infants, consider benefits relative to risks. Cephalosporins may accumulate in neonates. *Hypersensitivity:* Reactions range from mild to life-threatening. Administer drug with caution to penicillin-sensitive patients due to possible cross-reactivity. *Pseudomembranous colitis:* Should be considered in patients in whom diarrhea develops. *Renal impairment:* Use drug with caution in patients with renal impairment. Dosage adjustment based on renal function may be required. *Superinfection:* May result in bacterial or fungal overgrowth of non-susceptible microorganisms.

NURSING CONSIDERATIONS

Administration/Storage

- Reconstituted solution should be light yellow to amber. Do not administer if solution is cloudy or precipitate is present.
- When giving by IM route, inject deeply into large muscle (eg, upper outer quadrant of gluteus muscle or lateral thigh); massage well. Rotate injection sites.
- When giving by IV route, administer slowly over 3-5 min or further dilute with 50-100 ml D5W or 0.9% Sodium Chloride and infuse over 30 min. Change IV site q 48-72 hr.
- Reconstituted solution is stable for 24 hr at room temperature, 10 days when refrigerated and 14 days if frozen immediately after reconstitution.
- Thaw frozen solution completely at room temperature or under refrigeration before use. Do not force thaw. Do not refreeze.

Assessment/Interventions

- Obtain patient history, including drug history and any known allergies. Note renal impairment and allergy to cephalosporins or penicillins.
- Obtain specimens for culture and sensitivity before beginning therapy and periodically during treatment.
- Monitor renal function carefully during treatment.
- Monitor for signs of infection, especially fever, and for positive response to antibiotic therapy.
- Assess for signs and symptoms of anaphylaxis (shortness of breath, wheezing, laryngeal spasm). Have resuscitation equipment available.
- Assess for signs of superinfection, such as vaginitis or stomatitis.
- Assess for diarrhea with blood or pus, which may be symptom of pseudomembranous colitis. Symptoms may occur after antibiotic treatment.
- Monitor IV site for signs of infiltration, infection and thrombophlebitis.

OVERDOSAGE: SIGNS & SYMPTOMS

Seizures

Patient/Family Education

- Remind patient to check body temperature daily. If fever persists for more than a few days or if high fever (> 102°F) or shaking chills are noted, physician should be notified immediately.

- Advise patient to maintain normal fluid intake while using this medication.
- Instruct patient to report signs of superinfection: black "furry" tongue, white patches in mouth, foul-smelling stools, vaginal itching or discharge.

See Patient Guide, p. 113.

Cephradine

(SEFF-ruh-deen)

Velosef

Class: Antibiotic/cephalosporin

Action Inhibits mucopeptide synthesis in bacterial cell wall.

Indications
Oral: Treatment of infections of respiratory tract, urinary tract, skin and skin structure; treatment of otitis media due to susceptible strains of microorganisms.

Contraindications Hypersensitivity to cephalosporins.

Route/Dosage
ADULTS: PO 250 mg-1 g q 6-12 hr. CHILDREN: PO 25-100 mg/kg/day in equally divided doses q 6-12 hr (maximum 4 g/day).

Interactions
Probenecid: Inhibition of renal excretion of cephradine.

Lab Test Interferences
May cause false-positive urine glucose test results with Benedict's solution, Fehling's solution, or Clinitest tablets but not with enzyme-based tests (eg, Clinistix, Tes-tape); false-positive test results for proteinuria with acid and denaturization-precipitation tests; false-positive direct Coombs' test result in certain patients (eg, those with azotemia); false elevations in urinary 17-ketosteroid values; false-positive reactions in urinary protein tests that use sulfosalicylic acid.

Adverse Reactions
GI: Nausea; vomiting; diarrhea; colitis, including pseudomembranous colitis. *GU:* Renal dysfunction; pyuria; dysuria; reversible interstitial nephritis; hematuria; toxic nephropathy. *HEMA:* Eosinophilia; neutropenia; lymphocytosis; leukocytosis; decreased platelet function; anemia; aplastic anemia. *HEPA:* Hepatic dysfunction; abnormal liver function test results. *OTHER:* Hypersensitivity, including Stevens-Johnson syndrome, erythema multiforme, toxic epidermal necrolysis; candidal overgrowth; serum sickness–like reactions (eg, skin rashes, polyarthritis, arthralgia, fever).

Precautions
Pregnancy: Category B. *Lactation:* Excreted in breast milk. *Children:* Safety and efficacy for infants < 9 mo not established. *Hypersensitivity:* Reactions range from mild to life-threatening. Administer drug with caution to penicillin-sensitive patients due to possible cross-reactivity. *Pseudomembranous colitis:* Should be considered in patients in whom diarrhea develops. *Renal impairment:* Use drug with caution in patients with renal impairment. Renal function should be monitored and dosage adjusted. *Superinfection:* Drug may result in bacterial or fungal overgrowth of nonsusceptible microorganisms.

NURSING CONSIDERATIONS

Administration/Storage

- May administer without regard to meals. Administer with food or milk if GI upset occurs. Food slows but does not decrease absorption.
- Reconstituted oral suspension may be stored at room temperature for up to 7

days or in refrigerator for 14 days. Shake well before pouring.
- When drug is stored at room temperature, protect from light.

Assessment/Interventions
- Obtain patient history, including drug history and any known allergies. Note renal impairment and allergy to cephalosporins or penicillins.
- Obtain specimens for culture and sensitivity before beginning therapy and periodically during treatment.
- Monitor renal function carefully during therapy.
- Monitor for signs of infection, especially fever, and for positive response to antibiotic therapy.
- Assess for signs and symptoms of anaphylaxis (shortness of breath, wheezing, laryngeal spasm). Have resuscitation equipment available.
- Assess for signs and symptoms of superinfection, such as vaginitis or stomatitis.
- Assess for diarrhea with blood or pus, which may be symptom of pseudomembranous colitis. Symptoms may occur after antibiotic treatment.

OVERDOSAGE: SIGNS & SYMPTOMS
Seizures

Patient/Family Education
- Instruct patient to complete full course of therapy.
- Advise patient to take with food or milk if GI distress occurs.
- Remind patient to check body temperature daily. If fever persists for more than a few days or if high fever (> 102°F) or shaking chills are noted, physician should be notified immediately.
- Advise patient to maintain normal fluid intake while using this medication.
- Remind diabetic patient to use enzyme-based tests (eg, Clinistix or Tes-tape) for monitoring urine glucose because drug may give false results with other tests.
- Instruct patient to report these symptoms to physician: nausea, vomiting, diarrhea, skin rash, muscle or joint pain.
- Advise patient to report signs of superinfection: black "furry" tongue, white patches in mouth, foul-smelling stools, vaginal itching or discharge.
- Warn patient that diarrhea that contains blood or pus may be sign of serious disorders. Tell patient to seek medical care and not to treat at home.
- Instruct patient to seek emergency care immediately if wheezing or difficulty in breathing occurs.

See Patient Guide, p. 114.

Charcoal, activated

(CHAR-kole)

Actidose-Aqua, Actidose with Sorbitol, Charcoaid, Charcoaid 2000, Liqui-Char, SuperChar, ♣ *Charcodote*

Class: Antidote

Action Inhibits GI absorption.

Indications Emergency treatment of poisoning by most drugs and chemicals. **Unlabeled uses:** Treatment of diarrhea, stomach gas and excessive flatulence.

Contraindications None known. Ineffective for poisonings by cyanide, mineral acids and alkalis. Not particularly effective for poisonings by ethanol, methanol and iron salts.

Route/Dosage

Acute Intoxication

PO/Gavage tube 30-100 g (or 1 g/kg or approximately 5-10 times amount of poison ingested) as suspension (mixed with 6-8 oz water).

GI Dialysis

PO/Gavage tube 20-40 q 6 hr for 1-2

days; alternate aqueous suspension and sorbitol suspension.

Interactions
Food (milk, ice cream and sherbet): Decrease the absorptive capacity of drug. *Other medications*: May have decreased effectiveness due to absorption by activated charcoal (eg, oral acetylcysteine used as antidote for acetaminophen overdose). *Syrup of ipecac*: Inactivated due to absorption by activated charcoal. Do not administer together.

Lab Test Interferences
None well documented.

Adverse Reactions
GI: Vomiting; constipation or diarrhea; black stools. Sorbitol may cause loose stools and vomiting.

Precautions
Pregnancy: Pregnancy category undetermined. *Lactation*: Undetermined. *Children*: Use under physician's supervision so fluid and electrolyte balance can be monitored properly.

NURSING CONSIDERATIONS

Administration/Storage

- When inducing vomiting, do so before giving activated charcoal. When large doses of drugs have been ingested, remove as much of ingested poison as possible by gastric lavage.
- Note that patient may be intolerant of activated charcoal for 1-2 hr after ipecac-induced vomiting.
- Administer orally to conscious patients only.
- For comatose patients or patients with altered mental status, administer via nasogastric tube.
- Mix 30-100 g as a slurry with 6-8 oz water or use premixed solution with 12.5-50 g in sorbitol suspension.
- In acute poisoning, administer as soon as possible. Drug is most effective when given within 30 min of poisoning.
- Store in tightly closed container. Premixed suspension can be stored for up to 1 yr.

Assessment/Interventions

- Obtain patient history, including drug history and any known allergies, and note which medications were ingested and amounts ingested, if syrup of ipecac was given and if ingested material was acidic.
- Obtain a toxicology screen of urine and serum.
- Assess and monitor vital signs and neurologic signs.
- Assess mental status and LOC.
- Monitor airway, ECG and I&O.
- Observe for vomiting or diarrhea.
- Keep patient well hydrated.

Patient/Family Education

- This drug should *not* be used as antidote in home.
- Advise patient that stools will be black for several days.
- Advise patient that diarrhea may continue for 24-48 hr.

See Patient Guide, p. 115.

Chloral Hydrate

(KLOR-uhl HIGH-drate)

Aquachloral Supprettes, *Noctec*
Class: Sedative and hypnotic/ nonbarbiturate

Action Exact mechanism is unknown; can produce mild CNS depression.

Indications Management of short-term insomnia; sedation; adjunctive to anesthesia, analgesia; prevention or suppression of alcohol withdrawal symptoms (rectal). **Unlabeled uses:** Conscious sedation in pediatric dentistry.

Contraindications Hypersensitivity to chloral derivatives; severe renal or hepatic impairment; gastritis (oral forms); severe cardiac disease.

Route/Dosage

Insomnia

ADULTS: **PO/PR** 500 mg-1 g 15-30 min before bedtime. CHILDREN: **PO/PR** 50 mg/kg/day (up to 1 g per dose) for sleep.

Premedication

ADULTS: **PO** 500 mg-1 g 30 min before surgery.

Sedation

ADULTS: **PO** 250 mg tid after meals. CHILDREN: **PO/PR** 25 mg/kg/day; may be given in divided doses.

Dental Sedation

CHILDREN: 75 mg/kg; supplementation with nitrous oxide may provide better sedation than manufacturer's recommended dosage.

Interactions

Alcohol and other CNS depressants: May produce additive CNS depression. *Furosemide (IV):* Administration within 24 hr of chloral hydrate may lead to diaphoresis, hot flashes, tachycardia and hypertension. *Oral anticoagulants:* Anticoagulant effects may be increased, especially during first 2 wk. *Phenytoin:* May reduce effects of phenytoin.

Lab Test Interferences

May cause false-positive urine glucose test results with Benedict's solution or cupric sulfide tablets (eg, Clinitest), but not with enzyme-based tests (eg, Clinistix, Tes-tape); altered urinary 17-ketosteroid values when using the Reddy, Jenkins, and Thorn procedure; false-positive phentolamine test results; results of fluorometric tests for urine catecholamines may be altered (do not administer chloral hydrate 48 hr before this test).

Adverse Reactions

RESP: Respiratory depression. *CNS:* Somnambulism; ataxia; dizziness; headache; "hangover" effect. *GI:* Stomach pain; nausea; vomiting; diarrhea; flatulence; unpleasant taste in mouth. *HEMA:* Leukopenia; eosinophilia. *OTHER:* Hypersensitivity (rash, itching, erythema multiforme, fever).

Precautions

Pregnancy: Category C. *Lactation:* Excreted in breast milk. *Acute intermittent porphyria:* Attacks may be precipitated in susceptible patients. *Drug dependency:* May be habit forming. Use with caution in patients with history of drug or alcohol addiction. *GI disorders:* Avoid use in patients with esophagitis, gastritis or gastric or duodenal ulcers. *Skin/mucous membrane irritation:* Irritates skin and mucous membranes. *Tartrazine sensitivity:* Some products contain tartrazine, which can cause allergic-type reactions in some individuals.

NURSING CONSIDERATIONS

Administration/Storage

- Administer syrup or capsules with full glass of water or fruit juice to help prevent GI or renal problems. Chilling of syrup may lessen its unpleasant taste.
- Store at room temperature in tightly closed, light-resistant container.

Assessment/Interventions

- Obtain patient history, including drug history and any known allergies. Note history of drug abuse; allergic or hypersensitivity responses to chloral hydrate, tartrazine or aspirin; and history of cardiac or GI disease.
- Institute safety precautions (eg, use of siderails and having call bell within patient's reach).
- If signs of gastric, liver or renal dysfunction occur, notify physician.
- Observe patient for signs of alertness and signs of psychologic or physical dependence.

OVERDOSAGE: SIGNS & SYMPTOMS

Stupor, coma, pinpoint pupils, hypotension, slow or rapid and shallow respirations, hypothermia, muscle flaccidity; also: nausea, vomiting, gastritis, hemorrhagic gastritis and gastric necrosis caused by drug's corrosive action

Patient/Family Education

- Instruct patient to take medication exactly as prescribed. Warn that taking doses too close together could result in overdose. Missed doses should be omitted.
- Inform patient that effects of medication may not be noted until after 48 hr.
- Advise that medication will be discontinued gradually to prevent withdrawal symptoms, including CNS excitation with tremor, anxiety, hallucinations or delirium.
- Instruct patient to report these symptoms to physician: visual changes, irregular heartbeats or palpitations, yellowing of skin or eyes, rash or unusual bleeding or bruising, abdominal pains or gastrointestinal problems.
- Advise patient that drug may cause drowsiness or dizziness and to use caution when driving or performing other tasks requiring mental alertness.
- Caution patient to avoid intake of alcoholic beverages and other CNS depressants such as barbiturates and narcotics.
- Instruct patient not to take otc medications without consulting physician.

See Patient Guide, p. 116.

Chlorambucil

(klor-AM-byoo-sill)

Leukeran

Class: Antineoplastic/alkylating

Action Interacts with cellular DNA to produce cytotoxic cross-linkage.

Indications Palliation for chronic lymphocytic leukemia, malignant lymphomas including lymphosarcoma, giant follicular lymphoma and Hodgkin's disease. **Unlabeled uses:** Treatment of uveitis and meningoencephalitis associated with Behçet's disease; alternating therapy with corticosteroid in treating idiopathic membraneous nephropathy; treatment of rheumatoid arthritis.

Contraindications Patients with disease showing prior resistance to this agent; hypersensitivity to other alkylating agents.

Route/Dosage

Initial and Short Courses of Therapy

ADULTS: **PO** Usual dose 0.1-0.2 mg/kg/day for 3-6 wk. May be given as single daily dose.

Hodgkin's Disease

ADULTS: **PO** Usual dose 0.2 mg/kg/day.

Other Lymphomas or Chronic Lymphocytic Leukemia

ADULTS: **PO** Usual dose 0.1 mg/kg/day. (When lymphocytic infiltration of bone marrow is present or bone marrow is hypoplastic, do not exceed 0.1 mg/kg/day.)

Alternate Treatment of Chronic Lymphocytic Leukemia

ADULTS: **PO** Intermittent, biweekly or monthly "pulse" dosing with initial dose of 0.4 mg/kg; increase by 0.1 mg/kg based on response.

Interactions None well documented.

Lab Test Interferences None well documented.

Adverse Reactions

RESP: Bronchopulmonary dysplasia syndrome; pulmonary fibrosis; interstitial pneumonia. *CNS:* Tremors; muscle twitching; confusion; agitation;

ataxia; flaccid paralysis; peripheral neuropathy; seizures. *EENT:* Keratitis. *GI:* Nausea; vomiting; diarrhea. *GU:* Sterility; infertility (men); amenorrhea (women); sterile cystitis. *HEMA:* Bone marrow suppression, sometimes severe. *HEPA:* Hepatotoxicity with jaundice. *DERM:* Skin hypersensitivity, including erythema multiforme, toxic epidermal necrolysis, Stevens-Johnson syndrome. *OTHER:* Drug fever.

Precautions

Pregnancy: Category D. *Lactation:* Undetermined. *Children:* Safety and efficacy have not been established. *Bone marrow suppression:* Chlorambucil can severely suppress bone marrow function. It is dangerous to allow patient to go more than 2 wk without hematologic and clinical examination. *Carcinogenesis and leukemogenesis:* Because of its carcinogenic properties, do not give this drug for conditions other than chronic lymphatic leukemia or malignant lymphomas. *Fertility impairment:* Chlorambucil has caused chromatid or chromosome damage. Reversible and permanent sterility have occurred in both sexes. *Hypersensitivity:* There may be cross-sensitivity (skin rash) with other alkylating agents. *Radiation and chemotherapy:* Do not give drug at full dosage before 4 wk after full course of radiation or chemotherapy because of possible increased risk of bone marrow damage.

NURSING CONSIDERATIONS

Administration/Storage

- Administer drug either 1 hr before or 2 hr after meals.
- Store at room temperature in a dry place.

Assessment/Interventions

- Obtain patient history, including drug history and any known allergies.
- Observe for bleeding tendency (eg, nosebleeds, bleeding gums, easy bruising).
- Monitor Hbg and Hct, WBC with differential and platelets prior to therapy and then weekly during therapy. Notify physician if abnormalities occur.
- Monitor kidney and liver function and notify physician if abnormalities occur.
- If any bleeding occurs, notify physician.
- Monitor for signs of gout (uric acid level) and anemia.

OVERDOSAGE: SIGNS & SYMPTOMS

Pancytopenia, agitated behavior, ataxia, multiple grand mal seizures

Patient/Family Education

- Instruct patient to take medication as directed even if nausea occurs.
- Advise patient that nausea and vomiting may occur, but if they persist or occur shortly after dose is taken, patient should notify physician.
- Instruct patient to report any unusual bleeding or bruising, use care to avoid injury, use soft toothbrush, avoid medications that contain aspirin and use caution if taking anticoagulants.
- Caution patient to avoid exposure to infections and notify physician if signs of infection occur.
- Inform patient that bone marrow suppression may be delayed up to 3 wk and may last as long as 10 days after last dose.
- Discuss with patient the possibility of permanent sterility but advise to continue using birth control if sexually active and of childbearing age.
- Instruct patient to report these symptoms to physician: fever, nausea, vomiting, skin rash, chills, sore throat, cough, shortness of breath, seizures, amenorrhea, unusual lumps or masses, flank or stomach pain, joint pain, sores in mouth or on lips or yellow discoloration of skin or eyes.

See Patient Guide, p. 117.

Chloramphenicol

(KLOR-am-FEN-ih-kahl)

AK-Chlor, Chloromycetin, Chloromycetin Kapseals, Chloromycetin Otic, Chloroptic S.O.P., ♣ Diochloram, Ophtho-Chloram, Sopamycetin

Chloramphenicol Sodium Succinate

Chloromycetin Sodium Succinate

Chloramphenicol Palmitate

Chloromycetin Palmitate

Class: Antibiotic

Action Interferes with or inhibits microbial protein synthesis.

Indications

Systemic: Treatment of following types of infections caused by susceptible strains of specific microorganisms: serious systemic infections for which less potentially dangerous drugs are ineffective or contraindicated. *Topical:* Treatment of cystic fibrosis, superficial ocular infections, superficial infections involving external auditory canal, superficial skin infections; infection prophylaxis for minor cuts, wounds, burns and skin abrasions and for various gram-negative bacteria causing bacteremia and meningitis.

Contraindications

Oral use: Trivial infections (eg, colds, influenza, throat infections) or infections other than indicated; prophylaxis of systemic bacterial infections. *Ophthalmic use:* Epithelial herpes simplex keratitis; vaccinia; varicella; fungal disease of ocular structure; mycobacterial infections of eye; after uncomplicated removal of corneal foreign body. *Otic use:* Perforated tympanic membrane; when less potentially dangerous agents would be expected to be ineffective.

Route/Dosage

Systemic Infections

ADULTS: **PO/IV** 50 mg/kg/day in divided doses q 6 hr; may require up to 100 mg/kg/day initially for CNS infections. CHILDREN: **PO/IV** 50-75 mg/kg/day in divided doses q 6 hr; 50-100 mg/kg/day for meningitis. INFANTS & CHILDREN WITH IMMATURE METABOLIC PROCESSES: **PO/IV** 25 mg/kg/day. NEWBORNS: **PO/IV** Usually 25 mg/kg/day in 4 doses q 6 hr. NEONATES > 7 DAYS (> 2 KG): **PO/IV** 50 mg/kg/day in divided doses q 12 hr. NEONATES < 2 KG AND BIRTH-7 DAYS (> 2 KG): **PO/IV** 25 mg/kg qd.

Ophthalmic Infections

ADULTS & CHILDREN: **Ophthalmic** 1-2 gtt q 15-30 min initially for acute infections; then reduce frequency as infection is controlled.

Otic Infections

ADULTS & CHILDREN: **Otic** 2-3 gtt in ear tid.

Topical Infections

ADULTS & CHILDREN: **Topical** Apply 1-4 times daily to affected area.

Interactions

Anticoagulants: May enhance anticoagulation action. *Barbiturates:* May reduce effectiveness of chloramphenicol while barbiturate effects may be enhanced; effects may last days after barbiturates are withdrawn. *Ferrous salts:* May increase serum iron levels. *Hydantoins (eg, phenytoin):* May increase serum hydantoin levels, with possible toxicity; chloramphenicol levels may increase or decrease. *Rifampin:* May reduce chloramphenicol serum levels; effect may last days after rifampin is withdrawn. *Sulfonylureas:* May cause clinical manifestations of hypoglycemia. *Vitamin B_{12}:* May decrease hematologic effects of vitamin B_{12} in patients with pernicious anemia.

Lab Test Interferences

None well documented.

Adverse Reactions

CNS: Headache; mental confusion; delirium; mild depression; optic neuritis; peripheral neuritis. *GI:* Diarrhea; nausea; vomiting; glossitis; stomatitis. *HEMA:* Bone marrow depression; aplastic anemia; hypoplastic anemia;

thrombocytopenia; granulocytopenia. *DERM:* Topical use: Itching or burning; urticaria; angioneurotic edema; dermatitis. *OTHER:* Hypersensitivity reactions (eg, fever, rash, angioedema, urticaria, anaphylaxis); Gray syndrome. Topical use may produce same adverse reactions seen with systemic use.

Precautions

Pregnancy: Pregnancy category undetermined. *Lactation:* Excreted in breast milk. *Children:* Use drug with caution and in reduced dosages in premature and term infants to avoid Gray syndrome toxicity (toxic and potentially fatal reaction in premature infants and newborns). Symptoms of Gray syndrome generally appear in this sequence: abdominal distention with or without emesis; progressive pallid cyanosis; vasomotor collapse, frequently accompanied by irregular respiration; death within a few hours of onset (death occurs in 40% of patients within 2 days of initial symptoms). Other initial symptoms of Gray syndrome may include refusal to suck, loose green stools, flaccidity, ashen gray color, decreased temperature and refractory lactic acidosis. *Blood dyscrasias:* Serious and fatal blood dyscrasias can occur. *Inner ear infections:* Use systemic antibiotic therapy. *Ophthalmic ointment:* May retard corneal epithelial healing. *Renal or hepatic impairment:* Excessive blood levels of drug may occur; dosage adjustment may be required. Preexisting liver dysfunction may be significant risk factor for Gray syndrome. *Special risk patients:* Use drug with caution in patients with acute intermittent porphyria or G-6-PD deficiency. *Superinfection:* Use of antibiotics may result in bacterial or fungal overgrowth. Serious infections may need systemic treatment in addition to local treatment.

NURSING CONSIDERATIONS

Administration/Storage

Parenteral

- Chloramphenicol sodium succinate is intended for IV use only; it is ineffective when given via IM route.
- Give direct IV as 10% solution in Water for Injection or 5% Dextrose Injection over at least 1 min. Do not administer if cloudy. May also be diluted in 50-100 ml of D5W and administered over 30 min.
- Substitute oral administration as soon as possible.

Oral

- Administer orally in capsules and oral suspension with full glass of water on empty stomach at least 1 hr before or 2 hr after meals at evenly spaced intervals (q 6 hr) around clock.
- Administer with food if GI upset occurs.

Ophthalmic

- Have patient tilt head back. Place medication in conjunctival sac and close patient's eyes. Apply light finger pressure to lacrimal sac for 1 min after instillation.
- Do not touch tip of cap to eye, fingers or other surface.

Otic

- Avoid contact with eyes; for use in ear only.
- If ear drops are kept refrigerated, hold container in hand for a few minutes to warm to near body temperature.
- If drops are in suspension, shake well for 10 sec before using.
- Have patient lie on side or tilt affected ear up for ease of administration. Allow drops to run in, and keep ear tilted for about 2 min.
- Do not touch tip of cap to ear, fingers or other surface.

Topical

- Do not use in eyes. Topical preparation is for external use only.
- Cleanse affected area of skin prior to application unless otherwise instructed.
- Cover with sterile bandage if needed.

- Administer around clock at even intervals.

Assessment/Interventions

- Obtain patient history, including drug history and any known allergies. Note any renal or hepatic impairment.
- Determine baseline of infectious state: measure temperature; assess vital signs; examine appearance of wound, eye, ear, urine and stool; perform blood studies.
- Confirm diagnosis from cultures prior to administration of drug.
- Determine baseline CBC and platelet count and monitor every 2 days.
- Avoid concurrent therapy with other drugs that suppress bone marrow.
- Avoid repeat course of therapy if possible.
- Monitor serum levels of medication weekly. Therapeutic level peak is 5-20 mcg/ml; if level is higher, notify physician.
- If signs of anemia, leukopenia, reticulocytopenia or thrombocytopenia develop, notify physician.
- Observe patient daily for signs of bone marrow depression (eg, fatigue, sore throat, bleeding, aplastic anemia, hypoplastic anemia, thrombocytopenia, agranulocytosis) and Gray syndrome in infants.
- Discontinue drug at first sign of hematologic disorders attributable to chloramphenicol.

OVERDOSAGE: SIGNS & SYMPTOMS

Nausea, vomiting, unpleasant taste, diarrhea

Patient/Family Education

- Advise patient to take drug orally 1 hr before or 2 hr after meals. Explain that medication may be taken with food to avoid GI upset.
- Instruct patient to complete entire regimen even if feeling better.
- Emphasize importance of follow-up examinations because of possible complications from drug that can occur up to months after therapy is completed.
- Caution patient about not sharing prescription medications because of danger of side effects.
- Inform patient that ophthalmic solution may cause blurred vision or stinging for a few minutes after administration.
- Instruct patient that bitter taste that occurs after IV administration will subside 2-3 min after injection.
- Instruct patient to report these symptoms to physician: bleeding, fever, sore throat, itching, nausea, vomiting, diarrhea, bruising or numbness and weakness of hands or feet.
- Advise parents to report these symptoms to physician if they occur in infants: failure to feed, abdominal distention, drowsiness, blue or gray skin color or any problems in breathing.
- Instruct patient to report signs of further infection or worsening of current infection to physician.

See Patient Guide, p. 118-121.

Chlordiazepoxide

(klor-DIE-aze-ee-POX-ide)

Libritabs, Librium, Mitran, Reposans-10, ♣ *Solium*

Class: Antianxiety/benzadiazepine

Action Potentiates action of GABA to produce CNS depression.

Indications Management of anxiety disorders; relief of acute alcohol withdrawal symptoms; relief of preoperative apprehension and anxiety. **Unlabeled use:** Treatment of irritable bowel syndrome.

Contraindications Hypersensitivity to benzodiazepines; psychoses; acute narrow-angle glaucoma; shock; coma; acute alcohol intoxication.

Route/Dosage

Individualize dosage. Acute symptoms may be rapidly controlled IM or IV, with subsequent oral treatment (maximum 300 mg/day).

Mild to Moderate Anxiety

ADULTS: **PO** 5-10 mg tid or qid.

Severe Anxiety

ADULTS: **PO** 20-25 mg tid or qid. Initial dose: **IM/IV** 50-100 mg, then 25-50 mg tid or qid. ELDERLY OR DEBILITATED PATIENTS: **PO** 5 mg bid to qid. **IM/IV** 25-50 mg.

Preoperative Apprehension/Anxiety

ADULTS: **PO** 5-10 mg tid or qid on days preceding surgery. **IM** 50-100 mg 1 hr prior to surgery.

Acute Alcohol Withdrawal

ADULTS: **IM/IV** 50-100 mg; repeat q 2-4 hr prn. **PO** 50-100 mg, repeat prn (maximum oral or parenteral dose is 300 mg/day). CHILDREN (> 6 YR): **PO** 5-10 mg bid-qid; may be increased to 10 mg bid-tid. CHILDREN (> 12 YR): **IM** 0.5 mg/kg/day 6-8 hr.

Interactions

Alcohol and CNS depressants: Additive CNS depressant effects are possible. *Cigarette smoking, theophyllines:* May antagonize sedative effects. *Cimetidine, oral contraceptives, disulfiram, omeprazole:* May increase effects of chlordiazepoxide with excessive sedation and impaired psychomotor function. *Digoxin:* May increase serum digoxin concentrations.

Lab Test Interferences

None well documented.

Adverse Reactions

CV: Cardiovascular collapse; hypotension; hypertension; tachycardia; bradycardia; edema; phlebitis or thrombosis at IV sites. *CNS:* Drowsiness; confusion; ataxia; dizziness; fatigue; apathy; memory impairment; disorientation; anterograde amnesia; restlessness; headache; slurred speech; loss of voice; stupor; coma; euphoria; irritability; vivid dreams; psychomotor retardation; paradoxical reactions (eg, anger, hostility, mania, insomnia, muscle spasms). *EENT:* Visual or auditory disturbances; depressed hearing. *GI:* Constipation; diarrhea; dry mouth; coated tongue; nausea; anorexia; vomiting. *HEMA:* Blood dyscrasias including agranulocytosis; anemia; thrombocytopenia; leukopenia; neutropenia. *DERM:* Rash. *HEPA:* Abnormal liver function tests; hepatic dysfunction including hepatitis and jaundice. *OTHER:* Dependency/withdrawal syndrome.

Precautions

Pregnancy: Category D. Avoid especially in first trimester due to possible increased risk of congenital malformations. *Lactation:* Excreted in breast milk. *Children:* Initial dose should be small and gradually increased. Oral form not recommended in children < 6 yr; parenteral form not recommended in children < 12 yr. *Elderly or debilitated patients:* Initial dose should be small and gradually increased. Use with caution in patients with limited pulmonary reserve. *Dependency:* Prolonged use can lead to dependency. Withdrawal syndrome has occurred within 4-6 wk of treatment, especially if drug is abruptly discontinued. For discontinuation after long-term treatment, use caution and taper dosage. *Psychiatric disorders:* Not intended for patients with primary depressive disorder, psychosis or disorders in which anxiety is not prominent. Parenteral administration: Reserved primarily for acute states. *Renal or hepatic impairment:* Observe caution to avoid accumulation of drug. *Suicide:* Use with caution in patients with suicidal tendencies; do not allow patient access to large quantities of drug.

➤

NURSING CONSIDERATIONS

Administration/Storage

- Give oral form with food or milk to decrease GI irritation.
- Do not open capsules.
- Use parenteral solutions immediately after reconstitution. Discard unused portion.
- For intramuscular administration, reconstitute with diluent provided. Do not use diluent if opalescent or hazy. Agitate gently until dissolved. Give injection slowly deep in upper quadrant of gluteus maximus muscle.
- For intravenous administration, reconstitute with 5 ml sterile physiologic saline or Sterile Water for Injection. Do not use diluent for intramuscular form. Administer injection slowly over 1 min.
- Do not inject intra-arterially; intra-arterial injection may produce arteriospasm that can lead to gangrene.
- Keep powder form away from light. Store in refrigerator until reconstitution.

Assessment/Interventions

- Obtain patient history, including drug history and any known allergies. Consider cross-sensitivity with other benzodiazepines.
- Monitor BP, pulse rate and respiratory rate frequently when giving drug parenterally.
- Assist with ambulation and use siderails; drowsiness and orthostatic hypotension may occur early in therapy.
- Monitor CBC; blood dyscrasias occur rarely with long-term use.
- Monitor liver function during long-term therapy.
- Assess for ataxia and oversedation in elderly, debilitated patient.
- Monitor mental status: mood, sensorium, affect, sleep pattern, drowsiness, dizziness. Notify physician of mental status changes.
- Observe patient closely for 3 hr following parenteral administration; bed rest is preferred. Do not permit patient to drive or perform other potentially hazardous tasks.
- With treatment for alcohol withdrawal, assess for tremors, agitation, delirium and hallucinations.
- Monitor for parodoxical reactions: excitement, stimulation, acute rage.
- Restrict amount of medication available to patients with suicidal tendencies.
- Observe for physical dependency/withdrawal symptoms with long-term use: headache, muscle pain, weakness, nausea, vomiting, increased anxiety.
- Because of risk of apnea and cardiac arrest with parenteral administration, have resuscitative facilities available.

OVERDOSAGE: SIGNS & SYMPTOMS

Drowsiness, confusion, somnolence, impaired coordination, diminished reflexes, lethargy, ataxia, hypotonia, hypotension, hypnosis, coma, death

Patient/Family Education

- Instruct patient to take drug with food or milk to prevent GI irritation.
- Inform patient that drowsiness may be worse at beginning of therapy. Advise patient to use caution while driving or performing other tasks requiring mental alertness.
- Instruct patient to rise slowly, especially if elderly, to avoid fainting.
- Advise patient to report behavior changes, such as episodes of excitement, stimulation or acute rage, to physician.
- Inform patient receiving long-term therapy or taking high doses that withdrawal symptoms may occur if drug is suddenly discontinued.
- Advise patient to avoid intake of alcoholic beverages.
- Caution patient not to take otc medications without consulting physician.

See Patient Guide, p. 122.

Chlordiazepoxide/ Amitriptyline

(klor-DIE-aze-ee-POX-ide/am-ee-TRIP-tih-leen)

Limbitrol DS 10-25

Class: Psychotherapeutic combination

Action Amitriptyline blocks reuptake of serotonin and norepinephrine in CNS. Chlordiazepoxide potentiates effects of GABA in CNS.

Indications Treatment of moderate to severe depression associated with moderate to severe anxiety.

Contraindications Hypersensitivity to chlordiazepoxide or other benzodiazepines; hypersensitivity to amitriptyline or other tricyclic antidepressants; concomitant MAO inhibitor use; acute recovery phase of MI.

Route/Dosage

PO 1 tablet (10 mg chlordiazepoxide with 25 mg amitriptyline) tid or qid. May increase to 6 tablets daily if needed; some patients may respond to 1 tablet bid.

Interactions

Cimetidine, fluoxetine, haloperidol, phenothiazine antipsychotic compounds, oral contraceptives: May cause increased amitriptyline blood levels. *Cimetidine, oral contraceptives, disulfiram, fluoxetine, isoniazid, ketoconazole, metoprolol, propoxyphene, propranolol, valproic acid:* May increase chlordiazepoxide effects. *Clonidine:* May result in hypertensive crisis. *CNS depressants, alcohol:* Depressant effects may be additive. *Digoxin:* May increase digoxin serum levels. *Guanethidine:* May diminish antihypertensive effects. *MAO inhibitors:* May result in hypertensive crises, convulsions and death. *Oral anticoagulants:* May result in increased anticoagulant effect.

Lab Test Interferences

None well documented.

Adverse Reactions

CV: Hypotension; hypertension; tachycardia; palpitations; MI; arrhythmias; heart block; ECG changes; stroke. *RESP:* Difficult breathing. *CNS:* Hallucinations; hypomania; delusions; poor concentration; incoordination; tingling and paresthesias of extremities; extrapyramidal symptoms; syncope; changes in EEG patterns; dizziness; sedation; drowsiness; headache; lethargy; fatigue. *EENT:* Pupil dilation; blurred vision; nasal stuffiness; alteration in taste perception; parotid swelling. *GI:* Nausea; epigastric distress; vomiting; anorexia; diarrhea; black tongue; bloating; dry mouth; constipation. *GU:* Testicular swelling; decreased urinary frequency; menstrual irregularities; loss of bladder function; change in sex drive. *HEMA:* Bone marrow depression including agranulocytosis; eosinophilia; purpura; thrombocytopenia. *META:* Elevation or depression of glucose levels. *HEPA:* Jaundice; hepatic dysfunction; increased AST, ALT, alkaline phosphatase. *DERM:* Rash; urticaria; photosensitivity; edema of face and tongue; pruritus. *OTHER:* Weight gain or loss; paradoxical sweating; gynecomastia; breast enlargement and galactorrhea (women); syndrome of inappropriate antidiuretic hormone secretion.

Precautions

Pregnancy: Pregnancy category undetermined. *Lactation:* Excreted in breast milk. *Children:* Not recommended in children < 12 yr. *Elderly or debilitated patients:* Unit dosage to smallest effective amount to decrease risk of ataxia, oversedation, confusion or anticholinergic effects. *Special risk patients:* Use with caution in patients with history of seizures, urinary retention, urethral spasm, angle-closure glaucoma or increased intraocular pressure, cardiovascular disorders and hepatic or renal impairment; hyperthyroid patients or those receiving thyroid medication; schizophrenic or paranoid patients.

NURSING CONSIDERATIONS

Administration/Storage

- If patient has been taking MAO inhibitor, wait 2 wk before beginning limbitrol therapy. Cautiously begin treatment with reduced dosage.
- Therapy may begin with 1 tablet at bedtime with dosage titrated upward as tolerance to CNS depressant effect develops.
- Administer with food or water to reduce gastric irritation.
- Give larger portion of total daily dose at bedtime.
- Store in moisture-resistant container at room temperature.

Assessment/Interventions

- Obtain patient history, including drug history and any known allergies, especially to drug, amitriptyline or other benzodiazepines.
- Evaluate medical history for potential risk of drug or alcohol abuse or suicide.
- If elective surgery is planned, drug should be discontinued several days before surgical procedure.
- If patient is addiction prone or suicidal, remain with patient while patient takes tablet. Observe for signs of hoarding.
- Closely monitor patients with history of hyperthyroidism or patients taking thyroid medication.
- Monitor BP and pulse during initial therapy.
- If patient is undergoing long-term treatment, perform periodic blood counts and liver function studies.

OVERDOSAGE: SIGNS & SYMPTOMS

Drowsiness, temporary confusion, visual hallucinations, hypothermia, tachycardia, arrhythmias, CHF, dilated pupils, convulsions, hypotension, stupor, coma, agitation, hyperactive reflexes, muscle rigidity, vomiting, hyperpyrexia

Patient/Family Education

- Instruct patient to avoid intake of alcoholic beverages and other CNS depressants because additive effects can cause dangerous level of sedation and CNS depression.
- Advise patient that drug may cause drowsiness and to use caution while driving or performing other tasks requiring mental alertness.
- Instruct patient not to discontinue medication abruptly or change dosage without consulting with physician because withdrawal symptoms can occur.
- Caution patient to avoid excessive exposure to sunlight and to use sunscreen or wear protective clothing to avoid photosensitivity reaction.
- Advise patient that dry mouth may occur and that it may be relieved by taking sips of water frequently or sucking on hard sugarless candy or gum.
- Caution patient not to take any otc medications without consulting physician.

See Patient Guide, p. 123.

Chlorhexidine Gluconate

(klor-HEX-ih-deen GLUE-koe-nate)

Dyna-Hex, Dyna-Hex 2, Exidine, Exidine-2 Scrub, Exidine-4 Scrub, Hibiclens, Hibiclens Antiseptic/Antimicrobial Skin Cleanser, Hibistat, Hibistat Germicidal Hand Rinse, Hibistat Towelettes, Peridex; ✤ *Hexifoam, Hibidil, Hibitane, Spectro Gram*

Class: Antiseptic/germicide

Action Provides antimicrobial effect against a wide range of microorganisms.

Indications Surgical scrub; skin cleanser; preoperative skin preparation; skin wound cleanser; hand rinse; oral rinse for gingivitis. **Unlabeled**

use: Treatment of acne vulgaris. **Orphan drug use:** Amelioration of oral mucositis associated with cytoreductive therapy for bone marrow transplant candidates.

Contraindications Standard considerations.

Route/Dosage

Skin Use

5 ml is applied to skin and worked into lather.

Oral Rinse for Gingivitis

15 ml (1 capful) bid for 30 seconds, morning and evening after toothbrushing. Expectorate after rinsing; do not swallow.

Interactions None well documented.

Lab Test Interferences

None well documented.

Adverse Reactions

EENT: Deafness; transient parotitis, altered taste perception. *DERM:* Irritation; dermatitis; photosensitivity; sensitization and generalized allergic reactions, especially in genital area. *OTHER:* Staining of teeth and oral surfaces; increased calculus formation; minor irritation and superficial desquamation of oral mucosa.

Precautions

Pregnancy: Category B (oral rinse). Pregnancy category undetermined for skin use. *Lactation:* Undetermined.

NURSING CONSIDERATIONS

Administration/Storage

- For surgical wash, scrub, or bacteriostatic cleansing: wet hands with warm water and squeeze 5 ml into palm, add water, work up lather, apply lather to area being cleansed and rinse thoroughly.
- For oral rinse: swish in mouth for 30 seconds after toothbrushing and expectorate.
- For surgical hand scrub: wet hands and use nail cleaner under fingernails and to clean cuticles. Wet hands and forearms to elbows with warm water, apply lather, scrub for 3 minutes and rinse thoroughly. Scrub for additional 3 minutes, rinse and dry hands and forearms with sterile towel.
- Keep medication out of ears, eyes and mouth. Serious and permanent eye injury and deafness may occur if used improperly.
- Do not use this medication routinely on wounds involving more than superficial layers of skin.
- Avoid contact with meninges.
- Do not freeze.
- Store at room temperature.
- Prolonged direct exposure to strong light may cause brownish surface discoloration but does not affect action. Shake to disperse color.

Assessment/Interventions

- Obtain patient history, including drug history and any known allergies.
- Monitor for allergic reactions (urticaria, bronchospasm, cough, shortness of breath).
- Monitor skin and mouth for irritation.

OVERDOSAGE: SIGNS & SYMPTOMS

Gastric distress, alcohol intoxication

Patient/Family Education

- Inform patient that staining of teeth, dental work, tongue and oral tissue may occur. Staining does not adversely affect health and can usually be removed by professional techniques.
- Caution patient that taste perception may be altered during treatment; permanent taste alteration has not been noted.
- Inform patient that oral rinse contains alcohol.
- Instruct patient to avoid having medication come into contact with ears

and eyes, which could cause permanent damage.
- Instruct patient not to swallow product but to expectorate after oral rinsing.
- Advise patient to avoid eating 2-3 hr after treatment.

See Patient Guide, p. 124.

Chloroquine

(KLOR-oh-kwin)

Chloroquine Phosphate

Aralen Phosphate

Chloroquine Hydrochloride

Aralen HCl

Class: Anti-infective/antimalarial

Action Inhibits parasite growth, possibly by concentrating within parasite acid vesicles, raising pH.

Indications Prophylaxis and treatment of acute attacks of malaria caused by *Plasmodium vivax, P malariae, P ovale* and susceptible strains of *P falciparum*; extraintestinal amebiasis. **Unlabeled uses:** Treatment of rheumatoid arthritis, systemic and discoid lupus erythematosis, porphyria cutanea tarda, scleroderma, pemphigus, lichen planus, polymyositis and sarcoidosis.

Contraindications Retinal or visual field changes.

Route/Dosage

Doses are listed in base equivalents. (Chloroquine phosphate, 500 mg equals 300 mg base; chloroquine hydrochloride, 50 mg equals 40 mg base.)

Acute Malaria

CHLOROQUINE PHOSPHATE: ADULTS: Initial dose: **PO** 600 mg, then 300 mg 6 hr later and 300 mg qd for 2 days. CHILDREN: Initial dose: **PO** 10 mg/kg, then 5 mg/kg 6 hr later and 5 mg/kg qd for 2 days. CHLOROQUINE HYDROCHLORIDE: ADULTS: Initial dose: **IM** 160-200 mg then repeat dose in 6 hr if needed (maximum 800 mg base total dose in first 24 hr). CHILDREN: 5 mg/kg/dose; repeat dose in 6 hr (maximum 10 mg base/kg/24 hr; do not exceed 5 mg/kg as single parenteral dose).

Malaria Suppression

ADULTS: **PO** 300 mg base. CHILDREN: 5 mg/kg/dose (maximum 300 mg base) weekly. Begin 1-2 wk prior to exposure and continue for 4 wk after leaving endemic area. If suppressive therapy is not begun prior to exposure, double initial loading dose and give in 2 divided doses 6 hr apart.

Extraintestinal Amebiasis

CHLOROQUINE PHOSPHATE: ADULTS: **PO** 600 mg base/day for 2 days, then 300 mg base/day for 2-3 wk. CHLOROQUINE HYDROCHLORIDE: ADULTS: **IM** 4-5 ml (160-200 mg base)/day for 10-12 days.

Interactions

Cimetidine: May increase chloroquine serum concentration. *Kaolin aluminum or magnesium trisilicate antacids:* May decrease GI absorption of chloroquine. *Rabies vaccine:* Concomitant administration of intradermally administered rabies vaccine and chloroquine may result in diminished antibody response to vaccine. In this situation CDC recommends administering rabies vaccine intramuscularly.

Lab Test Interferences

None well documented.

Adverse Reactions

CV: Hypotension; ECG changes. *CNS:* Headache; neuropathy; seizures; psychotic episodes. *EENT:* Visual disturbances; retinal damage and deafness with prolonged high-dose use; tinnitus. *GI:* Anorexia; nausea; vomiting; diarrhea; abdominal cramps. *HEMA:* Agranulocytosis; blood dyscrasias; aplastic anemia. *HEPA:* Hepatitis. *DERM:* Pruritus; pigment changes; skin eruptions. *OTHER:* Muscle weakness.

Precautions

Pregnancy: Category D. *Lactation:* Excreted in breast milk. *Children:* Especially sensitive to adverse effects; do not exceed recommended dose. *G-6-PD deficiency:* May induce hemolysis in presence of infection or stressful condition. *Muscular weakness:* May need to discontinue therapy if muscle weakness occurs. *Psoriasis or porphyria:* May be exacerbated. *Retinopathy:* Irreversible retinal damage has occurred. *Special risk patients:* Monitor patients with hepatic disease or alcoholism or taking other hepatotoxic medications for evidence of worsening liver function such as bleeding.

NURSING CONSIDERATIONS

Administration/Storage

- Administer with food or milk.
- If taken once weekly, take on same day of week.
- Store in airtight, light-resistant container at room temperature.

Assessment/Interventions

- Obtain patient history, including drug history and any known allergies.
- Review history for blood disorders, eye or vision problems, G-6-PD deficiency, liver disease, alcoholism, porphyria or psoriasis.
- Arrange for a complete eye examination to establish baseline values.
- Perform baseline assessment for signs and symptoms of infection.
- Provide small, frequent meals if GI distress occurs.
- Arrange for and monitor periodic CBCs.
- If sore throat, fever, weakness, fatigue, unusual bleeding or bruising occurs, notify physician.
- Perform periodic neuromuscular examinations, and notify patient if knee and ankle reflexes are weak.

OVERDOSAGE: SIGNS & SYMPTOMS

Headache, drowsiness, visual disturbances, cardiovascular collapse, seizures, respiratory and cardiac arrest, death

Patient/Family Education

- Remind patient to take medication with food to minimize GI irritation.
- Stress importance of compliance with full course of therapy. If used for suppression, drug must be taken at least 1 wk before entering and for 4 wk after leaving endemic area.
- Caution patient to drink alcoholic beverages sparingly because of increased GI irritation and higher risk of liver damage.
- Stress importance of eye examinations q 3-6 mon during prolonged daily therapy.
- Inform patient that drug may cause rusty or brown discoloration of urine.
- Advise use of dark glasses in bright light to reduce risk of ocular damage.
- Instruct patient to report these symptoms to physician: blurring or change in vision, buzzing or difficulty hearing, muscle weakness, rash, vomiting or stomach pain, difficulty breathing or swallowing.

See Patient Guide, p. 125.

Chlorotrianisene

(klor-oh-try-AN-ih-seen)
TACE
Class: Estrogen

Action Promotes growth and development of female reproductive system and secondary sex characteristics; inhibits ovulation and prevents postpartum breast engorgement;

overrides stimulatory effects of testosterone.

Indications Prevention of postpartum breast engorgement; management of moderate to severe vasomotor symptoms associated with menopause; treatment of atrophic vaginitis, kraurosis vulvae, female hypogonadism, and inoperable, progressing prostatic carcinoma; palliation of symptoms of metastatic breast cancer.

Contraindications Breast cancer (except in patients being treated for metastatic disease); estrogen-dependent neoplasia; abnormal genital bleeding of undetermined etiology; history of or active thrombophlebitis or thromboembolic disorders; known or suspected pregnancy.

Route/Dosage

Postpartum Breast Engorgement

ADULTS: PO 12 mg qid for 7 days, or 50 mg every 6 hr for 6 doses; give first dose within 8 hr after delivery.

Symptoms Associated With Menopause

ADULTS: PO 12-25 mg/day cyclically for 30 days; course may be repeated.

Atrophic Vaginitis/Kraurosis Vulvae

ADULTS: PO 12-25 mg/day cyclically for 30-60 days.

Female Hypogonadism

ADULTS: PO 12-25 mg/day cyclically for 21 days.

Prostatic Carcinoma

ADULTS: PO 12-25 mg/day given chronically.

Interactions

Antidepressants, tricyclic: Chlorotrianisene may alter effects and increase toxicity of these agents. *Barbiturates or rifampin:* May decrease chlorotrianisene concentration. *Corticosteroids:* Clearance of corticosteroids may be reduced. *Dantrolene:* Increased risk of hepatotoxicity. *Hydantoins:* Loss of seizure control; decreased estrogenic effects may occur.

Lab Test Interferences

Endocrine and liver function test results may be affected; possible increased prothrombin time and platelet aggregability; increased thyroid-binding globulin; impaired glucose tolerance; decreased serum folate concentration; increased serum triglyceride, phospholipid and cholesterol concentrations.

Adverse Reactions

CV: Thrombosis; hypertension; thrombophlebitis; pulmonary embolism; MI. *CNS:* Headache; migraine; dizziness; chorea; depression. *EENT:* Steepening of corneal curvature; intolerance to contact lenses. *GI:* Nausea; vomiting; abdominal cramps; bloating; colitis; acute pancreatitis. *GU:* Increased risk of endometrial carcinoma; breakthrough bleeding; dysmenorrhea; amenorrhea; vaginal candidiasis; premenstrual-like syndrome; increased size of uterine fibromyomata; hemolytic uremic syndrome. *HEPA:* Cholestatic jaundice; hepatic adenoma. *DERM:* Chloasma; melasma; erythema nodosum or multiforme; scalp hair loss; hirsutism; urticaria; dermatitis. *OTHER:* Increase or decrease in weight; reduced glucose tolerance; edema; changes in libido; breast tenderness; porphyria; gynecomastia.

Precautions

Pregnancy: Category X. *Lactation:* Excreted in breast milk. *Children:* Safety and efficacy not established. *Calcium and phosphorus metabolism:* Use with caution in patients with metabolic bone diseases. *Fluid retention:* Use with careful observation when conditions that might be affected by this factor are present (eg, asthma, cardiac or renal dysfunction, epilepsy). *Gallbladder disease:* Risk of gallbladder disease may increase in women receiving postmenopausal estrogens. *Hepatic function impairment:* Estrogen metabolism may be impaired; use with caution. *Induction of malignant neoplasms:* May increase risk of endometrial or other carcinomas.

Tartrazine sensitivity: May cause allergic reaction in susceptible patients.

NURSING CONSIDERATIONS

Administration/Storage

- Administer first dose within 8 hr after delivery for prevention of postpartum breast engorgement.
- Give cyclically if used for postmenopausal problems or hypogonadism.

Assessment/Interventions

- Obtain patient history, including drug history and any known allergies.
- Assess patient's risk factors for estrogen-induced adverse reactions.
- Review results of electrolyte testing periodically, with close attention to calcium and phosphorus levels.
- Assess for fluid retention, especially in patients with respiratory, cardiac or renal dysfunction.
- Check blood sugar levels periodically.
- Measure blood pressure frequently, and review results of serum lipid measurements and liver function tests.
- Closely monitor patients with diabetes because decreased glucose tolerance may occur.
- Assess patients taking antidepressants for signs of toxicity.
- Closely monitor patients taking hydantoins for seizure control, because there may be reduced effectiveness.
- Check results of liver and endocrine tests, and notify physician of any abnormal results or trends.
- Remember that triglyceride levels and prothrombin time may be falsely increased and that patients taking barbituates, rifampin or other enzyme inducers may have decreased chlorotrianisene levels.

OVERDOSAGE: SIGNS & SYMPTOMS

Withdrawal bleeding in women, nausea, vomiting

Patient/Family Education

- Caution patient that this medication must not be taken during pregnancy or when pregnancy is possible. Advise patient to use reliable form of birth control while taking this drug.
- Instruct patient to have regular physical examinations and to notify physician of any change in vision, GI or GU function or other concerns.
- Caution patient to avoid exposure to sunlight and to use sunscreen or wear protective clothing to avoid photosensitivity reaction.
- Teach patient with diabetes how to check blood sugar.
- Teach female patients how to perform breast self-exam, and encourage regular or monthly examinations.
- Advise patient to follow low-sodium diet.
- Instruct patient to report these symptoms to physician: pain in groin or calves, sharp chest pain or sudden shortness of breath, abnormal vaginal bleeding, missed menstrual period or suspected pregnancy, lump in breast, sudden severe headache, dizziness or fainting, vision or speech disturbance, weakness or numbness in leg or arm, severe abdominal pain, depression, yellowing of skin, edema (swelling).
- Caution patient not to take otc medications without consulting physician.

See Patient Guide, p. 126.

Chlorpheniramine Maleate

(klor-fen-AIR-uh-meen MAL-ee-ate)

Aller-Chlor, Chlo-Amine, Chlor-Pro, Chlor-Trimeton, Chlorate, Chlortab-4, Chlortab-8, Chlortab-12, Pfeiffer's Allergy, Phenetron, Telachlor, Teldrin, ✤ *Chlor-Tripolon, Chlor-Tripolon Repetabs*

Class: Antihistamine/alkylamine

Action Competitively antagonizes histamine at H_1 receptor sites.

Indications Symptomatic relief of perennial and seasonal allergic rhinitis; relief of vasomotor rhinitis and allergic conjunctivitis; temporary relief of runny nose and sneezing due to common cold; treatment of allergic and nonallergic pruritic symptoms; relief of mild, uncomplicated urticaria and angiodema; amelioration of allergic reactions to blood or plasma; adjunctive therapy in anaphylactic reactions.

Contraindications Hypersensitivity to antihistamines; narrow-angle glaucoma; stenosing peptic ulcer; symptomatic prostatic hypertrophy; asthmatic attack; bladder neck obstruction; pyloroduodenal obstruction; MAO therapy; use in newborn or premature infants and in nursing mothers.

Route/Dosage

Symptomatic Allergic Conditions

ADULTS & CHILDREN > 12 YR: **PO** 4 mg q 4-6 hr (immediate-release form) or 8-12 mg at bedtime or q 8-12 hr (sustained release form) (maximum 24 mg/24 hr). **SC/IM/IV** 5-20 mg as single dose (maximum 40 mg/24 hr): CHILDREN 6-12 YR: **PO** 2 mg q 4-6 hr (immediate-release form) or 8 mg at bedtime or during day as indicated (sustained release form) (maximum 12 mg/24 hr). CHILDREN 2-6 YR: **PO** (only tablet or syrup; sustained release not recommended) 1 mg q 4-6 hr (maximum 4 mg/24 hr).

Allergic Reactions to Blood or Plasma

ADULTS: **SC/IM/IV** 10-20 mg as single dose (maximum 40 mg/24 hr).

Anaphylaxis

ADULTS: **IV** 10-20 mg as single dose.

Interactions

Alcohol and CNS depressants: May cause additive CNS depressant effects. MAO *inhibitors:* May increase anticholinergic effects of chlorpheniramine.

Lab Test Interferences

Skin testing procedures: Antihistamines may prevent or diminish otherwise positive reaction to dermal reactivity indicators.

Adverse Reactions

CV: Orthostatic hypotension; palpitations; bradycardia; tachycardia; reflex tachycardia; extrasystoles; faintness. *RESP:* Thickening of bronchial secretions; chest tightness; wheezing; nasal stuffiness; dry nose and throat; sore throat; respiratory depression. *CNS:* Drowsiness (often transient); sedation; dizziness; faintness; disturbed coordination; nervousness; restlessness. *GI:* Dry mouth; epigastric distress; anorexia; nausea; vomiting; diarrhea; constipation; change in bowel habits. *GU:* Urinary frequency or retention; dysuria. *HEMA:* Hemolytic anemia; thrombocytopenia; agranulocytosis. *META:* Increased appetite; weight gain. *OTHER:* Hypersensitivity reactions; photosensitivity.

Precautions

Pregnancy: Category B. Do not use during third trimester. *Lactation:* Contraindicated in nursing mothers. *Children:* Overdosage may cause hallucinations, convulsions and death. Antihistamines may diminish mental alertness. In young child, they may produce paradoxical excitation. Contraindicated in newborn or premature infants. Sustained release form not recommended in children < 6 yr. *Elderly patients:* Greater likelihood of dizziness, excessive sedation, syncope, toxic confusional states and hypotension in patients > 60 yr. Dosage reduction may be required. *Special risk patients:* Use drug with caution in patients with predisposition to urinary retention, history of bronchial asthma, increased IOP, hyperthyroidism, cardiovascular disease or hypertension. Avoid in patients with sleep apnea. *Hepatic impairment:* Use drug with caution in patients with cirrhosis or other liver disease. *Hypersensitivity reactions:* May occur. Have epinephrine 1:1000 immediately available. *Respiratory disease:* Generally not recommended to treat lower respiratory tract symptoms including asthma.

NURSING CONSIDERATIONS

Administration/Storage

- Administer with food or milk to decrease GI upset.
- Instruct patient not to chew or crush sustained release tablets; have patient swallow tablet whole.
- Instruct patient to chew chewable tablets and not to swallow tablet whole.
- Administer 10 mg/ml solution intravenously, intramuscularly or subcutaneously.
- Administer 100 mg/ml solution intramuscularly or subcutaneously only; do not administer intravenously.
- Administer IV solution undiluted in 10 mg dose over at least 1 min.
- Store at room temperature. Syrup and injectable forms should be protected from light.

Assessment/Interventions

- Obtain patient history, including drug history and any known allergies.
- Note baseline vital signs and monitor throughout therapy.
- Monitor I&O. Note any urinary retention or problems with voiding.
- Notify physician if patient has history of asthma.
- If signs of allergy or difficulty breathing occur, notify physician.
- Monitor breath sounds and report abnormalities to physician.

OVERDOSAGE: SIGNS & SYMPTOMS

Diminished mental alertness, ataxia, hallucinations, convulsions, death

Patient/Family Education

- Caution patient to avoid intake of alcoholic beverages or other CNS depressants.
- Instruct patient to notify physician if blurred vision occurs.
- Advise patient to use good oral hygiene, to take sips of water frequently, suck on ice chips, sugarless hard candy or chew sugarless gum if dry mouth occurs.
- Advise patient that concomitant administration of MAO inhibitors may prolong and intensify effects of medication.
- Instruct patient to maintain adequate fluid intake to avoid thickening of respiratory secretions.
- Caution patient to avoid exposure to sunlight and to use sunscreen or wear protective clothing to avoid photosensitivity reaction.
- Advise patient that drug may cause drowsiness and to use caution while driving or performing other tasks requiring mental alertness.
- Advise patient to carry Medi-Alert identification noting allergic condition.

See Patient Guide, pp. 127.

Chlorpromazine HCl

(klor-PRO-muh-zeen HIGH-droe-KLOR-ide)

Ormazine, *Thorazine*, *Thorazine Concentrate*, *Thorazine Spansules*, ♣ *Largactil*
Class: Antipsychotic/phenothiazine; antiemetic

Action Effects apparently due to dopamine receptor blockade in CNS.

Indications Management of psychotic disorders and manic phase of manic-depressive disorder; relief of anxiety and restlessness prior to surgery; adjunct in treatment of tetanus; management of acute intermittent porphyria, severe behavioral and conduct disorders in children; control of nausea and vomiting; relief of intractable hiccups. **Unlabeled uses:** Treatment of phencyclidine psychosis; treatment of migraine headaches (IM or IV forms).

Contraindications Comatose or severely depressed states; allergy to product or other phenothiazines; presence of large amounts of other CNS depressants; bone marrow depression; blood dyscrasias; liver damage; cerebral arteriosclerosis; coronary artery disease; severe hypotension or hypertension; subcortical brain damage.

Route/Dosage

Adults

PSYCHIATRIC (OUTPATIENT): **IM** 25 mg for prompt control; may repeat in 1 hr. **PO** 25-50 mg tid after initial regimen. May initiate oral dosing with 10 mg tid-qid and adjust individually; up to 800 mg/day may be needed. PSYCHIATRIC (INPATIENT): **PO** 25 mg tid; increase as needed; usually 400 mg/day. **IM** 25 mg initially; may give additional 25-50 mg in 1 hr. Increase gradually until controlled. Up to 2000 mg/day may be needed but generally not for extended periods. ACUTE INTERMITTENT PORPHYRIA: **PO** 25-50 mg; **IM** 25-50 mg tid-qid. TETANUS: **IM** 25 to 50 mg tid-qid; **IV** 25-50 mg diluted to at least 1 mg/ml and administered at rate of 1 mg/min. NAUSEA AND VOMITING: **PO** 10-25 mg q 4-6 hr prn. **PR** 50-100 mg q 6-8 hr prn. **IM** 25 mg. If no hypotension, may give 25-50 mg q 4-6 hr prn. INTRACTABLE HICCUPS: **PO** 25-50 mg tid-qid. **IM** May give 25-50 mg if symptoms persist 2-3 days **IV** May use slow infusion if hiccups persist.

Children > 6 Mo

PSYCHIATRIC (OUTPATIENT): **PO** 0.5 mg/kg q 4-6 hr prn; **PR** 1 mg/kg q 6-8 hr prn **IM** 0.5 mg/kg q 6-8 hr prn. PSYCHIATRIC (INPATIENT): **PO** Start low and increase gradually; 50-200 mg/day may be needed in severe cases or in older children. **IM** *Up to 5 years:* Do not exceed 40 mg/day. *5-12 years:* Do not exceed 75 mg/day if possible. TETANUS: **IM/IV** 0.5 mg/kg q 6-8 hr. When giving IV, dilute to at least 1 mg/ml and administer at rate of 1 mg over 2 minutes. In children ≤ 23 kg, do not exceed 40 mg/day; 23-45 kg, do not exceed 75 mg/day if possible. NAUSEA AND VOMITING: **PO** 0.55 mg/kg q 4-6 hr. **PR** 1.1 mg/kg q 6-8 hr prn. **IM** 0.55 mg/kg q 6-8 hr prn. Do not exceed 40 mg/day if < 5 yrs or 75 mg/day if 5-12 yrs.

Interactions

Alcohol: May cause increased CNS depression and may precipitate extrapyramidal reaction. *Anticholinergics:* May reduce therapeutic effects of and increase anticholinergic effects of chlorpromazine; may lead to tardive dyskinesia. *Barbiturate anesthetics:* May increase frequency and severity of neuromuscular excitation and hypotension. *Beta-blockers:* May result in increased plasma levels of beta-blocker and chlorpromazine. *Epinephrine*, *norepinephrine:* Actions of these drugs may be decreased or reversed. *Lithium:* May cause disorienting unconsciousness and extrapyramidal effects. *Meperidine:* May result in excessive sedation and hypotension. *Metrizamide:* Risk of seizure may increase.

Lab Test Interferences
Chlorpromazine may discolor urine (pink to red-brown). False-positive pregnancy test results may occur (less likely with a serum test). Increases in protein-bound iodine have been reported. False-positive phenylketonuria test results may occur.

Adverse Reactions
CV: Orthostatic hypotension; hypertension; tachycardia; bradycardia; syncope; cardiac arrest; circulatory collapse; ECG changes. *RESP:* Laryngospasm; bronchospasm; dyspnea, aspiration pneumonia. *CNS:* Faintness; dizziness; extrapyramidal side effects (eg, pseudoparkinsonism; tardive dyskinesia); muscle spasms; motor restlessness; headache; weakness; tremor; fatigue; slurring; insomnia; vertigo; seizures; sedation; neuroleptic malignant syndrome. *EENT:* Pigmentary retinopathy; glaucoma; photophobia; blurred vision; increased IOP; mydriasis. *GI:* Dry mouth; dyspepsia; constipation; adynamic ileus (with possible complications resulting in death). *GU:* Urinary retention and hesitancy; impotence; sexual dysfunction; menstrual irregularities. *HEMA:* Agranulocytosis; eosinophilia; leukopenia; hemolytic anemia; thrombocytopenic purpura. *HEPA:* Jaundice. *DERM:* Photosensitivity; skin pigmentation; dry skin; exfoliative dermatitis; urticarial rash; maculopapular hypersensitivity reaction; seborrhea; eczema. *META:* Altered cholesterol levels. *OTHER:* Increased appetite and weight; polydipsia; breast enlargement; galactorrhea; heat stroke/hyperpyrexia; sudden death.

Precautions
Pregnancy: Safety not established. *Lactation:* Excreted in breast milk. *Children:* Do not use in children < 6 mo unless considered lifesaving. Do not use in conditions for which specific children's dosage not established. *Elderly:* More susceptible to enhanced effects; consider lower dose. *Special risk patients:* Use caution in patients with cardiovascular disease or mitral insufficiency, history of glaucoma, EEG abnormalities or seizure disorders, prior brain damage, hepatic or renal impairment.

NURSING CONSIDERATIONS

Administration/Storage
- Store all forms at room temperature and avoid exposure to direct sunlight, excessive heat, or cold. Keep liquid concentrate in amber or opaque bottle.
- Give with food to avoid gastric irritation. Tablets may be crushed, but capsules should not be opened, crushed or chewed.
- Make certain that patient swallows oral preparations.
- Mix concentrate with juice, soft drink or semisolid food immediately prior to administration.
- If concentrate is spilled on skin or clothing, rinse area immediately with water to prevent or reduce skin irritation.
- Give deep IM injection. Solution may be slightly yellow without affecting potency. If skin irritation is a problem, dilute with normal saline or 2% procaine.
- Caution patient to remain recumbent for approximately 30 min following IM injection.
- Monitor BP frequently during IV infusion.

Assessment/Interventions
- Obtain patient history, including drug history and any known allergies.
- Identify last day of menses, and assess for possible pregnancy, use of contraceptives and whether patient is currently breastfeeding.
- Assess daily for changes in mental status.
- Notify physician of any signs or symptoms of possible adverse reactions.
- Assess lying and standing BP, vital

signs, and weight and compare to baseline values.
- Document orthostatic hypotension by routinely recording lying and standing BP.
- Document signs of anticholinergic-related effects such as dry mouth, blurred vision, constipation and urinary retention. Offer sugarless hard candy or gum and sips of water if dry mouth is a problem.
- Weigh patient weekly and monitor intake and output.

OVERDOSAGE: SIGNS & SYMPTOMS

CNS depression, hypotension, extrapyramidal symptoms, agitation, restlessness, convulsions, fever, hypothermia, hyperthermia, coma, autonomic reactions, ECG changes, cardiac arrhythmias

Patient/Family Education

- Instruct patient to report these symptoms to physician immediately: sore throat, fever, easy bruising, unusual bleeding, muscular rigidity, breathing difficulty, rapid heart beat, yellow skin or sclera, skin rash.
- Remind patient to continue medication even if symptoms subside because symptoms may recur if medication is discontinued. Caution patient not to stop taking medication abruptly.
- Explain that drug may cause drowsiness and to avoid intake of alcoholic beverages as well as any otc medications that also may cause drowsiness. Remind patient to use caution when driving or performing other tasks that require mental alertness.
- Instruct patient to consult physician before taking other medications including nonprescription drugs.
- Explain that dry mouth may be relieved by rinsing mouth with warm water, sucking on sugarless hard candy or gum and taking frequent sips of water.
- Remind patient to dress warmly in cold weather and avoid extended exposure to either very hot or very cold temperatures, as body temperature is harder to maintain with this drug.
- Explain that medication may cause increased sensitivity to sunlight and that sunscreen and/or protective clothing should be worn until sun tolerance is known.
- Inform patient that dizziness or lightheadedness may be experienced when rising to a sitting or standing position.
- Tell patient that a pink or red-brown urine discoloration is a harmless effect of the medication.
- Tell patient to carry a card or Medi-Alert bracelet at all times that lists the name and dosage of this medication.

See Patient Guide, p. 128.

Chlorpropamide

(klor-PRO-puh-mide)

Diabinese, ♣ *APO-Chlorpropamide*

Class: Antidiabetic/sulfonylurea

Action Decreases blood glucose by stimulating insulin release from pancreas.

Indications Adjunct to diet to lower blood glucose in patients with non-insulin-dependent diabetes mellitus (type II) whose hyperglycemia cannot be controlled by diet alone. **Unlabeled use:** Control of neurogenic diabetes insipidus.

Contraindications Hypersensitivity to sulfonylureas; diabetes complicated by ketoacidosis with or without coma; sole therapy for insulin-independent (type I) diabetes mellitus; diabetes when complicated by pregnancy.

Route/Dosage

Adults

Initial dose: **PO** 250 mg/day in single dose.

Elderly

Initial dose: **PO** 100-125 mg/day in single dose. Maintenance: **PO** 100-250 mg/day in single dose.

Severe Diabetic Adults

PO up to 500 mg/day; avoid doses > 750 mg/day.

Interactions

Androgens, anticoagulants, chloramphenicol, clofibrate, fenfluramine, methyldopa, MAO inhibitors, phenylbutazone, probenecid, salicylates, sulfonamides, tricyclic antidepressants, urinary acidifiers: May increase hypoglycemic effect. *Beta-blockers, corticosteroids, diazoxide, hydantoins, rifampin, thiazide diuretics, urinary alkalinizers:* May decrease hypoglycemic effect.

Lab Test Interferences

Liver function tests: Drug causes elevated results. *BUN and creatinine:* Drug causes mild to moderate elevations.

Adverse Reactions

CV: Increased risk of cardiovascular mortality when compared with patients treated with diet alone. *CNS:* Dizziness; vertigo. *EENT:* Tinnitus. *GI:* GI disturbances (eg, nausea, epigastric fullness, heartburn). *HEMA:* Leukopenia; thrombocytopenia; aplastic anemia; agranulocytosis; hemolytic anemia; pancytopenia; hepatic porphyria. *HEPA:* Cholestatic jaundice; elevated liver function tests. *DERM:* Allergic skin reactions; eczema; pruritus; erythema; urticaria; morbilliform or maculopapular eruptions; lichenoid reactions; photosensitivity. *META:* Hypoglycemia; syndrome of inappropriate secretion of antidiuretic hormone with water retention and dilutional hyponatremia, especially in patients with CHF or hepatic cirrhosis. *OTHER:* Disulfiramlike reaction; weakness; paresthesia; fatigue; malaise.

Precautions

Pregnancy: Category C. Insulin is recommended to maintain blood glucose levels during pregnancy. Prolonged severe neonatal hypoglycemia can occur if sulfonylureas are administered at time of delivery. If administering to pregnant patient, discontinue 2 days-4 wk before expected date of delivery. *Lactation:* Excreted in breast milk. *Children:* Safety and efficacy not established. *Elderly or debilitated patients:* Particularly susceptible to hypoglycemic action. Hypoglycemia can be difficult to recognize in elderly. *Hepatic and renal impairment:* Use drug with caution and monitor liver and renal function frequently.

NURSING CONSIDERATIONS

Administration/Storage

- Administer once a day.
- Give with food or 30 min before meal if drug causes GI upset.
- When discontinuing chlorpropamide and switching to another oral hypoglycemic agent, exercise caution for 2 wk; prolonged action of chlorpropamide may provoke hypoglycemia.
- Store in cool environment in tightly closed container.

Assessment/Interventions

- Obtain patient history, including drug history and any known allergies. Note presence of hepatic or renal impairment and nature of patient's diabetic illness.
- Check blood sugar levels frequently and observe for symptoms of hypoglycemia or hyperglycemia and report to physician.
- Be aware that hypoglycemia may be difficult to recognize in elderly patients or patients taking beta-blockers.
- When patients with impaired liver or renal function are receiving this drug, check liver and renal function test results frequently.
- Observe for evidence of possible water retention (especially in pa-

tients with CHF) and report to physician.

- If cholestatic jaundice occurs, discontinue drug and notify physician.

OVERDOSAGE: SIGNS & SYMPTOMS

Hypoglycemia, tingling of lips and tongue, hunger, nausea, lethargy, confusion, agitation, nervousness, tachycardia, sweating, tremor, convulsions, stupor, coma

Patient/Family Education

- Explain that this medication will not cure disease.
- Emphasize that drug must be taken on daily basis and should not be discontinued abruptly.
- Tell patient that drug may cause GI upset and to take it with food if GI upset occurs.
- Teach patient to self-monitor blood glucose.
- Inform patient that physician should be contacted if symptoms of hypoglycemia occur (fatigue, excessive hunger, profuse sweating, numbness of extremities).
- Instruct patient to notify physician if symptoms of hyperglycemia occur (excessive thirst or urination, urinary glucose or ketones).
- Tell patient to report constipation, nausea, vomiting, drowsiness, dizziness, fever, sore throat, rash and unusual bruising or bleeding to physician.
- Inform patient that this drug is not substitute for exercise and diet control; patient must follow prescribed regimens of diet, exercise and personal hygiene.
- Instruct patient to inform all physicians involved in patient's care that patient is taking this drug.
- Advise patient not to take any medication (including otc) or drink alcoholic beverages without consulting physician.
- Caution patient to avoid exposure to sunlight and to use sunscreen or wear protective clothing to avoid photosensitivity reaction.
- Advise patient that drug can cause dizziness and to use caution while driving or performing other tasks requiring mental alertness.
- Remind patient to wear Medi-Alert identification.

See Patient Guide, p. 129.

Chlorthalidone

(klor-THAL-ih-dohn)

Hygroton, Thalitone

Class: Thiazide diuretic

Action Inhibits reabsorption of sodium and chloride in proximal portion of distal convoluted tubules.

Indications Reduction of edema associated with CHF, hepatic cirrhosis, renal dysfunction, corticosteroid and estrogen therapy; management of hypertension. **Unlabeled uses:** Treatment of calcium nephrolithiasis, osteoporosis, diabetes insipidus.

Contraindications Hypersensitivity to thiazides, related diuretics or sulfonamide-derived drugs; anuria; renal decompensation.

Route/Dosage

Edema

ADULTS: **PO** 50-200 mg daily or on alternate days.

Hypertension

ADULTS: **PO** 25-100 mg daily. Doses > 25 mg/day potentiate potassium excretion but do not benefit sodium excretion or BP reduction.

Interactions

Allopurinol: Concurrent use may increase incidence of hypersensitivity reactions to allopurinol. *Amphotericin B, corticosteroids:* May intensify potassium depletion. *Anticholinergics:* May increase chlorthalidone absorption. *Anticoagulants:* May diminish anticoagulant effects. *Bile acid sequestrants:* May reduce chlorthalidone absorption. Give chlorthalidone ≥ 2 hr before bile acid sequestrant. *Calcium salts:* Hypercalcemia may develop. *Diazoxide:* May cause hyperglycemia. *Digitalis glycosides:* Diuretic-induced hypokalemia and hypomagnesemia may precipitate digitalis-induced arrhythmias. *Lithium:* May decrease renal excretion of lithium. *Loop diuretics:* Synergistic effects may result in profound diuresis and serious electrolyte abnormalities. *Methenamines, nonsteroidal anti-inflammatory drugs:* May decrease effectiveness of chlorthalidone. *Sulfonylureas, insulin:* May decrease hypoglycemic effect of sulfonylureas.

Lab Test Interferences

Increased serum bilirubin levels. Serum magnesium levels in uremic patients may be increased.

Adverse Reactions

CNS: Dizziness; lightheadedness; vertigo; headache; paresthesias; weakness; restlessness; insomnia. *EENT:* Xanthopsia (yellow vision). *GI:* Anorexia; gastric irritation; nausea; vomiting; abdominal pain or cramping; bloating; diarrhea; constipation; pancreatitis. *GU:* Impotence; reduced libido. *HEMA:* Leukopenia; thrombocytopenia; agranulocytosis; aplastic or hypoplastic anemia. *HEPA:* Jaundice. *DERM:* Purpura; photosensitivity; rash; urticaria; necrotizing angiitis; vasculitis; cutaneous vasculitis; exfoliative dermatitis; toxic epidermal necrolysis. *META:* Hyperglycemia; glycosuria; hyperuricemia; fluid and electrolyte imbalances. *OTHER:* Muscle cramps or spasms.

Precautions

Pregnancy: Category B. *Lactation:* Excreted in breast milk. *Children:* Safety and efficacy not established. *Hepatic function impairment:* Minor alterations of fluid and electrolyte balance may precipitate hepatic coma; use with caution. *Hypersensitivity:* May occur in patients with or without history of allergy or bronchial asthma; cross-sensitivity with sulfonamides also may occur. *Renal function impairment:* May precipitate azotemia; use with caution. *Lipids:* May cause increased concentrations of total serum cholesterol, total triglycerides and LDL in some patients. *Postsympathectomy patients:* Antihypertensive effects may be enhanced.

NURSING CONSIDERATIONS

Administration/Storage

- Administer drug early in AM so that diuresis will occur during day rather than night.
- Give with meals or milk to avoid GI upset.

Assessment/Interventions

- Obtain patient history, including drug history and any known allergies.
- Assess serum electrolytes and digitalis level (if appropriate) periodically.
- Closely monitor blood sugar, complete blood count and platelets.
- Review triglyceride and cholesterol levels periodically.

OVERDOSAGE: SIGNS & SYMPTOMS

Orthostatic hypotension, dizziness, drowsiness, syncope, potassium depletion, nausea, vomiting, lethargy, coma, GI irritation, GI hypermobility, seizures

Patient/Family Education

- Teach patient signs and symptoms of hypokalemia (weakness, cramps, nausea, and dizziness), especially if patient is taking digitalis.
- Explain diuretic effects of drug so patient is aware of expected and potential outcomes.
- Instruct patient to follow low-sodium diet to enhance action of medication.
- If high-potassium diet is recommended by physician, help patient

identify appropriate meal plans or potassium supplements.
- Teach patient to record weight daily at a consistent time and to notify physician if weight fluctuates ± 5 pounds.
- Tell patient to notify physician of salt or water retention occurs (eg, swelling of feet, ankles, calves).
- Caution patient to avoid exposure to sunlight and to use sunscreen or wear protective clothing to avoid photosensitivity reaction.
- Advise patient to avoid sudden position changes to prevent orthostatic hypotension. Have patient get up slowly and dangle feet before getting out of bed.
- Caution patient not to take any otc medications without consulting physician.

See Patient Guide, p. 130.

Chlorzoxazone

(klor-ZOX-uh-zone)

Paraflex, Parafon Forte DSC, Remular-S

Class: Skeletal muscle relaxant/centrally acting

Action Action may be related to its sedative properties or to inhibition of reflex arcs at spinal cord and subcortical levels of brain.

Indications Relief of discomfort associated with painful musculoskeletal conditions.

Contraindications Standard considerations.

Route/Dosage
ADULTS: **PO** Initial (for acute pain): 500 mg tid-qid; increase to 750 mg if needed. As improvement occurs, reduce dose; 250 mg tid-qid is usually sufficient.

Interactions
Alcohol and other CNS depressants: Additive CNS depressant effects may occur.

Lab Test Interferences
None well documented.

Adverse Reactions
CNS: Drowsiness; dizziness; lightheadedness; malaise; overstimulation. *GI:* GI disturbances. *GU:* Urine discoloration (orange or purple red). *HEPA:* Drug-induced hepatitis. *DERM:* Allergic-type skin rashes; petechiae. *OTHER:* Hypersensitivity (eg, angioneurotic edema; anaphylaxis).

Precautions
Pregnancy: Pregnancy category undetermined. *Lactation:* Undetermined. *Hepatic impairment:* Avoid use in patients with liver impairment; discontinue if signs of dysfunction occur. *Hazardous tasks:* May impair ability to perform tasks requiring mental or physical coordination or dexterity, including driving. Drowsiness is very common.

NURSING CONSIDERATIONS

Administration/Storage
- Give with meals to avoid GI upset.
- Discuss dosage adjustments with physician according to patient's response.

Assessment/Interventions
- Notify physician if patient is pregnant or nursing.
- Obtain patient history, including drug history and any known allergies.
- Monitor skin and sclera for jaundice.
- Monitor liver function throughout therapy.
- Report signs of liver dysfunction to physician.

OVERDOSAGE: SIGNS & SYMPTOMS
Nausea, vomiting, diarrhea, drowsiness, dizziness, lightheadedness, malaise, sluggishness, loss of muscle tone, decreased deep tendon reflex, respiratory depression

Patient/Family Education

- Instruct patient to inform physician of any urticaria, redness or itching.
- Tell patient to report to physician any yellowing of skin or eyes.
- Advise patient that drug may cause drowsiness and to use caution while driving or performing other tasks that require mental alertness.
- Advise patient to avoid intake of alcoholic beverages and other medications that cause drowsiness while taking product.
- Advise patient to notify physician before discontinuing medication.
- Inform patient to take a missed dose as soon as possible, unless several hours have passed. Advise patient not to double doses.
- Inform patient urine may turn orange or purple-red while taking this medication.
- Instruct patient to take with meals to avoid GI upset.

See Patient Guide, p. 131.

Cholestyramine

(koe-less-TIE-ruh-meen)

Questran, Questran Light
Class: Antihyperlipidemic/bile acid sequestrant

Action Increases removal of bile acids from body by forming insoluble complexes in intestine, which are then excreted in feces. As body loses bile acids, it converts cholesterol from blood to bile acid, thus lowering serum cholesterol.

Indications Reduction of serum cholesterol in patients with primary hypercholesterolemia; relief of pruritus associated with partial biliary obstruction. **Unlabeled uses:** Treatment of antibiotic-induced pseudomembranous colitis, bile salt–mediated diarrhea and digitalis toxicity.

Contraindications Hypersensitivity to bile acid sequestering resins; complete biliary obstruction.

Route/Dosage
ADULTS: PO 4 g 1-6 times/day; generally given 3-4 times/day.

Interactions
Acetaminophen, amiodarone, corticosteroids, digitalis glycosides, methotrexate, some NSAIDs (eg, piroxicam), propranolol, thiazide diuretics, thyroid, ursodiol, warfarin and other drugs: Cholestyramine may interfere with the absorption of many drugs, especially those listed. *Fats and fat-soluble vitamins A, D, E and K:* Cholestyramine may interfere with normal fat absorption and digestion; consider supplementation with these vitamins and with folic acid. *Iopanoic acid:* Coadministration may result in abnormal cholecystography.

Lab Test Interferences
Increased serum phosphorus and chloride; decreased serum sodium and potassium.

Adverse Reactions
GI: Constipation (can be severe and at times accompanied by fecal impaction); aggravation of hemorrhoids; abdominal pain and distention; GI bleeding; belching; flatulence; nausea; vomiting; diarrhea; heartburn; anorexia; steatorrhea. *HEMA:* Bleeding tendencies related to vitamin K deficiency; folic acid deficiency. *DERM:* Rash; irritation of skin, tongue, and perianal area. *META:* Fat-soluble vitamin deficiencies; hyperchloremic acidosis and increased urinary calcium excretion; osteoporosis.

Precautions
Pregnancy: Safety not estab-

lished. *Lactation:* Undetermined. *Children:* Safety and efficacy not established. *Carcinogenesis:* Incidence of intestinal tumors in studies was greater in cholestyramine-treated rats than in controls; relevance to clinical practice is not known.

NURSING CONSIDERATIONS

Administration/Storage

- Administer cholestyramine separate from other drugs. Give other drugs 1 hr before or 4-6 hr after cholestyramine.
- In general, give medication before meals.
- Never administer dry powder without liquid. Use any noncarbonated fluid.
- Instruct patient to chew tablets thoroughly. Follow with full glass of water.

Assessment/Interventions

- Obtain patient history, including drug history and any known allergies.
- Document serum cholesterol and triglycerides levels.
- Monitor electrolyte balance, and notify physician of increased serum phosphorus and chloride, decreased serum sodium and potassium.

OVERDOSAGE: SIGNS & SYMPTOMS

GI obstruction

Patient/Family Education

- In general, instruct patient to take medication before meals.
- Advise patient to take any other medications, including otc medications, 1 hr before or 4-6 hr after taking cholestyramine.
- Instruct patient to use dry powder form to mix with fluid (2-6 oz) according to packet directions.
- Teach patient how to implement any vitamin and mineral supplementation recommended by physician.
- Help patient identify appropriate meal plans that supply adequate sodium and potassium and are low in phosphorus.
- Tell patient to take prune juice, fruits and vegetables and good fluid intake on a regular basis to avoid constipation. If constipation or other GI upset occurs and is bothersome, instruct patient to notify physician.
- Advise patient to follow regular exercise routine.
- Instruct patient to adhere to diet low in fats and to participate in weight management program if appropriate.
- Advise patients with phenylketonuria that 5 g dose of Questran Light contains aspartame equivalent to 16.8 mg of phenylalanine.
- Instruct patient to report these symptoms to physician: constipation, flatulence, nausea, heartburn, abnormal bleeding.

See Patient Guide, p. 132.

Cimetidine

(sigh-MET-ih-deen)

Tagamet, ♣ *Apo-Cimetidine, Novocimetine, Nu-Cimet, Peptol*

Class: Histamine H_2 antagonist

Action Reversibly and competitively blocks histamine at H_2 receptors, particularly those in gastric parietal cells, leading to inhibition of gastric acid secretion.

Indications Management of duodenal ulcer; treatment of gastroesophageal reflux disease, including erosive esophagitis; therapy for benign gastric ulcer; treatment of pathologic hypersecretory conditions; prevention of upper GI bleeding. **Unlabeled uses:** Prevention of aspiration pneumonia and stress ulcers; herpesvirus infection; chronic idiopathic urticaria; anaphylaxis (relieves dermatologic symptoms only); dyspepsia; used before anesthesia to prevent aspiration pneumonitis; to treat hyperparathyroidism and to control secondary hyperparathyroidism in chronic hemodialysis patient; treatment of chronic viral warts in children.

Contraindications Hypersensitivity to cimetidine or other H_2 antagonists.

Route/Dosage

Duodenal Ulcer (Active)

ADULTS: PO 800 mg at bedtime for 4 to 6 weeks. ALTERNATE REGIMENS PO 300 mg qid w/meals and at bedtime or 400 mg bid. MAINTENANCE THERAPY PO 400 mg at bedtime.

Active Benign Gastric Ulcer

ADULTS: PO 800 mg at bedtime.

Gastroesophageal Reflux Disease

ADULTS: PO 1600 mg daily in divided doses (800 mg or 400 mg) for 12 weeks, although some patients may require chronic therapy.

Pathologic Hypersecretory Conditions

ADULTS: PO 300 mg qid w/meals and at bedtime. If needed, 300 mg doses may be given more often (maximum 2400 mg/day).

Prevention of Upper GI Bleeding

ADULTS: Continuous IV infusion of 50 mg/hr. For hospitalized patients with pathologic hypersecretory conditions or intractable ulcers, or patients unable to take PO medication. *Usual dose:* IM/IV 300 mg q 6 h to 8 h (maximum 2400 mg/day).

Interactions

Antacids, anticholinergics, metoclopramide: May decrease absorption of cimetidine. *Benzodiazepines, caffeine, calcium channel blockers, carbamazepine, chloroquine, labetalol, lidocaine, metoprolol, metronidazole, moricizine, pentoxifylline, phenytoin, propranolol, quinidine, quinine, sulfonylureas, theophyllines, triamterene, tricyclic antidepressants, warfarin:* Cimetidine may reduce metabolism and increase serum concentration and pharmacologic/toxic effects of these drugs. *Carmustine:* Bone marrow toxicity may be enhanced. *Cigarette smoking:* Reversed cimetidine's effects on suppression of nocturnal gastric secretion. *Ferrous salts, indomethacin, fluconazole, ketoconazole, tetracyclines:* Cimetidine may decrease absorption of these drugs. *Hydantoins:* Hydantoin levels may increase. *Narcotic analgesics:* Toxic effects (eg, respiratory depression) may be increased. *Procainamide:* Levels of procainamide and its active metabolite may increase. *Tocainide:* Cimetidine may decrease the pharmacologic effects of tocainide.

Lab Test Interferences

None well documented.

Adverse Reactions

CV: Cardiac arrhythmias. *RESP:* Bronchospasm. *CNS:* Headache; somnolence; fatigue; dizziness; confusional states; hallucinations. *GI:* Diarrhea. *GU:* Impotence; loss of libido. *DERM:* Exfoliative dermatitis or erythroderma; alopecia; rash; erythema multiforme; epidermal necrolysis. *OTHER:* Gynecomastia; hypersensitivity reactions; transient pain at injection site; reversible exacerbation of joint symptoms with preexisting arthritis, including gouty arthritis.

Precautions

Pregnancy: Category B. *Lactation:* Excreted in breast milk. *Children:* Safety and efficacy not established. *Elderly:* May have reduced renal function; decreased clearance may occur. *Renal function impairment:* Decreased clearance may occur; reduced dosage may be needed. *Hepatic function impairment:* Use caution; decreased clearance may occur. *Hypersensitivity:* Rare cases of anaphylaxis have occurred as well as rare episodes of hypersensitivity. *Gastric malignancy:* Symptomatic relief with cimetidine does not preclude gastric malignancy. *Antiandrogenic effect:* Gynecomastia, especially in patients treated for pathologic hypersecretory states may occur. *Rapid IV administration:* Has been followed by rare instances of cardiac arrhythmias and hypotension. *Reversible CNS effects:* Mental confusion, agitation, psychosis, depression, anxiety, hallucinations and disorientation have occurred, predominantly in severely ill patients. Advanced age and pre-existing liver or renal disease appear to be contributing factors.

NURSING CONSIDERATIONS

Administration/Storage

- Administer medication with or before meals and at bedtime for maximum effect.
- Administer IM dose undiluted. Dilute IV dose (300 mg) in 0.9% normal saline, D5W or other compatible solution to a total of 20 ml. Inject slowly over no less than 5 min.
- For intermittent IV infusion, dilute 300 mg in at least 50 ml of compatible solution; infuse over at least 20 min. (Continuous IV infusion is usually preceded by a loading dose.)
- Do not add drugs or additives to mixture. Stop other in-line drugs while administering, and flush lines before and after administration.
- Do not allow equipment containing aluminum to come in contact with the solution.
- Use only compatible solutions for admixture: 0.9% normal saline, 5% and 10% Dextrose in Water, lactated Ringer's solution, 5% sodium bicarbonate.
- Product may be added to standard TPN solutions.
- Store premixed products at room temperature. Discard any unused mixed solutions after 48 hr.

Assessment/Interventions

- Obtain patient history, including drug history and any known allergies.
- Establish baseline vital signs.
- Avoid administering antacids within 1 hr of medication.
- Review periodic monitoring of serum concentrations and clinical effects for other drugs affected by cimetidine.
- Renal/liver function studies and blood counts are all especially important in elderly.
- Assess patient for abdominal pain, confusion and GI bleeding (blood in stools or emesis).
- Assess gastric pH q 8 hr, when possible.

Patient/Family Education

- Counsel patients to stop smoking, since smoking reduces ulcer-healing efficacy of cimetidine.
- Instruct patients to keep appointments for laboratory testing and physician follow-up.
- Advise patients not to take otc medications without consulting physician.
- Instruct patients to report to physician immediately any black tarry stools, coffee-ground emesis, abdominal pain or confusion.
- Counsel patients regarding need for lifestyle changes, stress reduction programs and dietary modifications (eg, avoid spicy foods and alcohol).

See Patient Guide, p. 133.

Ciprofloxacin

(sip-ROW-FLOX-uh-sin)

Cipro, Cipro IV, Ciloxan
Class: Antibiotic/fluoroquinolone

Action Interferes with microbial DNA synthesis.

Indications Treatment of infections of lower respiratory tract, skin and skin structure, bone and joint, urinary tract, gonorrhea, chancroid and infectious diarrhea caused by susceptible strains of specific organisms; typhoid fever; uncomplicated cervical and urethral gonorrhea. **Ophthalmic use:** Treatment of corneal ulcers and conjunctivitis due to susceptible organisms. **Unlabeled uses:** Treatment of pulmonary exacerbations associated with cystic fibrosis; management of malignant external otitis, "traveler's" diarrhea, mycobacterial infections, cat scratch fever and chronic prostatitis.

Contraindications Hypersensitivity to fluoroquinolones or quinolones. *Ophthalmic use:* Epithelial herpes simplex keratitis; vaccinia; varicella; fungal disease of ocular structure; mycobacterial infections of eye.

Route/Dosage

Urinary Tract

ADULTS: **PO** 250-500 mg or **IV** 200-400 mg q 12 hr.

Respiratory Tract; Bone and Joint; Skin and Skin Structure

ADULTS: **PO** 500-750 mg or **IV** 400 mg q 12 hr.

Infectious Diarrhea

ADULTS: **PO** 500 mg q 12 hr.

Ocular Infections

ADULTS: *Topical:* Acute infection: 1-2 drops q 15-30 min; moderate infection: 1-2 drops 4-6 times daily.

Typhoid Fever

ADULTS: **PO** 500 mg q 12 hr.

Urethral/Cervical Gonoccocal Infections

ADULTS: **PO** 250 mg as a single dose.

Interactions

Antacids; iron salts; zinc salts; sucralfate; didanosine: May decrease oral absorption of fluoroquinolone. Stagger administration times. *Anticoagulants:* May increase effect of warfarin; monitor prothrombin time. *Antineoplastic agents:* Fluoroquinolone serum levels may be decreased by cyclophosphamide, cytarabine, daunorubicin, doxorubicin, mitoxantrone and vincristine. *Azlocillin:* Decreased clearance of ciprofloxacin. *Caffeine:* Clearance of caffeine is reduced. *Cimetidine:* May interfere with fluoroquinolone elimination and increase effect. *Cyclosporine:* Nephrotoxic effects of cyclosporine may be increased; monitor renal function. *Probenecid:* Decreased ciprofloxacin renal clearance. *Theophylline:* Decreased clearance and increased plasma levels of theophylline may result in toxicity; monitor theophylline level.

Lab Test Interferences

Increased ALT, AST, LDH, alkaline phosphatase, serum bilirubin; increased serum creatinine and BUN; increased triglycerides and cholesterol.

Adverse Reactions

CNS: Headache. *EENT* (ophthalmic use): Lid margin crusting; foreign body sensation; itching; conjunctival hyperemia; decreased vision; sensitivity reactions (eg, transient irritation, burning, stinging, inflammation, angioneurotic edema, dermatitis). Ophthalmic use may produce same adverse effects seen with systemic use. *GI:* Diarrhea; nausea; vomiting; abdominal pain/discomfort. *DERM:* Rash. *OTHER:* Abnormal taste; photosensitivity.

Precautions

Pregnancy: Category C. *Lactation:* Excreted in breast milk. *Children:* Do not use in children < 18 yr. *Convulsions:* CNS stimulation can occur; use with caution in patients with known or suspected CNS disorders. *Renal function impairment:* Reduced clearance may occur; adjust dose downward accordingly in patients with creatinine clearance < 50 ml/min. Refer to manufacturer's package insert for dose calculations. *Hypersensitivity reactions:* Serious and potentially fatal reactions have occurred. Discontinue drug if allergic reaction occurs. *Pseudomembranous colitis:* Consider possibility in patients with diarrhea. *Superinfection:* Use of antibiotics may result in bacterial or fungal overgrowth. Do not use topically in deep-seated ocular infections. *Photosensitivity:* Moderate to severe reactions have occurred with some fluoroquinolones; avoid excessive sunlight and discontinue therapy if phototoxicity occurs. *Crystalline precipitate:* A white crystalline precipitate in superficial portion of corneal defect may occur; reaction is generally self-limiting and does not appear to affect outcome.

NURSING CONSIDERATIONS

Administration/Storage

- Give oral preparation 2 hours after meals; if necessary may be taken with food. Avoid concurrent use of dairy products, antacids, iron- or zinc-containing products, such as multivitamins, with ciprofloxacin.
- For IV infusion dilute before administration to final concentration of 1 to 2 mg/ml.
- Refrigerate or store at room temperature and use within 14 days.
- Infuse over 60 min in a large vein to reduce risk of venous irritation.
- For ophthalmic application, have patient tilt head back, pull lower lid out to make pocket, then place medication in conjunctival sac. Then, without touching patient's eyes, close them. Apply light finger pressure on lacrimal sac for 1 min following application.

Assessment/Interventions

- Obtain patient history, including drug history and any known allergies.
- Monitor I&O.
- Monitor for signs of anaphylaxis (pharyngeal or facial edema, dyspnea, urticaria and itching, hypotension).
- Assess patency of IV site and observe for signs of phlebitis frequently during therapy.
- Monitor signs of infection throughout course of treatment.
- Notify physician if symptoms of pseudomembranous colitis occur (loose or foul-smelling stools) or if symptoms of CNS stimulation occur (tremor, restlessness, confusion and hallucinations).

Patient/Family Education

- Instruct patient to drink sufficient fluids to ensure adequate urinary output.
- Inform patient that tablets may be taken orally without regard to meals, although manufacturer recommends 2-hour interval after meals.
- Caution patient to avoid exposure to sunlight, and to use sunscreens or protective clothing until tolerance is determined.
- Instruct patient to report signs of bacterial or fungal overgrowth (black, furry appearance of tongue, vaginal itching or discharge, loose or foul-smelling stools).
- Caution patient that drug may cause dizziness or lightheadedness and to use caution while driving or performing other tasks requiring mental alertness.
- Caution patients against doubling a dose to "catch up" unless advised by a physician. Instruct patient to contact physician if more than one dose is missed.
- Emphasize importance of completing entire dose regimen.
- Advise patient not to take any otc medications without consulting physician.

See Patient Guide, pp. 134-135.

Cisapride

(SIS-uh-PRIDE)

Propulsid

Class: GI stimulant

Action GI prokinetic agent that enhances release of acetylcholine at myenteric plexus. Increases lower esophageal sphincter pressure and lower esophageal peristalsis; accelerates gastric emptying of liquids and solids.

Indications Symptomatic treatment of patients with nocturnal heartburn caused by gastroesophageal reflux disease.

Contraindications Active GI hemorrhage; mechanical GI obstruction or perforation; concomitant administration of itraconazole, ketoconazole, miconazole IV fluconazole, erythromycin, clarithromycin or troleandomycin.

Route/Dosage
ADULTS: PO 10-20 mg qid at least 15 min before meals and at bedtime.

Interactions
Anticholinergics: May compromise beneficial effect of cisapride. *Anticoagulants:* Coagulation times may increase. *Azole antifungals:* Inhibits the metabolism of cisapride. *H_2 antagonists:* Cimetidine (but not ranitidine) may increase cisapride levels. Also, cisapride may increase absorption of these H_2 antagonists. *Itraconazole, ketoconazole, miconazole IV or troleandomycin:* Serum cisapride concentrations may be elevated, increasing risk of life-threatening cardiac arrhythmias. *Macrolide troleandromycin:* Inhibits the metabolism of cisapride. *Narrow therapeutic ratio drugs or other drugs that require careful titration:* Follow patient closely. Accelerated gastric emptying produced by cisapride could affect rate of absorption of other drugs.

Lab Test Interferences
None well documented.

Adverse Reactions
CV: Tachycardia palpitations. *RESP:* Rhinitis; sinusitis; upper respiratory tract infection; coughing. *CNS:* Headache; somnolence; insomnia; anxiety; nervousness; seizure; extrapyramidal effects. *EENT:* Abnormal vision. *GI:* Diarrhea; abdominal pain; nausea; constipation; flatulence; dyspepsia; rumbling; bloating. *GU:* Urinary tract infection; increased frequency of micturition. *HEMA:* Thrombocytopenia; leukopenia; aplastic anemia; pancytopenia; granulocytopenia. *HEPA:* Elevated liver enzymes; hepatitis. *DERM:* Rash; pruritus. *OTHER:* Pain; arthralgia; fever; viral infection.

Precautions
Pregnancy: Category C. *Lactation:* Excreted in breast milk. *Children:* Safety and efficacy not established. *Arrhythmias:* Serious arrhythmias have been reported in patients taking cisapride with other drugs that inhibit cisapride metabolism. Some of these events have been fatal. *QT prolongation:* Avoid or use with caution in patients with conditions associated with QT prolongation (eg, congenital prolonged QT syndrome, uncorrected electrolyte disturbances, patient taking medications known to prolong QT interval).

NURSING CONSIDERATIONS

Administration/Storage

- Give oral preparations at least 15 min before meals and at bedtime.
- Store at room temperature. Protect tablets from moisture. Protect 20 mg tablets from light.

Assessment/Interventions

- Obtain patient history, including drug history and any known allergies.
- Note results of serum drug concentrations. Absorption rate of other drugs could be affected because of accelerated gastric emptying.
- Monitor results of platelet and WBC testing.
- Notify physician of tachycardia, headache, nausea, upset stomach, rash, diarrhea/constipation, or symptoms of urinary tract infection.

OVERDOSAGE: SIGNS & SYMPTOMS
Retching; rumbling/gurgling noises, flatulence, stool frequency, urinary frequency

Patient/Family Education

- Instruct patient to take medi-

cation at least 15 min before meals or bedtime.

- Teach patient to be aware that other medications may have increased effects while this drug is being taken.
- Advise patient not to use alcohol or benzodiazepines during therapy without physician approval.

See Patient Guide, p. 136.

Cisplatin (CDDP)

(SIS-plat-in)

Platinol, Platinol-AQ

Class: Antineoplastic/alkylator

Action Inorganic heavy metal coordination complex that produces cross-links in DNA; cell cycle nonspecific.

Indications Palliative therapy of metastatic testicular tumors, metastatic ovarian tumors and advanced bladder cancer after surgery or radiotherapy. Combination therapy with other antineoplastics may be required.

Contraindications Preexisting renal impairment; myelosuppression; hearing impairment; history of allergy to platinum-containing compounds.

Route/Dosage
For IV use only.

Metastatic Testicular Tumors
IV 20 mg/m^2/day for 5 days (days 1 to 5) q 3 wk for 3-4 courses; combination therapy recommended.

Metastatic Ovarian Tumors
As single agent: **IV** 100 mg/m^2 q 4 wk.

In Combination Therapy
IV 50 mg/m^2 once q 3-4 wk (day 1) followed by doxorubicin.

Advanced Bladder Cancer
As single agent: **IV** 1 dose 50 to 70 mg/m^2 q 3-4 wk. For heavily pretreated patients, give an initial dose of 50 mg/m^{2}repeated q 4 wk.

Repeat Courses
Do not give a repeat course until certain laboratory values (eg, serum creatinine, BUN, platelets, WBCs) and auditory acuity are acceptable.

Renal Impairment
Dosage adjustment in patients with renal impairment has been suggested but not clearly defined.

Interactions
Aluminum: Do not use needles or IV sets containing aluminum parts because aluminum displaces platinum from cisplatin molecule, causing loss of potency with presence of black precipitate. *Aminoglycosides (gentamicin, amikacin):* May increase nephrotoxicity. *Loop diuretics (ethacrynic acid, furosemide):* May cause additive ototoxicity. *Phenytoin:* Combination chemotherapy (including cisplatin) may reduce phenytoin plasma levels.

Lab Test Interferences
None well documented.

Adverse Reactions
CV: Vascular toxicities (MI, cardiovascular accidents) have occurred in combination therapy. *CNS:* Peripheral and autonomic neuropathy; seizures; taste loss; Lhermitte's sign. *EENT:* Optic neuritis, papilledema and cerebral blindness (usually reversible); blurred vision; altered color perception; tinnitus; high frequency hearing loss; vestibular toxicity. *GI:* Marked nausea and vomiting in nearly all patients, usually beginning 1-6 hours after administration and lasting for 24 hours or longer. *GU:* Nephrotoxicity; renal insufficiency; renal tubular damage. *HEMA:* Myelosuppression with leukopenia; thrombocytopenia; anemia; hemolysis. *DERM:* Rash. *META:* Hypomagnesemia; hypocalcemia; hyponatremia; hypokalemia and hypophosphatemia; increased plasma iron; syndrome of inappropriate antidiuretic hormone secretion. *OTHER:* Tetany; hyperuri-

cemia; anaphylactic reactions; anorexia; elevated ALT.

Precautions

Pregnancy: Category D. *Lactation:* Undetermined. *Children:* Safety and efficacy not established. *Hypersensitivity:* Anaphylactic-like reactions have occurred, including facial edema, wheezing, bronchoconstriction, tachycardia and hypotension. *Nephrotoxicity:* Dose-related and cumulative renal insufficiency is major dose-limiting toxicity. At high doses nephrotoxicity may be irreversible. Toxicity usually is noted 1-2 weeks after administration, with elevated BUN, serum creatinine and serum uric acid levels and reduced creatinine clearance. These should be closely monitored along with magnesium, calcium and potassium levels. Renal function must return to normal before another dose is given. Administration by slow IV infusion (over 6-8 hours) with IV hydration and mannitol diuresis may reduce renal toxicity. *Neuropathies:* Severe peripheral neuropathies have occurred in patients given higher doses or greater dose frequencies than recommended or after prolonged (4-7 mo) treatment. These may be irreversible and are seen as paresthesias in a stocking-glove distribution, areflexia and loss of proprioception and vibratory sensation. Loss of motor function (especially gait) has occurred. Discontinue drug when symptoms are first observed. *Ototoxicity:* May occur after single dose and is manifested by tinnitus, high-frequency hearing loss or decreased ability to hear normal conversation. Children (especially < 12 years old) may be more susceptible. Effects are cumulative. Perform audiometry before every dose.

NURSING CONSIDERATIONS

Administration/Storage

- Wear disposable gloves when preparing solutions. Wash immediately with soap and water if drug accidently contacts skin or mucosa.
- Dissolve contents of 10 and 50 mg vials with 10 or 50 ml of Sterile Water for Injection, respectively. Resulting solutions contain 1 mg/ml.
- Dilute reconstituted drug in 2 L of D5W in ½ or ⅓ Normal Saline containing 37.5 g of mannitol, and infuse over 6 to 8 hr.
- Store at room temperature. Use within 20 hr.

Assessment/Interventions

- Obtain patient history, including drug history and any known allergies.
- Document CBC, results of renal and liver function and electrolyte tests prior to initiation of therapy.
- Assess for fever, chills, sore throat and any other signs of infection.
- Assess patency of IV site frequently during therapy.
- Hydrate patient prior to initial dose with 1 to 2 L of fluid infused for 8 to 12 hr. Maintain adequate hydration and monitor urine output during the following 24 hr.
- Administer antiemetic 30-60 min prior to initiating therapy, to control nausea and vomiting. Continue antiemetics as necessary throughout treatment.
- Monitor for signs of anaphylaxis (facial edema, wheezing, tachycardia, hypotension).
- Monitor I&O and specific gravity of urine frequently.

OVERDOSAGE: SIGNS & SYMPTOMS

Kidney failure, liver failure, deafness, ocular toxicity (eg, retinal detachment), myelosuppression, nausea, vomiting, neuritis, death

Patient/Family Education

- Instruct patient to report pain at IV site immediately.
- Caution patient to avoid crowds and anyone with known infection.
- Advise patient to immediately report signs of neurotoxicity (tingling,

numbness, tremors of extremities) or other problems such as decreased urine output, weight gain, edema, anorexia, nausea, and vomiting.

- Instruct patient to report these symptoms to physician: tinnitus or hearing loss.

No patient monograph available.

Cladribine (2-Chlorodeoxyadenosine; CdA)

(KLAD-rih-BEAN)

Leustatin

Class: Antineoplastic

Action Cytotoxic to actively dividing and quiescent lymphocytes and monocytes, inhibiting both DNA synthesis and repair.

Indications Treatment of hairy cell leukemia. **Unlabeled uses:** Treatment of advanced cutaneous T-cell lymphomas, chronic lymphocytic leukemia, non-Hodgkin's lymphoma, acute myeloid leukemia, autoimmune hemolytic anemia, mycosis fungoides or Sezary syndrome.

Contraindications Standard considerations.

Route/Dosage
IV 0.09 mg/kg/day as continuous infusion for 7 consecutive days. Deviations from this regimen are not advised.

Interactions
D5W: Do not use dextrose as diluent because of increased degradation of cladribine.

Lab Test Interferences
None well documented.

Adverse Reactions
CV: Edema; tachycardia. *CNS:* Fatigue; headache; malaise; dizziness; insomnia; motor weakness. *RESP:* Abnormal breath or chest sounds; cough; shortness of breath. *GI:* Nausea; decreased appetite; vomiting; diarrhea; constipation; abdominal pain. *GU:* Renal dysfunction. *HEMA:* Neutropenia; anemia; thrombocytopenia; decreased CD_4 cell counts (lymphocyte subset); bone marrow hypocellularity; purpura; petechiae; epistaxis. *DERM:* Rash; injection site reactions; pruritus; pain; erythema. *OTHER:* Fever; infection; chills, diaphoresis; trunk pain.

Precautions
Pregnancy: Category D. *Lactation:* Undetermined. *Children:* Safety and efficacy not established. *Bone marrow suppression:* Common adverse effect. Careful hematologic monitoring is recommended. Administer only with supervision of experienced physician. *Fever:* Common adverse effect. Evaluate benefits vs risks before giving to patients with active infection. *Mutagenesis:* DNA damage is expected. *Nephrotoxicity/neurotoxicity:* May occur with high doses. *Renal or hepatic impairment:* Use caution.

NURSING CONSIDERATIONS

Administration/Storage

- Wear disposable gloves and protective garments.
- Use large peripheral vein for rapid dilution of medication. Do not use veins in hand.
- Use infusion pump to control rate. Adjust rate accordingly for patient with cardiovascular impairment.
- Refer to Haz Mat manual for proper procedure in event of spill. If required, complete unusual occurrence form.
- If accidental exposure to skin or mucus membranes occurs, wash area with copious amounts of water.
- Do not mix with other IV drugs, additives or use common IV line.
- Administer promptly or refrigerate for no more than 8 hr after dilution.
- Dilute only with designated diluent (0.9% sodium chloride with or with-

out benzyl alcohol preservative) with strict aseptic technique and environmental precautions. Discard any unused portion in approved manner.

- Do not heat, microwave or refreeze.
- Refrigerate unopened vials and protect from light. Freezing may form precipitate that will resolubilize by slow warming to room temperature and shaking vigorously.

Assessment/Interventions

- Obtain patient history, including drug history and any known allergies.
- Document baseline CBC and differential and renal and liver function test results.
- Anticipate fever. Empiric antibiotics may be indicated.
- If fatigue occurs, allow for frequent periods of rest; assist with activities of daily living to conserve patient's energy.
- Protect patient from exposure to potential sources of infection.
- If WBC < 1000 mm^2, place patient in protective isolation.
- If nausea occurs, provide small, frequent meals and frequent mouth care. Arrange for antiemetic if severe.
- Provide emotional support.
- Evaluate home care needs and refer to supportive services if indicated.
- Monitor renal and hepatic function.
- Anticipate bone marrow depression. Monitor CBC and differential.
- Assess carefully for signs of preexisting infection.
- Assess IV line for patency and infusion site for signs of infiltration, inflammation or thrombophlebitis, and change infusion site every 3 days unless peripherally inserted central catheter (PICC) or central line is used.
- If platelet count < 50,000, institute safety precautions to prevent bleeding. Monitor for unusual bleeding or bruising; check all urine, stool or emesis for blood; assess for sudden headache.

OVERDOSAGE: SIGNS & SYMPTOMS

Irreversible neurological damage, acute renal failure, severe bone marrow suppression

Patient/Family Education

- Stress importance of maintaining good nutrition by eating small, frequent meals. A soft, bland diet is appropriate if mouth sores are present. Encourage frequent mouth care.
- Advise patient that activity may need to be adjusted to provide for periods of rest.
- Stress importance of avoiding contact with people with infections. Encourage frequent handwashing and avoiding crowds.
- Caution patient to avoid activities or sports that could cause bruising or injury.
- Warn patient not to get immunizations unless physician has approved.
- Remind patient that routine laboratory tests and clinical assessments are vital to monitor progress, response to therapy and potential toxicity and to keep all scheduled appointments.
- Inform patient that adverse effects such as nausea, poor appetite and fatigue may occur.
- Instruct patient to report these symptoms to physician: fever, chills, sore throat, shortness of breath, difficulty swallowing, unusual bleeding or bruising or black, tarry stools.

No patient monograph available.

Clarithromycin

(kluh-RITH-row-MY-sin)

Biaxin

Class: Antibiotic/macrolide

Action Inhibits microbial protein synthesis.

Indications Treatment of infections of respiratory tract, skin and skin structure; treatment of disseminated atypical mycobacterial infections caused by susceptible strains of specific microorganisms. Prevention of disseminated *Mycobacterium avium* complex disease in patients with advanced HIV infection. CHILDREN: Acute otitis media.

Contraindications Hypersensitivity to erythromycin or any macrolide antibiotic. Patients receiving terfenadine who have pre-existing cardiac abnormalities or electrolyte disturbances.

Route/Dosage
ADULTS & CHILDREN ≥ 12 YR: **PO** 250-500 mg q 12 hr for 7-14 days; use 500 mg q 12 hr for prevention and treatment of mycobacterial infections. CHILDREN: **PO** 7.5 mg/kg q 12 hr for 10 days. Maximum dose for treatment and prevention of mycobacterial infections is 500 mg bid.

Interactions
Antihistamines, nonsedating (eg, terfenadine): Antihistamine blood level concentrations may increase, and serious cardiovascular side effects, including arrhythmias and death, may occur. *Carbamazepine:* May increase blood level concentrations of carbamazepine; recommend monitoring levels. *Cyclosporine:* Elevated cyclosporine levels with increased risk of toxicity. *Digoxin:* Elevated serum digoxin levels. *Theophylline*: May increase theophylline plasma concentration; recommend monitoring levels. *Tacrolimus:* Increased plasma levels with increased risk of toxicity.

Lab Test Interferences
None well documented.

Adverse Reactions
CNS: Headache; dizziness; insomnia; nightmares; vertigo. *GI:* Diarrhea; nausea; vomiting; abnormal taste; dyspepsia; abdominal pain/discomfort; glossitis; stomatitis; oral moniliasis; vomiting. *GU:* Elevated BUN. *HEMA:* Elevated PT. *DERM:* Rash. *CV:* Ventricular arrhythmias. *HEPA:* Hepatitis; jaundice. *EENT:* Hearing loss; tinnitus; abnormal sense of smell. *OTHER:* Urticaria; hypersensitivity; anaphylaxis; Stevens-Johnson syndrome.

Precautions
Pregnancy: Category C. *Lactation:* Undetermined. Other drugs of this class are excreted in breast milk. *Children:* Safety and efficacy in children <6 months of age not established. *Children:* Indicated for use in children only for mycobacterial infections; safety in children < 20 mo not established. *Pseudomembranous colitis:* Consider possibility in patients in whom diarrhea develops. *Renal or hepatic impairment:* Use cautiously and adjust dose in patients with severe renal impairment. No dosage adjustment necessary if patient has impaired hepatic function but normal renal function.

NURSING CONSIDERATIONS

Administration/Storage

- Administer with full glass of water.
- Give drug at evenly spaced intervals.
- Do not store liquid preparation in refrigerator. Discard 14 days after reconstitution.

Assessment/Interventions

- Obtain patient history, including drug history and any known allergies. Consider cross-sensitivity with other macrolides.
- Monitor serum levels of theophylline and carbamazepine, because clarithromycin may increase these drug levels.
- Notify physician if patient develops headache, abdominal pain, abnormal taste, diarrhea, nausea or vomiting.

OVERDOSAGE: SIGNS & SYMPTOMS

Nausea, vomiting, diarrhea

Patient/Family Education

- Instruct patient not to take

nonsedating antihistamines unless discussed with physician or pharmacist.

- Tell patient that if dose is missed not to double dose and to continue on schedule. If more than one dose is missed, tell patient to contact physician.
- Instruct patient to report these symptoms to physician: diarrhea, stomach pain.

See Patient Guide, p. 137.

Clemastine Fumarate

(KLEM-ass-teen FEW-muh-rate)

Tavist, Tavist-1

Class: Antihistamine/ethanolamine

Action Competitively antagonizes histamine at H_1 receptor sites.

Indications Symptomatic relief of perennial and seasonal allergic rhinitis, vasomotor rhinitis and allergic conjunctivitis; temporary relief of runny nose and sneezing caused by common cold; treatment of allergic and nonallergic pruritic symptoms; control of mild, uncomplicated urticaria and angioedema.

Contraindications Hypersensitivity to antihistamines; narrow-angle glaucoma; stenosing peptic ulcer; symptomatic prostatic hypertrophy; asthmatic attack; bladder neck obstruction; pyloroduodenal obstruction; MAO inhibitor therapy; use in newborn or premature infants and in nursing women.

Route/Dosage

ADULTS & CHILDREN > 12 YR: **PO** 1.34 mg bid to 2.68 mg tid (maximum 8.04 mg/day). DERMATOLOGIC CONDITIONS: **PO** 2.68 mg tid.

Interactions

Alcohol, CNS depressants: May cause additive CNS depressant effects. *MAO inhibitors:* May increase anticholinergic effects of clemastine fumarate.

Lab Test Interferences

Skin testing procedures: Drug may prevent or diminish otherwise positive reaction to dermal reactivity indicators.

Adverse Reactions

CV: Orthostatic hypotension; palpitations; bradycardia; tachycardia; arrythmias. *RESP:* Thickening of bronchial secretions; chest tightness; wheezing; nasal stuffiness; dry mouth, nose and throat; sore throat; respiratory depression. *CNS:* Drowsiness (often transient); sedation; dizziness; faintness; disturbed coordination. *EENT:* Blurred vision; tinnitus. *GI:* Epigastric distress; nausea; vomiting; diarrhea; constipation. *HEMA:* Hemolytic anemia; thrombocytopenia; agranulocytosis. *META:* Increased appetite; weight gain. *OTHER:* Hypersensitivity reactions; photosensitivity.

Precautions

Pregnancy: Category B. *Lactation:* Contraindicated in nursing mothers. *Children:* Safety and efficacy in children < 12 yr not established. *Elderly or debilitated patients:* At increased risk of dizziness, excessive sedation, syncope, toxic confusional states and hypotension. Dosage reduction may be required. *Hepatic impairment:* Use with caution in patients with cirrhosis or other liver disorders. *Special risk patients:* Use drug with caution in patients predisposed to urinary retention, history of bronchial asthma, increased intraocular pressure, hyperthyroidism, cardiovascular disease or hypertension. Avoid use in patients with history of sleep apnea.

NURSING CONSIDERATIONS

Administration/Storage

- Administer drug whole. If patient cannot take whole tablet, administer syrup form.
- Administer drug with food to avoid GI irritation.
- Store at room temperature.

Assessment/Interventions

- Obtain patient history, including drug history and any known allergies, especially to antihistamines.
- Determine whether there is history of glaucoma, ulcer, asthma or urinary tract obstruction.
- Notify physician if patient has history of hypertension or other cardiovascular disorders or is taking MAO inhibitor.

OVERDOSAGE: SIGNS & SYMPTOMS
CNS depression, hallucinations, convulsions, cardiovascular collapse

Patient/Family Education

- Instruct patient not to take drug for 4 days before allergy testing.
- Caution elderly patients that with this drug signs of CNS depression will be more pronounced.
- Instruct patient to report these symptoms to physician: difficulty breathing or problems voiding.
- Advise patient to take sips of water frequently, suck on ice chips or sugarless hard candy or chew sugarless gum if dry mouth occurs.
- Instruct patient to avoid intake of alcoholic beverages or other CNS depressants.
- Advise patient that drug may cause drowsiness and to use caution while driving or performing other tasks requiring mental alertness.
- Caution patient to avoid exposure to sunlight and to use sunscreen or wear protective clothing to avoid photosensitivity reaction.

See Patient Guide, p. 138.

Clindamycin

(KLIN-duh-MY-sin)

Clindamycin Phosphate
Cleocin Phosphate, Cleocin T, ♣ *Dalacin C Phosphate, Dalacin T Topical*

Clindamycin Hydrochloride
Cleocin, Cleocin Pediatric

Clindamycin Palmitate Hydrochloride
♣ *Dalacin C*

Class: Antibiotic/lincosamide

Action Suppresses bacterial protein synthesis.

Indications Treatment of serious infections caused by susceptible strains of specific microorganisms; treatment of acne vulgaris (topical use); treatment of bacterial vaginosis (vaginal use). **Unlabeled uses:** Treatment of CNS toxoplasmosis in AIDS patients, *Pneumocystis carinii* pneumonia and acute pelvic inflammatory disease; treatment of rosacea (topical).

Contraindications Hypersensitivity to lincosamides or any product component; treatment of minor bacterial or viral infections; history of regional enteritis, ulcerative colitis or antibiotic-associated colitis.

Route/Dosage
ADULTS: **PO** 150-450 mg q 6 hr. **IM/IV** 0.6-2.7 g/day divided into 2-4 doses. Do not use > 600 mg in single IM injection. CHILDREN: CLINDAMYCIN HYDROCHLORIDE: **PO** 8-20 mg/kg/day divided into 3-4 doses. CLINDAMYCIN PALMITATE HYDROCHLORIDE: **PO** 8-25 mg/kg/day divided into 3-4 doses. CHILDREN > 1 MO: **IM/IV** 20-40 mg/kg/day divided into 3-4 equal doses. NEONATES < 1 MO: **IM/IV** 15-20 mg/kg/day divided into 3-4 equal doses.

Acute Pelvic Inflammatory Disease
ADULTS: **IV** 900 mg q 8 hr with gentamicin. After discharge from hospital continue with doxycycline 100 mg bid for 10 days or oral clindamycin 450 mg 5 times daily for 10-14 days.

Acne
ADULTS: **Topical** Apply thin film to affected area bid.

Vaginosis
ADULTS: **Intravaginal** 1 applicatorful preferably at bedtime for 7 days.

Interactions

Erythromycin: May cause antagonism. *Kaolin-pectin antidiarrheals:* May delay absorption of clindamycin. *Nondepolarizing neuromuscular blockers:* May enhance actions of blockers. INCOMPATIBILITIES: Ampicillin, phenytoin sodium, barbiturates, aminophylline, magnesium sulfate, calcium gluconate.

Lab Test Interferences

None well documented.

Adverse Reactions

CV: Hypotension, cardiopulmonary arrest. *GI:* Diarrhea; colitis, including pseudomembranous colitis; nausea; vomiting; abdominal pain; esophagitis; anorexia. *GU:* Azotemia; oliguria; proteinuria; cervicitis or vaginitis (with intravaginal form of drug). *HEMA:* Neutropenia; leukopenia; agranulocytosis; thrombocytopenic purpura. *HEPA:* Jaundice; liver function test abnormalities. *DERM:* Hypersensitivity (eg, skin rash, urticaria, erythema multiforme, some cases resembling Stevens-Johnson syndrome). *OTHER:* Pain after injection; induration and sterile abscess after intramuscular injection; thrombophlebitis after intravenous infusion; anaphylaxis. Topical or vaginal use may theoretically produce adverse effects seen with systemic use as a result of absorption.

Precautions

Pregnancy: Oral, parenteral: Category B. Clindamycin does cross the placenta. Topical, intravaginal: Category B. *Lactation:* Excreted in breast milk. *Children:* Monitor organ system functions in newborns and infants; parenteral form may contain benzyl alcohol, which can cause gasping syndrome in premature infants. *Colitis:* Drug can cause severe and possibly fatal colitis characterized by severe persistent diarrhea, severe abdominal cramps and possibly passage of blood and mucus. Mild cases may respond to drug discontinuation. More severe cases may need fluid, electrolyte and protein supplementation, corticosteroids and other antibiotics. Consider possibility of pseudomembranous colitis *Elderly or debilitated patients:* May not tolerate diarrhea well (dehydration). *Hypersensitivity:* Use drug with caution in patients with asthma or significant allergies. *Meningitis:* Drug does not diffuse into CSF. Do not use to treat meningitis. *Mineral oil:* Vaginal cream contains mineral oil, which may weaken latex rubber condoms or diaphragms. *Renal or hepatic impairment:* Use drug with caution in patients with severe renal or hepatic disease with severe metabolic aberrations. *Tartrazine sensitivity:* Some products contain tartrazine, which may cause allergic-type reactions in susceptible individuals.

NURSING CONSIDERATIONS

Administration/Storage

- Administer capsules with full glass of water or with food.
- Give via deep IM injection. Do not administer more than 600 mg in single IM injection. Rotate injection sites.
- For IV infusion, dilute in 50-100 ml D5W or normal saline and infuse over 1 hr. Concentration should not exceed 18 mg/ml.
- Administer over 10-60 min (not to exceed 30 mg/min). Do not infuse as intravenous bolus.

- Do not infuse more than 1200 mg in 1 hr.
- Do not apply topical solution to abraded skin or mucous membranes.
- Keep vaginal cream and topical solution out of eyes.
- Store reconstituted clindamycin palmitate (pediatric oral solution) at room temperature for up to 2 wk. Do not refrigerate (causes thickening).

Assessment/Interventions
- Obtain patient history, including drug history and any known allergies. Check for renal or hepatic impairment, GI disease, asthma or significant allergies.
- When administering drug to newborns or infants, monitor organ system functions.
- With long-term therapy monitor liver and kidney function tests and blood counts.
- Report symptoms of colitis (severe diarrhea, severe abdominal cramps, passage of blood or mucus) to physician immediately. Symptoms may occur up to several wk after cessation of therapy.
- Be alert for the possibility of bacterial or fungal overgrowth on nonsusceptible organisms, especially yeasts.

Patient/Family Education
- Advise patient to take capsules with full glass of water or with food.
- Instruct patient using vaginal cream not to engage in sexual intercourse during treatment.
- Advise patients using vaginal cream that if they do engage in sexual intercourse not to use rubber or latex birth control devices (condoms, cervical caps or diaphragms) for 72 hr after treatment. Vaginal cream contains mineral oil, which may weaken latex rubber condoms or diaphragms.
- Teach patient to be careful to keep vaginal cream and topical solution out of eyes.
- Instruct patient not to apply topical solution to abraded skin or mucous membranes.
- Advise patient to notify physician if hypersensitivity reaction occurs (skin rash, urticaria, erythema multiforme) or if symptoms of disease being treated worsen.
- Instruct patient to notify physician if diarrhea develops; patient should not try to treat with otc medications. (Taking Lomotil [diphenoxylate compound] may prolong and worsen diarrhea.)

See Patient Guide, pp. 139-141.

Clofibrate

(kloe-FIH-brate)

Atromid-S

Class: Antihyperlipidemic

Action Lowers serum levels of triglycerides and very low density lipoproteins by mechanism not well established. Serum cholesterol and low density lipoproteins are lowered less predictably and less effectively.

Indications Management of primary type III hyperlipidemia not responding to dietary changes. May be considered in adults with very high serum triglycerides (types IV and V hyperlipidemia) who present risk of abdominal pain and pancreatitis and who do not respond to diet modification.

Contraindications Pregnancy; breastfeeding; clinically significant hepatic or renal dysfunction; primary biliary cirrhosis.

Route/Dosage
PO 2 g qd in 2-4 divided doses.

Interactions
Anticoagulants, oral: Hypoprothrombinemic effects may be enhanced. Anticoagulant dosage may need to be reduced. *Furosemide:* Diuretic effect may be increased. *Insulin, sulfonylureas:* Clofibrate may increase their effects, resulting in hypoglycemia. *Probenecid:*

May increase the therapeutic and toxic effects of clofibrate.

Lab Test Interferences

None well documented.

Adverse Reactions

CV: Increased or decreased angina; cardiac arrhythmias; swelling and phlebitis at xanthoma site. *CNS:* Fatigue; dizziness; headache. *GI:* Nausea; cholelithiasis; cholecystitis; reactivation of peptic ulcer; vomiting; diarrhea; dyspepsia; abdominal distress. *GU:* Impotence; decreased libido; renal dysfunction (dysuria, hematuria, proteinuria, decreased urine output) increased creatinine phosphokinase; hyperkalemia. *HEMA:* Leukopenia; anemia, eosinophilia; agranulocytosis. *HEPA:* Hepatomegaly; increased transaminases (AST, ALT); bromosulfophthalein; increased thymolturbidity. *DERM:* Skin rash; alopecia, dry skin; dry, brittle hair; allergic reactions. *OTHER:* Myalgia (muscle cramps, aches, weakness); flu-like symptoms; arthralgia; weight gain.

Precautions

Pregnancy: Category X. *Lactation:* Contraindicated in nursing women. *Children:* Safety and efficacy not established. *Carcinogenesis/mutagenesis:* Because of hepatic tumorigenicity in rodents and possible increased risk of malignancy and cholelithiasis in humans, use only as indicated. Discontinue if significant response is not obtained. *Response to therapy:* Clofibrate is not useful for hypertriglyceridemia of type I hyperlipidemia and has little effect on elevated cholesterol levels. *Special risk patients:* Use with caution in patients with history of jaundice, hepatic disease or peptic ulcer.

NURSING CONSIDERATIONS

Administration/Storage

- Give with meals if any GI upset occurs.
- Administer daily dosage in 2-4 divided doses.

Assessment/Interventions

- Obtain patient history, including drug history and any known allergies.
- Document WBC and Hct/Hgb as available.
- Document baseline cholesterol and triglyceride levels and monitor changes.
- Monitor results of liver function liver enzyme tests.
- If patient is taking anticoagulants, monitor prothrombin time for assistance in determining appropriate dose. Also monitor for signs of bleeding.
- If patient on phenytoin, monitor for signs of toxicity such as nystagmus, ataxia, slurred speech or blurred vision.
- If patient is taking insulin or sulfonylureas, assess for signs and symptoms of hypoglycemia.
- Notify physician if patient experiences chest pain, shortness of breath, irregular heartbeat, nausea, vomiting, fever, chills, hematuria, sore throat, decreased urine output, swollen lower extremities or flu-like symptoms.

Patient/Family Education

- Caution patient that this medication must not be taken during pregnancy or when pregnancy is possible. Advise patient to use reliable form of birth control while taking this drug.
- Teach patient importance of compliance with drug therapy because if trigylcerides do not decrease significantly in 3 mo drug should be discontinued. If patient takes clofibrate for xanthoma tuberosum, patient must take for at least 1 yr to achieve therapeutic effect.
- Explain necessity of strict adherence to diet of low fat, low cholesterol and low triglycerides.

- Advise patient to restrict alcohol intake.
- Tell patient to engage in regular exercise routine and, if appropriate, to join a weight management program.
- Instruct patients with diabetes to monitor own blood glucose level through fingersticks.

See Patient Guide, p. 142.

Clomiphene Citrate

(KLOE-mih-feen SIH-trate)

Clomid, Milophene, Serophene

Class: Ovulation stimulant

Action Induces ovulation in selected anovulatory women.

Indications Treatment of ovulatory failure in women desiring pregnancy when partner is fertile and potent. **Unlabeled use:** Treatment of male infertility.

Contraindications Liver disease; history of liver dysfunction; abnormal bleeding of undetermined origin; pregnancy.

Route/Dosage

Initial Therapy

PO 50 mg/day for 5 days.

Second and Third Courses

PO 100 mg/day for 5 days.

Interactions None well documented.

Lab Test Interferences None well documented.

Adverse Reactions *CV:* Vasomotor flushes. *CNS:* Headache, dizziness; lightheadedness. *EENT:* Visual symptoms; blurring spots or flashes; diplopia; photophobia. *GI:* Abdominal pain/discomfort; distension; bloating; nausea; vomiting. *HEPA:* Sulfobromophthalein retention. *GU:* Abnormal uterine bleeding; abnormal ovarian enlargement, luteal cyst formation. *OTHER:* Breast tenderness.

Precautions *Pregnancy:* Category X. *Lactation:* Undetermined. *Multiple pregnancy:* May increase chance for multiple pregnancies. *Ophthalmologic effects:* May cause blurring of vision.

NURSING CONSIDERATIONS

Administration/Storage

- Administer initially over 5 days at approximately 50 mg/day. Follow with second course of 100 mg/day for 5 days.

Assessment/Interventions

- Obtain patient history, including drug history and any known allergies.
- Monitor liver function tests before beginning therapy and throughout therapy in patients at risk for hepatotoxicity.
- Notify physician if patient experiences abdominal pain, abnormal uterine bleeding, visual changes or jaundice.

Patient/Family Education

- Caution patient that this medication must not be taken during pregnancy or when pregnancy is possible. Advise patient to use reliable form of birth control while taking this drug.
- Counsel patient and partner in purpose of scheduling clomiphene citrate, sexual intercourse and ovulation time to be successful in achieving pregnancy.
- Advise female patient that increased midcycle ovarian discomfort may be experienced and can assist her in planning intercourse.
- Instruct patient of importance of well-balanced diet, mild exercise routine, and avoidance of drugs, caffeine and alcohol while attempting to achieve pregnancy.

- Inform patient of possibility for multiple pregnancies.
- Explain that medication may cause dizziness, hot flashes, headache, nausea and weight gain but that these effects will subside after medication is stopped.
- Instruct patient to report these symptoms to physician: abnormal uterine bleeding, yellowish skin or eyes, blurred vision.
- Advise patient to use caution while driving or using heavy equipment because blurring of vision can occur.

See Patient Guide, p. 143.

Clomipramine HCl

(kloe-MIH-pruh-meen HIGH-droe-KLOR-ide)

Anafranil

Class: Tricyclic antidepressant

Action Inhibits reuptake of serotonin in CNS.

Indications Relief of obsessive-compulsive disorder. **Unlabeled uses:** Treatment of panic disorder or chronic pain (migraine, chronic tension headache, diabetic neuropathy, tic douloureux, cancer pain, peripheral neuropathy, postherpetic neuralgia, arthritic pain).

Contraindications Hypersensitivity to any tricyclic antidepressant. Not to be given in combination with or within 14 days of treatment with MAO inhibitor. Not to be given during acute recovery phases of MI.

Route/Dosage
ADULTS: Initial dose: **PO** 25 mg/day; gradually increase dose to 100 mg/day during first 2 wk. Dose may then be gradually increased to maximum of 250 mg/day. CHILDREN (≥ 10 YR): Initial dose: **PO** 25 mg/day; gradually increase dose to 3 mg/kg/day or 100 mg/day (whichever is less) during first 2 wk; then slowly increase dose to maximum 3 mg/kg/day or 200 mg/day (whichever is less).

Interactions
Anticholinergics: Effects may be increased. *Barbiturates, charcoal:* May increase effects of clomipramine. *Cimetidine, fluoxetine, haloperidol, phenothiazine antipsychotics, oral contraceptives:* May increase effects of clomipramine. *Clonidine:* May result in hypertensive crisis. *CNS depressants:* Depressant effects may be additive. *Guanethidine:* Antihypertensive effects may be decreased. MAO *inhibitors:* Sweating, convulsions and death may occur.

Lab Test Interferences
None well documented.

Adverse Reactions
CV: Orthostatic hypotension; hypertension; tachycardia; palpitations; arrhythmias; ECG changes. *RESP:* Pharyngitis; rhinitis; sinusitis; laryngitis; cough. *CNS:* Hyperthermia; confusion; hallucinations; delusions; nervousness; restlessness; agitation; panic; insomnia; nightmares; mania; exacerbation pf psychosis; drowsiness; dizziness; weakness; fatigue; emotional lability; aggressive reaction; seizures. *EENT:* Conjunctivitis; blurred vision; dilated pupils; increased intraocular pressure; tinnitus; nasal congestion; peculiar taste in mouth. *GI:* Nausea; vomiting; anorexia; GI distress; diarrhea; flatulence; dry mouth; constipation. *GU:* Impotence; sexual dysfunction; ejaculation failure; urinary tract infection; vaginitis; cystitis; dysmenorrhea; amenorrhea; urinary retention or hesitancy. *HEMA:* Bone marrow depression including agranulocytosis; eosinophilia; purpura; thrombocytopenia; leukopenia; anemia. *HEPA:* Hepatitis; elevated liver function tests. *DERM:* Rash; pruritus; photosensitivity; dry skin; acne; itching; dermatitis. *META:* Elevation or depression of glucose levels. *OTHER:* Numbness; tremors; breast enlargement; nonpuerperal lactation; extrapyramidal symptoms (pseu-

doparkinsonism, movement disorders, akathisia); vestibular disorder; muscle weakness; significant weight gain; hypothyroidism.

Precautions

Pregnancy: Category C. Neonatal withdrawal symptoms have been reported. *Lactation:* Excreted in breast milk. *Children:* Not recommended for children < 10 yr. *Special risk patients:* Use with caution in patients with history of seizures, urinary retention, urethral or ureteral spasm, angle-closure glaucoma or increased intraocular pressure, hepatic or renal impairment or cardiovascular disorders; hyperthyroid patients or those receiving thyroid medication and schizophrenic or paranoid patients.

NURSING CONSIDERATIONS

Administration/Storage

- During titration phase administer drug in divided doses daily with meals to lessen GI side effects.
- After titration, give daily dose at bedtime with large glass of water to minimize daytime sedation.
- Do not administer drug to patients who have taken MAO inhibitors within past 14 days.
- Supervise medication intake when prescribed for psychiatric patients.
- Store at room temperature. Protect from moisture.

Assessment/Interventions

- Obtain patient history, including drug history and any known allergies.
- Assess patient's physical and psychological condition monthly.
- Dosage must be gradually decreased before discontinuation.
- Monitor liver function, ECG, blood sugars (in patients with diabetes) and blood counts (CBC with differential) as needed.
- Monitor body weight monthly.
- Watch for anticholinergic effects; flushing, dry mouth, dilated pupils and hyperpyrexia.
- If there is urinary elimination problem, signs of neuroleptic malignant syndrome or drop in BP of 20 mm Hg, withhold medication and notify physician.
- If arrhythmia or increase in heart rate develop, notify physician.
- Discontinue medication immediately if patient demonstrates increased agitation or paranoid delusions.

OVERDOSAGE: SIGNS & SYMPTOMS

Confusion, hallucinations, agitation, cardiac arrhythmias, dilated pupils, seizures, flushing, dry mouth, fever, tachycardia, cardiac arrest, coma, respiratory depression, cyanosis, hypotension, shock, sweating

Patient/Family Education

- Instruct patient to keep weekly record of weight and to decrease caloric intake if necessary.
- Teach patient how to monitor BP and heart rate.
- Instruct patient on oral hygiene habits to prevent and treat dry mucous membranes.
- Advise patient to increase fluid intake.
- Instruct patient not to discontinue taking drug abruptly.
- Inform male patients of possible impotence or ejaculation failure.
- Caution patient to avoid sudden position changes to prevent orthostatic hypotension.
- Instruct patient to avoid intake of alcoholic beverages or other CNS depressants.
- Advise patient that drug may cause drowsiness and to use caution while driving or performing other tasks requiring mental alertness.
- Caution patient to avoid exposure to sunlight and to use sunscreen or wear protective clothing to avoid photosensitivity reaction.
- Instruct patient not to take otc medications without notifying physician.

See Patient Guide, p. 144.

Clonazepam

(kloe-NAY-ze-pam)

Klonopin, *Rivotril*

Class: Anticonvulsant/benzodiazepine

Action Potentiates action of GABA, inhibitory neurotransmitter, resulting in increased neuronal inhibition and CNS depression, especially in limbic system and reticular formation.

Indications Treatment of Lennox-Gastaut syndrome; management of akinetic and myoclonic seizures and absence seizures unresponsive to succinimides. **Unlabeled uses:** Treatment of restless legs syndrome, parkinsonian dysarthria, acute manic episodes of bipolar affective disorder, multifocal tic disorders and neuralgias; adjunctive therapy for schizophrenia.

Contraindications Hypersensitivity to benzodiazepines; psychoses; acute narrow-angle glaucoma; significant liver disease; shock; coma; acute alcohol intoxication.

Route/Dosage

ADULTS: Initial dose: **PO** 1.5 mg/day in 3 divided doses. Increase by 0.5-1 mg q 3 days until seizures are adequately controlled (maximum 20 mg/day). INFANTS & CHILDREN (≤ 10 YR OR 30 KG): Initial dose: **PO** 0.01-0.03 mg/kg/day in 2-3 divided doses. Increase by 0.25-0.5 mg q 3 days until maintenance dose of 0.1-0.2 mg/kg has been reached.

Interactions

Alcohol and CNS depressants: May cause additive CNS depressant effects. *Cimetidine, oral contraceptives, disulfiram:* May cause effects of clonazepam to increase, with excessive sedation and impaired psychomotor function. *Digoxin:* May increase serum digoxin concentrations. *Omeprazole:* May increase *Theophyllines:* May antagonize sedative effects.

Lab Test Interferences

None well documented.

Adverse Reactions

CV: Cardiovascular collapse; hypotension; phlebitis or thrombosis at intravenous sites. *CNS:* Drowsiness; confusion; ataxia; dizziness; lethargy; fatigue; apathy; memory impairment; disorientation; anterograde amnesia; restlessness; headache; slurred speech; aphonia; stupor; coma; euphoria; irritability; vivid dreams; psychomotor retardation; paradoxic reactions (eg, anger, hostility, mania, insomnia, muscle spasms). *EENT:* Visual and auditory disturbances; depressed hearing. *GI:* Constipation; diarrhea; dry mouth; coated tongue; excessive salivation; nausea; anorexia; vomiting. *GU:* Dysuria; enuresis; nocturia; urinary retention. *HEMA:* Blood dyscrasias including agranulocytosis; anemia; thrombocytopenia; leukopenia; neutropenia. *HEPA:* Hepatic dysfunction, including hepatitis and jaundice; elevated LDH, ALT, AST and alkaline phosphatase. *DERM:* Rash. *OTHER:* Dependence/withdrawal syndrome (eg, confusion, abnormal perception of movement, depersonalization, muscle twitching, psychosis, paranoid delusions, seizures).

Precautions

Pregnancy: Safety not established. Avoid drug, especially during first trimester, because of possible increased risk of congenital malformation. Not recommended during labor and delivery. *Lactation:* Excreted in breast milk. *Children:* Initial dose should be small and gradually increased. Long-term use may cause adverse effects such as possibly delayed mental or physical development. *Elderly or debilitated patients:* Initial dose should be small and gradually increased. Give drug with extreme care to elderly or very ill patient with limited respiratory reserve. *Psychiatric disorders:* Not intended for use in patients with primary depressive disorder, psychosis or disorders in which anxiety is not prominent. *Renal or hepatic impairment:* Use drug with caution to avoid accumulation. *Seizure:* In patients with multiple seizure types, drug may increase incidence or precipitate onset of grand mal seizures. *Suicide:* Use drug with caution in patients with suicidal tendencies; do not allow patient access to large quantities.

NURSING CONSIDERATIONS

Administration/Storage

- Give with food or milk to decrease GI upset.
- Do not administer with antacid; give at least 1 hr apart.
- If possible, divide daily dose into three equal doses. If doses are unequal, give largest dose at bedtime.
- Parenteral administration should be reserved primarily for acute states.
- Observe patient for up to 3 hr after parenteral administration.
- Do not inject drug intra-arterially; intra-arterial injection may produce arteriospasm that can lead to gangrene.
- Store at room temperature.

Assessment/Interventions

- Obtain patient history, including drug history and any known allergies.
- Assess renal studies: urinalysis, BUN, urine creatinine.
- Assess blood studies (CBC and platelets) prior to and regularly throughout therapy.
- Evaluate hepatic studies: ALT, AST, bilirubin, creatinine, alkaline phosphatase.
- Patient should undergo ophthalmic examination before, during and after therapy.
- Observe for drowsiness, ataxia, confusion, especially in elderly or debilitated patient.
- Drowsiness and dizziness may occur early in therapy; assist with ambulation, use siderails.
- Provide gum, hard candy and frequent sips of water to relieve dry mouth.
- Because of risk of apnea and cardiac arrest, resuscitative facilities should be available.
- Monitor drug levels during therapy. Therapeutic level is 20-80 mg/ml.
- Monitor for blood dyscrasias: observe for fever, sore throat, bruising, rash, jaundice.
- Monitor mental status: mood, sensorium, affect, oversedation, sleep pattern, drowsiness, behavioral changes (especially in children; eg, inattention in school). Report changes to physician.
- Monitor seizure activity and record. Take seizure precautions as needed.
- Abrupt withdrawal, particularly in long-term, high-dose therapy, may cause status epilepticus, vomiting, diarrhea, and sweating; monitor patient carefully.

OVERDOSAGE: SIGNS & SYMPTOMS

Somnolence, confusion, diminished reflexes, coma

Patient/Family Education

- Instruct patient to take drug with food or milk to decrease GI upset.
- Tell patient not to take drug within 1 hr of antacid.
- Instruct patient to keep record of seizure activity and report to physician.
- Encourage patient to carry identification card or Medi-Alert bracelet that indicates diagnosis and drug dosage.
- If patient is child, advise parents to supervise child's play and watch for inattention.
- Caution patient not to stop taking medication abruptly.
- Advise patient to contact physician immediately if serious side effects (eg, changes in mental status) occur.
- Instruct patient to rise slowly or faint-

ing may occur, especially in elderly patients.

- Advise patient to avoid intake of alcoholic beverages or other CNS depressants.
- Advise patient that drug may cause drowsiness and to use caution while driving or performing other tasks requiring mental alertness.

See Patient Guide, p. 145.

Clonidine HCl

(KLOE-nih-DEEN HIGH-droe-KLOR-ide)

Catapres, Catapres-TTS-1, Catapres-TTS-2, Catapres-TTS-3, ♣ *APO-Clonidine, Dixarit, Nu-Clonidine*

Class: Antihypertensive/antiadrenergic, centrally acting

Action Stimulates central alpha-adrenergic receptors to inhibit sympathetic cardioaccelerator and vasoconstrictor centers.

Indications Management of hypertension. **Unlabeled uses:** Treatment of constitutional growth delay in children, diabetic diarrhea, Gilles de la Tourette syndrome, hypertensive urgencies, menopausal flushing, postherpetic neuralgia and diagnosis of pheochromocytoma; ulcerative colitis; reduction of allergen-induced inflammatory reactions in patients with extrinsic asthma; facilitation of smoking cessation; alcohol withdrawal; and methadone/opiate detoxification. **Orphan drug use:** Epidural use for relief of cancer pain.

Contraindications Hypersensitivity to clonidine or any component of adhesive layer of transdermal system.

Route/Dosage

Hypertension

ADULTS: Initial dose: **PO** 0.1 mg bid; maintenance dose: increase by increments of 0.1-0.2 mg/day until desired response is achieved (maximum 2.4 mg/day in divided doses). **SL** 0.2-0.4 mg/day. **Transdermal** 0.1 mg patch weekly initially; titrate to determine best response. Dosage > two 0.3 mg patches does not improve efficacy. CHILDREN: **PO** 5-25 mcg/kg/day in divided doses given q 6 hr; increase dose as necessary at 5-7 day intervals.

Interactions

Alcohol, CNS depressants: Clonidine may enhance depressant effects. *Beta-adrenergic blocking agents:* May increase potential for rebound hypertension when clonidine therapy is discontinued. *Tricyclic antidepressants:* May reduce effect of clonidine.

Lab Test Interferences

None well documented.

Adverse Reactions

CV: CHF; orthostatic symptoms; palpitations; tachycardia; bradycardia. *CNS:* drowsiness; dizziness; sedation; nightmares; insomnia; nervousness or agitation; headache; fatigue. *EENT:* Itching, burning or dry eyes; retinal degeneration; dry nasal polyps. *GI:* Dry mouth; constipation; anorexia; nausea; vomiting. *GU:* Impotence; decreased libido; nocturia; difficulty in micturition; urinary retention. *DERM:* Rash; urticaria; erythema (with transdermal form); transient localized skin reactions; pruritus. *META:* Weight gain; gynecomastia; transient elevations in blood glucose or serum creatinine phosphokinase. *OTHER:* Increased sensitivity to alcohol; pallor; muscle weakness; muscle or joint pain; cramps of lower limbs; weakly positive Coombs' test.

Precautions

Pregnancy: Category C. *Lactation:* Excreted in breast milk. *Elderly or debilitated patients:* Reduced dosage may be required. *Perioperative considerations:* Continue clonidine therapy to within 4 hr of surgery and resume as soon as possible thereafter. *Rebound hypertension:* Discontinue therapy by reducing dose gradually over 2-4 days to avoid rapid increase in BP. *Sensitization to transdermal clonidine:* Generalized skin rash may develop in patients with localized reaction to patch if they are switched to oral clonidine.

NURSING CONSIDERATIONS

Administration/Storage

Oral

- Administer in divided doses every 12 hr.
- Store tablets in tightly closed light-resistant container at room temperature.

Transdermal

- Each transdermal system has two parts: (1) patch containing active drug and (2) adhesive overlay. Apply patch to hairless area of intact skin on upper arm or torso as directed. Then apply adhesive overlay to ensure good adhesion of patch.
- Do not alter or trim patch.
- Change patch every 7 days.
- Alternate sites of patch application to prevent skin irritation.
- Before discarding old patch, fold adhesive edges together.

Assessment/Interventions

- Obtain patient history, including drug history and any known allergies.
- Assess BP and apical pulse before administering drug. If systolic BP is < 90 mm Hg or pulse is < 60 bpm, withhold drug and notify physician.
- Weigh patient daily and record weight.
- Note any rash or skin irritation when removing patch.
- Observe for fluid retention and weight gain.
- In diabetic patients, monitor blood glucose levels.
- Monitor BP and pulse during initial therapy.
- If drug is being given to patients who have undergone prior beta-blocker therapy, be alert for signs of rebound hypertensive crisis (agitation, headache, tachycardia, sweating, flushing).

OVERDOSAGE: SIGNS & SYMPTOMS

Bradycardia, hypotension, CNS depression, respiratory depression, constricted pupils, seizures, lethargy, agitation, vomiting

Patient/Family Education

- Instruct diabetic patients to monitor blood glucose levels.
- Tell patient to adhere to any fluid or dietary restrictions given by physician.
- Caution patient not to stop taking medication abruptly.
- Advise patient on long-term therapy to have regular eye examinations to monitor for retinal degeneration.
- Inform patient that fatigue and constipation may be experienced for few wk after drug therapy is begun.
- Instruct patient to report these symptoms to physician: respiratory distress, constricted pupils, tremors, impotence or decreased libido.
- Advise patient to take sips of water frequently, suck on ice chips or sugarless hard candy or chew sugarless gum if dry mouth occurs.
- Caution patient to avoid sudden position changes to prevent orthostatic hypotension. Suggest to patient to dangle legs at bedside before standing.
- Advise patient that drug may cause drowsiness and to use caution while driving or performing other tasks requiring mental alertness.
- Instruct patient not to take otc medications without consulting physician.

See Patient Guide, p. 146.

Clorazepate Dipotassium

(klor-AZE-uh-PATE DIE-poe-TASS-ee-uhm)

Gen-XENE, Tranxene, Tranxene-SD, Tranxene-SD Half Strength, ♣ *Novoclopate*

Class: Antianxiety/benzodiazepine

Action Potentiates action of GABA, inhibitory neurotransmitter, resulting in increased neuronal inhibition and CNS depression, especially in limbic system and reticular formation.

Indications Management of anxiety disorders; relief of acute alcohol withdrawal symptoms; adjunctive therapy in management of partial seizures. **Unlabeled use:** Treatment of irritable bowel syndrome.

Contraindications Hypersensitivity to benzodiazepines; psychoses; acute narrow-angle glaucoma.

Route/Dosage

Anxiety

ADULTS: **PO** 30-60 mg/day in divided doses. SINGLE BEDTIME DOSING: Initial dose: **PO** 15 mg.

Elderly or Debilitated Patients

Initial dose: **PO** 7.5-15 mg/day.

Maintenance

ADULTS: **PO** 22.5 mg/day as single dose alternative once patient is stabilized with 7.5 mg tid; do not use 22.5 mg in single dose to initiate therapy. 11.25 mg tablet may be given as single dose q 24 hr.

Acute Alcohol Withdrawal

ADULTS: DAY 1: Initial dose: **PO** 30 mg, then 30-60 mg in divided doses. DAY 2: 45-90 mg in divided doses. DAY 3: 22.5-45 mg in divided doses. DAY 4: 15-30 mg in divided doses. Then gradually reduce to 7.5-15 mg/day; discontinue when patient is stable.

Partial Seizures

ADULTS & CHILDREN > 12 YR: Maximum initial dose: 7.5 mg tid; increase by no more than 7.5 mg/wk (maximum 90 mg/day). CHILDREN 9-12 YR: Maximum initial dose: 7.5 mg bid; increase by no more than 7.5 mg/wk (maximum 60 mg/day).

Interactions

Alcohol and CNS depressants: Possible additive CNS depressant effects. *Cimetidine, oral contraceptives, disulfiram:* May increase effects of clorazepate, with excessive sedation and impaired psychomotor function. *Digoxin:* May increase serum digoxin concentrations. *Omeprazole:* May increase clorazepate serum levels and enhance effects. *Theophyllines:* May antagonize sedative effects.

Lab Test Interferences

None well documented.

Adverse Reactions

CV: Cardiovascular collapse; hypotension. *CNS:* Drowsiness; confusion; ataxia; dizziness; lethargy; fatigue; apathy; memory impairment; disorientation; anterograde amnesia; restlessness; nervousness; headache; slurred speech; loss of voice; stupor; coma; euphoria; irritability; vivid dreams; psychomotor retardation; paradoxical reactions (eg, anger, hostility, mania, insomnia, muscle spasms). *EENT:* Blurred vision; diplopia. *GI:* Constipation; diarrhea; dry mouth; coated tongue; nausea; anorexia; vomiting. *HEMA:* Blood dyscrasias. *HEPA:* Hepatic dysfunction, including hepatitis and jaundice; elevated lactate dehydrogenase, alanine aminotransferase, aspartate aminotransferase and alkaline phosphatase. *DERM:* Rash. *OTHER:* Dependence/withdrawal syndrome.

Precautions

Pregnancy: Pregnancy category undetermined. *Lactation:* Excreted in breast milk. *Children:* Initial dose should be small and gradually increased. Not recommended in children < 9 yr. *Elderly or debilitated patients:* Initial dose should be small and gradually increased. *Dependence:* Prolonged use may lead to dependence. Withdrawal syndrome has occurred within 4-6 wk of treatment, especially if abruptly discontinued. Use caution and taper dosage. *Psychiatric disorders:* Not intended for use in patients with primary depressive disorder, psychosis or disorders in which anxiety is not prominent. *Renal or hepatic impairment:* Observe caution to avoid accumulation of drug.

NURSING CONSIDERATIONS

Administration/Storage

- Administer drug with food or milk to avoid GI irritation.
- Crush tablets if patient is unable to swallow tablets whole.
- Store at room temperature.

Assessment/Interventions

- Obtain patient history, including drug history and any known allergies.
- Assist patient with ambulation during initial therapy due to drowsiness and dizziness, especially if patient is elderly. Use siderails.
- Assess level of anxiety, what precipitates anxiety and whether drug controls symptoms.
- Observe for drowsiness, ataxia, and confusion, especially in elderly and debilitated.
- Give gum, hard candy, frequent sips of water to alleviate dry mouth.
- Monitor CBC; blood dyscrasias occur rarely with long-term use.
- Monitor liver function throughout long-term therapy.
- Monitor I&O and serum creatinine to assess renal function.
- Monitor mental status: mood, sensorium, affect, sleep pattern, drowsiness, dizziness. Notify physician of changes.
- Monitor for physical dependence and withdrawal symptoms after long-term use: increased anxiety, headache, muscle pain, weakness, nausea, vomiting. When patient is discontinuing therapy, gradually decrease dosage over 4-8 wk to prevent withdrawal symptoms, especially in patients with history of seizures or epilepsy.
- Assess for alcohol withdrawal symptoms: hallucinations, delirium, irritability, agitation, tremors.
- Assess for seizure control and type, duration and intensity of convulsions.
- Monitor BP, pulse and respiratory rate frequently in treatment of alcohol withdrawal.

OVERDOSAGE: SIGNS & SYMPTOMS

Drowsiness, confusion, somnolence, impaired coordination, diminished reflexes, lethargy, ataxia, hypotonia, hypotension, hypnosis, coma

Patient/Family Education

- Advise patient to take drug with food or milk to decrease GI irritation.
- Inform patient that drug may be habit forming and advise that patient discuss use with physician.
- Caution patient to rise slowly or fainting may occur, especially if patient is elderly. Drowsiness may be increased during initial therapy.
- Encourage patient to carry identification (Medi-Alert) indicating medication usage if taking drug for seizure disorder.
- Suggest to patient to keep log of seizure activity and report to physician.
- Emphasize that medication must not be discontinued abruptly after long-term use.
- Instruct patient to avoid intake of alcoholic beverages or other CNS depressants.
- Advise patient that drug may cause drowsiness and to use caution while driving or performing other tasks requiring mental alertness.

See Patient Guide, p. 147.

Clotrimazole

(kloe-TRIM-uh-zole)

Femcare, Gyne-Lotrimin, Lotrimin, Lotrimin AF, Mycelex, Mycelex-7, Mycelex-G, ♣ *Canesten, Clotrimaderm, Myclo*

Class: Topical/antifungal

Action Inhibits yeast growth by increasing cell membrane permeability in susceptible fungi.

Indications
Topical use: Treatment of tinea pedis (athlete's foot), tinea cruris (jock itch), tinea corporis (ringworm), candidiasis and tinea versicolor. *Oral use (troche):* Treatment of oropharyngeal candidiasis; prophylaxis of oropharyngeal candidiasis in specific groups of immunocompromised patients. *Vaginal use:* Treatment of vulvovaginal candidiasis.

Contraindications Standard considerations.

Route/Dosage

Oropharyngeal Candidiasis

ADULTS & CHILDREN > 3 YR: **PO** 1 10 mg troche (lozenge) dissolved slowly in mouth 5 times/day for 14 days.

Prophylaxis

PO 1 10 mg troche dissolved slowly in mouth tid.

Dermal Infections

Topical cream: Apply thin layer to affected and surrounding areas bid, AM and PM. **Topical lotion:** Apply thin layer to affected areas twice daily.

Vaginal Infections

WOMEN & GIRLS > 12 YR: **Intravaginal** Insert 1 applicatorful (5 g) of cream or 1 100 mg tablet at bedtime for 7-14 days (treatment for 14 days may yield higher cure rate), or insert 1 500 mg tablet one time only, preferably at bedtime.

Interactions None well documented.

Lab Test Interferences
None well documented.

Adverse Reactions
EENT: Unpleasant mouth sensations (troche). *GI:* Nausea (troche); vomiting; abdominal cramps; bloating. *HEPA:* Abnormal liver function test results. *DERM: Topical and vaginal products:* Erythema; stinging; blistering; peeling; edema; pruritus; urticaria; burning; general skin irritation; rash.

Precautions
Pregnancy: Category C (troches); Category B (topical and vaginal use). *Lactation:* Undetermined. *Children:* Safety not established in children < 3 yr. *Recurrent infections:* May indicate underlying medical cause, including diabetes or HIV infection. *Systemic or ophthalmic infections:* Do not use for these conditions.

NURSING CONSIDERATIONS

Administration/Storage

- Ensure that patient dissolves troche slowly in mouth over 15-30 min.
- Apply topical cream or solution to affected and surrounding areas. Wear latex gloves for application.
- Store drug at room temperature. Do not freeze.

Assessment/Interventions

- Obtain patient history, including drug history and any known allergies.
- *Troche:* Assess for nausea and vomiting, abdominal cramps, discomfort or unpleasant mouth sensations.
- *Topical and vaginal products:* Assess for blistering, edema, pruritus, burning or rash.
- Patients with diabetes mellitus, patients taking antibiotics, oral contraceptives or steroids and people with decreased immunity may experience recurrent vaginal candidiasis.

Patient/Family Education

- Instruct patient to practice birth control by refraining from sexual intercourse. Caution patient to avoid use of oral contraceptives.
- Teach pregnant woman in second and third trimesters to manually insert tablets (not to use applicator).
- Instruct patient in good hygiene practice (eg, handwashing before and after each application) and methods of preventing spread of fungus to other parts of body and to others in household (especially if ringworm or athlete's foot is source of infection).
- Emphasize importance of avoiding contact of medication with eyes.
- Explain to patient using vaginal cream or tablets that to reduce risk of reinfection it is important to refrain from sexual intercourse during therapy.
- Instruct patient to stop using medication if burning or blistering occurs and to contact physician.
- Advise patient to use medication continuously, even during menses. Emphasize that tampons should not be used.
- Tell patient that if symptoms do not improve in 1 wk, to discontinue medication and notify physician.

See Patient Guide, pp. 148-150.

Clozapine

(KLOE-zuh-PEEN)

Clozaril

Class: Antipsychotic

Action Interferes with dopamine binding at D_1 and D_2 receptors in CNS; antagonizes adrenergic, cholinergic, histaminergic and serotonergic neurotransmission.

Indications Management of severely and chronically mentally ill schizophrenic patients who have not responded to or cannot tolerate standard antipsychotic drug treatment.

Contraindications History of clozapine-induced agranulocytosis or severe granulocytopenia; myeloproliferative disorders; simultaneous administration with other agents known to cause bone marrow suppression; severe CNS depression or comatose states.

Route/Dosage

Cautious titration and divided dosage schedule are recommended. ADULTS: Initial dose: **PO** 25 mg qd or bid; increase by 25-50 mg/day up to 300-450 mg/day within 2 wk. May then increase dose in increments ≤ 100 mg once or twice weekly. Usual dosage: 300-600 mg/day (maximum 900 mg/day).

Interactions

Agents that suppress bone marrow: Risk or severity of bone marrow suppression may be increased. *Anticholinergics:* Anticholinergic effects may be potentiated. *Antihypertensives:* Hypotensive effects may be potentiated. *Cimetidine:* May increase blood levels of clozapine. *CNS drugs:* Use with caution because of CNS effects of clozapine. *Phenytoin:* May decrease blood levels of clozapine. *Protein-bound drugs (eg, warfarin, digoxin):* Clozapine may cause increase in plasma concentrations of these drugs.

Lab Test Interferences

None well documented.

Adverse Reactions

CV: Tachycardia; hypotension; hypertension; angina; ECG changes. *RESP:* Shortness of breath. *CNS:* Drowsiness; dizziness; headache; tremors; syncope; disturbed sleep; nightmares; restlessness; akinesia; agitation; seizures; rigidity; akathisia; confusion; fatigue; insomnia; hyperkinesia; weakness; lethargy; incoordination; slurred speech; depression; epileptiform movements; anxiety. *EENT:* Visual disturbances; nasal congestion; sore tongue; throat discomfort. *GI:* Constipation; nausea; abdominal discomfort; heartburn; vomiting; diarrhea; anorexia; dry mouth. *GU:* Urinary abnormalities; incontinence; abnormal ejaculation; urinary urgency or frequency; urinary retention. *HEMA:* Leukopenia; decreased WBC; neutropenia; agranulocytosis; eosinophilia. *HEPA:* Liver test abnormalities. *DERM:* Rash; sweating. *META:* Weight gain. *OTHER:* Excessive salivation; fever; muscle weakness; back, neck or leg pain; muscle spasms or pain.

Precautions

Pregnancy: Category B. *Lactation:* May be excreted in breast milk. *Children:* Safety and efficacy in children < 16 yr not established. *Elderly or debilitated patients:* Lower doses required. At high risk for anticholinergic and hypotensive effects. *Special risk patients:* Use great caution in patients with narrow-angle glaucoma, enlarged prostate or history of seizures. Greater likelihood of seizure at higher doses. *Agranulocytosis:* This very serious and life-threatening adverse reaction has been associated with clozapine. WBC with differential count must be performed weekly. Drug will not be dispensed by pharmacy without these tests demonstrating acceptable results. *ECG changes:* Some patients experience ECG repolarization changes during treatment. Several have experienced significant cardiac events including ischemic changes, MI, nonfatal arrhythmias and sudden, unexplained death. *Neuroleptic malignant syndrome:* This potentially fatal condition has been reported in association with antipsychotic drugs. Signs and symptoms include hyperpyrexia, muscle rigidity, altered mental status, irregular pulse or BP, tachycardia, diaphoresis, cardiac arrhythmias. *Orthostatic hypotension:* This may occur throughout therapy but is especially common during titration phase. *Seizures:* Use with caution in patients having history of seizures or other predisposing factors. *Tardive dyskinesia:* This syndrome of potentially irreversible, involuntary dyskinetic movements has occurred with other antipsychotic agents. Incidence is highest among elderly, especially women. *Withdrawal of medication:* For planned discontinuation of therapy, gradually reduce dosage over 1-2 wk.

NURSING CONSIDERATIONS

Administration/Storage

- Administer clozapine in divided doses and titrate it cautiously to minimize toxic effects.
- Observe patient carefully to ensure medication is actually taken.
- Administer tablets with food or milk to decrease GI irritation.
- Clozapine is available only in 1-wk supply through Clozaril Patient Management System, which combines drug management with laboratory studies for agranulocytosis.

Assessment/Interventions

- Obtain patient history, including drug history and any known allergies.
- If seizures occur, institute precautions and notify physician.
- Relieve anticholinergic effects by offering chipped ice, sugarless gum or hard candy and fluids.
- Give a high-fiber diet to prevent constipation.
- Monitor patient's mental status throughout therapy.
- Monitor lying, sitting and standing BP and pulse during titration.
- Monitor patient's temperature. Temperature elevations sometimes occur within first 3 wk of treatment. Such elevations are usually benign but may indicate underlying infection or developing agranulocytosis.
- Assess for adverse reactions to drug (seizures, agranulocytosis).
- Assess for side effects (sedation, dizziness, hypotension, constipation, increased salivation).
- Notify physician if extrapyramidal side effects occur; be prepared to discontinue or reduce dosage and

give antiparkinson drugs for these symptoms.

OVERDOSAGE: SIGNS & SYMPTOMS

Excessive salivation, hypotension, drowsiness, delirium, coma, seizures, tachycardia, respiratory depression

Patient/Family Education

- Advise patient to change positions slowly and to sit up 1 to 2 min before standing to minimize hypotension.
- Encourage patient to maintain high-fiber, high-fluid diet to prevent constipation.
- Teach patient that psychiatric symptoms will not improve until after several weeks of therapy.
- Inform patient of risk of seizures and importance of taking medication as prescribed.
- Stress the importance of regular follow-up care, including laboratory studies for agranulocytosis (CBC).
- Teach patient to recognize and report signs of urinary retention, an anticholinergic effect.
- Instruct patient to report these symptoms to physician: lethargy, weakness, fever, sore throat, malaise, mucous membrane ulceration or other possible signs of infection.
- Teach patient to take sips of water frequently, suck on ice chips or sugarless hard candy or chew sugarless gum if dry mouth occurs.
- Instruct patient to avoid intake of alcoholic beverages or other CNS depressants.
- Advise patient that drug may cause drowsiness and to use caution while driving or performing other tasks requiring mental alertness.
- Instruct patient not to take otc medications without consulting physician.

See Patient Guide, p. 151.

Codeine

(KOE-deen)

Available as generic only

Class: Narcotic analgesic; antitussive

Action Stimulates opiate receptors in the CNS; also causes respiratory depression, peripheral vasodilation, inhibition of intestinal peristalsis, stimulation of the chemoreceptors that cause vomiting, increased bladder tone and suppression of cough reflex.

Indications Relief of mild to moderate pain; cough suppression.

Contraindications Hypersensitivity to opiates; upper airway obstruction; respiratory compromise; acute asthma; diarrhea caused by poisoning or toxins.

Route/Dosage

Analgesic

ADULTS: **IM/slow IV/PO/SC** 15-60 mg q 4-6 hr (maximum 360 mg/day). CHILDREN (≥ 1 YR): **IM/PO/SC** 0.5 mg/kg q 4-6 hr.

Antitussive

ADULTS **PO** 10-20 mg q 4-6 hr (maximum 120 mg/day). CHILDREN (6-12 YR): **PO** 5-10 mg q 4-6 hr (maximum 60 mg/day). CHILDREN (2-6 YR): **PO** 2.5-5 mg q 4-6 hr (maximum 30 mg/day).

Interactions

CNS depressants, (eg, tranquilizers, sedatives and alcohol): Causes additive CNS depression.

Lab Test Interferences

Amylase and lipase determination: Increased levels for up to 24 hr after administration.

Adverse Reactions

CV: Hypotension; orthostatic hypotension; bradycardia; tachycardia; shock. *RESP*: Laryngospasm; depression of cough reflex; respiratory depression. *CNS*: Lightheadedness; dizziness; sedation; disorientation; incoordination; euphoria; delirium. *EENT*: Miosis. *GI*:

Nausea; vomiting; constipation; abdominal pain; anorexia; biliary tract spasm. *GU:* Urinary retention or hesitancy. *DERM:* Sweating; pruritus; urticaria. *OTHER:* Tolerance; psychological and physical dependence with chronic use.

Precautions

Pregnancy: Category C. *Lactation:* Excreted in breast milk. *Children:* Do not give IV to children < 12 yr. Children are more sensitive to effects of drug. *Elderly patients:* More sensitive to effects of drug. *Special risk patients:* Use with caution in patients with myxedema, acute alcoholism, history of drug abuse potential, acute abdominal conditions, ulcerative colitis, decreased respiratory reserve, head injury or increased intracranial pressure, hypoxia, supraventricular tachycardia, depleted blood volume circulatory shock, hypothyroidism and urinary/bowel elimination problems. *Dependency:* Codeine has abuse potential. *Renal or hepatic impairment:* Duration of action may be prolonged; may need to reduce dose.

NURSING CONSIDERATIONS

Administration/Storage

- Administer oral medication with food or milk to avoid GI irritation.
- Protect injectable forms from excessive exposure to light.
- Codeine is two thirds as effective given orally as parenterally.

Assessment/Interventions

- Obtain patient history, including drug history and any known allergies. Patients with sulfite sensitivity have increased risk of allergy with certain injectable codeine products.
- Assess degree of pain before and after administration.
- Monitor pulmonary status and heart rhythm after administration.
- Monitor bowel movements and inform physician of significant pattern change.
- If respiratory compromise or increased sedation develop, withhold medication and notify physician.

OVERDOSAGE: SIGNS & SYMPTOMS

Miosis, respiratory and CNS depression, circulatory collapse, seizures, cardiopulmonary arrest, death

Patient/Family Education

- Instruct patient on self-assessment of pain and on how and when to administer medication.
- Advise patient to increase fluid intake to relieve constipation and to take stool softener or mild laxative as needed.
- Advise patient to take medication with food if GI upset occurs and to monitor for GI irritation.
- Explain that codeine may be habit forming.
- Caution patient to avoid sudden position changes to prevent orthostatic hypotension.
- Instruct patient to avoid intake of alcoholic beverages or other CNS depressants.
- Advise patient that drug may cause drowsiness and to use caution while driving or performing other tasks requiring mental alertness.
- Instruct patient not to take otc medications without contacting physician.

See Patient Guide, p. 152.

Colchicine

(KOHL-chih-seen)

Available as generic only

Class: Analgesic/gout

Action Inhibits inflammation and reduces pain and swelling associated with gouty arthritis.

Indications Treatment of chronic gouty arthritis when complicated by frequent, recurrent acute attacks of gout; relief of pain associated with acute attacks; reduction of incidence of attacks. *Note:* Colchicine will not prevent progression of gout. **Unlabeled uses:** Familial Mediterranean fever; hepatic cirrhosis; primary biliary cirrhosis; primary amyloidosis; Behçet's disease; pseudogout caused by chondrocalcinosis; skin manifestations of scleroderma; psoriasis; palmoplantar pustulosis; dermatitis herpetiformis. **Orphan drug use:** Chronic progressive multiple sclerosis.

Contraindications Serious GI, renal, hepatic or cardiac disorders; blood dyscrasias.

Route/Dosage

Acute Gouty Arthritis

ADULTS: Initial dose (give at first warning of attack): **PO** 1-1.2 mg; then 0.5-1.2 mg q 1-2 hr until pain is relieved or nausea, vomiting or diarrhea occurs. Total dose usually is 4-8 mg. Wait 3 days before initiating second course of therapy.

Prophylaxis

ADULTS: **PO** 0.5 or 0.6 mg/day for 3-4 days/wk or qd if > 1 attack/yr.

Surgical Patients

ADULTS: **PO** 0.5 or 0.6 mg tid for 3 days before and 3 days after surgery.

Prophylaxis or Maintenance of Recurrent or Chronic Gouty Arthritis

PO 0.5-1 mg 1-2 times/wk

Parenteral Use

IV only; do not give via SC or IM route.

ADULTS: ACUTE ATTACKS: **IV** 2 mg over 2-5 min; may repeat with 0.5 mg q 6 hr until satisfactory response is achieved; do not exceed total of 4 mg/24 hr. PROPHYLAXIS OR MAINTENANCE: **IV** 0.5-1 mg qd or bid. *Note:* Oral form is preferable for prophylaxis and maintenance.

Interactions None well documented.

Lab Test Interferences

May cause false-positive results in urine tests for RBCS and hemoglobin.

Adverse Reactions

GI: Nausea; vomiting; diarrhea; abdominal pain. *HEMA:* Bone marrow depression with aplastic anemia; agranulocytosis, leukopenia or thrombocytopenia (long-term therapy). *HEPA:* Elevated alkaline phosphatase and AST. *DERM:* Dermatoses; purpura; alopecia. *OTHER:* Reversible azoospermia; myopathy; peripheral neuritis.

Precautions

Pregnancy: Oral form: Category C. Parenteral form: Category D. *Lactation:* Undetermined. *Children:* Safety and efficacy not established. *Elderly patients:* Administer with great caution to elderly and debilitated patients. *GI effects:* Drug may cause nausea, vomiting, diarrhea and abdominal pain that may aggravate preexisting peptic ulcer or spastic colon. Discontinue drug if these symptoms appear. *Hepatic function impairment:* Increased colchicine toxicity may occur. *Injection:* Severe local irritation occurs if drug is given by SC or IM route. *Myopathy and neuropathy:* Myoneuropathy may occur and cause weakness in patients with impaired kidney function; serum creatine kinase may be elevated. Usually resolves in 3-4 wk after drug withdrawal. *Vitamin B_{12} malabsorption:* Colchicine induces reversible malabsorption of vitamin B_{12} with long-term use.

NURSING CONSIDERATIONS

Administration/Storage

Parenteral

- Reconstitute with 0.9% Sodium Chloride (without preservatives) only.
- Administer parenterally via IV route only. Considerable irritation and tissue damage may occur if leakage into surrounding tissue occurs.

Oral

- Store tablets in airtight, light resistant container.

Assessment/Interventions

- Obtain patient history, including drug history and any known allergies.
- Monitor serum uric acid and creatinine throughout therapy.
- Check blood counts periodically in patients undergoing long-term therapy.
- Monitor for phlebitis and extravasation.
- Assess for signs of toxicity: abdominal pain, alopecia, nausea, vomiting, diarrhea, myopathy or peripheral neuritis. Notify physician immediately if these signs occur.
- Assess for signs of vitamin B_{12} deficiency: anemia and paresis of extremities.

OVERDOSAGE: SIGNS & SYMPTOMS

Nausea, severe abdominal pain, vomiting, diarrhea, shock, ST segment elevation, paralysis, respiratory failure, liver damage, renal failure, leukopenia, thrombocytopenia, coagulopathy, alopecia, stomatitis

Patient/Family Education

- Instruct patient to take colchicine regularly to prevent acute attacks.
- Instruct patient not to exceed 8 mg in course of therapy for acute attack. To minimize cumulative toxicity, patient should wait 3 days before starting second course.
- Advise patient with gout to drink at least 2000 ml of fluid daily, unless contraindicated.
- Reinforce physician's instructions about weight loss, diet and alcohol intake.
- Advise patient to have extra supply of drug on hand in case physician gives instructions to increase dosage.
- Instruct patient to stop taking drug if nausea, vomiting, diarrhea or abdominal pain occurs, especially if patient has history of spastic colon or ulcers.

See Patient Guide, p. 153.

Colestipol Hydrochloride

(koe-LESS-tih-pole HIGH-droe-KLOR-ide)

Colestid

Class: Antihyperlipidemic/bile acid sequestrant

Action Increases removal of bile acids from body by forming insoluble complexes in intestine, which are then excreted in feces. As body loses bile acids, it converts cholesterol from blood to bile acids, thus lowering serum cholesterol.

Indications Reduction of cholesterol in patients with primary hypercholesterolemia who do not respond adequately to diet. **Unlabeled use:** Treatment of digitalis toxicity.

Contraindications Hypersensitivity to bile acid sequestering resins; complete biliary obstruction.

Route/Dosage

ADULTS: Tablets **PO** 2-16 gm/day given once or in divided doses. Start with 2 gm once or twice daily and increase in amounts of 2 gm, once or twice daily at 1- or 2-month intervals. ADULTS: Granules **PO** 5-30 gm/day given once or in divided doses. Start with 5 gm once or twice daily and increase in amounts of 5 gm daily over 1-2 month intervals.

Interactions *Digitalis glycosides, furosemide, gemfibrozil, hydrocortisone, penicillin G, phosphate supplements, propanolol, tetracyclines, thiazide diuretics, fat soluble vitamins (ie, A, D, E, K)*: Absorption of these drugs may be decreased.

Lab Test Interferences None well documented.

Adverse Reactions *EENT*: Difficulty swallowing. *GI*: Constipation; abdominal pain and cramping; intestinal bloating; flatulence; indigestion; heartburn; diarrhea; nausea; vomiting; bloody hemorrhoids and stools; esophageal obstruction. *HEMA*: Bleeding tendencies related to vitamin K deficiency. *HEPA*: Elevated liver function tests. *DERM*: Rash; urticaria. *META*: Fat soluble vitamin deficiencies.

Precautions *Pregnancy*: Category undetermined. *Lactation*: Undetermined. *Children*: Safety and efficacy not established.

NURSING CONSIDERATIONS

Administration/Storage

- Administer before meals.
- Do not administer simultaneously with other medicines. Administer other medications 1 hr before or 4-6 hours after colestipol.
- Tablets are large and may be difficult to swallow.
- Swallow each tablet whole. Do not cut, crush or chew tablets.
- Drink plenty of fluids as the tablets are swallowed.
- Granulated form of medication should not be taken dry. Mix well in at least 90 ml of liquids of any type (except alcoholic beverages), soups, cereal or pulpy fruits. Colestipol will not dissolve.
- Rinse glass with small amount of beverage to ensure that all the medication is consumed.
- Store granules and tablets at room temperature.

Assessment/Interventions

- Obtain patient history.
- Monitor for signs of increased bleeding tendencies, such as swollen joints, ecchymotic areas and petechiae.
- Assess for bowel function, particularly pre-existing problems with constipation that may worsen with its use.
- Document serum cholesterol and triglyceride levels.
- Provide diet high in fiber; increase fluids to 2-3 L unless contraindicated. If constipation develops, notify physician.
- Obtain baseline serum total and LDL-C, and triglyceride levels.

OVERDOSAGE: SIGNS & SYMPTOMS

GI obstruction

Patient/Family Education

- Instruct patient to take medication before meals.
- Advise patient to take any other medications, including over-the-counter medications, 1 hr before or 4-6 hrs after taking colestipol.
- Advise patient regarding proper mixing of granules.
- Advise patient to implement any vitamin and mineral supplementation recommended by healthcare provider.
- Advise patient to drink prune juice, eat fruit and vegetables, and maintain good fluid intake on a regular basis to avoid constipation.
- Advise patient to notify healthcare provider if GI side effects (eg, constipation, cramping, heartburn, bloating, gas) become bothersome.
- Instruct patient in lifestyle changes (eg, low fat diet, regular exercise, weight reduction) that facilitate cholesterol/triglyceride control.

- Advise patient that lab tests will be required to monitor therapy. Be sure to keep appointments.

See Patient Guide, p. 154.

Colfosceril Palmitate (Synthetic Lung Surfactant; Dipalmitoylphosphatidylcholine; DPPC)

(kahl-FOSE-uhr-ILL PAL-mih-TATE)

Exosurf Neonatal

Class: Lung surfactant

Action Replaces deficient endogenous pulmonary surfactant and reduces surface tension.

Indications Prevention of neonatal respiratory distress syndrome (RDS) in infants with birth weight of < 1350 g; treatment of established hyaline membrane disease at all gestational ages. **Orphan drug use:** Adult RDS.

Contraindications Standard considerations.

Route/Dosage

NEONATES & INFANTS: **Intratracheal** Prevention: 5 ml/kg/instillation as soon as possible after birth; second and third doses: approximately 12-24 hr later to infants remaining on mechanical ventilation. Rescue: 5 ml/kg/instillation at confirmation of RDS diagnosis; repeat 5 ml/kg 12 hr later (if infant remains on mechanical ventilation).

Interactions None well documented.

Lab Test Interferences None well documented.

Adverse Reactions

RESP: Oxygen desaturation; pulmonary hemorrhage, nosocomial pneumonia; apnea; mucous plugs. *CNS:* Intraventricular hemorrhage.

Precautions Drug should be administered only by trained personnel in closely supervised setting. *Pulmonary hemorrhage:* Occurred more commonly in infants weighing < 700 g.

NURSING CONSIDERATIONS

Administration/Storage

- For intratracheal administration only.
- Reconstitute immediately before use, if possible, with Sterile Water for Injection. Do not use solutions that contain preservatives or buffers. Gently swirl or shake suspension before administration.
- Do not use suspensions if persistent large flakes or particles are present.
- Administer by instillation into trachea via side port on special adapter of endotracheal tube without interrupting mechanical ventilation.
- Before administering, assure proper placement of ET tube. Recheck during and after administration. If suctioning is required, allow patient's condition to stabilize before administering. Suctioning should be done before instillation and then no less than 2 hr after administration.
- Store unreconstituted powder at room temperature in a dry place.

Assessment/Interventions

- Obtain patient history, including drug history and any known allergies.
- Determine infant's weight, because accuracy is important for dosing.
- Maintain continuous ECG and trancutaneous oxygen saturation monitoring during administration; arterial BP monitoring is desirable.
- Maintain continuous bedside monitoring for at least 30 min after administration.
- Perform frequent blood gas monitor-

ing after administration to prevent hypocarbia and hyperoxia.

- If chest expansion improves significantly after administration, reduce peak ventilator inspiratory pressures immediately. Do not wait for blood gas confirmation.
- Do not suction for 2 hr after administration unless airway is obstructed. Be alert for possible mucus plugs. Replace ET tube immediately if suctioning is unsuccessful.
- Monitor heart rate, color, respirations (rate, quality), facial expression, endotracheal tube patency and oximeter during and after administration.
- Continually monitor oxygen and carbon dioxide levels and be prepared to adjust ventilator appropriately.

Patient/Family Education

- Explain use and benefits of medication and its possible side effects.
- Advise family of infant's condition and offer frequent updates.

No patient monograph available.

Corticotropin (Adrenocorticotropic hormone; ACTH)

(core-tih-koe-TROE-pin)

ACTH, ACTH-40, ACTH-80, Acthar

Class: Adrenal cortical steroid

Action Stimulates adrenal cortex to produce and secrete adrenocortical hormones (corticosteroids and glucocorticoids).

Indications Diagnostic testing of adrenocortical function; treatment of nonsuppurative thyroiditis, hypercalcemia associated with cancer, acute exacerbations of multiple sclerosis, tuberculous meningitis when accompanied by antituberculous chemotherapy, trichinosis with neurologic or myocardial involvement, and treatment of glucocorticoid responsive rheumatic, collagenous, dermatologic, allergic, ophthalmic, respiratory, hematologic, neoplastic and GI diseases. **Unlabeled use:** Treatment of infantile spasms.

Contraindications Scleroderma; osteoporosis; systemic fungal infections; ocular herpes simplex; recent surgery; history or presence of peptic ulcer; CHF; hypertension; sensitivity to porcine proteins; conditions accompanied by primary adrenocortical insufficiency or adrenocortical hyperfunction. IV administration is contraindicated, except in treatment of idiopathic thrombocytopenic purpura or diagnostic testing of adrenocortical function.

Route/Dosage

Rapid-acting Injection

ADULTS: **IM/SC** 20 U qid. DIAGNOSTIC TESTS: **IV** 10-25 U dissolved in 500 ml of D5W infused over 8 hr. ACUTE EXACERBATIONS OF MULTIPLE SCLEROSIS: **IM** 80-120 U/day for 2-3 wk. INFANTILE SPASMS: **IM** 20-40 U qd or 80 U qod for 3 mo or 1 mo after seizures stop.

Repository Injection

IM/SC 40-80 U q 24-72 hr. Not suitable for IV use.

Interactions

Anticholinesterases: Effects of these agents may be antagonized in myasthenia gravis. *Barbiturates:* May decrease effects of corticotropin.

Lab Test Interferences

May decrease I^{131} uptake; possible suppression of skin test reactions; falsely decreased urinary estradiol and estriol concentrations with Brown method; falsely decreased urinary estrogen concentrations with colorimetry and fluorometry.

Adverse Reactions

CV: Hypertension; CHF; necrotizing angiitis. *CNS:* Convulsions; vertigo; headache; increased intracranial pressure with papilledema; pseudotumor cerebri. *EENT:* Posterior subcapsular cataracts; increased IOP; glaucoma with possible optic nerve damage; exophthalmos. *GI:* Pancreatitis; ulcerative esophagitis; abdominal distention; peptic ulcer. *DERM:* Impaired wound healing; petechiae and ecchymoses; increased sweating; hyperpigmentation; thin, fragile skin; facial erythema; acne. *META:* Negative nitrogen balance because of protein catabolism; fluid and electrolyte disturbances (eg, sodium and fluid retention, potassium and calcium loss, hypokalemic alkalosis); antibody production and loss of stimulatory effect of ACTH with prolonged use. *OTHER:* Infection; musculoskeletal disturbances (eg, weakness, myopathy, loss of muscle mass, osteoporosis, vertebral compression fractures, pathologic fracture of long bones, aseptic necrosis of femoral and humeral heads); endocrine abnormalities (menstrual irregularities, growth suppression in children, hirsutism, cushingoid state, glucose intolerance, decreased carbohydrate tolerance, increased requirement for insulin or oral hypoglycemic agent in diabetic patients, secondary adrenocortical and pituitary unresponsiveness.

Precautions

Pregnancy: Category C. *Lactation:* Undetermined. *Children:* Because prolonged use inhibits skeletal growth, careful monitoring is necessary. *Fluid and electrolyte balance:* Drug may elevate BP, cause salt and water retention and increase potassium and calcium excretion. *Immunosuppression:* Live vaccine immunization is usually contraindicated, especially with high doses of corticotropin. *Infection:* Drug may mask signs of infection; resistance to infection may be decreased. *Long-term administration:* May lead to irreversible adverse effects. Complications are dependent on dose and duration of treatment. Prolonged use increases risk of hypersensitivity reactions and ocular effects. *Sensitivity to porcine proteins:* Perform skin testing in patients with suspected sensitivity to porcine proteins. Observe for sensitivity reactions during or after administration. *Stress:* Increased dosage of rapid-acting corticosteroid may be needed before, during and after stressful situations.

NURSING CONSIDERATIONS

Administration/Storage

- Medication may be given via IV, IM or SC route. Do not use IV route except in treatment of idiopathic purpura or diagnostic testing of adrenocortical function.
- If patient is sensitive to porcine proteins, skin tests must be performed before administration.
- Standard tests for adrenal responsiveness to corticotropin are performed via same route that will be used for administration of drug.

Corticotropin for Injection

- Check product label to be certain that medication is for IV use.
- Reconstitute powder in Sterile Water for Injection or Sterile Sodium Chloride for Injection. Use only enough diluent so that dose is contained in 1-2 ml of solution.
- Rotate vial while drawing into syringe.
- Refrigerate reconstituted solution and use within 24 hr.

Corticotropin Repository Injection

- Note that this form is for IM or SC use only, *not* for IV administration.
- Store repository corticotropin injection in refrigeration.

Assessment/Interventions

- Obtain patient history, including drug history and any known allergies.
- Observe patient for possible hypersensitivity reaction. Have epinephrine 1:1000 available for emergency use.

- Take patient's vital signs and monitor throughout therapy.
- Monitor I&O and weight.
- Monitor serum potassium and sodium levels.
- In patients with diabetes, monitor blood glucose frequently because dosage of insulin or oral hypoglycemic agent may need to be increased.
- Assess for recurrent symptoms, which may result from sudden withdrawal of medication after prolonged use.
- If any of these signs occur, report them to physician: fluid retention, muscle weakness, abdominal pain, seizures or headache; adrenal insufficiency (fatigue, anorexia, nausea, vomiting, diarrhea, weight loss, weakness and dizziness); visual disturbances; cushingoid symptoms.

Patient/Family Education

- Counsel patient to follow dietary regimen carefully (eg, salt restriction or potassium supplementation).
- Advise patient to avoid receiving live virus vaccinations while taking this medication.
- Instruct patient to have periodic eye examinations while taking medication as long-term therapy.
- If patient has diabetes, instruct to monitor blood glucose regularly throughout therapy since dosage of insulin or oral hypoglycemic agent may need to be increased.
- Advise patient to contact physician before discontinuing medication.
- Instruct patient to notify physician at first sign of infection: prolonged cold symptoms, sore throat, weight gain, GI upset, heart irregularities, delayed wound healing or changes in mood behavior.
- Tell patient to report these symptoms to physician: fluid retention, muscle weakness, abdominal pain, seizures or headaches.
- Instruct patient not to take otc medications without consulting physician.

See Patient Guide, p. 155.

Cortisone (Cortisone Acetate)

(CORE-tih-sone)

Cortone Acetate

Class: Corticosteroid

Action As short-acting glucocorticoid; depresses formation, release and activity of endogenous mediators of inflammation; has some salt-retaining properties.

Indications Treatment of primary or secondary adrenal cortex insufficiency; rheumatic disorders; collagen diseases; dermatologic diseases; allergic states; allergic and inflammatory ophthalmic processes; respiratory diseases; hematologic disorders; neoplastic diseases; edematous states (caused by nephrotic syndrome); GI diseases; multiple sclerosis; tuberculous meningitis; trichinosis with neurologic or myocardial involvement.

Contraindications Systemic fungal infections; administration of live virus vaccines in patients receiving immunosuppressive doses.

Route/Dosage

ADULTS: PO 25-300 mg/day. Use lowest possible effective dose. ALTERNATE-DAY THERAPY: Provides at least twice usual daily dosage of short- to intermediate-acting medication.

Interactions

Anticholinesterases: Drug may antagonize anticholinesterase effects in myasthenia gravis. *Anticoagulants, oral:* Drug may increase or decrease anticoagulant dose requirements. *Barbiturates:* May decrease pharmacologic effect of cortisone. *Phenytoin:* May decrease therapeutic efficacy of cortisone. *Rifampin:* May decrease therapeutic efficacy of cortisone. *Salicylates:* Drug may reduce serum levels and efficacy of salicylates.

Troleandomycin: May increase effects of cortisone.

Lab Test Interferences

False-negative nitroblue tetrazolium test.

Adverse Reactions

CV: Thromboembolism or fat embolism; thrombophlebitis; necrotizing angiitis; cardiac arrhythmias or ECG changes; syncopal episodes; hypertension; myocardial rupture after recent MI; CHF. *CNS:* Convulsions; increased intracranial pressure with papilledema; vertigo; headache; neuritis/paresthesias; psychosis; fatigue; insomnia. *EENT:* Cataracts; increased IOP; glaucoma; exophthalmos. *GI:* Pancreatitis; abdominal distention; ulcerative esophagitis; nausea; vomiting; increased appetite and weight gain; peptic ulcer; small bowel and large bowel perforation, especially in inflammatory bowel disease. *GU:* Increased or decreased motility and number of spermatozoa. *HEMA:* Leukocytosis. *DERM:* Impaired wound healing; petechiae and ecchymoses; erythema; lupus erythematosus–like lesions; suppression of skin test reactions; subcutaneous fat atrophy; purpura; hirsutism; acneiform eruptions; allergic dermatitis; urticaria; angioneurotic edema; perineal irritation; hyperpigmentation or hypopigmentation. *META:* Sodium and fluid retention; hypokalemia; hypokalemic alkalosis; metabolic alkalosis; increased serum cholesterol; hypocalcemia; hypothalamic-pituitary-axis suppression; endocrine abnormalities (decreased T_3, T_4 and ^{131}I uptake, menstrual irregularities, cushingoid state, growth suppression in children, increased sweating, decreased carbohydrate tolerance, hyperglycemia, glycosuria, increased insulin or sulfonylurea requirements, manifestations of latent diabetes mellitus, negative nitrogen balance because of protein catabolism, hirsutism). *OTHER:* Musculoskeletal effects (eg, muscle weakness, myopathy, tendon rupture, osteoporosis, aseptic necrosis of femoral and humeral heads, spontaneous fractures; anaphylactoid reactions; aggravation or masking of infections; malaise.

Precautions

Pregnancy: Pregnancy category undetermined. *Lactation:* Excreted in breast milk. *Children:* Observe growth and development of infants and children undergoing prolonged therapy. *Elderly patients:* May require lower doses. *Adrenal suppression:* Prolonged therapy may lead to hypothalmic-pituitary-adrenal suppression. Withdraw gradually after prolonged therapy. *Cardiovascular disease:* Use with caution in patients with recent MI. *Fluid and electrolyte balance:* Drug can cause elevated BP, salt and water retention, increased potassium and calcium excretion. Dietary salt restriction and potassium supplementation may be necessary. *Hepatitis:* Drug may be harmful in chronic active hepatitis that is positive for hepatitis B surface antigen. *Hypersensitivity:* Anaphylactoid reactions have occurred rarely. *Infections:* Drug may mask signs of infection and decrease host-defense mechanisms that prevent dissemination of infection. *Ocular effects:* Use cautiously in ocular herpes simplex because of possible corneal perforation. *Peptic ulcer:* Drug may contribute to peptic ulceration, especially in large doses. *Renal impairment:* Use cautiously. *Stress:* Increased dosage of rapid-acting corticosteroid may be needed before, during and after stressful situations.

NURSING CONSIDERATIONS

Administration/Storage

- Administer with meals or snacks to avoid GI irritation.
- Give single daily dose or alternate-day dose before 9 AM to obtain maximum benefit.
- Space multiple doses evenly throughout day.

- When giving large doses of cortisone, administer antacids between meals.
- Store at room temperature in tightly closed container. Protect from heat and freezing.

Assessment/Interventions

- Obtain patient history, including drug history and any known allergies.
- Note any sensitivity to sulfites, tartrazine and aspirin.
- Be prepared for emergency treatment of hypersensitivity reaction.
- Obtain baseline weight, vital signs, chemistry profile, 2 hr postprandial blood glucose and chest x-ray.
- Monitor I&O and weight daily. Observe for edema, and report steady weight gain to physician.
- Monitor renal function throughout therapy.
- Monitor for development of steroid psychosis, manifested by changes in mood behavior.
- If patient has diabetes, monitor blood glucose frequently.
- Monitor drug withdrawal carefully. Drug must be discontinued gradually to avoid adrenal insufficiency.
- Observe for signs of infection: depression, malaise, anorexia and delayed healing.
- Observe growth and development of infants and children undergoing prolonged therapy.
- Report signs of adrenal insufficiency to physician: fatigue, anorexia, nausea, vomiting, diarrhea, weight loss, weakness and dizziness.
- Report signs of cushingoid symptoms to physician.

OVERDOSAGE: SIGNS & SYMPTOMS

Acute adrenal insufficiency caused by too rapid withdrawal: fever, myalgia, arthralgia, malaise, anorexia, nausea, desquamation of skin, orthostatic hypotension, dizziness, fainting, dyspnea, hypoglycemia

Cushingoid changes from chronic use of too large dose: moonface, central obesity, striae, hirsutism, acne, eccymoses, fluid and electrolyte imbalance, hypertension, osteoporosis, myopathy, sexual dysfunction, diabetes, hyperlipidemia, peptic ulcer

Patient/Family Education

- Instruct patient to take with meals to avoid GI upset.
- Tell patient to take single daily dose before 9 AM.
- Instruct patient to monitor weight daily and to report steady gain to physician.
- Inform patients with diabetes to monitor blood glucose regularly.
- Instruct elderly patients undergoing long-term therapy to have BP, blood glucose and electrolytes checked every 6 mo.
- Advise patient to avoid receiving live virus vaccine during therapy.
- Instruct patients undergoing long-term therapy to have an annual eye examination and to carry ID card.
- For discontinuation after long-term therapy, instruct patient to adhere to tapering schedule.
- Advise patient to notify physician before discontinuing medication.
- Instruct patient to report these symptoms to physician: cold, infection or prolonged sore throat; change in vision; swelling of extremities; weakness; black tarry stools; irregular heartbeat; menstrual irregularities; changes in mood or behavior; fatigue; anorexia; nausea; vomiting; diarrhea; weight loss.

See Patient Guide, p. 156.

Cosyntropin (Synthetic Corticotropin, Synthetic ACTH)

(koe-sin-TROE-pin)
Cortrosyn
Class: Adrenal cortical steroid

Action Exhibits full corticosteroidogenic activity of natural ACTH, stimulating adrenal cortex to produce and secrete adrenocortical hormones.

Indications Diagnostic testing of adrenal function.

Contraindications Standard considerations.

Route/Dosage
ADULTS: **IM/IV (direct injection)** 0.25-0.75 mg. IV infusion: 0.25 mg in D5W or 0.9% saline administered at 0.04 mg/hr over 6 hr. CHILDREN ≤ 2 YR: **IM/IV** 0.125 mg often will be sufficient.

Interactions
Anticholinesterases: May antagonize anticholinesterase effects in myasthenia gravis. *Barbiturates:* May decrease pharmacologic effect of cosyntropin. *Hydantoins:* May increase clearance and decrease therapeutic efficacy of cosyntropin.

Lab Test Interferences
None well documented.

Adverse Reactions
OTHER: Rare hypersensitivity.

Precautions
Pregnancy: Category C. *Lactation:* Undetermined. *Hypersensitivity:* Exhibits slight immunologic activity but is less likely to cause reactions than natural ACTH.

NURSING CONSIDERATIONS

Administration/Storage
- Before administration, be prepared to treat possible acute hypersensitivity reaction.
- Administer by IM route, direct IV injection or IV infusion.
- Reconstitute 0.25 mg vial with 1 ml of 0.9% Sodium Chloride for Injection.
- Administer reconstituted drug via IM route or by direct IV injection over 2 min or further dilute in D5W or normal saline and infuse over 4-8 hr.
- Do not allow cosyntropin to mix with blood or plasma infusions.
- Reconstituted preparations should not be retained.

Assessment/Interventions
- Obtain patient history, including drug history and any known allergies. Note hypersensitivity to natural corticotropin.
- Measure plasma cortisol concentrations prior to and 30-60 min after administration. Collect blood sample of 6-7 ml in heparinized tube.
- Alternatively, measure urinary steroids before and after IV infusion.

Patient/Family Education
- Explain purpose of the test.
- Emphasize importance of lab tests.
- Instruct patients taking corticosteroids or aldosterone to omit doses on day of test.

See Patient Guide, p. 157.

Cromolyn Sodium (Disodium Cromoglycate)

(KROE-moe-lin SO-dee-uhm)
Crolom, Gastrocrom, Intal, Nasalcrom, ♣ *Nalcrom, Rynacrom*
Class: Respiratory inhalant

Action Stabilizes mast cells, which release histamine and other mediators of allergic reactions.

Indications
Inhalation: Prophylaxis of severe bronchial asthma; prevention of exer-

cise-induced asthma; prevention of acute bronchospasm induced by environmental pollutants and known antigens. *Nasal solution:* Prevention and treatment of allergic rhinitis. *Oral:* Treatment of mastocytosis. *Ophthalmic:* Treatment of vernal keratoconjunctivitis, vernal conjunctivitis and vernal keratitis. **Unlabeled uses:** *Oral form:* Symptoms of food allergies; eczema; dermatitis; ulceration; urticaria pigmentosa; chronic urticaria; hay fever; and postexercise bronchospasm.

Contraindications Standard considerations.

Route/Dosage

Bronchial Asthma

ADULTS & CHILDREN (≤ 5 YR FOR CAPSULES, ≥ 2 YR FOR SOLUTION): **Nebulization** Initially 20 mg inhaled qid at regular intervals. ADULTS & CHILDREN > 5 YR: **Aerosol** 2 metered sprays (1600 mcg) inhaled qid at regular intervals.

Prevention of Acute Bronchospasm

ADULTS: 2 metered dose sprays or 20 mg via inhaled capsule or nebulizer (10-15 min but no longer than 60 min) before exposure to precipitating factor.

Seasonal or Perennial Rhinitis

ADULTS & CHILDREN > 6 YR: **Nasal solution with spray device** Begin treatment prior to contact with allergen and continue throughout exposure period. One spray (5.2 mg) in each nostril 3-6 times/day at regular intervals.

Mastocytosis

ADULTS: **PO** 200 mg qid ½ hr before meals and at bedtime. CHILDREN 2-12 YR: **PO** 100 mg qid ½ hr before meals and at bedtime (maximum 40 mg/kg/day). *Note:* Decrease in dosage maintenance levels is done gradually, except with major complication. Abrupt withdrawal may result in increased asthma symptoms. TERM INFANTS-2 YR: **PO** 20 mg/kg/day in 4 divided doses (maximum 30 mg/kg/day). PREMATURE TO TERM INFANTS: Not recommended.

Vernal keratoconjunctivitis, vernal conjunctivitis and vernal keratitis ADULTS: **SOLN** 1 or 2 drops in each eye 4 to 6 times/day at regular intervals.

Interactions None well documented.

Lab Test Interferences

None well documented.

Adverse Reactions

RESP: Cough; wheezing; bronchospasm. *CNS:* Dizziness; headache. *EENT:* Lacrimation; nasal stinging, burning or irritation; sneezing; nasal congestion; bad taste; swollen parotid gland; dry or irritated throat. *GI:* Nausea; substernal burning; diarrhea (oral form). *GU:* Dysuria; urinary frequency. *DERM:* Rash; urticaria; angioedema. *OTHER:* Joint pain and swelling. *OPHTHALMIC:* Stinging; burning; watery eyes; itchy eyes; dryness around the eye; puffy eyes; eye irritation; and styes.

Precautions

Pregnancy: Category B. *Lactation:* Undetermined. *Children:* Capsules: Use not recommended in children < 5 yr. Aerosol: Safety and efficacy not established in children < 5 yr. Nebulizer: Safety and efficacy not established in children < 2 yr. Nasal solution: Safety and efficacy not established in children < 6 yr. *Acute asthma:* Do *not* use for acute asthma attack. Effects depend on regular administration. *Aerosol:* Use with caution in patients with coronary artery disease or cardiac arrhythmias because of propellants in this preparation. *Bronchospasm:* Cough or bronchospasm may follow inhalation. *Eosinophilic pneumonia:* If signs of this condition occur, therapy will need to be discontinued. *Hepatic or renal function impairment:* Decreased dose is recommended. *Hypersensitivity:* Severe anaphylactic reactions may occur.

NURSING CONSIDERATIONS

Administration/Storage

Oral

- Open and dissolve capsule contents completely in ½ glass of hot water. While stirring, add equal amount of cold water. Administer all of liquid. Do not mix with juice, milk or foods.
- Administer ½ hr before meals and at bedtime.
- Do *not* use oral capsules for inhalation.
- Store in airtight, light-resistant container at room temperature.

Inhalation

- Administer when patient's airway is clear for inhalation. Do *not* administer during acute asthmatic attack.

Nebulizer Solution/Inhalation Capsules

- Instruct patient to close eyes during inhalation to prevent accidental contact with eyes.
- If bronchodilating inhalant is also prescribed, give bronchodilator 5-15 min before cromolyn to enhance drug delivery. Have patient exhale completely, place mouthpiece between lips and inhale deeply and rapidly, hold breath for few seconds, remove mouthpiece, then exhale. Repeat until entire dose is taken.

Aerosol

- Store away from heat and direct sunlight. Protect from freezing. Do not puncture, break or burn container.
- Use spacer (eg, Aero chamber) to enhance delivery of drug.
- Inhalation capsules: Store in tight, light-resistant container. Avoid storing in moist environment (eg, bathroom).

Nasal

- Clear patient's nasal passages before administering spray. Have patient inhale medication through nose.
- Hold container upright. Use pumping motion to force solution mist into nasal passages.
- Store in airtight, light-resistant container.

Ophthalmic Solution

- The effectiveness of cromolyn therapy is dependent on its administration at regular intervals, as directed.
- Patient may experience a transient stinging or burning sensation following instillation of cromolyn.

Assessment/Interventions

- Obtain patient history, including drug history and any known allergies.
- Evaluate therapeutic effectiveness by decrease in frequency or severity of clinical symptoms or decrease in need for concomitant therapy over period of 4 wk.
- Notify physician if these signs occur: wheezing or coughing after inhalation or stinging effect after nasal instillation; joint pain; severe wheezing, difficulty breathing, chills, sweating or chest pain, which may indicate eosinophilic pneumonia.

Patient/Family Education

- Explain that cromolyn is used for prevention, not treatment, of acute asthma attacks.
- Give patient clear instructions about what to do during an acute asthma attack.
- Teach patient correct use of administration device (see instructions in package). Have patient demonstrate its use.
- Emphasize that inhalation capsules are not to be swallowed.
- Explain that oral capsules are oversized to prevent powder from spilling when capsule is opened. Remind patient to dissolve powder in water only and to drink entire contents of solution.
- Advise patient to minimize exposure to known allergens or precipitating factors.
- Instruct patient with cold or exercise-induced asthma to use medication at least 10-15 min before exposure but no longer than 1 hr.
- Advise patient to rinse mouth or gar-

gle after oral inhalation to prevent throat irritation.

- If patient is taking concurrent bronchodilators or corticosteroids, stress importance of not discontinuing abruptly, particularly systemic corticosteroids.
- Advise patient that effectiveness of therapy is dependent on administration at regular intervals. Maximum effectiveness may take 4 wk.
- Caution patient not to discontinue abruptly unless advised to do so by physician.
- Instruct patient to report these symptoms to physician: increased difficulty in breathing, increased wheezing, difficulty in swallowing, joint pain or swelling, severe headache.
- Patient should not wear contact lenses while using cromolyn ophthalmic solution.

See Patient Guide, pp. 158-161.

Cyanocobalamin (Vitamin B_{12})

(sigh-an-oh-koe-BAL-uh-min)

Crystamine, Cyanoject, Cyomin, Ener-B, Rubesol-1000, Rubramin PC, ✤ *Rubramin*

Class: Blood modifier/vitamin

Action Involved in protein synthesis; essential to growth, cell reproduction, hematopoiesis and nucleoprotein and myelin synthesis.

Indications Treatment of vitamin B_{12} deficiency caused by malabsorption syndrome of various causes (eg, pernicious anemia, GI pathology, fish tapeworm infestation, malignancy of pancreas or bowel, gluten enteropathy, small bowel bacterial overgrowth, gastrectomy, accompanying folic acid deficiency); supplementation because of increased requirements (associated with pregnancy, thyrotoxicosis, hemolytic anemia, hemorrhage, malignancy and hepatic and renal disease); vitamin B_{12} absorption test (Schilling test).

Contraindications Hypersensitivity to cobalt, vitamin B_{12} or any component of these medications; hereditary optic nerve atrophy.

Route/Dosage

Recommended Dietary Allowance

ADULTS: **PO** 2 mcg/day. CHILDREN: **PO** 0.3-2 mcg/day.

Vitamin B_{12} Deficiency

ADULTS: **PO** 25-1000 mcg/day. **IM** or **deep SC** 30 mcg/day for 5-10 days followed by 100-200 mcg/mo.

Addisonian Pernicious Anemia

ADULTS: **IM** or **deep SC** 100 mcg/day for 6-7 days. If reticulocyte response occurs, give 100 mcg qod for 7 doses, then give 100 mcg q 3-4 days for 2-3 wk. After this regimen, give 100 mcg/mo for life.

Shilling Test Flushing Dose

ADULTS **IM** 1000 mcg (z-tract method preferred).

Interactions *Chloramphenicol:* Decreases hematologic effects of vitamin B_{12} in patients with pernicious anemia. *Colchicine, excessive alcohol intake (> 2 wk) neomycin, time-released potassium, paraaminosalicylic acid:* Decreases GI absorption of vitamin B_{12}.

Lab Test Interferences *Methotrexate, pyrimethamine and most antibiotics:* May invalidate vitamin B_{12} diagnostic microbiological blood assays.

Adverse Reactions *With parenteral administration:* CV: Pulmonary edema; CHF; peripheral vascular thrombosis. *EENT:* Severe and rapid optic nerve atrophy. *GI:* Mild transient diarrhea. *DERM:* Itching; transitory exanthema; urticaria. *OTHER:* Hypersensitivity; pain at injection site; sensation of body swelling; hypokalemia; polycythemia vera.

Precautions
Pregnancy: Category C (parenteral). *Lactation:* Excreted in breast milk. *Children:* Some products contain benzyl alcohol, which has been associated with fatal "gasping syndrome" in premature infants. *Hypersensitivity:* Anaphylactic shock and death have been associated with parenteral use. *Hypokalemia:* Possibly fatal hypokalemia could occur as result of increased erythrocyte potassium requirements.

NURSING CONSIDERATIONS

Administration/Storage
- If patient is sensitive to cobalamins, perform an intradermal skin test prior to administering drug.
- Give IM injection or deep SC injection in large muscle mass.
- Parenteral administration is required in treatment of pernicious anemia.
- Protect parenteral vitamin B_{12} from light. Do not freeze.

Assessment/Interventions
- Obtain patient history, including drug history and any known allergies. Note any history of Leber's disease or sensitivity to cobalt and vitamin B_{12}.
- Obtain baseline reticulocyte counts, hematocrit, vitamin B_{12}, iron and folic acid levels and then repeat tests between 5th and 7th days of treatment.
- Obtain periodic hematology tests as long as patient is on therapy.
- Monitor serum potassium levels during the first 48 hr of treatment.
- Throughout treatment, monitor and report vision changes to physician.
- Report signs of hypersensitivity (urticaria, redness, itching) and hypokalemia (muscle weakness, heart irreguiarity) to physician.

Patient/Family Education
- Instruct patient with pernicious anemia of need to continue therapy throughout lifetime.
- Teach patient of need to maintain well-balanced diet. Remind patient of these good sources of vitamin B_{12}: seafood, egg yolks, organ meats, fortified breakfast cereals, meat, cheeses, milk and other dairy products.
- Advise patient that folic acid is not substitute for vitamin B_{12} but may be taken concurrently.
- Instruct vegetarians who do not use animal products of need for daily oral vitamin B_{12}.
- Inform patient with pernicious anemia of need to have periodic GI evaluations.
- Instruct patient to report these symptoms to physician: muscle weakness, shortness of breath, heart irregularity or vision disturbances.

See Patient Guide, pp. 162-163.

Cyclobenzaprine HCl

(SIGH-kloe-BEN-zuh-preen HIGH-droe-KLOR-ide)

Flexeril

Class: Skeletal muscle relaxant/centrally acting

Action Relieves skeletal muscle spasms of local origin without interfering with muscle function by acting within CNS at brain stem. Structurally and pharmacologically related to tricyclic antidepressants.

Indications Relief of muscle spasms associated with acute painful musculoskeletal conditions. **Unlabeled use:** Treatment of fibrositis.

Contraindications Use of MAO inhibitors or within 14 days of their discontinuation; acute recovery phase of MI; arrhythmias; heart block or conduction disturbances; CHF; hyperthyroidism.

Route/Dosage

ADULTS: PO 10 mg tid (maximum 60 mg/day). Do not use > 3 wk.

Interactions

Alcohol and other CNS depressants: May cause additive CNS depression. MAO *inhibitors:* May cause hyperpyretic crisis, severe convulsions and death.

Lab Test Interferences

None well documented.

Adverse Reactions

CV: Tachycardia; syncope; arrhythmias; vasodilation; palpitation; hypertension. *CNS:* Drowsiness; dizziness; fatigue; asthenia; headache; nervousness; convulsions; confusion. *EENT:* Blurred vision. *GI:* Dry mouth; nausea; constipation; dyspepsia; unpleasant taste. *HEMA:* Purpura; bone marrow depression; leukopenia; eosinophilia; thrombocytopenia. *DERM:* Sweating; skin rash; urticaria. *META:* Hypoglycemia; hyperglycemia.

Precautions

Pregnancy: Category B. *Lactation:* Undetermined. *Children:* Safety and efficacy in children < 15 yr not established. *Anticholinergic effects:* Use with caution in patients with urinary retention, angle-closure glaucoma and increased intraocular pressure.

NURSING CONSIDERATIONS

Administration/Storage

- Give with meals to avoid GI irritation.
- Do not give concomitantly with MAO inhibitors or within 14 days of last dose of MAO inhibitor.

Assessment/Interventions

- Obtain patient history, including drug history and any known allergies.
- Record any sensitivity to tricyclic antidepressants and cyclobenzaprine.
- Take vital signs as needed.
- Monitor for development of psychotic symptoms (eg, disorientation, depressed mood; anxiety; hallucinations.
- Obtain ECG if heart arrhythmia develops.

OVERDOSAGE: SIGNS & SYMPTOMS

Confusion, agitation, visual hallucinations, arrhythmia, CHF, hyperpyrexia, hyperactive reflexes, vomiting, drowsiness, stupor, coma, hypothermia, tachycardia, dilated pupils, seizures, hypotension

Patient/Family Education

- Inform patient that this medication makes injury temporarily feel better. Caution patient not to rush recovery and to avoid lifting or exercising too soon, which may further damage muscles.
- Caution patient to rise slowly from a sitting or standing position to avoid injury.
- Instruct patient to report these symptoms to physician: shortness of breath, palpitations, weight gain, heart irregularities, confusion, yellowing of skin or eyes, fever or difficulty urinating.
- Advise patient to take sips of water frequently, suck on ice chips or sugarless hard candy or chew sugarless gum if dry mouth occurs.
- Instruct patient to avoid intake of alcoholic beverages or other CNS depressants.
- Advise patient that drug may cause drowsiness and to use caution while driving or performing other tasks requiring mental alertness.
- Instruct patient not to take otc medications without consulting physician.

See Patient Guide, p. 164.

Cyclophosphamide

(sigh-kloe-FOSS-fuh-mide)

Cytoxan, Neosar ✦ *Procytox*

Class: Antineoplastic/alkylating

Action Metabolized into active alkylating metabolites, which may be involved with cross-linking of tumor cell DNA and interfering with growth of susceptible neoplasms and, to some extent, normal tissues. Has immunosuppressive activity.

Indications Treatment of malignant lymphoma, Hodgkin's disease, certain other lymphomas, multiple myeloma, certain leukemias, mycosis fungoides, neuroblastoma, ovarian adenocarcinoma, retinoblastoma and carcinoma of breast; secondary treatment of biopsy-proved "minimal change" nephrotic syndrome in children. Often used in combination therapy with other antineoplastic agents. **Unlabeled uses:** Treatment of variety of severe rheumatologic conditions including Wegener's granulomatosis, steroid-resistant vasculitis, severe progressive rheumatoid arthritis and systemic lupus erythematosus.

Contraindications Continued use in presence of severely depressed bone marrow function.

Route/Dosage

Malignant Disease

ADULTS & CHILDREN (WITHOUT HEMATOLOGIC DEFICIENCY): Initial dose: **IV:** 40-50 mg/kg in divided doses over 2-5 days. **Other IV regimens** 10-15 mg/kg q 7-10 days or 3-5 mg/kg twice weekly. **PO** 1-5 mg/kg/day.

Biopsy-proved "Minimal Change" Nephrotic Syndrome

CHILDREN: **PO** 2.5-3 mg/kg/day for 60-90 days.

Interactions

Anticoagulants: May increase anticoagulant effect. *Digoxin:* May reduce digoxin serum levels, especially when cyclophosphamide is used in combination with other neoplastic agents. *Succinylcholine:* May prolong neuromuscular blockage. *Thiazide diuretics:* May increase adverse effects of cyclophosphamide.

Lab Test Interferences

None well documented.

Adverse Reactions

CV: Massive doses have been associated with cardiotoxicity, including hemorrhagic cardiac necrosis, transmural hemorrhage and coronary artery vasculitis. *RESP:* Interstitial pulmonary fibrosis (with prolonged high doses). *GI:* Anorexia; nausea; vomiting; diarrhea; stomatitis; abdominal discomfort or pain. *GU:* Acute hemorrhagic cystitis; nonhemorrhagic cystitis; bladder fibrosis; urinary frequency; syndrome of inappropriate antidiuretic hormone (SIADH). *HEMA:* Leukopenia; thrombocytopenia; anemia. *DERM:* Alopecia (frequent but hair regrowth usually occurs); skin rash; pigment changes. *OTHER:* Amenorrhea, sterility, sexual dysfunction, gonodal atrophy (in boys).

Precautions

Pregnancy: Category D. *Lactation:* Excreted in breast milk. *Special risk patients:* Use cautiously in patients with renal or hepatic impairment, leukopenia, thrombocytopenia, tumor cell infiltration of bone marrow, previous radiation therapy, previous cytotoxic therapy or severe immunosuppression. Treatment may not be indicated or may need to be altered in patients who have infections or in whom infections develop. *Adrenalectomy patients:* Dose adjustment may be required. *Cardiac toxicity:* Has occurred in patients receiving high doses. Severe and sometimes fatal CHF has occurred within few days after first dose. *Carcinogenesis:* Secondary neoplasia has developed. *Fertility impairment:* May cause sterility in both sexes. *Wound healing:* Drug may interfere with normal wound healing.

NURSING CONSIDERATIONS

Administration/Storage

- Caution must be used in handling drug because of higher risk of fetal loss with occupational exposure.
- Antiemetic may be given before drug is administered to lessen nausea.
- Give tablet on empty stomach. If severe GI irritation occurs, administer with food.
- Use oral solution within 14 days of preparation and keep refrigerated.
- Use IV/IM solution prepared with Sterile Water for Injection within 24 hr when stored at room temperature. When stored in refrigerator, solution remains stable for 6 days. IV solution can be further diluted with D5W, normal saline or lactated Ringer's.

Assessment/Interventions

- Obtain patient history, including drug history and any known allergies. Note hypersensitivity to cyclophosphamide and history of cardiac disease.
- Obtain baseline BUN, creatinine, CBC and serum electrolytes. Monitor hematologic profile throughout therapy.
- Note other medications being taken, especially digoxin, thiazides, doxorubicin or succinylcholine.
- Encourage fluid intake.
- Monitor I & O throughout therapy.
- If hematuria or CHF occurs, notify physician.
- If leukocytes drop to < 2000 mm^3, notify physician.

Patient/Family Education

- Advise patient of childbearing age to use some form of contraception because of mutagenic potential of drug.
- Instruct patient to take oral medicine on an empty stomach; however, if severe GI irritation occurs, drug may be taken with food or milk.
- Advise patient to increase fluid intake and void frequently to help to prevent cystitis.
- Inform patient of the probability of hair loss and reassure patient that regrowth of hair can be expected, although it may be of a different color or texture.
- Explain that mouth sores may develop and that soothing mouth rinses may be used for relief.
- Instruct patient to report these symptoms to physician: unusual bleeding or bruisings, stomatitis, fever, chills, sore throat, cough, shortness of breath, joint pain, seizures, yellow skin or eyes or flank or stomach pain.

See Patient Guide, p. 165.

Cycloserine

(sigh-kloe-SER-een)

Seromycin

Class: Anti-infective/antitubercular

Action Inhibits cell wall synthesis in susceptible strains of certain microorganisms.

Indications Treatment of active pulmonary and extrapulmonary tuberculosis when organisms are susceptible (after failure of adequate treatment with primary medications); treatment of urinary tract infections caused by susceptible bacteria when conventional therapy has failed; treatment of Gaucher's disease.

Contraindications Epilepsy; depression; severe anxiety or psychosis; severe renal insufficiency; excessive concurrent use of alcohol.

Route/Dosage
ADULTS: **PO** 250-500 mg q 12 hr; start with 250 mg q 12 hr for first 2 wk (maximum 1 g/day). CHILDREN: **PO** 10-20 mg/kg/day administered in 2 equally divided doses (maximum 1 g/day).

Interactions
Alcohol: Increases possibility and

risk of epileptic episodes. Do not use together. *Isoniazid:* May increase cycloserine CNS side effects (eg, dizziness).

Lab Test Interferences

None well documented.

Adverse Reactions

CV: CHF. *CNS:* Convulsions; drowsiness; somnolence; headache; tremor; dysarthria; vertigo; confusion; loss of memory; psychoses with suicidal tendencies, behavior changes, hyperirritability, aggression, paresis; hyperreflexia; paresthesias; major and minor clonic seizures; coma; dizziness. *HEPA:* Elevated hepatic transaminase. *DERM:* Skin rash.

Precautions

Pregnancy: Category C. *Lactation:* Undetermined. *Children:* Safety and dosage not well established. *CNS toxicity:* Discontinue drug or decrease dosage if symptoms of CNS toxicity develop. May be increased with excessive alcohol consumption. Pyridoxine 200-300 mg/day may be given to prevent neurotoxic effects. *Renal impairment:* Weekly blood levels of drug should be determined and dosage adjusted to keep blood levels < 30 mcg/ml.

NURSING CONSIDERATIONS

Administration/Storage

- Administer with meals if GI irritation occurs.
- Store in airtight, light-resistant container at room temperature.

Assessment/Interventions

- Obtain patient history, including drug history and any known allergies.
- Review history for epilepsy, depression, severe anxiety or psychosis, renal insufficiency or excessive alcohol use.
- Review liver function, BUN, creatinine and CBC before beginning therapy.
- Obtain culture before treatment and verify susceptibility when results are available.
- Perform baseline assessment of signs and symptoms of infection.
- If patient has active and infectious tuberculosis, institute infection control measures.
- Monitor serum cycloserine levels at least weekly in patients receiving > 500 mg/day and in patients with reduced renal function or symptoms of toxicity. Blood levels should remain < 30 mcg/ml.
- Monitor CBC, liver and renal function studies.
- If allergic dermatitis or symptoms of CNS toxicity, convulsions, psychosis, depression, headache, tremor, vertigo, paresis or dysarthria develop, withhold medication and notify physician.
- If CNS alterations occur, institute safety precautions.
- In patients with tuberculosis, assess for therapeutic effectiveness by monitoring clinical signs and symptoms, sputum cultures or smears for acid-fast bacilli and chest x-rays.
- In patients with urinary tract infections, assess for therapeutic effectiveness by monitoring clinical signs and symptoms and urine cultures.

OVERDOSAGE: SIGNS & SYMPTOMS

CNS depression, drowsiness, mental confusion, headache, vertigo, hyperirritability, paresthesias, dysarthrias, psychosis, paresis, convulsions, coma

Patient/Family Education

- Instruct patient that if depression or suicidal thoughts occur, notify physician immediately.
- Stress importance of regular follow-up visits to physician for ongoing assessment.
- If patient does not have adequate family support system, refer patient to community health organization for monitoring and support.
- Instruct patient to report these symp-

toms to physician: rash, anxiety, restlessness, confusion or tremor.

- Caution patient to avoid intake of alcoholic beverages because of increased risk of seizures.
- Advise patient that drug may cause drowsiness and to use caution while driving or performing other tasks requiring mental alertness.

See Patient Guide, p. 166.

Cyclosporine (Cyclosporin A)

(SIGH-kloe-spore-EEN)

Sandimmune

Class: Immunosuppressive

Action Suppresses cell-mediated immune reactions and some humoral immunity, but exact mechanism is not known.

Indications Prophylaxis of organ rejection in kidney, liver and heart allogeneic transplants in conjunction with adrenal corticosteroid therapy; treatment of chronic rejection in patients previously treated with other immunosuppressive agents. **Unlabeled uses:** Prophylaxis in other transplant procedures; treatment of aplastic anemia, atopic dermatitis, Behçet's disease, biliary cirrhosis, Crohn's disease, rheumatoid arthritis, severe psoriasis, nephrotic syndrome, pulmonary sarcoidosis, pyoderma gangrenosum, ulcerative colitis, alopecia areata. **Orphan drug uses:** Ophthalmic form for treatment of keratoconjunctivitis sicca, use after keratoplasty and treatment of corneal melting syndrome.

Contraindications Hypersensitivity polyoxyethylated castor oil, which is present in concentrate for injection.

Route/Dosage

ADULTS & CHILDREN: **PO** 15 mg/kg/day (range 14-18 mg/kg/day) beginning 4-12 hr before transplantation. Continue for 1-2 wk postoperatively then taper dose by 5%/wk to maintenance level of 5-10 mg/kg/day. Lower doses may be used on basis of patient response, rejection rate and cyclosporine plasma concentrations. **IV** 5-6 mg/kg/day as single IV dose starting 4-12 hr before transplantation. Switch to oral form as soon as patient can tolerate.

Interactions

Amiodarone, diltiazem, fluconazole, imipenem-cilastatin, ketoconazole, macrolide antibiotics (eg, erythromycin), nicardipine: May increase cyclosporine concentrations. *Aminoglycosides, amphotericin B, NSAIDs, trimethoprim-sulfamethoxazole, melphalan, quinolones:* Additive nephrotoxicity possible. *Azathioprine, corticosteroids, cyclophosphamide, verapamil:* May cause additive immunosuppression, increasing risk of infection and malignancy. *Carbamazepine, hydantoins, phenobarbital, rifampin, rifabutin:* May decrease cyclosporine effects. *Digoxin:* May cause elevated digoxin concentrations and toxicity. *Etoposide:* May increase etoposide concentrations. *Lovastatin:* May cause severe myopathy or rhabdomyolysis; avoid concurrent use. *Metoclopramide:* Increases absorption of cyclosporine. *Potassium-sparing diuretics:* Causes hyperkalemic effects; avoid concomitant use.

Lab Test Interferences

None well documented.

Adverse Reactions

CV: Hypertension; MI. *CNS:* Tremor; convulsions; headache; confusion; flushing; ataxia; hallucinations; mania; depression; encephalopathy. *GI:* Gingival hyperplasia; diarrhea; nausea, vomiting; abdominal discomfort; anorexia; gastritis; peptic ulcer; hiccoughs. *GU:* Renal dysfunction. *HEMA:* Lymphoma; hemolytic anemia; leukopenia; anemia; thrombocytopenia. *HEPA:* Hepatotoxicity. *DERM:* Hirsutism; acne; brittle fingernails. *META:* Hyperglycemia; hyperkalemia; hyperuricemia.

OTHER: Paresthesia; gynecomastia; allergic reactions including anaphylaxis; cramps.

Precautions

Pregnancy: Category C. *Lactation:* Excreted in breast milk. *Children:* Although safety and efficacy have not been established, patients as young as 6 mo have received drug. May require higher doses than adults. *Absorption:* Absorption during long-term use is erratic. Patients with malabsorption may have difficulty achieving therapeutic concentrations with oral use. *Anaphylactic reactions:* Occur rarely with IV use. Have epinephrine 1:1000 and oxygen readily available. *Convulsions:* Have occurred, particularly in combination with high-dose methylprednisolone. *Nephrotoxicity:* Common adverse effect; may respond to decreased dose. *Renal impairment:* Requires close monitoring and possible dosage adjustment.

NURSING CONSIDERATIONS

Administration/Storage

- Give with adrenal corticosteroids but not with other immunosuppressive agents.

Intravenous

- Dilute parenteral solution immediately before use. Dilute each 1 ml (50 mg) concentrate in 20-100 ml of 0.9% Sodium Chloride for Injection or D5W. Observe for particulate matter and discoloration. Give IV infusion slowly over 2-6 hr.
- Store in glass container at room temperature. Protect from light. Solutions diluted with D5W are stable for 24 hr.

Oral

- Use calibrated pipettes for oral doses. Prepare solution in glass container just before administering to patient. Prepare with room-temperature white or chocolate milk or orange juice to improve flavor. Stir well and give to patient to drink. Do not use plastic utensils (drug binds to plastics). Do not allow mixture to stand before administering.
- Do not refrigerate or freeze. Use within 2 mo after opening.

Assessment/Interventions

- Obtain patient history, including drug history and any known allergies. Note hypersensitivity to cyclosporine or polyoxyethylated castor oil.
- Perform renal and hepatic function tests in conjunction with potassium and lipid level determinations before beginning treatment and periodically repeat tests during drug therapy.
- Assess vital signs initially and note hypertension, especially with children.
- Note any signs of infection (eg, fever, sore throat, tiredness), unusual bleeding, hematuria or bruising.
- Have emergency equipment available for IV drug administration and assess vital signs frequently (eg, q 5-10 min x 4) or according to hospital policy.
- Ensure medical asepsis and eliminate any potential sources of environmental contamination.
- Weigh patient daily and monitor I&O.

OVERDOSAGE: SIGNS & SYMPTOMS

Hepatotoxicity, nephrotoxicity

Patient/Family Education

- Instruct patient on necessity for frequent laboratory monitoring while taking medication.
- Instruct patient on proper technique for self-monitoring of BP and vital signs.
- Instruct patient to report any adverse reactions: infection (eg, fever, sore throat, fatigue, frequency, dysuria, cloudy urine), unusual bleeding (eg, hematuria, bleeding of gums, bruising), chest pain, headache, tremors or liver dysfunction (eg, abdominal pain, jaundice, dark urine, pruritus, light-colored stools).

- Direct patient to avoid contact with others who may have infections.
- Caution patient to avoid any trauma.
- Advise patient to use soft toothbrush, practice frequent oral hygiene and have regular dental checkups.
- Counsel patient on need for balanced diet and fluid intake according to specific physician orders.
- Advise patient to consult physician before any vaccinations.

See Patient Guide, p. 167.

Cyproheptadine HCl

(sip-row-HEP-tuh-deen HIGH-droe-KLOR-ide)

Periactin, ♣ *PMS-Cyproheptadine*
Class: Antihistamine/piperidine

Action Competitively antagonizes histamine at H_1 receptor sites. Also exhibits antiserotonin activity.

Indications Symptomatic relief of perennial and seasonal allergic rhinitis, vasomotor rhinitis, allergic conjunctivitis; temporary relief of runny nose and sneezing caused by common cold; management of allergic and nonallergic pruritic symptoms, mild skin manifestations of uncomplicated urticaria and angioedema and cold urticaria. **Unlabeled uses:** Appetite stimulation in underweight patients and in those with anorexia nervosa; treatment of vascular cluster headaches.

Contraindications Hypersensitivity to antihistamines; newborn or premature infants; nursing mothers; narrow-angle glaucoma; stenosing peptic ulcer; symptomatic prostatic hypertrophy; asthmatic attack; bladder neck obstruction; pyloroduodenal obstruction; MAO therapy.

Route/Dosage
ADULTS: **PO** 4 mg q 8 hr then 4-20 mg/day; not to exceed 0.5 mg/kg/day. CHILDREN: **PO** Total daily dosage 0.25 mg/kg or 8 mg/m^2. CHILDREN 7-14 YR: 4 mg bid or tid (max 16 mg/day). CHILDREN 2-7 YR: 2 mg bid or tid (max 12 mg/day).

Interactions
Alcohol, CNS depressants: May cause additive CNS depressant effects. *Fluoxetine:* Effects of fluoxetine may be reversed. *MAO inhibitors:* Anticholinergic effects of cyproheptadine may increase.

Lab Test Interferences
In skin testing procedures antihistamines may prevent or diminish otherwise positive reaction to dermal reactivity indicators.

Adverse Reactions
CV: Orthostatic hypotension; palpitations; tachycardia; reflex tachycardia; extrasystoles; faintness. *RESP:* Thickening of bronchial secretions; chest tightness; wheezing; nasal stuffiness; respiratory depression. *CNS:* Drowsiness (often transient); sedation; dizziness; faintness; disturbed coordination; confusion; restlessness; excitement; nervous tremor; paresthesias; convulsions; hallucinations. *EENT:* Dry mouth, nose and throat; sore throat. *GI:* Epigastric distress; nausea; vomiting; diarrhea; anorexia; constipation; change in bowel habits. *HEPA:* Jaundice. *HEMA:* Hemolytic anemia; thrombocytopenia; agranulocytosis. *DERM:* Photosensitivity; rash.

Precautions
Pregnancy: Category B. *Lactation:* Contraindicated in nursing women. *Children:* Safety and efficacy in children < 2 yr not established. *Elderly:* Dosage reduction may be required. *Special risk patients:* Use drug with caution in patients with predisposition to urinary retention, history of bronchial asthma, increased intraocular pressure, hyperthyroidism, cardiovascular disease or hypertension. *Hepatic impairment:* Use drug with caution in patients with cirrhosis or other liver disease. *Respiratory disease:* Generally not recom-

mended for treatment of lower respiratory tract symptoms including asthma.

Sedatives/CNS depressants: Avoid in patients with history of sleep apnea.

NURSING CONSIDERATIONS

Administration/Storage

- Administer medication with meals.
- Scored tablets may be crushed.
- Store in tight container at room temperature.

Assessment/Interventions

- Obtain patient history, including drug history and any known allergies.
- Assess baseline vital signs and lung sounds.
- For diabetic patients monitor blood glucose closely if taking sugar-based syrups.
- Monitor weight weekly for significant increases.
- Perform regular assessments and notify physician if patient exhibits signs of cardiovascular, neurologic or respiratory dysfunction (eg, cardiac arrhythmia, hypotension, increased drowsiness or agitation, confusion, chest tightness, wheezing).

OVERDOSAGE: SIGNS & SYMPTOMS

CNS depression, cardiovascular collapse, cardiovascular stimulation, seizures, hypotension, anticholinergic effects (dilated pupils, dry mouth, flushing), hyperthermia (especially in children), dystonic reactions, dizziness, ataxia, blurred vision

Patient/Family Education

- Instruct diabetic patients to monitor blood glucose closely if taking syrup preparations.
- Alert patients that syrup preparations contain alcohol, and advise against taking any additional alcoholic beverages or CNS depressants throughout therapy.
- Explain potential effects of chronic dryness of oral tissues and encourage patient to maintain good oral hygiene and obtain regular dental care.
- Explain that skin testing procedures may be affected if drug is not discontinued at least 4 days prior to test.
- Tell patient to report any adverse reactions, including changes in urinary habits, to physician.
- Instruct patient to take sips of water frequently, suck on ice chips or sugarless hard candy or chew sugarless gum if dry mouth occurs.
- Advise patient that drug may cause drowsiness and to use caution while driving or performing other tasks requiring mental alertness.
- Caution patients to avoid exposure to sunlight and prolonged exposure to extreme heat and to use sunscreen or wear protective clothing to avoid photosensitivity reaction.
- Instruct patient not to take otc medications without consulting physician.

See Patient Guide, p. 168.

Cytarabine (Cytosine Arabinoside; ARA-C)

(SIGH-tar-ah-bean)

Cytosar-U, ♣ *Cytosar*

Class: Antineoplastic/antimetabolite

Action Exhibits cell phase specificity, primarily killing cells undergoing DNA synthesis (S-phase); inhibits DNA polymerase.

Indications Induction and maintenance of remission in acute myelocytic leukemia, in single or combination chemotherapy of acute lymphocytic leukemia, and in meningeal leukemia (intrathecal administration).

Contraindications Standard considerations.

Route/Dosage

Acute Nonlymphocytic Leukemia

ADULTS & CHILDREN: **IV/SC** 100 mg/m^2/day by continuous infusion (days 1-7) or 100 mg/m^2 q 12 hr by IV injection (days 1-7). Administered in combination with other antineoplastic drugs.

Acute Lymphocytic Leukemia

Consult medical literature for current recommendations.

Refractory Acute Leukemia

ADULTS & CHILDREN: **IV/SC** 3 g/m^2 q 12 hr for 4-12 doses (repeated at 2-3 wk intervals) has been used.

Meningeal Leukemia

Intrathecal 5-75 mg/m^2 once daily for 4 days or once q 4 days.

Interactions

Digoxin: May decrease digoxin absorption for up to several days after chemotherapy is stopped. Digoxin capsules do not appear to be affected by cytarabine.

Lab Test Interferences

None well documented.

Adverse Reactions

RESP: Pneumonia; shortness of breath. *CNS:* Neuritis or neural toxicity; dizziness; headache. *EENT:* Conjunctivitis; sore throat. *GI:* Anorexia; nausea; vomiting; diarrhea; oral and anal inflammation or ulceration; bowel necrosis; abdominal pain; pancreatitis; esophageal ulceration; esophagitis. *GU:* Urinary retention; renal dysfunction. *HEMA:* Bone marrow suppression; anemia; leukopenia; thrombocytopenia; megaloblastosis and reduced reticulocytes. Cell count depression may be delayed and last for 12-24 days. *HEPA:* Jaundice; elevation of liver enzymes; hepatic dysfunction. *DERM:* Rash; skin ulceration; freckling; alopecia; pruritus; urticaria. *OTHER:* Fever; thrombophlebitis; bleeding; sepsis; cellulitis or thrombophlebitis at injection site; chest pain; anaphylaxis; edema; secondary infections; myalgia.

Precautions

Pregnancy: Category D. *Lactation:* Undetermined. *Benzyl alcohol:* May be contained in product diluent; may cause fatal "gasping syndrome" in premature infants. *Experimental doses:* Severe and sometimes fatal CNS, GI and pulmonary toxicity have occurred. Syndrome of sudden respiratory distress progressing to pulmonary edema and cardiomegaly are possible fatal reactions associated with high-dose therapy. *Hepatic impairment:* Use caution; reduce dose. *Hypersensitivity:* Cases of anaphylaxis with acute cardiopulmonary arrest have occurred. *Intrathecal route:* Carefully monitor for hematopoietic toxicity. Do not use a diluent with benzyl alcohol when giving drug intrathecally. *Myelosuppression:* Main toxic effect is bone marrow suppression with leukopenia, thrombocytopenia and anemia. For induction therapy, administer drug at facility capable of providing monitoring and treatment of potential drug toxicity.

NURSING CONSIDERATIONS

Administration/Storage

- For intrathecal administration or high doses of drug, reconstitute drug with preservative-free 0.9% Sodium Chloride for Injection; do not use diluent with benzyl alcohol.
- Administer initial doses in setting in which resuscitation equipment/supplies are readily available.
- Discard solution if slight haze develops.
- For intravenous infusion solutions, reconstituted cytarabine may be added to Bacteriostatic Water for Injection, D5W or 0.9% Sodium Chloride for Injection.
- Store reconstituted drug in glass or plastic disposable syringes at controlled room temperature for ≤ 48 hr.

Assessment/Interventions

- Obtain patient history, including drug history and any known allergies. Assess current immune status and cardiopulmonary, hematologic, hepatic, and renal function studies, including uric acid level.
- Determine patient's use of alcohol.
- Assess for baseline data on hematologic, hepatic, renal and neurologic functions.
- Provide protective/reverse isolation for immunosuppressed patient.
- Be alert for sudden changes in CNS status and possible cardiopulmonary distress.
- Check and record vital signs q 4 hr and prn.
- Monitor patient for any changes from predrug assessment findings.
- Monitor for signs and symptoms of inflammation (eg, at administration site) and infections of any kind.
- Monitor laboratory and pathology reports daily, especially for leukocyte and platelet counts and bone marrow studies.

OVERDOSAGE: SIGNS & SYMPTOMS

Irreversible CNS toxicity, death

Patient/Family Education

- Caution patient to avoid crowds and persons with known infections.
- Instruct patient to report unusual bleeding, use soft toothbrush and electric razor and avoid falls.
- Tell patient not to drink alcoholic beverages or take medications with aspirin.
- Advise patient to use contraceptive measures for at least 4 mo after conclusion of therapy.
- Instruct patient not to receive any vaccinations without advice of physician.
- Emphasize to patient the need for periodic laboratory tests to monitor side effects.

No patient monograph available.

Dacarbazine

(da-CAR-buh-zeen)

DTIC-Dome, Imidazole, ♣ *DTIC*

Class: Antineoplastic

Action Exact mechanism is unknown. Alkylation, inhibition of DNA synthesis, and interaction with sulfhydryl groups in proteins are proposed actions.

Indications Treatment of metastatic malignant melanoma; adjunctive therapy for Hodgkin's disease. **Unlabeled uses:** Adjunctive therapy for soft tissue sarcomas and neuroblastoma; treatment of malignant glucagonoma.

Contraindications Standard considerations.

Route/Dosage

Malignant Melanoma

ADULTS: **IV** 2-4.5 mg/kg/day for 10 days. Repeat q 4 wk. Alternatively: 250 mg/m^2/day for 5 days. Repeat q 3 wk.

Hodgkin's disease

ADULTS: **IV** 150 mg/m^2/day for 5 days or 375 mg/m^2/day on day 1, in combination with other drugs per protocol. Repeat q 15 days.

Interactions None well documented. INCOMPATIBILITIES: Do not mix with other drugs.

Lab Test Interferences

None well documented.

Adverse Reactions

CNS: Facial paresthesia; flu-like symptoms; myalgia; malaise. *GI:* Anorexia; nausea; vomiting; diarrhea. *HEMA:* Bone marrow depression; leukopenia; thrombocytopenia; anemia. *DERM:* Erythematous and urticarial rash; alopecia; photosensitivity; facial flushing. *OTHER:* Liver or renal function abnormalities.

Precautions

Pregnancy: Category C. *Lactation:* Undetermined. *Anaphylaxis:* May occur. *Extravasation:* Tissue damage and severe pain may occur after extravasation. *Hematopoietic depression:* Most common toxicity; careful monitoring required. *Hepatotoxicity:* Hepatic vein thrombosis and hepatocellular necrosis resulting in death have been reported in approximately 0.01% of patients.

NURSING CONSIDERATIONS

Administration/Storage

- Administer by IV route only.
- Give patient antiemetic 30 min before administering drug.
- Restrict food and fluids for 4-6 hr before administration to prevent nausea and vomiting.
- Reconstitute IV solution with Sterile Water for Injection. Drug may be further diluted with 5% dextrose or saline injection.
- Reconstituted drug may be stored for up to 8 hr at room temperature or up to 72 hr at 4°C (if further diluted with 5% dextrose or saline injection up to 24 hr at 4°C).

Assessment/Interventions

- Obtain patient history, including drug history and any known allergies. Note kidney disease, liver disease or blood dyscrasias.
- Ensure that baseline renal and hepatic function tests, as well as hemoglobin, hematocrit, WBC count, differential, reticulocyte and platelet counts, have been obtained before beginning therapy.
- Ensure that liver and renal function tests are repeated periodically.
- Monitor WBC, RBC and platelet levels frequently. Notify physician if hematopoietic depression develops.
- Monitor infusion site closely for extravasation. If present, stop infusion immediately and notify physician. Warm compresses can be used for inflammation at infusion site.
- Observe for nausea, vomiting, anorexia, diarrhea, rash, facial flushing, facial paresthesia, myalgia, malaise or alopecia. Notify physician if these occur.
- Observe for anaphylactic reactions.

Patient/Family Education

- Remind patient to restrict food and fluids for 4-6 hr before treatment.
- Advise patient that GI upset is common, but that tolerance usually develops quickly.
- Caution patient to avoid use of aspirin products or ibuprofen during therapy.
- Caution patient to avoid crowds and individuals with infections because drug may decrease resistance.
- Instruct patient to report these symptoms to physician: persistent GI complaints, rash, facial flushing, facial paresthesia, myalgia, malaise, vision changes or alopecia.
- Caution patient to avoid exposure to sunlight and to use sunscreen that blocks both UVA & UVB or wear protective clothing to avoid photosensitivity reaction.

See Patient Guide, p. 170.

Dactinomycin (Actinomycin D; ACT)

(DAK-tih-no-MY-sin)

Cosmegen

Class: Antineoplastic/antibiotic

Action Intercalates into DNA and inhibits messenger RNA synthesis, which stops cell division.

Indications Treatment of Wilms' tumor, rhabdomyosarcoma, choriocarcinoma, nonseminomatous testicular carcinoma, Ewing's sarcoma and sarcoma botryoides.

Contraindications Do not give at or near time of infection with chickenpox or herpes zoster; generalized infection may occur and could cause death.

Route/Dosage
ADULTS: **IV** 0.5 mg/day for maximum of 5 days; not to exceed 15 mcg/kg or 400-600 mcg/m^2 daily. CHILDREN: **IV** 0.015 mg/kg/day for 5 days; alternatively, total dose of **IV** 2.5 mg/m^2 given over 1 wk.

Interactions None well documented.

Lab Test Interferences
May interfere with bioassays for measuring antibacterial drug levels.

Adverse Reactions
EENT: Cheilitis; ulcerative stomatitis; pharyngitis; dysphasia. *GI*: Severe nausea; vomiting; abdominal pain; GI ulceration; anorexia; diarrhea. *HEPA*: Hepatitis; ascites; hepatomegaly; abnormal LFTs. *HEMA*: Bone marrow suppression; immunosuppression; thrombocytopenia; agranulocytosis; anemia; leukopenia; pancytopenia; aplastic anemia. *DERM*: Extravasation (can severely damage soft tissue); alopecia. *OTHER*: Fever; malaise; lethargy; fatigue; myalgia; hypocalcemia.

Precautions
Pregnancy: Category C. *Lactation*: Undetermined. *Children*: Not recommended in infants < 6 mo. *Radiation*: Combined dactinomycin-radiation therapy has variable effects; refer to prescribing information.

NURSING CONSIDERATIONS

Administration/Storage
- Avoid inhaling or contact with skin or eyes when mixing drug (use vertical flow laminar hood or gown, gloves and mask).

Assessment/Interventions
- Obtain patient history, including drug history and any known allergies.
- Document serum CBC and WBC before therapy and monitor throughout use of drug.
- Monitor infusion site for signs of extravasation. Change infusion sites as needed to prevent toxicity to soft tissues.
- Document increased fluid loss and decreased nutrition intake during entire course of treatment.
- Report elevated temperature to physician as soon as possible.
- Discontinue infusion if patient has burning and pain at administration site and evaluate site for potential complications such as needle or catheter obstruction or dislodgement and extravasation.
- Discontinue medication if patient has peripheral vascular changes distal to infusion site, and notify physician.
- Discontinue medication immediately if patient has significant respiratory changes, and notify physician.

Patient/Family Education
- Warn patient and family about temporary hair loss.
- Teach patient techniques for oral care to treat or prevent stomatitis.
- Tell patient to weigh weekly.
- Explain ways for patient to increase intake of fluid as tolerated.
- Explain why patient should avoid crowds and people with known, active infections.
- Reinforce basic hygiene information for patient and family.

No patient monograph available.

Dalteparin Sodium

(dal-TEH-puh-rin SO-dee-uhm)
Fragmin
Class: Anticoagulant

Action Inhibits reactions that lead to clotting.

Indications Prophylaxis of deep venous thrombosis in high risk patients undergoing abdominal surgery.

Contraindications Active major bleeding, thrombocytopenia, hypersensitivity to heparin or pork products.

Route/Dosage
ADULTS: **SC** 2500 units starting 1-2 hrs before surgery and continuing QD for 5-10 days. Do not give IM.

Interactions
Anticoagulants; Platelet Inhibitors: Increased risk of bleeding.

Lab Test Interferences
Aminotransferase (AST and ALT): Drug caused increased concentrations.

Adverse Reactions
HEMA: Thrombocytopenia; hematoma; bleeding. *HEPA:* Serum transaminase elevation rarely associated with increased bilirubin. *OTHER:* Injection site pain/hematoma; allergic reactions (pruritus, rash, fever); skin necrosis; anaphylactoid reactions.

Precautions
Pregnancy: Category B. *Lactation:* Undetermined. *Children:* Safety and efficacy not established. *Thrombocytopenia:* Use very cautiously in patients with history of heparin-induced thrombocytopenia. *Units:* Cannot be exchanged on a unit per unit basis with other types of heparin. *Bleeding risk:* Avoid use in patients at risk for bleeding (eg severe hypertension, severe liver or kidney disease, platelet defects, etc.) or shortly after brain, spinal or ophthalmological surgery.

NURSING CONSIDERATIONS

Administration/Storage
- Do not mix with other injections or infusions until compatibility is determined.
- Do not administer by IM injection.
- Inspect all preparations for particulate matter prior to administration.
- Vary injection site daily.
- Store at room temperature.

Assessment/Interventions
- Obtain patient history.
- Assess for signs of bleeding or bruising.
- Assess patient for signs of renal or hepatic insufficiency.
- During the course of treatment, monitor complete blood counts, including platelet count, and stool occult blood tests.

OVERDOSAGE: SIGNS & SYMPTOMS
Hemorrhagic complications

Patient/Family Education
- Instruct patient to report any signs of bleeding immediately.

See Patient Guide, p. 171.

Danazol

(DAN-uh-ZOLE)
Danocrine, ♣ *Cyclomen*
Class: Hormone

Action Suppresses pituitary-ovarian axis by inhibiting output of pituitary gonadotropins; has weak, dose-related androgenic activity with no estrogenic or progestational activity.

Indications Treatment of endometriosis; symptomatic treatment of fibrocystic breast disease; prevention of attacks of hereditary angioedema. **Unlabeled uses:** Treatment of precocious puberty, gynecomastia and menorrhagia; treatment of idiopathic immune thrombocytopenia, lupus-associated thrombocytopenia and autoimmune hemolytic anemia.

Contraindications Pregnancy; lactation; undiagnosed abnormal genital bleeding; markedly impaired hepatic, renal or cardiac function.

Route/Dosage

Endometriosis

ADULTS **PO** 800 mg/day in 2 divided doses.

Fibrocystic Breast Disease

ADULTS **PO** 100-400 mg/day in 2 divided doses.

Hereditary Angioedema

ADULTS **PO** 200 mg bid-tid.

Interactions *Anticoagulants:* May increase anticoagulant effects. *Carbamazepine:* May increase carbamazepine concentration. *Cyclosporine:* May increase cyclosporine levels, thus increasing risk of nephrotoxicity. *Insulin:* Diabetic patients may need increased insulin doses.

Lab Test Interferences May interfere with tests for determination of testosterone, androstenedione and dehydroepiandrosterone levels.

Adverse Reactions *GI:* Gastroenteritis. *HEPA:* Jaundice; elevated liver function test results; hepatic dysfunction. *DERM:* Acne; mild hirsutism; oily skin or hair. *OTHER:* Edema; decreased breast size; deepening of voice; weight gain; flushing; sweating; vaginitis; nervousness; emotional lability; amenorrhea; anovulation; breakthrough bleeding.

Precautions *Pregnancy:* Category X. Advise patient that this medication must not be taken during pregnancy or when pregnancy is possible. Instruct patient to use reliable form of birth control when taking this medication. *Lactation:* Drug contraindicated in nursing women. *Androgenic effects:* May not be reversible even when drug is discontinued. *Carcinoma of breast:* Should be exluded before treatment of fibrocystic breast disease. *Fluid retention:* Carefully observe patients who cannot tolerate edema (eg, epilepsy, cardiac/renal dysfunction, migraine). *Hepatic dysfunction:* May occur; observe patient, monitor liver function tests periodically. *Long-term experience:* Limited. Similar drugs have been associated with serious toxicity (eg, cholestatic jaundice, peliosis hepatitis). Use lowest effective dose and consider decreasing dose or withdrawing therapy periodically.

NURSING CONSIDERATIONS

Administration/Storage

- Initiate therapy during menstruation or after negative pregnancy test result.
- Give medication with food or milk to minimize GI irritation.
- When treating endometriosis, dosage should be titrated down to lowest dose sufficient to maintain amenorrhea and therapeutic response.
- Store drug in closed, light-resistant container at room temperature.

Assessment/Interventions

- Obtain patient history, including drug history and any known allergies.
- Review pregnancy test results to be certain that pregnancy has been ruled out before starting drug therapy.
- CBC and serum electrolytes should be performed before drug therapy is initiated.
- Monitor patient closely for masculin-

izing effects and changes in sexuality pattern.

- Monitor patient for signs of liver dysfunction (eg, liver function test changes, jaundice, nausea, vomiting, dark amber urine).
- Monitor patient's mental status: affect, mood, behavioral changes, aggression, sleep disturbances, depression.
- Semen should be checked for volume, viscosity, sperm count and motility q 3-4 mo.
- Perform ongoing assessment of patient's fluid balance (I&O, daily weight). Note edema or weight gain > 2 lb/wk. Report findings to physician.
- Observe for signs of hypercalcemia: GI symptoms, polydipsia, polyurea, increased calcium levels, decreased muscle tone.

Patient/Family Education

- Caution patient that this medication must not be taken during pregnancy or when pregnancy is possible. Advise patient to use reliable form of birth control while taking this drug.
- Remind patient to take medication with food or milk to minimize GI upset.
- Instruct patient to notify physician if masculinizing effects occur (eg, abnormal facial hair or other fine body hair growth, deepening of voice, acne, clitoral enlargement, testicular atrophy, decrease in breast size). Inform patient that most of these side effects will cease after drug is discontinued; however, some changes may be irreversible (eg, permanent voice changes have occurred due to structural changes in larynx).
- Inform patient to notify physician if change in libido should occur because this may indicate toxicity.
- Instruct patient to eat low-sodium diet to prevent fluid retention and to notify physician of any signs of edema.
- Advise women being treated for fibrocystic breast disease to notify physician of any nodule that persists or enlarges during treatment. Review proper technique for breast self-examination.
- Caution patient not to discontinue drug abruptly.
- Advise patient to notify physician of irregular menses. Explain that amenorrhea usually occurs but that menstruation usually resumes 2-3 mo after termination of therapy.
- Explain that drug-induced anovulation is reversible within 2-3 mo of discontinuation of therapy.

See Patient Guide, p. 172.

Dantrolene Sodium

(dan-troe-LEEN SO-dee-uhm)

Dantrium; Dantrium Intravenous

Class: Skeletal muscle relaxant/direct acting

Action Affects contraction of muscle at site beyond myoneural junction and directly on muscle itself; believed to interfere with calcium release from sarcoplasmic reticulum. Affects CNS, causing drowsiness, dizziness and generalized weakness.

Indications Control of spasticity associated with spinal cord injury, stroke, cerebral palsy or multiple sclerosis; prophylaxis, treatment and postcrisis therapy of malignant hyperthermia. **Unlabeled uses:** Management of exercise-induced muscle pain, neuroleptic malignant syndrome, heat stroke.

Contraindications Active hepatic disease; muscle spasm resulting from rheumatic disorders; where spasticity is used to sustain upright posture and balance in locomotion or to obtain or maintain increased function.

Route/Dosage

Chronic Spasticity

ADULT: **PO** Initial dose: 25 mg q day; increase at 4-7 day intervals to 25 mg bid-qid, up to max of 100 mg bid-qid if necessary. CHILDREN: **PO** Initial dose: 0.5 mg/kg bid; increase to 0.5 mg/kg tid-qid, then by increments of 0.5 mg/kg, up to 3 mg/kg bid-qid, if necessary. Maximum 100 mg qid.

Malignant Hyperthermia

ADULTS & CHILDREN: PREOPERATIVE PROPHYLAXIS: **PO** 4-8 mg/kg/day in 3 or 4 divided doses for 1 or 2 days prior to surgery with last dose given 3-4 hours before surgery or **IV** 2.5 mg/kg approximately 1¼ hours before anesthesia. Infused over 1 hour. May repeat during surgery, if needed. Treatment: **IV** 1 mg/kg by continuous rapid push; evaluate and repeat as needed until cumulative total dose is ≤ 10 mg/kg. POST-CRISIS FOLLOW-UP: **PO** 4-8 mg/kg/day in 4 divided doses for 1-3 days to prevent recurrence. If IV route must be utilized, start with ≥ 1 mg/kg, as needed.

Interactions

Estrogens: Women receiving these may be at increased risk for hepatotoxicity. *Verapamil:* Hyperkalemia and myocardial depression possible.

Lab Test Interferences

None well documented.

Adverse Reactions

Due to oral administration except where otherwise indicated. *CV:* Tachycardia; erratic blood pressure; phlebitis. *RESP:* Pleural effusion with pericarditis; pulmonary edema (IV). *CNS:* Drowsiness; dizziness; weakness; general malaise; fatigue; speech disturbances; seizures; headache; lightheadedness; insomnia, mental depression or confusion; increased nervousness. *EENT:* Visual disturbance, diplopia, alteration of taste. *GI:* Diarrhea; constipation; bleeding; anorexia; dysphagia; gastric irritation; abdominal cramps. *GU:* Increased urinary frequency; hematuria; crystalluria; difficult erection; urinary incontinence; nocturia; dysuria; urinary retention. *HEPA:* Hepatitis. *DERM:* Abnormal hair growth; acne-like rash; pruritus; urticaria (IV); exzematoid eruption; sweating; erythema (IV). *OTHER:* Myalgia; backache; chills; fever; feeling of suffocation; excessive tearing; thrombophlebitis (IV).

Precautions

Pregnancy: Category C (parenteral). *Lactation:* Undetermined. *Children:* Safety in children < 5 yr not established. *Special risk patients:* Use drug with caution in patients with impaired pulmonary function (especially COPD) or cardiac function. *Hepatic effects:* Fatal and nonfatal liver disorders may occur; use drug with caution in patients with pre-existing hepatic impairment and in females and patients > 35 yr. *Long-term use:* Safety and efficacy not established; use only if significant pain or disability is present or nursing care is reduced. Consider carcinogenicity risk and liver damage with long-term use. Discontinue therapy if no benefit within 45 days. *Malignant hyperthermia:* Supportive care should be foremost in treatment (ie, concurrent with dantrolene therapy).

NURSING CONSIDERATIONS

Administration/Storage

- Ensure good IV site using large peripheral vein; medication is very irritating to tissues.
- Reconstitute powder for IV infusion in 60 ml of sterile water *without* bacteriostatic agent.
- Shake until solution is clear.
- Store at room temperature for up to 6 hr. Protect from direct light.

Assessment/Interventions

- Obtain patient history, including drug history and any known allergies.
- Assess neuromuscular status before and during therapy.
- Assess family's anesthesia history.

Ask specifically about crises or deaths in operating room.

- Assess for constipation, and auscultate bowel sounds regularly.
- Encourage patient to increase fluid and fiber intake during therapy.
- Keep emergency equipment nearby to treat respiratory depression.
- Measure and document intake and output.
- Monitor infusion site regularly for potential complications.
- If weakness or dizziness develops, keep side rails up and supervise ambulation.
- If difficulty swallowing develops, implement safety precautions with meals and medications.

Patient/Family Education

- Teach patient and family the name, action, administration and side effects of dantrolene.
- Emphasize importance of follow-up exams and laboratory work to monitor drug therapy.
- Instruct patient to report these symptoms to physician: weakness, malaise, fatigue, nausea, diarrhea, skin rash, itching, bloody or black tarry stools or yellowish discoloration of skin.
- Instruct patient to avoid intake of alcoholic beverages or other CNS depressants.
- Advise patient that drug may cause drowsiness and to use caution while driving or performing other tasks requiring mental alertness.
- Caution patient to avoid exposure to sunlight and to use sunscreen or wear protective clothing to avoid photosensitivity reaction.

See Patient Guide, pp. 173-174.

Daunorubicin HCl

(DAW-no-RUE-bih-sin HIGH-droe-KLOR-ide)

Cerubudine

Class: Antineoplastic/antibiotic/anthracycline

Action Inhibits nucleic acid synthesis.

Indications In combination with other approved anticancer drugs, induction of remission in adult acute nonlymphocytic leukemia (myelogenous, monocytic, erythroid); induction of remission in acute lymphocytic leukemia of children and adults.

Contraindications Standard considerations.

Route/Dosage

Acute Nonlymphocytic Leukemia

ADULTS < 60 YR: **IV** 45 mg/m^2 on days 1, 2 and 3 of first course and days 1 and 2 of subsequent courses in combination with other approved anticancer drugs. May require up to 3 induction courses. ADULTS > 60 YR: **IV** 30 mg/m^2 on days 1, 2 and 3 of first course and days 1 and 2 of subsequent courses. May require up to 3 induction courses.

Acute Lymphocytic Leukemia

ADULTS: **IV** 45 mg/m^2 on days 1, 2 and 3. CHILDREN ≥ 2 YR: **IV** 25 mg/m^2 on day 1 q wk. May require 4-6 courses of treatment. CHILDREN < 2 YR: **IV** Dosage is based on weight instead of BSA.

Interactions None well documented. INCOMPATIBILITIES: Do not mix with other drugs or heparin unless specific data are available.

Lab Test Interferences None well documented.

Adverse Reactions *CV:* CHF. *CNS:* Fever; chills. *EENT:* Mucositis. *GI:* Nausea; vomiting; diarrhea. *GU:* Red urine discoloration may occur transiently. *HEMA:* Myelosuppression. *DERM:* Reversible alopecia; tissue necrosis. *META:* Hyperuricemia.

Precautions

Pregnancy: Category D. *Lacta-*

tion: Undetermined. *Bone marrow suppression:* Severe myelosuppression occurs in all patients; avoid use in patients with preexisting drug-induced bone marrow suppression. *Cardiac toxicity:* Potentially fatal cardiac toxicity may occur, particularly with high cumulative dosage, previous doxorubicin therapy or preexisting cardiac disease. *Hepatic or renal function impairment:* Dosage adjustment is needed. *IV infusion:* Give daunorubicin into rapidly flowing IV infusion. *Never* give via IM or SC route. If extravasation occurs, severe local tissue necrosis will result.

NURSING CONSIDERATIONS

Administration/Storage

- Use IV route only. *Never* administer via IM or SC route.
- Do not mix with heparin or other drugs.
- Reconstitute with 4 ml of Sterile Water for Injection to obtain solution of 5 mg/ml.
- Dilute desired dose in syringe of 10-15 ml of normal saline.
- Inject into tubing or Y-site of rapidly flowing infusion of D5W or normal saline.
- Protect solution from sunlight.
- Reconstituted solution will remain stable 24 hr at room temperature and 48 hr if refrigerated.

Assessment/Interventions

- Obtain patient history, including drug history and any known allergies.
- Monitor cardiac and respiratory status: BP, pulse, ECG, respiration.
- Monitor CBC, differential and platelet count throughout therapy.
- Monitor renal function studies: BUN, serum uric acid, electrolytes, urine uric acid levels.
- Monitor liver function studies during therapy: AST, ALT, bilirubin, serum phosphatase.
- Monitor I&O, appetite and nutritional intake. Encourage fluid intake to 2-3 L/day.
- Observe for signs of infection. Take patient's temperature q 4 hr and check for sore throat.
- Assess IV insertion site frequently. If pain or irritation occurs at site, discontinue infusion and restart in another vein to avoid damage to subcutaneous tissue. Notify physician immediately. Apply ice to site.
- Observe for bleeding: hematuria, guaiac stools and emesis, bruising, petechiae, bleeding gums.
- Assess patient for signs of CHF: peripheral edema, dyspnea, rales/crackles, weight gain, jugular vein distention.
- If stomatitis occurs, have patient rinse mouth tid-qid with water; brush teeth with soft brush, sponge brush or cotton-tipped applicator and use unwaxed dental floss.
- Assess patient for jaundice, dark urine, clay-colored stools, pruritus, abdominal pain, fever, diarrhea.

Patient/Family Education

- Explain that drug is likely to cause hair loss but that recovery will begin within 2-3 mo after drug is discontinued.
- Warn patient that urine and body fluids may be red-orange for 1-2 days after administration of drug but this effect is temporary.
- Instruct patient to drink up to 2-3 L/day of fluids, unless contraindicated.
- Instruct patient to inspect oral mucosa regularly and to report any bleeding, white spots or ulcerations in mouth.
- Instruct patient to avoid crowds and people with infections during myelosuppression and to report any signs of infection (fever, chills, sore throat) to physician.
- Advise patient to avoid foods with citric acid or hot or rough texture if mucositis is present.

- Instruct patient to report these symptoms to physician: irregular heart rhythm, shortness of breath or fluid retention in lower extremities.

No patient monograph available.

Desipramine HCl

(dess-IPP-ruh-meen HIGH-droe-KLOR-ide)

Norpramin, Pertofrane

Class: Tricyclic antidepressant

Action Inhibits reuptake of norepinephrine and serotonin in CNS.

Indications Relief of symptoms of depression. **Unlabeled uses:** Facilitation of cocaine withdrawal; treatment of panic and eating disorders (eg, bulimia nervosa).

Contraindications Hypersensitivity to any tricyclic antidepressant. Not to be given in combination with or within 14 days of treatment with an MAO (monoamine oxidase) inhibitor. Do not give during acute recovery phases of MI.

Route/Dosage

ADULTS: **PO** 100-300 mg/day. May be given in divided doses or once daily at bedtime. ELDERLY AND ADOLESCENT PATIENTS: **PO** 25-150 mg/day.

Interactions

Barbiturates, carbamazepine, charcoal: May decrease desipramine effects. *Cimetidine, fluoxetine, haloperidol, quinidine, oral contraceptives, phenothiazine antipsychotics:* May increase desipramine effects. *Clonidine:* May result in hypertensive crisis. *CNS depressants:* CNS and respiratory effects may be increased. *MAO inhibitors:* Hyperpyretic crises, severe convulsions and death may occur if administered together or within 14 days of each other.

Lab Test Interferences

None well documented.

Adverse Reactions

CV: Orthostatic hypotension; hypertension; tachycardia; palpitations; arrythmias; ECG changes; hypertensive episodes during surgery; stroke; heart-block; CHF. *RESP:* Pharyngitis, rhinitis; sinusitis; bronchospasm; cough. *CNS:* Confusion; disturbed concentration; hallucinations; delusions; nervousness; numbness; tremors; extrapyramidal symptoms (pseudoparkinsonism; movement disorders; akathisia); restlessness; agitation; panic; insomnia; nightmares; mania; exacerbation of psychosis; drowsiness; dizziness; weakness; fatigue; emotional lability; seizures. *EENT:* Conjunctivitis; blurred vision; increased intraocular pressure; mydriasis; tinnitus; nasal congestion; peculiar taste in mouth. *GI:* Nausea; vomiting; anorexia; GI distress; diarrhea; flatulence; dry mouth; constipation. *GU:* Impotence; sexual dysfunction; nocturia; urinary frequency; urinary tract infection; vaginitis; cystitis; urinary retention or hesitancy. *HEPA:* Hepatitis; jaundice. *HEMA:* Bone marrow depression including agranulocytosis; eosinophilia; purpura; thrombocytopenia; leukopenia. *DERM:* Rash; pruritus; photosensitivity reaction; dry skin; acne; itching; sweating. *META:* Elevation or depression of blood sugar levels. *OTHER:* Breast enlargement.

Precautions

Pregnancy: Pregnancy category undetermined. *Lactation:* Excreted in breast milk. *Children:* Not recommended in children < 12 yr. *Special risk patients:* Use drug with caution in patients with history of seizures, urinary retention, urethral or ureteral spasm, angle-closure glaucoma, increased intraocular pressure, or cardiovascular disorders; in patients receiving thyroid medication and in patients who have hepatic or renal impairment, schizophrenia or paranoia.

NURSING CONSIDERATIONS

Administration/Storage

- Administer in equal doses or one dose at bedtime.

Assessment/Interventions

- Obtain patient history, including drug history and any known allergies.
- Document serum bilirubin, alkaline phosphatase and blood glucose levels throughout therapy.
- Assess and document baseline behaviors and psychological status.
- Notify physician and discontinue medication immediately if patient has increased agitation and/or paranoid delusions.
- Document body weight monthly.
- Notify physician and withhold medication if there is a blood pressure drop of 20 mmHg or if heart arrhythmia or increase in heart rate develops.
- Inform physician if patient has urinary elimination problems.

OVERDOSAGE: SIGNS & SYMPTOMS

Confusion, agitation, hallucinations, seizures, status epilepticus, clonus, choreoathetosis, hyperactive reflexes, positive Babinski's signs, coma, cardiac arrhythmias, renal failure, flushing, dry mouth, dilated pupils, hyperpyrexia

Patient/Family Education

- Instruct patient to keep weekly record of weight.
- Teach patient how to take BP and heart rate.
- Explain missed medication procedure: less than 2 hrs, take medication; more than 2 hrs, wait until next scheduled dose. Do not double doses.
- Teach proper techniques for oral hygiene to help prevent/treat dry mucous membranes.
- Tell patient to increse fluid intake.
- Inform male patient of possible sexual dysfunction.
- Tell patient of possible difficult urination.
- Instruct patient to avoid intake of alcoholic beverages or other CNS depressants.
- Advise patient that drug may cause drowsiness and to use caution while driving or performing other tasks requiring mental alertness.

See Patient Guide, p. 175.

Desmopressin Acetate (1-Deamino-8-D-Arginine Vasopressin)

(DESS-moe-PRESS-in ASS-uh-TATE)

DDAVP, Stimate

Class: Posterior pituitary hormone

Action Has antidiuretic effect that decreases urinary volume and increases urine osmolality.

Indications Control of primary nocturnal enuresis; control of central cranial diabetes insipidus; maintenance of hemostasis in patients with hemophilia A and type I von Willebrand's disease during surgery and postoperatively. **Unlabeled use:** Treatment of chronic autonomic failure.

Contraindications Standard considerations.

Route/Dosage

Primary Nocturnal Enuresis

ADULTS & CHILDREN ≥ 6 YR: **Intranasal** 20 mcg (0.2 ml) at bedtime.

Central Cranial Diabetes Insipidus

ADULTS: **Intranasal** 0.1-0.4 qd. **IV/SC** 0.5-1 ml qd in 2 divided doses. **PO** 0.05 mg bid adjusted for adequate diurnal rhythm (range 0.1-1.2 mg/day divided). CHILDREN > 12 YR: **IV/SC** 0.5-1 ml qd in 2 divided doses. CHILDREN 3 MO-12 YR: **Intranasal** 0.05-0.3 ml qd. CHILDREN: **PO** 0.05 mg/day.

Hemophilia A, Type I von Willebrand's Disease

ADULTS & CHILDREN > 12 YR: **IV** 0.3 mcg/kg over 15-30 min. *Intranasal:* 1 spray/nostril for a total of 300 mcg. PATIENTS <50 KG: 150 mcg (single spray).

Interactions

Carbamazepine; chlorpropamide: May potentiate antidiuretic effects of desmopressin.

Lab Test Interferences

None well documented.

Adverse Reactions

CV: *Intranasal*—Slight elevation in blood pressure; facial flushing. *Stimate*—Chest pain; palpitations; tachycardia; edema. CNS: *Intranasal*—Headache. *Stimate*—Somnolence; dizziness; insomnia; agitation. EENT: *Intranasal*—Rhinitis; nosebleed; sore throat. *Stimate*—Itchy or light-sensitive eyes. GI: *Intranasal*—Nausea; mild abdominal cramps. *Stimate*—Dyspepsia; vomiting. RESP: *Intranasal*—Cough; upper respiratory infection. GU: *Intranasal*—Vulval pain. *Stimate*—Balanitis. HEPA: *Injection*—Elevated liver function test. DERM: *Injection*—Local erythema; swelling; pain. OTHER: *Stimate*—Chills; warm feeling; pain.

Precautions

Pregnancy: Category B. *Lactation:* Undetermined. *Children:* Infants and children require careful fluid intake restriction to prevent possible hyponatremia and water intoxication. Safety and efficacy of intranasal form have not been established in children < 3 mo. Safety and efficacy of parenteral form for control of diabetes insipidus have not been established for children < 12 yr. *Elderly patients:* Elderly patients should ingest only enough fluid to satisfy thirst; water intoxication and hyponatrenemia are possible. *Special risk patients:* Use drug with caution in patients with coronary artery insufficiency or hypertensive cardiovascular disease. Use with caution in patients with conditions associated with fluid and electrolyte imbalance (eg, cystic fibrosis). These patients are prone to hyponatremia. Use with caution in patients predisposed to thrombus formation. Rare thrombotic events have occurred in these patients. *Decrease in plasma osmolality:* An extreme decrease in plasma osmolality occurs rarely and may result in seizures and coma. *Hypersensitivity:* Rare severe allergic reactions have been reported. Anaphylaxis has occurred with IV administration.

NURSING CONSIDERATIONS

Administration/Storage

- For intranasal administration, ensure that nasal passages are intact, clean and free of obstruction before administration of drug. Calibrated plastic tube is provided in nasal tube delivery system. Draw solution up into this tube and insert into nostril. Place opposite end of tube in mouth and blow into tube to deliver medication.
- Cranial surgery, changes in nasal mucosa and nasal packing can compromise intranasal delivery. In this situation parenteral therapy should be considered.
- Refrigerate both nasal and injectable solutions.

Assessment/Interventions

- Obtain patient history, including drug history and any known allergies.
- Obtain baseline and ongoing measurements of both urine and plasma osmolality when treating patient with diabetes insipidus.
- Check coagulation status prior to treating patients with hemophilia A and type I von Willebrand's disease.

Coagulation testing may include factor VIII coagulant activity, factor VIII antigen, ristocetin cofactor, activated PTT and skin bleeding time.
- Monitor I&O closely and accurately when drug is administered to very young and elderly. Fluid restriction in infants, children and elderly is required to prevent possible hyponatremia and water intoxication.
- Continually assess patient for signs of fluid intoxication including lungs, extremities (edema), weight or jugular venous distention.

OVERDOSAGE: SIGNS & SYMPTOMS
Headache, abdominal cramps, nausea, facial flushing

Patient/Family Education
- Instruct patient on proper intranasal administration techniques and have patient or family demonstrate ability to perform.
- Remind patient receiving drug intranasally to frequently inspect nasal passages.
- Explain that it is important to reduce fluid intake when therapy is initiated to decrease chance of water intoxication.
- Instruct patient to report these symptoms to physician: headache, shortness of breath, heartburn, nausea, abdominal cramps or vulvar pain.

See Patient Guide, pp. 176-177.

Dexamethasone

(DEX-uh-METH-uh-sone)

Aeroseb-Dex, Decadron, Decaspray, Dexameth, Dexone, Hexadrol

Dexamethasone Acetate

Dalalone DP, Dalalone LA, Decadron-LA, Decaject-L.A., Dexacen LA-8, Dexasone-L.A., Dexone LA, Solurex LA

Dexamethasone Sodium Phosphate

AK-Dex, Dalalone, Decadron Phosphate, Decadron Phosphate Respihaler, Decadron Phosphate Turbinaire, Decaject, Dexacen-4, Dexasone, Dexone, Hexadrol Phosphate, Maxidex, Solurex, ♣ *Diodex, PMS-Dexamethasone, R.O. Dexsone*

Action Synthetic long-acting glucocorticoid that depresses formation, release and activity of endogenous mediators of inflammation including prostaglandins, kinins, histamine, liposomal enzymes and complement system. Also modifies body's immune response.

Indications Testing of adrenal cortical hyperfunction; management of primary or secondary adrenal cortex insufficiency, rheumatic disorders, collagen diseases, dermatologic diseases, allergic states, allergic and inflammatory ophthalmic processes, respiratory diseases, hematologic disorders, neoplastic diseases, cerebral edema associated with primary or metastatic brain tumor, craniotomy or head injury, edematous states (caused by nephrotic syndrome), GI diseases, multiple sclerosis, tuberculous meningitis, trichinosis with neurologic or myocardial involvement. *Intra-articular or soft tissue administration:* Short-term adjunctive treatment for such conditions as synovitis of osteoarthritis, rheumatoid arthritis, acute gouty arthritis, posttraumatic osteoarthritis. *Intralesional administration:* Treatment for such conditions as keloids, psoriatic plaques, discoid lupus erythematosus, alopecia areata. *Topical:* Treatment of inflammatory and pruritic manifestations of corticosteriod-responsive dermatoses. *Oral inhalation:* Treatment of corticosteroid-responsive and bronchial asthma bronchospastic states. *Intranasal:* Treatment of allergic or inflammatory nasal conditions, nasal polyps (excluding those originating within sinuses). *Ophthalmic:* Treatment of steroid-responsive inflammatory conditions of palpebral and bulbar conjunctiva, lid, cornea and anterior segment of globe. **Unlabeled uses:** Treatment of acute mountain sickness, bacterial meningitis, bronchopulmonary dysplasia in preterm infants; diagnosis of depression; treatment of hirsutism and use as antiemetic.

Contraindications Systemic fungal infections; IM use in idiopathic thrombocytopenic purpura; administration of live virus vaccines; topical monotherapy in primary bacterial infections; intranasal use in untreated localized infections involving nasal mucosa; ophthalmic use in acute superficial herpes simplex keratitis, fungal diseases of ocular structures, vaccinia, varicella and ocular tuberculosis.

Route/Dosage
All dosages shown are for adults unless indicated otherwise.

Dexamethasone
Initial dose: **PO** 0.75-9 mg/day. SUPPRESSION TESTS: Cushing's syndrome: **PO** 1 mg at 11 PM. Alternate: **PO** 0.5 mg q 6 hr for 48 hr. To distinguish Cushing's syndrome–caused pituitary ACTH excess from other causes: **PO** 2 mg q 6 hr for 48 hr. ACUTE MOUNTAIN SICKNESS: **PO** 4 mg q 6 hr. ANTI-EMETIC: **PO** 16-20 mg. DIAGNOSIS OF DEPRESSION: **PO** 1 mg. HIRSUTISM: **PO** 0.5-1 mg/day.

Dexamethasone Acetate
SYSTEMIC: **IM** 8-16 mg; may repeat in 1-3 wk. INTRALESIONAL: **IM** 0.8-1.6 mg. INTRA-ARTICULAR AND SOFT TISSUE: **IM** 4-16 mg; may repeat at 1-3 wk intervals.

Dexamethasone Sodium Phosphate
SYSTEMIC: **IV/IM** 0.5-9 mg/day. CEREBRAL EDEMA: **IV** 10 mg, then **IM** 4 mg q 6 hr until maximum response. BRAIN TUMORS: **IV/IM** 2 mg bid-tid. UNRESPONSIVE SHOCK: **IV** 1-6 mg/kg as single injection; or 40 mg followed by repeated IV injections q 2-6 hr. BACTERIAL MENINGITIS: **IV** 0.15 mg/kg q 6 hr. BRONCHOPULMONARY DYSPLASIA: *PRETERM INFANTS:* **IV** 0.5 mg/kg. INTRA-ARTICULAR, INTRALESIONAL OR SOFT TISSUE: LARGE JOINTS: 2-4 mg. SMALL JOINTS: 0.8-1 mg. BURSAE: 2-3 mg. TENDON SHEATHS: 0.4-1 mg. SOFT TISSUE INFILTRATION: 2-6 mg. GANGLIA: 1-2 mg. TOPICAL: Apply sparingly to affected areas bid-qid. ORAL INHALATION: ADULTS: 3 inhalations tid-qid. CHILDREN: 2 inhalations tid-qid. INTRANASAL: ADULTS: 2 sprays (168 mcg) into each nostril bid-tid. CHILDREN 6-12 YR: 1 or 2 sprays (84-168 mcg) into each nostril bid. OPHTHALMIC: SOLUTION: Instill 1-2 drops into conjunctival sac q 1 hr during day and q 2 hr during night. OINTMENT: Apply thin coating in lower conjunctival sac tid-qid.

Interactions
Aminoglutethimide: May decrease dexamethasone-induced adrenal suppression. *Anticholinesterases:* May antagonize anticholinesterase effects in myasthenia gravis. *Anticoagulants, oral:* May alter anticoagulant dose requirements. *Barbiturates:* May decrease effects of dexamethasone. *Hydantoins:* May increase clearance and decrease therapeutic efficacy of dexamethasone. *Rifampin:* May increase clearance and decrease therapeutic efficacy of dexamethasone. *Salicylates:* May reduce serum levels and efficacy of salicylates. *Troleandomycin:* May increase dexamethasone effects.

Lab Test Interferences
May cause increased urine glucose and serum cholesterol; decreased serum levels of potassium, T_3 and T_4; decreased uptake of thyroid ^{131}I; false-negative nitroblue-tetrazolium test; altered brain scan results; suppression of skin test reactions.

Adverse Reactions
CV: Thromboembolism or fat embolism; thrombophlebitis; necrotizing angiitis; cardiac arrhythmias or ECG changes; syncopal episodes; hypertension; myocardial rupture; CHF. *RESP:* Oral inhalation: Wheezing. *CNS:* Convulsions; increased intracranial pressure with papilledema (pseudotumor cerebri); vertigo; headache; neuritis; paresthesias; psychosis.

EENT: Posterior subcapsular cataracts; increased IOP; glaucoma; exophthalmos. Oral inhalation: Dry mouth; throat irritation; hoarseness; dysphonia; coughing. Intranasal: Nasal irritation; burning; stinging; dryness; epistaxis or bloody mucus; rebound congestion; sneezing, rhinorrhea; anosmia; loss of sense of taste; throat discomfort. Ophthalmic: Glaucoma with optic nerve damage; visual acuity and field defects; posterior subcapsular cataract formation; secondary ocular infections; transient stinging or burning. *GI:* Pancreatitis; abdominal distension; ulcerative esophagitis; nausea; vomiting; increased appetite and weight gain; peptic ulcer with perforation and hemorrhage; bowel perforation. *GU:* Increased or decreased number and motility of spermatozoa. *HEMA:* Leukocytosis. *DERM:* Impaired wound healing; thin fragile skin; petechiae and ecchymoses; erythema; lupus erythematosus–like lesions; subcutaneous fat atrophy; striae; hirsutism; acneiform eruptions; allergic dermatitis; urticaria; angioneurotic edema, perineal irritation; hyperpigmentation or hypopigmentation. Topical application: Burning; itching; irritation; erythema; dryness; folliculitis; hypertrichosis; pruritus; perioral dermatitis; allergic contact dermatitis; stinging, cracking and tightening of skin; secondary infections; skin atrophy; striae; miliaria; telangiectasia. *META:* Sodium and fluid retention; hypokalemia; hypokalemic alkalosis; metabolic alkalosis; hypocalcemia. *OTHER:* Musculoskeletal effects (eg, weakness, myopathy, muscle mass loss, osteoporosis, spontaneous fractures); endocrine abnormalities (eg, menstrual irregularities, cushingoid state, growth suppression in children sweating, decreased carbohydrate tolerance, hyperglycemia, glycosuria, increased insulin or sulfonylurea requirements in diabetics, anaphylactoid or hypersensitivity reactions); aggravation or masking of infections; malaise; leukocytosis; fatigue; insomnia. Intra-articular: Osteonecrosis; tendon rupture; infection; skin atrophy; postinjection flare; hypersensitivity; facial flushing. Topical use may theoretically produce adverse reactions seen with systemic use because of absorption.

Precautions

Pregnancy: Pregnancy category undetermined (systemic use); Category C (topical uses). *Lactation:* Excreted in breast milk. *Children:* May be more susceptible to adverse reactions from topical use than are adults. Observe growth and development of infants and children on prolonged therapy. *Elderly:* May require lower doses. *Adrenal suppression:* Prolonged therapy may lead to hypothalmic-pituitary-adrenal suppression. *Fluid and electrolyte balance:* Can cause elevated blood pressure, salt and water retention and increased potassium and calcium excretion. Dietary salt restriction and potassium supplementation may be needed. *Hepatitis:* May be harmful in chronic active hepatitis positive for hepatitis B surface antigen. *Infections:* May mask signs of infection. May decrease host-defense mechanisms to prevent dissemination of infection. *Ocular effects:* Use systemically with caution in ocular herpes simplex because of possible corneal perforation. *Ophthalmic use:* Prolonged use may result in glaucoma or other complications. *Peptic ulcer:* May contribute to peptic ulceration, especially in large doses. *Renal impairment:* Use cautiously; monitor renal function. *Stress:* Increased dosage of rapidly acting corticosteroid may be needed before, during and after stressful situations. *Sulfites:* Some products may contain sodium bisulfite, which may cause allergic-type reactions in some individuals. *Withdrawal:* Abrupt discontinuation may result in adrenal insufficiency. Discontinue gradually.

NURSING CONSIDERATIONS

Administration/Storage

- For IM injection, inject dexamethasone acetate deep into gluteal muscle. Avoid injection into deltoid, and rotate injection sites. Do not use SC route.
- Refer to package insert for directions on how to store particular form of dexamethasone.
- If ordered PO, administer in morning to coincide with body's normal secretion of cortisol.

Assessment/Interventions

- Obtain patient history, including drug history and any known allergies.
- Obtain baseline weight and vital signs.
- Assess involved system before and periodically during therapy.
- When used in child, periodically assess child's growth.
- Monitor intake and output.
- Assess patient regularly for signs of infection (delayed wound healing, WBC count) because steroids can mask other common signs of infection such as fever, swelling and redness.
- Notify physician if signs of fluid overload develop (peripheral edema, weight gain, rales/crackles, dyspnea).
- If emotional changes occur, such as depression, take safety measures such as suicide precautions.
- If side effects develop with long-term therapy, expect to change to alternate-day therapy. Check medication record and document well.

OVERDOSAGE: SIGNS & SYMPTOMS

Acute overdose: Fever, myalgia, arthralgia, malaise, anorexia, nausea, skin desquamation, orthostatic hypotension, dizziness, fainting, dyspnea, hypoglycemia.
Chronic: Cushingoid changes: Moonface, central obesity, striae, hirsuitism, acne, ecchymoses, hypertension, osteoporosis, myopathy, sexual dysfunction, diabetes, hyperlipidemia, peptic ulcer, infection, electrolyte and fluid imbalance

Patient/Family Education

- Caution patient that stopping drug abruptly is dangerous and may cause adrenal insufficiency.
- Explain rationale for tapering off medication when that time comes.
- Teach patient or family procedures for correctly administering specific form of drug (ophthalmic, inhalation, topical, etc.).
- Caution patient against receiving immunizations while drug is being taken.
- Advise patient on long-term therapy to carry medication identification card or to wear bracelet. In case of emergency, this information is important for treatment.
- Instruct patient to avoid people with infections, particularly respiratory.
- If form patient is receiving is intranasal, instruct him/her to clear nasal passages of secretions before administering drug.
- If topical, advise patient not to use occlusive dressings such as plastic wrap more than 12 hours a day. Occlusion may lead to sweat retention and bacterial and fungal infections. Remember that tight-fitting plastic diapers on infants may also be occlusive.
- Teach patient to take oral forms with meals or snacks if GI irritation occurs.
- Review guidelines for missed doses of particular product with patient.

- Teach patient on long-term therapy how to keep a weight record.
- Instruct patient to inform other physicians that he/she is taking a steroid.
- Review signs of infection and remind patient that fever, swelling and redness may be masked in infection.
- Review possible side effects of dexamethasone with patient and instruct him/her to report these to physician.

See Patient Guide, pp. 178-179.

Dextroamphetamine Sulfate

(DEX-troe-am-FET-uh-meen SULL-fate)

Dexedrine, Ferndex, Oxydess II, Spancap No. 1

Class: CNS stimulant/amphetamine

Action Activates noradrenergic neurons causing CNS and respiratory stimulation; stimulates satiety center in brain causing appetite suppression.

Indications Treatment of narcolepsy, attention deficit disorder with hyperactivity; adjunct therapy for short-term (ie, few weeks) exogenous obesity when alternative therapy has been ineffective.

Contraindications Advanced arteriosclerosis; symptomatic cardiovascular disease; moderate to severe hypertension; hyperthyroidism; hypersensitivity to or idiosyncratic reactions to sympathomimetic amines; glaucoma; agitated states; history of drug abuse; concurrent use or within 14 days of monoamine oxidase (MAO) inhibitor use.

Route/Dosage

Narcolepsy

ADULTS (> 12 YR): **PO** 10 mg/day; may increase weekly by 10 mg to maximum of 60 mg/day in divided doses. CHILDREN (6-12 YR): **PO** 5 mg/day; may increase weekly by 5 mg to maximum of 60 mg/day in divided doses.

Attention Deficit Disorder

CHILDREN ≥ 6 YR: **PO** 5 mg/day; may increase weekly by 5 mg to maximum of 40 mg/day in divided doses. Usual range is 0.1-0.5 mg/kg/dose q morning. CHILDREN 3-5 YR: **PO** 2.5 mg/day; may increase weekly by 2.5 mg. Usual range is 0.1-0.5 mg/kg/dose q morning.

Exogenous Obesity

ADULTS ≥ 12 YR: **PO** 5-10 mg 30-60 min before meals, up to 30 mg/day. Long-acting form: 10-15 mg q morning.

Interactions *Guanethidine:* Amphetamines may decrease effectiveness. MAO *inhibitors, furazolidone:* Hypertensive crisis and intracranial hemorrhage may occur. *Tricyclic antidepressants:* May decrease amphetamine effect. *Urinary acidifiers (ammonium chloride, ascorbic acid):* May decrease amphetamine levels. *Urinary alkalinizers (acetazolamide, sodium bicarbonate):* May increase amphetamine levels.

Lab Test Interferences Plasma and urinary steroid levels may be altered.

Adverse Reactions *CV:* Palpitations; tachycardia; hypertension; arrhythmias. *CNS:* Nervousness; tremors; dizziness; insomnia, euphoria; headache. *EENT:* Dry mouth; unpleasant taste. *GI:* Diarrhea; constipation; anorexia. *GU:* Impotence. *DERM:* Urticaria.

Precautions *Pregnancy:* Category C. *Lactation:* Excreted in breast milk. *Children:* Do not use as anorectic agent in children < 12 yr. Not recommended for attention deficit disorder in children < 3 yr. *Drug dependence:* Amphetamines have been extensively abused. *Tartrazine sensitivity:* Some products contain tartrazine, which may cause allergic reactions in susceptible individuals.

Tolerance: May occur; do not exceed recommended dose to overcome this.

NURSING CONSIDERATIONS

Administration/Storage

- Limit patient's access to medication.
- Give medication 30-45 min before meals. Give sustained release tablets once daily in morning.
- Do not crush or open sustained-release tablets.

Assessment/Interventions

- Obtain patient history, including drug history and any known allergies.
- Assess baseline nutritional status.
- Document any abnormal behavior.
- Document monthly measurement of physical growth in children.
- Document weight weekly.
- Notify physician and withhold medication if blood pressure increases by 20 mm Hg or if heart arrhythmias or increase in heart rate develops.

OVERDOSAGE: SIGNS & SYMPTOMS

Restlessness, tremor, hyperreflexia, confusion, hallucinations, panic, fatigue, depression, convulsions, coma, arrhythmias, hypertension, hypotension, circulatory collapse, nausea, vomiting, diarrhea, abdominal cramps

Patient/Family Education

- Instruct patient to take medication early in morning and, if possible, to take last dose at bedtime.
- Tell patient to record body weight weekly.
- Instruct patient/family to measure height monthly if patient is child.
- Tell patient to limit intake of coffee, tea, cocoa, chocolate and caffeinated soft drinks.
- Explain importance of good oral hygiene to prevent or treat dry mouth and breath odor changes.
- Instruct patient to be aware of increased agitation, palpitations, and dizziness and to take precautions while performing tasks that require physical coordination or mental alertness.

See Patient Guide, p. 180.

Dextromethorphan Hydrobromide

(DEX-troe-meth-OR-fan HIGH-droe-BROE-mide)

Children's Hold, Delsym, Hold DM, Pertussin CS, Robitussin Cough Calmers, Robitussin Pediatric, Scot-Tussin DM Cough Chasers, St. Joseph Cough Suppressant, Sucrets Cough Control, Suppress, Trocal, ♣ *Koffex DM, Robidex*

Class: Antitussive/nonnarcotic

Action Suppresses cough by central action on cough center in medulla.

Indications Management of nonproductive cough.

Contraindications Standard considerations.

Route/Dosage

Liquid, Lozenges, and Syrup

ADULTS & CHILDREN > 12 YR: **PO** 10-30 mg q 4-8 hr (maximum 120 mg/24 hr). CHILDREN 6-12 YR: **PO** 5-10 mg q 4 hr *or* 15 mg q 6-8 hr (maximum 60 mg/24 hr). CHILDREN 2-6 YR: 2.5-7.5 mg of syrup q 4-8 hr (maximum 30 mg/24 hr). CHILDREN < 2 YR: Use as directed by physician.

Sustained Action Liquid
ADULTS: PO 60 mg q 12 hr. CHILDREN 6-12 YR: PO 30 mg q 12 hr. CHILDREN 2-5 YR: PO 15 mg q 12 hr.

Interactions
MAO *inhibitors:* Hypotension, hyperpyrexia, nausea, myoclonic jerks and coma may develop after co-administration.

Lab Test Interferences
None well documented.

Adverse Reactions Nausea, drowsiness or dizziness.

Precautions
Pregnancy: Undetermined. *Lactation:* Undetermined. *Chronic cough:* Do not use for persistent or chronic cough (eg, smoking, asthma, emphysema) or when cough is accompanied by excessive secretions. Persons with high fever, rash, persistent headache, nausea or vomiting should use only under medical supervision. *Drug abuse and dependence:* Anecdotal reports of abuse have increased. However, abuse and dependency potential is undetermined.

NURSING CONSIDERATIONS

Administration/Storage
- Store liquids, lozenges and syrups at room temperature and out of reach of children.

Assessment/Interventions
- Obtain patient history, including drug history and any known allergies. Note any respiratory problems and smoking history.
- Assess type of cough (dry or productive), severity and progression.
- Assess baseline vital signs including fever.
- Do not administer for persistent or chronic cough, > 7 days, or when cough is accompanied by excessive secretions.
- Monitor blood glucose levels in diabetic patients.

OVERDOSAGE: SIGNS & SYMPTOMS
Children: Ataxia, respiratory depression, convulsions
Adults: Altered sensory perception, dysphoria and slurred speech

Patient/Family Education
- Alert patient that many products contain alcohol.
- Instruct patient to notify physician before taking medication with other prescriptions (eg, MAO inhibitors).
- Inform diabetic patients that base may contain sucrose or other sugars.
- Encourage increased fluid intake to thin secretions.
- Teach patients how to cough and breathe deeply to maximize respiratory efforts.
- Explain to parents not to give lozenges to young children.

See Patient Guide, p. 181.

Diazepam

(DIE-aze-uh-pam)
Valium, Valrelease, Zetran, ♣ *Diazemuls, Vivol*
Class: Antianxiety/benzodiazepine/anticonvulsant

Action Potentiates action of GABA; inhibitory neurotransmitter, resulting in increased neural inhibition and CNS depression, especially in limbic system and reticular formation.

Indications Management of anxiety disorders; relief of acute alcohol withdrawal symptoms; relief of preoperative apprehension and anxiety and reduction of memory recall; treatment of muscle spasms, convulsive disorders and status epilepticus. **Unlabeled uses:** Treatment of irritable bowel syndrome; relief of panic attack.

Contraindications Hypersensitivity to benzodiazepines; psychoses; acute narrow-angle glaucoma; shock; coma; acute alcohol intoxication; use in children < 6 mo; lactation.

Route/Dosage
Individualize dosage; increase cautiously. ADULTS & CHILDREN: Usual recommended dose **IM/IV** 2-20 mg, depending on indication and severity. In acute conditions injection may be repeated within 1 hr, but q 3-4 hr is usually satisfactory. Dosage and route vary with indication and age. Usual daily dose: CHILDREN ≥ 6 MO: **PO** 1-2.5 mg tid or qid initially; increase gradually as needed and tolerated.

Anxiety
ADULTS: **PO** 2-10 mg bid-qid. **IM/IV** 2-10 mg; repeat in 3-4 hr if needed.

Acute Alcohol Withdrawal
ADULTS: **PO** 10 mg tid-qid first 24 hr; then 5 mg tid-qid prn. **IM/IV** 10 mg; then 5-10 mg in 3-4 hr if needed.

Skeletal Muscle Spasm
ADULTS: **PO** 2-10 mg tid-qid. **IM/IV** 5-10 mg; then 5-10 mg in 3-4 hr if needed. Larger doses may be necessary in tetanus.

Tetanus
CHILDREN ≥ 5 YR: **IM/IV** 5-10 mg; repeat q 3-4 hr prn. INFANTS & CHILDREN 1 MO-5 YR: **IM/IV** 1-2 mg slowly; repeat q 3-4 hr prn.

Anticonvulsant Adjunct
ADULTS: **PO** 2-10 mg bid-qid. ELDERLY OR DEBILITATED PATIENTS: Initial dose: **PO** 2-2.25 mg qd-bid; increase gradually.

Status Epilepticus and Severe Recurrent Convulsive Disorders
ADULTS: **IM/IV** (IV preferred) 5-10 mg initially; then 5-10 mg at 10-15 min intervals (maximum total dose 30 mg). If needed, repeat in 3-4 hr. CHILDREN ≥ 5 YR: **IM/IV** 1 mg q 2-5 min (maximum total dose 10 mg). If needed, repeat in 2-4 hr. INFANTS & CHILDREN 1 MO-5 YR: **IM/IV** 0.2-0.5 mg slowly q 2-5 min (maximum total dose 5 mg).

Sedation/Muscle Relaxation
ADULTS: **IM/IV** 2-10 mg/dose q 3-4 hr as needed. CHILDREN ≥ 6 MO: **PO** 0.12-0.8 mg/kg/day in divided doses. **IM/IV** 0.04-0.2 mg/kg/dose q 2-4 hr (maximum 0.6 mg/kg in 8 hr period.

Preoperative (Anxiety and Tension)
ADULTS: **IM** 10 mg before surgery.

Cardioversion (Anxiety and Tension)
ADULTS: **IM/IV** 5-15 mg 10-15 min before procedure.

Interactions
Cimetidine, oral contraceptives, disulfiram: May increase effects of diazepam, with excessive sedation and impaired psychomotor function. *Digoxin:* May increase serum digoxin concentrations. *Omeprazole:* May increase diazepam levels and enhance effects. *Theophyllines:* May antagonize sedative effects. INCOMPATIBILITIES: Diazepam interacts with plastic containers and IV tubing, significantly decreasing availability of drug delivered. Do not mix or dilute with other solutions or drugs in syringe or infusion container.

Lab Test Interferences
None well documented.

Adverse Reactions
CV: Cardiovascular collapse; bradycardia; tachycardia; hypertension; palpitations; edema; hypotension; phlebitis or thrombosis at IV sites. *CNS:* Drowsiness; confusion; ataxia; dizziness; lethargy; fatigue; apathy; memory impairment; disorientation; anterograde amnesia; restlessness; headache; slurred speech; loss of voice; stupor, coma; euphoria; irritability; vivid dreams; psychomotor retardation; paradoxical reactions (eg, anger, hostility, mania, insomnia, muscle spasms). *EENT:* Visual or auditory disturbances; depressed hearing. *GI:* Constipation; diarrhea; dry mouth; coated tongue; nausea; anorexia; vomiting. *HEMA:* Blood dyscrasias including agranulocytosis, anemia,

thrombocytopenia, leukopenia, neutropenia. *HEPA*: Hepatic dysfunction including hepatitis and jaundice; abnormal LFTs. Dependency/withdrawal symptoms.

Precautions

Pregnancy: Category D. Avoid drug especially during first trimester due to possible increased risk of congenital malformations. *Lactation*: Excreted in breast milk. *Children*: Initial dose should be small and gradually increased. Oral form not recommended in patients < 6 mo; parenteral form not recommended in infants < 30 days. *Elderly or debilitated patients*: Initial dose should be small and gradually increased. Give with extreme care to elderly patients with limited pulmonary reserve. *Dependency*: Prolonged use can lead to dependency. Withdrawal syndrome has occurred within 4-6 wk of treatment, especially if abruptly discontinued. For discontinuation after long-term treatment, use caution and taper dosage. *Parenteral administration*: Reserved primarily for acute states. *Psychiatric disorders*: Not intended for use in patients with primary depressive disorder, psychosis or disorders in which anxiety is not prominent. *Renal or hepatic impairment*: Observe caution to avoid accumulation of drug. *Seizures*: Tonic status epilepticus has been precipitated in patients treated for petit mal or variant status. *Suicide*: Use drug with caution in patients with suicidal tendencies; do not allow patient access to large quantities of drug.

NURSING CONSIDERATIONS

Administration/Storage

- Crush tablets if patient is unable to swallow tablets whole (unless sustained-release).
- Instruct patient to swallow sustained release capsules whole.
- Do not give oral form within 1 hr of antacids.
- Administer oral solution alone or mix with juices or water. When administering Intensol (concentrated oral solution), mix with liquid or semiliquid food such as water, juices, carbonated soda, puddings and applesauce. Use calibrated dropper provided only. Stir Intensol into liquid or food. Entire mixture must be consumed immediately; do not store solution for future use.
- For IV administration, administer injection slowly—no more than 5 mg (1 ml)/min. Slow injection reduces risk of venous thrombosis, phlebitis, local irritation, swelling and vascular impairment. In children, administer injection slowly over 3 min to reduce risk of apnea and hypersomnolence. Do not use small veins of hand or wrist. Avoid intra-arterial injection or extravasation, which may produce arteriospasm that can lead to gangrene. Do not mix or dilute with other solutions or drugs.
- If unable to perform direct IV administration, inject slowly through infusion tubing or Y-site as close as possible to IV site.
- IV route is preferred in convulsing patients.
- For IM administration, inject deeply into muscle.

Assessment/Interventions

- Obtain patient history, including drug history and any known allergies.
- Monitor BP (lying, standing), pulse rate and respiratory rate. Notify physician of significant change in systolic BP or respiratory depression with concomitant use of narcotic analgesics.
- Monitor respiratory rate q 5-15 min during IV administration.
- Monitor CBC; blood dyscrasias rarely occur.
- Monitor liver function during long-term use.
- Provide sugarless gum or hard candy and frequent sips of water to relieve dry mouth.

- Assess level of anxiety, what precipitates anxiety and if drug controls symptoms.
- Assess for alcohol withdrawal symptoms: hallucinations, delirium, irritability, agitation, tremors.
- Assess for seizure control and type, duration and intensity of convulsions.
- Assess mental status: mood, sensorium, affect, sleep pattern, drowsiness dizziness. Report changes in mental status to physician.
- Observe patient closely for 3 hr following parenteral administration.
- Assess for physical dependency/withdrawal symptoms: headaches, muscle pain, weakness, nausea and vomiting after long-term use.
- Assess for suicidal tendencies; restrict amount of drug available to patient.
- Because of risk of apnea and cardiac arrest with parenteral administration, have resuscitative facilities available.

OVERDOSAGE: SIGNS & SYMPTOMS

Hypotension, respiratory or cardiac arrest, drowsiness, confusion, somnolence, impaired coordination, diminished reflexes, lethargy, ataxia, hypotonia, hypnosis, coma, death

Patient/Family Education

- Advise patient not to take within 1 hr of antacid.
- Remind patient to take with food or milk to decrease GI irritation.
- Instruct patient to avoid intake of alcoholic beverages or other CNS depressants (sleeping pills, antihistamines, narcotics) unless specifically ordered by physician.
- Caution patient to avoid sudden position changes to prevent orthostatic hypotension or fainting may occur, especially if patient is elderly.
- Advise patient that drowsiness is worse at beginning of treatment.
- Caution patient that drug may be habit-forming and advise that patient discuss use with physician.
- Encourage patient to carry identification (Medi-Alert bracelet) indicating medication usage if taking drug for seizure control.
- Advise patient that drug may cause drowsiness and to use caution while driving or performing other tasks requiring mental alertness.

See Patient Guide, p. 182.

Diazoxide, Oral

(DIE-aze-OX-ide)

Proglycem

Class: Glucose-elevating agent

Action Produces prompt dose-related increase in blood glucose by inhibiting pancreatic insulin release.

Indications Management of hypoglycemia caused by hyperinsulinism in adults with inoperable islet cell adenoma or carcinoma or extrapancreatic malignancy, in infants and children with leucine sensitivity, islet cell hyperplasia, nesidioblastosis, extrapancreatic malignancy, islet cell adenoma or adenomatosis.

Contraindications Hypersensitivity to thiazides; functional hypoglycemia.

Route/Dosage

ADULTS & CHILDREN: **PO** 3-8 mg/kg/day in 2-3 equal doses q 8-12 hr. INFANTS & NEWBORNS: **PO** 8-15 mg/kg/day in 2-3 equal doses q 8-12 hr.

Interactions

Antihypertensive agents: Enhanced antihypertensive effect. *Hydantoins:* Possible loss of seizure control. *Sulfonylureas:* Decreased pharmacologic effects of both drugs. *Thiazide diuretics:* Increased hyperglycemic and hyperuricemic effects of diazoxide; hypotension.

Lab Test Interferences

Hypoglycemia and hyperuricemia

produced by diazoxide may affect assessment of these metabolic states. Increased renin secretion and IgG concentrations and decreased cortisol secretion may occur. False-negative insulin response to glucagon may occur.

Adverse Reactions

CV: Tachycardia; palpitations; hypotension; transient hypertension; chest pain. *CNS:* Headache; weakness; malaise; anxiety; dizziness; insomnia; polyneuritis; paresthesia; extrapyramidal signs; fever. *EENT:* Transient cataracts; subconjunctival hemorrhage; ring scotoma; blurred vision; diplopia; lacrimation. *GI:* Anorexia; nausea; vomiting; abdominal pain; ileus; diarrhea; transient loss of taste; acute pancreatitis; pancreatic necrosis. *GU:* Azotemia; decreased creatinine clearance; reversible nephrotic syndrome; decreased urinary output; hematuria; albuminuria; glycosuria. *HEMA:* Thrombocytopenia with or without purpura; transient neutropenia; eosinophilia; decreased hemoglobin or hematocrit; excessive bleeding; decreased IgG. *DERM:* Hirsutism of lanugo type on forehead, back, and limbs; skin rash; pruritus; monilial dermatitis; herpes; loss of scalp hair. *META:* Hyperglycemia; increased serum uric acid; gout; galactorrhea; breast lump enlargement; increased AST and alkaline phosphatase. *OTHER:* Sodium and fluid retention; advance in bone age.

Precautions

Pregnancy: Category C. *Lactation:* Undetermined. *Labor:* May cause cessation of uterine contractions. *Blood levels:* May be higher with liquid than with capsule formulation; use caution when changing dosage forms. *Fluid retention:* May precipitate CHF in patients with compromised cardiac reserve. *Ketoacidosis and nonketotic hyperosmolar coma:* May occur with recommended doses. *Renal impairment:* May have decreased protein binding of diazoxide resulting in increased hypotensive effect.

NURSING CONSIDERATIONS

Administration/Storage

- Shake oral suspension well before administering.
- Store at room temperature. Protect suspension from light.

Assessment/Interventions

- Obtain patient history, including drug history and any known allergies. Note cardiac or renal impairment.
- Ensure that baseline laboratory tests have been obtained before beginning therapy.
- Monitor BP (lying, standing) for hypotensive effect, especially if patient is taking antihypertensive agent.
- Monitor blood and urine glucose and ketones carefully until stabilized, usually within 1 wk.
- Monitor I&O and weight at least weekly to monitor fluid retention.
- Monitor for signs of CHF: peripheral edema, dyspnea, rales/crackles, fatigue, weight gain, jugular vein distention. Notify physician immediately if these occur.
- Observe for signs of hirsutism.
- If ecchymosis, petechiae, or hemorrhage occur, notify physician immediately. Drug may need to be discontinued.

OVERDOSAGE: SIGNS & SYMPTOMS

Hypotension, hyperglycemia

Patient/Family Education

- Instruct patient to take medication as directed at same time each day. Warn patient not to switch from capsule to suspension without notifying physician.
- Review symptoms of hypoglycemia and hyperglycemia with patient and family.
- Advise patient to follow prescribed diet, medication and exercise regi-

men to prevent hypoglycemic or hyperglycemic reactions.
- Instruct patient to monitor blood glucose, urine glucose and ketones daily.
- Instruct patient to report these symptoms to physician: bruising, bleeding or fluid retention.
- Caution patient to avoid sudden position changes to prevent orthostatic hypotension. Inform patient that hirsutism is common side effect but should be reversed when drug is discontinued.
- Instruct patient not to take otc medications without consulting physician.

See Patient Guide, p. 183.

Diazoxide, Parenteral

(DIE-aze-OX-ide)

Hyperstat

Class: Agent for hypertensive emergencies

Action Relaxes smooth muscle in peripheral arterioles, thus reducing blood pressure.

Indications Short-term emergency reduction of blood pressure in severe, nonmalignant and malignant hypertension in hospitalized patients.

Contraindications Dissecting aortic aneurysm; hypersensitivity to thiazides or other sulfonamide derivatives; treatment of compensatory hypertension, such as that associated with aortic coarctation or arteriovenous shunt. Diazoxide is ineffective against hypertension caused by pheochromocytoma.

Route/Dosage
ADULTS: **IV** 1-3 mg/kg (maximum 150 mg in single injection) by rapid injection. May repeat at 5-15 min intervals until satisfactory reduction in blood pressure. May repeat at intervals of 4-24 hr until oral therapy can be initiated. Do not use for more than 10 days.

Interactions
Antihypertensive agents: Enhanced antihypertensive effect. *Highly protein-bound agents:* Higher blood levels of these agents may occur as a result of displacement by diazoxide. *Hydantoins:* Possible loss of seizure control. *Sulfonylureas:* Hyperglycemia may occur. *Thiazide diuretics:* May increase hyperuricemic, hyperglycemic, and antihypertensive effects of diazoxide.

Lab Test Interferences
Hyperglycemia and hyperuricemia produced by diazoxide may affect assessment of these metabolic states. Increased renin secretion and IgG concentrations and decreased cortisol secretion may occur. May cause false-negative insulin response to glucagon.

Adverse Reactions
CV: Sodium and water retention; hypotension to shock levels; congestive heart failure; edema; myocardial ischemia (angina, arrhythmias, ECG changes); supraventricular tachycardia; palpitations; bradycardia. *CNS:* Dizziness; weakness; cerebral ischemia; cerebral infarction (unconsciousness, convulsions, paralysis, confusion, focal neurologic deficit); sweating; flushing and feelings of warmth; transient neurologic findings (eg, headache, lethargy, somnolence, euphoria, ringing in ears, momentary hearing loss). *GI:* Nausea; vomiting; acute pancreatitis; diarrhea; abdominal discomfort. *DERM:* Cellulitis or phlebitis at site of extravasation; warmth or pain along course of injected vein. *META:* Hyperglycemia; hyperosmolar coma; hyperuricemia. *OTHER:* Hypersensitivity reactions; papilledema.

Precautions
Pregnancy: Category C. *Lactation:* Undetermined. *Special risk patients:* Diabetic patients may need treatment for hyperglycemia. Use with care in patients with impaired cerebral or cardiac

circulation in whom rapid reduction in BP might be deleterious. Observe caution when reducing severely elevated BP. *Fluid and electolyte balance:* Because of sodium and water retention, with possible edema and congestive heart failure, concomitant use of diuretic may be needed. However, thiazide diuretics may potentiate diazoxide's antihypertensive, hyperglycemic and hyperuricemic actions.

NURSING CONSIDERATIONS

Administration/Storage

- Administer IV, not SC or IM, over ≤ 30 sec.
- Have patient remain supine during IV administration.
- Protect liquid solution from light. Do not freeze.

Assessment/Interventions

- Obtain patient history, including drug history and any known allergies.
- Obtain baseline BP and pulse before therapy. Monitor BP and pulse frequently.
- Monitor for hyperglycemia in the diabetic patient.
- If signs of cerebral ischemia occur, such as slowed mental processes or anxiety, help patient into supine position, elevate patient's legs and notify physician.
- If signs of CHF (edema, dyspnea, weight gain, jugular vein distension) occur, notify physician.
- If headache occurs, administer analgesics as prescribed by physician.
- If nausea or vomiting occurs, offer small frequent feedings and fluids. Give antiemetic if ordered.

OVERDOSAGE: SIGNS & SYMPTOMS
Hypotension, hyperglycemia

Patient/Family Education

- Emphasize importance of follow-up exams and blood testing to assure effectiveness and to minimize adverse reactions.
- Tell patient to report adverse reactions to physician.
- Caution patient to avoid sudden position changes to prevent orthostatic hypotension.
- Instruct patient not to take otc medications without consulting physician.

No patient monograph available.

Diclofenac

(die-KLOE-fen-ak)

Cataflam, Voltaren, Votaren-XR
Class: Analgesic/NSAID

Action Decreases inflammation, pain and fever, probably through inhibition of cyclooxygenase activity and prostaglandin synthesis.

Indications Treatment of rheumatoid arthritis, ankylosing spondylitis, osteoarthritis. Potassium salt is also approved for management of pain and primary dysmenorrhea, when prompt pain relief is needed. *Ophthalmic:* Treatment of postoperative inflammation after cataract removal. **Unlabeled uses:** Treatment of biliary colic, dysmenorrhea, enuresis, glomerular disease, gout, migraine headache, renal colic.

Contraindications Sensitivity to aspirin or any NSAID; soft contact lenses (ophthalmic).

Route/Dosage

Osteoarthritis
PO 100-150 mg/day in divided doses.

Rheumatoid Arthritis
PO 150-200 mg/day in divided doses.

Ankylosing Spondylitis
PO 100-125 mg/day in divided doses; may give additional 25 mg at bedtime.

Analgesia and Primary Dysmenorrhea (Potassium Salt Only)
PO 50 mg tid; may give initial dose of 100 mg if needed.

Ophthalmic
1 drop of 0.1% solution in affected eye qid.

Interactions
Cyclosporine: May increase nephrotoxicity. *Digoxin:* May increase digoxin serum concentrations. *Diuretics:* May inhibit diuretic and antihypertensive effects. *Lithium:* May decrease lithium clearance. *Methotrexate:* May increase methotrexate levels. *Warfarin:* May increase risk of gastric erosion and bleeding.

Lab Test Interferences
May prolong bleeding time.

Adverse Reactions
CV: Edema; water retention; hypertension; CHF. *RESP:* Breathing difficulties in aspirin-sensitive individuals. *CNS:* Headache; vertigo; drowsiness; dizziness. *EENT:* Ophthalmic; transient stinging and burning tinnitus. *GI:* Diarrhea; vomiting; abdominal pain; dyspepsia; peptic ulcer; GI bleeding. *GU:* Acute renal failure, nephrotic syndrome. *HEMA:* Fall in hemoglobin; bruising; prolonged bleeding time; thrombocytopenia purpura; anemia. *DERM:* Rash; urticaria; fasciitis; photosensitivity. *OTHER:* Hypersensitivity reactions. Ophthalmic use may cause bleeding tendencies and other effects associated with systemic use, due to absorption.

Precautions
Pregnancy: Category B. *Lactation:* Undetermined. *Children:* Safety and efficacy not established. *Elderly:* Increased risk of adverse reactions. *GI effects:* Serious GI toxicity (eg, bleeding, ulceration, perforation) can occur at any time, with or without warning symptoms. *Renal effects:* Acute renal insufficiency; interstitial nephritis; hyperkalemia; hyponatremia and renal papillary necrosis may occur.

NURSING CONSIDERATIONS

Administration/Storage
- Administer after meals or with food to minimize gastric irritation.
- Do not administer antacids within 2 hours of giving enteric-coated diclofenac because antacids may destroy enteric coating.

Assessment/Interventions
- Obtain patient history, including drug history and any known allergies.
- Assess arthritic pain and limitations of movement before and after administration (pain location and intensity).
- If given for eye inflammation after surgery, assess for changes.
- Notify physician of any signs of GI bleeding.
- Monitor and document I&O.
- Monitor for GI problems and guaiac stool.
- Review baseline CBC, BUN and creatinine.
- If photosensitivity occurs, provide protective measures (sunscreens, clothing) until tolerance is developed.
- If blood pressure rises to hypertensive range, notify physician.

OVERDOSAGE: SIGNS & SYMPTOMS
Acute renal failure, nausea, vomiting, drowsiness

Patient/Family Education
- Teach name, expected action, method of administration and potential side effects of diclofenac.
- Tell patient to take medication with meals or food to minimize gastric irritation.
- Review signs and symptoms of GI irritation and bleeding.
- Advise patient to avoid alcohol, aspi-

rin and any other drugs that cause GI irritation and bleeding.
- Tell patient that drug may cause drowsiness and to avoid driving or performing other tasks requiring mental alertness if drowsiness or dizziness occurs.
- Teach patient proper technique for instilling eye drops.
- If patient is taking enteric-coated form, caution patient about avoiding use of antacids.
- Advise patient not to take otc analgesics while taking this medication.

See Patient Guide, p. 184-186.

Dicloxacillin Sodium

(DIE-klox-uh-SILL-in SO-dee-uhm)
Dycill, Dynapen, Pathocil
Class: Antibiotic/penicillin

Action Inhibits bacterial cell wall mucopeptide synthesis.

Indications Treatment of infections due to penicillinase-producing staphylococcal infection.

Contraindications Hypersensitivity to penicillins.

Route/Dosage
ADULTS & CHILDREN > 40 KG: **PO** 125-250 mg q 6 h. CHILDREN < 40 KG: **PO** 12.5-25 mg/kg/day divided in equal doses q 6 h.

Interactions
Contraceptives, oral: May reduce efficacy of oral contraceptives. *Food:* Antibacterial action may be reduced. *Tetracyclines:* May impair bactericidal effects of dicloxacillin.

Lab Test Interferences
May cause false-positive urine glucose test results with Benedict's Solution, Fehling's Solution, or Clinitest tablets but not with enzyme-based tests (e.g., Clinistix, Tes-tape); false-positive direct Coombs' test results in certain patient groups; false-positive protein reactions with sulfosalicylic acid and boiling test, acetic acid test, biuret reaction and nitric acid test but not with bromphenol blue test (Multistix).

Adverse Reactions
CNS: Dizziness; fatigue; insomnia; reversible hyperactivity; seizures. *EENT:* Laryngospasm; laryngeal edema; itchy eyes. *GI:* Glossitis; stomatitis; gastritis; sore mouth or tongue; dry mouth; furry tongue; black "hairy" tongue; abnormal taste sensation; anorexia; nausea; vomiting; abdominal pain or cramps; diarrhea or bloody diarrhea; rectal bleeding; flatulence; enterocolitis; pseudomembranous colitis. *GU:* Interstitial nephritis (eg, oliguria, proteinuria, hematuria, hyaline casts, pyuria); nephropathy. *HEMA:* Anemias; thrombocytopenia; eosinophilia; leukopenia; granulocytopenia; neutropenia; bone marrow depression; agranulocytosis; reduced hemoglobin or hematocrit; prolonged bleeding and prothrombin time; altered lymphocyte count; increased monocytes, basophils, platelets. *HEPA:* Transient hepatitis; cholestatic jaundice. *DERM:* Urticaria; dermatitis; vesicular eruptions; erythema multiforme; rashes. *META:* Elevated serum alkaline phosphatase and hypernatremia; reduced serum potassium, albumin, total proteins and uric acid. *OTHER:* Hypersensitivity reactions that may lead to death; vaginitis; hyperthermia.

Precautions
Pregnancy: Category B. *Lactation:* Excreted in breast milk. *Hypersensitivity:* Reactions range from mild to life-threatening. Administer cautiously to cephalosporin-sensitive patients due to possible cross-reactivity. *Superinfection:* May result in bacterial or fungal overgrowth of nonsusceptible organisms. *Pseudomembranous colitis:* Consider possibility in patients with diarrhea.

NURSING CONSIDERATIONS

Administration/Storage

- Obtain specimens for culture before initiating antibiotic therapy.
- Capsules can be opened and contents mixed with small amount of food or fluid, but patient may experience bad taste.
- Give on empty stomach (30 min-1 hr before meal or 2 hr after a meal).
- Give with full glass of water, not juice or carbonated beverage.
- If stored at room temperature, discard reconstituted oral solution after 7 days; after 14 days if refrigerated. Do not freeze.
- Always give in divided doses throughout day to maintain steady state.

Assessment/Interventions

- Obtain patient history, including drug history and any known allergies.
- Assess signs of infection before and during therapy (fever, vital signs, appearance of wounds, WBC).
- If signs of anaphylaxis (rash, pruritus, laryngeal edema, wheezing) occur, discontinue drug and notify physician immediately.

Patient/Family Education

- Instruct patient to take antibiotic on empty stomach before (30 min-1 hr) meals or after (2 hr) meals with full glass of water.
- Explain that doses should be scheduled evenly spaced throughout day and night to maintain adequate drug levels.
- Teach patient signs of sensitivity reaction and appropriate steps to take if they occur.
- Tell patient to discard any liquid solution after 7 days when stored at room temperature or after 14 days of refrigeration.
- Instruct patient to shake bottle before measuring pediatric suspension and to use a medication cup or other calibrated device for accurate dosing.
- Teach patient signs of superinfection, which can occur with any antibiotic (black, furry tongue, vaginal itching) and tell patient to notify physician if any occur.
- Instruct patient never to share antibiotic prescriptions with others.
- Advise patient to follow complete course of therapy, even if feeling better.

See Patient Guide, p. 187.

Dicyclomine HCl

(die-SIGH-kloe-meen HIGH-droe-KLOR-ide)

Antispas, Bemote, Bentyl, Byclomine, Dibent, Neoquess, Spasmoject,
✤ *Bentylol*

Class: Anticholinergic; antispasmodic

Action Relieves smooth muscle spasm of GI tract through anticholinergic effects and direct action on GI smooth muscle.

Indications Treatment of functional bowel/irritable bowel syndrome (irritable colon, spastic colon, mucous colitis). **Unlabeled use:** Intestinal colic in children > 6 mo.

Contraindications Narrow-angle glaucoma; adhesions between iris and lens; obstructive uropathy; obstructive disease of GI tract; paralytic ileus; intestinal atony of elderly or debilitated patient; severe ulcerative colitis; toxic megacolon complicating ulcerative colitis; hepatic or renal disease; tachycardia; myocardial ischemia; unstable cardiovascular status in acute hemorrhage; myasthenia gravis; infants < 6 mo.

Route/Dosage

ADULTS: Initial dose: **PO** 80 mg/day in 4 equally divided doses. Increase to 160 mg/day in 4 equally divided doses. **IM** 80 mg/day in 4 divided doses.

Interactions

Amantadine, tricyclic antidepressants: May cause increased anticholinergic side effects. *Atenolol, digoxin:* May increase pharmacologic effects of these drugs. *Phenothiazines:* May reduce antipsychotic effectiveness.

Lab Test Interferences

None well documented.

Adverse Reactions

CV: Palpitations; tachycardia. *CNS:* Headache; flushing; nervousness; drowsiness; weakness; dizziness; confusion; insomnia; fever (especially in children); mental confusion or excitement (especially in elderly, even with small doses); CNS stimulation (restlessness, tremor); lightheadedness. *EENT:* Blurred vision; mydriasis; photophobia; cycloplegia; increased IOP; dilated pupils; nasal congestion. *GI:* Dry mouth; altered taste perception; nausea; vomiting; dysphagia; heartburn; constipation; bloated feeling; paralytic ileus. *GU:* Urinary hesitancy and retention; impotence. *DERM:* Severe allergic reactions including anaphylaxis, urticaria and dermal manifestations; local irritation following injection. *OTHER:* Suppression of lactation; decreased sweating.

Precautions

Pregnancy: Category B. *Lactation:* Excreted in breast milk. *Children:* Safety and efficacy have not been established. Contraindicated in infants < 6 mo. In infants, serious respiratory symptoms, seizures, syncope, pulse rate fluctuation, muscular hypotonia, coma and death have been reported. *Elderly or debilitated patients:* Elderly patients may react with excitement, agitation, drowsiness, and other untoward manifestations to even small doses. *Special risk patients:* Use with caution in patients with autonomic neuropathy, hyperthyroidism, hypertension, coronary heart disease, CHF, hiatal hernia, prostatic hypertrophy. *Anticholinergic psychosis:* Reported in sensitive individuals and may include confusion, disorientation, short-term memory loss, hallucinations, dysarthria, ataxia, coma, euphoria, decreased anxiety, fatigue, insomnia, agitation and mannerisms, and inappropriate affect. *Diarrhea:* May be symptom of incomplete intestinal obstruction, especially in patients with ileostomy or colostomy. Treatment of diarrhea with drug is inappropriate and possibly harmful. *Gastric ulcer:* May delay gastric emptying rate and complicate therapy. *Heat prostration:* Can occur in presence of high environmental temperature.

NURSING CONSIDERATIONS

Administration/Storage

- For parenteral administration, give only intramuscularly. Drug is not for IV use.
- Administer drug 30 min before meals.
- Store in tightly closed container at room temperature and protect from light. Injection fluid should be clear.

Assessment/Interventions

- Obtain patient history, including drug history and any known allergies.
- Assess baseline vital signs.
- Monitor I&O.
- Ask patient if difficulty in voiding is a problem.
- Assess hydration status (eg, skin turgor, mucous membranes, stool consistency, frequency) and bowel sounds.
- Monitor patient for changes in vital signs and sensorium (eg, fever, tachycardia, confusion, anxiety).

OVERDOSAGE: SIGNS & SYMPTOMS

Circulatory failure, vomiting, abdominal distention, muscle weakness, anxiety, stupor, blurred vision, photophobia, dilated pupils, urinary retention

Patient/Family Education

- Instruct patient not to take any

otc medications without consulting physician.

- Advise contact lens wearers to use lubricating solutions.
- Warn patients to avoid direct sunlight and any heat extremes (eg, exercise in hot weather, saunas, prolonged activity in hot weather).
- Instruct patient to take sips of water frequently, suck on ice chips or sugarless hard candy or chew sugarless gum if dry mouth occurs.
- Alert patients to pay special attention to fever, decreased ability to sweat and changes in bowel or bladder habits.
- Advise elderly patients to report eye pain to physician or ophthalmologist and to undergo testing for glaucoma.
- Advise patient that drug may cause drowsiness and to use caution while driving or performing other tasks requiring mental alertness.
- Tell patient to report any difficulty in swallowing to physician.

See Patient Guide, p. 188.

Didanosine (ddI; dideoxyinosine)

(die-DAN-oh-SEEN)

Videx

Class: Anti-infective/antiviral

Action Inhibits replication of HIV by interfering with DNA synthesis.

Indications Advanced HIV infection in patients with intolerance or significant clinical or immunologic deterioration during zidovudine therapy.

Contraindications Standard considerations.

Route/Dosage

ADULTS (< 60 KG): **PO** 125 mg (as 2 tablets) or 167 mg (powder for suspension q 12 hr. ADULTS (> 60 KG): **PO** 200 mg (as 2 tablets) or 250 mg (powder for suspension) q 12 hr. CHILDREN: **PO** 100-300 mg/m^2/day bid as oral powder for suspension. Reduce dose by 20% for tablets. Children < 1 yr should receive 1-tablet dose; those > 1 yr should get a 2-tablet dose.

Interactions

Drugs that cause peripheral neuropathy or pancreatitis: Increased risk of these toxicities. *Food:* Reduces absorption of didanosine by as much as 50%. *Fluoroquinolones, tetracyclines:* Do not administer within 2 hr of didanosine. *Ketaconazole, dapsone, and other drugs whose absorption can be affected by gastric acidity:* Administer at least 2 hr before didanosine.

Lab Test Interferences

None well documented.

Adverse Reactions

RESP: Pneumonia; dyspnea; cough; epistaxis; hypoventilation; sinusitis. *CNS:* Peripheral neuropathy; asthenia; headache; pain; myopathy; seizure. *EENT:* Retinal depigmentation. *GI:* Pancreatitis; diarrhea; abdominal pain; nausea; vomiting; anorexia; dry mouth. *HEMA:* Leukopenia, thrombocytopenia, granulocytopenia, and decreased hemoglobin. *HEPA:* Hepatic failure. *DERM:* Rash; pruritis; alopecia; sweating. *OTHER:* Chills, fever; infection; sarcoma.

Precautions

Pregnancy: Category B. *Lactation:* Undetermined. *Special diets:* Each tablet contains 22.5 mg phenylalanine and 265 mg sodium; single-dose powder packet contains 1380 mg sodium. *Mutagenesis:* May be genotoxic. *Renal or hepatic impairment:* Dosage may need to be reduced. Hepatic failure has occurred in pediatric patients. *Pancreatitis:* Major toxicity; has been fatal. Should be considered if patient develops abdominal pain, nausea, vomiting or lab test abnormalities. *Peripheral neuropathy:* Occurs frequently; may be dose-related.

NURSING CONSIDERATIONS

Administration/Storage

- Give on an empty stomach.
- Have patients chew tablets or manually crush or disperse tablets in water (2 tablets per 1 oz water).
- When dispersing tablets in water, stir until uniform dispersion occurs, then have patient drink entire amount immediately.
- When preparing buffered powder for oral suspension, do not use fruit juice or other acid-containing liquid. Stir until completely dissolved in 4 oz liquid, then have patient drink entire amount immediately.
- Pediatric powder for oral suspension is first mixed with purified water to obtain concentration of 20 mg/ml, then mixed with antacid to obtain final concentration of 10 mg/ml.
- Pediatric oral solution admixture may be stored for up to 30 days if refrigerated. Shake well before use.

Assessment/Interventions

- Obtain patient history, including drug history and any known allergies. Note renal or liver impairment, history of pancreatitis and prior response to zidovudine therapy.
- Ensure that liver and renal function tests are obtained before beginning drug therapy and repeat periodically.
- Notify physician if diarrhea develops in patient receiving oral solution. Switching to tablets may alleviate symptoms.
- If patient has abdominal pain, nausea or vomiting, or has elevated amylase or liver function test results, contact physician and withhold drug until pancreatitis can be excluded.
- Observe for symptoms of peripheral neuropathy (distal numbness, tingling, pain in feet or hands) or evidence of opportunistic infections. Notify physician if these occur.
- Monitor uric acid levels closely for possible asymptomatic hyperuricemia.
- Monitor body temperature to detect possible infection.
- Document any change in vision in pediatric patients. Dilated examination should be performed every 6 mo.

Patient/Family Education

- Advise patient to take drug on empty stomach and to chew or crush tablets.
- Inform patient that drug does not completely eliminate HIV virus and therefore does not reduce risk of transmitting HIV. Appropriate precautions must be continued.
- Emphasize that drug does not cure AIDS or AIDS-related complex (ARC) and that significant changes in health should be reported to physician.
- Instruct patient to report these symptoms to physician: abdominal pain, diarrhea, nausea, vomiting, tingling pain or numbness in hands or feet, fever, sore throat or flulike symptoms.
- Advise patient to avoid intake of alcoholic beverages or taking otc medications without notifying physician.

See Patient Guide, p. 189.

Diethylpropion HCl

(die-ETH-uhl-PRO-pee-ahn HIGH-droe-KLOR-ide)

Tenuate, Tenuate Dospan, Tepanil, Tepanil Ten-Tab

Class: CNS stimulant/anorexiant

Action Stimulates satiety center in brain, causing appetite suppression.

Indications Short-term (8-12 weeks) adjunct to diet plan to reduce weight.

Contraindications Advanced arteriosclerosis; symptomatic cardiovascular disease; moderate to severe hypertension; hyperthyroidism; hypersensitivity to sympathomimetic amines; glaucoma; agitated states; history of drug abuse; concurrent with or within 14 days of MAO inhibitor use; coadministration with other CNS stimulants.

Route/Dosage

ADULTS: PO 25 mg tid, 1 hr before meals. Sustained release tablets: 75 mg once daily, in midmorning.

Interactions

Guanethidine: May decrease hypotensive effect. *MAO inhibitors, furazolidione:* Hypertensive crisis and intracranial hemorrhage may occur. *Tricyclic antidepressants:* May decrease anorexiant effect.

Lab Test Interferences

None well documented.

Adverse Reactions

CV: Palpitations; tachycardia; arrhythmias; hypertension; hypotension. *CNS:* Overstimulation; dizziness; insomnia; euphoria; tremor; headache. *EENT:* Mydriasis; blurred vision. *GI:* Dry mouth; unpleasant taste; nausea; diarrhea; constipation; stomach pain. *GU:* Dysuria; urinary frequency; impotence; menstrual disturbances. *HEMA:* Bone marrow depression; agranulocytosis; leukopenia. *DERM:* Excessive sweating; flushing. *OTHER:* Hair loss; myalgia; gynecomastia; allergic reactions (eg, urticaria; rash; erythema).

Precautions

Pregnancy: Category B. *Lactation:* Excreted in breast milk. *Children:* Not recommended in children < 12 yr. *Cardiovascular effects:* May cause or aggravate hypertension or arrhythmias. *Convulsions:* Diethylpropion may aggravate; dose titration or discontinuance may be necessary. *Drug dependence:* Related to amphetamine; has abuse potential. *Tolerance:* May occur.

NURSING CONSIDERATIONS

Administration/Storage

- Give medication 1 hr before meals. Give sustained release tablets once daily at midmorning.
- Do not crush or open sustained release tablets.

Assessment/Interventions

- Obtain patient history, including drug history and any known allergies.
- Assess physical and psychological status throughout therapy.
- Measure patient's weight weekly.
- Notify physician and withhold medication if there is a BP increase of 20 mm Hg or if heart dysrhythmia and/or increase in heart rate develop.

OVERDOSAGE: SIGNS & SYMPTOMS

Restlessness, tremor, hyperreflexia, fever, tachypnea, dizziness, panic, aggression, hallucinations, seizure, coma, arrhythmias, hypotension, hypertension, death

Patient/Family Education

- Explain potential for increased agitation, palpitations, and dizziness and identify precaution to take when performing tasks that require physical coordination and/or mental concentration.
- Tell patient to record weight weekly.
- Explain that drug will make patient feel less hungry and thus make it easier to adhere to diet but that weight loss will occur only with calorie reduction and increased physical activity.
- Instruct patient on missed medication procedure: if less than 2 hr, take medication; if greater than 2 hr, wait until next scheduled dose. Do not double up on medication.
- Advise patient to limit intake of coffee, tea, cocoa, chocolate and caffeinated soft drinks.
- Identify techniques to prevent and/or treat dry mouth.

See Patient Guide, p. 190.

Diethylstilbestrol (DES)

(die-ETH-uhl-still-BESS-trahl)

Available as generic only

Class: Estrogen

Diethylstilbestrol Diphosphate

Stilphostrol, ♣ *Honvol*

Action Promotes growth and development of female reproductive system and secondary sex characteristics; inhibits ovulation and prevents postpartum breast engorgement; overrides stimulatory effects of testosterone; inhibits implantation of fertilized ovum if administered within 72 hr of coitus.

Indications Palliation in breast cancer (inoperable, progressing) in postmenopausal women and in men; palliation in prostatic carcinoma (inoperable, progressing). **Unlabeled use:** Postcoital contraceptive.

Contraindications Undiagnosed abnormal genital bleeding; thrombophlebitis or thromboembolic disorders; estrogen-dependent neoplasia; breast cancer (except in patients being treated for metastatic disease); known or suspected pregnancy; lactation.

Route/Dosage

Prostate Cancer

ADULTS: **PO** 1-3 mg/day initially; dosage usually reduced to 1 mg/day. DES diphosphate is given **PO** 50 mg tid with doses as high as 1 g/day for advanced prostate cancer; **IV** 500 mg initially and followed by 1 g/day for 5 or more days (250-500 mg dose may be used for maintenance).

Breast Cancer

ADULTS: **PO** 15 mg/day given chronically for at least 3 mo.

Postcoital Contraceptive

ADULTS: **PO** 25 mg bid for 5 days; start therapy no later than 72 hr after intercourse.

Interactions

Barbiturates, rifampin: May decrease DES concentration. *Corticosteroids:* May reduce clearance of corticosteroids. *Hydantoins:* May cause loss of seizure control or decreased estrogenic effects. INCOMPATIBILITIES: Diethylstilbestrol diphosphate is incompatible with calcium gluconate, fentanyl citrate, droperidol, gantamicin.

Lab Test Interferences

None well documented.

Adverse Reactions

CV: Thrombosis; thrombophlebitis; elevated BP; pulmonary embolism; MI. *CNS:* Headache; migraine; dizziness; depression. *EENT:* Intolerance to contact lenses. *GI:* Nausea; vomiting; abdominal cramps; bloating; colitis; acute pancreatitis. *GU:* Increased risk of endometrial carcinoma; breakthrough bleeding; dysmenorrhea; amenorrhea; vaginal candidiasis; premenstrual-like syndrome; increased size of uterine fibromyomata; hemolytic uremic syndrome. *HEPA:* Cholestatic jaundice. *DERM:* Chloasma; melasma; erythema nodosum or multiforme; scalp hair loss; hirsutism; urticaria; dermatitis. *OTHER:* Increase or decrease in weight; reduced glucose tolerance; edema; changes in libido; breast tenderness; acute intermittent porphyria.

Precautions

Pregnancy: Category X. *Lactation:* Excreted in breast milk. Contraindicated in nursing women. *Children:* Safety and efficacy not established; consider effects on epiphyseal closure. *Calcium and phosphorus metabolism:* Use with caution in patients with metabolic bone diseases. *Fluid retention:* Use drug with caution when conditions that might be affected by this factor are present (eg, asthma, cardiac or renal dysfunction, epilepsy). *Gallbladder disease:* Risk of gallbladder disease may increase in women receiving postmenopausal estrogens. *Hepatic impairment:* Metabolism may be impaired; use with caution.

Induction of malignant neoplasms: May increase risk of endometrial or other carcinomas. *IV administration of diethylstilbestrol diphosphate:* Indicated only for prostatic carcinoma.

NURSING CONSIDERATIONS

Administration/Storage

- When administering parenteral solution, give 0.5 g dissolved in 250 ml saline solution or D5W IV. On subsequent days give 1 g dissolved in 250-500 ml of saline solution or D5W. During first 15 min, administer drug slowly (20-30 gtt/min) then adjust flow rate to deliver remainder in 1 hr.
- Parenteral solution may be stored at room temperature and away from direct light for approximately 5 days. Do not use if solution appears cloudy or if precipitate is present.
- Administer oral form with food to minimize nausea. Do not allow patient to crush or chew tablets.

Assessment/Interventions

- Obtain patient history, including drug history and any known allergies prior to initiation of estrogen therapy. Examination should include evaluation of BP, breasts, abdomen, pelvic organs and Pap smear.
- Assess patient's response to drug therapy to obtain maximum effectiveness at lowest possible dose.
- Perform complete history and physical examination q 6-12 mo during estrogen therapy.
- Assess patient frequently for adverse reactions to drug.
- Monitor BP regularly.

OVERDOSAGE: SIGNS & SYMPTOMS

Anorexia, nausea, vomiting, abdominal cramps, diarrhea, withdrawal vaginal bleeding

Patient/Family Education

- Caution patient that this medication must not be taken during pregnancy or when pregnancy is possible. Advise patient to use reliable form of birth control while taking this drug.
- Instruct patient to report these symptoms to physician: change in menstrual flow, abnormal vaginal bleeding, vaginal infection, unusual vaginal secretions, painful menstruation, nausea, vomiting, stomach cramps, bloating, diarrhea, headache, migraine, dizziness, fainting, depression, weakness, seizures, unusual body movements, excessive hair growth, itching, rash, hives, skin discoloration including yellowing, weight loss or gain, breast tenderness and/or enlargement, breast milk secretion, pain in groin or calves, chest pain, shortness of breath, vision problems, abnormal blood glucose, fluid retention, high BP, or change in sex drive.
- Caution patient to avoid exposure to sunlight and to use sunscreen or wear protective clothing to avoid photosensitivity reaction.
- Reassure male patient that with discontinuation of therapy, sex drive should return and secondary female sex characteristics (eg, breast enlargement) should disapper.
- Inform patient of possibility of contact lens intolerance and suggest that patient wear glasses during therapy if this effect occurs.
- Caution patient against cigarette smoking, which increases risk of thrombosis.

See Patient Guide, p. 191.

Diflunisal

(die-FLOO-nih-sal)

Dolobid

Class: Analgesic/salicylate

Action Decreases inflammation and relieves pain by inhibiting prostaglandin synthesis and release.

Indications Relief of mild to moderate pain, rheumatoid arthritis and osteoarthritis.

Contraindications Hypersensitivity to NSAIDs or aspirin.

Route/Dosage

Mild to Moderate Pain

ADULTS: **PO** 500-1000 mg for first dose, then 250-500 mg q 8-12 hr.

Arthritis

ADULTS: **PO** 250-500 mg bid. Maximum dose: **PO** 750 mg bid.

Interactions

Antacids: Decreased plasma concentration of diflunisal. *Cyclosporine:* Increased nephrotoxic effect of cyclosporine possible. *Methotrexate:* Life-threatening methotrexate toxicity possible. *Warfarin:* Prothrombin time may increase; increased risk of bleeding.

Lab Test Interferences

May falsely elevate salicylate serum concentrations.

Adverse Reactions

CV: Peripheral edema. *RESP:* Bronchospasm. *CNS:* Headache; somnolence; insomnia; dizziness. *EENT:* Angioedema; tinnitus. *GI:* Nausea; dyspepsia; GI pain; diarrhea; GI bleeding. *GU:* Renal impairment; interstitial nephritis; dysuria. *HEMA:* Thrombocytopenia; agranulocytosis; hemolytic anemia. *HEPA:* Jaundice. *DERM:* Rash; erythema multiforme; photosensitivity. *OTHER:* Anaphylaxis; hypersensitivity syndrome (eg, fever, chills, rash, liver or kidney dysfunction, leukopenia, thrombocytopenia, eosinophilia, DIC).

Precautions

Pregnancy: Category C. *Lactation:* Excreted in breast milk. *Children:* Not recommended for children < 12 yr. May increase risk of Reye's syndrome; do not use if varicella infection or flu symptoms are suspected. *Fluid retention:* Use with caution in patients with CHF, hypertension or other conditions associated with fluid retention. *History of peptic ulcer:* Use carefully and closely monitor for GI bleeding or peptic ulcer; monitor patients with GI disease closely.

NURSING CONSIDERATIONS

Administration/Storage

- Do not crush or allow patient to chew tablets.
- Administer with milk or food to minimize gastric irritation, give patient generous amounts of water or other fluids to increase gastric emptying.

Assessment/Interventions

- Obtain patient history, including drug history and any known allergies.
- Assess pain prior to and after administration of medication.
- Monitor I&O. Notify physician if signs of renal dysfunction occur (decreased urine output, elevated BUN, elevated creatinine).
- Include hepatic function in each assessment and notify physician if any signs or symptoms of hepatic dysfunction are noted (fatigue, jaundice, abdominal pain, elevated liver enzymes, dark urine).

OVERDOSAGE: SIGNS & SYMPTOMS

Drowsiness, vomiting, nausea, diarrhea, hyperventilation, tachycardia, sweating, tinnitus, disorientation, decreased urine output, cardiorespiratory arrest, stupor and coma; may lead to death

Patient/Family Education

- Advise patient to swallow tablets whole and not to chew or crush them.
- Explain that relief of arthritis may not occur for 1 wk to several weeks.
- Caution patients against taking products with aspirin or acetaminophen concurrently with diflunisal unless directed by physician.
- Warn patient that this medication can precipitate Reye's syndrome.
- Advise patients to avoid exposure to sunlight and to use sunscreens or wear protective clothing to avoid photosensitivity reaction until tolerance is determined.
- Inform patients that first dose tends to have slower onset of pain relief than other drugs with comparable effects.
- Instruct patients to report immediately any signs of nephrotoxicity including decreased urine output, weight gain, edema, anorexia, nausea and vomiting.
- Advise patients with history of GI problems to notify physician if abdominal pain, melena or hematemesis develops during therapy.
- Advise patient to report degree of pain relief to physician.

See Patient Guide, p. 192.

Digitoxin

(dih-jih-TOX-in)

Crystodigin, ♣ *Digitaline*

Class: Cardiac glycoside

Action Enhances force and velocity of myocardial systolic contractions, increasing refractory period of atrioventricular (AV) node and increasing total peripheral vascular resistance.

Indications Treatment of CHF, atrial fibrillation, atrial flutter, paroxysmal atrial tachycardia, cardiogenic shock.

Contraindications Ventricular fibrillation; ventricular tachycardia, unless congestive failure occurs that is not due to digitalis; digitalis toxicity; beriberi heart disease; hypersensitive carotid sinus syndrome.

Route/Dosage

ADULTS: Loading dose, rapid: PO 0.6 mg initially, followed by 0.4 mg then 0.2 mg at 4-6 hr intervals; slow digitalization: PO 0.2 mg bid for 4 days. Maintenance: PO 0.05-0.3 mg daily. CHILDREN < 1 YR: Digitalizing dose: PO 0.045 mg/kg. CHILDREN 1-2 YR: PO 0.04 mg/kg. CHILDREN > 2 YR: PO 0.03 mg/kg (0.75 mg/m^2). Children's maintenance dose is one tenth digitalizing dose. NEONATES/PREMATURE/IMMATURE INFANTS: Individualize dosage. In premature and immature infants, adjust dosage carefully, dividing total dose into 3 or more portions given at 6 hr intervals.

Interactions

Charcoal, activated: May reduce absorpton of digitoxin. *Cholestyramine, colestipol, rifampin:* Therapeutic effects of digitoxin may be decreased. *Diuretics:* May lead to digitalis-induced arrhythmia. *Propylthiouracil, methimazole, quinidine, thyroid hormones, verapamil:* May lead to digitalis toxicity.

Lab Test Interferences

None well documented.

Adverse Reactions

HEMA: Eosinophilia; thrombocytopenia. *DERM:* Skin rash. *OTHER:* Allergy; gynecomastia. Mild toxic symptoms may occur with therapeutic doses (see Overdosage: Signs & Symptoms).

Precautions

Pregnancy: Category C. *Lactation:* Excreted in breast milk. *Children:* Newborns show varying tolerance. Premature and immature infants are particularly sensitive; reduce and individualize dose. *Elderly:* Exercise care in dosing. *Cardiovascular disease:* Reduced dose may be required if electrical conversion of arrhythmia is performed. Advanced or complete heart block may develop in patients with incomplete heart block if digitoxin is given. If heart failure develops in patients with acute MI, severe pulmonary disease or severe carditis, it may be necessary to digitalize patients cautiously with low doses. Unless cardiac failure is severe, avoid digitoxin in patients with idiopathic hypertrophic subaortic stenosis. *Digitalis toxicity:* May resemble arrhythmia being treated. If possible, withhold digitoxin until digitalis toxicity is ruled out. Serum drug concentrations may be helpful. *Hepatic impairment:* May need to reduce dose. *Hypercalcemia, hypomagnesemia:* May predispose patient to digitalis toxicity. *Hypokalemia:* May sensitize myocardium to digitalis and may reduce positive inotropic effects.

NURSING CONSIDERATIONS

Administration/Storage

- Tablets can be crushed and administered with food or fluids if patient has difficulty swallowing. Otherwise, food intake does not need to be considered when scheduling doses.
- Do not administer concurrently with any drug that reduces absorption, such as kaolin, pectin or antacids.
- Store in tightly closed container at room temperature, unless otherwise specified by manufacturer.

Assessment/Interventions

- Obtain patient history, including drug history and any known allergies.
- Assess patient's baseline apical heart rate and rhythm before starting cardiac glycoside treatment. Apical pulse should then be checked for 1 full min before administering each dose.
- Monitor patient's serum digitoxin levels as prescribed. Draw blood preferably immediately before administering maintenance dose. Toxic concentration of digitoxin is > 35 ng/ml.
- Monitor liver function studies to detect liver dysfunction, and monitor serum electrolytes, especially potassium, calcium and magnesium concentrations.
- Assess for and document signs of improvement in patient's condition: decreased edema, weight loss, elimination of basilar crackles, increased urine output.
- Notify physician if apical pulse rate is < 60 bpm in adult, < 70 bpm in child or < 90 bpm in infant as well as presence of other identified signs or symptoms of drug toxicity.
- Measure and document patient's daily fluid intake and output.
- Weigh patient daily before breakfast.
- Apply "Heart Medicine" label to medication container to avoid self-administration error related to look-alike drug.

OVERDOSAGE: SIGNS & SYMPTOMS

May involve signs and symptoms of the following: *GI tract* (eg, anorexia, nausea, vomiting, diarrhea); *nervous system* (eg, headache, weakness, apathy, drowsiness, visual disturbances such as blurred, yellow or green vision, halo effect), depression, confusion, restlessness, disorientation, seizures, EEG abnormalities; delirium, hallucinations, neuralgia and psychosis; *cardiovascular system* (eg, ventricular tachycardia, premature ventricular contractions, paroxysmal and nonparoxysmal nodal rhythms, AV dissociation, accelerated nodal rhythm and premature atrial contraction with block, atrial fibrillation, ECG changes, all alterations in cardiac rate and rhythm). Conduction disturbances are common manifestations of toxicity in children

Patient/Family Education

- Teach patient to take his/her own pulse before each dose of medication. Advise patient to notify physician if pulse rate is < 60 bpm, or if there is change in pulse regularity or signs and symptoms of toxicity.

- Educate patient/family to recognize and report worsening signs of congestive heart failure: cough, shortness of breath, weight gain of 1 to 2 lb/day or 5 lb/week, edema, anorexia and nausea.

See Patient Guide, p. 193.

Digoxin

(dih-JOX-in)

Lanoxicaps, Lanoxin

Class: Cardiac glycoside

Action Increases force and velocity of myocardial systolic contraction (positive inotropic action), slows heart rate and decreases conduction through atrioventricular node.

Indications Treatment of CHF, atrial fibrillation, atrial flutter, paroxysmal atrial tachycardia, cardiogenic shock.

Contraindications Ventricular fibrillation; ventricular tachycardia except in certain cases; digitalis toxicity; beriberi heart disease; hypersensitivity to digoxin; some cases of hypersensitive carotid sinus syndrome.

Route/Dosage
ADULTS: Rapid digitalization with loading dose: **IV** 0.4-0.6 mg or **PO** 0.5-0.75 mg in previously undigitalized patients; additional doses may be given cautiously at 6-8 hr intervals (**IV** 0.1-0.3 mg or **PO** 0.125-0.375 mg) until clinical response is achieved; thereafter adjust dosage based on levels (usual range 0.125-0.5 mg/day as single daily dose). In previously digitalized patients, adjust dosage in proportion to ratio of desired vs current serum levels. INFANTS & CHILDREN: Rapid digitalization with loading dose: Individualize dosage. Usual pediatric doses are listed at end of section.

Interactions
Amiodarone, anticholinergics, benzodiazepines, ACE inhibitors, diltiazem, erythromycin, indomethacin, quinidine, quinine, tetracycline, verapamil: May increase digoxin serum levels. *Antacids, antineoplastics, cholestyramine, colestipol, kaolin/pectin, metoclopramide:* May decrease absorption and effect of digoxin. *Penicillamine:* May decrease effect of digoxin. *Potassium-sparing diuretics:* May alter effect of digoxin. *Thiazide or loop diuretics:* May increase effect of digoxin. *Thyroid hormones, thioamines:* May decrease effect of digoxin.

Lab Test Interferences
None well documented.

Adverse Reactions
CV: Arrhythmias (supraventricular arrhythmias are more common in infants and children), including ventricular tachycardia and premature ventricular contractions. *CNS:* Headache; weakness; apathy; drowsiness; mental depression; confusion; disorientation. *EENT:* Visual disturbances (blurred vision, halo effect). *GI:* Anorexia; nausea; vomiting, diarrhea.

Precautions
Pregnancy: Category C. *Lactation:* Excreted in breast milk. *Children:* Newborns show varying tolerance. Premature and immature infants are particularly sensitive; reduce and individualize dose as needed. *Elderly:* Use with caution; renal clearance likely to be reduced. *Cardiovascular disease:* Electrical conversion of arrhythmias may require dose reduction. *Digitalis toxicity:* Anorexia, nausea and vomiting may be associated with toxicity or CHF. Arrhythmias for which digoxin is indicated may also be a reflection of toxicity. *Impaired renal function:* Excretion may be decreased, leading to digoxin accumulation and toxicity; adjust dosage. *Electrolyte imbalance:* Maintain normal serum potassium, calcium, and magnesium levels. *Lanoxicaps:* Have greater bio-

availability than standard tablets. The 0.2 mg capsule is equivalent to 0.25 mg tablet; the 0.1 mg capsule, to 0.125 mg tablet; the 0.05 mg capsule, to 0.0625 mg tablet.

Usual Pediatric Digitalizing and Maintenance Dosages with Normal Renal Function Based on Lean Body Weight

Age	Digitalizing Dose (mcg/kg) PO	Digitalizing Dose (mcg/kg) IV	Daily Maintenance Dose as % of Loading Dose (mcg/kg in 2-3 divided doses)
Premature	20-30	15-25	20%-30%
Term	25-35	20-30	25%-35%
1-24 mo	35-60	30-50	25%-35%
2-5 yr	30-40	25-35	25%-35%
5-10 yr	20-35	15-30	25%-35%
>10 yr	10-15	8-12	25%-35%

NURSING CONSIDERATIONS

Administration/Storage

- Administer IM doses deep into gluteal muscles and massage well to reduce painful, local reactions. IM route should be avoided; use only when other routes not available.
- Do not use solutions that are discolored or contain precipitate if dilution for IV administration is desired.
- For IV administration, digoxin injection may be diluted (up to fourfold) with normal saline, D5W or Sterile Water for Injection. Infuse slowly, over 5 min or longer.
- Do not mix digoxin solution with other drugs.
- Before administering loading dose, determine if patient has taken digoxin or other digitalis preparation in past 2 weeks.

Assessment/Interventions

- Obtain patient history, including drug history and any known allergies.
- Monitor apical pulse for 1 full min before administering. Withhold dose and notify physician if pulse rate is < 60 bpm in adult, < 70 bpm in child, or < 90 bpm in infant.
- Assess for peripheral edema and auscultate lungs for rales/crackles before and throughout therapy.
- Plan for dosage adjustments when changing from parenteral to oral (and vice versa) route of administration.
- Notify physician if signs of toxicity occur (abdominal pain, anorexia, nausea, vomiting, visual disturbance, bradycardia, ECG changes, arrhythmias, headache, seizure). Be prepared to administer digoxin antibodies (digoxin-immune Fab) for severe overdose toxicity.
- Measure and record patient's daily weight and I&O.
- Monitor serum electrolyte levels, renal and hepatic function studies, and digoxin serum levels and report changes to physician.

OVERDOSAGE: SIGNS & SYMPTOMS

May involve signs and symptoms of the following: *GI tract* (eg, anorexia, nausea, vomiting, diarrhea); *nervous system* (eg, headache, weakness, apathy, drowsiness, visual disturbances such as blurred, yellow or green vision, halo effect), depression, confusion, restlessness, disorientation, seizures, EEG abnormalities; delirium, hallucinations, neuralgia and psychosis; *cardiovascular system* (eg, ventricular tachycardia, PVCs, paroxysmal and nonparoxysmal nodal rhythms, AV dissociation, accelerated nodal rhythm and premature atrial contraction with block, atrial fibrillation, ECG changes, all alterations in cardiac rate and rhythm). Conduction disturbances are common manifestations of toxicity in children.

Patient/Family Education

- Instruct patient to take digoxin at same time each day to ensure steady-state dosing and to contact physician for instructions if dose is missed.
- Teach patient and family name, action, administration, side effects and toxic effects of particular digoxin preparation.
- Emphasize importance of regular follow-up exams to determine effectiveness and to monitor for toxicity.
- Caution patient to avoid otc medications without consulting physician. Antacids and antidiarrheals, for example, slow absorption of digoxin.
- Teach patient and family to take pulse and to seek physician's advice for rates lower than 60 bpm or higher than 100 bpm (adults).
- Help patient identify ways to supplement potassium intake if prescribed by physician.

See Patient Guide, p. 194.

Dihydroergotamine Mesylate

(DIE-high-droe-err-GOT-uh-meen MEH-sih-LATE)

D.H.E. 45

Class: Analgesic/migraine/ergotamine derivative

Action Constricts peripheral and cranial blood vessels, depresses central vasomotor centers and reduces extracranial blood flow.

Indications Abortion or prevention of vascular headaches such as migraine, migraine-variant and cluster headache.

Contraindications Hypersensitivity to ergot alkaloids hepatic or renal impairment; severe pruritus; coronary artery disease; uncontrolled peripheral vascular disease; hypertension; sepsis; use during pregnancy, lactation or in women who may become pregnant; concurrent vasoconstrictor therapy.

Route/Dosage

ADULTS: **IM** 1 mg at first sign of headache; repeat q hr until symptomatic relief is achieved; do not exceed 3 mg IM per single migraine attack. If a more rapid effect is desired, give IV to maximum of 2 mg (maximum 6 mg/wk).

Interactions

Beta-blockers, macrolide antibiotics (eg, erythromycin), vasoconstrictors (eg, epinephrine): Can increase peripheral ischemia, cyanosis and numbness caused by ergot alkaloids. *Nitrates (eg, nitroglycerin)*: May oppose effects of nitrates.

Lab Test Interferences

None well documented.

Adverse Reactions

CV: Pulselessness; precordial distress or pain; transient tachycardia or bradycardia; raised arterial pressure; coronary vasoconstriction. *GI:* Nausea;

vomiting; abdominal pain. *OTHER:* Numbness and tingling of fingers and toes; muscle pain in extremities; weakness in legs; localized edema; itching. Drug has oxytocic and spasmolytic properties.

Precautions

Pregnancy: Category X. *Lactation:* Excreted in breast milk and may inhibit lactation. Drug can cause symptoms of ergotism in infant. *Children:* Safety and efficacy not established. *Dependence/withdrawal syndrome:* Has occurred with other ergot alkaloids; therefore recommended dosage should not be exceeded.

NURSING CONSIDERATIONS

Administration/Storage

- IM route is preferred. Do not mix with any other drug in syringe or solution.
- For IM administration, inject at first sign of headache. To determine minimal effective dose, adjust dose for several headaches and then use minimal effective dose at onset of subsequent attacks.
- For rapid effect, administer IV. May be given undiluted; give 1 mg or fraction thereof over 1 min.
- After drug is administered, have patient lie supine and relax for few min, preferably in quiet, darkened room.
- Avoid prolonged administration or excessive dosage because of danger of ergotism and gangrene.
- Protect ampules from light and heat.

Assessment/Interventions

- Obtain patient history, including drug history and any known allergies.
- Determine history of hypersensitivity to dihydroergotamine and ergotamine derivatives.
- Obtain baseline vital signs, with special attention to pulse and BP.
- Evaluate mental status and peripheral neurocirculatory status (eg, sensation, edema, color, weakness).
- Prepare drug in syringe that is free of other drugs and solutions and administer drug undiluted.
- Obtain baseline assessment of pain severity.
- Monitor for changes in vital signs, especially pulse and BP.
- Monitor for changes in mental status (eg, confusion, drowsiness).
- Monitor for effectiveness of headache relief with pain assessments every 15 min and for minimal effective dose.
- Check neurocirculatory status of extremities, especially distally (eg, pulse, warmth, color).

OVERDOSAGE: SIGNS & SYMPTOMS

Nausea, vomiting, leg weakness, pain in limb muscles, numbness and tingling of toes, precordial pain, changes in heart rate and BP, localized edema, itching, peripheral ischemia, gangrene, confusion, depression, drowsiness, convulsions

Patient/Family Education

- Caution patient that this medication must not be taken during pregnancy or when pregnancy is possible. Advise patient to use reliable form of birth control while taking this drug.
- Teach patient to measure or rate drug effectiveness (eg, use analog or other validated rating scale).
- Instruct patient to take drug at first sign of impending headache and not to exceed maximum dosage.
- Advise patient to relax in supine position in quiet, darkened room after drug administration.
- Tell patient to inform physician if diagnosed with any peripheral vascular disease.
- Instruct patient to report these symptoms to physician: pain, itching, weakness, tingling, edema, pallor, coolness, numbness (especially in distal extremities), chest discomfort or pain or any change in mental status

such as drowsiness, light-headedness, syncope or seizures.

- Advise patient to avoid intake of alcoholic beverages, smoking and exposure to cold because these vasoconstrictors may further impair peripheral circulation and cause or aggravate migraine headache.

See Patient Guide, p. 195.

Diltiazem HCl

(dill-TIE-uh-zem HIGH-droe-KLOR-ide)

Cardizem, Cardizem CD, Cardizem SR, Dilacor XR, Novo-Diltazen, Syn-Diltiazen, ♣ *APO-Diltiaz, Nu-Diltiaz*

Class: Calcium channel blocker

Action Inhibits movement of calcium ions across cell membrane in systemic and coronary vascular smooth muscle; slows calcium ion movement across cell membranes in both cardiac muscle and cardiac pacemaker cells, decreasing sinoatrial and atrioventricular (AV) conduction.

Indications
Oral form: Treatment of angina pectoris due to coronary artery spasm; chronic stable angina (classic effort-associated angina; Prinzmetal variant); essential hypertension (sustained released form only). *Parenteral form:* Treatment of atrial fibrillation or flutter; paroxysmal supraventricular tachycardia. **Unlabeled use:** Treatment of Raynaud's syndrome.

Contraindications Sick sinus syndrome; second- or third-degree AV block; except with functioning pacemaker; hypotension with systolic pressure < 90 mm Hg; acute MI; pulmonary congestion.

Route/Dosage
ADULTS: **PO** 120-360 mg/day in 4 divided doses. Sustained or controlled release forms may be given once or twice daily. *Dilacor XR (for angina):* Adjust dosage to each patient's needs, starting with a dose of 120 mg once daily, which may be titrated to doses of up to 480 mg once daily. Titration may be carried out over a 7 to 14 day period. **IV** Initial bolus of 0.25 mg/kg (average dose 20 mg) given over 2 min. May repeat after 15 min with 0.35 mg/kg (average dose 25 mg) given over 2 min. Subsequent boluses are titrated to response. Continuous infusion of 10 mg/hr may be started immediately after bolus dose (20 or 25 mg). Titration to response is done within range of 5-15 mg/hr. Infusion for longer than 24 hr is not recommended.

Interactions
Beta-blockers: May have additive negative inotropic and chronotropic effects. *Carbamazepine:* Carbamazepine levels may increase. *Cimetidine, ranitidine:* Diltiazem levels may be increased. *Cyclosporine:* Cyclosporine levels and toxicity may increase. *Encainide:* Encainide levels may increase. *Other antihypertensive agents:* May have additive effects.

Lab Test Interferences
None well documented.

Adverse Reactions
CV: Peripheral edema; hypotension (especially during initial treatment or with dose increases); bradycardia; angina; AV block; abnormal ECG; arrhythmias. *CNS:* Dizziness, lightheadedness; headache; weakness; shakiness; somnolence; asthenia. *GI:* Nausea; vomiting; constipation; abdominal discomfort; cramps; dyspepsia; dry mouth. *HEMA:* Leukopenia. *DERM:* Dermatitis; photosensitivity; petechiae; rash; hair loss; erythema multiforme; Stevens-Johnson syndrome. *OTHER:* Flushing; micturation disorder; gingival hyperplasia; gynecomastia; joint pain.

Precautions
Pregnancy: Category C. *Lactation:* Excreted in breast milk. *Children:* Safety and efficacy not established. *CHF:* Use with caution. *Hepatic or renal impairment:* Use with caution. Dosage

may need to be decreased. *Withdrawal syndrome:* Abrupt withdrawal may cause increased frequency and duration of angina. Dosage is tapered gradually.

NURSING CONSIDERATIONS

Administration/Storage

- Oral doses may be given with meals if GI irritation occurs.
- Keep injectable solutions under refrigeration.

Assessment/Interventions

- Obtain patient history, including drug history and any known allergies.
- Monitor BP and pulse periodically throughout therapy.
- Monitor ECG frequently during IV administration. Be alert for evidence of AV block.
- Measure I&O and weight during therapy.
- Assess for fluid overload: edema, rales, dyspnea, weight gain, jugular vein distention. Notify physician if these signs occur.
- Assess lab studies for renal and hepatic function with long-term therapy. Consider dosage adjustment if hepatic dysfunction is present.
- If patient is receiving cardiac glycosides (eg, digoxin) concurrently monitor serum digoxin levels. If signs of digitalis toxicity occur, notify physician.
- If dizziness occurs, institute safety precautions for falls. Have patient sit up for a few minutes before rising.

OVERDOSAGE: SIGNS & SYMPTOMS

Bradycardia, hypotension, high-degree AV block, heart failure

Patient/Family Education

- Teach patient to take pulse. Emphasize importance of doing so regularly while taking medication.
- Remind patient to swallow sustained release capsules whole.
- Caution patient to avoid sudden position changes to prevent orthostatic hypotension.
- Notify physician if irregular heart beat, shortness of breath, swelling of the hands and feet, pronounced dizziness, constipation, nausea or hypotension develop.
- Advise patient of importance of regular use of this medication. If dose is missed but remembered shortly after it was scheduled, missed dose should be taken. However, if time is close to next scheduled dose, missed dose should be skipped.
- Counsel patient to avoid intake of alcoholic beverages and otc medications without consulting physician.

See Patient Guide, p. 196.

Dimenhydrinate

(die-men-HIGH-drih-nate)

Calm-X, Dimetabs, Dommanate, Dramamine, Dramanate, Dramojet, Dymenate, Hydrate, Nico-Vert, Triptone, Vertab, Wehamine

Class: Antiemetic and antivertigo/anticholinergic

Action Directly inhibits labyrinthine stimulation for up to 3 hr.

Indications Prevention and treatment of motion sickness, dizziness, nausea, vomiting. **Unlabeled uses:** Treatment of Meniere's disease, nausea and vomiting of pregnancy, postoperative nausea and vomiting.

Contraindications Use in neonates; allergic reactions to diphenhydramine.

Route/Dosage

Motion Sickness

ADULTS: **PO** 50-100 mg 30 min prior to travel, followed by 50-100 mg q 4-6 hr (maximum 400 mg/day). **IM** 50 mg prn. **IV** 50 mg in 10 ml of Sodium Chloride for Injection administered over 2 min. CHILDREN (6-12 YR): **PO** 25-50 mg q 6-8 hr (maximum 150 mg/day). **IM** 1.25 mg/kg qid (maximum 300 mg/day). CHILDREN (2-6 YR): **PO** Up to 12.5-25 mg q 6-8 hr (maximum 75 mg/day). **IM** 1.25 mg/kg qid (maximum 300 mg/day).

Interactions

Alcohol, CNS depressants: Enhances CNS depressant effects. *Aminoglycosides:* May mask signs of aminoglycoside-related ototoxicity. *Anticholinergic drugs:* Causes additive anticholinergic effects. INCOMPATIBILITIES: Ammonium chloride, amobarbital, butorphanol, chlorpromazine, glycopyrrolate, heparin, hydrocortisone, hydroxyzine, midazolam, pentobarbital, phenobarbital, phenytoin, prednisolone, prochlorperazine, promethazine, tetracycline, theophylline, thiopental, trifluoperazine.

Lab Test Interferences

May cause false elevation in serum theophylline levels.

Adverse Reactions

CV: Palpitations; hypotension; tachycardia. *RESP:* Tightness of chest; wheezing; thickening of bronchial secretions. *CNS.* Sedation; hallucinations; delirium; drowsiness; confusion, nervousness; restlessness; headache; insomnia; tingling, heaviness and weakness of hands; vertigo; dizziness; lassitude; excitation. *EENT:* Diminished night vision; decreased color discrimination; exacerbation of narrow-angle glaucoma; blurred vision; diplopia; nasal stuffiness; dryness of nose and throat. *GI:* Nausea; vomiting; diarrhea; GI distress; constipation; anorexia; dry mouth. *GU:* Prostatic enlargement; difficult or painful urination. *DERM:* Fixed drug eruption; photosensitivity. *OTHER:* Anaphylaxis.

Precautions

Pregnancy: Category B. *Lactation:* Excreted in breast milk. *Children:* Safety and efficacy in children < 2 yr not established. *Special risk patients:* Use caution in patients with asthma, prostatic hypertrophy, narrow-angle glaucoma, stenosing peptic ulcer, cardiac arrhythmias. *Hypersensitivity:* Previous reactions to diphenhydramine.

NURSING CONSIDERATIONS

Administration/Storage

- Administer with food or milk to minimize nausea or GI distress.
- When administering drug IM, use Z-track method to avoid SC irritation.
- When administering drug IV, confirm correct catheter or needle placement. Note that this drug should never be given intra-arterially.

Assessment/Interventions

- Obtain patient history, including drug history and any known allergies.
- Assess drug history for concomitant use of other CNS depressants, alcohol and nonprescription CNS depressants, which could have additive effect.
- Take safety precautions if drowsiness or dizziness occurs.
- Assess patient's nutritional status, weigh patient daily and monitor I&O if drug is given to stop or prevent nausea and vomiting.
- If a paradoxical effect occurs (insomnia, CNS stimulation), notify physician.
- If visual or auditory disturbances occur (blurred vision/tinnitus, hearing loss), notify the physician.

> **OVERDOSAGE: SIGNS & SYMPTOMS**
>
> Drowsiness, hallucinations, convulsions, coma, respiratory depression

Patient/Family Education

- Advise patient to take medication 30 to 60 min before activity that may produce nausea or motion sickness.

- Instruct patient to report these symptoms to physician: drowsiness, nervousness, dry mouth, insomnia, constipation and blurred vision.
- If dimenhydrinate is being given as antiemetic, instruct patient to report nausea and vomiting to the physician.
- Instruct patient to take sips of water frequently, suck on ice chips or sugarless hard candy or chew sugarless gum if dry mouth occurs and to relieve constipation with increased fiber in diet and good hydration.
- Caution patient to avoid intake of alcoholic beverages or other CNS depressants.
- Advise patient that drug may cause drowsiness and to use caution while driving or performing other tasks requiring mental alertness.

See Patient Guide, p. 197.

Dinoprostone (PGE_2; Prostaglandin E_2)

(DIE-no-PROSTE-ohn)

Cervidil, Prepidil, Prostin E_2

Class: Prostaglandin/cervical ripening; abortifacient

Action Stimulates gravid uterus to contract; also stimulates smooth muscle of GI tract.

Indications
Gel: Cervical ripening in pregnant women at or near term with need for labor induction. *Vaginal suppositories:* Termination of pregnancy from 12-20 wk.

Contraindications Hypersensitivity to prostaglandins; patients in whom oxytocic drugs are contraindicated or when prolonged contractions of uterus are considered inappropriate; ruptured membranes; placenta previa; unexplained vaginal bleeding during current pregnancy; when vaginal delivery is not indicated; acute pelvic inflammatory disease; active cardiac, pulmonary, renal or hepatic disease.

Route/Dosage
Cervical Ripening
ADULTS: **Intravaginal Gel** 0.5 mg (contents of one syringe); may repeat dose 6 hr later if necessary (maximum dose 1.5 mg (3 syringes)/24 hr). **Intravaginal Insert** 10 mg (1 insert). Releases approximately 0.3 mg/hr over 12 hr. Remove insert upon onset of active labor or 12 hr after insertion.

Termination of Pregnancy
ADULTS: **Intravaginal** 1 suppository (20 mg) high into vagina. Repeat at 3-5 hr intervals until abortion occurs. Do not give continuously for > 2 days.

Interactions
Oxytocic agents: May augment effect of other oxytocic agents; avoid concomitant use.

Lab Test Interferences
None well documented.

Adverse Reactions
CV: Transient fall in BP; syncope; dizziness; arrhythmias. *RESP:* Bronchospasm; coughing; dyspnea; wheezing. *CNS:* Headache; flushing; anxiety; tension; hot flashes; paresthesia; weakness. *GI:* Anorexia; nausea; vomiting; diarrhea. *GU:* Uterine contractile abnormality; endometritis; uterine rupture; uterine pain; amnionitis; premature rupture of membranes; vaginal pain; warm feeling in vagina. *EENT:* Blurred vision; eye pain. *OTHER:* Back pain; muscular cramps; fever; chills; joint inflammation; breast tenderness; diaphoresis; rash; leg cramps; dehydration. *Fetal effects:* Fetal heart rate abnormalities; bradycardia; deceleration; sepsis; depression (1 min Apgar <7); acidosis.

Precautions
Pregnancy: Category C. Contraindicated if fetus in utero has reached

viability stage except when cervical ripening is indicated. *Lactation:* Undetermined. *Special risk patients:* Use with caution in patients with asthma, glaucoma, or raised intraocular pressure, hypotension or hypertension, cardiovascular or renal or hepatic dysfunction, anemia, jaundice, diabetes, epilepsy, compromised uterus, infected endocervical lesions; acute vaginitis.

NURSING CONSIDERATIONS

Administration/Storage

- Store suppository and insert in freezer. Store gel in refrigerator. Bring both to room temperature just prior to use, do not use external sources of heat (eg, hot water bath or microwave oven) to decrease warming time.
- Carefully examine vagina to determine degree of effacement and appropriate length of endocervical catheter to be used for application of gel (10 mm if 50% effaced, 20 mm if no effacement).
- Patient should be in dorsal position for administration and remain supine for 15-30 min after administration.
- Prevent contact of this drug with skin. Use of latex gloves followed by thorough hand washing with soap and water are recommended.
- Drug should be used in hospital setting only.

Assessment/Interventions

- Obtain patient history, including drug history and any known allergies.
- Perform physical assessment to determine baseline vital signs and fetopelvic relationships.
- Perform careful uterine and fetal monitoring throughout use of dinoprostone.
- Wait at least 6-12 hr after administration of gel before using IV oxytocin, a dosing interval of at least 30 minutes is recommended after removal of insert.
- Monitor patient closely for adverse reactions including nausea, vomiting or diarrhea.
- Monitor vital signs frequently during administration, noting especially any increase in temperature and hypertension or hypotension.
- Monitor for hypersensitivity reactions such as bronchospasms, cardiac arrhythmias or seizures. Notify physician should any of these symptoms occur.

OVERDOSAGE: SIGNS & SYMPTOMS

Uterine hypercontractility, uterine hypertonus

Patient/Family Education

- Inform patient of expected action and possible adverse reactions with drug.
- Inform patient that uterine contractions are expected and that if pain from contractions becomes severe, physician will be notified to obtain order for analgesic.
- Instruct patient to report these symptoms to nurse immediately: nausea, vomiting, difficulty breathing, chest pain or headache.

No patient monograph available.

Diphenhydramine HCl

(die-fen-HIGH-druh-meen HIGH-droe-KLOR-ide)

AllerMax, Banophen, Belix, Benadryl, Benahist, Ben-Allergin-50, Benoject, Benylin Cough, Bydramine Cough, Compoz Nighttime Sleep Aid, Diphen Cough, Diphenacen-50, Genahist, Gen-D-phen, Hydramine, Hydramyn, Hyrexin-50, Maximum Strength Sleepinal, Maximum Strength Unisom SleepGels, Nidryl, Nytol, Phendry, Sleep-Eze 3, Sleepwell 2-nite, Sominex, Tusstat, Twilite, Uni-

Bent Cough, Wehdryl, ♣ *Allerdryl, Sleep-eze D*
Class: Antihistamine/ethanolamine

Action Competitively antagonizes histamine at H_1 receptor sites.

Indications Symptomatic relief of perennial and seasonal allergic rhinitis, vasomotor rhinitis and allergic conjunctivitis; temporary relief of runny nose and sneezing caused by common cold; relief of allergic and nonallergic pruritic symptoms; treatment of urticaria and angioedema; amelioration of allergic reactions to blood or plasma; adjunct to epinephrine and other standard measures in anaphylaxis; relief of uncomplicated allergic conditions of immediate type when oral therapy is impossible or contraindicated (parenteral form); treatment and prophylactic treatment of motion sickness; nighttime sleep aid; management of parkinsonism (including drug-induced) in elderly who are intolerant of more potent agents, in mild cases in other age groups and in combination with centrally acting anticholinergics; control of cough from colds or allergy (syrup formulations).

Contraindications Hypersensitivity to antihistamines; narrow-angle glaucoma; stenosing peptic ulcer; symptomatic prostatic hypertrophy; asthmatic attack; bladder neck obstruction; pyloroduodenal obstruction; monoamine oxidase (MAO) inhibitor therapy; history of sleep apnea; use in newborn or premature infants and in nursing women.

Route/Dosage
ADULTS: **PO** 25-50 mg q 6-8 hr. **IV/IM** 10-100 mg if required (maximum 400 mg/day). CHILDREN (> 10 KG): **PO** 12.5-25 mg tid or qid or 5 mg/kg/day or 150 mg/m^2/day (maximum 300 mg/day). **IM/IV** 5 mg/kg/day or 150 mg/m^2/day (max 300 mg) in 4 divided doses.

Motion Sickness
ADULTS: Initial dose: **PO** 25-50 mg 30 min before exposure to motion followed by repeat doses 3-4 times/day for duration of exposure. CHILDREN: Initial dose: 12.5-25 mg 30 min before exposure to motion; repeat dosage pattern same as for adults.

Nighttime Sleep Aid
ADULTS: **PO** 50 mg at bedtime.

Cough Suppressant (Syrup)
ADULTS: **PO** 25 mg q 4 hr (maximum 150 mg/24 hr). CHILDREN (6-12 YR): **PO** 12.5 mg q 4 hr (maximum 75 mg/24 hr). CHILDREN (2-6 YR): **PO** 6.25 mg q 4 hr (maximum 25 mg/24 hr).

Interactions
Alcohol, CNS depressants: May cause additive CNS depression. MAO *inhibitors:* May increase anticholinergic effects. INCOMPATIBILITIES: Injectable form is incompatible with dexamethasone sodium phosphate, furosemide, iodipamide meglumine, parenteral barbiturates and phenytoin.

Lab Test Interferences
Skin tests: Antihistamines may prevent or diminish otherwise positive reaction to dermal reactivity indicators.

Adverse Reactions
CV: Orthostatic hypotension; palpitations; bradycardia; tachycardia; reflex tachycardia; extrasystoles; faintness. *RESP:* Thickening of bronchial secretions; chest tightness; wheezing; respiratory depression. *CNS:* Drowsiness (often transient); sedation; dizziness; faintness; disturbed coordination. *EENT:* Nasal stuffiness; dry mouth, nose and throat; sore throat. *GI:* Epigastric distress; nausea; vomiting; diarrhea; constipation; change in bowel habits. *HEMA:* Hemolytic anemia; thrombocytopenia; agranulocytosis. *META:* Increased appetite, weight gain. *OTHER:* Hypersensitivity reactions; photosensitivity.

Precautions
Pregnancy: Category B. *Lactation:* Excreted in breast milk. *Children:*

Contraindicated in newborn and premature infants. Overdosage may cause hallucinations, convulsions and death. Antihistamines may diminish mental alertness. In young children drug may produce paradoxical excitation. Use with caution in children < 2 yr. *Elderly and debilitated patients:* Greater risk of dizziness, excessive sedation, syncope, toxic confusional states and hypotension in patients > 60 yr. Dosage reduction may be required. *Special risk patients:* Use with caution in patients predisposed to urinary retention, prostatic hypertrophy, history of bronchial asthma, increased intraocular pressure, hyperthyroidism, cardiovascular disease or hypertension. *Hepatic impairment:* Use with caution in patients with cirrhosis or other liver diseases. *Hypersensitivity reactions:* May occur. Have epinephrine 1:1000 immediately available. *Respiratory disease:* Generally not recommended to treat lower respiratory tract symptoms including asthma. *Sulfites:* Some diphenhydramine products may contain sulfites as preservatives and aspartame as sweetener. Avoid in sulfite-allergic patients and in patients with phenylketonuria, respectively.

NURSING CONSIDERATIONS

Administration/Storage

- If patient is prone to excessive salivation (eg, postencephalitic patients), administer drug after meals. If mouth dries excessively, administer drug before meals.
- Syrup formulations are used only for control of cough.
- If drug is prescribed for motion sickness, administer first dose 30 min prior to exposure to motion.
- Give IM injection deep in muscle.
- Do not administer drug for at least 2 days before skin allergy testing.
- Store in tightly closed containers at room temperature.
- Store injection formulation in light-resistant container and protect from light.

Assessment/Interventions

- Obtain patient history, including drug history and any known allergies. Be alert for conditions that may place patient at greater risk for adverse effects (eg, bronchial asthma, glaucoma or prostatic hypertrophy).
- Be prepared to institute supportive treatment (advanced life support) in event of severe adverse reaction or overdose.
- Observe patient for adverse reactions to medication such as dry mouth, headaches, disorientation, drowsiness, tachycardia, shortness of breath, nausea, skin rash, urinary retention, constipation or increase in BP.
- If administering medication to children or elderly, be alert to fact that they are more likely to experience side effects and paradoxical reactions such as excitement, irritability and sleeplessness.
- Explain that drowsiness may occur at first but will lessen or disappear during long-term therapy.

OVERDOSAGE: SIGNS & SYMPTOMS

Circulatory collapse, cardiac arrest, respiratory depression or arrest, toxic psychosis, coma, stupor, seizures, ataxia, anxiety, incoherence, hyperactivity, combativeness, anhidrosis, fever, hot, dry, flushed skin, dry mucous membranes, dysphagia, decreased bowel sounds, dilated and sluggish pupils

Patient/Family Education

- Instruct patient not to discontinue long-term therapy without consulting physician.
- Warn patient using topical medication to avoid excessive application to skin eruptions.
- Instruct patient to report these symptoms to physician: excessive drowsiness or dry mouth, GI upset, constipation, blurred vision, rash, hives, difficulty breathing, difficulty urinat-

ing, confusion, fainting or irregular heart rate.

- Encourage patient to take sips of water frequently, suck on ice chips or sugarless hard candy or chew sugarless gum if dry mouth occurs.
- Instruct patient to avoid intake of alcoholic beverages or other CNS depressants.
- Advise patient that drug may cause drowsiness and to use caution while driving or performing other tasks requiring mental alertness.

See Patient Guide, p. 198.

Diphenoxylate HCl/Atropine Sulfate

(die-fen-OX-ih-late HIGH-droe-KLOR-ide/AT-troe-peen SULL-fate)

Logen, Lomanate, Lomotil, Lonox

Class: Antidiarrheal

Action Diphenoxylate, related to meperidine, decreases motility of GI tract. Atropine discourages deliberate overdosage of diphenoxylate.

Indications Adjunctive therapy in treatment of diarrhea.

Contraindications Obstructive jaundice; diarrhea associated with pseudomembranous enterocolitis or enterotoxin-producing bacteria; narrow-angle glaucoma; use in children < 2 yr.

Route/Dosage

ADULTS: Initial dose: **PO** 5 mg qid. Individualize dose. CHILDREN 2-12 YR: **PO** 0.3-0.4 mg/kg/day in 4 divided doses.

Interactions

Alcohol, barbiturates, CNS depressants, tranquilizers: May increase depressant action *Monoamine oxidase (MAO) inhibitors:* May precipitate hypertensive crisis.

Lab Test Interferences

None well documented.

Adverse Reactions

CV: Tachycardia. *CNS:* Dizziness; drowsiness; sedation; headache; malaise; lethargy; restlessness; euphoria; depression; numbness of extremities; confusion. *GI:* Dry mouth; anorexia; nausea; vomiting; abdominal discomfort; paralytic ileus; toxic megacolon; pancreatitis; constipation. *GU:* Urinary retention. *DERM:* Pruritus; angioneurotic edema; urticaria; dry skin and mucous membranes; flushing. *OTHER:* Swelling of gums; anaphylaxis; hyperthermia.

Precautions

Pregnancy: Category B. *Lactation:* Excreted in breast milk. *Children:* Contraindicated in children < 2 yr. Greater risk of atropinism, especially with Down syndrome. *Diarrhea:* Do not give for diarrhea associated with organisms that penetrate the intestinal mucosa (ie, *Salmonella, Shigella*), acute Crohn's disease or pseudomembranous colitis caused by antibiotic therapy. Notify physician and discontinue therapy for abdominal distention or other untoward symptoms. *Fluid/electrolyte imbalance:* Dehydration may contribute to adverse effects, especially in young children. If dehydration or electrolyte imbalance occurs, may need to discontinue therapy until condition is corrected. *Hepatic impairment:* Use with extreme caution; may precipitate hepatic coma.

NURSING CONSIDERATIONS

Administration/Storage

- May administer drug with food if GI irritation occurs.
- Administer liquid form to children 2-12 yr.
- Tablets may be crushed and administered with fluid.
- Store in tightly closed, light-resistant container at room temperature.

Assessment/Interventions

- Obtain patient history, including drug history and any known allergies. Note if patient is currently using MAO inhibitors (discontinuation may be necessary).
- Assess frequency and consistency of stools before and throughout therapy.
- Assess skin turgor and monitor fluid and electrolyte status during therapy.
- If signs of dehydration occur (poor skin turgor, decreased urine output, orthostatic hypotension, pulse changes, weight loss), notify physician.
- If signs and symptoms of toxic megacolon occur (abdominal pain, distention), notify physician.

OVERDOSAGE: SIGNS & SYMPTOMS

Dry skin and mucous membranes, mydriasis, restlessness, flushing, hyperthermia, tachycardia, lethargy, coma, nystagmus, pinpoint pupils, respiratory depression

Patient/Family Education

- Advise patient to continue taking drug until diarrhea has stopped for 24-36 hr. Discontinuing medication earlier may result in relapse or return of diarrhea.
- Instruct patient to notify physician if fever and palpitations occur or when diarrhea persists or becomes malodorous or bloody.
- Tell patient to take sips of water frequently, suck on ice chips or sugarless hard candy or chew sugarless gum if dry mouth occurs.
- Instruct patient to avoid intake of alcoholic beverages or other CNS depressants.
- Advise patient that drug may cause drowsiness and to use caution while driving or performing other tasks requiring mental alertness.

See Patient Guide, p. 199.

Diphtheria/Tetanus Toxoids/Acellular Pertussis Vaccine (DTaP)

(diff-THEER-ee-uh/TET-ah-nus toxoids/ay-SELL-you-luhr per-TUSS-iss vaccine)

Acel-Imune, Tripedia

Class: Vaccine, inactivated bacteria

Action Diphtheria and tetanus toxoids induce antibodies against toxins made by *Corynebacterium diphtheriae* and *Clostridium tetani*. Pertussis vaccine protects against *Bordetella pertussis*.

Indications Induction of active immunity against diphtheria, tetanus and pertussis administered as fourth or fifth dose in children 15 mo-7th birthday. Recipients must be previously immunized with 3 or 4 doses of whole-cell DTP (DTwP).

Contraindications Children who recovered from culture-confirmed pertussis; history of serious adverse reactions to previous dose of pertussis-containing vaccine; immediate anaphylactic reaction or encephalopathy occurring within 7 days after any DTP vaccination. (If contraindication to pertussis-vaccine component occurs, substitute diphtheria and tetanus toxoids for pediatric use [DT] for each of remaining doses.)

Route/Dosage

Ensure that patient's immunization history includes at least 3 doses of DTwP vaccine without adverse side effects.

Fourth Dose

CHILDREN 15-18 MO: **IM** 0.5 ml at least 6 mo after third DTwP dose.

Fifth Dose

CHILDREN 4-6 YR: **IM** 0.5 ml.

Interactions

Anticoagulants: Give DTaP with caution to persons on anticoagulant therapy. *Immunosuppressants*: May reduce vaccine's effectiveness. *Influenza vaccine*: To attribute causality of adverse reactions, do not give influenza vaccine within 3 days of pertussis vaccination.

Lab Test Interferences

None well documented.

Adverse Reactions

RESP: Upper respiratory infection or rhinitis. *GI*: Diarrhea or loose stools; vomiting. *DERM*: Rash. *OTHER*: Fever. Causal association exists between DTwP and acute encephalopathy, shock and unusual shock-like state, anaphylaxis and protracted, inconsolable crying; whether this association also occurs with DTaP administration is presently unknown. *OTHER*: *Local effects*: erythema; tenderness; induration. Chills; fatigue; myalgia; arthralgia.

Precautions

Pregnancy: Category C. *Lactation*: Undetermined. *Children*: Contraindicated for children < 15 mo or > 7 yr. *Febrile illness or acute infection*: Defer immunization during course of illness. Minor respiratory illness such as mild upper respiratory infection is usually not reason to defer immunization. *Immunodeficiency*: Defer immunization, if possible, until immunocompetency is restored. *Thrombocytopenia or coagulation disorder that would contraindicate IM injection*: Give vaccine with caution.

NURSING CONSIDERATIONS

Administration/Storage

- Administer drug by IM route only. Anterolateral aspect of thigh or deltoid muscle of upper arm is preferred. Do not inject in gluteal area or other areas with major nerve trunk.
- May administer vaccine with trivalent oral polio, injectable polio, *Haemophilus b*, hepatitis B, varicella, and measles, mumps and rubella virus vaccines.
- Always record manufacturer's name and vaccine lot number in child's permanent record file, along with date of administration, name, address and title of person administering vaccine.
- Shake vial well to ensure uniform suspension before withdrawing dose. If clumps remain after vigorous agitation, discard vial and contents. Rotate vial in palm to bring contents to room temperature before administration.
- Refrigerate vials; do not freeze. Discard frozen vaccine.

Assessment/Interventions

- Obtain patient history, including drug history and any known allergies.
- Check patient's immunization history to ensure that at least 3 doses of DTwP vaccine have previously been given. Give DTaP at least 6 mo after third DTP dose.
- Review patient's medical history for conditions that would contraindicate DTaP vaccine (children who have recovered from culture-confirmed pertussis, history of serious adverse reactions to previous dose of DTaP, hypersensitivity to any component of vaccine, anaphylactic reaction or encephalopathy occurring within 7 days after any DTP vaccination).
- Take child's temperature to determine if infection is present.
- Defer immunization during course of any febrile illness or acute infection. Minor respiratory illness such as mild upper respiratory infection is not usually reason to defer immunization.
- Give any DTP injection with caution to children with thrombocytopenia or any coagulation disorder in whom IM injection may be contraindicated.
- When child returns for next dose in series of either pertussis or any DTP vaccine, question child's parent or guardian about side effects to previous dose. If any serious side effects are noted, additional pertussis vaccine may not be appropriate. Consult with

child's pediatrician and continue childhood immunization with bivalent diphtheria and tetanus toxoids for pediatric use if recommended.

- There are no data on whether prophylactic use of antipyretic drugs (eg, acetaminophen) can decrease risk of febrile convulsions. Acetaminophen may reduce incidence of postvaccination fever. Immunization Practices Advisory Committee and American Academy of Pediatrics suggest administering appropriate dose of acetaminophen (based on age) at time of vaccination and q 4-6 hr to children at higher risk for seizures than general population (ie, children with personal or family history of seizures).

Patient/Family Education

- Inform parent of name, action, administration and side effects of DTaP.
- Provide parent with immunization history record and record this immunization in patient's medical record.
- Instruct patient to give acetaminophen for fever or local pain.
- If patient still requires 5th dose, inform parent of immunization schedule (5th dose: 4-6 yr).
- Advise parent to check with local school board; some school systems require that children receive 5th dose before entrance into kindergarten or elementary school.

No patient monograph available.

Diphtheria/Tetanus Toxoids/Whole-Cell Pertussis Vaccine (DTwP)

(diff-THEER-ee-uh/TET-ah-nus toxoids/whole cell per-TUSS-iss vaccine)

DTwP, Tri-Immunol

Class: Vaccine, inactivated bacteria

Action Diphtheria and tetanus toxoids induce antibodies against toxins made by *Corynebacterium diphtheriae* and *Clostridium tetani*. Pertussis vaccine protects against *Bordetella pertussis*.

Indications Induction of active immunity against diphtheria, tetanus and pertussis for children.

Contraindications Children who recovered from culture-confirmed pertussis; history of serious adverse reactions to previous dose of pertussis-containing vaccine; immediate anaphylactic reaction or encephalopathy occurring within 7 days after any DTP vaccination. (If contraindication to pertussis-vaccine component occurs, substitute diphtheria and tetanus toxoids for pediatric use [DT] for each of the remaining doses.)

Route/Dosage

CHILDREN: **IM** 0.5 ml at 2 mo, 4 mo, 6 mo, and 12-18 mo and 4-6 yr.

Interactions

Anticoagulants: Give DTwP with caution to persons on anticoagulant therapy. *Influenza vaccine:* To attribute causality of adverse reactions, do not give influenza vaccine within 3 days of pertussis vaccination. *Immunosuppressants:* May reduce efficacy of vaccine. If possible, deter giving vaccine until immunocompetency returns.

Lab Test Interferences

None well documented.

Adverse Reactions

RESP: Upper respiratory infection or rhinitis. *GI:* Diarrhea or loose stools; vomiting. *DERM:* Rash. *OTHER:* Fever; irritability. Although very rare, causal association exists between DTwP and acute encephalopathy, shock and unusual shocklike state, anaphylaxis and protracted, inconsolable crying; pain, redness and induration at injection site.

Precautions

Pregnancy: Category C. *Lactation:* Undetermined. *Children:* Contraindicated in children < 6 wk or > 7 yr;

do not reduce or divide dose for infants or children. *Children with thrombocytopenia or any coagulation disorder in whom IM injection may be contraindicated:* Give vaccine with caution. *Febrile illness or acute infection:* Defer immunization during course of illness. Minor respiratory illness such as mild upper respiratory infection is not usually reason to defer immunization. *Hypersensitivity:* Review patient history for possible sensitivity. Have epinephrine 1:1000 immediately available. *Infections:* Do not use DTwP for treatment of actual infection.

NURSING CONSIDERATIONS

Administration/Storage

- Administer drug by IM route only. Anterolateral aspect of thigh or deltoid muscle of upper arm is preferred. Do not inject in gluteal area or other areas with major nerve trunk.
- May administer vaccine with trivalent oral polio, injectable polio, *Haemophilus b*, hepatitis B, varicella, and measles, mumps and rubella virus vaccines.
- Always record the manufacturer's name and vaccine lot number in child's permanent record file, along with date of administration, name, address and title of person administering vaccine.
- Shake vial well to ensure uniform suspension before withdrawing dose. If clumps remain after vigorous agitation, discard vial and contents. Rotate vial in palm to bring contents to room temperature before administration.
- Refrigerate vials; do not freeze. Discard frozen vaccine.

Assessment/Interventions

- Obtain patient history, including drug history and any known allergies.
- Review patient's medical history for conditions that would contraindicate DTwP vaccine (children who have recovered from culture-confirmed pertussis, history of serious adverse reactions to previous dose of DTwP, hypersensitivity to any component of vaccine, anaphylactic reaction or encephalopathy occurring within 7 days after any DTP vaccination).
- Take child's temperature to determine if infection is present.
- Defer immunization during course of any febrile illness or acute infection. Minor respiratory illness such as mild upper respiratory infection is not usually reason to defer immunization.
- Give any DTP injection with caution to children with thrombocytopenia or any coagulation disorder in which IM injection may be contraindicated.
- When child returns for next dose in series of either pertussis or any DTP vaccine, question child's parent or guardian about serious side effects with previous dose. If any side effects that contraindicate additional pertussis vaccine are noted, consult with child's pediatrician and continue childhood immunization with bivalent diphtheria and tetanus toxoids (DT) if recommended.
- There are no data on whether prophylactic use of antipyretic drugs (eg, acetaminophen) can decrease risk of febrile convulsions. Acetaminophen may reduce incidence of postvaccination fever. Immunization Practices Advisory Committee and American Academy of Pediatrics suggest administering appropriate dose of acetaminophen (based on age) at the time of vaccination and q 4-6 hr to children at higher risk for seizures than general population (ie, children with personal or family history of seizures).

Patient/Family Education

- Inform parent of name, action, administration and side effects of DTwP.
- Provide parent with immunization

history record and record this immunization in patient's medical record.
- Instruct parent to give acetaminophen for fever and local pain.
- If patient will require further doses, review immunization schedule with parent and arrange for return visits as necessary.
- Advise parent to check with local school board; some school systems require that children receive complete series of vaccinations before entrance into kindergarten or elementary school.

No patient monograph available.

Dipyridamole

(DIE-pih-RID-uh-mole)
Persantine, Persantine IV,
♣ *Novodipiradol*
Class: Antiplatelet

Action Inhibits platelet adhesion; lengthens abnormally shortened platelete survival.

Indications Adjunct to warfarin and similar anticoagulants in prevention of postoperative thromboembolic complications following cardiac valve replacement. **Unlabeled uses:** Alone and in combination with aspirin: prevention of myocardial reinfarction and reduction of mortality after MI.

Contraindications Standard considerations.

Route/Dosage

Antiplatelet

ADULTS: PO 75-100 mg qid.

Interactions

Adenosine: May inhibit adenosine metabolism, producing profound bradycardia.

Lab Test Interferences
None well documented.

Adverse Reactions

CV: Oral use: Hypotension; angina. Intravenous use: Chest pain; angina pectoris; ECG abnormalities; hypotension; hypertension; arrhythmia; palpitations; ventricular tachycardia; bradycardia; MI; atrioventricular block; syncope; orthostatic hypotension; atrial fibrillation; supraventricular tachycardia; ventricular arrhythmia; heart block; cardiomyopathy. *RESP:* Intravenous use: Shortness of breath. *CNS:* Oral use: Dizziness; headache. Intravenous use: Headache; dizziness; fatigue. *GI:* Oral use: Diarrhea; vomiting; abdominal distress. Intravenous use: Nausea. *DERM:* Oral use: Rash, pruritus. Intravenous use: Paresthesia. *OTHER:* Flushing.

Precautions

Pregnancy: Category B. *Lactation:* Excreted in breast milk. *Children:* Safety and efficacy in children < 12 yr not established. *Hypotension:* In presence of hypotension, drug can cause peripheral vasodilatation. Use cautiously in patients with hypotension.

NURSING CONSIDERATIONS

Administration/Storage

- Administer oral medication in divided doses throughout day.
- Administer drug with full glass of water at least 1 hr before meals for faster absorption.
- Store in tight, light-resistant containers.

Assessment/Interventions

- Obtain patient history, including drug history and known allergies.
- Review patient's medication record for other anticoagulants that may have additive effect (eg, warfarin, aspirin) that may be desired.
- Assess lung sounds during therapy for asthma-like symptoms, which are indications of hypersensitivity.
- If hypotension occurs with IV infusion, place patient in supine position.
- Monitor bleeding times before and during therapy.

- If headache occurs, give prescribed analgesic.
- If dizziness and weakness occur, keep side rails up and supervise ambulation.
- Notify physician immediately if breathing difficulty occurs. Place patient in sitting position.

OVERDOSAGE: SIGNS & SYMPTOMS
Hypotension

Patient/Family Education
- Instruct patient to take dipyridamole 1 hr before meals with full glass of water.
- Stress importance of follow-up laboratory tests to monitor effectiveness of medication or potential for bleeding.
- Advise patient that if dizziness or syncope occurs not to perform activities that might lead to falling.
- Instruct patient to report these symptoms to physician: unusual bleeding or bruising.

See Patient Guide, p. 200.

Dirithromycin

(die-RITH-row-MY-sin)
Dynabac
Class: Antibiotic/macrolide

Action Interferes with microbial protein synthesis.

Indications Treatment of acute bacterial infection of chronic bronchitis, secondary bacterial infection of acute bronchitis, community-acquired pneumonia, pharyngitis/tonsillitis, and uncomplicated skin and skin structure infections caused by susceptible organisms.

Contraindications Hypersensitivity to erythromycin or any macrolide antibiotic.

Route/Dosage
ADULTS & CHILDREN ≥ 12 YR: PO 500 mg once daily for 7-14 days.

Interactions
Terfenadine: Since cardiotoxicity and death have occurred with other macrolide antibiotics, monitor patient during concurrent use; however, available clinical data indicate that there is no interaction. *Theophylline:* Slight decrease in theophylline serum concentrations may occur.

Lab Test Interferences
None well documented.

Adverse Reactions
RESP: Increased cough; shortness of breath. *CNS:* Headache; dizziness; vertigo; insomnia. *GI:* Abdominal pain; nausea; diarrhea; vomiting; dyspepsia; flatulence. *HEMA:* Increased platelet count; eosinophilia; increased segmented neutrophils. *DERM:* Rash; pruritus; urticaria. *META:* Decreased bicarbonate. *OTHER:* Increased serum potassium; pain; weakness; increased CPK.

Precautions
Pregnancy: Category C. *Lactation:* Undetermined. *Children:* Safety and efficacy in children < 12 yr not established. *Pseudomembranous colitis:* Consider possibility in patients who develop diarrhea. *Superinfection:* Prolonged use of antibiotics may result in bacterial or fungal overgrowth of nonsusceptible microorganisms.

NURSING CONSIDERATIONS

Administration/Storage
- Take tablets with food or within 1 hour after eating. Food helps increase absorption.
- Swallow each tablet whole. Do not cut, crush or chew tablets.
- Drink plenty of fluids as tablets are swallowed.
- Store at room temperature.

Assessment/Interventions

- Obtain patient history.
- Obtain baseline lab work including albumen, CBC, WBC with diff, platelet count and total protein.
- Monitor for signs and symptoms of superinfections.
- Monitor for diarrhea, nausea, vomiting and abdominal cramping.
- Assess infection for indications of effectiveness of medication.

> **OVERDOSAGE: SIGNS & SYMPTOMS**
> Nausea, vomiting, epigastric distress, diarrhea

Patient/Family Education

- Instruct patient to take medication with food or within 1 hr after meals.
- Instruct patient to notify healthcare provider if rash develops or difficulty breathing occurs.
- Stress to patient that entire course of therapy must be completed, and not to stop taking medication when feeling better.
- Warn patient that if infection does not seem to improve after 5 days, to notify healthcare provider.
- Instruct patient to drink 2-3 liters of fluid per day while taking oral antibiotics.

See Patient Guide, p. 201.

Disopyramide

(DIE-so-PIR-uh-mide)

Norpace, Norpace CR, ♣ *Rythmodan, Rythmodan-LA*

Class: Antiarrhythmic

Action Decreases rate of diastolic depolarizations rate; decreases upstroke velocity; increases action potential duration; prolongs refractory period.

Indications Suppression and documented prevention of ventricular arrhythmias considered to be life threatening. **Unlabeled use:** Treatment of paroxysmal supraventricular tachycardia.

Contraindications Cardiogenic shock; pre-existing second- or third-degree atrioventricular block (if no pacemaker present); congenital Q-T prolongation; sick sinus syndrome.

Route/Dosage

ADULTS: **PO** 400-800 mg/day in 4 divided, evenly spaced doses. CHILDREN (12-18 YR): **PO** 6-15 mg/kg/day in divided doses. CHILDREN (4-12 YR): **PO** 10-15 mg/kg/day in divided doses. CHILDREN (1-4 YR): **PO** 10-20 mg/kg/day in divided doses. CHILDREN (< 1 YR): **PO** 10-30 mg/kg/day in divided doses.

Severe Refractory Ventricular Tachycardia

May give **PO** up to 400 mg q 6 hr.

With Cardiomyopathy or Cardiac Decompensation

Limit to **PO** 100 mg q 6-8 hr initially.

Renal/Hepatic Impairment

ADULTS: **PO** 100 mg q 6 hr; increase to q 8-24 hr for patients with deteriorating renal function.

Interactions

Antiarrhythmic agents: May cause widened QRS and prolonged QT. *Erythromycin:* May cause increased disopyramide plasma levels. *Hydantoins:* May decrease disopyramide serum levels, half-life and bioavailability. *Rifampin:* May decrease disopyramide serum levels.

Lab Test Interferences

None well documented.

Adverse Reactions

CV: Hypotension; CHF; edema; shortness of breath; syncope; chest pain. *CNS:* Dizziness; fatigue; headache; nervousness. *EENT:* Blurred vision; dry nose, eyes, throat. *GI:* Nausea; pain; bloating; gas; anorexia; vomiting; diarrhea; dry mouth; constipation. *GU:* Urinary retention, frequency and urgency; impotence; urinary hesitancy. *DERM:* Rash; dermatoses; itching. *OTHER:* Muscle weakness; malaise; aches and pains; hypokalemia; weight gain; elevated cholesterol and triglycerides; hypoglycemia.

Precautions

Pregnancy: Category C. *Lactation:* Excreted in breast milk. *Anticholinergic activity:* Use with extreme caution in patients with urinary retention, glaucoma or myasthenia gravis. *Conduction abnormalities:* Use with caution in patients with bundle branch block or Wolff-Parkinson-White syndrome. *Heart block:* Reduce dose if first-degree block occurs; drug may need to be discontinued if heart block continues. *Heart failure/hypotension:* May cause or aggravate CHF or produce severe hypotension, especially in patients with depressed systolic function. *Potassium imbalance:* Disopyramide may be ineffective in hypokalemia and have enhanced toxicity in hyperkalemia. *Renal or hepatic impairment:* Dosage should be reduced.

NURSING CONSIDERATIONS

Administration/Storage

- Have patient swallow capsules whole.
- Administer doses 6 hr apart (12 hr apart for extended release form).
- Adjust dosage according to physiologic effect and serum levels.
- Store capsules in light-resistant container.

Assessment/Interventions

- Obtain patient history, including drug history and any known allergies.
- Assess apical/radial heart rate.
- Obtain baseline 12-lead ECG.
- Correct hypokalemia before giving drug.
- Assess I&O.
- Monitor patient weight daily.
- Monitor plasma levels and therapeutic response.
- Monitor serum electrolytes.
- If blood pressure drop of 20 mm Hg occurs, notify physician immediately.
- If heart arrhythmia or increase in heart rate develops, notify physician immediately.
- If serum potassium level is higher than recommended level, notify physician.
- If serum level of drug is higher than therapeutic level, notify physician.
- If patient has urinary elimination problems, notify physician.

OVERDOSAGE: SIGNS & SYMPTOMS

Loss of consciousness, cardiac arrhythmias, loss of spontaneous respiration, death

Patient/Family Education

- Instruct patient how to take own BP and heart rate.
- Tell patient to keep weekly record of weight and report any change ≥ 2 lb to physician.
- Instruct patient to increase roughage in diet.
- Inform patient about possibility of urinary elimination problems and instruct to notify physician if problems persist.
- Instruct patient not to crush or chew capsules.
- Advise patient about possibility of hypoglycemia and to be alert for cold sweats, drowsiness, confusion, anxiety and cool, pale skin.
- Instruct patient to take sips of water frequently, suck on ice chips or sugarless hard candy or chew sugarless gum if dry mouth occurs.
- Caution patient to avoid sudden position changes to prevent orthostatic hypotension.
- Instruct patient to avoid intake of alcoholic beverages or other CNS depressants.
- Advise patient that drug may cause

drowsiness and to use caution while driving or performing other tasks requiring mental alertness.

See Patient Guide, p. 202.

Disulfiram

(die-SULL-fih-ram)

Antabuse

Class: Antialcoholic

Action Produces intolerance to alcohol by blocking oxidation of acetaldehyde by enzyme aldehyde dehydrogenase, resulting in high blood levels of acetaldehyde and unpleasant physical symptoms.

Indications Aid in management of alcoholism in selected patients who want to remain in state of enforced sobriety.

Contraindications Hypersensitivity to thiuram derivatives used in pesticides and rubber vulcanization; severe myocardial disease or coronary occlusion; psychoses; patients receiving or who have recently received metronidazole, paraldehyde, alcohol or alcohol-containing products.

Route/Dosage

ADULTS: **PO** 500 mg qd (single dose) initially for 1-2 wk. Maintenance dose: **PO** 125-500 mg qd (maximum 500 mg/day).

Interactions

Alcohol: Causes severe alcohol-intolerance reaction. Symptoms include flushing, throbbing in head and neck, respiratory difficulty, nausea, vomiting, sweating, thirst, chest pain, palpitations, shortness of breath, tachycardia, hypotension, syncope, weakness, vertigo, blurred vision and confusion. In severe reactions there may be respiratory depression, cardiovascular collapse, unconsciousness, convulsions and death. *Anticoagulants:* Disulfiram may increase anticoagulant effect. *Antidepressants, tricyclic:* May produce acute organic brain syndrome. *Benzodiazepines:* Disulfiram decreases plasma clearance of benzodiazepines metabolized by oxidation. *Hydantoins:* Disulfiram may increase serum hydantoin levels. *Isoniazid:* Acute behavioral and coordination changes. *Metronidazole:* May cause patients to exhibit acute toxic psychosis or confusional state. One or both agents may need to be discontinued. *Theophyllines:* Disulfiram may inhibit metabolism and increase effect of theophyllines.

Lab Test Interferences

None well documented.

Adverse Reactions

CNS: Drowsiness; fatigue; headache; depression; restlessness; psychotic reactions. *EENT:* Metallic or garlic-like aftertaste. *HEPA:* Hepatotoxicity; hepatitis. *DERM:* Skin eruptions. *OTHER:* Peripheral neuropathy; polyneuritis; optic or retrobulbar neuritis; arthropathy; impotence.

Precautions

Pregnancy: Undetermined. *Lactation:* Undetermined. *Special risk patients:* Use with caution in patients with diabetes mellitus, hypothyroidism, epilepsy, cerebral damage, chronic and acute nephritis and hepatic cirrhosis or insufficiency. *Disulfiram-alcohol reaction:* Avoid alcohol in all forms, including alcoholic beverages, vinegars, liquid medications such as cough syrups or tonic, some sauces and aftershave products. Do not give disulfiram within 12 hr of drinking alcohol. Reactions can occur up to 2 wk after discontinuing disulfiram. *Ethylene dibromide:* Patients receiving disulfiram should not be exposed to ethylene dibromide or its vapors; toxic interaction resulting in tumors and death has occurred in research animals. *Hypersensitivity.* Evaluate patients with history of rubber contact dermatitis for hypersensitivity to thiuram derivatives. *Intoxication:* Never give drug to intoxicated patient or without patient's knowledge.

NURSING CONSIDERATIONS

Administration/Storage

- Do not administer until patient has abstained from alcohol for at least 12 hr.
- May crush or mix tablets with liquid.
- May administer at bedtime if sedative effect is experienced.
- Store medication at room temperature in amber-colored bottle.

Assessment/Interventions

- Obtain patient history, including drug history and any known allergies. Perform physical and psychosocial assessment to determine patient's readiness to initiate this type of drug therapy.
- Obtain baseline chemistry (specifically AST, ALT) and blood and urine alcohol level with follow-up testing (10-14 days) to detect hepatic dysfunction. Perform CBC and SMA-12 test q 6 mo.
- Evaluate history to ensure patient has not ingested any form of alcohol within 12 hr prior to initiation of therapy (including cough syrups, tonics and vinegars).
- For treatment of severe reaction to alcohol, be prepared to institute supportive measures to restore BP and to treat shock. Other measures may include oxygen, vitamin C administered intravenously in massive doses (1 g) and ephedrine sulfate. Intravenous antihistamines may also be used.
- Monitor potassium levels, especially in patients receiving digitalis, because hypokalemia has been reported.

OVERDOSAGE: SIGNS & SYMPTOMS

Lethargy, vomiting, tachypnea, seizures, ketosis, coma

Patient/Family Education

- Explain that disulfiram will not cure alcohol dependence and should be used in conjunction with psychotherapy.
- Advise patient that even trace amounts of alcohol in some food products or alcohol absorbed through skin (eg, aftershave lotion) can precipitate reaction.
- Inform patient of all effects that will occur if alcohol is ingested while taking this medication.
- Advise patient and family that some alcohol-disulfiram reactions can have serious effects on heart and respiratory systems that may require immediate emergency treatment.
- Instruct patients to read all product labels or consult pharmacist about alcohol content of all liquid medications before choosing one.
- Instruct patient to carry Medi-Alert identification while taking this drug. Information should include physician's phone number or name of medical facility that should be contacted in case of reaction.
- Caution patient that prolonged disulfiram therapy does not produce tolerance to alcohol but increased sensitivity.
- Advise patient that drug may cause drowsiness and to use caution while driving or performing other tasks requiring mental alertness.
- Explain that alcohol-disulfiram reactions may occur for several weeks after discontinuation of therapy.

See Patient Guide, p. 203.

Dobutamine

(doe-BYOOT-uh-meen)

Dobutrex

Class: Vasopressor

Action Stimulates $beta_1$-receptors in heart, causing more complete and forceful contractions (inotropy) without significantly increasing heart rate or BP.

Indications Treatment of cardiac decompensation caused by organic heart disease or cardiac surgical procedures. **Unlabeled use:** Congenital heart disease in children undergoing diagnostic cardiac catheterization.

Contraindications Idiopathic hypertrophic subaortic stenosis.

Route/Dosage

ADULTS: **IV infusion** 2.5-10 mcg/kg/min; titrate to desired response; increase in heart rate > 10% may develop in rate > 20 mcg/kg/min; rates up to 40 mcg/kg/min are rarely used. Duration of therapy up to 72 hr without decrease in clinical effectiveness may be used.

Interactions

Beta-blockers: May antagonize beta receptor–stimulating activity of dobutamine. *Furazolidone, methyldopa, rauwolfia alkaloids:* Hypertension may result. *Guanethidine:* May increase pressor response. *Halogenated hydrocarbon anesthetics:* May increase risk of arrhythmias by sensitizing cardiac tissue to sympathomimetic agents. *Tricyclic antidepressants:* May potentiate effect of dobutamine; use combination with caution. INCOMPATIBILITIES: Chemically incompatible with sodium bicarbonate or other alkaline solutions.

Lab Test Interferences None well documented.

Adverse Reactions

CV: Increased systolic BP; increased heart rate; chest pain; increased number of premature ventricular beats. *RESP:* Dyspnea. *CNS:* Headache; tingling sensations; paresthesia. *GI:* Nausea; vomiting. *OTHER:* Phlebitis; local inflammation after infiltration; leg cramps.

Precautions

Pregnancy: Safety not established. *Lactation:* Undetermined. *Children:* Safety and efficacy not established. *Special risk patients:* Use with extreme caution after myocardial ischemia. Avoid use in uncorrected hypovolemic states unless used as temporary emergency measure to maintain coronary and cerebral flow. *Cardiovascular effects:* May greatly increase BP and heart rate, especially with preexisting hypertension. Dose reduction may reverse effects. May precipitate or exacerbate ventricular ectopic activity. *Hypokalemia:* Mild hypokalemia may occur. *Sulfite sensitivity:* Use caution in sulfite-sensitive individuals; some preparations contain sodium bisulfite.

NURSING CONSIDERATIONS

Administration/Storage

- Administer by IV infusion only. Use electronic infusion device to monitor infusion rate.
- Reconstitution/dilution is done in two stages.
- First, more concentrated solution can be kept under refrigeration for 48 hr or at room temperature for 6 hr.
- Before administration, solution is further diluted to typical concentration of 0.25-1 mg/ml (250-1000 mcg/ml). Final concentration should not exceed 5 mg/ml. This solution should be used within 24 hr.
- Solution may have pink color, because of slight oxidation, but this effect does not indicate loss of potency.
- Do not freeze solution because crystallization may occur.

Assessment/Interventions

- Obtain patient history, including drug history and any known allergies.
- Monitor vital signs, ECG, cardiac output, pulmonary capillary wedge pressure, central venous pressure and urinary output carefully throughout infusion.
- Monitor potassium levels to detect possible hypokalemia.
- Monitor patency and placement of IV catheter to reduce risk of extravasation and phlebitis.
- If patient has diabetes, monitor blood glucose level. Report significant increase to physician.

OVERDOSAGE: SIGNS & SYMPTOMS

Excessive hypertension, tachycardia, nausea, vomiting, tremor, headache, chest pain

Patient/Family Education

- Instruct patient to report these symptoms to physician: pain or discomfort at IV site, any anginal pain.

No patient monograph available.

Docusate Sodium (Dioctyl Sodium Sulfosuccinate; DSS)

(DOCK-you-sate SO-dee-uhm)

Colace, Diocto, Disonate, Doxinate, Dioeze, DOK, DOS Softgels, DSS, Modane Soft, Pro-Sof, Regulax SS, Regutol, ✤ *Colax-S, Doxate-S, Regulex, Selax, Silace*

Docusate Calcium (Dioctyl Calcium Sulfosuccinate)

DC Softgels, Pro-Cal-Sof, Sulfalax Calcium, Surfak Liquigels, ✤ *Colax-C, Doxate-C*

Docusate Potassium (Dioctyle Potassium Sulfosuccinate)

Dialose, Diocto-K, Kasof, Perestan

Class: Laxative/fecal softener

Action Facilitates stool softening by detergent activity.

Indications Short-term treatment of constipation; prophylaxis in patients who should not strain during defecation (eg, after anorectal surgery, myocardial infarction).

Contraindications Nausea, vomiting or other symptoms of appendicitis; acute surgical abdomen; fecal impaction; intestinal obstruction; undiagnosed abdominal pain; coadministration with mineral oil.

Route/Dosage

Docusate Sodium

ADULTS & CHILDREN > 12 YR: **PO** 50-500 mg. CHILDREN 6-12 YR: **PO** 40-120 mg. CHILDREN 3-6 YR: **PO** 20-60 mg. CHILDREN < 3 YR: **PO** 10-40 mg.

Docusate Calcium

ADULTS: **PO** 240 mg. CHILDREN ≥ 6 YR & ADULTS WITH MINIMAL NEEDS: **PO** 50-150 mg.

Docusate Potassium

ADULTS: **PO** 100-300 mg. CHILDREN ≥ 6 YR: **PO** 100 mg at bedtime.

Interactions

Mineral oil: Docusate may increase absorption of mineral oil from GI tract, leading to toxicity.

Lab Test Interferences

None well documented.

Adverse Reactions

CV: Palpitations. *CNS:* Dizziness; fainting. *GI:* Excessive bowel activity (griping, diarrhea, nausea, vomiting); perianal irritation; bloating; flatulence; abdominal cramping. *OTHER:* Sweating; weakness.

Precautions

Pregnancy: Category C (docusate sodium). *Lactation:* Undetermined. *Abuse/dependence:* Long-term use may lead to laxative dependence, fluid and electrolyte imbalances, steatorrhea, osteomalacia and vitamin and mineral deficiencies. *Fluid and electrolyte imbalance:* Excessive laxative use may lead to significant fluid and electrolyte imbalance.

Rectal bleeding or failure to respond: May indicate serious condition that may require further medical attention.

NURSING CONSIDERATIONS

Administration/Storage

- Administer each dose with full glass of water.
- Do not open or otherwise alter capsules.
- Do not give within 1 hr of other drugs or antacids, milk or histamine H_2 blockers.
- Do not administer for > 1 wk without follow-up evaluation.
- Store capsules at room temperature. Protect liquid preparations from light.

Assessment/Interventions

- Obtain patient history, including drug history and any known allergies.
- Assess patient's bowel regimen to determine nonpharmacologic interventions for bowel evacuation.
- Review patient's diet history for medical restriction of sodium. If sodium restriction is present, docusate sodium should not be used.
- Document daily I&O.
- Evaluate and document patient's response to stool softener, noting and reporting any adverse reactions such as nausea, vomiting, abdominal cramping or diarrhea.
- Monitor patient frequently for signs and symptoms of dehydration and electrolyte imbalance such as weakness, dizziness, confusion, palpitations, thirst or decreased urine output.

Patient/Family Education

- Tell patient to drink full glass of water with each dose.
- Instruct patient to swallow tablets whole and not to chew them.
- Instruct patient not to use mineral oil while taking this drug.
- Teach patient other methods of stimulating regular bowel evacuation: attempt to evacuate bowels at same time each day; drink 6-8 full glasses of water; eat high-fiber diet; exercise daily; respond to urge for bowel movement as soon as possible.
- Explain that liquid forms, excluding syrup, may be mixed with fruit juice or milk to mask unpleasant taste.

See Patient Guide, p. 204.

Dopamine HCl

(DOE-puh-meen HIGH-droe-KLOR-ide)

Dopastat, Intropin, ♣ *Revimine*

Class: Vasopressor

Action Stimulates $beta_1$ receptors in heart, causing more complete and forceful contractions (inotropy). Also acts on alpha receptors (dose dependent) and has dopaminergic effects.

Indications Correction of hemodynamic imbalances present in shock after MI; trauma, endotoxic septicemia, surgery and renal failure or imbalances in conditions of chronic refractory cardiac decompensation (eg, CHF).

Contraindications Pheochromocytoma; uncorrected tachyarrhythmias; ventricular fibrillation.

Route/Dosage

ADULTS: **IV** Initial dose: 2-5 mcg/kg/min with incremental changes of 5-10 mcg/kg/min at 10-15 min intervals until adequate response is noted. Most patients are maintained at < 20 mcg/kg/min. If dosage exceeds 50 mcg/kg/min, assess renal function frequently.

Interactions

Furazolidone, methyldopa, rau-

wolfia alkaloids: Hypertension may result. *Guanethidine:* Antihypertensive effects of guanethidine may be negated. *Monoamine oxidase inhibitors:* May greatly increase pressor response from dopamine. *Phenytoin:* Severe hypotension and bradycardia may result after concomitant administration with dopamine. *Tricyclic antidepressants:* May decrease pressor response from dopamine. INCOMPATIBILITIES: Chemically incompatible with alkaline solutions (drug is inactivated).

Lab Test Interferences
None well documented.

Adverse Reactions
CV: Ectopic beats; tachycardia; anginal pain; palpitation; hypotension; vasoconstriction; ventricular arrhythmias (at high doses); hypertension. *RESP:* Dyspnea. *CNS:* Headache; anxiety. *EENT:* Dilated pupils (at high doses). *GI:* Nausea; vomiting. *GU:* Decreased urine output. *OTHER:* Gangrene of extremities.

Precautions
Pregnancy: Category C. *Lactation:* Undetermined. *Children:* Safety and efficacy not established. *Special risk patients:* Do not give in presence of uncorrected tachyarrhythmias or ventricular fibrillation. *Extravasation:* Avoid by infusing into large vein and monitoring infusion carefully. *Sulfite sensitivity:* Use caution in sulfite-sensitive individuals; some commercial preparations contain sodium bisulfite.

NURSING CONSIDERATIONS

Administration/Storage

- Administer by IV infusion only. Metering device is essential for controlling rate of flow.
- Dopamine is potent drug. Dilute before use if not prediluted.
- Dilute medication just prior to administration. Solution is stable for 24 hr after dilution.
- Do not use if solution is discolored.
- Store at room temperature and protect from light. Discard dissolved solution.

Assessment/Interventions

- Obtain patient history, including drug history and any known allergies.
- Monitor vital signs and ECG closely throughout therapy.
- Monitor I&O regularly. Notify physician promptly if urine output decreases.
- Monitor IV rate for free flow throughout administration.
- Monitor central venous pressure or pulmonary wedge pressure if possible during infusion.
- Observe infusion site for extravasation. If extravasation occurs, treat by infiltrating the area with 10-15 ml of normal saline containing 5-10 mg of phentolamine.
- Notify physician immediately if these signs occur: significant changes in vital signs, ECG changes (arrhythmias, tachycardia); deterioration of peripheral pulses and cold, mottled extremities.

OVERDOSAGE: SIGNS & SYMPTOMS
Hypertension

Patient/Family Education

- Instruct patient to inform nurse immediately if these signs occur: chest pain, dyspnea, numbness, tingling or burning of extremities and discomfort at IV site.

No patient monograph available.

Dornase Alfa (Recombinant Human Deoxyribonuclease; DNase)

(DOR-nace AL-fuh)

Pulmozyme

Class: Respiratory inhalant/enzyme

Action Cleaves DNA released by neutrophils that are mobilized to respiratory tract in response to infection, reducing viscoelasticity of purulent lung secretions, increasing airflow and decreasing risk of infection.

Indications Treatment of cystic fibrosis.

Contraindications Hypersensitivity to Chinese hamster ovary cell products.

Route/Dosage

ADULTS & CHILDREN > 5 YR: **Inhalation** 2.5 mg once daily by oral inhalation via nebulizer; patients > 21 yr and those with baseline forced vital capacity > 85% benefit from 2.5 mg bid.

Interactions None well documented.

Lab Test Interferences

None well documented.

Adverse Reactions

CV: Chest pain. *RESP:* Hoarseness; pharyngitis; laryngitis. *EENT:* Conjunctivitis; sore throat; voice alterations; hoarseness. *DERM:* Rash.

Precautions

Pregnancy: Category B. *Lactation:* Undetermined. *Children:* Safety and efficacy in children < 5 yr not established.

NURSING CONSIDERATIONS

Administration/Storage

- Use in conjunction with standard therapies for cystic fibrosis.
- Discard solution if cloudy or discolored.
- Discard unused portions of ampules.
- Do not dilute or mix drug with other drugs in nebulizer.
- Keep refrigerated and protected from strong light. Storing at room temperature for < 24 hr does not adversely affect product.

Assessment/Interventions

- Obtain patient history, including drug history and any known allergies.
- Assess patient's ability to clear secretions. Provide assistance with coughing, positioning (semi-Fowler's or sitting upright) and suctioning.
- Provide hydration to liquefy secretions and replace fluids.
- Perform auscultation to determine quality of breath sounds. Note characteristics of cough and sputum.
- Perform chest physiotherapy (percussion and postural drainage) as ordered.

Patient/Family Education

- Teach patient to follow manufacturer's instructions on use and maintenance of nebulizer and compression system.
- Instruct patient in proper administration and storage of drug.
- Tell patient that drug may cause sore throat, voice alterations or hoarseness and to inform physician if these or any other symptoms become bothersome.
- Inform patient that benefits of treatment may not become apparent for months.
- Emphasize importance of avoiding contraction of respiratory infections.

See Patient Guide, p. 205.

Dorzolamide Hydrochloride

(dore-ZOLE-uh-mide HIGH-droe-KLOR-ide)

Trusopt

Class: Carbonic anhydrase inhibitor

Action Inhibits carbonic anhydrase enzyme, reducing rate of aqueous humor formation and thus lowering intraocular pressure (IOP).

Indications Treatment of elevated IOP in patients with ocular hypertension or open-angle glaucoma.

Contraindications Hypersensitivity to other sulfonamides.

Route/Dosage
ADULTS: **Ophthalmic** One drop in affected eye(s) tid.

Interactions
None well documented.

Lab Test Interferences
None well documented.

Adverse Reactions
CNS: Headache. *EENT:* Ocular burning, stinging or discomfort; superficial punctate keratitis; blurred vision; tearing; conjunctivitis; ocular dryness; photophobia; ocular allergic reaction. *OTHER:* Nausea; bitter taste.

Precautions
Pregnancy: Category C. *Lactation:* Unknown. *Children:* Safety and efficacy not established. *Renal impairment:* Not recommended for use in patients with severe renal impairment. *Hepatic impairment:* Use with caution. *Contact lenses:* Do not administer while wearing soft contact lenses; preservative may be absorbed by soft contact lenses. *Concomitant use of oral carbonic anhydrase inhibitors:* Not recommended. *Bacterial keratitis:* Can occur by using contaminated eye drops.

NURSING CONSIDERATIONS

Administration/Storage

- Wash hands before and after using.
- To avoid contamination, do not touch tip of container to any surface or to eye structures.
- Administer only to affected eye.
- Gently apply pressure over nasolacrimal drainage system for 1-2 min after administration.
- Replace cap after administration and keep tightly closed when not in use.
- If used concomitantly with other topical ophthalmic drug products, wait 10 min between administering medications.
- Do not use with soft contact lenses. They may absorb the preservative.
- Other therapeutic interventions should be used in conjunction with dorzolamide in the treatment of acute narrow angle glaucoma.
- Store at room temperature, protected from light.

Assessment/Interventions

- Obtain patient history.
- Obtain baseline lab work including electrolytes and RBCs.
- Note baseline intraocular pressure before starting medication.

OVERDOSAGE: SIGNS & SYMPTOMS

Electrolyte imbalance, acidotic state, possible CNS effects

Patient/Family Education

- Instruct patient in proper administration of eye drop medications.
- Instruct patient about the need to keep the tip of the dropper clean to prevent eye infections.
- Inform patient that eye drops commonly produce transient stinging or discomfort upon administration, and to notify healthcare provider if they are severe.
- Stress need to return to healthcare provider frequently for monitoring of eye pressure.

- Inform patient not to wear soft contact lenses while using this medication.
- Inform patient that they may experience a bitter taste in mouth immediately after administration.
- Explain the need to be cautious when driving or participating in activities requiring close hand-eye coordination.
- Instruct patient to notify the health-care provider if any symptoms of eye infection (ie, burning, redness, itching, possible discharge) occur.

See Patient Guide, p. 206.

Doxapram HCl

(DOX-uh-pram HIGH-droe-KLOR-ide)

Dopram

Class: CNS stimulant/analeptic

Action Increases depth of respirations (tidal volume) by stimulating respiratory center in CNS; respiratory rate may increase slightly. May elevate BP by increasing cardiac output. Respiratory depression from opiates is reversed without affecting pain relief.

Indications Reversal of respiratory depression caused by anesthesia (other than muscle relaxants) or drug overdose; temporary measure for acute respiratory failure in patients with COPD who are not undergoing mechanical ventilation. **Unlabeled uses:** Low doses of doxapram have been used in the treatment of apnea of prematurity when methylxanthines have failed.

Contraindications Use in newborns (contains benzyl alcohol); seizures; muscle paresis; epilepsy or other convulsive states; flail chest; head injury; pneumothorax; acute asthma; pulmonary fibrosis; other conditions that restrict chest wall, respiratory muscles or alveolar expansion; severe hypertension; CVA.

Route/Dosage

Anesthesia-induced Respiratory Depression

ADULTS: **Bolus IV injection** 0.5-1 mg/kg (single dose not to exceed 1.5 mg/kg). Can be given as multiple IV injections q 5 min (not to exceed total dose of 2 mg/kg). **IV infusion** Initial rate: 5 mg/min until satisfactory respiratory response is noted. Maintenance rate: 1-3 mg/min. Maximum total infusion dose is 4 mg/kg.

Drug-induced CNS Depression

ADULTS: Maximum daily dose is 3 g. **Bolus IV injection** Priming dose is 2 mg/kg. Repeat in 5 min. Depending on response, may give q 1-2 hr. **Intermittent IV infusion** Priming dose is 2 mg/kg. If respirations improve, give by IV infusion at 1-3 mg/min. Discontinue after 2 hr or if patient awakens.

Acute Hypercapnia from COPD

ADULTS: **IV infusion** 2 mg/ml with initial rate of 1-2 mg/min; may increase to maximum of 3 mg/min; discontinue after 2 hr.

Interactions

Cyclopropane, enflurane, halothane: To prevent arrhythmias, wait at least 10 min after stopping these anesthetics before giving doxapram. *MAO inhibitors, sympathomimetics:* Increased risk of hypertension. *Muscle relaxants:* Residual effects may be temporarily masked by doxapram. INCOMPATIBILITIES: Do not add to or give with alkaline solutions such as aminophylline, thiopental or sodium bicarbonate.

Lab Test Interferences

None well documented.

Adverse Reactions

CV: Arrhythmias; tachycardia; increased BP; tightness in chest; chest pain; phlebitis. *RESP:* Laryngospasm; bronchospasm; rebound hypoventilation; cough; hiccoughs; dsypnea. *CNS:* Seizures; paresthesia; increased reflexes; disorientation; dizziness; involuntary movements. *EENT:* Mydriasis. *GI:* Nausea; vomiting; diarrhea; desire to defecate. *GU:* Urinary incontinence and retention; elevation of BUN. *HEMA:* Hemolysis (with rapid infusion). *OTHER:* Flushing; feelings of warmth; sweating.

Precautions

Pregnancy: Category B. *Lactation:* Undetermined. *Children:* Safety and efficacy not established in children < 12 yr. Doxapram contains benzl alcohol, which has been associated with fatal "gasping syndrome" in premature infants. *COPD patients:* Do not increase infusion rate in severely ill patients; drug may increase work of breathing. *Drug-induced CNS and respiratory depression:* Used as adjunct to supportive care. *Postanesthesia:* Do not use as antidote for opiates or neuromuscular blockers.

NURSING CONSIDERATIONS

Administration/Storage

- Ensure that patent airway has been established before administration.
- Do not give in conjunction with mechanical ventilation.
- Have readily available oxygen, IV barbiturates (eg, Valium) and resuscitative equipment.
- Allow 10 min after administration of anesthetic before starting infusion.
- Rotate injection sites to avoid skin irritation.
- For intermittent infusion, dilute 250 mg in 250 ml of D5W, D10W or 0.9% normal saline for concentration of 1 mg/ml. Dilute 400 mg in 180 ml of IV fluid for 2 mg/ml concentration.
- Store at room temperature.

Assessment/Interventions

- Obtain patient history, including drug history and any known allergies. Note any history of seizure disorder.
- Assess BP, pulse, deep tendon reflexes, neurologic status, ECG and ABGs before infusion and q 30 min during infusion.
- Institute seizure precautions before administering drug.
- Assess for poststimulation respiratory depression for at least 30 min-1 hr after patient becomes alert.
- Monitor respiratory status. Position patient on side in slightly elevated position to prevent aspiration.
- Monitor BP and deep tendon reflexes to prevent overdosage.
- Monitor patient's CBC since rapid infusion can cause hemolysis.
- If ABGs deteriorate, notify physician immediately. Drug may need to be discontinued and mechanical ventilation started.
- Check infusion site regularly for extravasation, skin irritation and signs of thrombophlebitis.

OVERDOSAGE: SIGNS & SYMPTOMS

Severe hypertension, tachycardia, hyperactive reflexes or seizures

Patient/Family Education

- Instruct patient/family to notify physician immediately if shortness of breath worsens.

No patient monograph available.

Doxazosin Mesylate

(DOX-uh-ZOE-sin MEH-suh-late)

Cardura

Class: Antihypertensive/antiadrenergic, peripherally acting

Action Selectively blocks postsynaptic alpha-1-adrenergic receptors, resulting in dilation of arterioles and veins.

Indications Treatment of hypertension, alone or in combination with other agents; treatment of benign prostatic hyperplasia (BPH). **Unlabeled use:** Treatment of CHF with concurrent digoxin and diuretic therapy.

Contraindications Hypersensitivity to prazosin or terazosin.

Route/Dosage

Hypertension

ADULTS: **PO** Initial: 1 mg qd. Maintenance: Based on standing BP response, may increase to 2 mg and thereafter to 4, 8 and 16 mg.

Benign Prostatic Hyperplasia

ADULTS: **PO** 1 mg/daily for initial dose. *Maintenance*—Increase to 2 mg, and thereafter to 4 and 8 mg once daily, which is the maximum dose for BPH. Recommended titration interval is 1 to 2 weeks.

Interactions None well documented.

Lab Test Interferences

None well documented.

Adverse Reactions

CV: Palpitations; orthostatic hypotension; hypotension; arrhythmia; chest pain. *RESP:* Dyspnea. *CNS:* Depression; dizziness; decreased libido; sexual dysfunction; nervousness; paresthesia; somnolence; headache; anxiety; insomnia; asthenia; ataxia; hypertonia. *EENT:* Abnormal vision; conjunctivitis; tinnitus; rhinitis; epitaxis; pharyngitis. *GI:* Nausea; vomiting; dry mouth; diarrhea; constipation; abdominal discomfort or pain; flatulence. *GU:* Incontinence; polyuria. *DERM:* Pruritus; rash; sweating. *OTHER:* Shoulder, neck, back or extremity pain; arthritis; joint or muscle pain; gout; arthralgia; vertigo; edema; facial edema; flushing.

Precautions

Pregnancy: Category B. *Lactation:* Excreted in breast milk. *Children:* Safety and efficacy not established. *"First-dose" effect:* Marked hypotension (especially orthostatic) and syncope may occur at 2-6 hr after first few doses, after reintroduction, with rapid increase in dosing or after addition of another antihypertensive. *Hepatic impairment:* Use drug with extreme caution. *Lipids:* Slight decrease in total serum cholesterol and LDL may occur as well as increase in HDL.

NURSING CONSIDERATIONS

Administration/Storage

- Have patient swallow tablet whole. Do not crush or allow patient to chew tablet.
- Give first dose at bedtime to decrease possibility of orthostatic hypotension, dizziness and syncope.
- Store at room temperature.

Assessment/Interventions

- Obtain patient history, including drug history and any known allergies. Note any history of liver failure.
- Record patient's weight daily.
- Monitor BP and pulse 2-6 hr after initial dose and each increase and daily throughout therapy.
- Monitor liver function tests, CBC, cholesterol, LDL, HDL, BUN, creatinine and triglycerides.
- Monitor I&O.
- Monitor for chest pain and arrhythmia. Notify physician if these signs are present.
- Monitor patient for nausea, vomiting, abdominal distention or pain.
- Monitor for edema. Check patient's feet and legs daily for swelling.
- Observe skin for rash or diaphoresis.

OVERDOSAGE: SIGNS & SYMPTOMS

Hypotension

Patient/Family Education

- Remind patient to take tablets whole, not to crush or chew tablets.
- Teach patient how to take BP. Advise to monitor weekly and to notify physician if significant changes occur.
- Emphasize importance of reducing risk factors: smoking cessation,

weight loss, discontinuation of dietary intake of fat, exercise.

- Caution patient not to discontinue medication, even if feeling well, unless directed by physician.
- Instruct patient to record weight 3 times/wk.
- Advise patient to report these symptoms to physician: nausea, vomiting or diarrhea; dizziness; chest pain or palpitations; swelling of feet or ankles.
- Caution patient to avoid sudden position changes 2-6 hr after taking medication to prevent orthostatic hypotension and syncope.
- Advise patient that drug may cause drowsiness and to use caution while driving or performing other tasks requiring mental alertness.
- Instruct patient not to take otc medications without consulting physician.

See Patient Guide, p. 207.

Doxepin HCl

(DOX-uh-pin HIGH-droe-KLOR-ide)

Adapin, Sinequan, Sinequan Concentrate, Zonalon, ♣ *Novo-Doxepin, Triadapin*

Class: Antianxiety/tricyclic antidepressant

Action Moderately blocks reuptake of norepinephrine and weakly blocks reuptake of serotonin; also produces antihistaminic and anticholinergic activity.

Indications Treatment of mental depression; anxiety. **Unlabeled uses:** Neurogenic pain; peptic ulcer disease. *Topical use:* Pruritus.

Contraindications Hypersensitivity to tricyclic antidepressants; use during acute recovery phase after MI; angle-closure glaucoma; risk of urinary retention; concomitant use with monoamine oxidase (MAO) inhibitor.

Route/Dosage

Mental Depression

ADULTS: **PO** Initial dose: 75 mg/day, increasing as tolerated. Maximum daily dose: 150 mg for outpatients, 300 mg for inpatients. Maximum single daily dose: 150 mg given at bedtime. FOR MILD CASES WITH ORGANIC DISEASE: **PO** 25-50 mg/day.

Pruritus

ADULTS: **Topical** Apply thin film qid with at least 3-4 hr between applications. Not recommended for > 8 days.

Interactions *Alcohol/CNS depressants:* CNS and respiratory depression may be potentiated. *Anticoagulants:* Anticoagulant action may increase. *Cimetidine:* May inhibit metabolism of doxepin, leading to increased concentrations. *Clonidine:* Concurrent use may lead to dangerous increases in BP. *Fluoxetine:* May increase serum concentrations of doxepin; effect may occur up to 5 wk after discontinuation of fluoxetine. *Guanethidine:* Hypotensive action may be inhibited. *MAO inhibitors:* Concurrent use may lead to severe seizures, hyperpyretic crisis and fatal reactions. Generally, allow 7-10 days between discontinuation of one drug and start of other. *Sympathomimetics (eg, dopamine, epinephrine):* Pressor response may increase or decrease; arrhythmias may occur.

Lab Test Interferences None well documented.

Adverse Reactions *CV:* Orthostatic hypotension; hypertension; fainting; tachycardia; arrhythmias; MI; heart block, precipitation of CHF; stroke. *RESP:* Brochospasms; dyspnea. *CNS:* Dizziness; drowsiness; headache; confusion; weakness; tremors; convulsions. *EENT:* Mydriasis; photophobia; blurred vision; increased IOP; unpleasant taste. *GI:* Nausea; constipation; dry mouth; paralytic ileus. *GU:* Urinary retention; nocturia; painful ejaculation; altered libido;

impotence; dysmenorrhea. *HEPA:* Hepatitis. *HEMA:* Agranulocytosis; eosinophilia; purpura; thrombocytopenia; leukopenia. *META:* Increased appetite; weight gain; syndrome of inappropriate secretion of antidiuretic hormone. *OTHER:* Hyperthermia. *Topical use:* Local burning or stinging; dry or tight skin. Results in significant plasma levels; drowsiness and other adverse effects are possible.

Precautions

Pregnancy: Oral form: Safety not established. *Lactation:* Excreted in breast milk. *Children:* Not recommended for children < 12 yr. *Special risk patients:* Use drug with caution in patients with history of seizures, urinary retention, urethral spasm, angle-closure glaucoma or increased IOP, cardiovascular disorders, hyperthyroidism (or those receiving thyroid medication), hepatic or renal impairment, schizophrenia or paranoia. *Topical use:* For external use only; do not use ophthalmically, orally or intravaginally. Because of absorption of drug, drowsiness often occurs.

NURSING CONSIDERATIONS

Administration/Storage

- Administer with meals or after meals to decrease GI upset.
- Have patient take capsule with full glass of water.
- If patient is unable to swallow capsule, open capsule and mix contents with food or fluids.
- Dilute concentrate with 120 ml of liquid (water, milk, fruit juice). Do not mix with carbonated beverages.
- If oversedation occurs when divided doses are given during day, administer total daily dose at bedtime.
- Do not prepare or store bulk dilutions.
- Store at room temperature in tight container and protect from sunlight.

Assessment/Interventions

- Obtain patient history, including drug history and any known allergies.
- Assess BP (lying, standing) and pulse q 4 hr. If systolic BP drops significantly, withhold drug and notify physician.
- Weigh patient weekly. Appetite may be increased.
- Monitor ECG before and during therapy, especially in elderly patients or patients with current cardiac condition or history of cardiac disease.
- Monitor blood studies: CBC, leukocytes and differential before and during therapy.
- Monitor liver function studies: AST, ALT, bilirubin and serum phosphatase.
- Monitor for urinary retention and constipation. Increase fluids and bulk in diet if constipation or urinary retention occurs.
- Assess patient's mental status: mood, sensorium, affect, suicidal tendencies, increased depression or panic.
- Observe for signs of extrapyramidal syndrome especially in elderly patients: rigidity, dystonia, akathisia.
- If drug was discontinued abruptly, observe patient for withdrawal symptoms: headache, nausea, vomiting, muscle pain, weakness.
- If drowsiness or dizziness occurs, assist patient with ambulation. Use siderails for safety, especially with elderly patients.

OVERDOSAGE: SIGNS & SYMPTOMS

Confusion, agitation, hallucinations, seizures, status epilepticus, clonus, choreoathetosis, hyperactive reflexes, positive Babinski's sign, coma, cardiac arrhythmias, renal failure, flushing, dry mouth, dilated pupils, hyperpyrexia

Patient/Family Education

- Emphasize that therapeutic effect may take up to 2-3 wk.
- Advise patient to monitor dietary intake because increased appetite may lead to weight gain.

- Instruct patient to increase fluid and bulk intake if constipation occurs.
- Explain that if daytime drowsiness occurs, patient should ask physician about taking total dose at bedtime. Explain that sedative effect tends to disappear with prolonged therapy.
- Caution patient not to stop taking drug abruptly since withdrawal symptoms may occur.
- Emphasize importance of follow-up appointments and lab tests.
- Instruct patient to report these symptoms to physician: urinary retention.
- Advise patient to take sips of water frequently, suck on ice chips or sugarless hard candy or chew sugarless gum if dry mouth occurs.
- Caution patient to avoid sudden position changes to prevent orthostatic hypotension.
- Instruct patient to avoid intake of alcoholic beverages or other CNS depressants.
- Advise patient that drug may cause drowsiness and to use caution while driving or performing other tasks requiring mental alertness.
- Caution patient to avoid exposure to sunlight and to use sunscreen or wear protective clothing to avoid photosensitivity reaction.

See Patient Guide, p. 208.

Doxorubicin HCl (ADR)

(DOX-oh-RUE-bih-sin HIGH-droe-KLOR-ide)

Adriamycin PFS, Adriamycin RDF, Rubex

Class: Antineoplastic/antibiotic/anthracycline

Action Inhibits nucleic acid synthesis by binding to DNA.

Indications Treatment of acute leukemias; lymphomas (Hodgkin's and non-Hodgkin's); Wilms' tumor; neuroblastoma; soft tissue and bone sarcomas; breast, ovarian, transitional cell bladder, thyroid, bronchogenic and gastric carcinomas.

Contraindications Marked myelosuppression induced by previous antitumor treatment or radiotherapy; preexisting heart disease; use in patients with complete cumulative doses of doxorubicin or daunorubicin from prior treatment.

Route/Dosage

For IV use only. All dosages shown are for adults unless indicated otherwise.

Recommended Dosage Schedule

IV 60-75 mg/m^2 as single injection at 21-day intervals.

Alternative Dose Schedules

IV 30 mg/m^2 on 3 successive days every 4 wk or 20 mg/m^2 once weekly.

Interactions

Digoxin: Digoxin levels may be reduced. INCOMPATIBILITIES: Incompatible with heparin, cephalothin and dexamethasone sodium phosphate. Do not mix with other drugs unless specific data are available.

Lab Test Interferences

None well documented.

Adverse Reactions

CV: CHF; facial flushing. *GI:* Nausea; vomiting; mucositis; anorexia; diarrhea. *GU:* Red urine discolorization. *HEMA:* Myelosuppression. *DERM:* Reversible alopecia; extravasation; hyperpigmentation of nailbeds and dermal creases. *META:* Hyperuricemia. *OTHER:* Hypersensitivity (eg, fever, chills, urticaria, anaphylaxis).

Precautions

Pregnancy: Safety not established. *Lactation:* Undetermined. *Cardiac toxicity:* Potentially irreversible fatal cardiac toxicity may occur, particularly with high cumulative dosage (> 550 mg/m^2 in adults, > 300 mg/m^2 in children > 2 yr, or > 10 mg/kg in children < 2 yr), use of other potentially cardiotoxic drugs (eg, daunorubicin, cyclophosphamide), preexisting cardiac disease or prior radiation exposure to area surrounding heart. *Extravasation:* Severe local tissue necrosis will result; administer only into freely flowing IV infusion. *Hepatic function impairment:* May increase toxicity; dosage reduction may be necessary. *Myelosuppression:* Severe hematologic toxicity may occur, resulting in superinfection or hemorrhage. Dose reduction or suspension of therapy may be required. *Necrotizing colitis:* Has occurred in patients taking certain combinations of doxorubicin and cytarabine. Condition may be severe, even fatal.

NURSING CONSIDERATIONS

Administration/Storage

- Practice safe handling of medication (eg, wear gloves and mask). Follow guidelines for disposal of antineoplastic agents (eg, proper disposal of needles, syringes, vials, and unused medication).
- Administer by IV route only. Do not give via IM or SC route.
- Dilute 10 mg vial with 5 ml, 20 mg vial with 10 ml, 50 mg vial with 25 ml, 100 mg vial with 50 ml and 150 mg with 75 ml of 0.9% Sodium Chloride to give final concentration of 2 mg/ml. Bacteriostatic diluents are not recommended.
- Administer doxorubicin slowly into tubing at Y-site of freely running IV infusion of normal saline or D5W.
- Do not administer in less than 3-5 min. Local erythematous streaking along vein and facial flushing may occur with too rapid administration.
- Administer drug into large vein. Phlebosclerosis may result if small veins are used or when single vein is used repeatedly.
- Do not mix with heparin, dexamethasone, cephalothin, aminophylline, 5FU or other drugs.
- Reconstituted solution is stable for 24 hr at room temperature and for 48 hr when refrigerated. Protect from sunlight. Discard unused portion.

Assessment/Interventions

- Obtain patient history, including drug history and any known allergies.
- Provide liquid diet; progress diet once nausea and vomiting have subsided.
- Assess IV insertion site frequently. If signs of extravasation are noted, restart in another vein. Notify physician immediately. Apply ice to site.
- Monitor cardiac and respiratory status: BP, pulse, ECG, respirations.
- Monitor CBC, differential and platelet count throughout therapy.
- Monitor renal function studies: BUN, serum uric acid, urine creatinine clearance, electrolytes.
- Monitor liver function studies during therapy: AST, ALT, bilirubin, serum phosphatase.
- Monitor I&O, appetite and nutritional intake. Encourage fluid intake to 2-3 L/day.
- Observe for signs of infection. Take patient's temperature q 4 hr, and check for sore throat.
- Assess for bleeding: hematuria, guaiac stools, bruising, petechiae, mucosa or orifices.
- Assess mouth q 8 hr for dryness, sores, ulceration, white patches, pain, bleeding, dysphagia. Mucositis may occur 5 to 10 days after initial dose.
- If stomatitis occurs, have patient rinse mouth tid-qid with water; brush teeth 2-3 times daily with soft brush or sponge brush or cotton-tipped applicator; and use unwaxed dental floss.
- Assess patient for signs of CHF: peripheral edema, dyspnea, rales/crackles, weight gain, jugular vein distention. May occur several weeks after therapy.
- Assess for jaundice, dark urine, clay-colored stools, pruitus, abdominal pain, fever, diarrhea.

OVERDOSAGE: SIGNS & SYMPTOMS

Acute overdose: Increased toxic effects of mucositis, leukopenia and thrombocytopenia. *Chronic overdose:* Increased risk of cardiomyopathy and CHF with cumulative dose > 550 mg/m^2 in adults, > 300 mg/m^2 in children > 2 yr or > 10 mg/kg in children < 2 yr

Patient/Family Education

- Explain that drug is likely to cause hair loss but that recovery will begin within 2-3 mo.
- Advise patient to exercise caution (eg, use gloves and needle box) in handling and disposal of solution.
- Tell patient or family members to wash with soap and water after skin contact with solution.
- Warn patient that urine and body fluids may be red-orange for 1-2 days after administration of drug but this effect is temporary.
- Instruct patient to drink 2-3 L of fluids daily, unless contraindicated, to prevent renal calculi.
- Tell patient to inspect oral mucosa regularly and to report any bleeding, white spots or ulcerations in mouth. Advise patient to use soft toothbrush or sponge brush 2-3 times daily.
- Instruct patient to avoid crowds and people with infection during myelosuppression and to report any sign of infection to physician: fever, chills, sore throat, cough.
- Advise patient to avoid foods with citric acid, hot or rough texture if mucositis is present.
- Instruct patient to report these symptoms to physician: irregular heart rhythm, shortness of breath or fluid retention in lower extremities.

See Patient Guide, p. 209.

Doxycycline

(DOX-ee-SIGH-kleen)

Doryx, Doxy 100, Doxy 200, Doxy-Caps, Doxychel Hyclate, Monodox, Vibramycin, Vibramycin IV, Vibra-Tabs, ♣ *Apo-Doxycin, Apo-Doxy, Novo-Doxylin*

Class: Antibiotic/tetracycline

Action Inhibits bacterial protein synthesis.

Indications Treatment of infections due to susceptible strains of gram-positive and gram-negative bacteria, *Rickettsiae, Mycoplasma pneumoniae;* treatment of trachoma and susceptible infections when penicillins are contraindicated; treatment of acute intestinal amebiasis, uncomplicated gonorrhea in adults; prophylaxis of malaria due to *Plasmodium falciparum*. **Unlabeled use:** Prevention of "traveler's diarrhea."

Contraindications Hypersensitivity to tetracyclines.

Route/Dosage

Infection

ADULTS & CHILDREN > 8 YR AND > 45 KG: **PO/IV** 200 mg day 1, then 100-200 mg qd in single or divided doses. CHILDREN > 8 YR AND < 45 KG: **PO/IV** 4.4 mg/kg day 1, then 2.2 mg/kg in single or two divided doses. CHILDREN > 8 YR: 2 mg/kg/day; do not exceed 100 mg/day.

Acute Gonococcal Infection

ADULTS & CHILDREN < 8 YR (AND ≥ 45 KG): **PO** 200 mg immediately, then 100 mg at bedtime day 1, then 200 mg qd for 3 days. *Single visit alternative:* **PO** 300 mg immediately, followed by 300 mg in 1 hr.

Primary/Secondary Syphilis

ADULTS (NONPREGNANT PENICILLIN-ALLERGIC): **PO/IV** 100 mg bid for 2 wk.

Chlamydia

ADULTS & CHILDREN ≥ 8 YR: **PO** 100 mg bid for 7 days.

Malaria Prophylaxis

ADULTS: **PO** 100 mg qd, beginning 1-2 days before travel and continuing for 4 wk after leaving area.

Interactions

Antacids containing aluminum, zinc, calcium, magnesium, bismuth salts, divalent/trivalent cations: May decrease oral absorption of doxycycline. *Barbiturates, carbamazepine, hydantoins:* May increase metabolism of and decrease effect of doxycycline. *Digoxin:* May increase digoxin serum levels. *Iron salts:* May decrease absorption of doxycycline. *Methoxyflurane:* Increased potential for nephrotoxicity exists; do not use together. *Penicillins:* May interfere with bactericidal action of penicillins.

Lab Test Interferences

False elevations of urinary catecholamine levels may occur due to interference with fluorescence test.

Adverse Reactions

CNS: Pseudotumor cerebri, manifested by headache and blurred vision. *GI:* Diarrhea; nausea; vomiting; abdominal pain or discomfort; anorexia; bulky, loose stools; sore throat; glossitis; anorexia. *DERM:* Rash; photosensitivity. *HEMA:* Hemolytic anemia; thrombocytopenia; neutropenia. *OTHER:* Hypersensitivity reactions (eg, urticaria, anaphylaxis, pericarditis).

Precautions

Pregnancy: Category D. *Lactation:* Excreted in breast milk. *Children:* Not recommended in children < 8 yrs; abnormal bone formation and tooth discoloration may result. *Anticoagulants:* May need to decrease dosage of anticoagulant. *Hepatic effects:* Doses > 2 g/day have been associated with liver failure; monitor function and avoid other hepatotoxic drugs. *Outdated product:* Do not use; degradation products of drug are highly nephrotoxic. *Photosensitivity:* May occur; avoid exposure to sunlight or ultraviolet light. *Prolonged use:* May result in thrombophlebitis; use oral form whenever reasonable. *Renal impairment:* Dosage reduction is required. *Superinfection:* Prolonged use may result in bacterial or fungal overgrowth.

NURSING CONSIDERATIONS

Administration/Storage

Oral

- Do not administer oral form with antacids.

Parenteral

- Do not inject via IM or SC route.
- Reconstitute vial contents with 10 ml of Sterile Water for Injection. Dilute further with D5W or normal saline to make concentration of 0.1-1 mg/ml.
- For solutions diluted with Lactated Ringer's Injection or 5% Dextrose in Lactated Ringer's, use within 6 hr of reconstitution. Discard any remaining solution.
- For solutions diluted with other preparations, store up to 72 hr before infusion. Complete infusion within 12 hr to ensure stability. Keep solution refrigerated and protect from light.

Assessment/Interventions

- Obtain patient history, including drug history and any known allergies.
- Review baseline WBC and BUN and monitor throughout therapy.
- Withhold drug and notify physician if GI disturbances develop.
- Monitor body temperature.
- Inform physician of signs/symptoms of superinfection.

Patient/Family Education

- Instruct patient not to take medication with antacids.
- Caution patient to avoid exposure to sunlight and to use sunscreen or wear protective clothing to avoid photosensitivity reaction.
- Explain rationale for and techniques for oral hygiene.
- Tell patient to increase fluid intake and to take medication after meals.
- Inform patient of possible skin rash (maculopapular or erythematous).

- Instruct patient to report any visual changes and any additional infections to physician.
- Explain missed medication procedure: < 2 hr, take medication; > 2 hr, wait until next scheduled dose. Do not double up on medication.

See Patient Guide, p. 210.

Dronabinol

(droe-NAB-ih-nahl)

Marinol

Class: Antiemetic/antivertigo; appetite stimulant

Action Principal psychoactive substance derived from cannabis (marijuana); mechanism by which it prevents nausea and vomiting is unknown.

Indications Control of chemotherapy-induced nausea and vomiting unresponsive to other antiemetics; appetite stimulation in AIDS cachexia.

Contraindications Hypersensitivity to marijuana or sesame oil.

Route/Dosage

Antiemetic

ADULTS & CHILDREN: **PO** 5 mg/m^2 1-3 hr before chemotherapy and q 2-4 hr after chemotherapy. Can give 4-6 doses/day and increase by 2.5 mg/m^2/dose; do not exceed 15 mg/m^2/dose.

Appetite Stimulation

ADULTS: **PO** 2.5 mg bid. Can give single daily dose of 2.5 mg to patients in whom adverse effects develop. Can increase by 2.5 mg/day; do not exceed 20 mg/day.

Interactions

Amphetamines, cocaine, sympathomimetics: Hypertension; tachycardia. *CNS depressants:* Increased CNS adverse effects.

Lab Test Interferences

None well documented.

Adverse Reactions

CV: Tachycardia; hypotension. *CNS:* Euphoria; dizziness; paranoid reaction; somnolence; seizures in patients with existing seizure disorders. *OTHER:* Tolerance, psychological and physical dependence with chronic use.

Precautions

Pregnancy: Category B. *Lactation:* Excreted in breast milk. *Children:* Not recommended in children with AIDS cachexia. *Elderly patients:* More sensitive to psychoactive effects. *Drug dependence:* Drug has abuse potential.

NURSING CONSIDERATIONS

Administration/Storage

- When given as appetite stimulant, administer bid before lunch and supper.
- Refrigerate capsules; do not freeze.

Assessment/Interventions

- Obtain patient history, including drug history and any known allergies. Note history of drug or alcohol abuse.
- Assess for nausea, vomiting, appetite, bowel sounds and abdominal pain before and after drug is administered.
- Monitor BP and pulse rate during therapy, especially in patients with hypotension or cardiac disease.
- Monitor I&O, hydration, nutritional status and weight regularly.
- Monitor side effects, which vary with each patient and are usually dose related. Side effects may be exacerbated in elderly, manic, depressive or schizophrenic patients.
- Administer IV fluids as ordered for severe nausea and vomiting.
- Assess for signs of withdrawal syndrome, including: irritability, restlessness, insomnia, hot flashes, sweating,

rhinorrhea, loose stools, hiccups, anorexia.
- Limit quantity of drug available to patient to amount necessary for single cycle of chemotherapy.
- Assist patient with ambulation. Implement safety measures (eg, siderails) to prevent falls, especially in elderly patients.

OVERDOSAGE: SIGNS & SYMPTOMS

Mild intoxication: Drowsiness, euphoria, heightened sensory awareness, altered time perception, reddened conjunctiva, dry mouth, tachycardia. *Moderate intoxication:* Memory impairment, depersonalization, mood alteration, urinary retention, reduced bowel motility. *Severe intoxication:* Decreased motor coordination, lethargy, slurred speech, postural hypotension. Apprehensive patients may experience panic reactions. Patients with seizure disorder may experience seizures

Patient/Family Education
- Instruct patient to take drug exactly as ordered by physician.
- Discuss psychoactive symptoms with patient and family. Symptoms may be minimized by providing quiet, supportive environment.
- Explain that signs of overdose (mood changes, confusion, hallucinations, depression, nervousness, fast or pounding heartbeat) may occur with increased doses.
- Instruct patient to make position changes slowly to prevent orthostatic hypotension.
- Advise patient and family that adult supervision is necessary as patient may experience drowsiness, dizziness, difficulty concentrating, and perceptual and coordination impairment.
- Instruct patient to avoid intake of alcoholic beverages, barbiturates and other CNS depressants.
- Advise patient that drug may cause drowsiness and to use caution while driving or performing other tasks requiring mental alertness.

See Patient Guide, p. 211.

Droperidol

(dro-PER-i-dahl)

Inapsine

Class: General anesthetic

Action Produces tranquilization, sedation and antiemetic effects as well as mild alpha-adrenergic blockade, resulting in hypotension and decreased peripheral vascular resistance.

Indications Tranquilization and reduction of incidence of nausea and vomiting in surgical and diagnostic procedures; premedication for and induction of general anesthesia; adjunctive use in regional anesthesia; combination therapy (with narcotics) in neuroleptanalgesia. **Unlabeled use:** Antiemetic in cancer chemotherapy.

Contraindications Hypersensitivity to butyrophenones.

Route/Dosage

Premedication

ADULTS: **IM** 2.5-10 mg 30-60 min preoperatively. CHILDREN 2-12 YR: **IM** 1-1.5 mg/9-11 kg/body weight.

Induction of General Anesthesia

ADULTS: **IV** ≤ 2.5 mg/9-11 kg. CHILDREN 2-12 YR: **IV** 1-1.5 mg/9-11 kg/body weight.

Maintenance of General Anesthesia

ADULTS: **IM** 1.25-2.5 mg.

Without General Anesthesia

ADULTS: **IM** 2.5-10 mg 30-60 min before procedure. Additional 1.25-2.5 mg doses may be given IV if needed.

Regional Anesthesia

ADULTS: **IM/slow IV** 2.5-5 mg.

Interactions
CNS depressants: Additive CNS depression may result. INCOMPATIBILITIES: Barbiturates are physically incompatible with droperidol.

Lab Test Interferences
None well documented.

Adverse Reactions
CV: Hypotension; tachycardia. *RESP:* Respiratory depression; bronchospasm; laryngospasm. *CNS:* Postoperative drowsiness; extrapyramidal effects (dystonia, akathisia and oculogyric crisis); restlessness; hyperactivity; anxiety; dizziness; postoperative hallucinations; mental depression. *OTHER:* Muscular rigidity; chills or shivering.

Precautions
Pregnancy: Category C. *Lactation:* Undetermined. *Children:* Safety and efficacy in children < 2 yr not established. *Special risk patients:* Decreased dose may be necessary. Use drug with caution in elderly, debilitated and hepatically or renally impaired patients.

NURSING CONSIDERATIONS

Administration/Storage
- If direct IV has been ordered, administer at slow rate (do not exceed 10 mg/30-60 sec).
- Store at room temperature and protect from light. Solution remains stable for 7-10 days.
- Compatible when mixed in syringe with atropine, butorphanol, chlorpromazine, fentanyl, glycopyrrolate, hydroxyzine, morphine, meperidine, perphenazine, promazine, promethazine, scopalamine.

Assessment/Interventions
- Obtain patient history, including drug history and any known allergies.
- Monitor vital signs and ECG throughout therapy. Observe for hypotension and tachycardia.
- Assess patient's respiratory status continuously. If patient is receiving narcotic analgesic concurrently, respiratory depression may occur.
- If patient experiences drowsiness, keep siderails up and assist with ambulation.
- If extrapyramidal symptoms (dystonia, hyperactivity, neck extension) occur, notify physician immediately.

OVERDOSAGE: SIGNS & SYMPTOMS
Extension of pharmacologic effects, including sedation and hypotension

Patient/Family Education
- Caution patient to avoid sudden changes in position to prevent orthostatic hypotension.
- Instruct patient to call for help before rising from bed.
- Advise patient to avoid intake of alcoholic beverages or other CNS depressants for at least 24 hr after treatment.

No patient monograph available.

Econazole Nitrate

(ee-CON-uh-zole NYE-trate)

Spectazole, ♣ *Ecostatin*
Class: Topical/antifungal

Action Increases cell membrane permeability in susceptible fungi.

Indications Treatment of tinea pedis (athlete's foot), tinea cruris (jock itch), tinea corporis (ringworm), cutaneous candidiasis, tinea versicolor.

Contraindications Standard considerations.

Route/Dosage
Tinea Pedis, Tinea Cruris, Tinea Corporis and Tinea Versicolor
ADULTS & CHILDREN: **Topical** Apply

sufficient quantity to cover affected areas once daily. Treat tinea versicolor, tinea cruris and tinea corporis for 2 wk and tinea pedis for 1 mo.

Cutaneous Candidiasis
ADULTS & CHILDREN: **Topical** Apply bid for 2 wk.

Interactions None well documented.

Lab Test Interferences
None well documented.

Adverse Reactions
DERM: Burning; itching; stinging; erythema.

Precautions
Pregnancy: Category C. *Lactation:* Undetermined.

NURSING CONSIDERATIONS

Administration/Storage
- Wash skin with soap and water and dry thoroughly prior to application.
- Cover treated area with sterile bandage if needed.

Assessment/Interventions
- Obtain patient history, including drug history and any known allergies.
- Assess condition of skin before beginning therapy and regularly throughout course of treatment. If burning, itching, stinging or erythema develops, notify physician.

Patient/Family Education
- Inform patient medication is for external use only.
- Teach patient to wash and dry skin before application.
- Teach patient and family name, desired action, technique of administration and potential side effects of medication.
- Advise patient to report signs of hypersensitivity such as rash, burning or redness.
- Instruct patient to use medication for length of treatment prescribed even if symptoms subside.

See Patient Guide, p. 212.

Edetate Calcium Disodium
(Calcium EDTA)

(EH-duh-tate KAL-see-uhm die-SO-dee-uhm)

Calcium Disodium Versenate
Class: Antidote

Action Calcium is displaced by heavy metals, such as lead, to form stable EDTA complexes that are excreted in urine.

Indications Treatment of acute and chronic lead poisoning and lead encephalopathy.

Contraindications Anuria; active renal disease; hepatitis.

Route/Dosage
ASYMPTOMATIC ADULTS: **IV** 5 ml ampule diluted with 250-500 ml normal saline or D5W. Administer dilution over at least 1 hr bid for up to 5 days. Interrupt therapy for 2 days; follow with 5 additional days if needed (maximum 50 mg/kg/day). SYMPTOMATIC ADULTS: **IV** 5 ml ampule diluted with 250-500 ml normal saline or D5W. Administer dilution over 2 hr. Give second daily infusion at least 6 hr after first. CHILDREN AND PATIENTS WITH OVERT OR INCIPIENT LEAD ENCEPHALOPATHY: **IM** 35 mg/kg bid q 8-12 hr for 3-5 days; give second course no sooner than 4 days later. Procaine or lidocaine may be added (for concentration of up to 0.5%) to minimize pain on injection.

Interactions None well documented.

Lab Test Interferences
None well documented.

Adverse Reactions

GU: Renal tubular necrosis.

Precautions

Pregnancy: Safety not established. *Lactation:* Undetermined. *Hydration:* Patients may be dehydrated from vomiting. Because drug is excreted in urine, establish urine flow by IV infusion before administering first dose; then restrict IV fluid to basal water and electrolyte requirements. *Lead encephalopathy:* Rapid infusion may be lethal in patients with cerebral edema, because of sudden increases in intracranial pressure. IM route is preferred. *Renal damage:* Discontinue if urinalysis reveals large renal epithelial cells, increasing numbers of red blood cells in urinary sediment or greater proteinuria.

NURSING CONSIDERATIONS

Administration/Storage

- Dilute 5 ml ampule in 250-500 ml of normal saline or D5W for IV administration.
- Use infusion pump to control rate of infusion. Infuse over at least 1 hr for asymptomatic adults. Infuse over at least 2 hr for symptomatic adults.
- Administer second daily infusion no sooner than 6 hr after first dose.
- Administer IM if patient is child or has lead encephalopathy. Inject deep into well-developed muscle, and rotate injection sites. Use procaine or lidocaine to minimize pain at injection site.
- Administer dimercaprol in separate injection site if used concurrently with edetate calcium disodium.
- Administer in courses of 3-5 days, with second course given no sooner than 2 days later if given IV or 4 days later if given IM.

Assessment/Interventions

- Obtain patient history, including drug history and any known allergies.
- Assess renal function prior to and during administration, including frequent urinalysis, BUN and creatinine.
- Document serum lead level prior to and during administration.
- Assess hydration status prior to administering drug.
- Assess for signs of increased intracranial pressure prior to and during IV administration.
- Obtain baseline and periodic ECG.
- Hydrate patient with IV infusion prior to administration because patient may be dehydrated from vomiting, and then reduce rate to basal fluid and electrolyte requirements.
- Maintain strict I&O measurement and daily weights. Do not administer unless patient has adequate urine output. Discontinue drug and notify physician if anuria develops.
- Monitor vital signs and assess for paresthesia, hypotension, arrhythmias, febrile reactions and histamine-like reaction including flushing, headache, sweating, sneezing, congestion and tachycardia.
- Wait 1 hour after administering dose before drawing serum lead sample.
- Notify physician and discontinue drug if urinalysis reveals renal damage, including large epithelial cells, increased protein, RBCs or BUN.
- Rehydrate in event of anuria and continue drug once urine flow resumes.
- Discontinue IV administration and notify physician if signs of increased intracranial pressure develop.
- Obtain ECG if patient complains of palpitations or heart rate irregularities.

OVERDOSAGE: SIGNS & SYMPTOMS

Cerebral edema, renal tubular necrosis

Patient/Family Education

- Explain method of administration and potential side effects.

- Instruct patient to notify physician immediately if side effects occur.
- Explain rationale for strict I&O measurement and how to assist.
- Refer to public health agency regarding potential sources of lead poisoning and assistance for family in proper removal.
- Provide appropriate referrals for child who has learning deficits resulting from lead poisoning.
- Teach signs of lead poisoning, including metallic taste in mouth, abdominal cramping, GI upset, decreased urine output, alteration in mentation, blue-black line along gum, paresthesia, seizures and coma. Instruct to notify physician if any of these signs appear.
- Counsel family in low-fat diet with adequate calcium, magnesium, zinc, iron and copper to prevent binding and storage of lead in body.
- Review follow-up schedule of appointments to monitor serum lead levels.

No patient monograph available.

Edetate Disodium (EDTA)

(EH-duh-tate die-SO-dee-uhm)

Chealamide, Disotate, Endrate

Class: Cardiovascular

Action Forms chelates with polyvalent metals, especially calcium, thus increasing their urinary excretion.

Indications Emergency treatment of hypercalcemia; control of ventricular arrhythmias associated with digitalis toxicity.

Contraindications Anuria.

Route/Dosage
ADULTS: **IV** 50 mg/kg/day (maximum 3 g/day). Usually administered in 5 consecutive daily doses followed by 2 days without medication, with repeated courses prn, for total of 15 doses. CHILDREN: **IV** 40 mg/kg/day (maximum 70 mg/kg/day) *or* 15-50 mg/kg/day (maximum 3 g/day) with 5 days between courses.

Interactions None well documented.

Lab Test Interferences
None well documented.

Adverse Reactions
CV: Transient drop in BP; adverse effects on myocardial contractility; thrombophlebitis. *CNS:* Transient circumoral paresthesia; numbness; headache. *GI:* Nausea; vomiting; diarrhea. *GU:* Nephrotoxicity; damage to reticuloendothelial system. *HEMA:* Thrombophlebitis; anemia. *DERM:* Exfoliative dermatitis; toxic skin and mucous membrane reactions. *META:* Electrolyte imbalances including hypocalcemia, hypokalemia, and hypomagnesemia; hyperuricemia. *OTHER:* Febrile reactions.

Precautions
Pregnancy: Category C. *Lactation:* Undetermined. *Special risk patients:* Use drug cautiously in patients with limited cardiac reserve or incipient congestive failure. *Diabetic patients:* Blood sugar and insulin requirements may be lower in insulin-dependent diabetic patients. *IV infusion:* Rapid IV infusion or high serum concentrations can cause a precipitous and potentially fatal drop in serum calcium. Do not exceed maximum dose or rate.

NURSING CONSIDERATIONS

Administration/Storage
- Do not confuse edetate disodium with edetate calcium disodium.
- Adults: Dissolve 50 mg/kg dose in 500 ml of D5W or 0.9% Sodium Chlo-

ride for Injection. Infuse over ≥ 3 hr.

- Children: Dissolve drug in sufficient volume of D5W or 0.9% Sodium Chloride for Injection to bring final concentration to ≤ 3%. Infuse over ≥ 3 hr.
- Store at room temperature.

Assessment/Interventions

- Obtain patient history, including drug history and any known allergies. Note previous history of renal disease or CHF.
- Because of potential for electrolyte disturbances, obtain appropriate laboratory determinations (electrolytes, calcium, renal function test).
- Adequately hydrate patient before administration.
- Assess patency of IV site frequently during therapy.
- Assist patient with ambulation.
- After infusion, have patient remain supine for short period because of possible orthostatic hypotension.
- Assess for allergic reaction: rash, urticaria. Withhold drug and notify physician if these signs occur.
- Monitor vital signs and I&O.
- Monitor rate of infusion closely.
- If signs or symptoms of hypocalcemia occur (circumoral numbness/tingling, positive Chvostek's or Trousseau's signs, tetany), notify physician.
- If signs or symptoms of cardiac dysfunction occur (tachycardia, arrhythmias, hypotension), notify physician.

OVERDOSAGE: SIGNS & SYMPTOMS

Drop in serum calcium

Patient/Family Education

- Advise patient to remain recumbent for 30 min after infusion because of possibility of orthostatic hypotension.
- Inform patient that breath may be odorous.

No patient monograph available.

Edrophonium Chloride

(eh-droe-FOE-nee-uhm KLOR-ide)

Enlon, Reversol, Tensilon

Class: Cholinergic muscle stimulant/anticholinesterase

Action Facilitates myoneural junction impulse transmission by inhibiting acetylcholine destruction by cholinesterase.

Indications Differential diagnosis of myasthenia gravis; adjunct in evaluating treatment of myasthenia gravis; evaluation of emergency treatment of myasthenic crises; reversal of neuromuscular blockade by curare, gallamine or tubocurarine; treatment of respiratory depression due to curare overdose.

Contraindications Hypersensitivity to anticholinesterases; mechanical intestinal and urinary obstruction.

Route/Dosage

Diagnosis of Myasthenia Gravis

ADULTS: **IM/IV** 10 mg. CHILDREN > 34 KG: **IV** 2 mg. If no response after 45 sec, may titrate up to 10 mg in increments of 1 mg q 30-45 sec. or **IM** 5 mg as single dose. CHILDREN < 34 KG: **IV** 1 mg. If no response after 45 sec, may titrate up to 5 mg in increments of 1 mg q 30-45 sec or **IM** 2 mg as single dose. INFANTS: **IV** 0.5 mg.

Evaluation of Myasthenia Gravis Treatment

ADULTS: **IV** 1-2 mg 1 hr after ingestion of treatment drug.

Crisis Test

ADULTS: **IV** When respiration is adequate, give 1 mg initially. If after 1 min patient is not further impaired, give additional 1 mg.

Curare Antagonist

ADULTS: **IV** 10 mg over 30-45 sec. Repeat prn up to maximum total dose of 40 mg.

Interactions

Corticosteroids: May antagonize anticholinesterases in myasthenia gravis, producing profound muscular depression. *Succinylcholine:* Neuromuscular blockade produced by succinylcholine may be either prolonged or antagonized.

Lab Test Interferences

None well documented.

Adverse Reactions

CV: Arrhythmia (especially bradycardia); hypotention; tachycardia; atrioventricular block; nodal rhythm; non-specific ECG changes; cardiac arrest; syncope. *RESP:* Increased tracheobronchial secretions; laryngospasm; bronchiolar constriction; respiratory paralysis; dyspnea; respiratory depression; respiratory arrest; bronchospasm. *CNS:* Convulsions; dysarthria; dysphonia; dizziness; loss of consciousness; drowsiness; headache. *EENT:* Lacrimation; miosis; spasm of accommodation; diplopia; conjunctival hyperemia; visual changes. *GI:* Increased salivary, gastric and intestinal secretions; nausea; vomiting; dysphagia; increased peristalsis; diarrhea; abdominal cramps; flatulence. *GU:* Urinary urgency, frequency and incontinence. *DERM:* Rash; urticaria; flushing. *OTHER:* Allergy and anaphylaxis; weakness; fasciculations; muscle cramps and spasms; arthralgia; diaphoresis.

Precautions

Pregnancy: Pregnancy category undetermined. *Lactation:* Undetermined. *Special risk patients:* Use with caution in patients with bronchial asthma, epilepsy, bradycardia, recent coronary occlusion, vagotonia, hyperthyroidism, cardiac arrhythmias or peptic ulcer. *Anticholinesterase insensitivity:* May develop.

NURSING CONSIDERATIONS

Administration/Storage

- Given IM or IV only.
- Store at room temperature.

Assessment/Interventions

- Obtain patient history, including drug history and any known allergies.
- Assess neuromuscular status before and frequently during therapy.
- Obtain baseline ECG and vital signs before therapy and monitor throughout administration.
- If ECG changes develop (supraventricular tachycardia), notify physician immediately.
- Take seizure precautions.
- Keep atropine available in syringe as antidote.
- Have respiratory support equipment available.

OVERDOSAGE: SIGNS & SYMPTOMS

Increasing parasympathomimetic action, cholinergic crisis, nausea, vomiting, diarrhea, sweating, increased bronchial and salivary secretions with resulting bronchial obstruction, bradycardia

Patient/Family Education

- Teach patient and family name, desired action, method of administration and potential side effects of edrophonium.
- Inform patient that effects of medication last up to 30 min after IM administration.
- Show patient and family how to assess and record changes in muscle strength.
- Advise patient that urinary urgency and frequency and increased GI motility and secretion will occur and should be reported to physician.

No patient monograph available.

Enalapril Maleate

(EH-NAL-uh-prill MAL-ee-ate)
Vasotec
Class: Antihypertensive/ACE inhibitor

Action Competitively inhibits angiotensin I–converting enzyme, preventing conversion of angiotensin I to angiotensin II, a potent vasoconstrictor. Clinical consequences include decreased sodium and fluid retention, decreased BP, and increased diuresis.

Indications Treatment of hypertension and symptomatic CHF in combination with diuretics and digitalis and asymptomatic left ventricular dysfunction after MI. **Unlabeled uses:** Treatment of diabetic nephropathy, childhood hypertension and hypertension related to scleroderma renal crisis.

Contraindications Standard considerations.

Route/Dosage

Hypertension

ADULTS: **PO** Initial dose: 2.5-5 mg/day. Titrate to desired BP control. Usual maintenance dose: 10-40 mg/day in single or twice daily doses.

Heart Failure

ADULTS: **PO** Initial dose: 2.5 mg/day or bid. Usual dose: 5-20 mg/day in two divided doses (maximum 40 mg/day).

Left Ventricular Dysfunction

ADULTS: **PO** Initial dose: 2.5 mg bid. Titrate to targeted daily dose of 20 mg in divided doses.

Interactions

Allopurinol: Greater risk of hypersensitivity possible with coadministration. *Antacids:* Enalapril bioavailability may be decreased. Separate administration times by 1 to 2 hours. *Capsaicin:* Cough may be exacerbated. *Digoxin:* Increased digoxin levels. *Indomethacin:* Hypotensive effects may be reduced, especially in low-renin or volume-dependent hypertensive patients. *Lithium:* Increased lithium levels and symptoms of lithium toxicity may occur. *Phenothiazine:* May increase pharmacological effect of phenothiazines. *Potassium preparations, potassium-sparing diuretics:* May increase serum potassium levels. *Rifampin:* Pharmacologic effects of enalapril may be decreased.

Lab Test Interferences

False elevation of liver enzymes, serum bilirubin, uric acid or blood glucose may occur.

Adverse Reactions

CV: Chest pain; myocardial infarction; hypotension; angina; orthostatic hypotension; tachycardia; syncope; vasculitis. *RESP:* Bronchitis; continuing cough; dyspnea. *CNS:* Headache; vertigo; dizziness; fatigue; asthenia. *GI:* Nausea; abdominal pain; vomiting; diarrhea. *GU:* Urinary tract infection. *HEMA:* Decreased hemoglobin and hematocrit; neutropenia; agranulocytosis; thrombocytopenia; pancytopenia; eosinophilia. *DERM:* Rash; photosensitivity. *META:* Hyperkalemia. *OTHER:* Fever; myalgia; arthralgia; arthritis.

Precautions

Pregnancy: Category D (second, third trimester); Category C (first trimester). *Lactation:* Excreted in breast milk. *Children:* Safety and efficacy not established. *Angioedema:* May occur. Use drug with extreme caution in patients with hereditary angioedema. *Cough:* Chronic dry cough may occur during treatment; higher incidence in women. *Hypotension/first-dose effect:* Significant decreases in blood pressure may occur after first dose, especially in severely salt- or volume-depleted patients or in those with heart failure; monitor closely for at least 2 hr after initial dose and during first 2 wk of therapy. Minimize risk by discontinuing diuretics, decreasing dose, or increasing salt intake approximately 1 wk prior to initiating enalapril. *Neutropenia and agranulocytosis:* Have occurred; risk appears greater with renal dysfunction, heart failure or immunosuppression; monitor WBC counts frequently. *Renal impairment:* Reduce dose and give less frequently. In renal insufficiency stable elevations in BUN and serum creatinine may occur because of inadequate renal perfusion; monitor renal function during first few weeks of therapy and adjust dosage.

NURSING CONSIDERATIONS

Administration/Storage

- May be administered without regard to meals.

Assessment/Interventions

- Obtain patient history, including drug history and any known allergies.
- Obtain baseline weight.
- Monitor patient's BP and pulse before therapy and regularly during treatment.
- Monitor I&O.
- If precipitous drop in BP develops, notify physician and administer with IV fluids or plasma volume expanders as prescribed.
- If signs of fluid overload develop (increase in weight, dyspnea, rales/crackles, jugular vein distention), notify physician immediately.
- If vertigo, dizziness or fatigue develops, notify physician.

OVERDOSAGE: SIGNS & SYMPTOMS

Hypotension

Patient/Family Education

- Teach patient and family name, desired action, method of administration and potential side effects of enalapril.
- Explain protocol for missed doses, and caution against taking missed dose with the next dose.
- Teach additional interventions for control of hypertension (weight reduction, exercise, stress management, stopping smoking).
- Inform patient of potential for temporarily altered impairment of taste sensation and for chronic cough.
- Instruct patient to make position changes slowly and to wait a few minutes before standing to minimize orthostatic hypertension.
- Teach patient and family how to measure BP and pulse.
- Emphasize importance of regular follow-up visits, and explain that hypertension is controlled, not cured.
- Instruct patient to report these symptoms to physician: rash, fever, chest pain, hives, or dyspnea.

See Patient Guide, p. 213.

Enalapril Maleate/ Hydrochlorothiazide

(EH-NAL-uh-prill MAL-ee-ate high-droe-klor-oh-THIGH-uh-zide)

Vaseretic 10-25

Class: Antihypertensive

Action Enalapril causes vasodilation and decreased blood pressure; hydrochlorothiazide causes loss of body water and increases urine output.

Indications Treatment of hypertension.

Contraindications Hypersensitivity to any component or to other sulfonamide-derived drugs; history of angioedema related to previous treatment with acetylcholinesterase (ACE) inhibitor; anuria.

Route/Dosage

ADULTS: PO 1-2 tablets (each containing 10 mg enalapril maleate and 25 mg hydrochlorothiazide) per day.

Interactions

Cholestyramine and colestipol resins: May bind to hydrochlorothiazide and decrease its bioavailability. *Diazoxide:* Hyperglycemia may occur. *Digitalis glycosides:* Arrhythmias may occur. *Indomethacin:* Hypotensive effects may be reduced. *Lithium:* Toxicity risk is greater; avoid use. *Loop diuretics:* Synergistic effects may cause profound diuresis and electrolyte abnormalities. *Potassium preparations, potassium-sparing diuretics:* May increase serum potassium levels. *Sulfonylureas:* May require dose adjustment.

Lab Test Interferences

PBI levels may be decreased without signs of thyroid disturbances; diagnostic interference with serum electrolyte levels, blood and urinary glucose levels, serum bilirubin levels and serum uric acid levels.

Adverse Reactions

CV: Hypotension; orthostatic effects; palpitations; tachycardia; chest pain. *RESP:* Chronic cough; dyspnea. *CNS:* Dizziness; headache; insomnia; nervousness; paresthesia; somnolence; vertigo; syncope. *EENT:* Tinnitus; dry mouth. *GI:* Nausea; diarrhea; abdominal pain; vomiting; dyspepsia; constipation; flatulence. *GU:* Impotence; decreased libido; urinary tract infections. *HEMA:* Neutropenia; agranulocytosis. *DERM:* Rash, pruritus. *META:* Hyperkalemia; hyponatremia; hypercalcemia; hypochloremic alkalosis; hypokalemia; gout; hypomagnesemia; hyperglycemia; increased triglyceride and cholesterol levels. *OTHER:* Angioedema; fatigue; weakness; muscle cramps; back pain; sweating.

Precautions

Pregnancy: Category D (second, third trimester); Category C (first trimester). *Lactation:* Excreted in breast milk. *Children:* Safety and efficacy not established. *Angioedema:* Angioedema of face, extremities, lips, tongue, glottis or larynx has been reported in patients treated with enalapril. Discontinue drug. *Bone marrow depression:* Other ACE inhibitors have caused bone marrow depression, particularly in patients with renal impairment and collagen vascular disease. Monitor hematopoietic system. *Diabetes:* Monitor closely, because adjustments may be needed in hypoglycemic agents. *Renal and hepatic impairment:* Use drug with caution in patients with renal disease and monitor renal function periodically; may precipitate azotemia; may alter renal function in susceptible individuals (incuding those with severe CHF). Use drug with caution in patients with impaired hepatic function or progressive liver disease, because changes in fluid and electrolyte balance can precipitate hepatic coma. *Systemic lupus erythematosus:* May be activated or exacerbated.

NURSING CONSIDERATIONS

Administration/Storage

- If patient is receiving diuretics keep patient under medical supervision for 2 hr after initial dose. Continue to monitor patient until blood pressure is stable for 1 hr.
- Give with food or milk if nausea occurs.
- Store at room temperature in sealed container.

Assessment/Interventions

- Obtain patient history, including drug history and any known allergies.
- Obtain baseline vital signs.
- Review baseline creatinine, BUN, magnesium, glucose, triglyceride, cholesterol, serum electrolytes and liver function test results.
- After initial dose, monitor vital signs for 2 hr until vital signs are stable for 1 hr.
- Assist patient with postural changes, and monitor orthostatic BP frequently during initial therapy and regularly thereafter.
- In diabetic patients, monitor blood glucose closely.
- Monitor I&O, serum electrolytes,

liver function test results, glucose and CBC.
- Assess for vertigo, somnolence, headache, nausea, abdominal pain.
- Notify physician if severe hypotension, chest pain or arrhythmia occur.

OVERDOSAGE: SIGNS & SYMPTOMS

Hypotension, orthostatic hypotension, dizziness, drowsiness, syncope, electrolyte abnormalities, hemoconcentration, confusion, muscular weakness, nausea, vomiting, depressed respiration, lethargy, coma

Patient/Family Education

- Advise patient to take with food or milk if nausea occurs.
- Caution patient that medication increases urination and to take as early in day as possible.
- Advise patient that lethargy may be experienced until body adjusts.
- Caution patient to take missed dose as soon as possible but not to take missed dose with next dose. If more than one dose is missed, tell patient to contact physician.
- Advise patient not to use salt substitutes unless approved by physician.
- Instruct patient to report these symptoms to physician: weakness, muscle cramps, dizziness, nausea, neck or facial swelling, faintness on standing, sore throat or dry, persistent cough.

See Patient Guide, p. 214.

Enalaprilat

(EH-NAL-uh-prill-at)

Vasotec IV

Class: Antihypertensive/ACE inhibitor

Action Competitively inhibits angiotensin I–converting enzyme, preventing conversion of angiotensin I to angiotensin II, a potent vasoconstrictor. Clinical consequences include decrease in sodium and fluid retention, decrease in blood pressure and increase in diuresis.

Indications Treatment of hypertension when oral therapy is not practical. **Unlabeled use:** Hypertensive emergencies.

Contraindications Standard considerations.

Route/Dosage

IN ADULT PATIENTS NOT TAKING DIURETICS: **IV** 1.25 mg over 5 min q 6 hr. IN ADULT PATIENTS TAKING DIURETICS: **IV** 0.625 mg over 5 min. If inadequate response after 1 hr, may repeat 0.625 mg. Give additional doses of 1.25 mg q 6 hr.

Interactions

Allopurinol: Greater risk of hypersensitivity possible with coadmistration. *Antacids:* Enalaprilat bioavailability may be decreased. Separate administration times by 1 to 2 hr. *Capsaicin:* Cough may be exacerbated. *Digoxin:* Increased digoxin levels. *Indomethacin:* Hypotensive effects may be reduced, especially in low-renin or volume-dependent hypertensive patients. *Lithium:* Increased lithium levels and symptoms of lithium toxicity may occur. *Phenothiazines:* May increase pharmacological effect of phenothiazines. *Potassium preparations, potassium-sparing diuretics:* May increase serum potassium levels. *Rifampin:* Pharmacologic effects of enalapril may be decreased.

Lab Test Interferences

False elevation of liver enzymes, serum bilirubin, uric acid or blood glucose may occur.

Adverse Reactions

CV: Chest pain; myocardial infarction; hypotension; angina; orthostatic hypotension; tachycardia. *RESP:* Bronchitis; cough; dyspnea. *CNS:* Headache; vertigo; dizziness; fatigue; asthenia; syncope. *GI:* Nausea; abdominal pain; vomiting; diarrhea. *GU:* Urinary tract infection. *HEMA:* Decreased hemoglobin and hematocrit; neutropenia;

agranulocytosis; thrombocytopenia; pancytopenia; eosinophilia. *DERM:* Rash; photosensitivity. *META:* Hyperkalemia. *OTHER:* Fever; myalgia; arthralgia; arthritis; vasculitis.

Precautions

Pregnancy: Category D (second, third trimester); Category C (first trimester). *Lactation:* Excreted in breast milk. *Children:* Safety and efficacy not established. *Angioedema:* May occur. Use extreme caution in patients with hereditary angioedema. *Cough:* Chronic severe cough may occur during treatment. *Hypotension/first-dose effect:* Significant decreases in blood pressure may occur following first dose, especially in severely salt- or volume-depleted patients or those with heart failure; monitor closely for at least 2 hr after initial dose and during first 2 wk of therapy. Minimize risk by discontinuing diuretics, decreasing dose or increasing salt intake approximately 1 wk prior to initiating enalaprilat. *Neutropenia and agranulocytosis:* Have occurred; risk appears greater with renal dysfunction, heart failure or immunosuppression; monitor WBC counts periodically. *Proteinuria:* May occur, especially in patients with prior renal disease or those receiving high doses. *Renal impairment:* Reduce dose and give less frequently. In renal insufficiency, stable elevations in BUN and serum creatinine may occur due to inadequate renal perfusion; monitor renal function during first few weeks of therapy and adjust dosage.

NURSING CONSIDERATIONS

Administration/Storage

- Dilute with 0.9% normal saline in D5W or 5% Dextrose in Lactated Ringer's.
- Give as slow IV infusion over 5 min.
- Store at room temperature and discard after 24 hr.

Assessment/Interventions

- Obtain patient history, including drug history and any known allergies.
- Obtain baseline vital signs, LFT results, serum bilirubin, uric acid, electrolytes, CBC, creatinine and BUN, and monitor these values throughout therapy.
- Monitor vital signs closely after initial dose, at least 2 hr and during first 2 wk of therapy. Peak effect with initial dose may be 4 hr after injection.
- Notify physician of any adverse reaction, including angioedema, chest pain, hypotension, tachycardia, dyspnea, bronchitis, vertigo, nausea or vomiting.

OVERDOSAGE: SIGNS & SYMPTOMS

Hypotension

Patient/Family Education

- Advise patient to notify nurse of any vertigo, chest pain, tachycardia, dyspnea, persistent cough, nausea or vomiting.
- Caution patient not to discontinue drug suddenly.

No patient monograph available.

Enoxacin

(en-OX-uh-SIN)

Penetrex

Class: Antibiotic/fluoroquinolone

Action Interferes with microbial DNA synthesis.

Indications Treatment of urinary tract infections caused by susceptible organisms; treatment of sexually transmitted disease caused by *Neisseria gonorrhoeae*.

Contraindications Hypersensitivity to fluoroquinolones.

Route/Dosage

Urinary Tract Infections

ADULTS: PO 200-400 mg q 12 hr for 7-14 days.

Sexually Transmitted Diseases

ADULTS: PO 400 mg as single dose.

Interactions *Antacids, iron salts, zinc salts, sucralfate, bismuth subsalicylate:* May decrease oral absorption of fluoroquinolone. *Caffeine:* Reduces clearance of caffeine. *Digoxin:* May increase digoxin levels. *Theophylline:* Can cause decreased clearance and increased plasma levels of theophylline, which may result in toxicity.

Lab Test Interferences None well documented.

Adverse Reactions *CNS:* Headache; dizziness; insomnia; vertigo. *EENT:* Tinnitus; unusual taste in mouth. *GI:* Diarrhea; nausea; vomiting; abdominal pain or discomfort; dyspepsia; heartburn. *DERM:* Pruritus; photosensitivity.

Precautions

Pregnancy: Category C. *Lactation:* Excreted in breast milk. *Children:* Contraindicated in children. *CNS disorders:* Use drug with caution in patients predisposed to seizures or with other CNS disorders. *Convulsions:* CNS stimulation can occur; use drug with caution in patients with known or suspected CNS disorders. *Hypersensitivity:* Serious and potentially fatal reactions have occurred. Discontinue drug if allergic reaction occurs. *Pseudomembranous colitis:* Consider possibility in patients in whom diarrhea develops subsequent to administration of antibacterial agents. *Renal impairment:* Reduced clearance may occur; dosage adjustment may be required. *Superinfection:* Use of antibiotics may result in bacterial or fungal overgrowth of nonsusceptible microorganisms.

NURSING CONSIDERATIONS

Administration/Storage

- Do not administer with antacids.
- Administer medication at least 1 hr before or 2 hr after meal.
- Encourage patient to increase fluid intake.

Assessment/Interventions

- Obtain patient history, including drug history and any known allergies.
- Determine baseline WBC and BUN.
- Assess renal and liver function.
- Monitor temperature.
- Monitor patient for signs and symptoms of hypersensitivity.
- Inform physician of signs and symptoms of superinfection (eg, black furry tongue, white patches in mouth, foul-smelling stool).
- If GI disturbances develop, withhold drug and notify physician.
- If photosensitivity occurs, withhold drug and notify physician.

OVERDOSAGE: SIGNS & SYMPTOMS

Renal failure

Patient/Family Education

- Instruct patient to take drug at least 1 hr before meals or 2 hr after meals.
- Advise patient not to take medication with antacids.
- Caution patient to avoid exposure to sunlight and to use sunscreen or wear protective clothing to avoid photosensitivity reaction.
- Instruct patient to increase fluid intake and to restrict or eliminate caffeine intake.
- Advise patient to report any visual changes, agitation or rash to physician.
- Instruct patient to report any additional infections after completion of medication to physician.
- Tell patient to notify physician if diarrhea develops.
- Advise patient that drug may cause

dizziness and lightheadedness and to use caution while driving or performing other tasks requiring mental alertness.

See Patient Guide, p. 215.

Enoxaparin Sodium

(eh-NOX-uh-par-in SO-dee-uhm)

Lovenox

Class: Anticoagulant

Action Causes higher anti-factor Xa to antithrombin activities (anti-factor IIa) ratio than heparin, which may prevent thrombosis.

Indications Prevention of deep vein thrombosis after hip replacement surgery. **Unlabeled use:** Prevention of thrombosis after knee replacement surgery.

Contraindications Hypersensitivity to enoxaparin, heparin or pork products; active major bleeding; thrombocytopenia associated with positive in vitro test for antiplatelet antibody in presence of enoxaparin.

Route/Dosage

ADULTS: **Deep SC** 30 mg bid.

Interactions

Anticoagulants, platelet inhibitors: Use enoxaparin with care. INCOMPATIBILITIES: Do not mix enoxaparin with other injections or infusions.

Lab Test Interferences

Transaminase determinations: Drug causes asymptomatic elevations in AST and ALT.

Adverse Reactions

HEMA: Hemorrhage; thrombocytopenia. *DERM:* Local erythema. *OTHER:* Local irritation and pain; hematoma.

Precautions

Pregnancy: Category B. *Lactation:* Undetermined. *Children:* Safety and efficacy not established. *Elderly and debilitated patients:* Delayed elimination of drug possible. Use drug with caution. *Special risk patients:* Use drug with caution in patients with bleeding diathesis, uncontrolled arterial hypotension, or history of recent GI ulceration and hemorrhage. *Hemorrhage:* Use drug with extreme caution in patients with conditions associated with increased risk of hemorrhage. *Interchangeability with heparin:* Cannot be used interchangeably (unit for unit) with heparin. *Renal impairment:* Delayed elimination of drug may occur. Use drug with caution.

NURSING CONSIDERATIONS

Administration/Storage

- Administer only by deep subcutaneous injection; enoxaparin cannot be administered via IM or IV injection.
- With patient lying down, administer drug by subcutaneous injection. Alternate administration between left and right anterolateral and posterolateral abdominal wall. Introduce whole length of needle into skin fold held between thumb and forefinger; hold skin fold throughout injection.
- Do not aspirate into syringe; do not rub site after injection. These activities may cause tissue damage and subcutaneous bleeding.
- Store at room temperature. Do not freeze.

Assessment/Interventions

- Obtain patient history, including drug history and any known allergies.
- Review patient's health history for any condition that could contraindicate enoxaparin (active major bleeding, thrombocytopenia, hypersensitivity to enoxaparin, heparin or pork products).
- Review patient's medication record

for use of drugs that present special risks when used with enoxaparin (anticoagulants, platelet inhibitors).
- Obtain bleeding disorder laboratory tests before administering enoxaparin to assess for bleeding disorder.
- Monitor patient for signs of bleeding throughout therapy.
- Perform periodic CBCs (including platelet count) and stool occult blood tests during course of treatment.
- If bleeding develops (epistaxis, hematuria, hematemesis, bloody or black tarry stools), notify physician immediately.
- If laboratory studies for coagulation and bleeding are abnormal, notify physician.

OVERDOSAGE: SIGNS & SYMPTOMS
Hemorrhage

Patient/Family Education
- Teach patient and family the name, action, administration and side effects of enoxaparin.
- Instruct patient to report any signs of bleeding immediately.
- Explain to patient rationale for follow-up examinations and laboratory studies to ensure effectiveness of medication and to monitor for side effects.
- If patient has home therapy, teach patient or family proper subcutaneous injection technique.
- Caution patient to take safety precautions to prevent cuts and bruising (eg, use electric razor, soft toothbrush, handrails).

See Patient Guide, p. 216.

Ephedrine

(eh-FED-rin)

Ephedrine Sulfate, Kondon's Nasal, Pretz-D, Vicks Vatronol

Class: Vasopressor; decongestant

Action Stimulates both alpha- and beta-receptors, causing increased heart rate, unchanged or augmented stroke volume, enhanced cardiac output and increased blood pressure. Causes relaxation of smooth muscle of bronchi and GI tract, stimulation of cerebral cortex and pupil dilation.

Indications
IM/IV/SC form: Treatment of acute hypotensive states; treatment of Adams-Stokes syndrome with complete heart block; stimulation of CNS to combat narcolepsy and depressive states; treatment of acute bronchospasm; treatment of enuresis; treatment of myasthenia gravis. *Nasal form:* Treatment of nasal congestion; promotion of nasal or sinus drainage; relief of eustachian tube congestion.

Contraindications Angle-closure glaucoma; patients anesthetized with cyclopropane or halothane; cases in which vasopressor drugs are contraindicated (eg, thyrotoxicosis, diabetes mellitus, hypertension of pregnancy); MAO inhibitor therapy.

Route/Dosage

Hypotension

ADULTS: **SC** 25-50 mg (**IM/IV** if rapid effect is needed). 10-25 mg may be given by IV push; may give additional doses at 5-10 min intervals (maximum 150 mg/24 hr). CHILDREN: **IV/SC** 3 mg/kg/day *or* 25-100 mg/m^2/day in 4-6 divided doses.

Nasal Congestion

ADULTS: **Nasal** 1-3 gtt or sprays q 3-4 hr.

Labor

ADULTS: **SC/IV/IM** prn to maintain BP ≤ 130/80 mm Hg.

Interactions
Guanethidine: May negate guanethidine's antihypertensive effects. *MAO inhibitors:* Increases pressor response from vasopressors significantly;

hypertensive crisis and intracranial hemorrhage are possible. *Rauwolfia alkaloids, methyldopa, furazolidone:* May result in hypertension. *Tricyclic antidepressants:* May potentiate pressor response. *Urinary acidifiers:* May increase elimination of ephedrine. *Urinary alkalinizers:* May decrease elimination of ephedrine. INCOMPATIBILITIES: Ephedrine is chemically incompatible with sodium bicarbonate; avoid admixture.

Lab Test Interferences

Amphetamine enzyme-multiplied immunoassay test (EMIT) assay: False-positive results may occur.

Adverse Reactions

CV: Palpitation; tachycardia; precordial pain; cardiac arrhythmias; hypertension. *RESP:* Shortness of breath. *CNS:* Headache; insomnia; sweating; nervousness; vertigo; confusion; delirium; restlessness; anxiety; tension; tremor; weakness; dizziness; hallucinations. *EENT:* Nasal use: local irritation; sneezing; rebound congestion. *GI:* Nausea; vomiting; anorexia; dry mouth. *GU:* Difficult and painful urination; urinary retention in males with prostatism; decreased urine formation (initial parenteral use). *OTHER:* Pallor.

Precautions

Pregnancy: Category C. *Labor:* Do not use when maternal BP exceeds 130/80 mm Hg; usage during delivery may cause acceleration of fetal heart rate. *Lactation:* Undetermined. *Asthma:* Use drug with caution. *Hypertension:* Drug may cause severe hypertension, resulting in intracranial hemorrhage, angina or potentially fatal arrhythmias, especially in patients with organic heart disease or those receiving drugs that sensitize myocardium. *Sulfite sensitivity:* Use nasal decongestant form of drug with caution.

NURSING CONSIDERATIONS

Administration/Storage

- For nasal spray, have patient keep head upright. Instruct patient to sniff hard for few min after administration.
- For nasal drops, have patient recline on bed and hang head over edge. Instill drops in nose. Instruct patient to remain in this position for several min and to turn head from side to side.
- Protect from light. Do not give unless solution is clear. Discard any unused medication.

Assessment/Interventions

- Obtain patient history, including drug history and any known allergies. Note any hypersensitivity to epinephrine or sulfites.
- Obtain baseline assessment of vital signs and monitor frequently.
- Determine baseline glucose for patients with diabetes mellitus.
- Monitor for nervousness and agitation.
- Monitor for nasal congestion.

OVERDOSAGE: SIGNS & SYMPTOMS

Convulsions, nausea, vomiting, chills, cyanosis, irritability, nervousness, fever, suicidal behavior, tachycardia, dilated pupils, blurred vision, opisthotonos, spasms, pulmonary edema, gasping respirations, coma, respiratory failure, personality changes

Patient/Family Education

- Caution patient to use topical decongestants only in acute states and not to use > 3-5 days.
- Inform patient that nasal burning or stinging may occur with nasal drops or spray.
- Caution patient not to share nasal spray container with others.
- Advise patient to notify physician if symptoms do not improve after 7 days.
- With topical decongestant form of drug, instruct patient to report these symptoms to physician: headache,

palpitations, tremors, sweating, faintness, insomnia or weakness.

- With subcutaneous form of drug, advise patient to notify physician of syncope, palpitations, weakness, agitation, dizziness or chest pain.
- Instruct patient to take sips of water frequently, suck on ice chips or sugarless hard candy or chew gum if dry mouth occurs.
- Caution patient not to take otc medications without consulting physician.

See Patient Guide, p. 217.

Epinephrine

(epp-ih-NEFF-rin)

Adrenalin Chloride, Ana-Guard, Ana-Kit, AsthmaNefrin, Bronitin Mist, Bronkaid Mist, Epifrin, Epinal, Epinephrine Pediatric, Epi-Pen, Epi-Pin Jr., Epi-Ez-Pen, Eppy/N, Glaucon, MicroNefrin, Nephron, Primatene Mist, Racepinephrine, S-2, SusPhrine, Vaponefrin, ♣ *Bronkaid Mistometer*

Class: Vasopressor

Action Stimulates both alpha- and beta-receptors (alpha-receptors at high doses; $beta_1$- and $beta_2$-receptors at moderate doses) within sympathetic nervous system. Relaxes smooth muscle of bronchi and iris and is antagonist of histamine.

Indications Treatment and prophylaxis of cardiac arrest and attacks of transitory atrioventricular heart block; treatment of Adams-Stokes syndrome; treatment of hay fever; relief of bronchial asthma; treatment of syncope due to heart block or carotid sinus hypersensitivity; symptomatic relief of serum sickness, urticaria and angioedema; relaxation of uterine musculature; anaphylaxis. *Ophthalmic solution:* Treatment of open-angle glaucoma. *Nasal solution:* Treatment of nasal congestion; relief of eustachian tube congestion. *Inhalation:* Temporary relief from acute paroxysms of bronchial asthma and other states; treatment of postintubation and infectious croup.

Contraindications Hypersensitivity to epinephrine; narrow-angle glaucoma; concomitant use during general anesthesia with halogenated hydrocarbons or cyclopropane; cerebral arteriosclerosis or organic brain damage; use with anesthesia for fingers and toes; use during labor; phenothiazine-induced circulatory collapse; MAO inhibitor therapy.

Route/Dosage

Cardiac Arrest

ADULTS: **IV/Endotracheal/Intracardiac** 0.5-1 mg (5-10 ml of 1:10,000 solution) q 5 min prn. Myocardial injection usually given in left ventricular chamber by trained personnel at dose of 0.3-0.5 mg.

Other IV Uses

ADULTS: **IV** 1 mg in 250 ml of D5W (4 mcg/ml) for infusion at 1-4 mcg/min (15-60 ml/hr).

Intraspinal Use

ADULTS: **Intraspinal** 0.2-0.4 ml of 1:1000 solution added to anesthetic spinal fluid mixture. Epinephrine 1:100,000 to 1:20,000 is usual concentration employed with local anesthetics.

Open-Angle Glaucoma

ADULTS: **Ophthalmic** 1 gH in affected eyes 2 times daily.

Nasal Congestion

ADULTS & CHILDREN ≥ 6 YR: **Nasal** Apply as drops, spray or with sterile swab as required.

Asthma

ADULTS & CHILDREN: **Inhalation** Individualize dosage. Start administration at first symptoms; wait 1-5 min between inhalations.

Interactions *Beta-blocking agents:* May decrease effects of these agents, resulting in hypertension. *Guanethidine:* May increase pressor response. *Oxytoxic drugs:* May cause severe persistent hypertension. *Rauwolfia alkaloids, methyldopa, furazolidone:* May cause hypertension. *Tricyclic antidepressants:* May potentiate epinephrine's vasopressive effects. INCOMPATIBILITIES: Epinephrine is unstable in alkaline solutions (eg, sodium bicarbonate); avoid admixture.

Lab Test Interferences

None well documented.

Adverse Reactions

CV: Cardiac arrhythmias and excessive hypertension; palpitations (especially in hyperthyroid and hypertensive patients); anginal pain in predisposed patients; cerebral and subarachnoid hemorrhage; flushing. *RESP:* Shortness of breath. *CNS:* Anxiety; headache; restlessness; tremor; weakness; hemiplegia; dizziness; insomnia. *EENT:* Topical ophthalmic use: Transient stinging, burning, conjunctival hyperemia, pain and allergic lid reaction. May also cause effects seen with systemic use due to absorption. Nasal use: Local irritation; sneezing; rebound congestion. *GI:* Nausea; vomiting. *GU:* Decreased urine formation with initial parenteral use. *OTHER:* Severe metabolic acidosis; pallor; urticaria; wheal and hemorrhage at site of injection; necrosis at injection site following repeated injections; sweating; transient elevations of blood glucose; elevated serum lactic acid.

Precautions

Pregnancy: Category C. *Labor:* Do not use when maternal BP exceeds 130/80 mm Hg; may delay second stage or induce uterine atony. *Lactation:* Excreted in breast milk. *Children:* Administer drug with caution. Syncope has occurred in asthmatic children. *Special risk patients:* Use drug with caution in elderly patients, patients with cardiovascular disease, pulmonary edema, hypertension, hyperthyroidism, diabetes, psychoneurotic illness, asthma, prefibrillatory rhythm, anesthetic cardiac accidents. *Cerebrovascular hemorrhage:* May result from overdosage or inadvertent IV injection. *Glaucoma:* Ophthalmic epinephrine for topical use only; not for injection or intraocular use. Evaluate anterior chamber angle by gonioscopy before using. Maculopathy with decreased visual acuity may occur in aphakic eye; if this occurs, discontinue drug. *Pulmonary edema:* May cause fatalities due to peripheral constriction or cardiac stimulation. *Sulfite sensitivity:* Use drug with caution in sulfite-sensitive individuals; some products contain sulfites.

NURSING CONSIDERATIONS

Administration/Storage

- Have patient wait 1 full min between inhalations if receiving drug via inhalation therapy.
- Do not use if solution appears discolored or contains any precipitate.
- Massage SC injection site to reduce vasoconstrictive effects.
- Rotate injection sites to avoid irritation.
- Protect from light, extreme heat or freezing. Store at room temperature.

Assessment/Interventions

- Obtain patient history, including drug history and any known allergies. Note any hypersensitivity to epinephrine or sulfites.
- Perform baseline assessment of vital signs, ECG, peripheral pulses, lung sounds, level of consciousness.
- Determine baseline glucose for patients with diabetes mellitus.
- Monitor vital signs frequently.
- Assess lung sounds for rhonchi, rales or wheezes.
- Monitor ECG, skin color, changes in mentation, tremors, nervousness and agitation.

OVERDOSAGE: SIGNS & SYMPTOMS

Precordial distress, vomiting, headache, shortness of breath, unusually elevated blood pressure, cerebrovascular hemorrhage, pulmonary arterial hypertension, pulmonary edema, ventricular hyperirritability, bradycardia, tachycardia, arrhythmias, extreme pallor, cold skin, metabolic acidosis, kidney failure

Patient/Family Education

- Caution patient to use topical decongestant form of drug only in acute states and to not use > 3-5 days.
- If indicated, teach patient how to self-administer epinephrine for anaphylactic reaction via auto-injector.
- Instruct patient to notify physician of insomnia, weakness or palpitations.
- Advise patient that nasal burning or stinging may occur with topical decongestant.
- Caution patient not to share nasal spray container with others.
- Advise patient to notify physician if symptoms do not improve after 7 days.
- If patient is being treated for glaucoma, advise patient to notify physician of prolonged blurred vision, headache, palpitation, tremors, sweating and faintness and to use caution while driving or performing hazardous tasks.
- Caution patient that stinging of eyes will occur on instillation of ophthalmic epinephrine solution in eyes.
- Advise glaucoma patient not to use drug while wearing soft contact lenses; discoloration of lens may result.
- If patient is receiving drug subcutaneously, advise patient to notify physician of syncope, palpitations, weakness and agitation.
- If patient is receiving drug through inhalation therapy, caution patient to notify physician if no relief from symptoms is gained. Advise patient to notify physician of dizziness or chest pain.

See Patient Guide, p. 218.

Epoetin Alfa (Erythropoietin; EPO)

(eh-POE-eh-tin AL-fuh)

Epogen, Procrit

Class: Recombinant human erythropoietin

Action Stimulates red blood cell production.

Indications Treatment of anemia related to chronic renal failure, zidovudine therapy in HIV-infected patients and nonmyeloid malignancies. **Unlabeled use:** Increased procurement of autologous blood in patients about to undergo elective surgery.

Contraindications Hypersensitivity to mammalian cell–derived products or human albumin, uncontrolled hypertension.

Route/Dosage

Chronic Renal Failure

ADULTS: **IV/SC** Initial dose: 50-100 U/kg 3 times weekly. Maintenance: Individually titrate.

Zidovudine-treated HIV-infected Patients

ADULTS: **IV/SC** Initial dose: 100 U/kg for 8 wk; increase by 50-100 U/kg 3 times weekly until appropriate maintenance dose is reached.

Nonmyeloid Malignancies

ADULTS: **SC** Initial dose: 150 U/kg 3 times weekly for 8 wk; if response not satisfactory, may increase up to 300 U/kg 3 times weekly.

Interactions None well documented. INCOMPATIBILITIES: Do not give with other drug solutions.

Lab Test Interferences None well documented.

Adverse Reactions

CV: Hypertension; tachycardia; clotted vascular access. *RESP:* Shortness of breath. *CNS:* Headache; seizures. *GI:* Nausea; vomiting; diarrhea. *OTHER:* Allergy, including anaphylaxis, skin rashes and urticaria; fever; paresthesia; arthralgia.

Precautions

Pregnancy: Category C. *Lactation:* Undetermined. *Children:* Safety and efficacy not established. *Hypersensitivity:* Anaphylactoid reactions, mild and transient skin rashes and urticaria may occur. *Seizures:* May occur; relationship to drug uncertain. *Thrombotic events:* During hemodialysis, patients may need increased anticoagulation to prevent clotting of vascular access.

NURSING CONSIDERATIONS

Administration/Storage

- When administering through IV tubing, flush the line with saline before and after administration of epoetin alfa.
- Do not shake vial.
- Use only one dose per vial; do not reenter vial.
- Discard unused portions.
- Refrigerate. Do not freeze or shake.

Assessment/Interventions

- Obtain patient history, including drug history and any known allergies. Note any hypersensitivity to human albumin or mammalian cell–derived products.
- Obtain baseline CBC, bleeding time, urinalysis, BUN, creatinine, electrolytes, serum iron, iron-binding capacity and serum ferritin.
- Obtain baseline vital signs.
- Note any history of hypertension, cardiovascular disease, seizures or porphyria.
- Monitor vital signs routinely.
- In chronic renal failure patients, determine hematocrit twice/wk until stabilized then for 2-6 wk with each dosage change; perform CBC with differential and platelet counts regularly; monitor electrolytes, uric acid and phosphorus regularly; monitor serum iron and iron-binding capacity; monitor potassium, BUN and creatinine.
- In zidovudine-treated HIV-infected patients, determine hematocrit once/wk until stabilized then periodically; monitor serum iron and iron-binding capacity; monitor potassium, BUN and creatinine.
- If rashes, urticaria or anaphylactic reactions occur, withhold medication immediately and notify physician.
- Iron indices, particularly serum ferritin and transferrin saturation, must be monitored. Almost all patients will eventually require supplemental iron to increase or maintain transferrin saturation to levels that will adequately support epoetin-stimulated erythropoiesis.
- Notify physician if hct increases > 4 points in 2-wk period or if hct does not increase 5-6 points after 8 wk of therapy.
- Notify physician if hct exceeds "target hct."
- Closely monitor patients with preexisting vascular disease.

OVERDOSAGE: SIGNS & SYMPTOMS

Polycythemia

Patient/Family Education

- Advise patient that the use of iron supplements and monitoring will probably be needed.
- Advise patient to have BP checked regularly.
- Instruct patient to notify physician if seizures, severe headache, shortness of breath, dyspnea, cough, nausea, vomiting or diarrhea occur.
- Inform patient that drug may be associated with risk of seizures during first 90 days of treatment and advise pa-

tient to avoid potentially hazardous activities during this period.

See Patient Guide, p. 219.

Ergoloid Mesylates (Dihydrogenated Ergot Alkaloids; Dihydroergotoxine)

(err-GO-loyd MEH-suh-lates)

Gerimal, Hydergine, Hydergine LC, Niloric

Class: Psychotherapeutic

Action Unknown; may increase brain metabolism, possibly increasing cerebral blood flow.

Indications Treatment of age-related decline in mental capacity, primary progressive dementia, Alzheimer's dementia, multi-infarct dementia and senile onset.

Contraindications Hypersensitivity to ergoloid mesylates or other ergot alkaloids; acute or chronic psychosis.

Route/Dosage
ADULTS: **PO/SL** 1-2 mg tid (up to 12 mg/day has been used).

Interactions None well documented.

Lab Test Interferences
None well documented.

Adverse Reactions
CV: Orthostatic hypotension; bradycardia. *GI:* Transient nausea; GI disturbances; sublingual irritation. *DERM:* Rash.

Precautions
Pregnancy: Pregnancy category undetermined. *Lactation:* Undetermined. *Children:* Safety and efficacy not established. *Special risk patients:* Administer drug with caution to patients with history of bradycardia or hypotension. *Liver impairment:* Elimination of drug may be affected.

NURSING CONSIDERATIONS

Administration/Storage

- Instruct patient to allow SL tablets to completely dissolve under tongue; do not allow patient to swallow, crush or chew tablet.
- Do not permit patient to eat, drink or smoke while SL tablet is dissolving.
- Store in tightly closed, light-resistant container at room temperature.

Assessment/Interventions

- Obtain patient history, including drug history and any known allergies.
- Potentially reversible and treatable conditions should be ruled out prior to use of ergoloid mesylates in treating age-related decline of mental capacity.
- Assess patient's mental status (alertness, memory, orientation, mood, emotional liability and self-care) prior to and during administration of drug.
- Monitor BP and pulse rate prior to initiation of therapy and at periodic intervals during therapy.
- Take appropriate safety measures if lightheadedness, weakness or changes in mental status develop.

OVERDOSAGE: SIGNS & SYMPTOMS

Headache, flushing, anorexia, nausea, vomiting, abdominal cramps, nasal congestion, impaired vision, dizziness, fainting

Patient/Family Education

- Teach patient how to decrease effects of orthostatic hypotention by rising slowly from supine position and dangling feet for few min before standing.
- Instruct patient to avoid alcohol consumption, which may enhance hypotensive effect.
- Caution patient not to take otc

cough, cold and allergy preparations that contain alcohol.

- Instruct patient to avoid excessive exposure to cold since temperature regulation may be impaired.
- Instruct patient to notify physician if adverse reactions occur.
- Advise patient/family that it may require 3-4 wk and up to 6 mo to determine clinical effectiveness of drug.

See Patient Guide, p. 220.

Erythromycin

(eh-RITH-row-MY-sin)

AK-Mycin, Akne-mycin, Del-Mycin, E-Base, E-Mycin, E.E.S., Eramycin, Erygel, Ery-sol, Ery-Tab, Eryc, EryPed, Erythrocin Stearate, Erythromycin Lactobionate, Ilosone, Ilotycin, PCE Dispertab, Robimycin, Wyamycin S, ♣ *Diomycin, Novorythro Encap*

Class: Antibiotic/macrolide

Action Interferes with microbial protein synthesis.

Indications

Oral/intravenous use: Treatment of infections of respiratory tract, skin and skin structure, and sexually transmitted diseases due to susceptible organisms; treatment of pertussis, diphtheria, erythrasma, intestinal amebiasis, conjunctivitis of newborn and Legionnaire's disease; prevention of attacks of rheumatic fever; prevention of bacterial endocarditis; treatment of acute otitis media (in combination with sulfisoxazole). *Ophthalmic use:* Treatment of superficial ocular infections due to strains of susceptible organism. *Topical use:* Infection prophylaxis in minor cuts, wounds, burns and skin abrasions; treatment of acne vulgaris. **Unlabeled uses:** Treatment of *Neisseria gonorrhoeae* in pregnancy; treatment of diarrhea caused by *Campylobacter jejuni*; as alternative to penicillin in selected infections.

Contraindications Hypersensitivity to erythromycin or any macrolide antibiotic; pre-existing liver disease (with estolate salt); epithelial herpes simplex keratitis; fungal disease of eye; vaccinia or varicella (ophthalmic use).

Route/Dosage

Systemic Use

ADULTS: **PO** 250-500 mg of base (400-800 mg ethylsuccinate) q 6 hr or 500 mg q 12 hr or 333 mg q 8 hr. **IV** 15-20 mg/kg/day; up to 4 g/day in very severe infections. CHILDREN: **PO** 30-50 mg/kg/day in divided doses.

Acute Ocular Infection

ADULTS & CHILDREN: **Ophthalmic** 0.5 inch ribbon of ointment placed in eye q 3-4 hr.

Mild to Moderate Ocular Infection

ADULTS & CHILDREN: **Ophthalmic** 0.5 inch ribbon of ointment placed in eye bid-tid.

Prophylaxis of Neonatal Gonococcal or Chlamydia Conjunctivitis

NEONATES: **Ophthalmic** 0.2-0.4 inch ribbon of ointment placed in each conjunctival sac at time of delivery.

Skin Infections

ADULTS & CHILDREN: **Topical** Apply 1-4 times daily to affected area.

Acne Vulgaris

ADULTS & CHILDREN: **Topical** Apply bid.

Interactions

Anticoagulants: May increase anticoagulant effects. *Antihistamines, nonsedating (eg, astemizole, terfenadine):* May increase antihistamine levels and cause serious adverse cardiovascular events, including ventricular arrhythmias and death. *Bromocriptine:* May increase serum bromocriptine levels. *Carbamazepine:* May result in serious carbamazepine toxicity. *Clindamycin, topical:* Antagonism may occur with topical erythromycin. *Cyclosporine:* May cause increased cyclosporine levels with renal toxicity. *Digoxin:* May cause increased digoxin levels. *Lovastatin:* Severe myopathy or rhabdomyolysis may occur. *Methylprednisolone:* May decrease clearance of methylprednisolone. *Theophyllines:* May increase theophylline plasma concentration.

Lab Test Interferences
None well documented.

Adverse Reactions
GI: Diarrhea; nausea; vomiting abdominal pain/cramping. *GU:* Vaginitis. *HEPA:* Hepatotoxicity (primarily with estolate salt). *DERM:* Rash; photosensitivity; erythema and peeling (topical use). *OTHER:* Venous irritation or phlebitis with IV administration.

Precautions
Pregnancy: Category B. *Lactation:* Excreted in breast milk. *Acne therapy:* Cumulative irritant effect may occur. *Hepatic impairment:* Use drug cautiously. Hepatic dysfunction, with or without jaundice, has occurred. Cholestatic hepatitis has occurred. *Hypersensitivity:* Serious reactions, including anaphylaxis, have occurred. *Ophthalmic ointments:* May slow corneal epithelial healing. *Ototoxicity:* May occur, especially in patients with renal or hepatic insufficiency and elderly patients and with administration of large doses. *Pseudomembranous colitis:* Consider possibility in patients in whom diarrhea develops. *Superinfection:* Prolonged use of antibiotics may result in bacterial or fungal overgrowth of nonsusceptible microorganisms.

NURSING CONSIDERATIONS

Administration/Storage

Oral

- Administer with full glass of water 1 hr before or 2 hr after meals. If GI upset is significant, give with food or milk. Do not crush tablets or allow patient to chew them.

Parenteral

- Use only Sterile Water for Injection for reconstitution. Do not use diluents containing preservatives or organic salts.
- Dilute reconstituted drug in 1-5 mg/ml in 0.9% Sodium Chloride. If D5W is used, buffer solution with Sodium Bicarbonate or neutralize (add 1 ml/100 ml of solution).
- Administer IV infusion at slow rate over 30-60 min to reduce venous irritation.
- Piggyback vial must be used within 8 hr of preparation if stored at room temperature or 24 hr if refrigerated.
- Frozen solution may be stored for 30 days. Thaw in refrigerator and use within 8 hr after thawing. Do not refreeze thawed solution.

Topical

- With topical use, cleanse affected area with 0.9% Sodium Chloride before application.
- For ophthalmic use, have patient tilt head back, pull lid down, place medication in conjunctival sac and have patient close eyes. Take care not to touch lids.

Assessment/Interventions

- Obtain patient history, including drug history and any known allergies. Note any hypersensitivity to macrolide antibiotics and history of liver disease, fungal disease or colitis.
- Culture and sensitivity testing should be done to determine organism sensitivity.
- Obtain baseline LFTs and CBC.
- Monitor LFTs routinely.
- Monitor I&O.
- Monitor for signs and symptoms of superinfection (ie, thrush, vaginal yeast, perianal irritation, vaginal discharge, black furry tongue).
- Monitor for diarrhea, nausea, vomiting or abdominal discomfort. Contact physician if these symptoms are persistent.
- If skin rash, respiratory distress or urti-

caria occur, stop infusion immediately and notify physician.

- Monitor IV site if using IV route. Change IV heparin locks q 3 days or per institution guidelines.
- If patient is undergoing oral anticoagulant therapy, monitor PT.

OVERDOSAGE: SIGNS & SYMPTOMS

Severe nausea, vomiting, diarrhea, epigastric distress, hearing loss, vertigo

Patient/Family Education

- Advise patient to take medication with full glass of water 1 hr before or 2 hr after meals. If extreme GI distress occurs, drug may be taken with food or milk.
- Inform patient that following ophthalmic administration, temporary blurring of vision or stinging may occur. Advise patient to notify physician if redness, irritation or pain persists or worsens. Instruct patient to use medication 1 hr before driving.
- Instruct patient to notify physician if nausea, vomiting, diarrhea, abdominal pain, jaundice, dark urine, pale stools, unusual fatigue or signs of superinfection occur.
- Instruct patient to follow complete course of therapy.
- When used topically for treatment of acne vulgaris, caution patient not to use otc peeling, abrasive agents or abrasive sponges because cumulative irritant effect may occur.
- When drug is used topically, advise patient to avoid exposure to sunlight and to use sunscreen or wear protective clothing to avoid photosensitivity reaction.

See Patient Guide, p. 221-223.

Erythromycin Ethylsuccinate/ Sulfisoxazole

(eh-RITH-row-MY-sin ETH-il-SUX-i-nate/sul-fih-SOX-uh-zole)

Eryzole, Pediazole

Class: Anti-infective

Action Erythromycin suppresses bacterial protein synthesis; sulfonamides interfere with bacterial folic acid synthesis.

Indications Treatment of acute otitis media in children caused by susceptible strains of *Haemophilus influenzae*.

Contraindications Hypersensitivity to chemically related drugs (sulfonylureas, thiazide and loop diuretics, carbonic anhydrase inhibitors, sunscreens containing PABA, local anesthetics) or salicylates; patients taking terfenadine or astemizole; porphyria; use in infants < 20 mo, pregnant women at term and women nursing infants < 2 mo.

Route/Dosage

CHILDREN: **PO** 50 mg/kg/day erythromycin and 150 mg/kg/day (maximum 6 gm/day) sulfisoxazole in equally divided doses qid for 10 days.

Interactions

Anticoagulants: May increase anticoagulant effects. *Antihistamines, nonsedating (eg, astemizole, terfenadine):* Erythromycin significantly alters metabolism of terfenadine. Rare cases of serious cardiovascular events including death have been reported. *Astemizole, bromocriptine, carbamazepine, disopyramide, hexobarbital, methylprednisolone, phenytoin:* May cause decreased metabolism and increased concentrations of these drugs. *Cyclosporine:* Erythromycin may interfere with metabolism while sulfonamides may decrease cyclosporine levels; both increase risk of nephrotoxicity. *Digoxin:* May increase digoxin levels. *Lovastatin:* Severe myopathy or rhabdomyolysis may occur. *Methotrexate:* Sulfonamides can displace methotrexate from protein-binding sites and increase free methotrexate levels. *Sulfonylureas:* Sulfisoxazole may potentiate hypoglycemic effects. *Theophyllines:* May increase theophylline plasma concentrations. *Thiopental:* May enhance anesthetic effects of thiopental.

Lab Test Interferences

Sulfosalicyclic acid turbidity test for urinary protein: Sulfisoxazole may produce false-positive results. *Urinary glucose test:* Sulfonamides may produce false-positive results when performed by Benedict's method. *Urobilistix test:* Sulfisoxazole may interfere with test results.

Adverse Reactions

CNS: Headache; peripheral neuropathy; dizziness; psychosis; hallucinations; depression; convulsions. *EENT:* Hearing loss (associated with high doses erythromycin and renal insufficiency). *GI:* Nausea; vomiting; abdominal pain/cramping; diarrhea; anorexia. *GU:* Crystalluria; hematuria; increased BUN and creatinine; nephritis; toxic nephrosis with oliguria. *HEPA:* Hepatic dysfunction; abnormal liver function test results; pseudomembranous colitis; GI hemorrhage; pancreatitis. *HEMA:* Leukopenia; agranulocytosis; aplastic anemia; thrombocytopenia; hemolytic anemia; purpura; eosinophilia; clotting disorders; methemoglobinemia. *DERM:* Urticaria; skin eruptions; pruritus; photosensitivity; anaphylaxis; erythema multiforme; toxic epidermal necrolysis; exfoliative dermatitis; angioedema; arteritis; vasculitis. *OTHER:* Fever; chills; arthralgias; myalgias; periarteritis nodosum; systemic lupus erythematosus; serum sickness.

Precautions

Pregnancy: Category C. *Lactation:* Both erythromycin and sulfisoxazole are excreted in breast milk. *Children:* Children < 2 mo should not be exposed (directly or through breast milk) to sulfonamides because of risk of kernicterus. *Special risk patients:* May aggravate weakness in patients with myasthenia gravis. Use drug with caution in patients with severe allergies or bronchial asthma. Dose-related hemolytic anemia may occur in patients with G-6-PD deficiency. *Fatalities:* Rare fatalities from severe reactions associated with hypersensitivity, agranulocytosis, aplastic anemia, blood dyscrasias, renal and hepatic damage, irreversible neuromuscular and CNS changes and fibrosing alveolitis have been reported with sulfonamides. *Hepatic or renal impairment:* Use drug with caution in patients with renal or hepatic impairment. Hepatotoxicity has been associated with erythromycin. *Ototoxicity:* May occur, especially in patients with renal or hepatic insufficiency and elderly patients and with administration of large doses. *Pseudomembranous colitis:* Consider possibility in patients with diarrhea. *Superinfection:* Prolonged use may result in bacterial or fungal overgrowth of nonsusceptible microorganisms.

NURSING CONSIDERATIONS

Administration/Storage

- Give with full glass of water 1 hr before or 2 hr after meals.
- If GI upset is significant, administer with food or milk.
- Shake oral suspension well. Refrigerate after opening. Discard unused portion after 14 days.

Assessment/Interventions

- Obtain patient history, including drug history and any known allergies. Note any hypersensitivity to erythromycin or macrolide antibiotics and history of liver disease, fungal disease or colic.
- Obtain baseline CBC, BUN, creatinine and liver function tests and monitor throughout therapy.
- Obtain culture and sensitivity before instituting drug regimen.
- Monitor for diarrhea, nausea, vomiting and abdominal discomfort. If severe, contact physician.

- Monitor I&O. Encourage oral intake of fluids.
- Monitor for signs and symptoms of superinfection: perianal irritation, black furry tongue or vaginal discharge.
- Notify physician of tachycardia, palpitations, syncope, cyanosis, seizures and hallucinations or any change in hearing.
- Notify physician if urticaria or anemia occur.

OVERDOSAGE: SIGNS & SYMPTOMS

Nausea, vomiting, diarrhea, hearing loss, vertigo, dizziness, headache, drowsiness, unconsciousness, toxic fever, acidosis, hemolytic anemia

Patient/Family Education

- Instruct patient/family to follow complete course of therapy.
- Advise patient to shake suspension well before using and refrigerate after opening.
- Tell patient to take drug with full glass of water 1 hr before or 2 hr after meals. If GI distress occurs, take with food or milk.
- Instruct patient to report these symptoms to physician: tachycardia, palpitations, syncope, cyanosis, seizures, hallucinations, shortness of breath, rash, bleeding, diarrhea, inability to void, urticaria, abdominal pain or signs of superinfection.
- Caution patient to avoid exposure to sunlight and to use sunscreen or wear protective clothing to avoid photosensitivity reaction.
- Instruct patient not to take otc medications without consulting physician.

See Patient Guide, p. 224.

Esmolol HCl

(ESS-moe-lahl HIGH-droe-KLOR-ide)

Brevibloc

Class: Beta-adrenergic blocker

Action Blocks beta-receptors primarily affecting cardiovascular system (decreases heart rate, contractility and BP) and lungs (promoting bronchospasm).

Indications Short-term management of supraventricular tachyarrhythmias and noncompensatory sinus tachycardia. **Unlabeled uses:** Treatment of caffeine toxicity; attenuation of cardiovascular responses to electroconvulsive therapy or induction of anesthesia; adjunct therapy for acute MI and unstable angina; treatment of thyroid storm.

Contraindications Sinus bradycardia; second- or third-degree heart block; CHF unless secondary to tachyarrhythmia treatable with beta-blockers; overt cardiac failure; cardiogenic shock.

Route/Dosage

ADULTS: Usual: **IV** 500 mcg/kg/min for 1 min; then infusion of 50-200 mcg/kg/min, which has been titrated to desired endpoint (eg, heart rate, BP) in 50 mcg/kg/min increments.

Interactions

Clonidine: May enhance or reverse antihypertensive effect; potentially life-threatening increases in BP may occur, especially on withdrawal. *NSAIDs:* Some agents may impair antihypertensive effect. *Prazosin:* Potential for and degree of orthostatic hypotension may be increased. *Verapamil:* Effects of both drugs may be increased. INCOMPATIBILITIES: 5% Sodium Bicarbonate Injection.

Lab Test Interferences

Antinuclear antibodies may develop; usually reversible on discontinuation. May interfere with glucose or insulin tolerance test results. May cause changes in serum lipid levels.

Adverse Reactions

CV: Hypotension; bradycardia; CHF; cold extremities; pallor; second-

or third-degree heart block. *RESP:* Bronchospasm; shortness of breath; wheezing. *CNS:* Insomnia; fatigue; dizziness; depression; lethargy; drowsiness; forgetfulness. *EENT:* Dry eyes; blurred vision; tinnitus; slurred speech; sore throat. *GI:* Nausea; vomiting; diarrhea; dry mouth. *GU:* Impotence; painful, difficult or frequent urination. *HEMA:* Agranulocytosis; thrombocytopenia purpura. *DERM:* Rash; hives; fever; alopecia. *OTHER:* Weight changes; facial swelling; muscle weakness; inflammation at infusion site.

Precautions

Pregnancy: Category C. *Lactation:* Undetermined. *Children:* Safety and efficacy not established. *Anaphylaxis:* Deaths have occurred; aggressive therapy may be required. *CHF:* Administer drug in patients with CHF controlled by digitalis and diuretics. Notify physician at first sign or symptom of CHF or other unexplained respiratory symptoms. *Diabetes mellitus:* May mask signs and symptoms of hypoglycemia (eg, tachycardia, BP changes). May potentiate insulin-induced hypoglycemia. *Nonallergic bronchospasm (eg, chronic bronchitis, emphysema):* Use caution in patients with bronchospastic diseases. *Peripheral vascular disease:* May precipitate or aggravate symptoms of arterial insufficiency. *Renal/hepatic impairment:* Reduced daily dose advised. *Thyrotoxicosis:* May mask clinical signs (eg, tachycardia) of developing or continuing hyperthyroidism. Abrupt withdrawal may exacerbate symptoms of hyperthyroidism, including thyroid storm.

NURSING CONSIDERATIONS

Administration/Storage

- Avoid concentrations > 10 mg/min in order to minimize venous irritation.
- 10 mg/ml vial does not need further dilution.
- Do not administer through butterfly needles.
- For IV administration, use 250 mg/ml solution diluted in 5% Dextrose Injection and 0.9% or 0.45% Sodium Chloride Injection, Lactated Ringer's Injection, and Potassium Chloride (40 mEq/L) in 5% Dextrose Injection or 0.9% or 0.45% Sodium Chloride Injection. To prepare solution remove 20 ml from 500 ml bottle of suitable infusion fluid and add 2 amps of 250 mg/ml solution of esmolol. Final concentration is 10 mg/ml.
- Do not mix with sodium bicarbonate.
- Store diluted solution at room temperature or under refrigeration. Discard after 24 hr.
- Use of esmolol infusion up to 24 hr is well documented. Limited data indicate that esmolol is well tolerated up to 48 hr.
- When converting patient to another agent, reduce esmolol infusion rate by 50% ½ hr after first dose of new drug. After second dose of new drug, if patient is stable for 1 hr, discontinue esmolol infusion.

Assessment/Interventions

- Obtain patient history, including drug history and any known allergies.
- Obtain baseline ECG and measure QT interval.
- Obtain baseline vital signs and weight.
- Auscultate and document baseline heart and lung sounds and monitor throughout therapy.
- Monitor vital signs frequently.
- Monitor I&O, BUN, creatinine, serum glucose, CBC, liver function tests and bilirubin throughout therapy.
- Assess patient for rashes, urticaria, shortness of breath, arthralgia and systemic lupus erythematosus syndrome.
- If reaction develops at infusion site, use alternative site.
- Notify physician if vomiting, abdominal distention, vertigo, bradycardia,

new ventricular arrhythmia, shock symptoms or signs of CHF occur.

- If patient is receiving digoxin, monitor digoxin levels and observe patient for digoxin toxicity.

OVERDOSAGE: SIGNS & SYMPTOMS

Hypotension, bradycardia, intraventricular conduction disturbances, shock

Patient/Family Education

- Caution patient to notify physician or nurse of any urticaria, shortness of breath, vertigo, syncope or inability to void.
- Advise diabetic patient to notify physician or nurse of hypoglycemic reaction symptoms.

No patient monograph available.

Estradiol

(ESS-truh-DIE-ole)

Estinyl, Estrace, Estraderm, ♣ *Estraderm 25*

Estradiol Valerate

Deladiol-40, Delestrogen, Dioval, Duragen, Estra-L, Gynogen L.A., Valergen

Estradiol Cypionate

depGynogen, Depogen, Depo-Estradiol, Dura-Estrin, Estra-D, Estro-Cyp, Estroject-L.A.

Class: Estrogen

Action Promotes growth and development of female reproductive system and secondary sex characteristics; affects release of pituitary gonadotropins; inhibits ovulation and prevents postpartum breast engorgement; conserves calcium and phosphorous and encourages bone formation; overrides stimulatory effects of testosterone.

Indications Management of moderate to severe vasomotor symptoms associated with menopause, female hypogonadism, female castration, primary ovarian failure, postpartum breast engorgement and atrophic conditions caused by deficient endogenous estrogen production; palliative treatment of metastatic breast or prostate cancer in selected women and men; prevention and treatment of osteoporosis.

Contraindications Breast cancer (except in patients being treated for metastatic disease); estrogen-dependent neoplasia; undiagnosed abnormal genital bleeding; thrombophlebitis or thromboembolic disorders associated with previous estrogen use; known or suspected pregnancy.

Route/Dosage

Vasomotor Symptoms

ESTRADIOL: ADULTS: **PO** 1-2 mg/day, adjust to control symptoms; cyclic therapy recommended. **Transdermal** 0.05 to 0.1 mg/day. Start with 0.05 mg system applied to skin twice weekly and adjust dose as necessary to control symptoms. VALERATE INJECTION: ADULTS: **IM** 10-20 mg q 4 wk. CYPIONATE INJECTION: ADULTS: **IM** 1-5 mg q 3-4 wk. ETHINYL ESTRADIOL: ADULTS: **PO** 0.02-1.5 mg/day cyclically.

Female Hypogonadism

ESTRADIOL: ADULTS: **PO** 1-2 mg/day, adjust to control symptoms, cyclic therapy recommended. **Transdermal** 0.05 to 0.1 mg/day. Start with 0.05 mg system applied to skin twice weekly and adjust dose as necessary to control symptoms. VALERATE INJECTION: ADULTS: **IM** 10-20 mg q 4 wk. CYPIONATE INJECTION: ADULTS: **IM** 1.5-2 mg q mo. ETHINYL ESTRADIOL: ADULTS: **PO** 0.05 mg 1-3 times/day during first 2 wk of theoretical menstrual cycle.

Vulva/Vaginal Atrophy Associated with Menopause, Female Castration, Primary Ovarian Failure

ESTRADIOL: ADULTS: **PO** 1-2 mg day; adjust to control symptoms; cyclic therapy recommended. **Transdermal** 0.05 to 0.1 mg/day. Start with 0.05 mg system applied to skin twice weekly and adjust dose as necessary to control symptoms. Give continuously in patients without intact uterus; otherwise give cyclically. VALERATE INJECTION: ADULTS: **IM** 10-20 mg q 4 wk. **Intravaginal** Insert: 2-4 mg qd intravaginally.

Prostatic Carcinoma
ESTRADIOL: ADULTS: **PO** 1-2 mg tid. VALERATE INJECTION: ADULTS: **IM** 30 mg or more q 1-2 wk. ETHINYL ESTRADIOL: ADULTS: **PO** 0.15-2 mg/day.

Breast Cancer
ESTRADIOL: ADULTS: **PO** 10 mg tid for at least 3 mo. ETHINYL ESTRADIOL: ADULTS: **PO** 1 mg tid.

Osteoporosis Prevention
ESTRADIOL: ADULTS: **PO** 0.5 mg/day (3 weeks on, 1 week off). **Transdermal** 0.05 to 0.1 mg/day. Start with 0.05 mg system applied to skin twice weekly and adjust dose as necessary to control symptoms.

Breast Engorgement Prevention
VALERATE INJECTION: ADULTS: **IM** 10-25 mg at end of first stage of labor.

Interactions

Antidepressants, tricyclic: Estradiol may alter effects and increase toxicity of these agents. *Barbiturates, rifampin:* May decrease estradiol concentration. *Corticosteroids:* Clearance of corticosteroids may be reduced. *Hydantoins:* Loss of seizure control or decreased estrogenic effects may occur.

Lab Test Interferences

Endocrine and liver function test results may be affected; possible decreased PT and increased platelet aggregability; decreased antithrombin III activity; increased thyroid-binding globulin and total T_4; impaired glucose tolerance; decreased serum folate concentration; increased serum triglyceride and phospholipid concentrations.

Adverse Reactions

CV: Thrombosis; thrombophlebitis; MI; elevated BP; pulmonary embolism. *CNS:* Headache; migraine; dizziness; depression. *EENT:* Intolerance to contact lenses. *GI:* Nausea; vomiting; abdominal cramps; bloating; colitis; acute pancreatitis. *GU:* Increased risk of endometrial carcinoma; breakthrough bleeding; dysmenorrhea; amenorrhea; vaginal candidiasis; premenstrual-like syndrome; increased size of uterine fibromyomata; hemolytic uremic syndrome. *HEPA:* Cholestatic jaundice. *DERM:* Chloasma; melasma; erythema nodosum or multiforme; scalp hair loss; hirsutism; urticaria; dermatitis. *META:* Hyperglycemia; hypercalcemia. *OTHER:* Pain at injection site; redness and irritation at site of transdermal system; increase/decrease in weight; reduced carbohydrate tolerance; edema; changes in libido; breast tenderness; acute intermittent porphyria; vaginal bleeding.

Precautions

Pregnancy: Category X. *Lactation:* Excreted in breast milk. *Children:* Safety and efficacy not established. *Calcium and phosphorus metabolism:* Use drug with caution in patients with metabolic bone diseases. *Fluid retention:* Use drug with careful observation when conditions that might be affected by this factor are present (eg, asthma, cardiac or renal dysfunction, epilepsy). *Gallbladder disease:* Risk of gallbladder disease may increase in women receiving postmenopausal estrogens. *Hepatic impairment:* Metabolism may be impaired; use drug with caution. *Induction of malignant neoplasms:* May increase risk of endometrial or other carcinomas. *Tartrazine sensitivity:* Some products contain tartrazine, which may cause allergic reaction in susceptible patients. *Unopposed estrogen administration (eg, without progesterone):* Increases risk of uterine cancer. Therefore, when using estrogens on long-term basis in women with intact uterus, consider cyclic therapy with progesterone (eg, estrogen on days 1-25 of mo with progesterone added for last 12 days) or daily coadministration of estrogen plus progesterone on daily basis. In women without uterus, use of cyclic therapy and/or therapy with progesterone is not necessary.

NURSING CONSIDERATIONS

Administration/Storage

- Apply skin patch to clean, dry skin on trunk of body, preferably on abdomen. Do not apply to breasts. Rotate application sites so that no site is used more than once/wk. Skin should not be oily, damaged or irritated. Avoid areas where clothing could dislodge patch.
- Apply patch immediately after opening pouch and removing protective liner.
- Press firmly with palm of hand for approximately 10 seconds. Be sure good contact is made, especially at edges. If patch falls off, attempt to reapply. New patch may be applied if necessary.
- Insert vaginal cream high in vagina (approximately ⅔ length of applicator).
- Administer IM injection deeply into muscle.

Assessment/Interventions

- Obtain complete patient history, including drug history and any known allergies.
- Monitor BP frequently.
- In patients with diabetes, monitor blood sugar and report changes to physician.
- Review documentation of breast, abdomen and pelvic examination. Review results of Pap test, which should be conducted at least annually.
- Watch for increased LFT results.

OVERDOSAGE: SIGNS & SYMPTOMS

Nausea, withdrawal bleeding in women

Patient/Family Education

- Caution patient that this medication must not be taken during pregnancy or when pregnancy is possible. Advise patient to use reliable form of birth control while taking this drug.
- Instruct patient to report these symptoms to physician: calf pain or burning sensation; severe headache; weakness or numbness of extremities; speech disturbances; dizziness; high BP; chest pain; severe abdominal pain; shortness of breath; vision changes; midcycle bleeding; breast fullness; contact lens intolerance; evidence of swelling; weight gain of more than 2 lb/wk.
- Instruct patient to avoid prolonged exposure to sunlight or other sources of UV light and to wear sunscreen and protective clothing until sun tolerance is determined.
- Encourage patient to stop smoking or to reduce number of cigarettes to less than 15/day while taking this drug because of increased risk of cardiovascular complications.
- Remind patient to have Pap test every 6-12 mo while undergoing therapy.
- Teach patient proper method of performing breast self-examination.

See Patient Guide, p. 225-227.

Estramustine Phosphate Sodium

(ESS-truh-muss-TEEN FOSS-fate SO-dee-uhm)

Emcyt

Class: Antineoplastic/nitrogen mustard and hormone

Action Chemically combines estradiol and nitrogen mustard. Appears to act as relatively weak alkylating agent and imparts weak estrogenic activity.

Indications Palliative treatment of metastatic or progressive prostate carcinoma.

Contraindications Hypersensitivity to estradiol or nitrogen mustard; active thrombophlebitis or thromboembolic disorders except when actual tumor is cause of thromboembolic phenomenon and benefits of therapy outweigh risk.

Route/Dosage

ADULTS: **PO** 14 mg/kg/day (ie, one 140 mg capsule for each 10 kg) in 3 or 4 divided doses (dosage range 10-16 mg/kg/day).

Interactions

Milk, milk products and calcium-rich foods or drugs: May impair absorption of estramustine.

Lab Test Interferences

None well documented.

Adverse Reactions

CV: Thrombophlebitis; CHF; edema; MI. *RESP:* Pulmonary emboli; shortness of breath; upper respiratory tract discharge; hoarseness. *CNS:* Cerebral vascular accident; lethargy; emotional lability; insomnia; headache; anxiety. *EENT:* Eye tearing. *GI:* Nausea; vomiting; diarrhea; anorexia; flatulence; GI bleeding; burning throat; thirst; minor GI upset. *HEMA:* Leukopenia; thrombocytopenia. *HEPA:* Abnormal liver function tests. *DERM:* Rash; pruritus; dry skin; fingertip skin peeling; easy bruising; flushing; hair thinning. *OTHER:* Leg cramps; chest pain; breast tenderness or mild enlargement.

Precautions

Pregnancy: Pregnancy category undetermined. *Lactation:* Undetermined. *Carcinogenesis, impairment of fertility, mutagenesis:* Estradiol and nitrogen mustard are mutagenic; advise use of contraception. *Elevated BP:* May occur; monitor periodically. *Glucose tolerance:* May be decreased; monitor diabetic patients. *Hepatic impairment:* Use drug with caution. *Thrombosis:* Risk of thrombosis, including MI, increases in men given estrogens for prostate cancer. Use caution in patients with prior clotting disorders, cerebral vascular or coronary artery disease.

NURSING CONSIDERATIONS

Administration/Storage

- Give capsule with water at least 1 hr before or 2 hr after meals.
- Do not divide or crush capsule.
- Do not administer with milk, milk products or calcium-rich drugs (eg, calcium-containing antacids).
- Keep refrigerated. Drug may be left unrefrigerated for 24-48 hr without affecting drug's potency.

Assessment/Interventions

- Obtain complete history, including drug history and any known allergies. Note current status of hepatic and cardiopulmonary function.
- Obtain baseline data of vital signs, especially BP, and determine glucose tolerance if patient is diabetic.
- Monitor for changes in cardiovasculopulmonary status, including fluid retention, hypertension and clotting disorders.
- Observe for carcinogenic potential of

drug, especially with long-term administration of drug.

OVERDOSAGE: SIGNS & SYMPTOMS

Exaggerated side effects

Patient/Family Education

- Instruct patient to store medication in refrigerator.
- Advise patient to take drug with water at least 1 hr before or 2 hr after meals.
- Caution patient not to take drug with milk, milk products, calcium-rich foods or otc drugs containing calcium (eg, Tums).
- Advise patient to use nonhormonal forms of contraception if patient is sexually active and has reproductive capability.
- Caution patient that hair loss may occur.
- Instruct patient to report these symptoms to physician: change in appetite, nutritional intake or other GI problems; chest pain or shortness of breath; leg cramps; upper respiratory discharge; hoarseness; changes in skin and scalp, including peeling skin of fingertips, easy bruising, flushing and thinning hair; lethargy; emotional lability; insomnia; headache; anxiety; tearing eyes; breast tenderness and mild to moderate breast enlargement.

See Patient Guide, p. 228.

Estrogens, Conjugated

(ESS-truh-janz, KAHN-juh-gay-tuhd)

PBM 200, PMP 400, Premarin, Premarin IV, ♣ *C.E.S., Congest*

Class: Estrogen

Action Promotes growth and development of female reproductive system and secondary sex characteristics; affects release of pituitary gonadotropins; inhibits ovulation and prevents postpartum breast engorgement; conserves calcium and phosphorous and encourages bone formation; overrides stimulatory effects of testosterone.

Indications Management of moderate to severe vasomotor symptoms associated with menopause; treatment of atrophic vaginitis, kraurosis vulvae, female hypogonadism, symptoms of female castration, and primary ovarian failure; prevention and treatment of osteoporosis; palliative treatment of metastatic breast cancer in selected women and men and prostatic carcinoma; treatment of postpartum breast engorgement and abnormal uterine bleeding (parenteral form).

Contraindications Breast cancer (except in patients being treated for metastatic disease); estrogen-dependent neoplasia; undiagnosed abnormal genital bleeding; thrombophlebitis or thromboembolic disorders associated with previous estrogen use; known or suspected pregnancy.

Route/Dosage

Vasomotor Symptoms, Female Castration, Primary Ovarian Failure

ADULTS: **PO** 1.25 mg/day.

Atrophic Vaginitis, Kraurosis Vulvae

ADULTS: **PO** 0.3-1.25 mg or more/day. **Intravaginal** Insert 2-4 g daily.

Female Hypogonadism

ADULTS: **PO** 2.5-7.5 mg/day in divided doses for 20 days, followed by 10-day rest period.

Prostatic Carcinoma

ADULTS: **PO** 1.25-2.5 mg tid.

Breast Cancer

ADULTS: **PO** 10 mg tid for at least 3 mo.

Osteoporosis

ADULTS: **PO** 0.625 mg/day (3 wk on estrogen, 1 wk off with progesterone therapy or daily if combined with progesterone).

Postpartum Breast Engorgement

ADULTS: **PO** 3.75 mg q 4 hr for 5 doses, *or* 1.25 mg q 4 hr for 5 days.

Abnormal Uterine Bleeding

ADULTS: **IV/IM** 25 mg; may repeat in 6-12 hr.

Interactions

Antidepressants, tricyclic: Estrogens may alter effects and increase toxicity of these agents. *Barbiturates, rifampin:* May decrease estrogen concentration. *Corticosteroids:* Clearance of corticosteroids may be reduced. *Hydantoins:* Loss of seizure control or decreased estrogenic effects may occur. INCOMPATIBILITIES: Infusion of conjugated estrogen with other agents is not recommended. Solution is compatible with normal saline, dextrose, and invert sugar solutions. It is not compatible with any solution with acidic pH.

Lab Test Interferences

Endocrine and liver function test results may be affected; possible decreased PT and increased platelet aggregability; increased thyroid-binding globulin and total T_4; impaired glucose tolerance; decreased serum folate concentration; increased serum triglyceride and phospholipid concentrations.

Adverse Reactions

CV: Thrombosis; thrombophlebitis; pulmonary embolism; MI; elevated BP. *CNS:* Headache; migraine; dizziness; depression. *EENT:* Intolerance to contact lenses. *GI:* Nausea; vomiting; abdominal cramps; bloating; colitis; acute pancreatitis. *GU:* Increased risk of endometrial carcinoma; breakthrough bleeding; dysmenorrhea; amenorrhea; vaginal candidiasis; premenstrual-like syndrome; increased size of uterine fibromyomata; hemolytic uremic syndrome. *HEPA:* Cholestatic jaundice. *DERM:* Chloasma; melasma; erythema nodosum/multiforme; scalp hair loss; hirsutism; urticaria; dermatitis. *META:* Hyperglycemia; hypercalcemia. *OTHER:* Increase or decrease in weight; reduced glucose tolerance; edema; changes in libido; breast tenderness; acute intermittent porphyria.

Precautions

Pregnancy: Category X. *Lactation:* Excreted in breast milk. *Children:* Safety and efficacy not established. *Calcium/phosphorus metabolism:* Use drug with caution in patients with metabolic bone diseases. *Fluid retention:* Use with careful observation when conditions that might be affected by this factor are present (eg, asthma, cardiac or renal dysfunction, epilepsy). *Gallbladder disease:* Risk of gallbladder disease may increase in women receiving postmenopausal estrogens. *Hepatic impairment:* Metabolism may be impaired; use drug with caution. *Induction of malignant neoplasms:* May increase risk of endometrial or other carcinomas. *Unopposed estrogen administration (eg, without progesterone):* Increases risk of uterine cancer. Therefore, when using estrogens on long-term basis in women with intact uterus, consider cyclic therapy with progesterone (eg, estrogen on days 1-25 of mo with progesterone added for last 12 days) or daily coadministration of estrogen plus progesterone on daily basis. In women without uterus, use of cyclic therapy and/or therapy with progesterone is not necessary.

NURSING CONSIDERATIONS

Administration/Storage

- Administer IM injection deeply into muscle.
- Administer IV injection slowly to avoid flushing.
- Insert vaginal cream high in vagina (about ⅔ length of applicator).
- Store vials for parenteral administration in refrigerator.
- Use reconstituted solution within a few hr.
- Reconstituted solution can be stored for 60 days in refrigerator.
- Do not use parenteral preparation if darkening or precipitation is noted.

Assessment/Interventions

- Obtain patient history, includ-

ing drug history and any known allergies.
- Monitor blood glucose level in diabetic patients.
- Include in physical assessment thorough documentation of BP, breast, abdomen and pelvic examination; review results of Pap smear, which should be conducted at least annually.

OVERDOSAGE: SIGNS & SYMPTOMS

Nausea, withdrawal bleeding in women

Patient/Family Education
- Caution patient that this medication must not be taken during pregnancy or when pregnancy is possible. Advise patient to use reliable form of birth control while taking this drug.
- Advise patient regarding importance of smoking cessation or reduction of intake to fewer than 15 cigarettes/day because of risk of cardiovascular complications.
- Teach patient proper method of performing breast self-examination.
- Advise patient to avoid exposure to sunlight or other sources of UV light. Sunscreens and/or protective clothing should be used until sun tolerance is determined.
- Instruct patient to report these symptoms to physician: pain in groin or calves; sharp chest pain or sudden shortness of breath; abnormal vaginal bleeding; breast lumps; sudden severe headache; dizziness or fainting; vision or speech problems; weakness or numbness in arm or leg; severe abdominal pain; yellowing of skin or eyes; severe depression.
- Remind patient to have Pap smear every 6-12 mo while undergoing therapy.

See Patient Guide, p. 229.

Estropipate (Piperazine Estrone Sulfate)

(ESS-troe-PIH-pate)

Ogen, Ortho-Est

Class: Estrogen

Action Promotes growth and development of female reproductive system and secondary sex characteristics; affects release of ovulation and prevents postpartum breast engorgement; conserves calcium and phosphorous and encourages bone formation; overrides stimulatory effects of testosterone.

Indications Management of moderate to severe vasomotor symptoms associated with menopause; female hypogonadism, female castration, primary ovarian failure and atrophic conditions caused by deficient endogenous estrogen production; prevention and treatment of osteoporosis.

Contraindications Breast cancer; estrogen-dependent neoplasia; undiagnosed abnormal genital bleeding; thrombophlebitis or thromboembolic disorders associated with previous estrogen use; known or suspected pregnancy.

Route/Dosage

Vasomotor Symptoms

ADULTS: PO 0.625-5 mg/day given cyclically.

Female Hypogonadism, Female Castration, Primary Ovarian Failure

ADULTS: PO 1.25-7.5 mg/day for 3 wk followed by 8-10 day drug-free period.

Osteoporosis

ADULTS: PO 0.625 mg/day for 25 days of 31-day cycle.

Atrophic Vaginitis, Kraurosis Vulvae

ADULTS: PO 0.625-5 mg/day. **Intravaginal** 2-4 g daily.

Interactions

Antidepressants, tricyclic: Estrogens may alter effects and increase toxicity of these agents. *Barbiturates, rifampin:* May decrease estropipate concentration. *Corticosteroids:* Clearance of corticosteroids may be reduced. *Hydantoins:* Loss of seizure control or decreased estrogenic effects may occur.

Lab Test Interferences
Endocrine and liver function test results may be affected; possible decreased PT and increased platelet aggregability; increased thyroid-binding globulin and total T_4; impaired glucose tolerance; decreased serum folate concentration; increased serum triglyceride and phospholipid concentrations.

Adverse Reactions
CV: Thrombosis; thrombophlebitis; increased BP; pulmonary embolism; MI. *CNS:* Headache; migraine; dizziness; depression. *EENT:* Intolerance to contact lenses. *GI:* Nausea; vomiting; abdominal cramps; bloating; colitis; acute pancreatitis. *GU:* Increased risk of endometrial carcinoma; breakthrough bleeding; dysmenorrhea; amenorrhea; vaginal candidiasis; premenstrual-like syndrome; increased size of uterine fibromyomata; hemolytic uremic syndrome. *HEPA:* Cholestatic jaundice. *DERM:* Chloasma; melasma; erythema nodosum/multiforme; scalp hair loss; hirsutism; urticaria; dermatitis. *META:* Hyperglycemia; hypercalcemia. *OTHER:* Increase or decrease in weight; edema; changes in libido; breast tenderness; acute intermittent porphyria.

Precautions
Pregnancy: Category X. *Lactation:* Excreted in breast milk. *Children:* Safety and efficacy not established. *Calcium and phosphorus metabolism:* Use drug with caution in patients with metabolic bone diseases. *Fluid retention:* Use drug with careful observation when conditions that might be affected by this factor are present (eg, asthma, cardiac or renal dysfunction, epilepsy). *Gallbladder disease:* Risk of gallbladder disease may increase in women receiving postmenopausal estrogens. *Hepatic function impairment:* Metabolism may be impaired; use drug with caution. *Induction of malignant neoplasms:* May increase risk of endometrial or other carcinomas. *Unopposed estrogen administration (eg, without progesterone):* Increases risk of uterine cancer. Therefore, when using estrogens on long-term basis in women with intact uterus, consider cyclic therapy with progesterone (eg, estrogen on days 1-25 of mo with progesterone added for last 12 days) or daily coadministration of estrogen plus progesterone on daily basis. In women without uterus, use of cyclic therapy and/or therapy with progesterone is not necessary.

NURSING CONSIDERATIONS

Administration/Storage

- Administer vaginal cream high in vagina (about ⅔ length of applicator).
- Give tablets with meal to decrease GI upset.

Assessment/Interventions

- Obtain patient history, including drug history and any known allergies.
- Include in physical assessments BP measurements, and examination of breasts, abdomen and pelvic organs. Review results of Pap test, which should be conducted at least annually.
- Monitor blood sugar in diabetic patients and report changes to health care provider.
- Be alert for changes in liver function test results and possible decreased PT.

OVERDOSAGE: SIGNS & SYMPTOMS

Nausea, withdrawal bleeding in women

Patient/Family Education

- Caution patient that this medication must not be taken during pregnancy or when pregnancy is possible. Advise patient to use reliable form of birth control while taking this drug.

- Instruct patient to report these symptoms to physician: pain in groin or calves; sharp chest pain or sudden shortness of breath; abnormal vaginal bleeding; breast lumps; sudden severe headache; dizziness or fainting; vision or speech problems; weakness or numbness of arms or legs; severe abdominal pain; yellowing of skin or eyes; or severe depression.
- Advise patient to stop smoking or to reduce number of cigarettes smoked to < 15/day because of increased risk of cardiovascular complications.
- Remind patient to have Pap smear every 6-12 mo while undergoing therapy.
- Teach patient proper method of breast self-examination.
- Advise patient to avoid prolonged exposure to sunlight or other sources of UV light. Sunscreens and protective clothing should be used until tolerance is determined.

See Patient Guide, p. 220-231.

Ethacrynic Acid (Ethacrynate)

(eth-uh-KRIN-ik acid)

Edecrin, Edecrin Sodium

Class: Loop diuretic

Action Inhibits reabsorption of sodium and chloride in proximal and distal tubules and in loop of Henle.

Indications Treatment of edema associated with CHF, hepatic cirrhosis or renal disease; treatment of ascites, congenital heart disease, nephrotic syndrome. **Unlabeled uses:** Treatment of glaucoma; treatment of nephrogenic diabetes insipidus, hypercalcemia.

Contraindications Anuria; infants; increasing azotemia; severe diarrhea; dehydration; electrolyte imbalance; hypotension.

Route/Dosage

ADULTS: **PO** 50-200 mg qd. **IV** 50 mg (0.5-1 mg/kg) qd. CHILDREN: **PO** 25 mg qd.

Interactions

Aminoglycosides: May increase auditory toxicity. *Cisplatin:* May cause additive ototoxicity. *Digitalis glycosides:* Electrolyte disturbances may predispose to digitalis-induced atrial and ventricular arrhythmias. *Lithium:* May increase plasma lithium levels and toxicity. *Nonsteroidal anti-inflammatory drugs:* May decrease effects of ethacrynic acid. *Salicylates:* May impair diuretic response in patients with cirrhosis and ascites. *Thiazide diuretics:* Synergistic effects may result in profound diuresis and serious electrolyte abnormalities.

Lab Test Interferences

None well documented.

Adverse Reactions

CV: Orthostatic hypotension; emboli. *CNS:* Apprehension; confusion; fatigue; malaise; vertigo; headache; dysphagia. *EENT:* Blurred vision; sense of ear fullness; tinnitus; hearing loss. *GI:* Anorexia; nausea; vomiting; diarrhea; pancreatitis; discomfort; pain; sudden watery, profuse diarrhea; bleeding. *GU:* Hematuria. *HEMA:* Neutropenia; thrombocytopenia; agranulocytosis; hyponatremia; hypokalemia; hypomagnesemia; hypocalcemia; hypercalciuria; hypovolemia. *HEPA:* Jaundice; abnormal LFTs. *DERM:* Rash. *META:* Acute gout; hyperuricemia; hyperglycemia. *OTHER:* Fever; chills; local irritation and pain with parenteral administration.

Precautions

Pregnancy: Category B. *Lactation:* Undetermined. *Children:* Safety and efficacy not established in infants (see Contraindications) and in children (IV). *Dehydration:* Excessive diuresis may cause dehydration and decreased blood volume with circulatory collapse and possible vascular thrombosis and embolism, especially in elderly. *Electrolyte imbalance:* May be more likely in patients receiving large doses with restricted salt intake. *Hepatic cirrhosis and ascites:* Sudden alterations of electrolyte balance may precipitate hepatic encephalopathy and coma. *Ototoxicity:* Associated with rapid injection, very large doses or concurrent use of other ototoxic drugs. *Photosensitivity:* May occur. *Systemic lupus erythematosus:* May be exacerbated or activated.

NURSING CONSIDERATIONS

Administration/Storage

- Administer drug PO or IV only. SC or IM injection causes local pain and irritation.
- To prepare IV solution, add 50 ml of D5W or normal saline. If solution is hazy or opalescent, do not use.
- For IV dose, administer drug slowly. Rotate injection sites to avoid thrombophlebitis.
- Discard reconstituted solution if not used within 24 hr.
- Do not administer drug with other drugs or with blood products.
- Do not give with other ototoxic drugs.
- Give oral medication after meal or with food to prevent GI upset.
- Avoid administering within 6-8 hr of bedtime to avoid nocturia.

Assessment/Interventions

- Obtain patient history, including drug history and any known allergies.
- Obtain baseline BUN, creatinine, potassium and sodium chloride and monitor daily.
- Closely monitor blood glucose.
- Monitor I&O and obtain daily weight.
- Assess patient for signs of GI bleeding.
- Monitor CBC and differential daily.
- Obtain BP and pulse before and during treatment, observing for orthostatic hypotension.
- Assess neurologic status prior to administering drug and during treatment.
- If severe, watery diarrhea occurs, report to physician.
- If signs of ototoxicity (ear fullness, tinnitus, vertigo, hearing loss) occur, slow rate of IV injection.
- If patient develops anuria, hematuria, increases in BUN or creatinine or significant changes in electrolytes, report to physician.
- If signs of dehydration develop (hypotension, tachycardia, postural hypotension, rapid weight loss, decreased filling pressures), notify physician.
- If patient shows change in LOC or mentation, notify physician.
- If patient is elderly or debilitated, observe for possible dehydration.

OVERDOSAGE: SIGNS & SYMPTOMS

Water loss, volume depletion, electrolyte depletion, circulatory collapse, vascular thrombosis and embolism, weakness, dizziness, confusion, anorexia, lethargy, vomiting, cramps

Patient/Family Education

- Tell patient to take drug with food or milk.
- Instruct patient to take drug in morning.
- Advise patient to avoid exposure to sunlight or UV light and to use sunscreen or wear protective clothing to avoid photosensitivity reaction.
- Caution patient to avoid sudden position changes to prevent orthostatic hypotension.
- Instruct patient to report these symptoms to physician: confusion or mood changes, increased thirst, dizziness, irregular heart beat, weakness or increased tiredness, diarrhea, blood in urine or stool, muscle weakness or cramps, sudden joint pain or any changes in hearing.
- Advise patients with diabetes mel-

litus to monitor blood glucose levels closely.

See Patient Guide, p. 232.

Ethchlorvynol

(eth-klor-VIH-nahl)

Placidyl

Class: Sedative and hypnotic/ nonbarbiturate

Action Unknown; produces CNS depressant effects similar to those of barbiturates.

Indications Short-term therapy in management of insomnia (up to 1 wk). **Unlabeled use:** Sedation.

Contraindications Porphyria.

Route/Dosage
ADULTS: **PO** 500-1000 mg at bedtime. If patient awakens in early morning, give additional 200 mg.

Interactions
Alcohol and CNS depressants: Enhances CNS depressant effects. *Anticoagulants:* May decrease anticoagulant activity.

Lab Test Interferences
None well documented.

Adverse Reactions
CV: Hypotension. *CNS:* Dizziness; facial numbness; paradoxical reaction (eg, excitement, restlessness). *EENT:* Blurred vision. *GI:* Nausea; vomiting; gastric upset; unpleasant taste in mouth. *HEMA:* Thrombocytopenia. *OTHER:* Hangover; muscle weakness; symptoms of acute toxicity (eg, low body temperature, shortness of breath, slow heart beat); symptoms of chronic toxicity (eg, confusion, slurred speech, double vision, tingling, trembling, staggering); hypersensitivity reactions (eg, rash, itching, cholestatic jaundice).

Precautions
Pregnancy: Category C. *Lactation:* Undetermined. *Children:* Safety and efficacy not established. *Elderly or debilitated patients:* Should receive smallest effective dose. *Dependency:* Do not administer for periods longer than 1 wk. Prolonged use may lead to tolerance or physical and psychological dependence; withdrawal symptoms (including intoxication, tremors, slurred speech, diplopia, muscle weakness) may occur after prolonged use. Use with caution or avoid in patients with history of drug/alcohol abuse. *Mental depression:* Use with caution in depressed patients with or without suicidal tendencies. *Renal and hepatic impairment:* Use with caution. *Tartrazine sensitivity:* Some products contain tartrazine, which may cause allergic-type reactions in susceptible individuals.

NURSING CONSIDERATIONS

Administration/Storage

- Obtain baseline vital signs before administering drug. If respiratory rate is < 12-14 breaths/min, do not administer medication.
- Administer with snack and full glass of water, milk or fruit juice to reduce potential giddiness and ataxia.
- Instruct patient to swallow capsule whole and not to chew.
- Supplemental dose of 200 mg may be given if patient reawakens during early morning hours following bedtime dose.
- Store in tightly closed, light-resistant container at room temperature.

Assessment/Interventions

- Obtain patient history, including drug history and any known allergies. Note use of CNS depressants or anticoagulants, drug or alcohol abuse, depression, suicidal tendencies, porphyria, renal or liver disease and hypersensitivity reactions, especially

to ethchlorvynol, aspirin and tartrazine.
- Assess usual sleep patterns, nature of sleep disturbance and drug effectiveness.
- Provide pain-relieving measures prior to administering drug to patient experiencing pain.
- Adjust dosage of anticoagulants at initiation and discontinuance of treatment.
- Enhance effectiveness of drug by encouraging usual sleep patterns and routines.
- Provide relaxing environment that facilitates sleep induction.
- Eliminate stimuli that inhibit sleep.
- Utilize safety precautions to prevent injury such as keeping bed in low position with siderails up.
- Inform patient to call for assistance when getting up in the night because patient may experience dizziness.
- Monitor coagulation laboratory results if patient is taking anticoagulants.
- Observe for side effects such as hypotension, dizziness, weakness, unpleasant aftertaste, hangover, vomiting or paradoxical reaction.
- In patients receiving daytime sedation, report appearance of mental confusion, hallucinations or drowsiness to physician.

OVERDOSAGE: SIGNS & SYMPTOMS

Respiratory depression, hypotension, somnolence, confusion, shock, constricted pupils, tachycardia, edema, hepatic dysfunction, coma

Patient/Family Education

- Instruct patient that drug is for short-term use only and that its use can lead to tolerance and physical and psychological dependency.
- Warn patient that if drug is taken > 2 wk, withdrawal symptoms may be experienced.
- Instruct patient on how drug should be taken and that it should be taken in prescribed dose only.
- Inform patient that some side effects can be reduced if drug is taken with food.
- If medication is to be taken at bedtime, remind patient to take before midnight. Explain that if medication is being used as sedative it should not be taken in middle of night or early in morning.
- Instruct patient to report these symptoms to physician: visual changes, irregular heart beats, chest pains, yellowing of skin and eyes, rash or unusual bleeding or bruising.
- Instruct patient to avoid intake of alcoholic beverages or other CNS depressants.
- Advise patient that drug may cause drowsiness and to use caution while driving or performing other tasks requiring mental alertness.

See Patient Guide, p. 233.

Ethosuximide

(ETH-oh-SUX-ih-mide)

Zarontin

Class: Anticonvulsant/succinimide

Action Elevates seizure threshold and suppresses paroxysmal spike and wave activity associated with lapses of consciousness common in absence (petit mal) seizures.

Indications Control of absence (petit mal) seizures.

Contraindications Hypersensitivity to succinimides.

Route/Dosage

ADULTS & CHILDREN ≥ 6 YR: **PO** 500 mg/day. Optimal dose for most children is 20 mg/kg/day. Maintenance therapy: Individualize dose. Increase daily dose slowly by 250 mg q 4-7 days until control is achieved with minimal side effects. Doses exceeding 1.5 g/day should be administered in divided doses under strict medical supervision. CHILDREN 3-6 YR: Initial dose: **PO** 250 mg/day.

Interactions

Hydantoins: May increase serum hydantoin levels. *Primidone:* Lower primidone and phenobarbital levels may occur.

Lab Test Interferences

None well documented.

Adverse Reactions

CNS: Drowsiness; headache; dizziness; euphoria; hiccups; irritability; hyperactivity; lethargy; fatigue; ataxia; psychological disturbances such as sleep disorders; night terrors; poor concentration; aggressiveness. *EENT:* Myopia. *GI:* Anorexia; GI upset; nausea; vomiting; cramps; epigastric and abdominal pain; weight loss; gum hypertrophy; tongue swelling. *GU:* Vaginal bleeding; microscopic hematuria. *HEMA:* Leukopenia; agranulocytosis; pancytopenia; bone marrow suppression; eosinophilia. *DERM:* Urticaria; Stevens-Johnson syndrome; systemic lupus erythematosus; pruritic erythematous rash; hirsutism.

Precautions

Pregnancy: Anticonvulsant drugs have been observed to increase the incidence of birth defects. *Hematologic effects:* Blood dyscrasias, including fatal cases, have occurred. Periodic blood counts should be done. *Hepatic or renal impairment:* Use caution and perform periodic function tests. *Lupus:* Cases of systemic lupus erythematosus have occurred. *Withdrawal:* Do not withdraw drug abruptly as this may precipitate absence (petit mal) status; proceed slowly when increasing or decreasing dose.

NURSING CONSIDERATIONS

Administration/Storage

- Dosage should be increased in small increments.
- If GI upset occurs, give with food or milk.
- Store capsules in tight containers and syrup in light-resistant containers at room temperature. Avoid freezing.

Assessment/Interventions

- Obtain patient history, including drug history and any known allergies.
- Assess location, duration and characteristics of seizure activity.
- Document baseline CBC, hepatic function and urinalysis, and monitor routinely throughout course of therapy.
- Observe frequently for occurrence of seizure activity and report findings to physician.
- Ensure that patient is protected from injury. Supervise and assist with ambulation if dizziness and drowsiness are problems. Pad siderails and head of bed with towels or blanket for patients who experience seizures during night.
- Assess patient's mood, behavior patterns and facial expressions. Patients with history of psychiatric disorders have an increased risk of developing behavioral changes.
- Observe for GI symptoms, drowsiness, ataxia, dizziness and other neurologic side effects.

OVERDOSAGE: SIGNS & SYMPTOMS

Acute overdose: Confusion; sleepiness; unsteadiness; flaccid muscles; coma with slow, shallow respiration; nausea and vomiting
Chronic overdose: Skin rash; confusion; ataxia; dizziness; drowsiness; irritability; poor judgment; periorbital edema; proteinuria; hepatic dysfunction; fatal bone marrow aplasia; hematuria; nephrosis

Patient/Family Education

- Instruct patient to take medi-

cation with food to minimize GI upset.

- Advise patient to carry wallet identification card or Medi-Alert bracelet, describing disease process and medication regimen, physician's name and telephone number.
- Emphasize importance of follow-up exams to monitor progress and side effects.
- Explain that medication may change color of urine to pink, red or red-brown, and assure that this is not harmful.
- Instruct patient to report these symptoms to physician: skin rash, sore throat, fever, unusual bleeding or bruising, swollen glands or pregnancy.
- Tell patient to avoid intake of alcoholic beverages or other CNS depressants.
- Advise patient that drug may cause drowsiness and to use caution while driving or performing other tasks requiring mental alertness.
- Instruct patient not to take otc medications without consulting physician.

See Patient Guide, p. 234.

Etidronate Disodium

(eh-TIH-DROE-nate die-SO-dee-uhm)

Didronel

Class: Hormone/biphosphonate

Action Inhibits normal and abnormal bone resorption; reduces bone formation.

Indications Treatment of symptomatic Paget's disease; prevention and treatment of heterotopic ossification; treatment of hypercalcemia of malignancy. **Unlabeled use:** Treatment of postmenopausal osteoporosis.

Contraindications Hypersensitivity to biphosphonates; patients with class Dc and higher renal functional impairment (serum creatinine > 5 mg/dl).

Route/Dosage

Paget's Disease

ADULTS: Initial treatment: **PO** 5-10 mg/kg/day (not to exceed 6 mo) or 11-20 mg/kg/day (not to exceed 3 mo). Reserve doses > 10 mg/kg/day for specific situations. Retreatment: Initiate only after etidronate-free period ≥ 90 days and if there is evidence of active disease.

Heterotopic Ossification from Spinal Cord Injury

ADULTS: **PO** 20 mg/kg/day for 2 wk followed by 10 mg/kg/day for 10 wk; total treatment period is 12 wk.

Heterotopic Ossification Complicating Total Hip Replacement

ADULTS: **PO** 20 mg/kg/day for 1 mo preoperatively followed by 20 mg/kg/day for 3 mo postoperatively.

Hypercalcemia

ADULTS: **IV** 7.5 mg/kg/day for 3 successive days given by slow infusion (over a period of at least 2 hr). Retreatment may be needed; wait at least 7 days between courses. Adjust dose for renal impairment. Regimen of oral etidronate (20 mg/kg/day for 30 days) may be started after last infusion.

Interactions None well documented.

Lab Test Interferences

Calcium supplements, antacids, foods: Products containing calcium and other multi-valent cations interfere with etidronate absorption.

Adverse Reactions

EENT: Metallic or altered taste; loss of taste. *GI:* Diarrhea; nausea; constipation; stomatitis; diarrhea in enterocolitis patients. *GU:* Abnormal elevations of serum creatinine and BUN; mild to moderate abnormalities in renal function. *OTHER:* Hypersensitivity (eg, angioedema, urticaria, rash, pruritus); increased or recurrent bone pain in

Paget's disease; hypocalcemia; fractures with excessive doses; convulsions; hypophosphatemia; hypomagnesemia.

Precautions
Pregnancy: Category B (oral); Category C (parenteral). *Lactation:* Undetermined. *Children:* Safety and efficacy not established. *Paget's disease:* Response may be slow and may continue for months after treatment has been discontinued. Dosage must not be prematurely increased or treatment prematurely reinitiated until patient has had at least 90-day etidronate-free interval. *GI disorders:* Use this drug with caution in patients with active upper GI problems such as dysphagia (difficulty swallowing); symptomatic esophageal diseases; gastritis; duodenitis or ulcers.

NURSING CONSIDERATIONS

Administration/Storage

- Have patient take drug on empty stomach 2 hr before meals.
- Administer oral medication as a single dose. If GI upset occurs, dose may be divided.
- To maximize absorption of drug, have patient avoid food high in calcium (eg, milk and milk products), vitamins with mineral supplements and antacids high in metals within 2 hr of dosing.
- Dilute daily intravenous dose in at least 250 ml of sterile normal saline.
- Slow IV infusion is important. Infuse diluted dose over ≥ 2 hr.
- Store diluted dose at room temperature no longer than 48 hr.
- Store intravenous medication away from excessive heat.

Assessment/Interventions

- Obtain patient history, including drug history and any known allergies. Note any hypersensitivity to biphosphonates.
- Record dates of any previous treatments with etidronate.
- Treatment of hypocalcemia includes intravenous calcium administration.
- Monitor serum calcium, phosphate, potassium, BUN and creatinine.
- Monitor renal status throughout treatment.

OVERDOSAGE: SIGNS & SYMPTOMS

Diarrhea, vomiting, hypocalcemia

Patient/Family Education

- Instruct patient to avoid eating 2 hr before and 2 hr after taking medication since absorption of drug is reduced by food.
- Advise patient to avoid vitamins, mineral supplements and antacids that are high in metals, especially calcium, iron, magnesium and aluminum.
- Instruct patient to maintain adequate intake of foods containing calcium and vitamin D within 2 hours of taking etidronate.
- Inform patient of transient effect of metallic or altered taste or loss of taste.
- Tell patient to report these symptoms to physician: rash, respiratory difficulty, GI upset, visual disturbances or jaundice.
- Instruct patient not to take any otc medications without consulting physician.

See Patient Guide, p. 235.

Etodolac

(EE-toe-DOE-lak)
Lodine
Class: Analgesic/NSAID

Action Decreases inflammation, pain and fever, probably through inhibition of cyclooxygenase activity and prostaglandin synthesis.

Indications Management of pain; management of signs and

symptoms of osteoarthritis. **Unlabeled uses:** Control of symptoms of rheumatoid arthritis; treatment of temporal arteritis.

Contraindications Patients in whom aspirin, iodides or any NSAID has caused allergic-type reactions.

Route/Dosage

Analgesia

ADULTS: **PO** 200-400 mg q 6-8 hr prn.

Osteoarthritis

ADULTS: **PO** 800-1200 mg/day initially in divided doses; followed by dosage adjustments within range of 600-1200 mg/day in divided doses (maximum 1200 mg/day).

Interactions

Anticoagulants: May increase prothrombin time. Watch for signs and symptoms of bleeding. *Beta blockers:* May decrease antihypertensive effect of beta blockers. *Lithium:* May increase lithium levels and effects. *Loop diuretics:* May decrease diuretic effect. *Methotrexate:* May increase methotrexate levels. *Salicylates:* Plasma concentrations of NSAIDs may be decreased when taken with salicylates. There is no therapeutic advantage to this combination, but adverse GI effects may be increased.

Lab Test Interferences

Serum uric acid levels: Drug may cause small decrease. *Urinary bilirubin test:* Drug may cause false-positive results. *Urinary dipstick tests:* Drug may cause results that are false positive for ketones.

Adverse Reactions

CV: Fluid retention; edema; hypertension; flushing; CHF; syncope; palpitations. *RESP:* Asthma. *CNS:* Dizziness; headaches; drowsiness; insomnia; asthenia; malaise; depression; nervousness. *EENT:* Blurred vision; photophobia; visual changes; tinnitus. *GI:* Dyspepsia; nausea; vomiting; diarrhea; indigestion; heartburn; abdominal pain; constipation; flatulence; gastritis; melena; dry mouth; anorexia; stomatitis; peptic ulcers. *GU:* Urinary frequency; dysuria. *HEMA:* Anemia; leukopenia; pancytopenia; thrombocytopenia; increased bleeding time; agranulocytosis; hemolytic anemia; neutropenia. *HEPA:* Jaundice; cholestatic jaundice; hepatitis. *DERM:* Rash, pruritus, Stevens-Johnson syndrome, hyperpigmentation; urticaria; purpura. *META:* Weight gain; hypouricemia. *OTHER:* Chills; fever.

Precautions

Pregnancy: Category C: *Lactation:* Undetermined. *Children:* Safety and efficacy not established. *Elderly or debilitated patients:* Increased risk of adverse reactions. *GI effects:* Serious GI toxicity (eg, bleeding, ulceration, perforation) can occur at any time, with or without warning symptoms. *Hypersensitivity:* May occur; use caution in aspirin-sensitive individuals because of possible cross-sensitivity. *Renal effects:* Acute renal insufficiency, interstitial nephritis, hyperkalemia, hyponatremia and renal papillary necrosis may occur. *Renal impairment:* Assess renal function before and during therapy.

NURSING CONSIDERATIONS

Administration/Storage

- Do not give more than 20 mg/kg to patients weighing ≤ 60 kg.
- Food delays peak action of medication by 1-4 hr.
- Give with food, milk or antacids if stomach upset occurs.
- Store at room temperature in tightly closed container. Protect from moisture.

Assessment/Interventions

- Obtain patient history, including drug history and any known allergies, especially to aspirin, iodides or other NSAIDs. Note history of GI bleeding.
- Assess location, duration and intensity of pain before and 60 min after administration.
- Monitor hematocrit and hemoglobin

levels in patients on long-term therapy.
- Monitor for signs of agranulocytosis (sore throat, fever).
- Monitor renal function.
- Monitor for edema and weight gain in patients with CHF and renal impairment.
- Monitor PT/APTT levels of patients taking anticoagulants.
- Monitor elderly patients carefully for possible adverse reactions.
- Review liver function test results, and report signs of hepatic dysfunction to the physician.
- Discontinue drug if hypersensitivity develops.
- Inform physician of decreased renal function, hyponatremia and hyperkalemia laboratory values.

OVERDOSAGE: SIGNS & SYMPTOMS

Respiratory depression, hypotension, epigastric pain, drowsiness, lethargy, GI irritation/bleeding, nausea, vomiting, tinnitus, sweating, acute renal failure

Patient/Family Education

- Advise patient to take medication with full glass of water and to remain upright for 15-30 min after administration.
- Encourage patients on long-term therapy to have regular eye examinations.
- Advise patient to inform physician or dentist of medication regimen before treatment or surgery.
- Instruct patient to report these symptoms to physician: rash, stomach problems, tinnitus, dizziness or visual disturbances, black tarry stools, increased bruises or bleeding.
- Caution patient not to use aspirin or other otc medications or drink alcoholic beverages while taking this medication.
- Advise patient that drug may cause drowsiness and to use caution while driving or performing tasks requiring mental alertness.
- Caution patient to avoid exposure to sunlight and to use sunscreen or wear protective clothing to avoid photosensitivity reaction.

See Patient Guide, p. 236.

Etoposide (VP-16-213)

(EH-toe-POE-side)

VePesid

Class: Antineoplastic/mitotic inhibitor

Action Causes lysis of cells entering mitosis; prevents cells from entering prophase; inhibits DNA synthesis.

Indications Combination therapy of refractory testicular tumors; combination therapy for small cell lung cancer. **Unlabeled uses:** Alone or in combination treatment of leukemias, lymphomas, Kaposi's and soft tissue sarcoma, neuroblastoma, choriocarcinoma, rhabdomyosarcoma, hepatocellular carcinoma and epithelial ovarian, non-small and small cell lung, testicular, gastric, endometrial and breast cancers.

Contraindications Hypersensitivity to teniposide.

Route/Dosage

Testicular Cancer

ADULTS: **IV** 50-100 mg/m^2/day for 3-5 days q 3-4 wk.

Small Cell Lung Cancer

ADULTS: **IV** 35-50 mg/m^2/day for 4-5 days q 3-4 wk. **PO** Twice the IV dose rounded to nearest 50 mg.

Interactions

Cyclosporine: May increase etoposide concentration, causing toxicity.

Lab Test Interferences

None well documented.

Adverse Reactions

CV: Hypotension. *CNS:* Peripheral neurotoxicity. *GI:* Nausea; vomiting; anorexia; diarrhea; stomatitis. *HEMA:* Myelosuppression. *HEPA:* Hepatic dysfunction. *DERM:* Alopecia. *OTHER:* Hypersensitivity, including anaphylactic reactions.

Precautions

Pregnancy: Category D. *Lactation:* Undetermined. *Children:* Safety and efficacy not established. *Anaphylaxis:* Serious reactions may occur; manifested by chills, fever, tachycardia, bronchospasm, shortness of breath, facial flushing, hypertension or hypotension. *Carcinogenesis/mutagenesis:* Carcinogenic and mutagenic potential exists. *Hypotension:* May occur with rapid intravenous injection; give by slow infusion (30-60 min or longer). *Myelosuppression:* Bone marrow suppression is most significant toxicity. May result in infection or bleeding; dose may need to be decreased if severe.

NURSING CONSIDERATIONS

Administration/Storage

- Dosage by IV or oral route may be adjusted if drug is used with other myelosuppressive agents or if patient has compromised bone marrow function because of previous radiation or chemotherapy.
- Give antiemetics 30-60 min before IV or oral administration to decrease chance of nausea or vomiting.
- Prepare solution in biologic cabinet. Skin reactions may occur with accidental exposure. Use gloves, gown and mask when handling. Discard equipment in designated containers.
- If solution comes in contact with skin or mucosa, wash immediately with soap and water.
- For intravenous administration, dilute with either D5W or 0.9% Sodium Chloride for Injection for final concentration of 0.2 or 0.4 mg/ml.
- Plastic devices made of acrylic or ABS have cracked and leaked when used with undiluted etoposide. This has not been reported with diluted solutions.
- Administer intravenous solution slowly over 30-60 min or longer.
- Discard solution if crystals or discoloration is present.
- Unopened vials are stable for 2 yr at room temperature. Diluted solutions (0.2 or 0.4 mg/ml) are stable for 96 and 48 hr, respectively, at room temperature under normal room fluorescent light in both glass and plastic containers.
- Refrigerate capsules. Do not freeze.

Assessment/Interventions

- Obtain patient history, including drug history and any known allergies.
- Determine whether patient is receiving cyclosporine and note last level.
- Obtain baseline BP prior to administration; monitor BP q 15 min during infusion.
- Assess CBC and differential and platelet count prior to and periodically during therapy.
- Have resuscitation equipment and epinephrine nearby during administration. If hypersensitivity reaction occurs, discontinue infusion and notify physician.
- Avoid taking temperature rectally. Avoid IM injections if possible.
- Apply pressure to intravenous insertion site for 10 min after infusion.
- Encourage fluid intake of 2-3 L/day to prevent formation of renal calculi and to preserve renal function.
- Monitor hematologic parameters and blood chemistry values (electrolytes, BUN, creatinine) frequently during therapy.
- Liver function studies (AST, ALT, LDH and bilirubin) and renal function studies (BUN, creatinine and creatinine clearance) should be monitored prior to and periodically

during therapy to detect hepatotoxicity and nephrotoxicity.
- During administration monitor patient carefully for symptoms of anaphylaxis (chills, fever, tachycardia, bronchospasm, shortness of breath, facial flushing, hypertension or hypotension).
- Monitor I&O. Report decrease in urine output, especially if < 30 ml/hr.
- Assess for signs of bleeding (bleeding gums, petechiae, blood in stool, urine or emesis).
- If hypotension occurs during administration, stop infusion and notify physician. After stabilizing BP with intravenous fluids and/or other measures, resume infusion at slower rate.
- Notify physician of any symptoms of infection.
- Notify physician of nausea and vomiting; administration of an antiemetic may be necessary.
- Notify physician if leukocyte count is < 1000/mm^3. Notify physician if platelet count is < 75,000/mm^3.

OVERDOSAGE: SIGNS & SYMPTOMS
Severe bone marrow depression

Patient/Family Education
- Instruct patient to take etoposide exactly as directed even if nausea or vomiting occurs. Advise patient to notify physician if vomiting occurs shortly after medication is taken.
- Caution patient to avoid crowds and persons with known infections, to be alert for signs of infection (fever, chills, sore throat) and to report these signs to physician immediately.
- Advise patient to be alert for signs of bleeding (bleeding gums, bruising, petechiae, blood in urine or stool, bloody emesis) and to use soft toothbrush and electric razor. Patient should notify physician if signs of bleeding occur.
- Advise patient to use sponge brush and rinse mouth with water after eating and drinking if redness or ulceration occur in mouth. Instruct patient to report these signs to physician.
- Advise patient with stomatitis to avoid spicy foods, alcohol and smoking.
- Caution patient not to receive any vaccinations without physician approval.
- Discuss with patient possibility of hair loss and explore ways to compensate (caps, hats, turbans, scarves, wigs). Assure patient that hair does return after therapy although hair may be of different texture or color.
- Instruct patient to report these symptoms to physician: abdominal pain, weakness, yellow skin or sclera, paresthesia, gait disturbance or breathing difficulties.
- Caution patient to avoid intake of alcoholic beverages or aspirin or aspirin-containing products.

See Patient Guide, p. 237.

Factor IX Complex

Konyne-HT, Profilnine, Proplex T, Proplex SX-T
Class: Antihemophilic

Action Restores hemostasis in patients with factor IX deficiency.

Indications Management of factor IX deficiency (hemophilia B, Christmas disease), bleeding episodes in patients with inhibitors to factor VIII; reversal of coumarin anticoagulant hemorrhage; prevention or control of bleeding in patients with factor VII deficiency (Proplex T only).

Contraindications Treatment of factor VII deficiency (except for Proplex T); liver disease with signs of intravascular coagulation or fibrinolysis.

Route/Dosage
ADULTS & CHILDREN: **IV** Dose based on patient condition, degree of deficiency and desired level of factor IX

to be achieved. *Dosing guideline*: 1 U/kg × body weight (kg) × desired increase (% of normal) factor VII deficiency: 0.5 U/kg × body weight (kg) × desired increase (% of normal), repeated q 4-6 h prn.

Hemarthroses

In hemophiliacs with inhibitors to factor VIII, **IV** 75 IU/kg. *Maintenance*: Usually, **IV** 10-20 IU/kg/day. Hemophilia A patients with inhibitors to factor VIII: **IV** 75 IU/kg as single dose followed by second dose in 12 hr if necessary.

Prophylaxis

In patients with Hemophilia B, **IV** 10-20 IU/kg 1-2 times/wk.

Interactions

Aminocaproic acid: May increase risk of thrombosis.

Lab Test Interferences

None well documented.

Adverse Reactions

CV: Thrombosis or disseminated intravascular thrombosis; changes in BP; MI (with high doses). *RESP:* Pulmonary embolism. *CNS:* Headache. *GI:* Nausea; vomiting. *DERM:* Flushing; urticaria. *OTHER:* Pyrogenic reactions (eg, fever and chills); tingling.

Precautions

Pregnancy: Category C. *Hepatitis and HIV infection:* Some risk due to preparation from pooled units of plasma. *Intravascular coagulation:* If signs of DIC occur, stop infusion promptly.

NURSING CONSIDERATIONS

Administration/Storage

- Use powder and diluent at room temperature when reconstituting.
- Gently swirl solution during reconstitution to prevent foaming. Infuse within 3 hr of reconstitution.
- Administer by IV infusion only.
- Start infusion within 3 hr after reconstitution.
- Maintain prescribed rate of infusion, (eg, Konyne-HT, 100 U/min; Profilnine, < 10 ml/min; Proplex T, < 3 ml/min.
- Store powdered form of drug in refrigerator. Do not freeze.
- Do not refrigerate reconstituted solution.

Assessment/Interventions

- Obtain patient history, including drug history and any known allergies. Note hepatitis B vaccination.
- In patients with major bleeding or those being prepared for surgery, monitor factor VII or IX assays daily prior to infusion.
- In patients receiving factor IX for prolonged periods, daily monitor factors II, IX and X.
- Assess BP and heart rate prior to and during infusion.
- Observe for signs of DIC, MI, pulmonary embolus and venous thrombosis.
- Monitor I&O and observe for hemolytic reaction.
- Stop infusion and notify physician if any of the following develops: tingling, urticaria, chills, fever, headache, flushing, nausea or vomiting, change in heart rate or BP. Infusion may be restarted at a slower rate when symptoms subside.
- Discontinue infusion if signs of DIC (eg, petechiae, oozing from puncture sites), tachycardia, tachypnea or joint pain develop, and notify physician.

Patient/Family Education

- Instruct patient to report any chills, headache, urticaria, tingling, flushing, or nausea and vomiting to nurse or physician.
- Tell patient to immediately report any chest pain/pressure or difficulty breathing.
- Caution patient to avoid activities that could lead to injury or bleeding.
- Instruct patient to report any signs of bleeding (petechiae, purpura, bleed-

ing gums or rectum, and blood in urine).
- Discuss questions concerning HIV and hepatitis risk.
- Instruct patient to report any signs or symptoms of AIDS or hepatitis.
- Review methods of preventing and stopping bleeding.
- Advise patient to carry identification/information regarding bleeding tendency.

No patient monograph available.

Famotidine

(fuh-MOE-tih-deen)

Pepcid

Class: Histamine H_2 antagonist

Action Reversibly and competitively blocks histamine at H_2 receptors, particularly those in gastric parietal cells, leading to inhibition of gastric acid secretion.

Indications Short-term treatment and maintenance therapy for duodenal ulcer, gastroesophageal reflux disease (GERD, including erosive or ulcerative disease), benign gastric ulcer, treatment of pathologic hypersecretory conditions. **Unlabeled uses:** Treatment of upper GI bleeding; prevention of stress ulcers; prior to anesthesia for prevention of pulmonary aspiration of gastric acid.

Contraindications Hypersensitivity to other H_2 antagonists.

Route/Dosage

Duodenal Ulcer (Active)

PO 40 mg at bedtime or 20 mg bid for 6-8 wk, maintenance: 20 mg at bedtime.

Benign Gastric Ulcer (Acute)

40 mg at bedtime.

GERD

ADULTS: 20 mg bid (maximum 6 wk). For esophagitis and accompanying symptoms due to GERD 20-40 mg bid (maximum 12 wk).

Pathologic Hypersecretory Conditions

ADULTS: Start at 20 mg q 6 hr, continued as clinically indicated; doses up to 160 mg q 6 hr have been used.

Severely Impaired Renal Function

(CCr < 10 ml/min) May need to reduce to 20 mg at bedtime or increase dosing interval to 36-48 hr. Parenteral: For hospitalized patients with pathologic hypersecretory conditions or intractable ulcers, or patients unable to take orally: 20 mg IV q 12 hr. Parenteral use in GERD not established.

Interactions

Ketoconazole: Effects of ketoconazole may be decreased.

Lab Test Interferences

None well documented.

Adverse Reactions

CV: Palpitations. *RESP:* Bronchospasm. *CNS:* Headache; somnolence; fatigue; dizziness; confusion; hallucinations; agitation or anxiety; depression; insomnia; paresthesias. *EENT:* Tinnitus; taste disorder; orbital edema; conjunctival injection. *GI:* Diarrhea; constipation; nausea; vomiting; abdominal discomfort; anorexia; dry mouth. *GU:* Impotence; loss of libido. *HEMA:* Thrombocytopenia. *DERM:* Alopecia; rash; pruritus; urticaria; acne; dry skin; flushing. *OTHER:* Arthralgia; transient pain at injection site; fever.

Precautions

Pregnancy: Category B. *Lactation:* Undetermined. *Children:* Safety and efficacy not established. *Elderly patients:* May have reduced renal function; decreased clearance may occur. *Gastric malignancy:* Symptomatic response to famotidine does not preclude gastric malignancy. *Hepatic function impairment:* Use caution; decreased clearance may occur. *Hypersensitivity:* Rare cases of anaphylaxis have occurred. *Renal function impairment:* Decreased clearance may occur; reduced dose may be needed.

NURSING CONSIDERATIONS

Administration/Storage

- To prepare for IV push, dilute 2 ml famotidine (solution containing 10 mg/ml) with 0.9% Sodium Chloride for Injection in 5-10 ml volume. Administer over 2 min.
- To prepare IV infusion, dilute 2 ml famotidine (solution containing 10 mg/ml) with 100 ml 5% dextrose. Other diluents that may be used include 0.9% Sodium Chloride for Injection, 10% dextrose, Lactated Ringer's Injection, or 5% sodium bicarbonate. Infuse over 15-30 min.
- Keep powder vials away from heat. After reconstitution store in the refrigerator, but do not freeze. Discard after 30 days.
- Store parenteral solutions in refrigerator. When mixed in polyvinyl chloride minibags stability is 14 days in refrigerator; if frozen, solution remains stable for 28 days and for 48 hr at room temperature.
- Administer with antacids if necessary.
- Medication may be mixable with TPN. Stability depends on solution used.

Assessment/Interventions

- Obtain patient history, including drug history and any known allergies.
- Monitor renal and hepatic function in elderly patients. Notify physician of any chnages in hepatic or renal function.
- Monitor fluid I&O for possible dosage adjustment.
- Give with antacids if necessary.

Patient/Family Education

- Instruct patient not to double up on medication if dose is missed, but to wait and take next scheduled dose on time.
- Tell patient to notify physician immediately of any black, tarry stool or "coffee-ground" vomit.
- Tell patient to notify physician of any shortness of breath, GI disturbances, bleeding, rash, dizziness or fever.
- Tell patient to shake suspension well before taking.

See Patient Guide, p. 239.

Felbamate

(FELL-buh-MATE)

Felbatol

Class: Anticonvulsant

Action May reduce seizure spread in generalized tonic-clonic or partial seizures and may increase seizure threshold in absence seizures.

Indications Monotherapy or adjunctive therapy in treatment of partial seizures with and without generalization in epileptic adults. Adjunctive therapy in treatment of partial and generalized seizures associated with Lennox-Gastaut syndrome in children.

Contraindications Standard considerations.

Route/Dosage

Because of reports of aplastic anemia, it has been recommended to stop use of this drug unless physician decides that withdrawal would cause greater risk.

Initial Monotherapy

ADULTS & ADOLESCENTS ≥ 14 YR: **PO** 1200 mg/day in 3 or 4 divided doses; increase in 600 mg increments q 2 wk to 2400 mg/day and then 3600 mg/day if indiciated.

Conversion to Monotherapy

ADULTS & ADOLESCENTS ≥ 14 YR: Initial dose: **PO** 1200 mg/day in 3 or 4 divided doses, reducing dose of other antiepileptic drugs by ⅓. At wk 2 increase felbamate to 2400 mg/day and at wk 3 increase to 3600 mg/day; continue to reduce dose of other antiepileptic drugs as indicated.

Adjunctive Therapy

ADULTS & ADOLESCENTS ≥ 14 YR: Initial dose: **PO** 1200 mg/day in 3 or 4 divided doses; reduce original dose of other antiepileptic drugs by 20%-33% for 1 wk. At wk 2 increase felbamate to 2400 mg/day and at wk 3 increase to 3600 mg/day if needed; reduce dosage of other antiepileptic drugs as clinically indicated. CHILDREN 2-14 YR WITH LENNOX-GASTAUX SYNDROME: Initial dose: **PO** 15 mg/kg/day in 3 or 4 divided doses while reducing other antiepileptic drugs by ≥ 20%. Increase felbamate by 15 mg/kg/day increments at weekly intervals up to 45 mg/kg/day; continue to reduce dosage of other antiepileptic drugs as needed.

Interactions

Antiepileptic drugs: Felbamate may increase blood levels of phenytoin and valproic acid and decrease blood levels of carbamazepine. Phenytoin or carbamazepine may increase clearance of felbamate.

Lab Test Interferences

None well documented.

Adverse Reactions

RESP: Upper respiratory tract infection; coughing. *CNS:* Insomnia; headache; anxiety; somnolence; dizziness; nervousness; tremor; abnormal gait; depression; paresthesia; ataxia; dry mouth; stupor; thinking abnormalities; emotional lability. *EENT:* Diplopia; abnormal vision; miosis; otitis media; rhinitis; sinusitis; taste perversion; pharyngitis. *GI:* Dyspepsia; vomiting; constipation; diarrhea; nausea; anorexia; abdominal pain; hiccoughs. *GU:* Urinary incontinence; intramenstrual bleeding; UTI. *HEMA:* Aplastic anemia; purpura; leukopenia. *HEPA:* Increased ALT and AST; acute liver failure. *DERM:* Acne; rash; pruritus. *OTHER:* Fatigue; weight decrease; facial edema; fever; chest pain; pain; hypophosphatemia; myalgia.

Precautions

Pregnancy: Category C. *Lactation:* Excreted in breast milk. *Children:* Safety and efficacy not established other than for adjunctive therapy of Lennox-Gastaut syndrome. *Elderly patients:* Use caution and start with low doses. Clinical experience is limited. *Aplastic anemia:* It is recommended that use of felbamate be suspended unless physician judges that patient's well-being is at greater risk if drug is discontinued. *Carcinogenesis:* Drug may have carcinogenic potential. *Discontinuation:* Withdraw drug slowly to avoid increased seizure frequency. *Hypersensitivity:* Administer drug with caution to patients with prior hypersensitivity reactions to carbamates. ***Pre-existing liver failure:* Eight cases of acute liver failure have occurred, including four deaths, in association with the use of felbamate. Evaluate patients prior to treatment initiation for evidence of pre-existing liver damage; avoid use in patients with pre-existing liver pathology. Once treatment is initiated, monitor ALT, AST, and bilirubin on a weekly basis. The drug should be withdrawn immediately in patients who develop lab findings indicating liver injury. *Aplastic anemia:* It is recommended that use of felbomate be suspended unless physician judges that patient's well-being is at a greater risk if drug is discontinued.**

NURSING CONSIDERATIONS

Administration/Storage

- Instruct patient to take tablet whole with full glass of water; do not crush.
- May administer tablet with food.
- Administer suspension if patient is unable to swallow tablets.
- Shake suspension prior to administration.
- Do not discontinue administration

suddenly because of the possibility of increased frequency of seizures.
- Store at room temperature in tightly closed container away from excessive heat, direct sunlight and moisture.

Assessment/Interventions
- Obtain patient history, including drug history and any known allergies. Note current status and frequency of seizures and use of other antiepileptic drugs, nonprescription drugs and social drugs (alcohol).
- Assess baseline data on patient's weight and hematologic and hepatic functions.
- Monitor for effectiveness; note any changes in seizure patterns and frequency.
- If seizures occur, protect patient from injury.
- Weigh patient weekly and record weight.
- Monitor serum levels of felbamate and/or other antiepileptic drugs as necessary.

Patient/Family Education
- Instruct patient to drink at least one full glass of water with each dose.
- Remind patient to take tablet whole; do not crush.
- Inform patient that tablet may be taken with food.
- Caution patient to not stop taking this medication suddenly because of possibility of increasing seizure frequency.
- Advise patient to avoid exposure to sunlight or sunlamps and to use sunscreen or wear protective clothing to avoid photosensitivity reaction.
- Instruct patient and family that if seizures occur, they should protect patient from injury.
- Inform patient to report these symptoms to physician: loss of appetite, nausea, vomiting, indigestion, constipation, diarrhea, weight loss/gain, anxiety, nervousness, tremors, dizziness, depression, chest pain, fever, headache, poor coordination, drowsiness, sleeplessness, edema (fluid retention), intramenstrual bleeding (women), dry mouth, vision problems and any changes in seizure activity.
- Advise patient that drug may cause drowsiness, dizziness and vision problems and to use caution while driving or performing other tasks requiring mental alertness.

See Patient Guide, p. 240.

Felodipine

(feh-LOW-dih-peen)

Plendil, *Renedil*

Class: Calcium channel blocker

Action Inhibits movement of calcium ions across cell membrane in systemic and coronary vascular smooth muscle, altering contractile process.

Indications Treatment of hypertension.

Contraindications Sick sinus syndrome; second- or third-degree atrioventricular (AV) block except with functioning pacemaker; hypotension with systolic pressure < 90 mm Hg.

Route/Dosage
PO 2.5-10 mg once daily. Maximum 20 mg once daily. Elderly rarely require > 10 mg qd.

Interactions
Barbiturates: Effects of felodipine may be decreased. *Carbamazepine*: Plasma levels of felodipine may be decreased, reducing effect. *Food*: Effects of felodipine may increase if given with grapefruit juice. *Histamine H_2 antagonists*: Cimetidine may increase effects of felodipine. *Hydantoins*: Serum felodipine levels may be decreased, reducing effects. *Other antihypertensive agents*: May have additive effects.

Lab Test Interferences

None well documented.

Adverse Reactions

CV: Peripheral edema; hypotension; syncope; AV block; MI; arrhythmias; angina; tachycardia. *RESP:* Nasal or chest congestion; sinusitis; rhinitis; pharyngitis; shortness of breath; wheezing; cough; sneezing; respiratory infections. *CNS:* Headache; dizziness; lightheadedness; nervousness; psychiatric disturbances; paresthesias; somnolence; asthenia; insomnia; anxiety; irritability. *GI:* Nausea; diarrhea; constipation; abdominal discomfort; cramps; dyspepsia; vomiting; dry mouth; thirst; flatulence. *GU:* Micturition disorders; sexual difficulties. *HEMA:* Epistaxis. *OTHER:* Muscle cramps, pain or inflammation; gingival hyperplasia.

Precautions

Pregnancy: Category C. *Lactation:* Undetermined. *Children:* Safety and efficacy not established. *Elderly patients:* May have greater hypotensive effects and increased risk of peripheral edema when dosage exceeds 20 mg/day. Monitor closely; doses > 10 mg usually not needed. *CHF:* Use with caution. *Hepatic impairment:* Use with caution in patients with impaired hepatic function or reduced hepatic blood flow. *Withdrawal syndrome:* Abrupt withdrawal may cause increased frequency and duration of angina. Taper dose gradually.

NURSING CONSIDERATIONS

Administration/Storage

- Do not crush tablet or allow patient to chew it.
- Give with food, if patient experiences GI upset.

Assessment/Interventions

- Obtain patient history, including drug history and any known allergies.
- Monitor BP frequently during dosage adjustment, especially for patients over 65 yr and patients with liver dysfunction.

OVERDOSAGE: SIGNS & SYMPTOMS

Hypotension, bradycardia, nausea, weakness, dizziness, slurred speech

Patient/Family Education

- Instruct patient not to crush or chew tablets.
- Teach patient and family member correct method of measuring BP.
- Explain that mild peripheral edema may occur within 2-3 wk after beginning therapy.
- Advise patient that drug may cause drowsiness and dizziness and to use caution while driving or performing other tasks requiring mental alertness.
- Instruct patient to avoid sudden position changes to prevent postural hypotension.
- Explain importance of proper oral hygiene and regular dental examinations to prevent gum disease.
- Tell patient not to double up medication if dose is missed, but to wait and take next scheduled dose on time.
- Instruct patient to report these symptoms to physician: irregular heart beat, increased frequency or severity of angina, shortness of breath, swelling of hands and feet, dizziness, constipation, nausea, unusual bleeding or bruising and hypotension.

See Patient Guide, p. 241.

Fenfluramine HCl

(fen-FLURE-uh-meen HIGH-droe-KLOR-ide)

Pondimin, ✤ *Ponderal*

Class: CNS stimulant/anorexiant

Action Stimulates satiety center in brain, causing appetite suppression.

Indications Short-term (8-12 wk) adjunct to diet plan to reduce weight. **Unlabeled use:** Treating autistic children with elevated serotonin levels.

Contraindications Hypersensitivity to sympathomimetic amines; alcoholism; advanced arteriosclerosis; symptomatic cardiovascular disease; moderate to severe hypertension; hyperthyroidism; glaucoma; agitated states; history of drug abuse; during or within 14 days of MAO inhibitor use; coadministration with other CNS stimulants; schizophrenia.

Route/Dosage

ADULTS: **PO** 20-40 mg tid, before meals.

Interactions

Anesthetics: Combined use has been associated with cardiac arrest. *Guanethidine:* May decrease hypotensive effect. *Insulin, sulfonylurea hypoglycemics:* May increase hypoglycemic effects. *MAO inhibitors and furazolidone:* Hypertensive crisis and intracranial hemorrhage may occur. *Tricyclic antidepressants:* May decrease anorexiant effect.

Lab Test Interferences None well documented.

Adverse Reactions

CV: Palpitations; tachycardia; arrhythmias; hypertension; hypotension. *CNS:* Overstimulation; dizziness; drowsiness; insomnia; euphoria; tremor; headache; psychosis; depression. *EENT:* Mydriasis; blurred vision. *GI:* Dry mouth; unpleasant taste; nausea; diarrhea; constipation; stomach pain. *GU:* Dysuria; urinary frequency; impotence; menstrual disturbances. *HEMA:* Bone marrow depression; agranulocytosis; leukopenia. *META:* Lowered blood glucose levels. *OTHER:* Hair loss; excessive sweating; flushing; myalgia; gynecomastia; allergic reactions (eg, urticaria, rash, erythema).

Precautions

Pregnancy: Category C. *Lactation:* Undetermined. *Children:* Not recommended for children < 12 yr. *Cardiovascular effects:* May cause or aggravate hypertension or arrhythmias. *Drug dependence:* Related to amphetamine; has abuse potential. *Surgical anesthesia:* Use of anesthetics has been associated with cardiac arrest. *Tolerance:* May occur.

NURSING CONSIDERATIONS

Administration/Storage

- Give medication 1 hr before meals.
- Administer last dose of day at least 6 hr before bedtime.
- Make dosage increases in small increments (ie, 1 tablet/day at weekly intervals).
- Store capsules in tight containers and syrup in light-resistant containers at room temperature. Avoid freezing.

Assessment/Interventions

- Obtain complete patient history, including drug history and any known allergies.
- Assess patient's mood, behavioral patterns and facial expressions. Patients with history of psychiatric disorder have increased risk of developing behavioral changes.
- Monitor hepatic and renal function.
- Monitor patient's weight for possible reduction.
- Evaluate baseline CBC and urinalysis, and monitor routinely throughout course of prolonged therapy.
- Implement protective measures, and

supervise and assist with ambulation if dizziness and drowsiness are problems.

- Observe for GI symptoms, drowsiness, ataxia, dizziness and other neurologic side effect, as they may indicate need for dosage adjustment.
- Observe for signs of withdrawal; abrupt discontinuation may precipitate ataxia, tremor, disturbed concentration, depression and hallucinations.

OVERDOSAGE: SIGNS & SYMPTOMS

Acute overdose: Confusion, sleepiness, unsteadiness, flaccid muscles, coma with slow, shallow respiration, nausea and vomiting. *Chronic overdose:* Skin rash, confusion, ataxia, dizziness, drowsiness, irritability, poor judgment, periorbital edema, proteinuria, hepatic dysfunction, fatal bone marrow aplasia, hematuria, nephrosis

Patient/Family Education

- Encourage patient to follow medically supervised weight reduction program.
- Instruct patient to avoid intake of alcoholic beverages or other CNS depressants.
- For patients who have had seizures, advise them to carry wallet identification or wear Medi-Alert bracelet describing disease process and medication regimen, physician's name and telephone number.
- Advise patient to take sips of water frequently, suck on ice chips or sugarless hard candy or chew sugarless gum to relieve dry mouth.
- Instruct patient to notify physician if skin rash, sore throat, fever, unusual bleeding or bruising, swollen glands or pregnancy occurs.
- Emphasize importance of follow-up exams to monitor progress and side effects.
- Advise patient that drug may cause drowsiness and to use caution while driving or performing other tasks requiring mental alertness.

See Patient Guide, p. 264.

Fenoprofen Calcium

(FEN-oh-PRO-fen KAL-see-uhm)

Nalfon

Class: Analgesic/NSAID

Action Decreases inflammation, pain and fever, probably through inhibition of cyclooxygenase activity and prostaglandin synthesis.

Indications Symptomatic relief for rheumatoid arthritis, osteoarthritis, mild to moderate pain. **Unlabeled uses:** Symptomatic relief for juvenile rheumatoid arthritis; migraine prophylaxis and treatment.

Contraindications Sensitivity to aspirin or other NSAIDs; preexisting renal disease.

Route/Dosage

Rheumatoid Arthritis/Osteoarthritis

PO 300-600 mg tid-qid; do not exceed 3.2 g/day.

Mild/Moderate Pain

PO 200 mg q 4-6 h prn.

Interactions

Anticoagulants: May increase risk of bleeding caused by gastric erosion. *Methotrexate:* May increase methotrexate levels.

Lab Test Interferences

False elevation in free and total serum T_3 as measured by Amerlex-M kit.

Adverse Reactions

CV: CHF; hypotension; hypertension; peripheral edema; fluid retention; vasodilation. *RESP:* Bronchospasm; laryngeal edema; hemoptysis;

shortness of breath. *CNS:* Dizziness; drowsiness; headaches; nervousness; anxiety; confusion. *EENT:* Visual disturbances; tinnitus; dry eyes. *GI:* Heartburn; dyspepsia; nausea; vomiting; diarrhea; constipation; increased or decreased appetite; indigestion; GI bleeding; ulceration. *GU:* Hematuria; proteinuria; renal insufficiency; glomerular and interstitial nephritis; acute renal failure with preexisting renal dysfunction. *HEMA:* Bone marrow depression; neutropenia; leukopenia; hypocoagulability. *DERM:* Pruritus; erythemia; urticaria. *META:* Hyperglycemia; hypoglycemia; hyponatremia.

Precautions

Pregnancy: Category B. *Lactation:* Undetermined. *Children:* Safety and efficacy not established. *Elderly patients:* Increased risk of adverse reactions. *Hypersensitivity:* Use caution in aspirin-sensitive individuals due to possible cross-sensitivity. *GI effects:* Serious GI toxicity (eg, bleeding, ulceration, perforation) can occur at any time, with or without warning symptoms. *Renal effects:* Acute renal insufficiency, interstitial nephritis, hyperkalemia, hyponatremia and renal papillary necrosis may occur.

NURSING CONSIDERATIONS

Administration/Storage

- Give with food, milk or antacids if GI upset occurs.

Assessment/Interventions

- Obtain patient history, including drug history and any known allergies.
- Assess baseline renal function, BP, blood glucose levels, prothrombin time and CBC prior to beginning therapy and monitor periodically during therapy.
- Monitor blood glucose closely in patients with diabetes.
- Assess for any visual disturbances. Notify physician if any visual changes occur.
- Assess auditory function during prolonged therapy in patients with impaired hearing.
- Report any CNS or respiratory disturbances to physician.
- Monitor PT if patient is concurrently taking anticoagulant.
- Evaluate for signs and symptoms of ulceration and bleeding if patient is on prolonged therapy.

OVERDOSAGE: SIGNS & SYMPTOMS

Drowsiness, dizziness, mental confusion, disorientation, lethargy, paresthesias, numbness, vomiting, gastric irritation, nausea, abdominal pain, headache, tinnitus, sweating, convulsions, blurred vision, elevations in serum creatine and BUN, hypotension, tachycardia

Patient/Family Education

- Instruct patient to take with food, milk or antacids if GI symptoms occur (eg, pain, nausea, anorexia). If symptoms persist, report to physician.
- Advise patient that improvement may occur in 2-3 days but 2-3 wk may be required.
- Inform patients taking anticoagulant concurrently to watch for signs and symptoms of bleeding or unusual bruising and report immediately to physician.
- Instruct patient to call physician if headaches or other CNS disturbances occur. If headaches persist despite dosage reduction, drug may be discontinued.
- Advise patient to avoid aspirin and alcoholic beverages while taking medication.
- Instruct patient that drug may cause drowsiness and to use caution while driving or performing other tasks re-

quiring mental alertness, coordination and dexterity.

- Instruct patient to report to physician any fever, rash, joint pain or any changes in urinary elimination including those associated with pain, discoloration or decreased amount.
- Advise patient to minimize exposure to sun and to use sunscreen or wear protective clothing outdoors until tolerance is determined.

See Patient Guide, p. 243.

Fentanyl Citrate

(FEN-tuh-nill SIH-trate)

Sublimaze

Class: Narcotic analgesic

Action A potent, short-acting, rapid-onset opiate agonist that relieves pain by stimulating opiate receptors in CNS; also causes respiratory depression, peripheral vasodilation, inhibition of intestinal peristalsis, sphincter of Oddi spasm, stimulation of chemoreceptors that cause vomiting, and increased bladder tone.

Indications Short-term analgesia before, during and after anesthesia; supplement to general or regional anesthesia; for administration with neuroleptic during anesthesia; anesthesia with oxygen for high-risk patients.

Contraindications Known intolerance to fentanyl.

Route/Dosage

Premedication

ADULTS: **IM** 0.05-0.1 mg 30-60 min before surgery. Elderly patients may need reduced dose.

Postoperative (Recovery Room)

IM/IV 0.05-0.1 mg for pain control, tachypnea or emergent delirium. May repeat in 1-2 hr.

Adjunct to Regional Anesthesia

IM/IV 0.05-0.1 mg; dose administered over 1-2 min prn.

Adjunct to General Anesthesia

See dosage information on the next page.

General Anesthesia

IV 0.05-0.1 mg/kg with oxygen and muscle relaxant. Maximum of **IV** 0.15 mg/kg. CHILDREN 2-12 YR: For induction and maintenance, reduce dose as low as **IV** 2-3 mcg/kg.

Interactions

Amiodarone: Profound bradycardia, sinus arrest and hypotension may occur. *Barbiturate anesthetics, other CNS depressants:* May have additive effects. Dose of fentanyl required will be less than usual.

Lab Test Interferences

Increased amylase and lipase may occur up to 24 hr after dose.

Adverse Reactions

CV: Hypotension; hypertension; bradycardia; tachycardia; chest wall rigidity. *RESP:* Laryngospasm; depression of cough reflex; respiratory depression; rebound respiratory depression postoperatively. *CNS:* Lightheadedness; dizziness; sedation; disorientation; incoordination; seizures. *GI:* Nausea; vomiting; constipation; abdominal pain. *GU:* Urinary retention or hesitancy. *DERM:* Sweating; pruritus; urticaria. *OTHER:* Skeletal muscle rigidity; tolerance; psychological and physical dependence with chronic use.

Precautions

Pregnancy: Category C. *Lactation:* Excreted in breast milk. *Children:* Not recommended for children under 2 yr. *Special risk patients:* Use with caution in elderly patients and patients with myxedema, acute alcoholism, acute abdominal conditions, ulcerative colitis, decreased respiratory reserve, head injury or increased intracranial pressure, hypoxia, bradycardia, supraventricular tachycardia, depleted blood volume or circulatory shock. *Hypoventilation:*

Naloxone and intubation equipment must be available. *Renal or hepatic impairment:* Duration of action may be prolonged; may need to reduce dose.

Adjunct to General Anesthesia

Depth of anesthesia	Total dose	Maintenance*
Low	0.002 mg/kg	Usually not needed
Moderate	0.002-0.02 mg/kg	0.025-0.1 mg IV/IM
High	0.02-0.05 mg/kg	0.025 mg to 50% of induction dose

*Given when vital signs indicate surgical stress/lightening of anesthesia.

NURSING CONSIDERATIONS

Administration/Storage

- Use medication immediately after dilution.
- Check calculated dose volume carefully.
- Administer IV dose slowly over 1-2 minutes.
- Store at room temperature and protect from light.

Assessment/Interventions

- Obtain patient history, including drug history and any known allergies.
- Assess pain type and intensity prior to administration; assess effectiveness of pain relief shortly after administration.
- Assess respiratory rate, heart rate and BP frequently. Report significant changes to physician.
- Assess for confusion; implement safety precautions as needed.
- Monitor GI, urinary and bowel function (urinary retention commonly occurs).
- Take precautions to prevent falls secondary to lightheadedness, dizziness, confusion and/or hypotension.
- Ensure that naloxone and intubation/airway management equipment are available in event of overdose.

OVERDOSAGE: SIGNS & SYMPTOMS

Miosis, respiratory depression, CNS depression, circulatory collapse, seizures, cardiopulmonary arrest, death

Patient/Family Education

- Instruct patient about adverse effects, and identify signs and symptoms that should be reported.
- Explain that lightheadedness and dizziness are frequently experienced and that transfer assistance should be used as needed.
- Instruct patient to avoid use of other CNS depressants or alcohol and to avoid driving after administration.
- Explain potential for tolerance with continued use.

See Patient Guide, p. 244.

Fentanyl Transdermal System

(FEN-tuh-nill)

Duragesic-25, Duragesic-50, Duragesic-75, Duragesic-100

Class: Narcotic analgesic

Action A potent, short-acting, rapid-onset opiate agonist that relieves pain by stimulating opiate receptors in CNS; also causes respiratory depression, peripheral vasodilation, inhibition of intestinal peristalsis, sphincter of Oddi spasm, stimulation of chemoreceptors that cause vomiting, and increased bladder tone.

Indications Management of chronic pain refractory to less potent agents.

Contraindications Hypersensitivity to fentanyl or adhesives.

Route/Dosage

PATIENTS WHO HAVE NOT TAKEN ANOTHER OPIATE CHRONICALLY (ADULTS): Give lowest dose (25 mcg/hr) initially. ELDERLY PATIENTS: May need reduced dose. PATIENTS WHO HAVE RECEIVED ANOTHER OPIATE CHRONICALLY (ADULTS): Calculate dose based on previous day's opiate requirement. Maximum pain relief does not occur until 24 hr after application; a short-acting opiate may be needed for breakthrough pain. Initial dose can be increased after 3 days. Further dosage increases should occur at not less than 6-day intervals. Patches should be replaced every 3 days; some patients require new patch every 2 days.

Interactions

Amiodarone: Profound bradycardia, sinus arrest and hypotension may occur. *Barbiturate anesthetics, other CNS depressants:* May have additive effects. Dosage of fentanyl required will be less than usual.

Lab Test Interferences

None well documented.

Adverse Reactions

CV: Hypotension; orthostatic hypotension; hypertension; bradycardia; tachycardia; chest pain. *RESP:* Laryngospasm; depression of cough reflex; dyspnea; hypoventilation. *CNS:* Lightheadedness; dizziness; sedation; disorientation; incoordination; headache; hallucinations; euphoria; depression; seizures. *GI:* Nausea; vomiting; constipation; abdominal pain; diarrhea; dyspepsia; dry mouth. *GU:* Urinary retention or hesitancy. *DERM:* Sweating; pruritus; urticaria; exfoliative dermatitis. *OTHER:* Tolerance; psychological and physical dependence with chronic use.

Precautions

Pregnancy: Category C. *Lactation:* Excreted in breast milk. *Children:* Do not use in children < 12 years, or < 18 years who weigh < 50 kg. *Special risk patients:* Use with caution in elderly patients or patients with myxedema, acute alcoholism, acute abdominal conditions, ulcerative colitis, decreased respiratory reserve, head injury or increased intracranial pressure, hypoxia, supraventricular tachycardia, depleted blood volume or circulatory shock. *Exposure to external heat:* Direct contact with heating pads, electric blankets, saunas or hot tubs could increase fentanyl absorption. *Fever:* May increase absorption of fentanyl; monitor for adverse reactions. *Renal or hepatic impairment:* Use with caution since fentanyl is renally and hepatically excreted.

NURSING CONSIDERATIONS

Administration/Storage

- Select dry, flat surface on chest or back for application. If excessive body hair is present, clip hair in affected area. Do not shave.
- Avoid applying to any irritated body area.

- After removing wrap, apply to skin using firm pressure for about 20 seconds. Be certain that edges are sealed. If gel accidentally comes in contact with skin, wash area with water.
- Remove after 72 hr; fold adhesive side in on itself and discard in toilet.
- Rotate application sites.
- If patch becomes loose, reinforce edges with tape. Do not completely cover patch with another occlusive dressing.

Assessment/Interventions

- Obtain patient history, including drug history and any known allergies.
- Assess respiratory rate, heart rate, and BP prior to administration and frequently during therapy, especially after dosage adjustment. Report significant alterations to physician.
- Assess pain type and intensity prior to administration and 24 hr after administration. Assess need for intermittent short-term analgesia until adequate pain control is achieved.
- Reassess 72 hr after administration to determine effectiveness of inital dose, and after every dosage adjustment.
- Assess for signs of developing tolerance.
- Monitor GI, urinary and bowel function.
- Take precautions to prevent falls, especially with initial dosages.
- If adverse reactions occur, remove patch and notify physician. Continue to monitor patient frequently for at least 12 hours.
- Assure that naloxone and intubation/airway management equipment are available.

OVERDOSAGE: SIGNS & SYMPTOMS

Miosis, respiratory depression, CNS depression, hypoventilation, circulatory collapse, seizures, cardiopulmonary arrest, death

Patient/Family Education

- Inform patient that maximal effect is not achieved for 3 days after initial application, and that supplemental analgesia may be needed.
- Instruct patient to self-monitor effectiveness of medication regularly and to report any significant change. Inform patient that tolerance may develop.
- Advise patient that patches are generally changed every 3 days, but that in some cases a change every 2 days is more effective.
- Explain adverse reactions, and identify signs and symptoms that should be reported. Inform patient that adverse reactions can persist for several hours after removal of patch.
- Explain measures to reduce constipation if present.
- Instruct patient to avoid driving or other potentially hazardous activities unless tolerant to the effects of the drug.
- Caution patient to avoid intake of alcoholic beverages or other CNS depressants.
- Explain potential for tolerance and abuse.
- Inform patient that withdrawal symptoms may be experienced when drug is discontinued and not to discontinue unless advised by physician.

See Patient Guide, p. 245.

Ferrous Salts

(FER-uhs salts)

Femiron, Feosol, Feostat, Feratab, Fergon, Fer-In-Sol, Fer-Iron, Fero-Gradumet Filmtab, Ferospace, Ferra-TD, Ferralet, Ferralet Slow Release, Ferralyn Lanacaps, Ferrous Sulfate, Fumasorb, Fumerin, Hemocyte, Ircon, Mol-Iron, Nephro-Fer, Simron, Slow-FE, Span-FF

Class: Iron product

Action Iron is major factor in oxygen transport and essential mineral component of hemoglobin, myoglobin and several enzymes.

Indications Prevention and treatment of iron-deficiency anemia. **Unlabeled use:** Use with epoetin to ensure hematologic response to epoetin.

Contraindications Hypersensitivity to any ingredient, hemosiderosis, hemolytic anemia.

Route/Dosage

Stated iron dose is for elemental iron. Dosage must be calculated based on salt form. Ferrous sulfate is 20% elemental iron. Ferrous sulfate, exsiccated, is approximately 30% elemental iron. Ferrous gluconate is approximately 12% elemental iron. Ferrous fumarate is 33% elemental iron. ADULT MALES: **PO** 10 mg. ADULT FEMALES 11-50 YR: **PO** 15 mg. ADULT FEMALES ≥ 51 YR: **PO** 10 mg; pregnancy: 30 mg; lactation: 15 mg.

Iron Replacement in Deficiency States

ADULTS: **PO** 100-200 mg tid. CHILDREN (2-12 YR): 3 mg/kg/day in 3-4 divided doses. CHILDREN (6 MO-2 YR): Up to 6 mg/kg/day in 3-4 divided doses. INFANTS: 10-25 mg qd in 3-4 divided doses.

Interactions

Antacids: May decrease iron absorption. *Chloramphenicol:* May increase serum iron concentrations. *Food:* May decrease iron absorption; eggs and milk decrease iron absorption. *Levodopa:* Effects of levodopa may be decreased. *Penicillamine:* Decreased absorption of penicillamine. *Quinolones:* Iron may decrease quinolone absorption. *Tetracyclines:* Absorption of both drugs may be decreased.

Lab Test Interferences

None well documented.

Adverse Reactions

GI: Irritation; anorexia; nausea; vomiting; diarrhea; constipation; dark stool. *OTHER:* Teeth staining with liquid formulation.

Precautions

GI effects: Discomfort, such as nausea, may be minimized by taking with food. *Sulfite sensitivity:* Some products contain sulfites, which cause allergic-type reactions in susceptible individuals. *Tartrazine sensitivity:* Some products contain tartrazine, which may cause allergic-type reactions in susceptible individuals.

NURSING CONSIDERATIONS

Administration/Storage

- Administer drug orally only.
- Do not crush sustained release tablets.
- Administer between meals for maximum absorption. Give with food or meals if GI upset occurs.
- When giving liquid preparation, dilute to decrease staining of teeth. Patient may drink through straw to avoid staining.

Assessment/Interventions

- Obtain patient history, including drug history and any known allergies.
- Document baseline Hbg, Hct, bilirubin and reticulocyte count and monitor at regular intervals.
- Monitor color of stool.
- If anorexia, nausea, vomiting, constipation or diarrhea develops, report to physician.
- Test stool for occult blood if bleeding is suspected.

OVERDOSAGE: SIGNS & SYMPTOMS

Lethargy, nausea, vomiting, abdominal pain, tarry stool, weak/rapid pulse, hypotension, dehydration, acidosis, coma, diffuse vascular congestion, pulmonary edema, shock, acidosis, convulsions, anuria, hypothermia, pyloric or antral stenosis, hepatic cirrhosis, CNS damage

Patient/Family Education

- Tell patient to take drug on an

empty stomach unless GI upset develops. Instruct patient to then take drug after meals or with food, but not to take with eggs or milk.
- Advise patient taking sustained release preparation not to chew, open or crush drug.
- Advise patient to dilute liquid iron preparations in water or juice, to drink through a straw and to rinse mouth after taking.
- Instruct patient not to take drug with antacids.
- Tell patient that drug may cause black stools, constipation or diarrhea and to report anorexia, nausea, vomiting or pronounced diarrhea or constipation.
- Identify foods to include for iron-rich diet.
- Warn patient that iron poisoning may occur if more than prescribed amount of medication is taken.

See Patient Guide, p. 246.

Filgrastim (G-CSF)

(fill-GRAH-stim)

Neupogen

Class: Colony-stimulating factor

Action Stimulates neutrophil production within bone marrow.

Indications Decrease incidence of infection, manifested by febrile neutropenia, in patients with nonmyeloid malignancies receiving myelosuppressive anticancer drugs; cancer patients receiving myelosuppressive chemotherapy; cancer patients receiving bone-marrow transplant; patients with severe chronic neutropenia (SCN); peripheral blood progenitor cell (PBPC) collection and therapy in cancer patients.

Contraindications Hypersensitivity to *Escherichia coli*–derived proteins.

Route/Dosage

Myelosuppressive chemotherapy

IV/SC: 5 mcg/kg/day as single daily injection; may increase in increments of 5 mcg/kg for each chemotherapy cycle.

Bone marrow transplant

IV/SC: 10 mcg/kg/day given as an IV infusion of 4 or 24 hours or as a continuous 24 hour SC infusion.

Severe chronic neutropenia

Congenital neutropenia: Starting dose: 6 mcg/kg twice daily SC every day. *Idiopathic or cyclic neutropenia:* Starting dose: 5 mcg/kg as a single injection SC every day. *Dose adjustments*—Chronic daily administration is required to maintain clinical benefit. ANC should not be used as the sole indication of efficacy. Individually adjust the dose based on the patients' clinical course as well as ANC. In the Phase III study, the target ANC was 1,500 to 10,000/mm^3. However, patients may experience clinical benefit with ANCs below this target range. Reduce the dose if the ANC is persistently more than 10,000/mm^3.

Interactions None well documented. INCOMPATIBILITIES: Precipitate may form if diluted with saline.

Lab Test Interferences

None well documented.

Adverse Reactions

HEMA: Leukocytosis. *OTHER:* Bone pain; reversible elevations in uric acid, LDH and alkaline phosphatase.

Precautions

Pregnancy: Category C. *Lactation:* Undetermined. *Cardiac events:* Monitoring patients with preexisting cardiac conditions is recommended. *Chronic administration:* Safety and efficacy not established. *Hematologic effects:* Regular monitoring of hematocrit and platelet count recommended due to possible increased risk of thrombocytopenia or anemia.

NURSING CONSIDERATIONS

Administration/Storage

- Do not give filgrastim 24 hr before or 24 hr after cytotoxic chemotherapy.
- Do not shake medication.
- Warm to room temperature before injection. Use within 24 hr.
- Use only one dose per vial, and do not reenter vial.
- Do not dilute with saline.
- Give IV injection, diluted in D5W, over 15-30 min.
- Store in refrigerator, but do not freeze. Discard any unused vial left at room temperature > 6 hr.

Assessment/Interventions

- Obtain complete patient history, including drug history and any known allergies.
- Monitor hematocrit, CBC and platelet count 2-3 times weekly.
- Document any hypotensive effects.
- Document CBC and platelet counts prior to chemotherapy and twice per week during therapy.
- Inform physician and discontinue dose if absolute neutrophil count > 10,000/mm^3.

OVERDOSAGE: SIGNS & SYMPTOMS

Leukocytosis

Patient/Family Education

- Instruct in proper techniques for administration and storage.
- Explain that most common adverse effect is bone pain.
- Explain importance of follow-up laboratory work as directed.
- Counsel patient on signs of thrombocytopenia (eg, bruising, petechiae, ecchymosis, epistaxis, bleeding from mucus membranes) and ways to avoid infection.

See Patient Guide, p. 247.

Finasteride

(fih-NASS-teer-IDE)

Proscar

Class: Androgen hormone inhibitor

Action Inhibits conversion of testosterone into 5-alpha-dihydrotestosterone, a potent androgen.

Indications Treatment of symptomatic benign prostatic hyperplasia (BPH). **Unlabeled uses:** Adjuvant monotherapy following radical prostatectomy; prevention of progression of first-stage prostate cancer; treatment of male-pattern baldness, acne and hirsutism.

Contraindications Use during pregnancy or lactation and use in children.

Route/Dosage
ADULTS: **PO** 5 mg q day.

Interactions None well documented.

Lab Test Interferences
Decreased prostate-specific antigen levels.

Adverse Reactions
GU: Impotence; decreased libido; decreased volume of ejaculate.

Precautions
Pregnancy: Category X. *Lactation:* Do not use in lactating women. *Children:* Not recommended for children. *Carcinogenesis, mutagenesis:* Based on animal studies, may have carcinogenic or mutagenic potential. *Duration of therapy:* Minimum of 6 mo therapy may be necessary to see effect. *Hepatic function impairment:* Use with caution. *Obstructive uropathy:* Carefully monitor patients with large residual urine volume or severely diminished urinary flow.

NURSING CONSIDERATIONS

Administration/Storage

- Do not allow women of childbearing age to handle crushed tablets.
- Store medication in tightly closed container and protect from light.

Assessment/Interventions

- Obtain patient history, including drug history and any known allergies.
- Document results of liver function tests prior to starting therapy.
- Carefully monitor I&O in patients with large residual urine volume or diminished urinary flow.
- Review prostate-specific antigen levels and document any sustained increase.

Patient/Family Education

- Inform patient that impotence, decreased libido or decreased volume of ejaculate may occur.
- Advise patient that contact with crushed tablet could be hazardous to pregnant females and that exposure also may occur via semen.
- Explain that partners of patients taking finasteride who are of childbearing age should use reliable method of contraception. Emphasize that drug may cause abnormalities of external genitalia of male fetus.
- Point out importance of regular follow-up by physician.

See Patient Guide, p. 248.

Flavoxate

(flay-voke-sate)

Urispas

Class: Urinary tract antispasmodic/ alkalinizer

Action Counteracts smooth muscle spasms of urinary tract.

Indications Symptomatic relief of dysuria, urgency, nocturia, suprapubic pain, frequency and incontinence associated with cystitis, prostatitis, urethritis, urethrocystitis/ urethrotrigonitis.

Contraindications Pyloric or duodenal obstruction; obstructive intestinal lesions or ileus; achalasia; GI hemorrhage; obstructive uropathies of lower urinary tract.

Route/Dosage

ADULTS & CHILDREN (> 12 YR): PO 100-200 mg 3-4 times daily.

Interactions None well documented.

Lab Test Interferences None well documented.

Adverse Reactions

CV: Tachycardia; palpitations. *CNS:* Nervousness; headache; drowsiness; mental confusion. *EENT:* Vertigo; blurred vision, ocular tension; disturbances in accommodation. *GI:* Nausea; vomiting; dry mouth. *GU:* Dysuria. *HEMA:* Eosinophilia; leukopenia. *DERM:* Urticaria and other dermatoses. *OTHER:* High fever.

Precautions

Pregnancy: Category B. *Lactation:* Undetermined. *Children:* Safety and efficacy in children < 12 yr not established. *Glaucoma:* Give cautiously to patients with suspected glaucoma.

NURSING CONSIDERATIONS

Administration/Storage

- Administer drug orally only.

Assessment/Interventions

- Obtain patient history, including drug history and any known allergies.
- Assess baseline mental status and monitor during therapy.

- Carefully monitor patients with glaucoma.
- Report to physician any problems such as visual disturbances, nausea or vomiting, dysuria, high fever, tachycardia, palpitations or mental status changes.

Patient/Family Education

- Caution patient against performing potentially hazardous activities until effects of product are well-tolerated.
- Instruct patient to take sips of water frequently, suck on ice chips or sugarless hard candy or chew sugarless gum if dry mouth occurs.
- Advise patient to report these symptoms to physician: persistent or worsening dry mouth, hives, rash, nausea or vomiting, unusual nervousness, vertigo, headache, drowsiness, confusion, high fever, dysuria, tachycardia, palpitations or vision problems.

See Patient Guide, p. 249.

Flecainide Acetate

(fleh-CANE-ide ASS-uh-TATE)

Tambocor

Class: Antiarrhythmic

Action Produces a dose-related decrease in intracardiac conduction in all parts of the heart; also has local anesthetic activity.

Indications Prevention of paroxysmal atrial fibrillation/flutter (PAF) associated with disabling symptoms; paroxysmal supraventricular tachycardias (PSVTs); prevention of documented life-threatening ventricular arrhythmias.

Contraindications Preexisting second- or third-degree atrioventricular (AV) block; right bundle branch block when associated with a left hemiblock (unless a pacemaker is present); recent MI; presence of cardiogenic shock.

Route/Dosage

PSVT, PAF

ADULTS: Initial dose: **PO** 50 mg q 12 hr, increasing by 50 mg bid q 4 days until efficacy is achieved. Maximum for PSVT: 300 mg/day.

Sustained Ventricular Tachycardia

ADULTS: Initial dose: **PO** 100 mg q 12 hr, increasing to 150 mg bid if needed. Maximum: 400 mg/day.

Interactions

Amiodarone: Increased flecainide plasma levels. *Cimetidine:* Increased bioavailability and clearance of flecainide. *Digoxin:* Increased digoxin plasma levels. *Propranolol:* Levels of either drug may be increased; additive negative inotropic effects. *Smoking:* Increased dosage may be required. *Urinary acidifiers:* Effects of flecainide may be decreased. *Urinary alkalinizers:* Effects of flecainide may be increased.

Lab Test Interferences

None well documented.

Adverse Reactions

CV: Arrhythmias; palpitations; chest pain; tachycardia; hypotension. *CNS:* Dizziness; insomnia; syncope; anxiety; ataxia; depression; hypoesthesia; malaise; paresthesia; vertigo; lightheadedness; faintness; headache; fatigue; asthenia; tremor; increased sweating; somnolence. *EENT:* Visual disturbances; tinnitus; diplopia. *GI:* Nausea; constipation; abdominal pain; vomiting; diarrhea; anorexia. *DERM:* Rash; flushing. *OTHER:* Fever; dyspnea.

Precautions

Pregnancy: Category C. *Lactation:* Excreted in breast milk. *Children:* Safety and efficacy in children < 18 yr not established. *Mortality:* In clinical trials, an excessive mortality rate was noted. *Cardiovascular disorders:* Use with caution in patients with arrhythmias, CHF, cardiomyopathy, low ejection fraction, and conduction abnormalities. Flecainide slows cardiac conduction in most patients to produce a dose-related increase in PR, QRS and QT intervals. Use with extreme caution in patients with sick sinus syndrome because drug may cause sinus bradycardia, sinus pause or sinus arrest. Flecainide increases endocardial pacing thresholds and may suppress ventricular escape rhythms in patients with pacemakers. *Hepatic impairment:* Do not use in patients with hepatic impairment unless benefits outweigh risks. *Potassium imbalances:* Effect of flecainide may be altered in patients with hypokalemia or hyperkalemia; condition should be corrected before administering flecainide.

NURSING CONSIDERATIONS

Administration/Storage

- May be given with or without food.
- Store at room temperature in tightly closed, light-resistant container.

Assessment/Interventions

- Obtain patient history, including drug history and any known allergies. Note recent MI.
- If patient has sustained ventricular tachycardia, initiate therapy in hospital and monitor rhythm.
- Ensure that baseline liver and kidney function tests have been obtained before beginning therapy.
- Ensure that baseline potassium level has been obtained before beginning therapy and monitor at regular intervals.
- Review baseline ECG to assess for second- or third-degree heart block or sick sinus syndrome. Monitor rhythm closely while initiating therapy.
- Measure PR, QRS and QT intervals before beginning therapy and monitor closely while initiating therapy.
- Monitor urinary pH while initiating therapy because pH alters drug elimination.
- In patient with pacemakers, determine pacing threshold before beginning therapy, at 1 wk and at regular intervals thereafter while receiving drug.
- Assess BP before initiating therapy and at regular intervals during treatment.
- Monitor trough plasma levels of drug at regular intervals.
- Monitor renal patients closely for toxic effects and assess plasma levels frequently.
- If patient is also receiving digoxin, monitor digoxin levels closely.
- Assess patient for signs and symptoms of CHF.
- If patient develops potassium imbalances, increased PR, QRS and QT intervals, chest pain, hypotension, or signs of CHF, notify physician immediately.

OVERDOSAGE: SIGNS & SYMPTOMS

Cardiac arrhythmias

Patient/Family Education

- Emphasize importance of taking drug as prescribed and not missing or adjusting dosage.
- Teach patient how to take pulse and instruct to do so daily.
- Instruct patient to report these symptoms to physician: diarrhea, abdominal pain, palpitations, chest pain, tachycardia, hypotension, dizziness, asthenia, tremor, tinnitus, somnolence, visual disturbances, fever, dyspnea or rash.
- Instruct patient in measuring and recording weight on daily basis.
- Offer family instruction in basic life support.
- Advise patient that drug may cause dizziness or drowsiness and to use caution while driving or performing other tasks requiring mental alertness.

See Patient Guide, p. 250.

Floxuridine

(flox-YUR-ih-deen)
FUDR
Class: Antineoplastic/antimetabolite

Action Interferes with DNA synthesis and to a lesser extent the formation of RNA. When given by continuous infusion its direct anabolism to FUDR-monophosphate is enhanced, thus increasing DNA inhibition.

Indications Palliative management of GI adenocarcinoma metastasized to liver in patients incurable by surgery or other means.

Contraindications Poor nutritional status; depressed bone marrow function; potentially serious infections.

Route/Dosage
ADULTS: **Intra-arterial** 0.1-0.6 mg/kg/day by continuous infusion. (Higher dose usually used for hepatic artery infusion.)

Interactions None well documented.

Lab Test Interferences
None well documented.

Adverse Reactions
CV: MI. *GI:* Nausea; vomiting; diarrhea; enteritis; stomatitis; duodenal ulcer; duodenitis; gastritis; bleeding; gastroenteritis; glossitis; pharyngitis; anorexia; cramps; abdominal pain. *HEMA:* Leukopenia; thrombocytopenia; anemia. *HEPA:* Possible intrahepatic and extrahepatic biliary sclerosis; acalculous cholecystitis. *DERM:* Alopecia; dermatitis; nonspecific skin toxicity; rash. *OTHER:* Localized erythema; fever; lethargy; malaise; weakness; local complications (eg, arterial aneurysm; arterial ischemia; arterial thrombosis; embolism; fibromyositis; thrombophlebitis; hepatic necrosis; abcess; infection or bleeding at catheter site; catheter blocked, displaced or leaking); hemorrhage from any site; interferences with BSP, prothrombin, total protein and sedimentation rate assays.

Precautions
Pregnancy: Category D. *Lactation:* Undetermined. *Children:* Safety and efficacy not established. *Special risk patients:* Use extreme caution in patients with impaired hepatic or renal function or history of high-dose pelvic irradiation or previous use of alkylating agents. Drug is not intended as adjuvant to surgery. *Combination Therapy:* Any therapy adding to stress of patient, interfering with nutrition or depressing bone marrow will increase toxicity. Caution patient that this medication should not be taken during pregnancy or when pregnancy is possible. Advise both male and female patients to use reliable form of birth control while taking this drug. *Toxicity:* Drug is highly toxic with narrow margin of safety. Careful supervision is required, because therapeutic response is unlikely to occur without some toxicity. Severe hematologic toxicity, GI hemorrhage and death may occur.

NURSING CONSIDERATIONS

Administration/Storage

- Administer by continuous intra-arterial infusion only, using an infusion pump. Administration should be done only by nurses educated in intra-arterial therapy.
- Reconstitute drug with 5 ml Sterile Water for Injection and dilute in D5W or Sodium Chloride for Injection according to volume ordered.
- Reconstituted vials are stable when refrigerated for up to 2 wk.
- Note that heparin and floxuridine are compatible and that heparin is often added to infusion to prevent thrombi.

Assessment/Interventions

- Obtain patient history, including drug history and any known allergies.
- Because of possible severe toxic reac-

tions, patient should be hospitalized for first course of therapy.

- Ensure that baseline CBC with differential has been obtained and monitor daily during treatment.
- Ensure that baseline BUN, creatinine and liver function tests have been performed before beginning therapy and monitor during treatment.
- Keep patient well hydrated and monitor fluid status during therapy.
- Assess infusion site for signs of infection or bleeding, especially in immunocompromised patients.
- If heparin is included in infusion, monitor partial thromboplastin time.
- If allergic reaction occurs, discontinue infusion and notify physician.
- If myocardial ischemia, stomatitis, esophopharyngitis, leukopenia (WBC count < 3500) or a rapidly falling WBC count, intractable vomiting, GI ulceration or bleeding, thrombocytopenia (platelets < 100,000), or hemorrhage occur, notify physician immediately.

OVERDOSAGE: SIGNS & SYMPTOMS

Nausea, vomiting, diarrhea, GI ulceration and bleeding, bone marrow depression

Patient/Family Education

- Explain that temporary hair loss may occur with therapy. Discuss coping strategies and use of wigs or scarves.
- Instruct patient to report any pain, redness, bleeding or creamy drainage at infusion site.
- Emphasize importance of maintaining adequate nutrition and fluid intake during treatment.
- Explain that contraceptive measures are recommended for men and women during therapy.
- Instruct patient to report these symptoms to physician: chills, nausea, vomiting, unusual bleeding or bruising, jaundice of skin or eyes, abdominal pain, flank or joint pain, or swelling of feet or legs.
- Advise patient that fever, weakness and diarrhea are common side effects but to notify physician if they become persistent problems.

See Patient Guide, p. 251.

Fluconazole

(flew-KOE-nuh-zole)

Diflucan

Class: Anti-infective/antifungal

Action Interferes with the formation of fungal cell membrane, causing leakage of cellular contents and cell death.

Indications Oropharyngeal and esophageal candidiasis; serious systemic candidal infections; cryptococcal meningitis.

Contraindications Standard considerations.

Route/Dosage

Oropharyngeal or Esophageal Candidiasis

ADULTS: **PO/IV** 200 mg first day, followed by 100 mg qd thereafter for minimum of 2 weeks for oropharyngeal candidiasis or 3 weeks for esophageal candidiasis. CHILDREN: **PO/IV** 6 mg/kg on first day, followed by 3 mg/kg qd thereafter for minimum of 2 weeks for oropharyngeal candidiasis or 3 weeks (at least 2 weeks after symptom resolution) for esophageal candidiasis.

Systemic Candidiasis or Cryptococcal Meningitis

ADULTS: **PO/IV** 400 mg first day, followed by 200 mg qd thereafter (400 mg may be used for meningitis) for minimum of 4 wk for candidiasis or for 10-12 wk after CSF culture is negative for initial meningitis; 200 mg qd for suppression of relapse of cryptococcal meningitis. CHILDREN: **PO/IV** *Candidemia and disseminated Candida infections*—6 to 12 mg/kg/day. *Cryptococcal meningitis*—12 mg/kg on first day, followed by 6 mg/kg/day (or 12 mg/kg/day based on medical judgment of patient's response). Recommended duration is 10 to 12 weeks after CSF becomes culture negative. *Suppression of relapse in AIDS patients*—6 mg/kg/day. NEONATES: Experience is limited to pharmacokinetic studies in premature newborns. Prolonged half-life has been noted. These children, in the first 2 weeks of life, should receive the same mg/kg dosage as other children, but administered every 72 hours. After the first two weeks, dose once daily.

Interactions

Anticoagulants (eg, warfarin): Anticoagulant effect may be increased. *Antihistamines, nonsedating (eg, terfenadine)*: Increased levels of antihistamine, with possible severe cardiotoxicity. *Cyclosporine*: Increased cyclosporine concentrations. *Hydantoins (eg, phenytoin)*: Increased hydantoin levels.

Lab Test Interferences

Elevated transaminase levels. *Coumadin*: Increased prothrombin time (PT) may occur in patient receiving warfarin.

Adverse Reactions

CNS: Headache; seizures. *GI*: Nausea; vomiting; abdominal pain; diarrhea. *HEMA*: Leukopenia; thrombocytopenia. *HEPA*: Hepatic reactions, including abnormal liver function test results, hepatitis, cholestasis, hepatic failure. *DERM*: Rash, exfoliative skin disorder.

Precautions

Pregnancy: Category C. *Lactation*: Excreted in breast milk. *Children*: Efficacy not established; some patients 3-13 yr have been treated safely with 3-6 mg/kg/day. *Anaphylaxis*: Has occurred rarely. *Dermatologic changes*: Exfoliative skin disorders have been reported. *Hepatic injury*: Patients with abnormal liver function test results should be monitored for development of more severe hepatic injury. *Immunocompromised patients*: To prevent relapse, patients with AIDS and cryptococcal meningitis usually require maintenance therapy. *Renal impairment*: Dosage reduction based on creatinine clearance may be necessary.

NURSING CONSIDERATIONS

Administration/Storage

- Do not administer if solution is cloudy or if precipitate is present.
- Do not add supplemental medications to IV infusion.
- Administer IV infusion at maximum rate of 200 mg/hr.

Assessment/Interventions

- Obtain patient history, including drug history and any known allergies. Note renal impairment and sensitivity to fluconazole or other azoles.
- Obtain baseline BUN and creatinine levels.
- Ensure that baseline liver function tests have been obtained and monitor at regular intervals during treatment.
- Assess skin for rashes before beginning therapy and q 8 hr during treatment.
- If patient is receiving anticoagulants, assess for bleeding. Monitor coagulation studies closely.
- For patients also receiving coumadin, monitor PT for possible increased levels.
- If patient develops signs and symptoms of liver disease or new rash during therapy, notify physician.

Patient/Family Education

- Emphasize importance of taking drug for full course of therapy, which may be several weeks.
- Tell patient that if dose is missed, it

should be taken as soon as possible. If close to next dose, do not double up; take next dose as scheduled.

- Instruct patient to report these symptoms to physician: nausea, vomiting, right upper quadrant abdominal pain, diarrhea, headache, rash.

See Patient Guide, p. 252.

Flucytosine

(flew-SITE-oh-seen)

Ancobon, 5-FC, 5-Fluorocytosine, ♣ *Ancotil*

Class: Anti-infective/antifungal

Action Exact mechanism is unknown; interferes with DNA and RNA synthesis. Active against *Candida* and *Cryptococcus*.

Indications Treatment of serious infections caused by susceptible strains of *Candida* or *Cryptococcus*. **Unlabeled use:** Treatment of Chromomycosis.

Contraindications Standard considerations.

Route/Dosage

ADULTS & CHILDREN > 50 KG: **PO** 50-150 mg/kg/day in divided doses q 6 hr.

Interactions

Amphotericin B: Increased therapeutic action and toxicity of flucytosine. *Cytosine:* Inactivates antifungal activity of flucytosine.

Lab Test Interferences

Interferes with creatinine value determinations with dry-slide enzymatic method (Kodak Ektachem analyzer); use Jaffe method.

Adverse Reactions

CV: Cardiac arrest. *RESP:* Respiratory arrest; chest pain; dyspnea. *CNS:* Ataxia; hearing loss; headache; sedation; confusion; fatigue; weakness; dizziness; vertigo, paresthesia; parkinsonism; peripheral neuropathy; pyrexia; hallucinations; psychosis. *GI:* Nausea; emesis; abdominal pain; diarrhea; anorexia; duodenal ulcer; GI hemorrhage. *GU:* Azotemia; creatinine and BUN elevation; crystalluria; renal failure; dry mouth. *HEMA:* Anemia; agranulocytosis; aplastic anemia; eosinophilia; leukopenia; pancytopenia; thrombocytopenia. *HEPA:* Hepatic dysfunction; jaundice; ulcerative colitis; increased bilirubin; elevated hepatic enzymes. *DERM:* Rash; pruritus; urticaria; photosensitivity. *META:* Hypoglycemia; hypokalemia.

Precautions

Pregnancy: Category C. *Lactation:* Undetermined. *Children:* Safety and efficacy not established. *Bone marrow depression:* Use with extreme caution in patients with bone marrow depression or those at risk (eg, hematologic disease, radiation treatment, other bone-marrow suppressant drugs). *Hepatic or renal impairment:* Use with extreme caution in patients with renal impairment. Adjust dose according to blood levels and monitor hepatic function.

NURSING CONSIDERATIONS

Administration/Storage

- Administer capsules a few at a time over 15 min to minimize GI upset.

Assessment/Interventions

- Obtain patient history, including drug history and any known allergies.
- Ensure that baseline liver function tests, BUN, and creatinine, electrolytes and glucose have been obtained before beginning therapy and monitor at regular intervals.
- Obtain baseline CBC with differential and repeat daily. Assess for bone marrow depression.

- Obtain specimens for culture and sensitivity before beginning therapy.
- Monitor BP at regular intervals during therapy. Assess for cardiovascular collapse.
- Monitor blood levels of drug closely in patient with impaired renal function.
- If patient has ataxia, hearing loss, headache, paresthesia, peripheral neuropathy, pyrexia, hallucinations, psychosis, laboratory evidence of liver or renal dysfunction, chest pain, or respiratory distress, notify physician immediately.

OVERDOSAGE: SIGNS & SYMPTOMS
Nausea, vomiting, diarrhea, CNS changes, leukopenia, thrombocytopenia, hepatitis

Patient/Family Education
- Instruct patient to take capsules a few at a time over a 15-min period with food.
- Instruct diabetic patients to monitor glucose closely.
- Instruct patient to report these symptoms to physician: sore throat, cough, unusual bleeding or bruising, petechiae, blood in urine, bleeding gums, abdominal pain, nausea, vomiting, change in color or consistency of stools, fever, yellow skin/eyes, ataxia, hearing loss, paresthesia, shaking, tingling, altered sensation, parkinsonism, peripheral neuropathy, hallucinations or psychosis, anorexia, increased fatigue, rash or itching.
- Warn patient to seek emergency care if respiratory distress or chest pain occur.
- Advise patient that drug may cause dizziness or vertigo and to use caution while driving or performing other tasks requiring mental alertness.
- Caution patient to avoid unnecessary exposure to sunlight and to use sunscreen and wear protective clothing to avoid photosensitivity reaction.

See Patient Guide, p. 253.

Fludarabine Phosphate

(flew-DAR-uh-BEAN FOSS-fate)
Fludara
Class: Antineoplastic/antimetabolite

Action Drug metabolite appears to inhibit DNA synthesis, which prevents cell replication.

Indications Treatment of B-cell chronic lymphocytic leukemia (CLL) in patients who have not responded to or progressed from at least one alkylating agent–containing regimen. **Unlabeled uses:** Non-Hodgkin's lymphoma (orphan drug status); macroglobulinemic lymphoma; prolymphocytic leukemia or polymphocytoid variant of CLL; mycosis fungoides; hairy-cell leukemia; Hodgkin's disease.

Contraindications Standard considerations.

Route/Dosage
ADULTS: **IV** Usual dose: 25 mg/m^2 over 30 min for 5 consecutive days; may repeat every 28 days. Adjust dosage based on drug toxicity. Administer 3 additional cycles after achieving maximal response.

Interactions None well documented.

Lab Test Interferences
None well documented.

Adverse Reactions
CV: Edema; pericardial effusion. *RESP:* Pneumonia; pulmonary hypersensitivity reaction (dyspnea, cough and interstitial pulmonary infiltrate). *CNS:* Weakness; fatigue; agitation; confusion; visual disturbances; coma; peripheral neuropathy. *GI:* Nausea; vomiting; anorexia; diarrhea; stomatitis; GI bleeding. *HEMA:* Myelosuppression (may be severe and cumulative, causing neutropenia, thrombocytopenia and anemia);

bone marrow fibrosis. *DERM:* Rash. *META:* Tumor lysis syndrome (possible hyperurecemia, hyperphosphatemia, hypocalcemia, metabolic acidosis, hyperkalemia, hematuria, urate crystaluria and renal failure). *OTHER:* Fever; chills; infection; malaise.

Precautions

Pregnancy: Category D. *Lactation:* Undetermined. *Children:* Safety and efficacy not established. *Bone marrow suppression:* Can severely suppress bone marrow function. *Tumor lysis syndrome:* Has been reported in patients with CLL with large tumor as early as first week of therapy. *Renal insufficiency:* Use with caution. *Toxicity:* At high doses in acute leukemia, severe neurologic effects, including delayed blindness, coma and death have occurred. Symptoms appeared 21 to 60 days after last dose. Although toxicity appears to be dose dependent, cumulative effect of chronic administration on CNS is unknown.

NURSING CONSIDERATIONS

Administration/Storage

- Avoid exposure by inhalation or by direct contact with skin or mucus membranes. Wear gloves, gown and mask while preparing or reconstituting medication. If contact occurs, wash thoroughly with soap and water; rinse eyes thoroughly with plain water.
- Reconstitute vial with 2 ml of Sterile Water for Injection. Each ml of resulting solution will contain 25 mg fludarabine phosphate, 25 mg mannitol and sodium hydroxide. Reconstituted solution may be further diluted in 100 or 125 ml of D5W or normal saline.
- Test patency of vein before beginning infusion. Monitor patient closely while medication is infusing and stop infusion any time vein patency is in question.
- Administer medication with infusion control device.
- Treat all equipment and unused drug as hazardous waste and dispose of according to facility's policy and procedure.
- Keep unopened vial refrigerated. Use within 8 hr of preparation.

Assessment/Interventions

- Obtain patient history, including drug history and any known allergies. Note CNS impairment and renal or hepatic insufficiency.
- Obtain baseline neurologic and respiratory assessment before beginning therapy.
- Ensure that baseline CBC with differential and liver and kidney function tests have been obtained before beginning therapy.
- Monitor hematologic profile prior to and regularly following each course of treatment.
- Monitor patient for evidence of pulmonary hypersensitivity reaction (dyspnea, cough).
- Assess for rash, edema, myalgia, weakness, stomatitis, pain and signs of infection after initiation of therapy.
- Observe for signs and symptoms of tumor lysis syndrome, often heralded by flank pain and hematuria.
- Use strict aseptic technique while providing care and use protective isolation during periods of leukopenia.
- Observe for any signs of abnormal bleeding from any site and inspect skin for ecchymotic and petechial areas during periods of thrombocytopenia.
- Notify physician if the following signs of severe toxicity occur: stomatitis or esophagopharyngitis; leukopenia; thrombocytopenia; intractable vomiting or diarrhea; GI ulceration and bleeding; hemorrhage; CNS changes.
- If patient displays a local or generalized reaction, stop IV infusion imme-

diately. Maintain venous access with sterile normal saline or D5W.

> **OVERDOSAGE: SIGNS & SYMPTOMS**
> Irreversible CNS toxicity characterized by delayed blindness, coma, and death; severe thrombocytopenia and neutropenia due to bone marrow suppression

Patient/Family Education

- Advise patient to maintain adequate food and fluid intake. Discuss the option of food supplements. (Low-residue diet will decrease diarrhea.)
- Caution patient to avoid persons with known infections during course of treatment.
- Instruct patient to check mucous membranes for signs of inflammation and ulceration. Discuss importance of oral hygiene in prevention of stomatitis.
- Advise patient to use electric razor for shaving and soft toothbrush or sponge-tipped "toothette"; avoid harsh temperatures; avoid drugs that interfere with platelet function (eg, aspirin, alcohol, cough medicine); and avoid rectal temperature-taking and enemas.
- If stomatitis occurs, instruct patient to rinse frequently with warm water or normal saline solution (1 teaspoon salt in 1 quart water) and to avoid extremely hot or cold foods, spices, highly acidic fluids and rough foods.
- Instruct patient to notify physician if mouth pain interferes with eating. Systemic or topical analgesics (eg, viscous lidocaine mouthwashes) may be ordered.
- Inform patient to report these symptoms immediately to physician: flank pain, blood in urine or excessive itching.
- Instruct patient to report these symptoms to physician: bleeding, bruising, hemorrhage, excessive fatigue, dyspnea, respiratory congestion or fever.
- Tell patient to consult physician if vomiting and/or diarrhea become persistent and are not relieved by prescribed medications.
- Instruct patient to contact physician if pain is not controlled with prescribed medication.
- Offer patient support in coping with diagnosis of cancer.

No patient monograph available.

Fludrocortisone Acetate

(flew-droe-CORE-tih-sone ASS-uh-TATE)

Florinef Acetate

Class: Mineralocorticoid

Action Exerts salt-retaining (mineralo-corticoid) activity by acting on renal distal tubules to enhance reabsorption of sodium and increasing urinary excretion of potassium, hydrogen and magnesium ions.

Indications Partial replacement therapy for primary and secondary adrenocortical insufficiency in Addison's disease; treatment of salt-losing adrenogenital syndrome. **Unlabeled use:** Treatment of severe orthostatic hypotension.

Contraindications Systemic fungal infections.

Route/Dosage

Addison's Disease

ADULTS & CHILDREN: PO 0.05-0.1 mg/day (range 0.1 mg 3 times/wk-0.2 mg/day). INFANTS: PO 0.1-0.2 mg/day.

Salt-Losing Adrenogenital Syndrome

ADULTS & CHILDREN: PO 0.1-0.2 mg/day.

Severe Orthostatic Hypotension

ADULTS: PO 0.1-0.4 mg/day.

Interactions

Amphotericin, potassium-losing diuretics: May increase potassium loss. Hy-

dantoins (eg, phenytoin), rifampin: Decreased fludrocortisone activity.

Lab Test Interferences

None well documented.

Adverse Reactions

CV: Edema; hypertension; CHF; heart enlargement. *DERM:* Brusiing; increased sweating; hives; rash. *OTHER:* Hypokalemic alkalosis. May also cause adverse reactions associated with glucocorticoids (eg, dexamethasone).

Precautions

Pregnancy: Category C. *Lactation:* Excreted in breast milk. *Children:* Safety and efficacy not established. *Addison's disease:* Patients with Addison's disease may exhibit exaggerated side effects; monitor closely for development of edema, significant weight gain or increases in BP. *Adrenal insufficiency:* May occur. Increased doses may be needed before, during or after stressful situations. *Electrolyte disturbances:* Sodium retention and potassium loss are increased by high sodium intake. Sodium restriction and potassium supplementation may be necessary. *Supplemental measures:* Patients receiving fludrocortisone may need supplemental measures (eg, glucocorticoids, electrolyte control) for optimal control of symptoms.

NURSING CONSIDERATIONS

Administration/Storage

- Store in tightly closed container at room temperature. Protect from light.

Assessment/Interventions

- Obtain patient history, including drug history and any known allergies. Note cardiovascular disorders and recent or present fungal infection or other systemic infections.
- Assess baseline psychological status before beginning therapy.
- Take pulse and BP and monitor daily during therapy.
- Ensure that chest x-ray and serum electrolyte levels have been obtained before beginning therapy and monitor frequently during treatment.
- Monitor weight gain and I&O during therapy.
- If signs of concurrent infection, significant increase in weight or BP, signs of hypokalemic alkalosis, dizziness, or severe headache occur, notify physician.

OVERDOSAGE: SIGNS & SYMPTOMS

Hypertension, edema, hypokalemia, excessive weight gain, increase in heart size

Patient/Family Education

- Instruct patient to take medication exactly as prescribed. If dose is missed, it should be taken as soon as possible. Do not double up if within several hours of next dose. Caution patient not to stop medication abruptly. Instruct patient to notify physician if more than one dose is missed or a dosage cannot be taken due to nausea and/or vomiting.
- Advise patient to reduce dietary sodium, which accelerates potassium loss, and to eat foods rich in potassium.
- Tell patient to notify physician when experiencing a stressful situation (eg, emotional upheavals, dental extractions, trauma, surgery or illness) as increased dosage may be needed.
- Instruct patient to report these symptoms to physician: increased or irregular heart beat, high BP, fluid retention, joint pain, muscle weakness, headache, dizziness, fever or unusual weight gain.
- Instruct patient to report euphoria, depression or other changes in mental status.
- Tell patient to be alert for spontaneous fractures and impaired wound healing.
- Advise patient of the importance of keeping follow-up visits.

See Patient Guide, p. 254.

Flumazenil

(flew-MAZ-ah-nil)

Romazicon

Class: Antidote

Action Antagonizes actions of benzodiazepines on CNS by blocking receptors.

Indications Complete or partial reversal of sedative effects of benzodiazepines where general anesthesia induced or maintained with benzodiazepines, where sedation produced with benzodiazepines for diagnostic or therapeutic procedures, and for the management of benzodiazepine overdose.

Contraindications Hypersensitivity to flumazenil or benzodiazepines; in patients given benzodiazepines for control of a potentially life-threatening condition (eg, status epilepitcus); in patients showing signs of serious cyclic antidepressant overdose.

Route/Dosage

Reversal of conscious sedation or in general anesthesia

ADULTS: **IV** 0.2 mg over 15 sec. If desired level of consciousness is not achieved in 45 sec, additional 0.2 mg doses can be administered at 60 sec intervals (maximum 1.0 mg). In event of resedation, repeat doses (0.2 mg/min—maximum 1.0 mg) at 20 min intervals as needed (maximum 3.0 mg/hr).

Management of suspected benzodiazepine overdose

ADULTS: **IV** 0.2 mg over 30 sec. If desired level of consciousness is not achieved in 30 sec, an additional dose of 0.3 mg over 30 sec can be administered. Further doses of 0.5 mg over 30 sec can be administered at 1 min intervals as needed (maximum 3.0 mg).

Interactions Toxic effects of other drugs taken in toxic doses may emerge with reversal of benzodiazepine effect.

Lab Test Interferences
None well documented.

Adverse Reactions
CV: Cutaneous vasodilation (sweating, flushing, hot flushes); palpitations. *CNS:* Convulsions; headache; dizziness; agitation; emotional lability; fatigue; paresthesia; insomnia; dyspnea; hypoesthesia. *EENT:* Visual field defect; diplopia; blurred vision. *GI:* Nausea; vomiting. *DERM:* Sweating. *RESP:* Hyperventilation. *OTHER:* Injection site pain; injection site reaction; dry mouth.

Precautions
Pregnancy: Category C. *Lactation:* Undetermined. *Children:* Safety and efficacy not determined. *Labor and delivery:* Not recommended; effects on newborn are unknown. *Seizures:* Reversal of benzodiazepine effects may be associated with the onset of seizures in certain high-risk populations including: concurrent major sedative-hypnotic drug withdrawal; recent therapy with repeated doses of parenteral benzodiazepines; myoclonic jerking or seizure activity prior to flumazenil in overdose cases; concurrent cyclic antidepressant poisoning. *Resedation/hypoventilation:* Flumazenil may not fully reverse postoperative airway problems or ventilatory insufficiency induced by benzodiazepines; its effects may wear off before the effects of many benzodiazepines. *Hepatic function impairment:* Elimination of flumazenil is reduced in patients with liver disease. *Intensive care unit:* Use of flumazenil to diagnose benzodiazepine-induced sedation in the ICU is not recommended due to the risk of adverse effects. *Head injury:* Use with caution in patients with head injury due to risk of precipitating convulsions or altering cerebral blood flow in patients receiving benzodiazepines. *Neuromuscular block-*

ing agents: Do not use flumazenil until effects of neuromuscular blocking agents have been fully reversed. *Psychiatric:* Flumazenil may provoke panic attacks in patients with a history of panic disorder. *Drug/alcohol dependence:* Use with caution in patients with alcoholism and other drug dependencies due to the increased frequency of benzodiazepine tolerance and dependence observed in these patient populations. *Overdose situations:* Flumazenil is intended as an adjunct to, not as a substitute for, proper management of overdose patients (eg, airway maintenance, decontamination, etc). *Benzodiazepine tolerance:* Flumazenil may cause benzodiazepine withdrawal symptoms in individuals who have been taking benzodiazepines long enough to have some degree of tolerance or physical dependence. *Ambulatory:* The effects of flumazenil may wear off before a long-acting benzodiazepine is completely cleared from the body.

NURSING CONSIDERATIONS

Administration/Storage

- For IV use only.
- Is compatible with D5W, LR and NS.
- Administer through a freely flowing IV in a large vein.
- In high-risk patients, administer smallest amount effective. Wait 6-10 min between trial dose administration in high-risk patients.
- Do not rush administration. Secure airway and IV access.
- If patient does not respond after 5 min of a cumulative dose of 5 mg, sedation is probably not due to benzodiazepines.
- Do not use if solution is discolored or has particulate matter.
- Stable for 24 hours at room temperature after mixing. Best if used just after mixing.

Assessment/Interventions

- Obtain patient history.
- Determine reason for use prior to administration (benzodiazepine overdose; reverse anesthesia; sedation). Use this information to select the proper dosing strategy.
- Monitor level of consciousness during and after administration.
- Resedation may take place in 15-30 min because half-life of many benzodiazepines is longer than flumazenil.
- Monitor patient during and after administration for seizure activity and respiratory or cardiac arrest.
- Monitor patient for confusion, agitation, emotional lability and perceptual distorting after administration.

Patient/Family Education

- Instruct patient that flumazenil does not reverse amnesia. Repeat patient instructions in post-procedure period.
- Warn patient that although they may feel alert at time of discharge, effects of benzodiazepines may reoccur, affecting their memory and judgement.
- Instruct patient to avoid activities requiring complete alertness, such as operating hazardous machinery or driving for at least 18 to 24 hours after discharge.
- Warn patients to avoid alcohol or over-the-counter drugs for at least 18-24 hours after discharge.

No patient monograph available.

Flunisolide

(flew-NIH-sole-ide)

AeroBid, AeroBid-M, Nasalide, ♣ *Bronalide*

Class: Corticosteroid

Action Has local anti-inflammatory activity on lung or nasal mucosa with minimal systemic effect. May decrease number and activity of cells involved in inflammatory response and enhance effect of other drugs or endogenous substances that aid in bronchodilation.

Indications
Inhalation: Control of bronchial asthma and related bronchospastic states for patients requiring chronic treatment with corticosteroids. *Intranasal:* Symptoms of perennial or seasonal rhinitis. **Unlabeled uses:** Treatment of serous otitis media in children and treatment of polyps.

Contraindications Primary treatment of status asthmaticus or acute asthma when intensive measures are required; systemic fungal infections; persistently positive *Candida albicans* sputum culture; untreated local infection of the nasal mucosa (intranasal use).

Route/Dosage
ADULTS & CHILDREN 6-15 YR: **Inhalation** 2 inhalations (500 mcg) bid. ADULTS: Do not exceed 4 inhalations bid (2 mg/day). CHILDREN: Do not exceed 2 inhalations bid. ADULTS: **Intranasal:** Initial dose: 2 sprays (50 mcg) in each nostril bid. Maximum: 8 sprays in each nostril daily. CHILDREN 6-14 YR: Initial dose: 1 spray (25 mcg) in each nostril tid or 2 sprays in each nostril bid. Maximum: 4 sprays in each nostril daily.

Interactions None well documented.

Lab Test Interferences
None well documented.

Adverse Reactions
RESP: Inhalation: Throat irritation; hoarseness; dysphonia; coughing; wheezing; pharyngeal fungal infections; pulmonary infiltrates. Intranasal use: Nasopharyngeal irritation; burning; stinging; rebound congestion; bronchial asthma; sneezing; rhinorrhea. *CNS: Inhalation, intranasal use:* Headache; lightheadedness. *GI:* Dry mouth. *DERM:* Rash. *Inhalation:* Facial edema. *META: Inhalation:* Suppression of hypothalamic-pituitary-adrenal (HPA) function. *OTHER:* Hypersensitivity reaction (eg, urticaria, angioedema, rash, bronchospasm).

Precautions
Pregnancy: Category C. *Lactation:* Undetermined. *Children:* Safety and efficacy in children < 6 yr not established. *Acute asthma:* Not indicated for rapid relief of bronchospasm. *Fungal infections:* Antifungal therapy and discontinuance of steroid may be necessary. *Hypersensitivity:* Immediate and delayed reactions have occurred. *Systemic effects:* Use cautiously in patients taking alternate-day prednisone; may increase likelihood of HPA suppression. Exceeding recommended dose may cause systemic effects.

NURSING CONSIDERATIONS

Administration/Storage

- Before nasal inhalation, have patient blow nose gently to clear nasal passages. A decongestant may be used 15 min before administration to ensure adequate penetration of spray if nasal passages are congested.
- Use bronchodilator before inhalation if bronchospasm is evident.
- Use spacer for metered-dose inhaler to enhance intrapulmonary deposition.
- Shake inhaler well before administration.
- Cleanse inhaler daily with warm water.
- Store at room temperature.

Assessment/Interventions

- Obtain patient history, including drug history and any known allergies. Note any untreated infections especially those involving nasal mucosa, unhealed ulcers in nasal septum, or active or quiescent tubercular infections of respiratory tract.
- If change is made from systemic (oral) to inhaled or intranasal corticosteroids, observe patient carefully for

signs of steroid withdrawal (eg, depression, joint pain), acute adrenal insufficiency or exacerbation of asthma. Notify physician if these occur.

- If signs of localized fungal infection or any alteration in nasal mucosa, recurrent epistaxis, significant increase in weight or BP, persistent dizziness or severe headache occur, notify physician.

Patient/Family Education

- Instruct patient to shake spray container or inhaler before using.
- Caution patient not to exceed prescribed dose.
- Review manufacturer's instructions with patient for correct use of nasal spray.
- Explain that effects of drug are not immediate. Benefit requires regular use and usually occurs after several days. Caution patient not to continue intranasal therapy beyond 3 wk if there is no improvement.
- Advise patient that dosage will be slowly tapered before stopping.
- Instruct patient to notify physician if more than one dose is missed or if a dosage cannot be taken due to persistent severe nasopharyngeal irritation.
- Inform patient that mild nasopharyngeal irritation, burning, stinging, and dryness are common side effects.
- If patient is using inhalation bronchodilator, instruct patient to use device 5 min before taking flunisolide.
- Advise patient to rinse mouth and brush teeth after using inhaler to prevent *Candida* infection.
- Advise patient to use spacer with metered-dose inhaler to maximize intrapulmonary deposition.
- Instruct patient to report these symptoms to physician: rebound congestion, loss of taste, persistent epistaxis or sneezing, infection, increased or irregular heart beat, high BP, fluid retention, joint pain, muscle weakness, headache, dizziness, weight gain, fungal infection of nose or throat.
- Advise patient to use with caution if sores or injuries occur in nasal passages. Drug may prevent or slow proper healing.

See Patient Guide, p. 255.

Fluorouracil (5-Fluorouracil; 5-FU)

(FLURE-oh-YUR-uh-sill)

Adrucil, Efudex, Fluoroplex

Class: Antineoplastic/antimetabolite

Action Inhibits DNA and RNA synthesis by blocking methylation reaction of deoxyuridilic acid, which is essential for cell division and growth.

Indications Systemic (by injection): Treatment of carcinoma of colon, rectum, breast, stomach, esophagus and pancreas. *Topical:* Treatment of multiple actinic or solar keratoses and superficial basal cell carcinoma. **Unlabeled uses:** *Systemic:* Cancer of liver, bladder, cervix, ovaries in combination with interferon alpha-2a recombinant for esophageal and advanced colorectal carcinoma (orphan drug status). *Topical:* Treatment of condylomata acuminata.

Contraindications Poor nutritional status; depressed bone marrow function; potentially serious infections.

Route/Dosage

Carcinoma

ADULTS: **IV** Initial dose: 12 mg/kg qd for 4 days (do not exceed 800 mg/day). If no toxicity, give 6 mg/kg on days 6, 8, 10, and 12. In special-risk patients or those with inadequate nutritional status, give 6 mg/kg/day for 3 days. If no toxicity, give 3 mg/kg/day on days 5, 7, and 9. Do not exceed 400 mg/day. Maintenance: Repeat dose of first course every 30 days after last day of previous course, when tolerated.

Actinic or Solar Keratoses
ADULTS: **Topical** Apply bid to cover lesions for 2-6 wk. Continue until inflammatory response reaches erosion, necrosis and ulceration stage (2-6 wk), then discontinue.

Superficial Basal Cell Carcinoma
ADULTS: **Topical** Apply 5% strength cream or solution bid for at least 3-6 wk; may require 10-12 wk.

Interactions

Cimetidine: May enhance effect of fluorouracil. *Leukovorin calcium:* Enhanced toxicity of fluorouracil.

Lab Test Interferences

Elevations in alkaline phosphatase, serum transaminase, serum bilirubin and LDH may occur.

Adverse Reactions

CV: MI; angina. *CNS:* Lethargy; malaise; weakness; acute cerebral syndrome; headache; disorientation; confusion; euphoria. *EENT:* Photophobia; lacrimation; decreased vision; nystagmus; diplopia; other visual changes; lacrimal duct stenosis; epistaxis. *GI:* Stomatitis; esophagopharyngitis; diarrhea; anorexia; nausea; vomiting; enteritis; cramps; duodenal ulcer; duodenitis; gastritis; glossitis; intra- and extra-hepatic biliary sclerosis; acalculus cholecystitis; GI ulceration; bleeding. *HEMA:* Leukopenia; thrombocytopenia; pancytopenia; agranulocytosis; anemia; thrombophlebitis. *DERM:* Alopecia; dermatitis; nonspecific skin toxicity; photosensitivity; nail changes; dry skin; fissuring; vein pigmentation; urticaria. *OTHER:* Anaphylaxis; generalized allergic reactions; fever. Topical use may cause pain; pruritis; hyperpigmentation; irritation; inflammation; burning; allergic contact dermatitis; scarring; soreness; tenderness; suppuration; scaling; swelling. Systemic adverse effects may also occur due to absorption.

Precautions

Pregnancy: IV form: Category D; *topical form:* Safety not established. *Lactation:* Undetermined. *Children:* Safety and efficacy not established. *Special risk patients:* Use extreme caution in patients with history of high-dose pelvic irradiation, prior use of alkylating agents, widespread bone marrow metastasis or impaired renal or hepatic function. Not intended as adjuvant to surgery. *Topical use:* Occlusive dressings will increase risk of inflammatory reactions in adjacent normal skin. There is increased absorption through ulcerated or inflamed skin. Note that 1%-2% products are for use in active keratosis on head and neck; 5% product is for solar keratosis on rest of body and for basal cell carcinoma. *Toxicity:* Highly toxic drug with narrow safety margin. Hospitalize patients during initial course of therapy due to possible toxicity. Discontinue if signs of toxicity occur (eg, stomatitis or esophagopharyngitis; rapidly falling WBC count; leukopenia (WBC $< 3500/mm^3$); intractable vomiting; diarrhea or frequent bowel movements; GI ulceration or bleeding; thrombocytopenia (platelets $< 100,000/mm^3$); hemorrhage). Any therapy that adds to patient stress, interferes with nutrition or depresses bone marrow function will increase toxicity.

NURSING CONSIDERATIONS

Administration/Storage

- Administer by IV route with or without dilution by direct injection or IV infusion with 5% Dextrose in Normal Saline. Administration over 2- to 8-hr period appears to reduce onset of toxicity.
- Test patency of vein prior to infusion and monitor closely while medication is infusing. Stop infusion if vein patency is in question.
- Administer antiemetic prior to IV medication administration to alleviate nausea and vomiting.
- Consult physician about pretreat-

ment preparation of lesion when administering topical medication.

- For topical use, apply 1%-2% products for solar keratosis on head and neck. Use 5% product for solar keratosis on other parts of body and for basal cell carcinoma.
- Apply topical medication using nonmetallic applicator or gloved fingers. Avoid occlusive dressings. A porous gauze dressing may be applied for cosmetic reasons without increasing normal skin inflammation.
- Avoid application of topical medication near eyes, nose, mouth and other mucosal areas (eg, rectum, vagina).
- Avoid exposure by inhalation or by direct contact with skin or mucus membranes for IV and topical medications. Always wear gloves while handling this medication. If contact occurs wash thoroughly with soap and water; rinse eyes thoroughly with plain water.
- Treat all equipment and unused drug as hazardous waste and dispose of according to facility's policy and procedure.
- Store at room temperature and protect from light and freezing.
- If precipitate forms in IV preparation due to exposure to low temperatures, heat to 60°C with vigorous shaking; cool to body temperature before using.
- Discard dark yellow solution.

Assessment/Interventions

- Obtain patient history, including drug history and any known allergies. Note renal or hepatic impairment; high-dose pelvic irradiation or previous use of alkylating agents; widespread involvement of bone marrow by metastatic tumors or preexisting coronary artery disease.
- Ensure that baseline CBC with differential and liver and kidney tests have been obtained before beginning therapy.
- Monitor hematologic profile (particularly WBC and platelet counts) prior to and regularly following each course of treatment.
- Inspect skin before applying topical medication.
- Assess for rash, edema, myalgia, weakness, stomatitis, pain, abnormal bleeding and signs of infection after initiation of IV therapy.
- Assess for local and systemic reactions from the application of topical medication.
- Observe for and report to physician if signs of severe toxicity occur.
- Use strict aseptic technique and protective isolation during periods of leukopenia.
- Discontinue medication immediately if patient's mental status changes (disorientation or confusion).
- Stop IV infusion immediately if patient displays local or generalized reaction. Maintain venous access with sterile normal saline or D5W.

Overdosage: Signs & Symptoms

Nausea, vomiting, diarrhea, GI ulceration and bleeding, bone marrow depression (thrombocytopenia, neutropenia, agranulocytosis)

Patient/Family Education

- Advise patient that with topical treatment, lesion usually responds in four stages: (1) early inflammation with erythema for several days; (2) severe inflammation with burning, stinging and vesiculation; (3) disintegration with erosion, ulceration, necrosis, pain, crusting and reepithelization; (4) healing with residual erythema and occasional temporary hyperpigmentation, over 1-2 wk.
- Advise patient to maintain adequate food and fluid intake. Discuss option of food supplements (Low-residue diet will decrease diarrhea.)
- Caution patient to avoid persons with known infections during course of treatment.
- Instruct patient to check mucous membranes for signs of inflammation and ulceration. Discuss importance

of oral hygiene in prevention of stomatitis.

- Advise patient to use electric razor for shaving and soft toothbrush or sponge-tipped "toothette"; avoid harsh temperatures; and avoid otc mouthwashes and drugs that interfere with platelet function (aspirin, alcohol, cough medicine, etc).
- If stomatitis occurs, instruct patient to rinse frequently with warm water or normal saline solution (1 teaspoon salt in 1 quart water) and to avoid extremely hot or cold foods, spices, highly acidic fluids and rough foods.
- Instruct patient to notify physician if mouth pain interferes with eating. Topical or systemic analgesics such as viscous lidocaine mouth washes may be ordered.
- Advise patient that pain, vomiting, diarrhea, fever and weakness may occur. Caution patient to consult physician if these become pronounced and are not relieved by prescribed medications.
- Instruct patient to report these symptoms to physician: chest pain, bleeding, excessive fatigue, persistent GI discomfort, excessive bruising, persistent headache, change in level of consciousness, yellowing of skin or eyes, swelling of feet or legs or disorientation.
- Instruct patient receiving topical or IV infusion therapy to avoid exposure to sunlight, and to use sunblock or wear protective clothing to avoid photosensitivity reaction. Explain that skin pigmentation may be increased and nail changes (discoloration, partial loss) may occur.

See Patient Guide, p. 256.

Fluoxetine HCl

(flew-OX-uh-teen HIGH-droe-KLOR-ide)

Prozac

Class: Antidepressant

Action Blocks reuptake of serotonin, enhancing serotonergic function.

Indications Depression; obsessive-compulsive disorder. **Unlabeled uses:** Obesity; bulimia nervosa.

Contraindications Concurrent use with, or within 14 days of discontinuation of, MAO inhibitor.

Route/Dosage
ADULTS: **PO** 20-80 mg/day. ELDERLY: **PO** 10-60 mg/day. Daily doses > 20 mg can be taken as either single morning dose or split into morning and noontime dose.

Interactions
Carbamazepine: Increased carbamazepine levels causing toxicity. *Cyproheptadine:* Decreased or reversed effects of fluoxetine. *Hydantoins (eg, phenytoin):* Increase hydantoin levels, causing toxicity. MAO *inhibitors (MAOIs):* Combination may lead to serious, possibly fatal reactions. Discontinue MAOI at least 14 days before starting fluoxetine; discontinue fluoxetine at least 5 wk before starting MAOI. *Tricyclic antidepressants:* Increased toxic effects of tricyclic antidepressant.

Lab Test Interferences
None well documented.

Adverse Reactions
CV: Hot flashes; palpitations; angina; heart block; cerebral ischemia; MI; ventricular arrhythmias. *RESP:* Flulike symptoms; bronchitis; rhinitis; yawning; coughing; asthma; pneumonia; apnea; lung edema; pleural effusion. *CNS:* Agitation; anxiety; nervousness; headache; insomnia; abnormal dreams; drowsiness; dizziness; tremor; fatigue; decreased libido; decreased concentration; seizures; delusions; hallucinations; coma. *EENT:* Visual disturbances. *GI:* Nausea; vomiting; diarrhea; dry mouth; anorexia; upset stomach; constipation; abdominal pain; change in taste. *GU:* Painful men-

struation; sexual dysfunction (decreased libodo); frequent micturition; urinary tract infection. *HEMA:* Blood dyscrasias; leukopenia; petechia; purpura; altered platelet function. *DERM:* Increased sweating; rash; itching; erythema multiform. *META:* Weight loss; hypoglycemia; hyponatremia. *OTHER:* Weakness; chills; joint or muscle pain; fever; hypersensitivity reaction.

Precautions

Pregnancy: Category B. *Lactation:* Excreted in breast milk. *Children:* Safety and efficacy not established. *Anorexia:* Weight loss and decreased appetite are more likely to occur with fluoxetine than with tricyclic antidepressants. *Diabetes mellitus:* May alter glycemic control. Insulin dosing may need adjustment. *Mania/hypomania:* Fluoxetine may precipitate mania/hypomania in susceptible patients. *Renal or hepatic impairment:* Use with caution. A lower or less-frequent dosing schedule may be required. *Seizures:* Use with caution in patients with history of seizures. *Suicide:* Depressed patients at risk should be supervised during initial drug therapy.

NURSING CONSIDERATIONS

Administration/Storage

- Administer oral medication with food to minimize GI upset.
- Ensure that patient swallows capsule to avoid hoarding for suicide attempt.
- Capsules may be emptied and mixed with food or juice if patient has difficulty swallowing.
- Administer medication no later than 6 hr before bedtime to prevent insomnia. Morning and early afternoon administration is advised.
- Store at room temperature. Avoid heat and moisture.

Assessment/Interventions

- Obtain patient history, including drug history and any known allergies. Note recent use of MAOIs; history of drug or alcohol abuse.
- Assess vital signs and weight before beginning therapy and at regular intervals thereafter.
- Assess mental status, mood changes, affect and suicidal tendencies daily.
- In patients with diabetes, monitor blood glucose levels before beginning and periodically during therapy.
- Assess for symptoms of blood dyscrasias: fever, sore throat, malaise, unusual bleeding, excessive bruising.
- Determine whether suicide precautions are advisable and implement them as necessary.
- Assist patient to ambulate and change positions to prevent postural hypotension.
- Weigh patient several times/wk on same scale at same time of day.
- Monitor I&O and evaluate bowel elimination.

OVERDOSAGE: SIGNS & SYMPTOMS

Nausea, vomiting, agitation, restlessness, hypomania, seizures

Patient/Family Education

- Instruct patient not to skip or double up on doses. Advise patient not to change dose except as directed by physician.
- Explain that improvement in mood and functioning may not be noted for several wk after initiation of drug therapy. Discuss fact that dosage may be increased or decreased by physician in effort to achieve optimal outcome.
- Instruct patient to avoid taking medication within 6 hr of bedtime as it may cause insomnia.
- Tell patient that doses > 20 mg can be taken as single dose or split into morning and noontime doses.
- Advise patient to take sips of water frequently, suck on ice chips or sugarless hard candy or chew sugarless gum if dry mouth occurs.
- Instruct patient to avoid sudden posi-

tion changes to prevent orthostatic hypotension.

- Advise patients with diabetes that drug may cause loss of glycemic control.
- Instruct patient to report these symptoms to physician: fever, malaise, unusual bleeding, excessive bruising, sore throat, persistent nausea or vomiting, severe headache, tachycardia, severe anorexia, weight loss.
- Advise patient to avoid caffeine as this may increase stimulant effect of drug.
- Advise patient to avoid intake of alcoholic beverages or other CNS depressants (eg, analgesics, sedatives, or antihistamines).
- Warn patient that drug may cause drowsiness and to use caution while driving or performing other tasks requiring mental alertness.
- Instruct patient not to take otc medications without consulting physician.
- Advise patient to carry Medi-Alert information at all times describing medications being taken.

See Patient Guide, p. 257.

Fluphenazine

(flew-FEN-uh-zeen)

Fluphenazine HCl
Permitil, Prolixin, ♣ *Moditen HCl*
Fluphenazine Enanthate
Prolixin Enanthate, ♣ *Moditen Enanthate*
Fluphenazine Decanoate
Prolixin Decanoate, ♣ *Modecate, Modecate Concentrate*
Class: Antipsychotic/phenothiazine; antiemetic

Action Blocks dopamine receptor in CNS.

Indications
Fluphenazine HCl: Management of psychotic disorders. *Fluphenazine decanoate and fluphenazine enanthate:* Long-acting parenteral depot products for long-term antipsychotic therapy. **Unlabeled uses:** Treatment of Tourette's syndrome; acute agitation in elderly; some symptoms of dementia; hyperactivity; hallucinations; suspiciousness; hostility and uncooperative behaviors; Huntington's chorea.

Contraindications Allergy to any phenothiazine; comatose or severely depressed states; concurrent use of large doses of other CNS depressants; bone marrow depression or blood dyscrasias; liver damage; cerebral arteriosclerosis; coronary artery disease; severe hypotension or hypertension; subcortical brain damage.

Route/Dosage
Fluphenazine HCl
ADULTS: **PO** 0.5-40 mg/day in divided doses. **IM** 2.5-10 mg/day in divided doses 6-8 hr apart.

Fluphenazine Decanoate or Enanthate
ADULTS: **IM/SC** Initial dose: 12.5-25 mg. Do not exceed 100 mg/dose. Usual dosing interval: 1-4 wk.

Interactions
Alcohol: Increased CNS depression; may precipitate extrapyramidal reaction. *Anticholinergics:* Reduced therapeutic effects and increased anticholinergic side effects of fluphenazine; may lead to tardive dyskinesia. *Barbiturate anesthetics:* Increased frequency and severity of neuromuscular excitation and hypotension. *Beta-blockers:* Increased plasma levels of both drugs. *Bromocriptine:* Effectiveness of bromocriptine may be reduced. *Guanethidine:* Hypotensive action may be inhibited. *Hydantoins (eg, phenytoin):* Increase or decrease in phenytoin levels. *Lithium:* May result in disorientation, unconsciousness and extrapyramidal symptoms. *Metrizamide:* Increased seizure risk.

Lab Test Interferences
False-positive pregnancy tests

may occur but are less likely with serum test. Increases in protein-bound iodine have been reported. Increased cephalin flocculation accompanied by altered liver function tests has been reported with fluphenazine enanthate. Discolored urine: pink to red-brown.

Adverse Reactions

CV: Orthostatic hypotension; hypertension; tachycardia; bradycardia; syncope; cardiac arrest; circulatory collapse; lightheadedness; faintness; dizziness; ECG changes; arrhythmias; CHF. *RESP:* Laryngospasm; bronchospasm; dyspnea. *CNS:* Pseudoparkinsonism; dyskinesia; motor restlessness; oculogyric crises; opisthotonos; hyperreflexia; tardive dyskinesia; headache; weakness; tremor; fatigue; slurring; insomnia; vertigo; seizures; drowsiness; hallucinations. *EENT:* Pigmentary retinopathy; glaucoma; photophobia; blurred vision; miosis; mydriasis; increased intraocular pressure; dry mouth or throat; nasal congestion. *GI:* Nausea; dyspepsia; constipation. *GU:* Menstrual irregularities; urinary hesitancy and retention; impotence; sexual dysfunction. *HEMA:* Agranulocytosis; eosinophilia; leukopenia; hemolytic anemia; thrombocytopenic purpura. *HEPA:* Jaundice. *DERM:* Photosensitivity; skin pigmentation; dry skin; exfoliative dermatitis; urticarial rash; maculopapular hypersensitivity reaction; seborrhea; eczema; jaundice. *META:* Decreased cholesterol. *OTHER:* Increases in appetite and weight; polydipsia; dysmenorrhea; breast enlargement; galactorrhea; increased prolactin levels; adynamic ileus (may result in death); neuroleptic malignant syndrome (NMS).

Precautions

Pregnancy: Pregnancy category undetermined. *Lactation:* Safety not established. *Children:* Not recommended in children < 12 yr. *Adolescents, elderly or debilitated patients:* More susceptible to effects; consider reduced dose. *Special risk patients:* Use with caution in patients with cardiovascular disease or mitral insufficiency, history of glaucoma, EEG abnormalities or seizure disorders, prior brain damage, hepatic or renal impairment and patients exposed to extreme heat or phosphorous insecticides. *Abrupt withdrawal:* Although this drug is not known to cause psychological or physical dependence, abrupt discontinuation of high-dose therapy has been associated with withdrawal symptoms (nausea, vomiting, dizziness, headache, tachycardia, insomnia, tremulousness). *NMS:* Potentially fatal condition that has occurred, most often with fluphenazine decanoate or enanthate. Signs and symptoms include hyperpyrexia, muscle rigidity, altered mental status, irregular pulse, fluctuating blood pressure, tachycardia and diaphoresis. *Pulmonary effects:* Cases of bronchopneumonia, some fatal, have occurred. *Sudden death:* Has been reported; predisposing factors may be seizures or previous brain damage. Flare-up of psychotic behavior may precede death. *Tardive dyskinesia:* Syndrome of potentially irreversible, involuntary body and facial movements may develop. Prevalence highest in elderly, especially women. Use smallest effective doses for shortest possible time period. *Tartrazine:* Some formulations contain tartrazine, which may cause allergic-type reactions in susceptible individuals.

NURSING CONSIDERATIONS

Administration/Storage

- Give with food to avoid GI irritation. Tablets may be crushed if patient has difficulty swallowing.
- Because antacids diminish drug absorption, give oral preparation at least 1 hr before or 1 hr after administration of antacid.
- Divided doses are usually given initially; however, once-daily dosing is very useful for maintenance and improves compliance.
- Mix hydrochloride concentrate only

with the following diluents: water, milk, carbonated orange or lemon-lime beverage or pineapple, orange, apricot, prune, grapefruit or tomato juice. Avoid caffeinated colas and drinks, tea and apple juice, because incompatibility may result.

- When giving by IM route, use deep, slow injection; massage well.
- Keep patient recumbent for at least ½ hr after IM injection to minimize hypotension.
- Potency of IM solution is not altered when solution is slightly yellowed.
- Store all forms at room temperature and avoid exposure to direct sunlight, excessive heat or cold.

Assessment/Interventions

- Obtain patient history, including drug history and any known allergies. Note sensitivity to this or other phenothiazines.
- Ensure that baseline lab tests (BUN, creatinine, electrolytes, CBC with differential, platelets, liver function tests and ophthalmic examination), vital signs and weight have been obtained before beginning therapy.
- Assess mental status, mood, behavior, activity and interest level daily. Side effects are most common during first few days of therapy.
- Weigh patient weekly and monitor I&O.
- Monitor for signs of tardive dyskinesias (involuntary movements of tongue, face, mouth or jaw). Notify physician if these signs occur.
- Monitor for extrapyramidal symptoms: akinesia, akathisia, pseudoparkinsonism, dystonias and occulogyric crisis. Notify physician if these occur.
- Monitor patient's bowel function. Encourage intake of food and fluid to prevent constipation.
- Assess for symptoms of blood dyscrasias: fever, sore throat, malaise, excessive bruising, unusual bleeding.
- Notify physician immediately if symptoms of neuroleptic malignant syndrome occur: rapid-onset muscular rigidity, akinesia, respiratory difficulty, hyperthermia.

Overdosage: Signs & Symptoms

Somnolence, coma, extrapyramidal symptoms, cardiac arrhythmias, fever, hypotension, seizures

Patient/Family Education

- Stress importance of taking medication even if patient feels that he or she no longer needs it. Symptoms may recur if medication is discontinued.
- Emphasize that drug is not addictive, but tell patient not to stop taking drug abruptly, because withdrawal symptoms may occur (nausea, vomiting, headache, insomnia, tremulousness, and tachycardia).
- Advise patient to dress warmly in cold weather and to avoid extended exposure to either very hot or very cold temperatures.
- Advise patient to carry card or wear Medi-Alert tag at all times listing name and dosage of medication.
- Explain that jaundice is common side effect, usually occurs between second and fourth weeks of treatment and is harmless.
- Tell patient that drug may cause urine to become pink or red-brown colored; this is harmless.
- Instruct patient to report these symptoms to physician: sore throat, fever, easy bruising, unusual bleeding, muscular rigidity, respiratory difficulty, tachycardia, yellow skin or sclera, skin rash, light-colored stools, vision changes, cellulitis, constipation, urinary retention.
- Tell patient to take sips of water frequently, suck on ice chips or sugarless hard candy or chew sugarless gum if dry mouth occurs.
- Advise patient that drug may cause drowsiness and to use caution while driving or performing tasks requiring mental alertness.
- Caution patient to avoid sudden posi-

tion changes to prevent dizziness or lightheadedness.

- Instruct patient to avoid intake of alcoholic beverages or other CNS depressants, which may precipitate extrapyramidal reactions.
- Caution patient to avoid exposure to sunlight and to use sunscreen or wear protective clothing to avoid photosensitivity reaction.
- Instruct patient not to take otc medications without consulting physician. Many drug interactions occur with this medication.

See Patient Guide, p. 258.

Flurazepam HCl

(flure-AZE-uh-pam HIGH-droe-KLOR-ide)

Dalmane, ♣ *Somnol*

Class: Sedative and hypnotic/benzodiazepine

Action Potentiates action of gamma-aminobutyric acid, an inhibitory neurotransmitter, resulting in increased neural inhibition and CNS depression, especially in limbic system and reticular formation.

Indications Treatment of insomnia.

Contraindications Hypersensitivity to benzodiazepines; pregnancy.

Route/Dosage

ADULTS: PO 15-30 mg at bedtime. ELDERLY OR DEBILITATED PATIENTS: PO 15 mg until individual response is determined.

Interactions

Alcohol, other CNS depressants: Additive CNS depressant effects; may continue several days after discontinuation. *Cimetidine, disulfiram, oral contraceptives, isoniazid, omeprazole:* Increased effects of flurazepam. *Digoxin:* Serum digoxin concentrations may increase. *Phenytoin:* Serum concentrations may be increased. *Rifampin:* Decreased effects of flurazepam. *Theophyllines:* May antagonize sedative effects.

Lab Test Interferences

None well documented.

Adverse Reactions

CV: Palpitations; chest pains; tachycardia; hypotension (rare). *RESP:* Shortness of breath. *CNS:* Dizziness; drowsiness; lightheadedness; staggering; ataxia; falling; lethargy; confusion; impaired memory; headache; weakness; paradoxical excitement; talkativeness; euphoria; apprehension; irritability; hallucinations; slurred speech; depression. *EENT:* Difficulty focusing; blurred vision; burning of eyes; taste alterations. *GI:* Heartburn; nausea and vomiting; diarrhea; constipation; anorexia; upset stomach; GI pain; dry mouth. *GU:* Urinary incontinence; urinary retention, hesitancy or urgency. *HEMA:* Leukopenia; granulocytopenia. *HEPA:* Elevated AST, ALT, bilirubin and alkaline phosphatase; hepatitis. *DERM:* Pruritus; rash. *OTHER:* Tolerance; physical and psychological dependence; body and joint pains; sweating; flushing.

Precautions

Pregnancy: Contraindicated. *Lactation:* Excreted in breast milk. *Children:* Not recommended in children < 15 yr. *Elderly or debilitated patients:* Increased side effects; start with lowest dose. *Anterograde amnesia:* Has occurred with similar drugs. Alcohol may increase risk. *Depression:* Administer with caution to severely depressed patients or those with suicidal tendencies. Signs and symptoms of depression may be intensified. *Renal or hepatic impairment:* Use with caution. Abnormal liver function tests and blood dyscrasias have occurred. *Withdrawal:* Withdrawal symptoms may occur after discontinuation of higher doses taken over long periods.

NURSING CONSIDERATIONS

Administration/Storage

- Administer at bedtime with fluid.
- Store at room temperature in light-resistant container.

Assessment/Interventions

- Obtain patient history, including drug history and any known allergies.
- Perform baseline neuro assessment and reassess with initiation of drug.
- Ensure that side rails are raised after administration.
- Assist patient with ambulation after drug administration.
- Assess vision before beginning drug therapy and monitor during initial treatment period.
- Ensure that baseline CBC, liver and kidney function tests have been obtained before beginning therapy and monitor at regular intervals.
- Assess for signs of bleeding (petechiae, bruising, oozing at puncture sites).
- Assess for right upper quadrant abdominal tenderness or jaundice.

OVERDOSAGE: SIGNS & SYMPTOMS

Somnolence, confusion, respiratory depression, apnea, hypotension, impaired coordination, slurred speech, seizures, coma

Patient/Family Education

- Caution patient that this medication must not be taken during pregnancy or when pregnancy is possible. Advise patient to use reliable form of birth control while taking this drug.
- Tell patient to take drug with full glass of water at bedtime.
- Emphasize importance of not exceeding recommended dosage. If symptoms do not improve within 2 to 3 days of beginning drug therapy or if tolerance develops, notify physician.
- Tell patient not to stop taking drug abruptly to avoid withdrawal symptoms. Explain that nighttime sleep may be disturbed for 1-2 nights after gradual discontinuation.
- Instruct patient to monitor weight and to report any excessive gain or loss.
- Advise patient to report these symptoms to physician: palpitations or chest pain, signs of bleeding, abdominal pain, jaundice, shortness of breath, rash, confusion, dizziness, nausea or vomiting.
- Instruct patient to take sips of water frequently, suck on ice chips or sugarless hard candy or chew sugarless gum if dry mouth occurs.
- Advise patient to avoid intake of alcoholic beverages or other CNS depressants.
- Advise patient that drug may cause drowsiness and to use caution while driving or performing other tasks requiring mental alertness.

See Patient Guide, p. 259.

Flurbiprofen

(FLURE-bih-PRO-fen)

Ansaid, ♣ *Froben, Froben SR*

Flurbiprofen Sodium

Ocufen

Class: Analgesic/NSAID

Action Decreases inflammation, pain and fever, probably through inhibition of cyclooxygenase activity and prostaglandin synthesis.

Indications

Systemic: Treatment of rheumatoid arthritis and osteoarthritis. *Ophthalmic:* Inhibition of intraoperative miosis. **Unlabeled uses:** Treatment of juvenile rheumatoid arthritis; migraine; dysmenorrhea; sunburn; mild to moderate pain; acute gout; ankylosing spondylitis; tendonitis; bursitis; inflammation after cataract surgery; uveitis.

Contraindications

Systemic/ophthalmic: Patients in whom aspirin, iodides, or any NSAID has caused allergic-type reactions; dendritic keratitis. *Ophthalmic:* Epithelial herpes simplex keratitis.

Route/Dosage

Rheumatoid Arthritis or Osteoarthritis

ADULTS: **PO** 200-300 mg in divided doses bid-qid; do not exceed 300 mg/day.

Dysmenorrhea

ADULTS: **PO** 50 mg qid.

Inhibition of Intraoperative Miosis

ADULTS: **Topical** 1 drop of 0.03% solution q 30 min beginning 2 hr before surgery.

Interactions

Beta-blockers: Decreased antihypertensive effect of beta-blocker. *Cyclosporine:* Increased risk of nephrotoxicity. *Lithium:* Increased levels and effects of lithium. *Loop diuretics:* Decreased diuretic effect. *Methotrexate:* Increased methotrexate levels. *Salicylates:* Increased risk of GI toxicity. *Warfarin:* Increased risk of gastric erosion and bleeding.

Lab Test Interferences

May prolong bleeding time.

Adverse Reactions

CV: CHF; hypotension; hypertension; peripheral edema; fluid retention; vasodilation. *RESP:* Bronchospasm; laryngeal edema; dyspnea; hemoptysis; shortness of breath. *CNS:* Dizziness; drowsiness; vertigo; headaches; nervousness; migraine; anxiety; confusion. *EENT: Systemic use:* Blurred vision; changes in color vision; hearing disturbances; taste changes. *Ophthalmic use:* Ocular irritation; transient stinging and burning of eyes. *GI:* Heartburn; dyspepsia; nausea; vomiting; anorexia; diarrhea; constipation; increased or decreased appetite; indigestion; GI bleeding; ulceration. *GU:* Hematuria; proteinuria; renal insufficiency; glomerular and interstitial nephritis; acute renal failure with pre-existing renal dysfunction. *HEMA:* Anemia; bone marrow depression; neutropenia; leukopenia; hypocoagulability. *DERM:* Pruritus; erythema; photosensitivity; urticaria. *OTHER:* Hyperglycemia; hypoglycemia; hyponatremia.

Precautions

Pregnancy: Category B (flurbiprofen); Category C (flurbiprofen sodium). *Lactation:* Excreted in breast milk. *Children:* Safety and efficacy not established. *Elderly:* Increased risk of adverse reactions. *GI effects:* Serious GI toxicity (eg, bleeding, ulceration, perforation) can occur at any time, with or without warning symptoms. *Hypersensitivity:* May occur; use caution in aspirin-sensitive individuals because of possible cross-sensitivity. *Renal effects:* Acute renal insufficiency, interstitial nephritis, hyperkalemia, hyponatremia and renal papillary necrosis may occur. *Renal impairment:* Assess function before and during therapy, because NSAID metabolites are eliminated renally.

NURSING CONSIDERATIONS

Administration/Storage

- Give with food, milk or antacids.
- Have patient remain in an upright position for 15-30 min after administration, if possible.
- Store at room temperature in tightly closed, light-resistant container.

Assessment/Interventions

- Obtain patient history, including drug history and any known allergies. Note hypersensitivity to aspirin products, renal impairment, ulcer disease or bleeding disorders.
- Monitor effectiveness of drug therapy by evaluating joint symptoms and pain regularly.
- For patients undergoing prolonged or high-dose therapy, monitor hemoglobin and renal and hepatic function.

- Be aware that effects of this drug may mask signs and symptoms of infection.

OVERDOSAGE: SIGNS & SYMPTOMS

Drowsiness, dizziness, mental confusion, disorientation, lethargy, numbness, vomiting, nausea, gastric upset, abdominal pain, headache, convulsions, renal failure, coma

Patient/Family Education

- Instruct patient to take medication as prescribed, not to skip a dose and not to double up doses if close to next dose.
- Advise diabetic patient to monitor blood glucose levels carefully during treatment.
- Warn patients about the potential for bleeding and the need to notify other health care professionals that drug is being taken.
- Instruct patient using ophthalmic preparation to use great care to prevent contamination of solution.
- Instruct patient to report these symptoms to physician: bleeding, bruising, dyspnea, edema (oral drug); burning or stinging, tearing, photophobia (ophthalmic drug).
- Advise patient that drug may cause drowsiness and to use caution while driving or performing other tasks requiring mental alertness.
- Tell patient to avoid intake of alcoholic beverages, aspirin or other otc medications without consulting physician.

See Patient Guide, pp. 260-261.

Flutamide

(FLEW-tuh-mide)

Eulexin, ♣ *Euflex*

Class: Antineoplastic/antiandrogen

Action Inhibits androgen uptake or nuclear binding of androgen in target tissues.

Indications In combination with gonadotropin-releasing hormone (GnRH now encompassing luteinizing hormone-releasing hormone; LH-RH) agonistic analogs (eg, leuprolide) for treatment of metastatic prostatic carcinoma (stage D2). Start both drugs simultaneously.

Contraindications Standard considerations.

Route/Dosage

ADULTS: PO 250 mg q 8 hr.

Interactions None well documented.

Lab Test Interferences

None well documented.

Adverse Reactions

CNS: Drowsiness; confusion; depression; anxiety; nervousness. *GI:* Diarrhea; nausea; vomiting; other GI disturbances. *GU:* Loss of libido; elevated creatinine; impotence. *HEMA:* Anemia; leukopenia; thrombocytopenia; hemolytic and macrocytic anemia. *HEPA:* Elevated AST, ALT, bilirubin; hepatitis; jaundice; cholestatic jaundice; hepatic encephalopathy; hepatic necrosis. *DERM:* Injection-site irritation; rash; photosensitivity. *OTHER:* Gynecomastia; edema; anorexia; neuromuscular symptoms; hypertension; pulmonary symptoms; hot flushes.

Precautions

Pregnancy: Category D.

NURSING CONSIDERATIONS

Administration/Storage

- Administer concurrently with GnRH agonist.

Assessment/Interventions

- Obtain patient history, including drug history and any known aller-

gies. Note hepatic or hematopoietic impairment.

- Ensure that CBC and liver and renal function tests have been performed before beginning combination therapy (flutamide with GnRH-agonists) and monitor periodically during treatment.
- Obtain baseline vital signs and perform neuromuscular and respiratory assessment before beginning therapy.

OVERDOSAGE: SIGNS & SYMPTOMS

Hypoactivity, piloerection, slow respiration, ataxia, lacrimation, anorexia, tranquilization, emesis, gynecomastia, breast tenderness, slight increase in AST

Patient/Family Education

- Inform patient that drug should be taken along with GnRH agonist (eg, leuprolide) and that drug therapy should not be interrupted without consulting physician.
- Advise patient to expect any of these reactions from combination therapy: hot flushes, loss of libido, impotence, diarrhea, nausea/vomiting, gynecomastia, GI disturbances.
- Instruct patient to report these symptoms to physician: excessive diarrhea or vomiting; lethargy, depression, nervousness, yellowish appearance to skin or eyes, excessive weakness, fever, bleeding, right upper abdominal pain or unexplained flu-like symptoms.

See Patient Guide, p. 262.

Fluvastatin

(FLEW-vah-stat-in)

Lescol

Class: Antihyperlipidemic/HMG-coenzyme A reductase inhibitor.

Action Increases rate at which body removes cholesterol from blood and reduces production of cholesterol in body by inhibiting enzyme that catalyzes early rate-limiting step in cholesterol synthesis; increases HDL; reduces LDL, VLDL and triglycerides.

Indications Reduction of elevated cholesterol and LDL cholesterol levels in patients with primary hypercholesterolemia (types IIa and IIb).

Contraindications Active liver disease or unexplained persistent elevations of liver function tests, pregnancy, lactation.

Route/Dosage

ADULTS: PO 20-40 mg qd at bedtime.

Interactions

Cholestyramine: Reduced absorption of fluvastatin if taken with or up to 4 hours after cholestyramine. *Cyclosporine, erythromycin, gemfibrozil, niacin:* Severe myopathy or rhabdomyolysis may occur with coadministration. *Digoxin:* Digoxin serum levels may be increased. *Cimetidine, ranitidine, omeprazole:* Fluvastatin serum levels may be increased. *Rifampicin:* Fluvastatin serum levels may be reduced.

Lab Test Interferences

None well documented.

Adverse Reactions

RESP: Upper respiratory infection; cough; bronchitis. *CNS:* Headache; dizziness; insomnia; fatigue. *EENT:* Rhinitis; sinusitis; pharyngitis. *GI:* Nausea; vomiting; diarrhea; abdominal pain/cramps; constipation; flatulence; dyspepsia. *DERM:* Rash; pruritis. *OTHER:* Muscle cramps/pain; back pain; arthropathy.

Precautions

Pregnancy: Category X. *Lactation:* Excreted in breast milk. Do not nurse while taking. *Children:* Safety and efficacy in children < 18 yr not established. *Liver dysfunction:* Use with caution in patients who consume substantial quantities of alcohol or who have a history of liver disease. *Liver function tests:* Perform liver function tests before initiating therapy, every 4-6 weeks during the first 3 months of therapy, every 6-12 weeks during the next 12 months (or after a dose increase) and periodically (eg, every 6 months) thereafter. *Skeletal muscle effects:* Rhabdomyolysis with renal dysfunction secondary to myoglobinuria has been reported with other drugs in this class. Temporarily withhold therapy in any patient experiencing an acute or serious condition predisposing to the development of renal failure secondary to rhabdomyolysis (eg, sepsis, hypotension, etc). The risk of myopathy with other drugs in this class was found to be increased if therapy with either cyclosporine, gemfibrozil, erythromycin or niacin is administered concurrently. Myopathy should be considered in any patient with diffuse myalgias, muscle tenderness or weakness, or marked elevations of CPK. *Endocrine effects:* Use caution when administering HMG-CoA reductase inhibitors with drugs that affect steroid levels or activity.

NURSING CONSIDERATIONS

Administration/Storage

- Swallow each tablet whole. Do not cut, crush or chew tablets.
- Drink plenty of fluids as the tablets are swallowed.
- May be taken with evening meal or on empty stomach.
- Store at room temperature.

Assessment/Interventions

- Obtain patient history.
- Ensure that blood cholesterol and triglyceride levels are assessed before beginning therapy and repeated periodically during treatment.
- Place patient on standard cholesterol-lowering diet before beginning therapy and continue diet during treatment.
- Ensure that liver function tests are performed q 4-6 wk during first 3 mo of therapy, q 6-8 wk during next 18 mo and q 6 mo thereafter.
- If elevated serum transaminase levels develop during treatment, repeat tests more frequently.
- If transaminase levels rise to 3 times upper limit of normal and are persistent, notify physician. Drug may be discontinued.
- If muscle tenderness or weakness develops during therapy, monitor CPK levels. Notify physician if CPK levels are markedly increased or if symptoms continue.

OVERDOSAGE: SIGNS & SYMPTOMS

None reported

Patient/Family Education

- Caution patient that this medication must not be taken during pregnancy or when pregnancy is possible. Advise patient to use reliable form of birth control while taking this drug.
- Advise patient to take medication with evening meal if possible.
- Explain importance of adhering to low-cholesterol, low-fat diet during treatment. Suggest consultation with nutritionist as needed.
- Instruct patient to report these symptoms to healthcare provider: unexplained muscle pain, tenderness or weakness, especially if accompanied by fever or malaise.
- Caution patient to avoid or decrease alcohol intake.
- Advise patient not to take any additional medications or supplementations without approval by healthcare provider.
- Emphasize importance of returning for follow-up liver function and blood cholesterol tests as instructed.
- Explain that this treatment must be continued over years.

See Patient Guide, p. 263.

Foscarnet Sodium (Phosphonoformic Acid)

(foss-CAR-net SO-dee-uhm)

Foscavir

Class: Anti-infective/antiviral

Action Inhibits replication of several viruses, including cytomegalovirus (CMV).

Indications Treatment of CMV retinitis in patients with AIDS.

Contraindications Standard considerations.

Route/Dosage

ADULTS: **IV** Initially 60 mg/kg/dose at constant rate over at least 1 hr q 8 hr for 2-3 wk. Adjust for clinical response and renal function. Maintenance dose: 90 mg/kg/day infused over 2 hr; individualized; maximum maintenance dose 120 mg/kg/day.

Interactions

Nephrotoxic drugs: Elimination of foscarnet may be impaired by drugs that inhibit renal tubular secretion. Increased potential for nephrotoxicity with aminoglycosides, amphotericin B and IV pentamidine. *Pentamidine:* Concomitant IV pentamidine may cause hypocalcemia. *Zidovudine:* Increased risk of anemia. INCOMPATIBILITIES: Do not give other drugs or supplements via same IV catheter.

Lab Test Interferences

None well documented.

Adverse Reactions

CV: Hypertension; palpitations; ECG abnormalities including sinus tachycardia, first-degree heart block, nonspecific ST-T segment changes; hypotension; flushing; cerebrovascular disorder. *RESP:* Coughing; dyspnea; pneumonia; respiratory disorders or insufficiency; pulmonary infiltrates; stridor; pneumothorax; hemoptysis; bronchospasm. *CNS:* Headache; paresthesia; dizziness; involuntary muscle contractions; hypoesthesia; neuropathy; seizures; depression; confusion; anxiety; tremor; ataxia; dementia; stupor; generalized spasms; sensory disturbances; meningitis; aphasia; abnormal coordination; leg cramps; EEG abnormalities; insomnia; somnolence; nervousness; amnesia; agitation; aggressive reaction; hallucination. *EENT:* Vision abnormalities; eye pain; conjunctivitis; sinusitis; rhinitis; taste perversions; pharyngitis. *GI:* Anorexia; nausea; diarrhea; vomiting; abdominal pain; constipation; dysphagia; dyspepsia; rectal hemorrhage; dry mouth; melena; flatulence; ulcerative stomatitis; pancreatitis. *GU:* Alterations in renal function, including decreased creatinine clearance, abnormal renal function; albuminuria; dysuria; polyuria; urethral disorder; urinary retention; urinary tract infections; acute renal failure; nocturia; abnormal albumin-globulin ratio; increased AST and ALT. *HEMA:* Anemia; bone marrow suppression; granulocytopenia; leukopenia; thrombocytopenia; platelet abnormalities; thrombosis; WBC abnormalities; lymphadenopathy. *DERM:* Rash; increased sweating; pruritus; skin ulceration; seborrhea; erythematous or maculopapular rash; skin discoloration; facial edema. *META:* Mineral and electrolyte imbalances, including hypo- or hypercalcemia, hypokalemia, hypomagnesemia, hypo- or hyperphosphatemia, hyponatremia; decreased weight; increased alkaline phosphatase, LDH, BUN; acidosis. *OTHER:* Fever; fatigue; rigors; asthenia; malaise; arthralgia or myalgia; cachexia; thirst; infection; sepsis; death; back or chest pain; edema; influenza-like symptoms; abscess; lymphoma-like disorders; sarcoma; injection site pain or inflammation.

Precautions

Pregnancy: Category C. *Lactation:* Undetermined. *Children:* Safety and efficacy not studied. Drug is deposited in teeth and bone. *Mineral and electrolyte imbalances:* Patients, especially those on concomitant drugs known to influence serum minerals or electrolytes or those with cardiac or neurological abnormalities, may experience changes in electrolytes (calcium, potassium, magnesium, phosphate) that could cause cardiac disturbances or seizures. Replacement therapy may be needed. *Renal impairment:* Major toxicity; occurs to some degree in most patients. If creatinine clearance drops below 0.4 ml/min/kg, drug should be discontinued. *Toxicity/local irritation:* Infuse into veins with adequate blood flow to permit rapid dilution and distribution and avoid local irritation. Drug is excreted in urine and may cause irritation or ulceration of penile or vulvovaginal epithelium.

NURSING CONSIDERATIONS

Administration/Storage

- Administer by IV infusion only, at rate not to exceed 1 mg/kg/min. Use infusion pump to prevent rapid or bolus injection.
- When administering through central vein, 24 mg/ml solution may be used. In peripheral veins, dilute with D5W or normal saline to 12 mg/ml.
- Administer only with normal saline or D5W; incompatible with many drugs and supplements.
- Do not use same tubing or catheter for any other drug or IV solution.
- Prehydrate patient with 0.9% sodium chloride to decrease chance of renal damage.
- Use prepared solutions within 24 hr of first entry into sealed bottle.

Assessment/Interventions

- Obtain patient history, including drug history and any known allergies. Note cardiac, neurologic or renal disorders.
- Ensure that baseline serum electrolyte levels (calcium, magnesium, potassium, phosphate) have been obtained before beginning therapy and repeat 2-3 times/wk during induction therapy and 1-2 times/wk during maintenance therapy.
- Ensure that baseline renal function tests have been obtained before beginning therapy and repeat 2-3 times/wk during induction therapy and 1-2 times/wk during maintenance therapy. Dosage will be adjusted or drug discontinued if creatinine clearance decreases.
- Assess renal function before and after administration in elderly patients.
- Monitor I&O and ensure that patient is well hydrated. Note urine pH.
- Monitor for anemia; obtain CBC frequently.
- Monitor for seizures, especially in patients with CNS disorder such as toxoplasmosis or HIV encephalopathy.
- Observe for fever, nausea, diarrhea, vomiting and headache. Report these and other common side effects to physician.
- If symptoms of electrolyte imbalance, such as complaints of perioral tingling, numbness in extremities or paresthesias occurs, notify physician immediately. Infusion may need to be discontinued and electrolyte supplementation initiated.

OVERDOSAGE: SIGNS & SYMPTOMS

Electrolyte disturbances, paresthesia, renal dysfunction, seizures, coma

Patient/Family Education

- Emphasize that drug does not cure CMV retinitis but may help prevent worsening of symptoms.
- Explain that drinking plenty of fluids and good hygiene may help reduce risk of genital irritation or ulceration.
- Instruct patient to report these symptoms to physician: perioral tingling, numbness in extremities, paresthesias, fever, nausea, diarrhea, vomiting, headache, increased or decreased frequency or amount of urination or other bothersome side effects.

- Caution patient not to take any otc medications without consulting physician. Explain that serious drug interactions may result.

See Patient Guide, p. 265.

Fosinopril Sodium

(FAH-sin-oh-PRILL SO-dee-uhm)

Monopril

Class: Antihypertensive/ACE inhibitor

Action Competitively inhibits angiotensin I-converting enzyme, preventing conversion of angiotensin I to angiotensin II, a potent vasoconstrictor that also stimulates release of aldosterone. Results in decrease in blood pressure, reduced sodium reabsorption and potassium retention.

Indications Hypertension; heart failure.

Contraindications Hypersensitivity to ACE inhibitors.

Route/Dosage

Hypertension

ADULTS: Initial dose: **PO** 10 mg qd. Maintenance dose: 20-80 mg/day; if inadequate response, consider dividing into two doses.

Heart Failure

ADULTS: Initial dose: **PO** 10 mg qd. Increase over several weeks. Usual range is 20-40 mg/day. Do not exceed 40 mg/day.

Interactions

Allopurinol: Increased risk of hypersensitivity reactions. *Antacids:* May decrease effects of fosinopril. *Capsaicin:* Cough may be exacerbated. *Digoxin:* May increase serum levels of digoxin. *Indomethacin:* Hypotensive effects may be reduced, especially in low-renin or volume-dependent hypertensive patients. *Lithium:* Increased lithium levels and symptoms of lithium toxicity may occur. *Phenothiazines:* May increase pharmacological effect of phenothiazines. *Potassium preparations, potassium-sparing diuretics:* May increase serum potassium levels.

Lab Test Interferences

Measurement of serum digoxin with DigiTab RIA kit may be falsely low. False elevation of liver enzymes, serum bilirubin, uric acid or blood glucose may occur.

Adverse Reactions

CV: Orthostatic hypotension. *RESP:* Cough. *CNS:* Headache; dizziness; fatigue. *GI:* Nausea; vomiting; diarrhea. *HEMA:* Hemoglobin decrease (transient); neutropenia; leukopenia; eosinophilia. *META:* Hyperkalemia; hyponatremia.

Precautions

Pregnancy: Category D (second, third trimester); Category C (first trimester). *Lactation:* Excreted in breast milk. *Children:* Safety and efficacy not established. *Angioedema:* May occur. Use extreme caution in patients with hereditary angioedema. *Hepatic impairment:* May result in elevated plasma levels; monitor carefully; reduce doses. *Hypotension/first-dose effect:* Significant decreases in BP may occur after first dose, especially in severely salt- or volume-depleted patients or those with heart failure; monitor closely for at least 2 hr after initial dose and during first 2 wk of therapy. Minimize risk by discontinuing diuretics, decreasing dose or increasing salt intake approximately 1 wk prior to initiating fosinopril. *Neutropenia and agranulocytosis:* Have occurred; risk appears greater in patients with renal dysfunction, heart failure or immunosuppression; monitor WBC counts frequently. *Proteinuria:* May occur, especially in patients with prior renal disease or those receiving high doses; generally within 6 mo. *Renal impairment:* Reduce dose and give less frequently. In renal insufficiency stable elevations in BUN and serum creatinine may occur because of inadequate renal perfusion; monitor renal function during first few weeks of therapy and adjust dosage.

NURSING CONSIDERATIONS

Administration/Storage

- May be administered with or without food.
- If patient is taking diuretic, it should be discontinued 2-3 days before initiation of fosinopril. If diuretic cannot be discontinued, reduced dose of fosinopril should be administered.

Assessment/Interventions

- Obtain patient history, including drug history and any known allergies. Note renal impairment, angioedema, immunosuppression, nutritional status, history of smoking and hypersensitivity to ACE inhibitors.
- Ensure that baseline serum electrolyte levels, BUN, serum creatinine levels, liver function tests, urine protein and CBC have been obtained before beginning therapy and monitor regularly during therapy.
- Obtain baseline BP and monitor at regular intervals. Compare with peak and trough blood levels at 2-6 hr after initial dose and then at 24 hr after. Observe for orthostatic changes.

OVERDOSAGE: SIGNS & SYMPTOMS

Hypotension

Patient/Family Education

- Instruct patient not to interrupt or stop medication or change dosage without consulting physician.
- Caution patient not to double up doses; if a dose is missed it should be taken as soon as possible, unless close to time of next dose. Consult physician if more than one dose is missed.
- Inform patient not to use salt substitute or potassium supplement without consulting physician.
- Emphasize importance of follow-up visits and frequent assessment of BP while taking drug.
- Advise patient that he or she may feel tired for first few days after starting medication. If tiredness increases and becomes a problem, notify physician.
- Explain that chronic cough may occur, especially in women. Instruct patient to avoid cough, cold or allergy medications and to notify physician.
- Advise patient that dizziness or lightheadedness may occur after first doses. Instruct patient to avoid sudden changes in posture, hot baths or showers and to call physician if symptoms become severe or if fainting occurs.
- Instruct patient to report these symptoms to physician: dizziness or fainting on arising, constant cough or any unusual symptoms or feelings; swelling of eyes, face, lips, tongue or throat; difficulty breathing, speaking (eg, hoarseness) or swallowing; signs of infection (eg, fever, sore throat).
- Advise patient to use caution while driving or performing other tasks requiring mental alertness.

See Patient Guide, p. 266.

Furosemide

(fyu-ROH-se-mide)

Lasix, ♣ *Lasix Special*

Class: Loop diuretic

Action Inhibits reabsorption of sodium and chloride in proximal and distal tubules and loop of Henle.

Indications Treatment of edema associated with CHF, hepatic cirrhosis and renal disease; hypertension.

Contraindications Hypersensitivity to sulfonylureas; anuria.

Route/Dosage

Edema

ADULTS: **PO** 20-80 mg/day as a single

dose; may titrate up to 600 mg/day. **IV/IM** 20-40 mg qd or bid.

Hypertension
ADULTS: **PO** 40 mg bid. Maximum dose: 6 mg/kg.

CHF and Chronic Renal Failure
ADULTS: **PO** Up to 2-2.5 g/day. **IV** Up to 2-2.5 g/day. Maximum IV bolus: 1 g/day over 30 min.

Acute Pulmonary Edema
ADULTS: **IV** 40 mg (over 1-2 min). If response not satisfactory within 1 hr, increase to 80 mg. INFANTS & CHILDREN: **PO** Usual dose: 0.5-2 mg/kg qd or bid. Maximum dose 6 mg/kg. **IV/IM** Usual dose: 1 mg/kg. Maximum dose 6 mg/kg.

Interactions
Aminoglycosides: May increase auditory toxicity. *Charcoal:* May reduce absorption of furosemide. *Cisplatin:* May cause additive ototoxicity. *Digitalis glycosides:* Electrolyte disturbances may predispose to digitalis-induced arrhythmias. *Lithium:* May increase plasma lithium levels and toxicity. *Nonsteroidal antinflammatory drugs:* May decrease effects of furosemide. *Phenytoin:* May reduce diuretic effects of furosemide. *Salicylates:* May impair diuretic response in patients with cirrhosis and ascites. *Thiazide diuretics:* Synergistic effects that may result in profound diuresis and serious electrolyte abnormalities. INCOMPATIBILITIES: *Gentamicin, milrinone or netilmicin in D5W or normal saline:* Do not add to furosemide solution; precipitate forms. *Highly acidic solutions of pH < 5.5:* Do not mix with furosemide solution.

Lab Test Interferences
None well documented.

Adverse Reactions
CV: Orthostatic hypotension; thrombophlebitis; chronic aortitis. *CNS:* Vertigo; headache; dizziness; paresthesia; restlessness; fever. *EENT:* Blurred vision; xanthopsia (yellow vision); tinnitus; hearing impairment. *GI:* Anorexia; nausea; vomiting; diarrhea; oral and gastric irritation; cramping; constipation; pancreatitis. *GU:* Urinary bladder spasm; interstitial nephritis; glycosuria. *HEMA:* Anemia; leukopenia; purpura; aplastic anemia; thrombocytopenia; agranulocytosis. *HEPA:* Jaundice; ischemic hepatitis. *DERM:* Photosensitivity; urticaria; pruritus; necrotizing angiitis (vasculitis, cutaneous vasculitis); exfoliative dermatitis; erythema multiforme; rash; occasionally, local irritation and pain with parenteral use. *META:* Hyperuricemia; hyperglycemia; hypokalemia; metabolic alkalosis. *OTHER:* Muscle spasm; weakness.

Precautions
Pregnancy: Category C. *Lactation:* Excreted in breast milk. *Children:* May increase incidence of patent ductus arteriosus in premature infants with respiratory distress syndrome, especially in first few weeks of life. *Dehydration:* Excessive diuresis may cause dehydration and decreased blood volume with circulatory collapse and possible vascular thrombosis and embolism, especially in elderly. *Diarrhea:* Furosemide solution vehicle contains sorbitol and may induce diarrhea, especially in children. *Hepatic cirrhosis and ascites:* Sudden alterations of electrolyte balance may precipitate hepatic encephalopathy and coma; monitor carefully. *Hypersensitivity:* Patients with known sulfonamide sensitivity may show allergic reactions to furosemide. *Ototoxicity:* Associated with rapid injection, severe renal impairment, very large doses or concurrent use of other ototoxic drugs. *Photosensitivity:* Photosensitization may occur. *Renal impairment:* If severe effects occur, may need to discontinue. If high-dose parenteral therapy is used, controlled IV infusion is advised. *Systemic lupus erythematosus:* May be exacerbated or activated.

NURSING CONSIDERATIONS

Administration/Storage

- Administer oral medication with food to prevent GI irritation.
- Administer qd dose in morning and bid doses at 8 AM and 2 PM to avoid nocturia and sleep disturbance.
- Do not exceed infusion rate of 4 mg/min in adults.
- Use infusion solutions mixed with cefoperazone sodium in 5% Dextrose within 24 hr if stored at room temperature and within 5 days if kept refrigerated.
- Do not use if discolored.
- Store medication at room temperature; avoid excessive exposure to light.

Assessment/Interventions

- Obtain patient history, including drug history and any known allergies. Note renal or hepatic impairment, systemic lupus erythematosus, hearing impairment or hypersensitivity to sulfonamides.
- Obtain baseline hearing evaluation.
- Ensure that baseline BP; apical pulse; weight; serum electrolyte, calcium, glucose, uric acid, CO_2, BUN and serum creatine levels; CBC; and liver and renal function tests have been obtained before beginning therapy and monitor regularly.
- Monitor I&O and weigh patient daily.
- Monitor renal function and notify physician if increasing azotemia, oliguria or increases in BUN or creatinine occur.
- Notify physician if sudden alteration in fluid and electrolyte status is noted.
- Monitor for signs and symptoms of hypokalemia.

OVERDOSAGE: SIGNS & SYMPTOMS

Acute profound water loss, volume and electrolyte depletion, dehydration, reduction of blood volume, circulatory collapse with possibility of vascular thrombosis and embolism

Patient/Family Education

- Instruct patient to take medication early in day to avoid disruption of sleep from increased urination and to take with food or milk to avoid GI upset.
- Teach patient to take and monitor pulse daily, especially if patient is taking cardiac drugs in addition to furosemide.
- Advise patient to eat diet high in potassium. Provide list of suggested foods (ie, baked potato, bananas, cantaloupe, avocados, dates, raisins, orange juice, peaches, watermelon, etc.).
- Emphasize importance of follow-up visits and frequent assessment of BP while taking drug.
- Advise patient to control hypertension through weight loss, sodium restriction and exercise.
- Explain to diabetic patients that drug may increase blood glucose levels and affect urine glucose test results and that glucose levels should be monitored carefully.
- For patients taking this medication to lower BP, explain that they may feel fatigued during first few weeks of therapy. Instruct patient to continue taking drug but to consult with physician if problem persists.
- Instruct patient to report these symptoms to physician: indication of weakness, dizziness, mental confusion, anorexia, lethargy, vomiting, cramps, persistent headache or fever, abdominal pain, diarrhea, rapid or irregular heart beat, yellowing of skin or eyes or dyspnea.
- Caution patient to avoid sudden position changes to prevent orthostatic hypotension.

- Advise patient to avoid exposure to sunlight and to use sunscreens or wear protective clothing to avoid photosensitivity reaction.
- Instruct patient not to take aspirin or otc medications without consulting physician.

See Patient Guide, p. 267.

Gabapentin

(GAB-uh-PEN-tin)
Neurontin
Class: Anticonvulsant

Action Mechanism unknown; gabapentin-binding sites have been found in neocortex and hippocampus areas of brain.

Indications Adjunctive therapy in treatment of partial seizures with or without secondary generalization in adults with epilepsy.

Contraindications Standard considerations.

Route/Dosage
ADULTS & CHILDREN > 12 YR: **PO** 900-1800 mg/day in divided doses tid. Initial dose: 300 mg on day 1 and titrate upward rapidly. To minimize CNS side effects, administer initial dose on day 1 at bedtime.

Interactions
Antacids: May reduce bioavailability of gabapentin. *Cimetidine:* Reduces renal clearance of gabapentin.

Lab Test Interferences
False-positive readings for Ames N-Multistix SG dipstick test when gabapentin is added to other antiepileptic drugs. Sulfosalicylic acid precipitation procedure is recommended instead.

Adverse Reactions
CV: Hypertension. *RESP:* Rhinitis; pharyngitis; coughing; pneumonia. *CNS:* Somnolence; dizziness; ataxia; tremor; nervousness; dysarthria; amnesia; depression; abnormal thinking; twitching; abnormal coordination; vertigo; hyperkinesia; parasthesia; reflex abnormality; hostility; anxiety. *EENT:* Diplopia; amblyopia; nystagmus; abnormal vision; gingivitis. *GI:* Dyspepsia; dry mouth or throat; constipation; dental abnormalities; increased appetite; anorexia; flatulence. *DERM:* Pruritus; abrasion; purpura. *OTHER:* Fatigue; weight increase; back pain; peripheral edema; impotence; leukopenia; vasodilation; asthenia; malaise; facial edema; arthralgia.

Precautions
Pregnancy: Category C. *Lactation:* Undetermined. *Children:* Safety and efficacy in children < 12 yr not established. *Elderly and debilitated patients:* Because of age-related renal impairment, dosage adjustment may be required. *Carcinogenesis:* May have carcinogenic potential. *Renal impairment:* Dose reduction recommended. *Serious adverse effects:* During clinical trials some patients experienced status epilepticus, and 8 sudden, unexplained deaths occurred. The association of these events with gabapentin use is unclear. *Withdrawal:* Do not discontinue antiepileptic drugs abruptly because of possible increased seizure frequency on drug withdrawal.

NURSING CONSIDERATIONS

Administration/Storage

- Administer medication with or without food and at least 2 hr after antacid administration.
- Administer initial dose on day 1 at bedtime to minimize CNS side effects.
- Titrate to effective dose given tid up to 1800 mg/day; maximum time between doses in tid schedule should not exceed 12 hr.
- Discontinue medication gradually over minimum of 1 wk.

- Store medication in tightly sealed container.

Assessment/Interventions

- Obtain patient history, including drug history and any known allergies. Note compromised renal function, compromised cardiovascular function and seizure pattern.
- Assess baseline vital signs.
- Evaluate for reduced renal clearance when administered concurrently with cimetidine.
- Withdraw medication gradually to avoid the possibility of increasing seizure frequency.

OVERDOSAGE: SIGNS & SYMPTOMS

Ataxia, labored breathing, ptosis, sedation, hypoactivity or excitation, double vision, slurred speech, drowsiness, lethargy, diarrhea

Patient/Family Education

- Instruct patient to take medication at least 2 hr after taking antacid.
- Explain that missed dose should be taken as soon as remembered but that 2 doses should not be taken together. Instruct patient to call physician if 2 or more doses are missed.
- Instruct patient to report these symptoms to physician: excessive fatigue or weakness, dizziness, somnolence, incoordination, tremor or other symptoms of CNS depression, change in normal behavior, weight gain, back pain, alterations in GI system, alteration in skin or mucous membranes, fluid retention, general body discomfort, anorexia, visual disturbances and impotence.
- Advise patient that drug may cause drowsiness and to use caution while driving or performing other tasks requiring mental alertness.

See Patient Guide, p. 268.

Gallium Nitrate

(GAL-ee-uhm NYE-trate)

Ganite

Class: Hormone

Action Exerts hypocalcemic effect by inhibiting calcium resorption from bone, possibly by stabilizing bone matrix, thereby reducing increased bone turnover.

Indications Treatment of symptomatic cancer-related hypercalcemia unresponsive to adequate hydration.

Contraindications Severe renal impairment (serum creatinine > 2.5 mg/dl).

Route/Dosage

ADULTS: **IV** 100-200 mg/m^2/day for 5 consecutive days.

Interactions

Nephrotoxic drugs (eg, aminoglycosides, amphotericin B): May increase risk for development of renal insufficiency.

Lab Test Interferences

None well documented.

Adverse Reactions

CV: Tachycardia; lower extremity edema; asymptomatic hypotension. *RESP*: Shortness of breath; rales and rhonchi; pleural effusion; pulmonary infiltrates. *EENT*: Acute optic neuritis; visual impairment; tinnitus. *GI*: Nausea or vomiting; diarrhea; constipation. *GU*: Increased BUN and creatinine; acute renal failure. *HEMA*: Anemia; leukopenia. *META*: Hypocalcemia; mild to moderate transient hypophosphatemia; decreased serum bicarbonate concentrations. *OTHER*: Lethargy; confusion; hypothermia; fever; paresthesia; skin rash.

Precautions

Pregnancy: Category C. *Lactation*: Undetermined. *Children*: Safety and efficacy not established. *Asymptomatic or mild to moderate hypocalcemia*: Occurs frequently. *Renal impairment*: Hypercalcemia in cancer patients is commonly associated with impaired renal function. *Visual and auditory disturbances:* Have occurred in some patients treated with multiple high doses of gallium combined with investigational anticancer drugs.

NURSING CONSIDERATIONS

Administration/Storage

- Dilute medication with 1 L of either 0.9% Sodium Chloride for Injection or D5W.
- Administer diluted solution daily by IV infusion over 24 hr.
- Maintain adequate hydration of patient.
- If serum calcium concentrations are lowered into normal range in < 5 days, treatment may be discontinued early.
- Mixed solution is stable for 48 hr at room temperature and for 7 days if refrigerated. Discard unused portion.

Assessment/Interventions

- Obtain patient history, including drug history and any known allergies. Note compromised renal or cardiovascular function.
- Carefully monitor infusion rate to maintain hydration while avoiding overhydration, especially in patients with compromised cardiovascular status.
- Assess baseline vital signs, BUN, CBC, serum creatinine, calcium, phosphate and bicarbonate levels.
- Obtain baseline respiratory, neurological, visual and auditory assessment.
- Take safety precautions with patient with increased neuromuscular irritability caused by hypocalcemia.
- Carefully evaluate patient with cancer-related hypercalcemia for renal insufficiency when there is concurrent use of gallium nitrate and other potentially nephrotoxic drugs (aminoglycosides, amphotericin B). If use of potentially nephrotoxic drug is indicated during therapy, discontinue gallium nitrate and continue hydration for several days after administering potentially nephrotoxic drug. Closely monitor serum creatinine and urine output during and after this period. Discontinue gallium nitrate therapy if serum creatinine level becomes > 2.5 mg/dl.
- Monitor serum creatinine, calcium and BUN continually during therapy. Monitor calcium and phosphorus levels daily and twice weekly, respectively.
- Evaluate patient for signs of hypocalcemia: tingling and numbness of fingers and circumoral region, painful tonic muscle spasms, facial spasms, grimacing, fatigue, laryngospasm, positive Trousseau's and Chvostek's signs, convulsions, palpitations and arrhythmias.
- Evaluate patient for signs of hypercalcemia: anorexia, lethargy, fatigue, nausea, vomiting, constipation, dehydration, renal insufficiency, impaired mental status, coma and cardiac arrest.

OVERDOSAGE: SIGNS & SYMPTOMS

Nausea, vomiting, renal insufficiency

Patient/Family Education

- Instruct patient and family members to report these symptoms to physician: numbness or spasms noted in extremities or face, increased or irregular heart rate, edema, excessive pain not relieved by prescribed medication, excessive weakness, breathing difficulty, fever, bleeding and seizures, visual or auditory impairment, nausea, vomiting, diarrhea, constipation, abnormal skin sensations, skin rash, chills, pain at injection site.

No patient monograph available.

Ganciclovir Sodium (DHPG)

(gan-SIGH-kloe-VIHR SO-dee-uhm)

Cytovene

Class: Anti-infective/antiviral

Action Inhibits cytomegalovirus (CMV) and other virus replication by competitive inhibition of viral DNA polymerases and direct incorporation into viral DNA.

Indications **IV:** Treatment of CMV retinitis in immunocompromised patients; prevention of CMV disease in organ transplant patients at risk for CMV. **Oral:** Alternative to the IV formulation for maintenance treatment of CMV retinitis in immunocompromised patients, including patients with AIDS, in whom retinitis is stable following appropriate induction therapy and for whom the risk of more rapid progression is balanced by the benefit associated with avoiding daily IV infusions. **Unlabeled use:** Treatment of other CMV infections (pneumonitis, gastroenteritis, hepatitis) in some immunocompromised patients.

Contraindications Hypersensitivity to acyclovir.

Route/Dosage

CMV Retinitis or Prevention in Transplant Recipients

ADULTS: **IV** Induction: 5 mg/kg over 1 hr q 12 hr for 14-21 days. Maintenance: 5 mg/kg over 1 hr qd or 6 mg/kg over 1 hr daily 5 days/wk (maximum 6 mg/kg over 1 hr). **Oral:** Following induction treatment, the recommended maintenance dose of oral ganciclovir is 1,000 mg 3 times daily with food. Alternatively, the dosing regimen of 500 mg 6 times daily every 3 hours with food, during waking hours, may be used.

Decreased Renal Function

ADULTS: **IV** Induction: 2.5 mg/kg q 12 hr (creatinine clearance 50-79 ml/min/1.73 m^2); 2.5 mg/kg q 24 hr (creatinine clearance 25-49 ml/min/1.73 m^2); 1.25 mg/kg q 24 hr (creatinine clearance < 25 ml/min/1.73 m^2). Maintenance: ½ induction dose. **Oral:** 1000 mg tid or 500 mg q3h, 6 times/day (creatine clearance 70 ml/min or greater); 1,500 mg qd or 500 mg tid (creatinine clearance 50 to 69 ml/min); 1,000 mg qd or 500 mg bid (creatinine clearance 25-49 ml/min); 500 mg qd (creatinine clearance 10 to 24); 500 mg three times per week, following hemodialysis (less than 10 ml/min).

Interactions

Amphotericin B, cyclosporine, nephrotoxic drugs: May increase serum creatinine. *Cytotoxic drugs:* May cause added toxicity. *Imipenem-cilastatin:* May cause generalized seizures. *Probenecid:* May reduce renal clearance and increase serum levels of ganciclovir. *Zidovudine:* Both zidovudine and ganciclovir can cause granulocytopenia; combination therapy at full dose may not be tolerated. INCOMPATIBILITIES: Do not mix with other drugs.

Lab Test Interferences

None well documented.

Adverse Reactions

CNS: Headache; confusion. *GU:* Renal toxicity. *HEMA:* Granulocytopenia; thrombocytopenia; anemia. *HEPA:* Abnormal liver function test results. *DERM:* Rash; phlebitis or pain at injection site. *OTHER:* Sepsis; fever.

Precautions

Pregnancy: Category C. *Lactation:* Undetermined. Advise against nursing during and for at least 72 hr after treatment. *Children:* Safety and efficacy not established. *Carcinogenesis:* Ganciclovir is potentially carcinogenic. *Cytopenia:* Use drug with caution in patients with preexisting cytopenias; granulocytopenia is common. *Hydration:* Administration should be accompanied by adequate hydration because ganciclovir is excreted by the kidneys. *Renal impairment:* Use drug cautiously and adjust dose. *Renal toxicity:* Carefully monitor renal function, especially when other nephrotoxic drugs are given. *Reti-*

nal detachment: Has occurred; relationship to drug undetermined.

NURSING CONSIDERATIONS

Administration/Storage

IV

- Reconstitute with 10 ml of Sterile Water for Injection (do not use bacteriostatic water or other solutions) and shake well to dissolve drug.
- Prepare infusion solution by mixing with 0.9% Sodium Chloride for Injection, D5W, Ringer's Injection or Lactated Ringer's Injection.
- Wear gloves, gown and mask while preparing solution.
- Use caution during administration to prevent personal exposure.
- Do not infuse at concentrations > 10 mg/ml.
- Use infusion pump to prevent rapid or bolus injection.
- Administer only into veins that permit rapid dilution and distribution.
- Do not administer to patients with absolute neutrophil count of < 500/mm^3 or platelet count of < 50,000/mm^3.
- Refrigerate infusion solution until use but not for more than 24 hr.
- Discard reconstituted drug if vial has particulate matter or is discolored.
- Reconstituted solution in vial is stable at room temperature for 12 hr; do not refrigerate.
- Dispose of unused drug with appropriate precautions for nucleoside analog cytotoxic agents.

Assessment/Interventions

- Obtain patient history, including drug history and any known allergies. Note history of cytopenia or impaired renal function.
- Obtain neutrophil and platelet counts before starting therapy, every 2 days during twice-daily dosing and weekly thereafter.
- Obtain daily neutrophil counts in patients with history of drug-induced leukopenia or in whom neutrophil counts are < 1000/mm^3 at initiation of treatment.
- Obtain serum creatinine or measure creatinine clearance at least q 2 wk.
- Be especially attentive to renal function of elderly.
- Be alert for evidence of new infection and report to physician.

OVERDOSAGE: SIGNS & SYMPTOMS

Neutropenia, emesis, hypersalivation, anorexia, bloody diarrhea, inactivity, cytopenia, elevated liver function test results, elevated BUN and serum creatinine, testicular atrophy, death

Patient/Family Education

- Give patient and family members instructions regarding handling of ganciclovir and proper disposal techniques when drug is to be administered at home.
- Inform patient that it is important to drink plenty of fluids.
- Teach patient being treated for CMV retinitis that drug is not cure, but it may help to keep symptoms from getting worse.
- Advise CMV retinitis patients to have regular ophthalmologic examinations at least q 6 wk during treatment.
- Instruct both male and female patients to use barrier form of contraception for at least 90 days after treatment because ganciclovir is potentially teratogenic.
- Explain to male patients that drug may cause temporary or permanent male infertility.
- Tell patient to avoid crowds and people with infections.
- Instruct patient to report these symptoms to physician: headache, mental status changes, rash, pain at injection site, fever, nausea, unusual bleeding or bruising, black tarry stools or other physical complaints.

See Patient Guide, p. 269.

Gemfibrozil

(gem-FIE-broe-ZILL)

Lopid

Class: Antihyperlipidemic

Action Decreases blood levels of triglycerides and VLDL by decreasing their production. Also decreases cholesterol and increases HDL.

Indications Treatment of hypertriglyceridemia in adult patients with type IV or V hyperlipidemia that presents risk of pancreatitis and does not respond to diet; reduction of coronary heart disease risk in type IIb patients who have low HDL levels (in addition to elevated LDL and triglycerides) and have not responded to other measures.

Contraindications Hepatic or severe renal dysfunction, including primary biliary cirrhosis; preexisting gallbladder disease.

Route/Dosage

ADULTS: **PO** 600 mg bid 30 min before morning and evening meals.

Interactions

Lovastatin: Increases risk of rhabdomyolysis. *Oral anticoagulants (eg, warfarin):* Anticoagulent effect may be increased.

Lab Test Interferences

None well documented.

Adverse Reactions

CV: Atrial fibrillation. *CNS:* Fatigue; vertigo; headache. *EENT:* Blurred vision. *GI:* Dyspepsia; abdominal pain; diarrhea; nausea; vomiting; constipation; acute appendicitis. *GU:* Impotence. *HEMA:* Anemia; leukopenia; bone marrow hypoplasia; eosinophilia. *HEPA:* Elevated liver function test results; cholestatic jaundice. *DERM:* Eczema; rash. *META:* Mild hyperglycemia. *OTHER:* Muscle pain or weakness; myositis; rhabdomyolysis; taste perversions.

Precautions

Pregnancy: Category B. *Lactation:* Undetermined. *Children:* Safety and efficacy not established. *Cholelithiasis:* Drug may increase cholesterol excretion into the bile, leading to cholelithiasis.

NURSING CONSIDERATIONS

Administration/Storage

- Administer 30 minutes before breakfast and supper.
- Store at room temperature in a tightly closed container.

Assessment/Interventions

- Obtain patient history, including drug history and any known allergies. Note preexisting kidney, liver or gallbladder disease or diabetes.
- Assess dietary intake of fats.
- Perform periodic blood counts during first 12 mo of administration.
- Obtain periodic determinations of serum lipids.
- Monitor liver studies.
- Assess for side effects, particularly abdominal pain, nausea and vomiting.

Patient/Family Education

- Inform patient of need to restrict dietary intake of fats; teach patient dietary restrictions to be followed.
- Emphasize importance of decreased cardiac risk factors: smoking, alcohol consumption, lack of exercise.
- Instruct patient to report these symptoms to physician: abdominal pain, persistent nausea and vomiting, bleeding and irregular heartbeat.
- Advise patient that drug may cause dizziness or blurred vision and to use caution while driving or performing other tasks requiring mental alertness.

See Patient Guide, p. 270.

Gentamicin

(JEN-tuh-MY-sin)

Garamycin, Garamycin Intrathecal, Garamycin Pediatric, Gentak, Genoptic, Genoptic S.O.P., Gentacidin, G-myticin, Jenamicin, ♣ Alcomicin, Cidomycin, Diogent

Class: Antibiotic/aminoglycoside

Action Inhibits production of bacterial protein, causing bacterial cell death.

Indications Short-term treatment of serious infections caused by susceptible strains of microorganisms, especially gram-negative bacteria; adjunct to systemic gentamicin in serious CNS infections (intrathecal); treatment of superficial ocular infections (ophthalmic); treatment of superficial skin infections, infection prophylaxis and aid to healing (topical).

Contraindications Long-term therapy (parenteral); epithelial herpes simplex keratitis, vaccinia, varicella, mycobacterial infections, fungal diseases (ophthalmic); hypersensitivity to aminoglycosides.

Route/Dosage

ADULTS: **IM/IV** 3-5 mg/kg/day in divided doses. For obese patients, base dose on estimate of lean body weight. CHILDREN: **IM/IV** 6-7.5 mg/kg/day (2-2.5 mg/kg q 8 hr). INFANTS & NEONATES: **IM/IV** 7.5 mg/kg/day (2.5 mg/kg q 8 hr). PREMATURE OR TERM NEONATES (< 1 WK): **IM/IV** 5 mg/kg/day (2.5 mg/kg q 12 hr) or 2.5 mg/kg q 18 hr or 3 mg/kg q 24 hr.

Prevention of Bacterial Endocarditis

ADULTS: **IM/IV** 1.5 mg/kg with ampicillin ½ hr before procedure (maximum 80 mg). CHILDREN: **IM/IV** 2 mg/kg with ampicillin ½ hr before procedure.

Superficial Skin Infections

ADULTS & CHILDREN: **Topical** Apply 1-4 times daily to infected area.

Ocular Infections

ADULTS & CHILDREN: **Topical** Apply 0.5-inch ribbon of ointment in each eye bid or tid or 1-2 gtt 4-6 times/day.

Interactions

Drugs with nephrotoxic potential (eg, amphotericin, cephalosporins, enflurane, methoxyflurane, vancomycin): May increase risk of nephrotoxicity. *Loop diuretics:* May increase risk of auditory toxicity. *Neuromuscular blocking agents:* May enhance effects of these agents. *Polypeptide antibiotics:* May increase risk of respiratory paralysis and renal dysfunction. INCOMPATIBILITIES: Do not mix beta-lactam antibiotics (eg, penicillins, especially ticarcillin and carbenicillin, cephalosporins) in IV solutions.

Lab Test Interferences

None well documented.

Adverse Reactions

RESP: Apnea; pulmonary fibrosis. *CNS:* Headache; dizziness; vertigo; encephalopathy; confusion; fever; lethargy; convulsions; muscle weakness and twitching; peripheral neuropathy; acute organic brain syndrome; depression; pseudotumor cerebri; increased CSF protein; arachnoiditis or burning at injection site after intrathecal administration. *EENT:* Blurred vision; tinnitus; hearing loss; mydriasis and conjunctival paresthesia (ophthalmic). *GI:* Nausea; vomiting. *GU:* Oliguria; proteinuria; increased serum creatinine and BUN; casts; Fanconi-like syndrome. *HEMA:* Anemia; eosinophilia; leukopenia; thrombocytopenia; granulocytopenia. *HEPA:* Elevated liver function test results. *DERM:* Rash; urticaria; itching; anaphylaxis; photosensitivity (topical). *OTHER:* Pain and irritation at injection site; splenomegaly; hypomagnesemia; hyponatremia; hypocalcemia; hypokalemia.

Precautions

Pregnancy: Category D (parenteral). Category C (ophthalmic). *Lactation:* Undetermined. *Children:* Use cautiously in premature infants and neonates because of renal immaturity. *Elderly or debilitated patients:* Drug levels and renal function must be monitored closely. *Burn patients:* Pharmacokinetics may be altered; serum levels must be closely monitored for dosing. *Hypomagnesemia:* Occurs often, especially in those with restricted diets or poor nutrition. *Neuromuscular blockade:* Potential curare-like effects may aggravate muscle weakness or cause neurotoxicity. Use with caution with anesthesia or muscle relaxants; in patients with neuromuscular disorders, hypomagnesemia, hypocalcemia and hypokalemia; and in neonates whose mothers received magnesium sulfate. *Sulfite sensitivity:* Some products contain sulfites. Do not use if there is history of hypersensitivity. *Toxicity:* Drug is associated with significant nephrotoxicity and ototoxicity. Use with particular caution in patients with renal impairment and elderly patients.

NURSING CONSIDERATIONS

Administration/Storage

- Do not premix with any other drugs; administer separately.
- For topical use, cleanse affected area of skin before applying ointment.
- For ophthalmic use, have patient tilt head back, place medication in conjunctival sac, and instruct patient to close eyes. Apply light finger pressure on lacrimal sac for 1 min after instillation.
- Store at room temperature.

Assessment/Interventions

- Obtain patient history, including drug history and any known allergies. Note sulfite sensitivity.
- Monitor renal function (serum creatinine, BUN, creatinine clearance) and 8th cranial nerve function.
- Peak and trough levels should be evaluated within 48 hr after initiating therapy and then q 3-4 days.
- If culture and sensitivity is ordered, obtain specimen prior to administration of drug.
- Keep patient well hydrated and monitor serum electrolytes.
- Withhold drug and notify physician if any of following symptoms occur: decreased urinary output, headache, dizziness, confusion, tinnitus, vertigo, hearing loss, vaginal itching or discharge.

OVERDOSAGE: SIGNS & SYMPTOMS

Nephrotoxicity, ototoxicity

Patient/Family Education

- With parenteral administration, instruct patient to report any changes in urinary output (decreased), hearing (ringing in ears, hearing loss), dizziness, tingling or numbness in hands and feet, growth on tongue and vaginal itch or discharge.
- For topical application, instruct patient to cleanse affected area of skin prior to application and to notify physician if rash or irritation develops or if condition worsens.
- For ophthalmic use, instruct patient in proper technique for instilling drops or ointment, emphasizing importance of avoiding contact between dispensing container and eyes. Inform patient that drug may cause temporary blurring of vision or stinging after administration. Advise patient to notify physician if stinging, itching or burning increase or if irritation or pain persists. Remaining ophthalmic preparation should be discarded after completion of therapy.
- Instruct patient to continue using medication for prescribed time, even after signs and symptoms have been relieved, to prevent recurrence.
- Caution patient to avoid exposure to sunlight and to use sunscreen or wear protective clothing to avoid photosensitivity reaction.

See Patient Guide, p. 271.

Glimepiride

(GLIE-meh-pie-ride)
Amaryl
Class: Antidiabetic/sulfonylurea

Action Decreases blood glucose by stimulating insulin release from pancreas. May also decrease hepatic glucose production as well as increase sensitivity to insulin.

Indications Adjunct to diet and exercise in type II diabetics whose hyperglycemia cannot be controlled by diet and exercise alone; in combination with insulin for type II diabetics with secondary failure to oral sulfonylureas.

Contraindications Hypersensitivity to sulfonylureas; diabetic ketoacidosis with or without coma.

Route/Dosage
ADULTS: **PO** 1-2 mg QD with breakfast or the first main meal of the day. Increase by 1-2 mg/dose. Titrate at 1-2 week intervals based on blood glucose response. Maintenance: 1 and 4 mg daily (maximum 8 mg/day). Combination therapy with insulin is appropriate for secondary failure to oral sulfonylureas. The same dosing recommendations apply.

Interactions
Alcohol: Produces disulfiram-like reaction (facial flushing, headache, breathlessness). *Chloramphenicol, clofibrate, dicumarol, fenfluramine, histamine H_2 antagonists, miconazole, monoamine oxidase inhibitors, probenecid, salicylates, sulfinpyrazone, sulfonamides, tricyclic antidepressants, urinary acidifiers:* May increase hypoglycemic effect. *Beta-blockers, cholestyramine, diazoxide, rifampin, thiazide diuretics, urinary alkalinizers:* May decrease hypoglycemic effect.

Lab Test Interferences
None well documented.

Adverse Reactions
CV: Although issue is controversial, oral sulfonylureas may have increased risk of cardiovascular morbidity when compared with patients treated with diet alone. *META:* Hypoglycemia. *CNS:* Dizziness. *EENT:* Blurred vision. *GI:* Nausea; vomiting; gastrointestinal pain; diarrhea. *DERM:* Allergic skin reactions (pruritus, erythema, urticaria, morbilliform or maculopapular rash); porphyria cutanea tarda; photosensitivity. *HEMA:* Leukopenia; agranulocytosis; thrombocytopenia; hemolytic anemia; aplastic anemia; pancytopenia. *HEPA:* Cholestatic jaundice; elevated liver function tests. *OTHER:* Headache; asthenia; hyponatremia with or without syndrome of inappropriate antidiuretic hormone (SIADH).

Precautions
Pregnancy: Category C. Insulin is recommended to maintain blood glucose levels during pregnancy. Prolonged severe neonatal hypoglycemia can occur if sulfonylureas are administered at time of delivery. *Lactation:* Undetermined. *Children:* Safety and efficacy not established. *Elderly and debilitated patients:* Increased risk for development of hypoglycemia. Hypoglycemia may be difficult to detect in elderly patients. *Hepatic and renal impairment:* Use with caution; lower doses may be adequate.

NURSING CONSIDERATIONS

Administration/Storage
- The dose should be given with breakfast or the first meal of the day.
- Store at room temperature.

Assessment/Interventions
- Obtain patient history.
- Assess patient for evidence of hypoglycemic reaction; hypoglycemia may be difficult to detect in the elderly.
- Note hepatic or renal impairment.

OVERDOSAGE: SIGNS & SYMPTOMS

Hypoglycemia, tingling of lips and tongue, hunger, nausea, lethargy, tachycardia, sweating, confusion, tremor, convulsions, stupor, coma

Patient/Family Education

- Instruct patient in signs, symptoms and treatment of hypoglycemic reaction.
- Review dietary and exercise guidelines for diabetes with patient.
- Instruct patient to take drug with breakfast.
- Teach patient to self-monitor urine or blood glucose.
- Instruct patient to inform all healthcare providers involved in his/her care that he/she is taking this drug and to carry medical identification (eg, Medi-Alert bracelet).
- Instruct patient to notify healthcare provider if symptoms of hypoglycemia occur (fatigue, excessive hunger, profuse sweating, numbness of extremities) or if blood glucose is below 60 mg/dl.
- Tell patient to notify healthcare provider if symptoms of hyperglycemia occur (excessive thirst or urination, urinary glucose or ketones).
- Instruct patient to report these symptoms to healthcare provider: Nausea, vomiting, diarrhea, heartburn, sore throat, rash, unusual bleeding or bruising, or other physical complaints.
- Advise patient not to take any medication, including OTC, or alcohol without consulting healthcare provider.
- Advise patient to avoid exposure to sunlight or sunlamps and to use sunscreen or wear protective clothing to avoid photosensitivity reaction.

See Patient Guide, p. 272.

Glipizide

(GLIP-ih-zide)

Glucotrol

Class: Antidiabetic/sulfonylurea

Action Decreases blood glucose by stimulating insulin release from pancreas and by increasing tissue sensitivity to insulin.

Indications Adjunct to diet to lower blood glucose in patients with non–insulin-dependent diabetes mellitus (type II) whose hyperglycemia cannot be controlled by diet alone.

Contraindications Hypersensitivity to sulfonylureas; diabetes complicated by ketoacidosis, with or without coma; sole therapy of insulin-dependent (type I) diabetes mellitus; diabetes when complicated by pregnancy.

Route/Dosage

ADULTS: PO 5 mg/day 30 min before breakfast. Dose should be adjusted in 2.5-5 mg/day increments based on blood glucose response. Divided doses may be given (maximum single daily dose 15 mg; maximum total daily dose 40 mg). ELDERLY OR PATIENTS WITH LIVER DISEASE: PO 2.5 mg/day initially.

Interactions

Alcohol: Produces disulfiram-like reactions (facial flushing, headache, breathlessness). *Androgens, chloramphenicol, clofibrate, fenfluramine, fluconazole, gemfibrozil, histamine H_2 antagonists, magnesium salts, methyldopa, monoamine oxidase, oral anticoagulants, phenylbutazone, probenecid, salicylates, sulfinpyrazone, sulfonamides, tricyclic antidepressants, urinary acidifiers:* Hypoglycemic effects may be increased. *Beta-blockers, cholestyramine, diazoxide, hydantoins, rifampin, thiazide diuretics, urinary alkalinizers:* May decrease hypoglycemic effect. *Food:* Absorption is delayed when taken with food. Give drug approximately 30 min before meal.

Lab Test Interferences

Mild to moderate elevations in BUN and creatinine.

Adverse Reactions

CV: May have increased risk of cardiovascular mortality when compared with patients treated with diet alone. *CNS:* Dizziness; vertigo. *EENT:* Tinnitus. *GI:* GI disturbances (eg, nausea, epigastric fullness, heartburn); diarrhea. *GU:* Mild diuresis; elevated BUN and creatinine. *HEPA:* Cholestatic jaundice; elevated liver function test results. *HEMA:* Leukopenia; thrombocytopenia; aplastic anemia; agranulocytosis; hemolytic anemia; pancytopenia; hepatic porphyria. *DERM:* Allergic skin reactions; eczema; pruritus; erythema; urticaria; morbilliform or maculopapular eruptions; lichenoid reactions; photosensitivity. *META:* Hypoglycemia. *OTHER:* Disulfiram-like reaction; weakness; paresthesia; fatigue; malaise.

Precautions

Pregnancy: Category C. Insulin is recommended to maintain blood glucose levels during pregnancy. Prolonged severe neonatal hypoglycemia can occur if sulfonylureas are administered at time of delivery. *Lactation:* Undetermined. *Children:* Safety and efficacy not established. *Elderly and debilitated patients:* Elderly and debilitated patients are particularly susceptible to hypoglycemic action. Hypoglycemia may be difficult to recognize in elderly. *Hepatic and renal impairment:* Use drug with caution and monitor liver and renal function frequently.

NURSING CONSIDERATIONS

Administration/Storage

- Dose can be divided if single dose is not effective. Also divide doses if patient is taking > 15 mg/day.
- Administer drug 30 min before meal; food delays absorption.
- If administering to pregnant patient, discontinue at least 1 mo before expected date of delivery.
- Store in tightly closed container at room temperature.

Assessment/Interventions

- Obtain patient history, including drug history and any known allergies. Note hepatic or renal impairment and nature of patient's diabetes (type I vs type II).
- Check blood sugars frequently and observe for symptoms of hypoglycemia or hyperglycemia and report to physician.
- Test urine for glucose and acetone at least three times daily during titration period; report results to physician.
- When patients with impaired liver or renal function are receiving this drug, check liver and renal function tests frequently.

OVERDOSAGE: SIGNS & SYMPTOMS

Prolonged hypoglycemia, tingling of lips and tongue, hunger, nausea, lethargy, yawning, confusion, agitation, nervousness, tachycardia, sweating, tremor, convulsions, stupor, coma

Patient/Family Education

- Remind patient that medication should be taken on empty stomach 30 min before meals.
- Teach patient to self-monitor blood glucose.
- Emphasize importance of following diabetic diet.
- Inform patient that this drug is not substitute for exercise and diet control and that patient should follow prescribed regimens.
- Instruct patient to inform all physicians involved in his/her care that they are taking this drug.
- Advise patient to carry identification stating that patient is diabetic.
- Inform patient that physician should be contacted if symptoms of hypoglycemia occur (fatigue, excessive hun-

ger, profuse sweating, numbness of extremities).

- Tell patient to notify physician if symptoms of hyperglycemia occur (excessive thirst or urination, urinary glucose or ketones).
- Instruct patient to report these symptoms to physician: nausea, vomiting, diarrhea, heartburn, sore throat, rash, unusual bruising or bleeding or other physical complaints.
- Advise patient not to take any medication (including otc) or alcohol without consulting physician.

See Patient Guide, p. 273.

Glucagon

(GLUE-kuh-gahn)

Available as generic only

Class: Glucose elevating

Action Elevates blood glucose concentrations (by stimulating production from liver glycogen stores), relaxes smooth muscle of GI tract, decreases gastric and pancreatic secretions in GI tract and increases myocardial contractility.

Indications Treatment of severe hypoglycemic reactions in diabetic patients when glucose administration is not possible or during insulin shock therapy in psychiatric patients; diagnostic aid in radiologic examination of stomach, duodenum, small bowel and colon when hypotonic state is advantageous. **Unlabeled uses:** Treatment of propranolol overdose, cardiovascular emergencies and GI disturbances associated with spasms.

Contraindications Standard considerations.

Route/Dosage

Hypoglycemia

ADULTS & CHILDREN: **SC/IM/IV** 0.5-1 mg. May give 1-2 additional doses if needed.

Insulin Shock Therapy

ADULTS: **SC/IM/IV** 0.5-1 mg after 1 hr of coma (larger doses have been used to reverse coma). Patient will usually awaken in 10-25 min. If no response, may repeat dose.

Diagnostic Aid

ADULTS & CHILDREN: **IM/IV** 0.25-2 mg depending on procedure and desired length of smooth muscle relaxation.

Interactions

Anticoagulants, oral: May increase hypoprothrombinemic effects, possibly with bleeding.

Lab Test Interferences

None well documented.

Adverse Reactions

GI: Nausea; vomiting. *OTHER:* Generalized allergic reactions, including urticaria, respiratory distress and hypotension.

Precautions

Pregnancy: Category B. *Lactation:* Undetermined. *Insulinoma/pheochromocytoma:* Administer cautiously to patient with history of insulinoma or pheochromocytoma.

NURSING CONSIDERATIONS

Administration/Storage

- Separate vial of diluting solution is supplied with vial of glucagon crystals. After dilution, solution should be clear; discard if not clear.
- After reconstitution, use solution immediately.
- Position patient on side during administration.
- If necessary, solution may be refrigerated for 48 hr after dilution. Date vial if it is to be used for multiple doses.
- Store unopened vials at room temperature.

Assessment/Interventions

- Obtain patient history, includ-

ing drug history and any known allergies. Note diabetes mellitus.
- Asssess patient's level of compliance with regimen of diabetes control and level of understanding. Obtain family input if patient is unable or unwilling to give this information.
- Initiate safety precautions to prevent injury caused by seizures, falling or aspiration.
- In event of vomiting when neurologic status is decreased, institute measures to maintain patent airway.
- Use fingerstick blood level test to quickly determine glucose level.
- Administer supplemental oral sources of carbohydrates if patient is alert and oriented and does not exhibit any swallowing difficulties.
- Assess for signs and symptoms of hypoglycemic reactions: neurologic alterations, sweating, hunger, weakness, headache, dizziness, tremor, irritability, tachycardia, anxiety.
- Assess blood glucose levels before, during and after administration.
- Assess for nausea and vomiting. Notify physician if vomiting occurs.

OVERDOSAGE: SIGNS & SYMPTOMS
Nausea, vomiting, hypokalemia

Patient/Family Education
- Review with patient and family correct technique for administering IV injections.
- Teach importance of early recognition and treatment of hypoglycemia. Inform patient about immediate use of oral carbohydrates and how to evaluate effectiveness. Teach importance of obtaining fingerstick blood level as soon as feasible.
- Instruct patient to obtain glucagon emergency kit. Instruct family about glucagon administration technique in presence of swallowing difficulties or other neurologic symptoms. Explain importance of notifying physician of such symptoms.
- Tell family to turn patient on side if patient loses consciousness.
- Advise family to administer food to patient after consciousness and swallowing function return.
- Teach patient ways to prevent hypoglycemia (medication administration, dietary modifications, activity) and measures to institute in event of acute illness.
- Emphasize importance of checking medication expiration dates monthly and having sufficient medication on hand.
- Instruct patient to carry medical history identification and quick source of carbohydrates at all times.

See Patient Guide, p. 274.

Glutethimide

(glue-TETH-ih-mide)
Doriden
Class: Sedative and hypnotic

Action Produces CNS depressant effects similar to those of barbiturates.

Indications Short-term relief of insomnia (up to 1 wk).

Contraindications Porphyria, renal impairment.

Route/Dosage
ADULTS: PO 250-500 mg at bedtime. May repeat once at least 4 hr later if needed. Maximum 1 g/day.

Interactions
Activated charcoal: May reduce absorption of glutethimide. *Alcohol and CNS depressants:* May produce additive CNS depressant effects. *Anticoagulants, oral:* May decrease anticoagulant effectiveness, monitor PT. *Anticholingerics/antidepressants:* May have additive anticholingeric effects, such as dry mouth, constipation, urinary retention.

Lab Test Interferences
Metyrapone test: Drug may interfere with results. *Phentolamine test:* Drug

may cause false-positive results. *Urinary 17-ketosteroid tests:* Drug may alter results.

Adverse Reactions

CNS: Headache; vertigo; hangover; drowsiness; dizziness; confusion; depression; paradoxical excitation. *EENT:* Blurred vision. *GI:* Nausea; dry mouth. *HEMA:* Blood dyscrasias (eg, thrombocytopenia, aplastic anemia, leukopenia). *DERM:* Rash; nocturnal diaphoresis.

Precautions

Pregnancy: Category C. *Lactation:* Excreted in breast milk. *Children:* Safety and efficacy not established. *Special risk patients:* Because of its anticholinergic activity, glutethimide may aggravate certain medical conditions such as glaucoma, cardiac arrhythmias, prostatic hypertrophy, bladder neck obstruction and peptic ulcers. Use drug with caution in patients with these conditions. *Abuse/dependence:* Excessive or prolonged use may produce tolerance or physical and psychological dependence. Use with caution in patients with history of drug or alcohol abuse, depression or suicidal tendencies.

NURSING CONSIDERATIONS

Administration/Storage

- Administer ½-1 hr before bedtime. Because glutethimide may have delayed effect, second dose should not be given until 4 hr after last dose.
- Store in tightly capped childproof container.

Assessment/Interventions

- Obtain patient history, including drug history and any known allergies. Note depression and suicidal tendencies.
- Asssess patient for dependence on drugs or alcohol. If signs of drug dependence develop, notify physician. Do not discontinue drug abruptly.
- If grogginess develops in morning, dose may need to be reduced.
- Assess patient's ability to walk (especially if elderly). Institute safety precautions (eg, siderails, supervised walking) as needed.
- If rash develops, notify physician.

OVERDOSAGE: SIGNS & SYMPTOMS

Diminished or absent peristalsis, severe hypotension, tonic muscular spasms, convulsions, hypothermia, CNS depression, dilation of pupils, inadequate ventilation, sudden apnea, depressed or lost deep tendon reflexes, depression or absence of corneal and pupillary reflexes, impairment of memory and ability to concentrate, impaired gait, ataxia, tremors, hyperreflexia, slurring of speech

Patient/Family Education

- Instruct patient to take safety precautions if dizziness or oversedation occur.
- Caution patient not to discontinue this drug abruptly. Withdrawal symptoms may occur if medicine is suddenly discontinued after more than 7 days of use.
- Advise patient to contact physician if rash develops.
- Instruct patient to notify physician if medication is ineffectual in promoting sleep.
- Caution patient not to smoke cigarettes.
- Instruct patient to avoid intake of alcoholic beverages or other CNS depressants.
- Explain that effects of this medication may have sudden onset. Remind

patient to use caution while driving or performing other tasks requiring mental alertness. Point out that there may be a residual or "hangover" effect the day after taking the medication.

See Patient Guide, p. 275.

Glyburide

(glie-BYOO-ride)

DiaBeta, Glynase PresTab, Micronase, ✤ *Euglucon, Gen-Glybe, Novo-Glyburide*

Class: Antidiabetic/sulfonylurea

Action Decreases blood glucose by stimulating insulin release from pancreas. May also decrease hepatic glucose production and/or increased response to insulin.

Indications Adjunct to diet to lower blood glucose in patients with non-insulin-dependent diabetes mellitus (type II) whose hyperglycemia cannot be controlled by diet alone.

Contraindications Hypersensitivity to sulfonylureas; diabetes complicated by ketoacidosis with or without coma; sole therapy of insulin-dependent diabetes mellitus (type I); diabetes when complicated by pregnancy.

Route/Dosage

Nonmicronized Form

ADULTS: **PO** 2.5-5 mg/day with breakfast or first main meal.

Patients More Sensitive to Hypoglycemic Drugs (eg, elderly or patients with renal or hepatic dysfunction)

ADULTS: **PO** 1.25 mg/day initially. Maintenance: 1.25-20 mg daily in single or divided doses (patients receiving > 10 mg/day may have better response to twice-daily dosing).

Micronized Form (Glynase PresTab)

ADULTS: **PO** 1.5-3 mg/day with breakfast or first main meal. Maintenance: 0.75-12 mg/day. Patients receiving > 6 mg/day have more satisfactory response to twice-daily dosing.

Interactions

Alcohol: Produces disulfiram-like reaction (facial flushing, headache, breathlessness). *Adrogens, chloramphenicol, clofibrate, dicumarol, fenfluramine, fluconazole, gemfibrozil, histamine H_2 antagonists, magnesium salts, methyldopa, monoamine oxidase inhibitors, phenylbutazone, probenecid, salicylates, sulfinpyrazone, sulfonamides, tricyclic antidepressants, urinary acidifiers:* May increase hypoglycemic effect. *Beta-blockers, cholestyramine, diazoxide, hydantoins, rifampin, thiazide diuretics, urinary alkalinizers.* May decrease hypoglycemic effect.

Lab Test Interferences

None well documented.

Adverse Reactions

CV: Although issue is controversial, oral sulfonylureas may have increased risk of cardiovascular mortality when compared with patients treated with diet alone. *CNS:* Dizziness; vertigo. *EENT:* Tinnitus. *GI:* Nausea, epigastric fullness; heartburn. *GU:* Mild diuresis; mild to moderate elevations in BUN and creatinine. *HEMA:* Leukopenia; thrombocytopenia; aplastic anemia; agranulocytosis; hemolytic anemia; pancytopenia; hepatic porphyria. *HEPA:* Cholestatic jaundice; elevated liver function test results. *DERM:* Allergic skin reactions; eczema; pruritus; erythema; urticaria; morbilliform or maculopapular eruptions; lichenoid reactions; photosensitivity. *META:* Hypoglycemia. *OTHER:* Disulfiram-like reactions; weakness; paresthesia; fatigue; malaise.

Precautions

Pregnancy: Category B. Insulin is recommended to maintain blood glucose levels during pregnancy. Prolonged severe neonatal hypoglycemia can occur if sulfonylureas are administered at time of delivery. *Lactation:* Undetermined. *Children:* Safety and efficacy not established. *Elderly and debilitated patients:* Elderly and debilitated patients are particularly susceptible to the hypoglycemic action. Hypoglycemia may be difficult to recognize in elderly. *Bioavailability:* Micronized glyburide (Glynase PresTab) and conventional (nonmicronized) glyburide formulations are not equivalent. *Hepatic and renal impairment:* Use drug with caution; lower doses may be adequate.

NURSING CONSIDERATIONS

Administration/Storage

- Administer with first main meal of day; patients taking large doses may require twice-daily dosing.
- Dose must be readjusted when switching between micronized and conventional (nonmicronized) formulations; they are not bioequivalent.
- If administering to a pregnant patient, discontinue at least 1 mo before expected date of delivery.
- Store in tightly capped container, and keep out of reach of children.

Assessment/Interventions

- Obtain patient history, including drug history and any known allergies.
- Note hepatic or renal impairment and the nature of the patient's diabetes (type I vs type II).
- Be aware that hypoglycemia may be difficult to recognize in elderly.
- Test urine for glucose and acetone at least three times daily during titration period, unless patient is already testing blood glucose. Report results to physician.
- When patients with impaired liver or renal function are receiving this drug, check liver and renal function tests frequently.
- Check blood sugars frequently and observe for symptoms of hypoglycemia or hyperglycemia and report to physician.

OVERDOSAGE: SIGNS & SYMPTOMS

Hypoglycemia, tingling of lips and tongue, hunger, nausea, lethargy, yawning, confusion, agitation, nervousness, tachycardia, sweating, tremor, convulsions, stupor, coma

Patient/Family Education

- Review with patient dietary guidelines for diabetes.
- Instruct patient to take drug with meals.
- Teach patient to self-monitor urine or blood glucose.
- Inform patient that this drug is not substitute for exercise and diet control and that patient should follow prescribed regimens.
- Instruct patient to inform all physicians involved in his/her care that he/she is taking this drug and to carry medical identification (eg, Medi-Alert bracelet).
- Instruct patient to notify physician if symptoms of hypoglycemia occur (fatigue, excessive hunger, profuse sweating, numbness of extremities) or if blood glucose is below 60 mg/dl.
- Tell patient to notify physician if symptoms of hyperglycemia occur (excessive thirst or urination, urinary glucose or ketones).
- Instruct patient to report these symptoms to physician: nausea, vomiting, diarrhea, heartburn, sore throat, rash, unusual bruising or bleeding or other physical complaints.
- Advise patient not to take any medication (including otc) or alcohol without consulting physician.

See Patient Guide, p. 276.

Glycerin (Glycerol)

(GLIH-suh-rin)

Fleet Babylax, Ophthalgan Ophthalmic, Osmoglyn, Sani-Supp

Class: Osmotic diuretic; laxative; ophthalmic

Action Reduces intraocular pressure by creating osmotic gradient between plasma and ocular fluids (oral form). Promotes bowel evacuation by local irritation and hyperosmotic actions (rectal form). Reduces edema and clears corneal haze by attracting water through semipermeable corneal epithelium (ophthalmic form).

Indications
Oral: Control of acute attack of glaucoma; reduction of intraocular pressure prior to and after ocular surgery. *Rectal:* Short-term treatment of constipation. *Ophthalmic:* Clearance of edematous corneas to facilitate ophthalmoscopic and gonioscopic examination in acute glaucoma, bullous keratitis and Fuchs' endothelial dystrophy. **Unlabeled use:** Reduction of intraocular and intracranial pressure via special IV preparations.

Contraindications
Oral form: Anuria, severe dehydration, frank or impending acute pulmonary edema, severe cardiac decompensation. *Rectal forms:* Nausea, vomiting, acute surgical abdomen, fecal impaction, intestinal obstruction, undiagnosed abdominal pain.

Route/Dosage
ADULTS: **PO** 1-2 g/kg 1-1½ hr prior to surgery. **PR** Insert 1 suppository (3 g) or 5-15 ml as rectal enema and retain 15 min. **Topical** 1-2 gtt instilled in eye(s) prior to examination. CHILDREN > 6 YR: **PR** Same as adults. CHILDREN 2-6 YR: **PR** 1-1.5 g suppository or 2-5 ml as rectal enema. CHILDREN < 2 YR: Use only on advice of physician.

Interactions None well documented.

Lab Test Interferences
None well documented.

Adverse Reactions
CV: Arrhythmias. *CNS:* Headache; confusion; disorientation; weakness; dizziness; fainting. *EENT:* Ophthalmic solution: Ocular pain and irritation. *GI:* Nausea; vomiting. Rectal form: Excessive bowel activity; abdominal cramps; bloating; flatulence. *DERM:* Rectal form: Perianal irritation; sweating. *META:* Dehydration; hyperosmolar nonketotic coma.

Precautions
Pregnancy: Category C. *Lactation:* Undetermined. *Children:* Do not administer enemas or suppositories to children < 2 yr. Safety and efficacy of other forms undetermined. *Elderly and debilitated patients:* Use with caution. *Special risk patients:* Use oral form with caution in patients with hypovolemia, confused mental states, CHF, diabetes mellitus and severe dehydration.

NURSING CONSIDERATIONS

Administration/Storage

- Administer 50% oral solution with 0.9% Sodium Chloride flavored with orange, lemon or lime juice or administer commercially prepared 50% or 75% flavored solution.
- Administer suppository high in rectum with patient lying down on side; encourage patient to retain suppository in rectum for at least 15 min.
- To administer rectal liquid, have patient lie on left side, insert stem of applicator into rectum with tip pointing toward navel, squeeze unit until nearly all liquid has been dispensed and remove applicator. Small amount of liquid may remain in unit.
- Ophthalmic solution may cause burning sensation in eye. Local anesthetic should be administered before instillation of drug.
- Store suppositories in cool location,

but do not freeze. Other formulations may be stored at room temperature.

Assessment/Interventions

- Obtain patient history, including drug history and any known allergies.
- Assess for nausea, vomiting, headache, altered neurologic status and dehydration.
- With ophthalmic form, assess for eye pain or discomfort.
- With rectal form, assess last bowel movement, use of laxatives, ability to retain suppository and effectiveness of drug regimen.
- Monitor I&O.
- Systemic administration will cause diuresis and possibly hypotension with dizziness. Institute safety precautions in presence of neurologic manifestations. Have patient maintain supine position after administration.
- With oral or ophthalmic forms, do not give hypotonic solutions after drug is administered.
- With rectal form, encourage fluid intake, fiber in diet and activity.

Patient/Family Education

- Inform patient of need to maintain supine position after administration of oral form of drug.
- With rectal form, advise patient about dangers associated with long-term laxative use. Instruct patient in alternative measures to encourage bowel movements (increase fluid intake, increase intake of dietary fiber, increase activity). Instruct patient to avoid laxative use in presence of abdominal pain, vomiting or nausea.

See Patient Guide, pp. 277-278.

Glycopyrrolate

(glie-koe-PIE-row-late)

Robinul, Robinul Forte

Class: Anticholinergic; antispasmodic

Action Exerts anticholinergic effects, resulting in GI smooth muscle relaxation, diminished volume and acidity of GI secretions and reduced pharyngeal, tracheal and bronchial secretions.

Indications

Oral: Adjunctive treatment of peptic ulcer. *Parenteral:* Preoperative administration for reduction of salivary, tracheobronchial and pharyngeal secretions, reduction of volume and acidity of gastric secretions and blockade of cardiac vagal inhibitory reflexes before and during induction of anesthesia and intubation; intraoperatively for counteraction of drug-induced or vagal traction reflexes with associated arrhythmias.

Contraindications Narrow-angle glaucoma; adhesions between iris and lens; obstructive uropathy; obstructive disease of GI tract; paralytic ileus; intestinal atony of elderly or debilitated patient; severe ulcerative colitis; toxic megacolon complicating ulcerative colitis; hepatic or renal disease; tachycardia; myocardial ischemia; unstable cardiovascular status in acute hemorrhage; myasthenia gravis.

Route/Dosage

Peptic Ulcer

ADULTS & CHILDREN > 12 YR: **PO** 1-2 mg bid or tid. **IM/IV** 0.1-0.2 mg tid or qid.

Preanesthetic Medication

ADULTS: **IM** 0.004 mg/kg 20 min-1 hr prior to anesthesia. CHILDREN < 12 YR: **IM** 0.0044-0.0088 mg/kg. CHILDREN < 2 YR: **IM** up to 0.0088 mg/kg.

Intraoperative Medication

ADULTS: **IV** 0.1 mg. May repeat at 2-3 min intervals. CHILDREN: **IV** 0.004 mg/kg (maximum 0.1 mg in single dose); may repeat at 2-3 min intervals.

Reversal of Neuromuscular Blockade

ADULTS & CHILDREN: **IV** 0.2 mg for each 1 mg neostigmine or 5 mg pyridostigmine. Administer simultaneously.

Interactions

Haloperidol: May cause decreased serum haloperidol levels, worsened schizophrenic symptoms and tardive dyskinesia. INCOMPATIBILITIES: Because stability of glycopyrrolate is questionable above pH of 6.0, do not combine in same syringe with methohexital sodium, chloramphenicol sodium succinate, dimenhydrinate, pentobarbital sodium, thiopental sodium, secobarbital sodium, sodium bicarbonate, diazepam, dexamethasone sodium phosphate or buffered solution of lactated Ringer's solution.

Lab Test Interferences

None well documented.

Adverse Reactions

CV: Palpitations; tachycardia; orthostatic hypotension. *CNS:* Headache; flushing; nervousness; drowsiness; weakness; dizziness; confusion; insomnia; fever (especially in children); mental confusion or excitement (especially in elderly, even with small doses); CNS stimulation (restlessness, tremor, hallucinations). *EENT:* Blurred vision; mydriasis; photophobia; cycloplegia; increased intraocular pressure; dilated pupils; nasal congestion. *GI:* Dry mouth; altered taste perception; nausea; vomiting; dysphagia; heartburn; constipation; bloated feeling; paralytic ileus. *GU:* Urinary hesitancy and retention; impotence. *DERM:* Severe allergic reactions including anaphylaxis, urticaria and dermal manifestations. *OTHER:* Suppression of lactation; decreased sweating.

Precautions

Pregnancy: Category B. *Lactation:* Undetermined. *Children:* Not recommended for treatment of peptic ulcer in children < 12 yr. *Elderly and debilitated patients:* May react with excitement, agitation, drowsiness and other untoward manifestations even with small doses. *Special risk patients:* Use with caution in patients with autonomic neuropathy, hepatic or renal disease, ulcerative colitis, hyperthyroidism, coronary heart disease, CHF, cardiac tachyarrhythmias, hypertension, prostatic hypertrophy, hiatal hernia associated with reflux esophagitis. *Anticholinergic psychosis:* Reported in sensitive individuals; may include confusion, disorientation, short-term memory loss, hallucinations, dysarthria, ataxia, coma, euphoria, anxiety, fatigue, insomnia, agitation and inappropriate affect. *Diarrhea:* May be symptom of incomplete intestinal obstruction, especially in patients with ileostomy or colostomy. Treatment of diarrhea with drug is inappropriate and possibly harmful. *Gastric ulcer:* May delay gastric emptying rate and complicate therapy. *Heat prostration:* Can occur in presence of high environmental temperature.

NURSING CONSIDERATIONS

Administration/Storage

- For IM administration give drug undiluted or mixed with D5W, D10W or 0.9% Sodium Chloride.
- May administer undiluted drug IV.
- Do not administer parenteral solution if cloudy.
- Store parenteral and oral formulations at room temperature.

Assessment/Interventions

- Obtain patient history, including drug history and any known allergies.
- Assess bowel sounds and frequency of bowel movements.
- Monitor I&O.
- Monitor vital signs closely, particularly heart rate and BP, during parenteral administration.
- Assess for side effects: palpitations, neurologic alterations, GI alterations.
- Assess urinary output and signs and symptoms of urinary retention.
- Assess for presence of abdominal pain.

OVERDOSAGE: SIGNS & SYMPTOMS

Dry mouth, thirst, vomiting, nausea, abdominal distention, difficulty swallowing, muscular weakness, paralysis, fever, coma, circulatory failure, rapid pulse and respiration, vasodilation, tachycardia with weak pulse, hypertension, hypotension, respiratory depression, palpitations

Patient/Family Education

- Instruct patient that constipation can occur and to institute preventive measures (increase fluids, increase bulk in diet, increase activity).
- Advise patient that urinary hesitancy or retention may be experienced. Instruct patient to assess urination patterns and to notify physician if urinary retention is experienced.
- Inform male patient that impotence is potential side effect and to report this symptom to physician.
- Because drug interferes with body's thermoregulation, instruct patient to avoid exposure to high environmental temperature to prevent heat prostration.
- Instruct patient to notify physician immediately if eye pain or increased sensitivity to light occurs. Emphasize importance of routine eye examinations throughout therapy.
- Inform patient that dry mouth is a normal side effect. Instruct patient to take sips of water frequently, suck on ice chips or sugarless hard candy or chew sugarless gum if dry mouth occurs.
- Caution patient to avoid sudden position changes to prevent orthostatic hypotension.
- Advise patient that drug may cause drowsiness and blurred vision and to use caution while driving or performing other tasks requiring mental alertness.

See Patient Guide, p. 279-280.

Gold Sodium Thiomalate

(gold SO-dee-uhm thigh-oh-MAL-ate)

Aurolate, Myochrysine

Class: Anti-inflammatory/antirheumatic/gold compound

Action Mechanism unknown; suppresses symptoms of rheumatoid arthritis and may slow progression of this disease.

Indications Symptomatic relief of active adult and juvenile rheumatoid arthritis not adequately controlled by other therapies. **Unlabeled uses:** Treatment of pemphigus and psoriatic arthritis.

Contraindications Previous severe reaction to gold compounds or other heavy metals; uncontrolled diabetes mellitus or CHF; severe debilitation; kidney disease; liver disease; severe hypertension; agranulocytosis or bleeding disorder; recent radiation exposure; systemic lupus erythematosus; urticaria; eczema.

Route/Dosage

ADULTS: **IM** As weekly injections: first wk, 10 mg; second wk, 25 mg; third and following wks, 25-50 mg until major clinical improvement or toxicity occurs. If cumulative dose reaches 1 g without improvement, use of gold therapy should be re-evaluated. Once improvement occurs, dose may be decreased or dosing interval increased. Maintenance therapy: 25-50 mg every other wk for 2-20 wk. On basis of response, dosage interval may be increased to every third and subsequently fourth wk (maximum dose per injection: 100 mg). CHILDREN: After test dose of 10 mg, give 1 mg/kg (maximum dose per injection: 50 mg). Dosage schedule similar to that for adults.

Interactions

Cytotoxic drugs, immunosuppressives (except steroids), phenylbutazone: May increase risk of blood dyscrasias. *Antimalarials, penicillamine:* Safety of combination antirheumatic therapy is unknown.

Lab Test Interferences None well documented.

Adverse Reactions May occur months after therapy is discontinued. *RESP:* Interstitial pneumonitis; pulmonary fibrosis. *EENT:* Stomatitis; corneal gold deposition; corneal ulceration; iritis; conjunctivitis; metallic taste. *Children:* Safety and efficacy in children under 6 has not been established. *GI:* Diarrhea; nausea; cholestatic jaundice; ulcerative enterocolitis; GI bleeding; difficulty swallowing; abdominal pain and cramping. *GU:* Nephrotic syndrome or glomerulitis with proteinuria and hematuria. *HEMA:* Anemia; thrombocytopenia; leukopenia; aplastic anemia. *DERM:* Dermatitis; pruritus; exfoliative dermatitis; angioedema; chrysiasis (gray-blue skin pigmentation). *OTHER:* Anaphylactoid reactions within minutes of injection, arthralgias for several days after injection, "nitritoid reaction" (vasomotor reaction with flushing, fainting, weakness, dizziness, sweating, nausea, vomiting, malaise and headache).

Precautions

Pregnancy: Category C. *Lactation:* Excreted in breast milk. *CNS:* Confusion; hallucinations; seizures. *Elderly or debilitated patient:* Use with caution. Tolerance to gold decreases with age. *Special risk patients:* Use with caution in patients with diabetes mellitus, CHF, history of blood dyscrasias, cardiovascular or cerebral circulation problems, skin rash, previous kidney or liver disease, marked hypertension, compromised circulation or inflammatory bowel disease.

NURSING CONSIDERATIONS

Administration/Storage

- Color of solution is pale yellow. Do not administer drug if drug has darkened in color or contains precipitate.
- Mix contents of vial thoroughly before withdrawing into syringe.
- Administer drug only by IM injection into upper outer quadrant of gluteus maximus muscle.
- Instruct patient to remain lying down for 10-15 min after injection.
- Store in light-resistant containers at room temperature.

Assessment/Interventions

- Obtain patient history, including drug history and any known allergies.
- Review patient's history for indications of uncontrolled diabetes mellitus, systemic lupus erythematosus, renal disease, inflammatory bowel disease, liver disease, granulocytopenia and previous hypersensitivity to medication.
- Review patient's laboratory values for indications of gold toxicity such as decreased hemoglobin, WBC < 4000 mm^3, platelets < 100,000-150,000/mm^3, granulocytes < 1500/mm^3, proteinuria and elevated liver enzymes.
- Prior to each injection, assess patient for early signs and symptoms of toxicity: pruritus, dermatitis, stomatitis, metallic taste in mouth, indigestion or diarrhea.
- Collect urine to test for proteinuria and sediment changes prior to each injection.
- Assess patient for possible nitritoid reaction (sweating, fainting, bradycardia, dizziness, flushing, nausea, vomiting, headaches and weakness) and hypersensitivity of allergic reactions (swelling of face, lips or eyelids, thickening of tongue, shortness of breath, rash, hypotension, tachycardia).
- If anaphylactic shock, syncope, bradycardia, thickening of the tongue, dysphagia, shortness of breath or angioneurotic edema occur

within minutes of injection, notify physician immediately.

- Exfoliative dermatitis, nephrosis, thrombocytopenia and leukopenia require cessation of gold treatment.
- Order laboratory test for CBC including platelet estimation before every other injection throughout treatment.
- Monitor patients with GI symptoms for GI bleeding.

OVERDOSAGE: SIGNS & SYMPTOMS

Hematuria, proteinuria, thrombocytopenia, granulocytopenia, fever, nausea, vomiting, diarrhea, skin lesions, urticaria, exfoliative dermatitis, severe pruritus

Patient/Family Education

- Explain that adverse reactions can occur any time during therapy, even months after drug has been discontinued.
- Caution patient to minimize exposure to sun and other sources of ultraviolet light (eg, sunlamp). Explain need to wear protective clothing outdoors.
- Advise patient of importance of continued assessment of disease status and monitoring of renal, hepatic and hematologic functions.
- Teach patient to perform good oral hygiene, including use of soft toothbrush and daily flossing. If mild stomatitis develops, isotonic sodium chloride and sodium bicarbonate solution can be used. Advise patient to avoid strong commercial mouthwashes and spicy or acidic foods.
- Inform patient that joint pain may continue for 1-2 days after injection but will usually decrease after first few injections. Therapeutic effects may not be seen until after 3-6 mo of treatment. Explain that drug will not reverse damage or cure disease but may slow or stop its progression.
- Instruct patient to report these symptoms to physician: dermatitis, pruritus, weakness, metallic taste, fatigue, hematuria, unusual bruising or ecchymosis, nose bleeds, sore mouth or dark-colored stools.

See Patient Guide, p. 281.

Gonadorelin Acetate

(go-NAD-oh-RELL-in ASS-uh-TATE)

Lutrepulse

Class: Gonadotropin-releasing hormone

Action Causes synthesis and release of luteinizing hormone and follicle-stimulating hormone.

Indications Treatment of infertility by induction of ovulation in women with primary hypothalamic amenorrhea.

Contraindications Any condition that could be exacerbated by pregnancy; ovarian cysts or causes of anovulation other than of hypothalamic origin; hormonally dependent tumors.

Route/Dosage

ADULTS: **IV** 5 mcg over pulse period of 1 min and pulse frequency of 90 min delivered via gonadorelin pump. Pump also can be programmed to deliver 2.5 mcg, 10 mcg and 20 mcg doses per pulse. Typically patients are treated for 21 days. If ovulation occurs, therapy is continued for 2 wk to maintain corpus luteum.

Interactions

Ovulation stimulators: Do not use concomitantly.

Lab Test Interferences

None well documented.

Adverse Reactions

GU: Multiple pregnancy; ovarian hyperstimulation. *HEMA:* Mild phlebitis. *DERM:* Local inflammation; hematoma at catheter site. *OTHER:* Anaphylaxis.

Precautions

Pregnancy: Category B. *Lactation:* Undetermined. *Children:* Safety and efficacy in children < 18 yr not established. *Multiple pregnancy*: Multiple pregnancy is possibility. Minimize risk by proper dosage and monitoring. *Ovarian hyperstimulation*: Drug may cause sudden, abnormal ovarian enlargement.

NURSING CONSIDERATIONS

Administration/Storage

- Reconstitute drug immediately prior to use.
- Dilute contents of vial with 8 ml of supplied diluent. Reconstituted solution should be clear, colorless and free of particulate matter.
- After dilution, transfer solution to plastic pump reservoir.
- An 8 ml solution generally supplies 7 consecutive days.
- To avoid sepsis, carefully monitor infusion area and change intravenous site and cannula every 48 hr.
- Store unopened vials at room temperature.

Assessment/Interventions

- Obtain patient history, including drug history and any known allergies.
- Monitor for anaphylactic reaction.
- Assess for irritation or signs of infection at infusion site. Check pump to make sure that it is delivering medication correctly.
- If ovarian enlargement, ascites, pleural effusion or phlebitis occurs, discontinue therapy and notify physician.
- Institute supportive therapy for local inflammation (ie, apply ice intermittently).

OVERDOSAGE: SIGNS & SYMPTOMS

Temporary reduction of pituitary responsiveness

Patient/Family Education

- Advise patient of importance of repeated ovarian ultrasonographic examinations and continued treatment in event of pregnancy.
- When indicated, instruct patient regarding reconstitution of solution and use of pump.
- Instruct patient about potential side effects (eg, local inflammation) and supportive therapy that can be undertaken.
- Inform patient of signs and symptoms of ovarian enlargement, ascites and pleural effusion and advise patient to notify physician immediately if these symptoms occur.

No patient monograph available.

Goserelin Acetate

(GO-suh-REH-lin ASS-uh-TATE)

Zoladex

Class: Gonadotropin-releasing hormone analog

Action Synthetic analog of gonadotropin-releasing hormone (GnRH) that acts as potent inhibitor of pituitary gonadotropin secretion.

Indications Alternative to orchiectomy or estrogen therapy in palliative treatment of advanced carcinoma of prostate; treatment of endometriosis.

Contraindications Hypersensitivity to GnRH, GnRH agonist analogs, D,L-lactic and glycolic acid polymer or acetic acid; pregnancy; breastfeeding or lactation.

Route/Dosage

ADULTS: SC 3.6 mg implant q 28 days into upper abdominal wall by sterile technique under physician supervision.

Interactions None well documented.

Lab Test Interferences

Diagnostic tests of pituitary-gonado-

tropic and gonadal functions: Results may be misleading. *Hypercalcemia in patients with bone metastases:* Drug may cause initial transient increase. *Testosterone:* Drug may cause initial transient increases in serum levels.

Adverse Reactions

CV: Hot flushes; CHF; arrhythmia; cerebrovascular accident; hypertension; MI; peripheral vascular disorder; chest pain. *RESP:* Upper respiratory tract infection; COPD. *CNS:* Pain; lethargy; dizziness; insomnia; anxiety; depression; headache. *GI:* Anorexia; nausea; constipation; diarrhea; ulcer; vomiting. *GU:* Sexual dysfunction; decreased erections; renal insufficiency; urinary obstruction; UTI. *HEMA:* Anemia. *HEPA:* Elevated liver function test results. *DERM:* Rash; sweating. *META:* Gout; hyperglycemia; hypercalcemia; hyperlipidemia; weight gain. *OTHER:* Edema; fever; chills; breast swelling or tenderness; initial worsening of prostatic carcinoma, including possible severe bone pain.

Precautions

Pregnancy: Category X. *Lactation:* Contraindicated. *Children:* Safety and efficacy not established. *Special risk patients:* Isolated cases of spinal cord compression and ureteral obstruction have been reported. Use with caution in patients prone to these problems. *Bone mineral density changes:* Decreases in vertebral trabecular bone mineral density have been observed; patients with certain risk factors (eg, alcohol or tobacco abuse, family history of osteoporosis) may be at additional risk. *Hypersensitivity:* Antibody formation to goserelin has been observed. Although no anaphylactic reactions have been reported, allergic reactions are theoretically possible. *Prostatic cancer worsening:* Drug initially causes transient increase in testosterone. Worsening of signs and symptoms of prostate cancer, such as bone pain, may occur during first few weeks of treatment.

NURSING CONSIDERATIONS

Administration/Storage

- Clean area of upper abdominal skin with alcohol swab. Use local anesthetic to numb skin.
- Aseptically stretch skin and inject subcutaneously into upper abdominal wall. Do not aspirate.
- If blood appears in syringe, do not inject implant. Instead, withdraw needle and discard syringe. Use new syringe at different site.
- Store at room temperature.

Assessment/Interventions

- Obtain patient history, including drug history and any known allergies.
- Assess presence of menstruation or breakthrough bleeding in women after therapy begins.
- Report increased bone pain, symptoms of spinal cord compression (paresthesias, numbness, tingling, loss of sphincter control, motor weakness), ureteral obstruction (pain, chills, fever, dysuria, oliguria), infection (fever, chills) and increase in liver enzymes (ALT, AST) to physician.

Patient/Family Education

- Explain to male patients that bone pain may intensify at beginning of therapy but will lessen over time. Discuss methods of pain management.
- Caution patient that this medication must not be taken during pregnancy or when pregnancy is possible. Advise patient to use reliable form of birth control while taking this drug.
- Warn female patients that menopausal state will be induced pharmacologically and to expect hot flushes and vaginal dryness.
- Inform patient that sexual dysfunction, decreased erections in men and infertility will occur. These side effects are probably reversible.

- Advise patient that gynecomastia may occur but will decrease when treatment is discontinued.
- Instruct male patients that worsening of symptoms of prostate cancer may occur during first few wk of treatment. Advise patient to notify physician if unable to void.
- Instruct patient to report these symptoms to physician: breakthrough bleeding or menstruation, vaginitis, shortness of breath, edema, chest pain, urinary problems, pain, dizziness, depression, nausea, fever and chills.
- Advise patient that drug may cause dizziness and to use caution while driving or performing other tasks requiring mental alertness until effects of drug are known.

See Patient Guide, p. 282.

Griseofulvin

(griss-ee-oh-FULL-vin)

Microsize

Fulvicin U/F, Grifulvin V, Grisactin, ♣ *Grisovin-FP*

Ultrasize

Fulvicin P/G, Gris-PEG, Grisactin Ultra

Class: Anti-infective/antifungal

Action Deposited preferentially into infected skin, which gradually sloughs off and is replaced by noninfected tissue; binds tightly to new keratin, which becomes highly resistant to fungal invasions.

Indications Treatment of ringworm infections of skin, hair and nails caused by susceptible fungi.

Contraindications Porphyria; hepatic disease.

Route/Dosage

ADULTS: PO 500-1000 mg microsize (330-750 mg ultramicrosize) in single or divided doses. May need to give for several weeks. CHILDREN: PO 11 mg microsize kg/day (125-500 mg) or 7.3 mg ultramicrosize/kg/day (82.5-330 mg).

Interactions

Alcohol: Effects of alcohol may be potentiated with tachycardia and flushing. *Anticoagulants:* Anticoagulant effect may be decreased. *Barbiturates:* May depress griseofulvin serum levels. *Oral contraceptives:* May cause loss of contraceptive effectiveness.

Lab Test Interferences

False elevation of vanillylmandelic acid test assayed by photometric tests but not with gas or thin layer chromatography method.

Adverse Reactions

CNS: Headache; fatigue; dizziness; insomnia; confusion; paresthesias. *EENT:* Oral thrush. *GI:* Nausea; vomiting; epigastric distress; diarrhea; GI bleeding. *GU:* Proteinuria. *HEMA:* Leukopenia; granulocytopenia. *HEPA:* Hepatic toxicity. *DERM:* Rash; urticaria. *META:* Interferes with porphyrin metabolism. *OTHER:* Angioneurotic edema.

Precautions

Pregnancy: Category C. *Lactation:* Undetermined. *Hypersensitivity:* Drug may need to be discontinued. Also, penicillin cross-sensitivity is possible, although some penicillin-sensitive patients have used without difficulty. *Lupus:* May excaberate lupus or lupus-like syndrome.

NURSING CONSIDERATIONS

Administration/Storage

- Administer with or after meals, particularly with fatty foods if not contraindicated.
- Generally administered on conjunction with topical agent.
- Do not interchange griseofulvin microsize with ultramicrosize because dosage is different.

- Store at room temperature in tightly closed containers.

Assessment/Interventions

- Evaluate skin condition prior to and throughout therapy.
- Institute general supportive measures to maintain skin integrity.
- Observe for signs of infection or re-infection.
- Institute safety precautions if dizziness or other neurologic alterations occur.

Patient/Family Education

- Advise patient to inspect skin for signs of improvement of infection or re-infection.
- Explain importance of good hygiene, particularly to affected areas.
- Inform patient that beneficial effects of drug may not be observable for weeks to months.
- Emphasize importance of continued follow-up examinations.
- Instruct patient to report these symptoms to physician: fever, sore throat or skin rash.
- Caution patient to avoid intake of alcoholic beverages or other CNS depressants.
- Advise patient that drug may cause dizziness and to use caution while driving or performing other tasks requiring mental alertness.
- Caution patient to avoid exposure to sunlight and to use sunscreen or wear protective clothing to avoid photosensitivity reaction.

See Patient Guide, p. 283.

Guaifenesin (Glyceryl Guaiacolate)

(GWHY-fen-ah-sin)

Amonidrin, Anti-Tuss, Breonesin, Diabetic Tussin EX, Fenesin, Gee-Gee, Genatuss, GG-Cen, Glyate, Glycotuss, Glytuss, GuiaCough CF, GuiaCough PE, Guiatuss, Halotussin, Humibid L.A., Humibid Sprinkle, Hytuss, Malotuss, Mytussin, Naldecon Senior EX, Pneumomist, Robitussin, Scot-tussin Expectorant, Uni-tussin, ♣ *Balminil Expectorant, Benylin-E, Resyl*

Class: Expectorant

Action May enhance output of respiratory tract fluid by reducing adhesiveness and surface tension, thus facilitating removal of viscous mucus and making nonproductive coughs more productive and less frequent. Efficacy not well documented.

Indications Symptomatic relief of respiratory conditions characterized by dry, nonproductive cough and use in presence of mucus in respiratory tract.

Contraindications Standard considerations.

Route/Dosage

ADULTS & CHILDREN ≥ 12 YR: **PO** 100-400 mg q 4 hr (maximum 2.4 g/day). LONG-ACTING TABLETS: **PO** 1-2 tablets q 12 hr. CHILDREN 6-12 YR: **PO** 100-200 mg q 4 hr (maximum 1.2 g/day). CHILDREN 2-6 YR: **PO** 50-100 mg q 4 hr (maximum 600 mg/day). LONG-ACTING TABLETS. **PO** ½ tablet q 12 hr.

Interactions None well documented.

Lab Test Interferences

May cause color interference with certain laboratory determinations of 5-hydroxyindoleacetic acid and vanillylmandelic acid. Discontinue use 48 hr before test.

Adverse Reactions

CNS: Dizziness; headache. *GI:* Nausea; vomiting. *DERM:* Rash; urticaria.

Precautions

Pregnancy: Category C. *Lactation:* Undetermined. *Persistent cough:* May indicate serious condition. Notify physician if cough persists for > 1 wk, tends to recur or is accompanied by high fever, rash or persistent headache.

NURSING CONSIDERATIONS

Administration/Storage
- Follow administration with glass of water.
- Store at room temperature.

Assessment/Interventions
- Obtain patient history, including drug history and any known allergies.
- Assess lung sounds, cough, sputum production and color.
- Maintain fluid intake to 2000 ml per day if no contraindications exist.
- Notify physician if these signs occur: high fever, rash or headaches; persistent cough.

Patient/Family Education
- Explain importance of maintaining increased fluid intake.
- Explain that expectorants are not recommended for some chronic cough conditions, such as cough associated with smoking, emphysema and asthma.
- Instruct patient to report these symptoms to physician: cough persisting for more than 1 wk or if recurring or accompanied by high fever; high fever; rash or headache.

See Patient Guide, p. 284.

Guanabenz Acetate

(GWAHN-uh-benz ASS-uh-TATE)
Wytensin
Class: Antihypertensive/antiadrenergic, centrally acting

Action Appears to stimulate central alpha$_2$-adrenergic receptors, inhibiting sympathetic outflow from brain to peripheral circulation.

Indications Treatment of hypertension.

Contraindications Standard considerations.

Route/Dosage
ADULTS: PO 4 mg bid initially; may increase by 4-8 mg daily every 1-2 wk; maximum dose 32 mg bid.

Interactions
CNS depressants: Increased sedation.

Lab Test Interferences
None well documented.

Adverse Reactions
CV: Chest pain; edema; arrhythmias; palpitations. *RESP:* Dyspnea. *CNS:* Drowsiness; dizziness; sedation; headache; sleep disturbances; anxiety. *EENT:* Blurred vision; nasal congestion; taste disorders. *GI:* Dry mouth; constipation; diarrhea; nausea; vomiting; abdominal discomfort. *GU:* Urinary frequency; disturbances of sexual function. *HEPA:* Increased liver enzymes. *DERM:* Rash; pruritus. *OTHER:* Gynecomastia; muscle or joint pain; weakness.

Precautions
Pregnancy: Category C. *Lactation:* Undetermined. *Children:* Safety and efficacy in children < 12 yr not established. *Special risk patients:* Use with caution in patients with severe coronary insufficiency, recent MI or cerebrovascular disease. *Sedation:* Occurs in large percentage of patients. *Withdrawal:* Do not discontinue therapy without consulting physician; drug must be withdrawn gradually to avoid rapid rise in BP.

NURSING CONSIDERATIONS

Administration/Storage
- Administer with food or milk.
- Store in tightly closed container in cool environment.

Assessment/Interventions
- Obtain patient history, including drug history and any known aller-

gies. Note any cardiovascular or cerebrovascular disease.

- Take patient's BP (lying, sitting, standing) and pulse before administering drug. Monitor periodically throughout therapy.
- Assess for dry mouth and follow treatment measures as necessary.
- Report these signs to physician immediately: hypotension, chest pain, arrhythmias, edema, dyspnea.

OVERDOSAGE: SIGNS & SYMPTOMS

Marked hypotension, somnolence, lethargy, irritability, miosis, bradycardia

Patient/Family Education

- Instruct patient and family member in proper technique for taking BP. Advise patient to check and record BP weekly.
- Advise patient to lie down if dizziness or blurred vision occurs.
- Explain that impotence may occur but is reversible. Tell patient to report to physician.
- Instruct patient not to discontinue drug abruptly.
- Counsel patient about benefits of weight reduction, exercise, reduction of alcohol and sodium, cessation of smoking.
- Instruct patient to report these symptoms to physician: headache, dizziness, weakness, blurred vision.
- Advise patient to take sips of water frequently, suck on ice chips or sugarless hard candy or chew sugarless gum if dry mouth occurs.
- Caution patient to avoid sudden position changes to prevent orthostatic hypotension.
- Instruct patient to avoid intake of alcoholic beverages or other CNS depressants.
- Advise patient that drug may cause drowsiness and to use caution while driving or performing other tasks requiring mental alertness.
- Instruct patient not to take otc medications without consulting physician.

See Patient Guide, p. 285.

Guanadrel Sulfate

(GWAHN-uh-drell SULL-fate)

Hylorel

Class: Antihypertensive/antiadrenergic, peripherally acting

Action Inhibits vasoconstriction by restraining norepinephrine release from nerve storage sites; depletion of norepinephrine causes relaxation of vascular smooth muscle, decreasing total peripheral resistance and venous return.

Indications Treatment of hypertension in patients not responding adequately to thiazide-type diuretic.

Contraindications Pheochromocytoma; concurrent use or use within 1 wk of monoamine oxidase (MAO) inhibitors; frank CHF.

Route/Dosage

ADULTS: **PO** 10 mg/day (5 mg bid) initially. Maintenance dose: 20-75 mg/day, usually in 2 divided doses; tid or qid dosing may be needed. In patients with renal impairment, dosage adjustment may be necessary.

Interactions

Alpha-blockers, beta-blockers, reserpine: Effects of guanadrel may be potentiated, resulting in excessive orthostatic hypotension and bradycardia. *Indirect-acting sympathomimetics (eg, ephedrine):* Reverse antihypertensive effect. MAO *inhibitors, phenothiazines, tricyclic antidepressants:* Inhibit antihypertensive effect.

Lab Test Interferences

None well documented.

Adverse Reactions

CV: Palpatations; chest pain; peripheral edema; orthostatic hypotension; syncope. *RESP:* Shortness of breath; coughing. *CNS:* Fatigue; headache; faintness; drowsiness; paresthesias; confusion; depression; sleep disorders. *EENT:* Dilated pupils; visual disturbances, glossitis. *GI:* Increased bowel movements; gas pain/indigestion; constipation; anorexia; nausea/vomiting; abdominal distress or pain. *GU:* Nocturia; urination urgency or frequency; ejaculation disturbances; impotence; hematuria; decreased urine output. *OTHER:* Excessive weight loss or gain; aching limbs; leg cramps; back or neckache; joint pain or inflammation; gangrene.

Precautions

Pregnancy: Category B. *Lactation:* Undetermined. *Children:* Safety and efficacy not established. *Asthma:* Drug may aggravate asthma because of depletion of catecholamines; drugs used to treat asthma may reduce hypotensive effect of guanadrel. *Surgery:* Discontinue 48-72 hr before elective surgery to prevent vascular collapse during anesthesia; for emergency surgery, preanesthetic and anesthetic agents are administered in reduced dosage.

NURSING CONSIDERATIONS

Administration/Storage

- Administer medication with food or milk.
- Store at room temperature.

Assessment/Interventions

- Obtain patient history, including drug history and any known allergies. Note any CHF, renal disease, asthma and pheochromocytoma.
- Take patient's BP (lying, sitting, standing) and pulse before administering drug. Monitor periodically throughout therapy.
- Assess for symptoms of CHF: edema, dyspnea, wet rales.
- Notify physician if any of these signs occur: hypotension, chest pain, bradycardia, edema, dyspnea, coughing, confusion, syncope, nausea, oliguria, hematuria, excessive weight loss or gain.

OVERDOSAGE: SIGNS & SYMPTOMS

Marked dizziness, blurred vision, syncope, orthostatic hypotension

Patient/Family Education

- Teach proper technique for taking BP. Advise patient to check BP weekly.
- Instruct patient not to discontinue drug abruptly.
- Advise patient about benefits of weight reduction, exercise, reduction of alcohol and sodium intake, cessation of smoking.
- Tell patient to lie down if dizziness or blurred vision occurs.
- Explain that impotence or ejaculation disturbance may occur but is reversible. Tell patient to report to physician.
- Instruct patient to report these symptoms to physician: headache, dizziness, myalgia, depression, chest pain, nausea, visual disturbances.
- Caution patient to avoid sudden position changes to prevent orthostatic hypotension.
- Caution patient to avoid intake of alcoholic beverages or other CNS depressants.
- Advise patient that drug may cause drowsiness and to use caution while driving or performing other tasks requiring mental alertness.
- Instruct patient not to take otc medications without consulting physician.

See Patient Guide, p. 286.

Guanethidine Monosulfate

(gwahn-ETH-ih-deen MAH-no-SULL-fate)

Ismelin

Class: Antihypertensive/antiadrenergic, peripherally acting

Action Interferes with release or distribution of norephinephrine from nerve endings, resulting in reduction in total peripheral resistance and both diastolic and systolic BP.

Indications Treatment of moderate and severe hypertension and renal hypertension, including that secondary to pyelonephritis, renal amyloidosis and renal artery stenosis. **Unlabeled use:** Reflex sympathetic dystrophy and causalgia.

Contraindications Known or suspected pheochromocytoma; frank CHF not related to hypertension; use of monoamine oxidase (MAO) inhibitors.

Route/Dosage

ADULTS: AMBULATORY: **PO** 10 mg qd initially; may increase by approximately 10 mg at 5-7 days; increase only if no decrease in standing BP is observed. Maintenance dose: 25-50 mg qd. HOSPITALIZED: **PO** 25-50 mg initially; increase by 25 or 50 mg/day or qod until desired response is obtained. Loading dose (for severe hypertension): Give at 6 hr intervals over 1-3 days, omitting nighttime dose. CHILDREN: **PO** 0.2 mg/kg/24 hr (6 mg/m^2/24 hr) as single oral dose initially; increase by increment of 0.2 mg/kg/24 hr every 7-10 days. Maximum: 3 mg/kg/24 hr.

Interactions

Anorexiants: May reverse hypotensive effect of drug. MAO *inhibitors:* May decrease effectiveness of guanethidine; discontinue MAO inhibitors > 1 wk before starting guanethidine therapy. *Phenothiazines:* May inhibit hypotensive effect. *Sympathomimetics (eg, ephedrine, epinephrine):* May reverse hypotensive effect of guanethidine; guanethidine may potentiate effects of sympathomimetics. *Tricyclic antidepressants:* May inhibit hypotensive effect of drug.

Lab Test Interferences

None well documented.

Adverse Reactions

CV: Bradycardia; orthostatic fluid retention; edema; angina. *RESP:* Dyspnea; asthma in susceptible individuals. *CNS:* Dizziness; weakness; lassitude; syncope; fatigue; muscle tremor; mental depression; chest paresthesias; ptosis; headache; confusion. *EENT:* Blurred vision; nasal congestion. *GI:* Nausea; vomiting; dry mouth; parotid tenderness; diarrhea (may be severe, requiring discontinuation of therapy); increase in bowel movements. *GU:* Inhibition of ejaculation; nocturia; urinary incontinence; priapism. *HEMA:* Anemia; thrombocytopenia. *OTHER:* Myalgia; weight gain; dermatitis; scalp hair loss; leg cramps.

Precautions

Pregnancy: Category C. *Lactation:* Excreted in breast milk. *Children:* Safety and efficacy not established. *Elderly patients:* More prone to side effects of guanethidine therapy, especially orthostatic hypotension. *Bronchial asthma:* May aggravate the hypersensitive condition of asthmatics because of further catecholamine depletion. *Cardiovascular disease:* Use cautiously in patients with coronary disease, recent MI or cerebral vascular disease, especially with encephalopathy; avoid use in patients with severe cardiac failure. *Fever:* May decrease dosage requirements. *Orthostatic hypotension:* Occurs frequently, especially during initial treatment and with postural changes. *Peptic ulcer:* Ulcers may be aggravated by relative increase in parasympathetic tone. *Preoperative withdrawal:* Withdrawal is recommended 2 wk prior to surgery to reduce risk of vascular collapse and cardiac arrest during anesthesia; during emergency surgery administer preanesthetic and anesthetic agents cautiously in reduced dosages and prepare for possible vascular collapse. *Renal impairment:* Use very cautiously, because hypotension may worsen renal impairment.

NURSING CONSIDERATIONS

Administration/Storage

- Administer with food or milk.
- Store in tightly closed container at room temperature. Keep out of reach of children.

Assessment/Interventions

- Obtain patient history, including drug history and any known allergies. Note any cardiovascular, cerebrovascular or peptic ulcer disease, asthma or pheochromocytoma.
- Take patient's BP (lying, sitting, standing) and pulse before administering drug. Monitor periodically throughout therapy.
- In patients with cardiac decompensation, monitor for weight gain and edema.
- Report these signs to physician immediately: hypotension, chest pain, edema, dyspnea, diarrhea, excessive weight loss or gain, CNS changes.

OVERDOSAGE: SIGNS & SYMPTOMS

Severe drowsiness, hypotension, bradycardia, severe diarrhea, nausea, vomiting, syncope

Patient/Family Education

- Instruct patient in proper technique for taking BP. Advise patient to check BP weekly.
- Caution patient not to get out of bed without help during period of dosage adjustment.
- Advise patient to lie down if dizziness or blurred vision occurs.
- Warn patient not to double up on doses.
- Instruct patient not to discontinue drug abruptly and not to stop taking drug because of feeling better.
- Counsel patient about benefits of weight reduction, exercise, reduction of alcohol and sodium intake and cessation of smoking.
- Explain that impotence and ejaculation disturbances may occur but is reversible. Tell patient to report to physician.
- Instruct patient to report these symptoms to physician: dizziness, diarrhea, confusion, depression, fever, sore throat.
- Caution patient to avoid sudden position changes to avoid orthostatic hypotension.
- Instruct patient to avoid intake of alcoholic beverages or other CNS depressants.
- Advise patient that drug may cause drowsiness and to use caution while driving or performing other tasks requiring mental alertness.
- Instruct patient not to take otc medications without consulting physician.

See Patient Guide, p. 287.

Guanfacine HCl

(GWAHN-fay-seen HIGH-droe-KLOR-ide)

Tenex

Class: Antihypertensive/antiadrenergic, centrally acting

Action Appears to stimulate central alpha$_2$-adrenergic receptors, with decreased sympathetic outflow, causing decrease in peripheral vascular resistance and reduction in heart rate.

Indications Treatment of hypertension. **Unlabeled use:** Amelioration of heroin withdrawal symptoms.

Contraindications Standard considerations.

Route/Dosage
ADULTS: PO 1 mg daily at bedtime; may increase gradually up to 3 mg daily.

Interactions
Alcohol, CNS depressants: Increased CNS depression. *Barbiturates, phenytoin:* Decreased guanfacine levels with loss of antihypertensive effect.

Lab Test Interferences
None well documented.

Adverse Reactions
CV: Chest pain; bradycardia; palpitations. *CNS:* Somnolence; drowsiness; dizziness; headache; sleep disturbances; insomnia; confusion; depression. *EENT:* Conjunctivitis; visual disturbance; tinnitus; rhinitis; taste perversion. *GI:* Dry mouth; constipation; diarrhea; nausea; abdominal discomfort; dyspnea. *GU:* Urinary incontinence; testicular disorder; decreased libido; impotence. *DERM:* Dermatitis; pruritus; sweating. *OTHER:* Paresthesia; paresis; leg cramps; hypokinesia.

Precautions
Pregnancy: Category B. *Lactation:* Excreted in breast milk. *Children:* Safety and efficacy in children < 12 yr not established. *Special risk patients:* Use with caution in patients with severe coronary insufficiency, recent MI, cerebrovascular disease or chronic renal or hepatic impairment. *Sedation:* Occurs in a large percentage of patients. *Withdrawal:* Do not discontinue therapy without consulting physician; drug must be withdrawn gradually to avoid rapid rise in BP (rebound hypertension).

NURSING CONSIDERATIONS

Administration/Storage
- Administer medication at bedtime.
- Give with food or milk if patient experiences stomach upset.
- Store in tightly closed container and protect from light.

Assessment/Interventions
- Obtain patient history, including drug history and any known allergies. Note cardiovascular, cerebrovascular renal or hepatic disease.
- Take patient's BP (lying, sitting, standing) and pulse before administering drug. Monitor periodically throughout therapy.
- Notify physician if these signs occur: hypotension, chest pain, palpitations, anemia, leukopenia, thrombocytopenia, edema, dyspnea, diarrhea.

OVERDOSAGE: SIGNS & SYMPTOMS

Severe drowsiness, hypotension, bradycardia

Patient/Family Education
- Instruct patient to take medication at bedtime.
- Teach patient proper technique for taking BP. Advise patient to check BP weekly.
- Instruct patient not to discontinue drug abruptly.
- Advise patient on benefits of weight loss, exercise, reduction of alcohol and sodium intake and cessation of smoking.
- Instruct patient to lie down if dizziness or blurred vision occurs.
- Explain that impotence may occur but is reversible. Tell patient to report to physician.
- Instruct patient to report these symptoms to physician: dizziness, constipation, headache, insomnia, nausea, sweating or weakness.
- Advise patient to take sips of water frequently, suck on ice chips or sugarless hard candy or chew sugarless gum if dry mouth occurs.
- Caution patient to avoid sudden position changes to avoid orthostatic hypotension.
- Instruct patient to avoid intake of alcoholic beverages or other CNS depressants.

- Advise patient that drug may cause drowsiness and to use caution while driving or performing other tasks requiring mental alertness.
- Instruct patient not to take otc medications without consulting physician.

See Patient Guide, p. 288.

Haemophilus b Conjugate Vaccine

(hem-AHF-ill-us)

HibTITER, OmniHIB, PedvaxHIB, ProHIBIT

Class: Vaccine, inactivated bacteria

Action Induces specific protective antibodies against *Haemophilus influenzae* type b (Hib).

Indications Induction of active immunity against Hib infection. Routine immunization of all infants beginning at age 2 mo is recommended.

Contraindications Hypersensitivity to any product component (some products contain thimerosal).

Route/Dosage

HibTITER

Beginning at 2 months of age, give 3 doses, 2 months apart, plus a booster dose at 15 months.

OmniHIB (or ActHIB)

Beginning at 2 months of age, give 3 doses, 2 months apart, plus a booster dose at 15-18 months.

PedvaxHIB

Beginning at 2 months of age, give 2 doses, 2 months apart, plus a booster dose at 12 months.

ProHIBIT

Beginning at 12 months of age, give 1 dose.

Interactions None well documented.

Lab Test Interferences

Diagnostic value of antigen detection (eg, with latex agglutination kits) may be diminished in suspected Hib disease within few days to 2 wk after immunization.

Adverse Reactions

CNS: Irritability; fever; restless sleep or convulsions. *GI:* Diarrhea; vomiting or loss of appetite. *GU:* Renal failure. *DERM:* Rash or hives. *OTHER:* Guillain-Barré syndrome; local erythema; swelling; tenderness; induration.

Precautions

Pregnancy: Category C. *Lactation:* Undetermined. *Children:* Prohibit is not recommended in children < 12 mo. Hibtiter and Pedvaxhib are not recommended in children < 2 mo. *Interchange:* In general, vaccination series begun with one brand of Hib vaccine should be completed with that brand unless specific information about interchangeability is available. *Anticoagulant therapy:* Administer Hib vaccine with caution to persons receiving anticoagulant therapy.

NURSING CONSIDERATIONS

Administration/Storage

- Administer intramuscular in outer aspect of vastus lateralis, midthigh or outer aspect of upper arm. Do not inject in gluteal area or near major nerve trunk.
- Do *not* inject via intravenous route.
- Inspect product for particulate matter and/or discoloration. If these conditions exist, do not administer vaccine.
- Keep vaccine refrigerated. Do not freeze.

Assessment/Interventions

- Obtain patient history, includ-

ing drug history and any known allergies.
- Interview parent or guardian about child's current health. If any febrile illness or active infection is present, vaccine administration may need to be delayed until after recovery. Also question parent or guardian about any allergies the child might have, specifically to any component of vaccine or previous reactions to vaccine.
- Assess for possible anaphylaxis.

Patient/Family Education

- Advise that acetaminophen (appropriate for age) may be given every 4 hr for low-grade fever. Emphasize that aspirin should *not* be given to children.
- Instruct parent or guardian to report any adverse effects after vaccine administration.
- Remind parent to keep child's immunization record up to date.

No patient monograph available.

Haloperidol

(HAL-oh-pehr-i-dahl)

Haldol, ♣ *Novoperidol*

Haloperidol Decanoate

Haldol Decanoate 50, Haldol Decanoate 100, ♣ *Haldol LA*

Class: Antipsychotic/butyrophenone

Action Has antipsychotic effect, apparently due to dopamine-receptor blockage in CNS.

Indications Management of psychotic disorders; control of Tourette's disorder in children and adults; management of severe behavioral problems in children; short-term treatment of hyperactive children. Long-term antipsychotic therapy (haloperidol decanoate). **Unlabeled uses:** Treatment of phencyclidine (PCP) psychosis; antiemetic.

Contraindications Severe toxic CNS depression or comatose states from any cause; Parkinson's disease.

Route/Dosage

Individualize dosage. ADULTS: **PO** 0.5-40 mg/day in divided doses; up to 100 mg/day in severe cases. ADULTS: **IM** 0.5-5 mg q 60 min; however, q 4-8 hr may be satisfactory.

Haloperidol Decanoate

ADULTS: **IM** (deep injection) Initial dose is 10-20 times oral dose. Usually given q 4 wk. CHILDREN 3-12 YR: **PO** Initially 0.5 mg/day. Increase in 0.5 mg increments every 5-7 days until therapeutic effect is achieved. Total dose divided and given bid or tid.

Interactions

Anesthetics, opiates, alcohol: May increase CNS depressant effects. *Anticholinergics:* May increase anticholinergic effects. May worsen schizophrenic symptoms, decrease haloperidol serum concentrations and lead to tardive dyskinesia. *Carbamazepine:* May decrease effects of haloperidol. *Lithium:* May induce disorientation, unconsciousness and extrapyramidal symptoms.

Lab Test Interferences

Pregnancy tests: False-positive results may occur; less likely to occur with serum test. *Protein-bound iodine:* Increases have been reported.

Adverse Reactions

CV: Orthostatic hypotension; hypertension; tachycardia; ECG changes. *RESP:* Laryngospasm; bronchospasm; increased depth of respiration. *CNS:* Tardive dyskinesia; tardive dystonia; insomnia; restlessness; anxiety; euphoria; agitation; drowsiness; depression; lethargy; headache; confusion; vertigo; seizures; exacerbation of psychotic symptoms; pseudoparkinsonism (eg, mask-like face, drooling, pill rolling, shuffling gait, inertia, tremors, cogwheel rigidity); muscle spasms; dyskinesia; akathisia; oculogyric crises; opisthotonos; hyperreflexia. *EENT:* Cataracts; retinopathy; visual disturbances; mydriasis; increased IOP; nasal congestion. *GI:* Dyspepsia; anorexia; diarrhea; hypersalivation; nausea; vomiting; dry mouth. *GU:* Impotence; sexual dysfunction; priapism; urinary hesitancy or retention. *HEMA:* Agranulocytosis; leukopenia; leukocytosis; anemia. *HEPA:* Jaundice; impaired liver function. *DERM:* Maculopapular and acneiform skin reactions; photosensitivity; hair loss. *OTHER:* Menstrual irregularities; breast enlargement; lactation; gynecomastia; hyperglycemia; hypoglycemia; hyponatremia; elevated prolactin levels; adynamic ileus (may lead to death).

Precautions

Pregnancy: Haloperidol: Safety not established. Haloperidol decanoate: Category C. *Lactation:* Excreted in breast milk. *Children:* Do not use in children < 3 yr. Intramuscular form not recommended in children. *Elderly or debilitated patients:* More susceptible to effects; consider lower dose. *Special risk patients:* Use drug with caution in patients with cardiovascular disease or mitral insufficiency, history of glaucoma, EEG abnormalities or seizure disorders, prior brain damage or hepatic or renal impairment. *Antiemetic effects:* Due to suppression of cough reflex, aspiration of vomitus possible. *CNS effects:* May impair mental or physical abilities, especially during first few days of therapy. *Hepatic effects:* Jaundice usually occurs between second and fourth wk of treatment and is considered hypersensitivity reaction. Usually reversible. *Neuroleptic malignant syndrome (NMS):* Has occurred and is potentially fatal. Signs and symptoms are hyperpyrexia, muscle rigidity, altered mental status, irregular pulse, irregular BP, tachycardia and diaphoresis. *Sensitivity to neuroleptic drugs:* May require lower dosage. *Sudden death:* Has been reported; predisposing factors may be seizures or previous brain damage. Flareup of psychotic behavior may precede death. *Tardive dyskinesia:* Syndrome of potentially irreversible, involuntary dyskinetic movements may develop. Prevalence is highest in elderly, especially women. Use smallest effective dose for shortest period of time needed. *Tartrazine sensitivity:* Note that tartrazine is a component of this product.

NURSING CONSIDERATIONS

Administration/Storage

- Dilute liquid in fruit juice.
- Observe patient carefully when administering to ensure medication is taken and not hoarded.
- Give with food or full glass of water to minimize GI irritation.
- Injectable form should be replaced by oral form as soon as possible.
- Protect liquid concentrate from light and store in opaque bottle.

Assessment/Interventions

- Obtain patient history, including drug history and any known allergies.
- Observe patient for extrapyramidal symptoms and tardive dyskinesia. Notify physician if symptoms develop.
- Assess patient's mental status throughout therapy.
- Evaluate CBC and liver function studies before and periodically throughout therapy.
- Assess I&O and bowel function frequently.
- Take safety precautions such as close patient supervision and removal of harmful objects from patient's environment.
- Increase bulk and fluids in patient's diet to minimize constipation.
- Keep the patient recumbent after intramuscular injection to reduce hypotension.

OVERDOSAGE: SIGNS & SYMPTOMS

CNS depression, somnolence, hypotension, extrapyramidal symptoms, hypertension, agitation, restlessness, convulsions, fever, hypothermia, hyperthermia, coma, autonomic reactions, ECG changes, cardiac arrhythmias

Patient/Family Education

- Caution patient to avoid exposure to sunlight and to use sunscreen or wear protective clothing to avoid photosensitivity reaction.
- Instruct patient to avoid intake of alcoholic beverages or other CNS depressants.
- Instruct patient to use mouth rinses, good oral hygiene and sugarless gum or candy to relieve dry mouth.
- Advise patient to avoid sudden position changes to prevent orthostatic hypotension.
- Instruct patient to report these symptoms to physician: drooling, tremors, shuffling gait, restlessness, muscle spasms, aching or numbness, weakness, impaired vision, sore throat, fever, bleeding or bruising, rash or jaundice.
- Inform patient of possibility of hair loss.
- Advise patient that drug may cause drowsiness and to use caution while driving or performing other tasks requiring mental alertness.

See Patient Guide, p. 289.

Heparin

(HEP-uh-rin)

Heparin Sodium, Heparin Sodium Lock Flush, Hep-Lock, Hep-Lock U/P, Heparin Lock Flush Preservative Free, ♣ *Calcilean, Hepalean, Hepalean-Lok, Heparin Leo*

Class: Anticoagulant

Action Inhibits reactions that lead to clotting.

Indications Prophylaxis and treatment of venous thrombosis and its extensions, pulmonary embolism, peripheral arterial embolism and atrial fibrillation with embolization; diagnosis and treatment of acute and chronic consumption coagulopathies (DIC); prevention of postoperative deep venous thrombosis and pulmonary embolism. **Unlabeled uses:** Prophylaxis of left ventricular thrombi and cerebrovascular accidents post-MI; treatment of myocardial ischemia; prevention of cerebral thrombosis in evolving strokes; adjunctive treatment of coronary occlusion with acute MI.

Contraindications Severe thrombocytopenia; uncontrolled bleeding (except due to DIC); patients in whom suitable blood coagulation tests cannot be performed.

Route/Dosage

ADULTS: **SC** 10,000-20,000 U as initial dose followed by 8000-20,000 U q 8-12 hr. **Intermittent IV** 10,000 U as initial dose followed by 5000-10,000 U q 4-6 hr. **IV infusion** 20,000-40,000 U/day. CHILDREN: **Intermittent IV** 50 U/kg as initial dose followed by 100 U/kg q 4 hr. **IV infusion** 50 U/kg as initial dose followed by 20,000 U/m^2/24 hr.

Low-dose Prophylaxis

SC 5000 U 2 hr before surgery and q 8-12 hr thereafter for 7 days or until patient is fully ambulatory, whichever is longer.

Surgery of Heart and Blood Vessels

ADULTS: 300-400 U/kg.

Blood Transfusion

Add 400-600 U/100 ml of whole blood.

Clearing Intermittent Infusion Sets

10-100 U/ml.

Laboratory Samples

Add 70-150 U/10-20 ml of whole blood.

Interactions

Dipyridamole, hydroxychloroquine,

NSAIDs, salicylates: May cause increased risk of bleeding. INCOMPATIBILITIES: Heparin is acidic and incompatible with many drugs.

Lab Test Interferences

Aminotransferase (AST and ALT): Drug causes increased concentrations.

Adverse Reactions

HEMA: Hemorrhage; thrombocytopenia. *DERM:* Necrosis; transient alopecia; urticaria. *OTHER:* Hypersensitivity (chills, fever, urticaria, asthma, rhinitis, lacrimation, headache, nausea, vomiting, shock); anaphylactoid reactions; allergic vasospastic reactions, including painful ischemia, cyanotic limbs; osteoporosis; priapism; rebound hyperlipidemia on discontinuation.

Precautions

Pregnancy: Category C. *Lactation:* Not excreted in breast milk. *Elderly or debilitated patients:* Higher incidence of bleeding in women > 60 yr. *Benzyl alcohol sensitivity:* Benzyl alcohol, used as preservative in some products, is associated with fatal gasping syndrome in premature infants. *Intramuscular use:* Avoid intramuscular use because of local irritation, erythema, pain, hematoma or ulceration. *Hypersensitivity:* Generalized hypersensitivity can occur. Reactions range from mild to severe. *Hemorrhage:* Hemorrhage can occur at virtually any site. Use heparin with extreme caution in patients at increased risk of hemorrhage. *Hyperlipidemia:* Heparin administration may cause hyperlipidemia in patients with dysbetalipoproteinemia (type III).

NURSING CONSIDERATIONS

Administration/Storage

- Heparin is strongly acidic and is incompatible with many drugs. Avoid mixing any drug with heparin unless specifically advised by physician.
- Avoid intramuscular administration.
- Subcutaneous administration should be deep, preferably into fatty layers of abdomen. Use small-gauge needle to minimize tissue trauma. Bunch up tissue without pinching and insert needle at 90-degree angle to skin. Inject slowly.
- Do not aspirate patient to check entry into blood vessel. Apply gentle pressure to puncture site for about 1 min; do not massage. Rotate injection sites frequently and keep record.
- Intravenous administration may be given undiluted over 1 min.
- For intravenous infusion, dilute prescribed amount in 0.9% Sodium Chloride for Injection, D5W, or Ringer's Injection solution. Use infusion pump to ensure accuracy.
- For heparin locks, inject diluted heparin solution of 10-100 U (0.5-1 ml).
- To prevent incompatibility of heparin with medication, flush heparin lock set with Sterile Water for Injection or 0.9% Sodium Chloride for Injection before and after medication is administered.
- Store at room temperature. Protect from freezing.
- Inspect all preparations for particulate matter prior to administration. Also inspect for discoloration; note that slight discoloration does not alter potency.

Assessment/Interventions

- Obtain patient history, including drug history and any known allergies.
- Monitor vital signs. Report fever, drop in blood pressure, rapid pulse, and other signs and symptoms of hemorrhage to physician.
- Baseline blood coagulation tests, hemoglobin, hematocrit, RBC and platelet counts should be performed before therapy is initiated.
- Monitor I&O during early therapy. Heparin may have diuretic effect beginning 36-48 hr after initial dose and last 36-48 hr after termination of therapy.

- Assess for signs of bleeding and hemorrhage. Venipuncture sites may require pressure to prevent bleeding and hematoma formation.
- Assess for evidence of additional or increased thrombosis.
- Observe injection sites for hematomas, ecchymosis and inflammation.
- Activated partial thromboplastin time (APTT) and activated coagulation time (ACT) are coagulation tests commonly used to monitor heparin therapy. Dosage is adjusted to keep APTT between 1½ and 2 times normal control level. ACT is ideally 2 to 3 times control value in sec.
- During dosage adjustment periods, draw blood for coagulation tests ½ hr before each scheduled subcutaneous or intermittent intravenous dose.
- Follow agency protocol for heparin administration, particularly when "piggybacking" heparin with other drugs.
- Inform all personnel caring for patient that patient is receiving anticoagulant therapy.
- Avoid intramuscular injections of other medication because hematomas may develop.
- In patients requiring long-term anticoagulation therapy, oral anticoagulation therapy should be instituted. To ensure continuous anticoagulation, continue full heparin therapy for several days after PT has reached therapeutic range. Heparin can then be stopped without tapering.
- Monitor patient frequently for signs of infiltration, to see that tubing is not kinked, to ensure that tubing is properly positioned in pump and to check all connections for leakage.
- Construct flow chart indicating dates, coagulation time determinations, Hct, leukocyte and platelet counts, heparin doses and urine and stool tests for occult blood.
- Make accurate observations of clinical response.

OVERDOSAGE: SIGNS & SYMPTOMS

Bleeding, nosebleeds, hematuria, tarry stools, easy bruising or petechiae

Patient/Family Education

- Caution patient to avoid intramuscular injections.
- Advise patient to avoid activities that carry risk of injury.
- Instruct patient to use soft toothbrush and electric razor.
- Caution patient to avoid aspirin and aspirin-containing medications.
- Advise patient to report unusual bruising or bleeding (nosebleeds, bleeding gums) or tarry stools to physician immediately.
- Instruct patient to inform physicians and dentists of use of this medication before treatment or surgery.
- Inform patient of potential for hair loss. Explain that this effect may occur several months after heparin therapy is started. Reassure patient that if alopecia occurs, hair growth will return after drug has been discontinued.
- Advise patient to carry identification card or to wear a medication identification bracelet (ie, Medi-Alert) that indicates heparin therapy.
- Inform female patients that menstruation may be somewhat increased and prolonged. Usually this effect is not contraindication to therapy if bleeding is not excessive and there is no underlying pathologic condition.
- Advise patient that smoking and alcohol may alter response to heparin and therefore are not advised.
- Inform patient that abrupt withdrawal of heparin may precipitate increased coagulability.

See Patient Guide, p. 290.

Hepatitis B Immune Globulin (HBIG)

(hep-uh-TIGHT-iss)

H-BIG, Hep-B-Gammagee, HyperHep

Class: Immune serum

Action Directly neutralizes hepatitis B virus.

Indications For passive, transient prevention of hepatitis B infection after viral exposure via needlestick or mucous membrane contact; prevention of hepatitis B in infants born to HBsAg-positive mothers. Most effective when used within 7 days of exposure.

Contraindications None well documented.

Route/Dosage

ADULTS & CHILDREN: **IM** 0.06 ml/kg (usually 3-5 ml). Administer as soon as possible after exposure and repeat 28-30 days later. NEWBORNS OF HBSAG-POSITIVE MOTHERS: **IM** 0.5 ml. Administer first HBIG dose as soon as possible, preferably < 12 hr after birth. Also give hepatitis B vaccine. If hepatitis B vaccine is declined, repeat HBIG at 3 and 6 mo of age.

Interactions

Anticoagulants: Give HBIG with caution to persons receiving anticoagulant therapy. *Vaccines:* To avoid inactivating vaccines containing live viruses (except measles vaccine) or bacteria, give live vaccines 3 mo after HBIG.

Lab Test Interferences

None well documented.

Adverse Reactions

Other: Local pain and tenderness at injection site; urticaria; angioedema; anaphylactic reactions.

Precautions

Pregnancy: Category C. *Lactation:* Undetermined.

NURSING CONSIDERATIONS

Administration/Storage

- Inspect solution for particulate matter and discoloration before administration.
- Administer intramuscularly, preferably in gluteal or deltoid muscle in adults and children. In newborns administer intramuscularly in anterolateral thigh. Do not give intravenously.
- Always record manufacturer's name and lot number on vial in patient's permanent record file along with date of administration, name and title of person administering injection.
- Refrigerate vials. Do not freeze.

Assessment/Interventions

- Obtain complete history, including drug history and any known allergies.
- Check patient's immunization history to verify that administration regimen is being followed.
- Review patient's medical history for history of serious adverse reactions to previous dose of HBIG.
- Monitor for hypersensitivity and/or anaphylaxis. Epinephrine should always be available to counteract any possible reactions.

OVERDOSAGE: SIGNS & SYMPTOMS

Pain, tenderness

Patient/Family Education

- Instruct parent that all at-risk infants should be vaccinated as soon after birth as possible and again at 3 mo.
- Instruct patient that therapy is useful as postexposure prophylaxis as soon after exposure as possible (preferably within 7 days.)
- Provide patient or parent with immunization history record and record this injection in patient's medical records.
- Instruct patient to give analgesic for

local pain. Avoid giving aspirin to children.

- Inform parent or patient of schedule for vaccination program if necessary.

No patient monograph available.

Hepatitis B Vaccine

(hep-uh-TIGHT-iss)

Engerix-B, Recombivax HB

Class: Vaccine, inactivated virus

Action Induces specific antibodies against hepatitis B virus.

Indications Induction of active immunity against hepatitis B virus among persons of all ages who are currently or who will be at increased risk of infection with this virus. Routine vaccination is recommended for infants and adolescents.

Vaccination is also indicated for those at high risk of exposure to or development of hepatitis B virus (ie, health care personnel, dentists, oral surgeons, patients and staff in hemodialysis units and hematology/oncology units, patients requiring frequent or large-volume blood transfusions or clotting factor concentrates, residents and staff of institutions for mentally handicapped, household and other intimate contacts of persons with persistent hepatitis B antigenemia, infants born to HBsAg-positive mothers, populations with high incidence of hepatitis B virus [Alaskan Eskimos, Indochinese refugees, Haitian refugees], persons at increased risk due to their sexual practices [prostitutes, persons who repeatedly contract STDs, homosexually active men, persons with multiple sexual partners], morticians, embalmers, prisoners, users of illicit injectable drugs, police and fire department personnel who render first aid or medical assistance).

Contraindications Hypersensitivity to yeast or any other component of vaccine.

Route/Dosage

Preexposure and Postexposure Hepatitis B Prophylaxis

ADULTS > 19 YR: Recombivax HB: **IM** 10 mcg at 0, 1 and 6 mo; Engerix-B: **IM** 20 mcg at 0, 1 and 6 mo. ADOLESCENTS 11-19 YR: Recombivax HB: **IM** 5 mcg at 0, 1 and 6 mo; Engerix-B: **IM** 10 mcg at 0, 1 and 6 mo. INFANTS & CHILDREN < 11 YR: Recombivax HB: **IM** 2.5 mcg at 0, 1 and 6 mo; Engerix-B: **IM** 10 mcg at 0, 1 and 6 mo. INFANTS OF HBSAG-POSITIVE MOTHERS: Recombivax HB: **IM** 5 mcg at 0, 1 and 6 mo; Engerix-B: **IM** 10 mcg at 0, 1 and 6 mo. DIALYSIS AND IMMUNOCOMPROMISED PATIENTS: Recombivax HB: **IM** 40 mcg at 0, 1 and 6 mo; Engerix-B: **IM** 40 mcg at 0, 1 and 6 mo. Booster dose may be considered for patients undergoing dialysis if anti-Hbs level is < 10 mIU/ml 1-2 mo after third dose.

Interactions None well documented.

Lab Test Interferences
None well documented.

Adverse Reactions
CNS: Fatigue; weakness; headache; malaise; dizziness. *EENT:* Earache; pharyngitis. *RESP:* Upper respiratory infection. *GI:* Nausea; diarrhea. *OTHER:* Fever; pain, tenderness, pruritus, induration, erythema, ecchymosis, swelling, warmth or nodule formation at injection site.

Precautions
Pregnancy: Category C. *Lactation:* Undetermined. *Elderly patients:* Hepatitis B immunogenicity may be reduced in patients > 40 yr. *Hypersensitivity:* Anaphylaxis and symptoms of immediate hypersensitivity have occurred within hours of administering vaccine. *Immunosuppressed patients:* May require larger doses and may not respond to

vaccine. *Infection:* Delay use of hepatitis B vaccine in presence of serious active infection except when withholding vaccine entails greater risk. *Severely compromised cardiopulmonary status:* Administer vaccine with caution. *Unrecognized hepatitis B infection:* May be present at time of vaccination and vaccine may not prevent hepatitis B because of long incubation period.

NURSING CONSIDERATIONS

Administration/Storage

- Administer intramuscularly in deltoid muscle in adults. In infants and young children administer intramuscularly in anterolateral thigh. Avoid gluteal injection into buttock, which may result in less than optimal immune response.
- May administer vaccine subcutaneously in patients who are at risk of hemorrhage following intramuscular injection (eg, persons with hemophilia or thalassemia). However, subcutaneous route may produce less than optimal response and may lead to increased incidence of local reactions.
- Always record manufacturer's name and vaccine lot number in patient's permanent record file along with date of administration, name and title of person administering vaccine.
- Have epinephrine 1:1000 available in case of laryngospasms.
- Use vaccine as supplied. No dilution or reconstitution is necessary. Note that vaccine is slightly opaque, white suspension.
- Refrigerate unopened and open vials. Do not freeze. Freezing destroys potency.

Assessment/Interventions

- Obtain complete history, including drug history and any known allergies.
- Review patient's medical history for history of serious adverse reactions to previous dose of hepatitis B vaccine.
- Check patient's immunization history to verify that administration regimen is being followed.
- Consider delaying immunization during course of serious active infection.
- Monitor for hypersensitivity and/or anaphylaxis. Epinephrine should always be available to counteract any possible reactions.

Patient/Family Education

- Instruct patient or parent that for vaccine to be effective, all series of injections must be completed.
- Provide patient or parent with immunization history record and record of this immunization in patient's medical records.
- Instruct parent to give antipyretics for fever and/or analgesics (eg, acetaminophen) for local pain.
- Inform patient or parent of immunization schedule.

No patient monograph available.

Hetastarch (Hydroxyethyl Starch; HES)

(HET-uh-starch)

Hespan

Class: Plasma expander

Action Produces expansion of plasma volume. Does not have oxygen-carrying capacity or contain plasma protein, so it is not blood or plasma substitute.

Indications Adjunct therapy for plasma volume expansion in shock due to hemorrhage, burns, surgery, sepsis or other trauma; adjunct in leukapheresis to improve harvesting and increase yield of granulocytes.

Contraindications Severe bleeding disorders; severe cardiac failure; renal failure with oliguria or anuria.

Route/Dosage

Plasma Volume Expansion

ADULTS: **IV** 500-1000 ml/day; dosage does not usually exceed 1500 ml/day.

Leukapheresis

ADULTS: **IV** 250-700 ml.

Interactions None well documented.

Lab Test Interferences

May alter coagulation and result in transient prolongation of prothrombin time (PT), partial thromboplastin time (PTT), bleeding and clotting times, decreased Hct and excessive plasma protein dilution; increases indirect bilirubin concentrations.

Adverse Reactions

CNS: Headache. *EENT:* Submaxillary and parotid glandular enlargement. *GI:* Vomiting. *DERM:* Itching. *OTHER:* Anaphylactoid reactions (eg, periorbital edema, urticaria, wheezing, mild temperature elevation); chills; mild influenza-like symptoms; muscle pain; peripheral edema of lower extremities.

Precautions

Pregnancy: Category C. *Lactation:* Undetermined. *Children:* No data available. *Special risk patients:* Due to possibility of circulatory overload, special care should be taken when administering to patients with renal impairment, at risk of pulmonary edema or with CHF. *Hypersensitivity:* May cause anaphylactoid reactions.

NURSING CONSIDERATIONS

Administration/Storage

- Administer by intravenous infusion only.
- Store at room temperature.
- Do not use if solution is turbid deep brown or if crystalline precipitate forms.

Assessment/Interventions

- Obtain complete history, including drug history and any known allergies.
- Assess for bleeding disorders and severe cardiac failure with oliguria or anuria.
- Take baseline vital signs and hematologic parameters before administration of drug.
- Check vital signs q 5 min for first 30 min following administration.
- Monitor urinary output. If output does not increase, report to physician.
- Monitor CVP during infusion to assess for circulatory overload (elevated CVP, rales/crackles, shortness of breath during and after administration).
- Report prolonged PT, PTT, bleeding and clotting times, decreased Hct, decreased plasma proteins to physician.
- Report anaphylactoid reactions (eg, periorbital edema, urticaria, wheezing, fever), chills, muscle pain, peripheral edema to physician.
- During leukapheresis, monitor CBC, differential WBC count, Hgb, Hct, PT and PTT.

Patient/Family Education

- Instruct patient to report these symptoms to physician: itching, dyspnea, chills, myalgia, headache, vomiting and glandular enlargement.

No patient monograph available.

Hyaluronidase

(high-uhl-yur-AHN-ih-dase)

Wydase

Class: Enzyme

Action Hydrolyzes hyaluronic acid to temporarily decrease viscosity of cellular cement and promote diffusion of injected fluids, localized transudates or exudates, thus facilitating their absorption.

Indications Adjuvant treatment to increase absorption and dispersion of other injected drugs; hypodermolysis; adjunct in subcutaneous urography for improving resorption of radiopaque agents. Adjunct therapy when intravenous administration cannot be accomplished, particularly in infants and small children.

Contraindications Injection into or around infected or acutely inflamed area; injection into area known or suspected to be cancerous.

Route/Dosage
ADULTS: **SC/IM/Intradermal** 150 U. Drug is added to injection solutions or injected subcutaneously. CHILDREN < 3 YR: Limit volume of single clysis to 200 ml. PREMATURE INFANTS OR NEONATES: Do not exceed 25 ml/kg/day. Rate should not exceed 2 ml/min.

Interactions
Local anesthesia: Hastens onset of analgesia and tends to reduce swelling caused by local infiltration, but under spread of local anesthetic solution increases absorption of drug, which shortens duration of action of drug and tends to increase incidence of systemic reaction. INCOMPATIBILITIES: Do not add to solution containing another drug without consulting appropriate references for chemical or physical incompatibilities.

Lab Test Interferences
None well documented.

Adverse Reactions
CV: Cardiac fibrillation. *DERM*: Hypersensitivity reactions, including urticaria and anaphylactic-like reactions.

Precautions
Pregnancy: Category C. *Lactation*: Undetermined. *Children*: Drug may be added to small volumes of solution (up to 200 ml) such as small clysis for infants or solutions of drugs for subcutaneous injection.

NURSING CONSIDERATIONS

Administration/Storage
- Preliminary intradermal skin test for hypersensitivity should be performed.
- Reconstitute 150 U and 1500 U vial with 1 and 10 ml, respectively, of 0.9% Sodium Chloride for Injection to yield 150 U/ml.
- Store unconstituted powder in dry place.
- Keep reconstituted solution refrigerated. Discard after 24 hr.

Assessment/Interventions
- Obtain patient history, including drug history and any known allergies (including thiomensol)
- Check for compatibility and interactions before adding drug to solution containing another drug.
- If itching, rash, hives or difficulty in breathing occur, discontinue drug and notify physician.

OVERDOSAGE: SIGNS & SYMPTOMS

Local edema, urticaria, erythema, chills, nausea, vomiting, dizziness, tachycardia, hypotension

Patient/Family Education
- Instruct patient to report these symptoms to physician: pain at injection site, itching, difficulty in breathing or dizziness.

No patient monograph available.

Hydralazine HCl

(high-DRAL-uh-zeen HIGH-droe-KLOR-ide)

Apresoline, *Nu-Hydral*
Class: Antihypertensive/vasodilator

Action Directly relaxes vascular smooth muscle to cause peripheral vasodilation, decreasing arterial BP and peripheral vascular resistance.

Indications Treatment of essential hypertension (oral form). Treatment of severe essential hypertension (parenteral form). **Unlabeled uses:** Reduction of overload in treatment of CHF, severe aortic insufficiency and after valve replacement.

Contraindications Coronary artery disease; mitral valvular rheumatic heart disease.

Route/Dosage
Adjust individually. ADULTS: **PO** Begin with 10 mg qid for 2-4 days; then 25 mg qid for 3-5 days; then 50 mg qid (maximum 300 mg/day). **IV/IM** 20-40 mg repeated prn. CHILDREN: **PO** 0.75 mg/kg/day in 4 divided doses initially; increase gradually over 3-4 wk to maximum of 7.5 mg/kg/day or 200 mg/day. **IV/IM** 0.1-0.2 mg/kg/dose q 4-6 hr prn.

Interactions
Beta-blockers: May increase effect of hydralazine or effect of beta-blockers. *NSAIDs:* Effects of hydralazine may be decreased.

Lab Test Interferences
None well documented.

Adverse Reactions
CV: Palpitations; tachycardia; angina pectoris; edema. *CNS:* Headache; peripheral neuritis with paresthesias, numbness and tingling; dizziness; tremors; depression; disorientation; anxiety. *EENT:* Lacrimation; conjunctivitis. *GI:* Anorexia; nausea; vomiting; diarrhea; constipation. *HEMA:* Blood dyscrasias; decreased hemoglobin; decreased RBC; leukopenia; agranulocytosis. *OTHER:* Hypersensitivity (eg, rash, urticaria, pruritus, fever, chills, arthralgia, eosinophilia); systemic lupus erythematosus.

Precautions
Pregnancy: Category C. *Lactation:* Excreted in breast milk. *Children:* Safety and efficacy have not been established by controlled clinical trials, but there is experience with its use. *Lupus erythematosus:* Drug may produce clinical picture similar to that with systemic lupus erythematosus (eg, arthralgia, dermatoses, fever, splenomegaly), including glomerulonephritis, when > 50 mg/day is given for long periods. Symptoms usually reverse when drug is discontinued, but treatment may be required. *Renal impairment:* Use drug with caution in patients with advanced renal damage. *Tartrazine sensitivity:* Some of these products contain tartrazine, which can cause allergic-type reactions in susceptible individuals, especially those who have aspirin hypersensitivity.

NURSING CONSIDERATIONS

Administration/Storage
- Administer oral form of drug with food.
- Use parenteral form immediately after drawn into syringe.
- Parenteral solution discolors after contact with metal filter.
- Store at room temperature.

Assessment/Interventions
- Obtain complete history, including drug history and any known allergies. Note use of other medications (particularly beta-blockers and NSAIDs), coronary artery disease, mitral valvular rheumatic heart disease, renal impairment, lupus erythematosus, pregnancy, lactation.
- Monitor BP prior to and frequently during intravenous administration.

- Monitor CBC and antinuclear antibody titer.
- Monitor for orthostatic hypotension.
- If decreased hemoglobin or RBC, leukopenia, agranulocytosis or purpura occur, report to physician.
- If symptoms of lupus erythematosus or positive antinuclear antibody titer occur, notify physician.
- If hypotension occurs during therapy, caution patient to sit or lie down (with head in low position). Discontinue drug and notify physician.

OVERDOSAGE: SIGNS & SYMPTOMS

Hypotension, tachycardia, headache, flushing, MI, myocardial ischemia, cardiac arrhythmias, profound shock

Patient/Family Education

- Instruct patient to take medication with meals to enhance absorption.
- Caution patient to avoid abrupt discontinuation of drug to prevent sudden increase in BP.
- Encourage patient to make lifestyle changes: weight reduction, sodium and alcohol restriction, discontinuance of smoking, regular exercise and behavior modification.
- Advise patient to monitor BP and weight regularly.
- Instruct patient to report sudden weight gain caused by fluid retention.
- Advise patient to follow physician's orders for monitoring of CBC and other laboratory values.
- Advise patient to avoid sudden changes in position or very hot baths to avoid orthostatic hypotension.
- Caution patient not to take otc medications without consulting physician.
- Instruct patient to report these symptoms to physician: prolonged tiredness, muscle or joint pain, chest pain, fever, numbness or tingling of hands or feet, or rash.
- Explain that drug may cause drowsiness and to use caution when driving or performing other tasks requiring mental alertness.

See Patient Guide, p. 291.

Hydrochlorothiazide (HCTZ)

(high-droe-klor-oh-THIGH-uh-zide)

Esidrix, Ezide, Hydro-Par, HydroDIURIL, Oretic, ♣ Apo-Hydro

Class: Thiazide diuretic

Action Enhances excretion of sodium, chloride and water by interferring with transport of sodium ions across renal tubular epithelium.

Indications Adjunctive therapy for edema associated with CHF, hepatic cirrhosis, renal dysfunction, and corticosteroid and estrogen therapy; treatment of hypertenson. **Unlabeled uses:** Prevention of formation and recurrence of calcium nephrolithiasis; therapy for nephrogenic diabetes insipidus.

Contraindications Hypersensitivity to thiazides, related diuretics or sulfonamide-derived drugs; anuria; renal decompensation.

Route/Dosage

Edema

ADULTS: **PO** 25-100 mg/day. Rarely patients may require 200 mg/day.

Hypertension

ADULTS: **PO** 25-50 mg/day as single dose or 2 divided doses. INFANTS < 6 MO: **PO** Up to 3.3 mg/kg/day in 2 doses. INFANTS 6 MO-2 YR: **PO** 12.5-37.5 mg daily in 2 doses. CHILDREN 2-12 YR: **PO** 37.5-100 mg daily in 2 doses.

Interactions

Bile acid sequestrants: May reduce thiazide absorption; give thiazide ≥ 2 hr before resin. *Diazoxide:* May cause hyperglycemia. *Digitalis glycosides:* Diuretic-induced hypokalemia and hypomagnesemia may precipitate digitalis-induced arrhythmias. *Lithium:* May decrease renal excretion of lithium.

Loop diuretics: Synergistic effects may result in profound diuresis and serious electrolyte abnormalities. *Sulfonylureas, insulin:* May decrease hypoglycemic effect of sulfonylureas. May need to increase dosage of sulfonylureas or insulin.

Lab Test Interferences

Drug may decrease serum protein-bound iodine levels without signs of thyroid disturbance. May cause diagnostic interference of serum electrolyte levels, blood and urine glucose levels, serum bilirubin levels and serum uric acid levels. Drug may increase serum magnesium levels in uremic patients. Drug may cause increased concentrations of total serum cholesterol, total triglycerides and LDL.

Adverse Reactions

CV: Orthostatic hypotension. *RESP:* Respiratory distress; pneumonitis; pulmonary edema. *CNS:* Dizziness; lightheadedness; vertigo; headache; paresthesias; weakness; restlessness; insomnia. *EENT:* Blurred vision; xanthopsia (yellow vision). *GI:* Anorexia; gastric irritation; nausea; vomiting; abdominal pain or cramping; bloating; diarrhea; constipation; pancreatitis; sialadenitis. *GU:* Impotence; reduced libido; interstitial nephritis. *HEMA:* Leukopenia; thrombocytopenia; agranulocytosis; aplastic or hypoplastic anemia; hemolytic anemia. *HEPA:* Jaundice. *DERM:* Purpura; photosensitivity; rash; urticaria; necrotizing angiitis, vasculitis, cutaneous vasculitis; alopecia; exfoliative dermatitis; toxic epidermal necrolysis; erythema multiforme; Stevens-Johnson syndrome. *META:* Hyperglycemia; glycosuria; hyperuricemia; electrolyte imbalance. *OTHER:* Muscle cramp or spasm; fever; anaphylactic reactions.

Precautions

Pregnancy: Category B. *Lactation:* Excreted in breast milk. *Children:* Safety and efficacy have not been established in controlled clinical studies. *Hepatic impairment:* Minor alterations of fluid and electrolyte balance may precipitate hepatic coma; use drug with caution. *Hypersensitivity:* May occur in patients with or without history of allergy or bronchial asthma; cross-sensitivity with sulfonamides may also occur. *Lupus erythematosus:* Exacerbation or activation may occur. *Postsympathectomy patients:* Drug may enhance antihypertensive effects. *Renal impairment:* Drug may precipitate azotemia; use drug with caution.

NURSING CONSIDERATIONS

Administration/Storage

- If drug is administered as single dose, give in morning.
- Administer drug with food or milk to minimize GI irritation.
- Store tablets in tightly closed container at room temperature.

Assessment/Interventions

- Obtain patient history, including drug history and any known allergies. Note hypersensitivity to thiazides, oral antidiabetics and sulfonamides.
- Weigh patient daily.
- Monitor I&O and check for fluid retention.
- Monitor BP lying and standing.
- Monitor serum potassium, sodium, calcium, magnesium, blood pH, ABGs, uric acid.
- Monitor renal nonprotein nitrogen, BUN, creatinine and liver (ALT, activated clotting time) function tests.
- Monitor blood and urine glucose levels of diabetic patients.
- Observe closely for anaphylaxis (eg, shortness of breath, rash, edema) after first dose.
- Report rising nonprotein nitrogen, BUN, creatinine or liver enzyme levels to physician.
- Report muscle weakness, cramps, nausea, blurred vision, dizziness and potassium levels < 3.5 to physician.

OVERDOSAGE: SIGNS & SYMPTOMS

Orthostatic or general hypotension, tachycardia, shock, weakness, syncope, confusion, dizziness, electrolyte abnormalities, potassium deficiency, vomiting, nausea, lethargy, cramps of calf muscles, thirst, polyuria, anuria

Patient/Family Education

- Tell patient to take medication early in day with food or milk.
- Instruct patient to monitor weight daily.
- Advise patient to avoid exposure to sunlight and to use sunblock or wear protective clothing to avoid photosensitivity reaction.
- Instruct diabetic patients to report increased levels of blood glucose to physician.
- Caution patient to avoid intake of alcoholic beverages.
- Instruct patient not to take otc medications without physician approval.
- Caution patient to rise slowly from lying or sitting position and to lie down if blurred vision or dizziness occurs.
- Tell patient to report these symptoms to physician: GI disturbances, decrease in urinary output, jaundice, muscle cramps, weakness, nausea, blurred vision or dizziness.
- Instruct patient to drink 2-3 L of fluids daily unless contraindicated by physician.
- Advise patient that drug may cause dizziness and blurred vision and to use caution while driving or performing other tasks requiring mental alertness.
- Tell patient that therapeutic effect may require 2-3 wk.

See Patient Guide, p. 292.

Hydrochlorothiazide/ Triamterene (HCTZ/Triamterene)

(high-droe-klor-oh-THIGH-uh-zide/try-AM-tur-een)

Maxzide-25MG, Dyazide, Maxzide

Class: Diuretic combination

Action Hydrochlorothiazide inhibits reabsorption of sodium and chloride in ascending loop of Henle and early distal tubules. Triamterene interferes with sodium reabsorption at distal tubule. Combination provides additive diuretic activity and antihypertensive effects and minimizes potassium depletion.

Indications Treatment of edema or hypertension in patients who have or are at risk of developing hypokalemia.

Contraindications Anuria; renal decompensation; severe hepatic disease; hypersensitivity to thiazides, triamterene, or sulfonamide-derived drugs; patients receiving spironolactone, amiloride, or potassium supplements; hyperkalemia; metabolic or respiratory acidosis.

Route/Dosage

ADULTS: **PO** 1-2 tablets or capsules daily.

Interactions

Angiotensin-converting enzyme inhibitors: May result in severely elevated serum potassium levels. *Allopurinol:* May increase incidence of hypersensitivity reactions to allopurinol. *Amantadine:* May increase amantadine plasma levels and risk for adverse effects. *Anticoagulants:* May diminish anticoagulant effects. *Bile acid sequestrants:* May reduce thiazide absorption; give thiazide ≥ 2 hr before sequestrant. *Diazoxide:* May cause hyperglycemia. *Digitalis glycosides:* Diuretic-induced hypokalemia and hypomagnesemia may precipitate digitalis-induced arrhythmias. *Indomethacin:* May cause rapid progression into acute renal failure. *Lithium:* May decrease renal excretion of lithium; monitor lithium levels. *Loop diuretics:*

May cause synergistic effects that may result in profound diuresis and serious electrolyte abnormalities. *Methenamines, NSAIDS:* May decrease effectiveness of thiazide. *Potassium preparations:* May severely increase serum potassium levels, possibly resulting in cardiac arrhythmias or cardiac arrest. Monitor serum potassium closely if potassium is administered concurrently. *Sulfonylureas, insulin:* May decrease hypoglycemic effect of sulfonylureas. May need to adjust dosage of sulfonylureas or insulin.

Lab Test Interferences

May interfere with the fluorescent measurement of quinidine serum levels. May decrease serum protein-bound iodine levels without signs of thyroid disturbance.

Adverse Reactions

CV: Orthostatic hypotension. *CNS:* Dizziness; lightheadness; vertigo; headache; paresthesias; weakness; restlessness; insomnia; fatigue. *EENT:* Blurred vision; xanthopsia (yellow vision). *GI:* Anorexia; gastric irritation; nausea; vomiting; abdominal pain or cramping; bloating; diarrhea; constipation; pancreatitis; sialadenitis; dry mouth. *GU:* Impotence; reduced libido; interstitial nephritis; azotemia; elevated BUN and creatinine. *HEMA:* Leukopenia; thrombocytopenia; agranulocytosis; aplastic or hypoplastic anemia; hemolytic anemia; megaloblastic anemia. *HEPA:* Jaundice; liver enzyme abnormalities. *DERM:* Purpura; photosensitivity; rash; urticaria; necrotizing angiitis, vasculitis, cutaneous vasculitis; alopecia; exfoliative dermatitis; toxic epidermal necrolysis; erythema multiforme; Stevens-Johnson syndrome. *META:* Hyperglycemia; glycosuria; hyperuricemia; hyperkalemia; electrolyte imbalance; hypochloremia; hyponatremia. *OTHER:* Muscle cramp or spasm; fever; anaphylactic reactions.

Precautions

Pregnancy: Category C. *Lactation:* Excreted in breast milk. *Children:* Safety and efficacy have not been established. *Electrolyte imbalances and BUN increase:* Hyperkalemia (serum potassium > 5.5 mEq/L), hyponatremia, hypochloremia and increases in BUN may occur. *Hematologic effects:* Triamterene is weak folic acid antagonist and may contribute to megaloblastosis. *Hepatic impairment:* Minor alterations of fluid and electrolyte balance may precipitate hepatic coma; use drug with caution. *Hypersensitivity:* May occur in patients with or without history of allergy or bronchial asthma; cross-sensitivity with sulfonamides may also occur. *Lipids:* May affect total serum cholesterol, total triglycerides and LDL in some patients. *Postsympathectomy patients:* Antihypertensive effects may be enhanced. *Renal impairment:* May precipitate azotemia or hypermagnesemia; use drug with caution. *Renal stones:* Triamterene has been found in renal stones; use drug with caution in patients with histories of stone formation.

NURSING CONSIDERATIONS

Administration/Storage

- Administer as morning dose.
- Give with food or milk.
- Administer every other day to decrease electrolyte imbalance.
- Store in tightly closed container at room temperature.

Assessment/Interventions

- Obtain patient history, including drug history and any known allergies.
- Weigh patient daily.
- Measure I&O.
- Monitor patient's BP with patient lying down and standing.
- Monitor serum potassium, calcium, magnesium, sodium, ABGs, uric acid.
- Monitor renal (nonprotein nitrogen,

BUN, creatinine) and liver (ALT, AST) function tests.

- Monitor blood glucose levels in diabetic patients.
- Observe closely for anaphylaxis (shortness of breath, rash, edema) after first dose.
- Report muscle weakness, cramps, nausea, blurred vision or dizziness to physician.

OVERDOSAGE: SIGNS & SYMPTOMS

Orthostatic or general hypotension, tachycardia, syncope, electrolyte abnormalities, potassium deficiency, vomiting, nausea, shock, weakness, confusion, dizziness, cramps of calf muscles, thirst, polyuria, anuria, lethargy

Patient/Family Education

- Instruct patient to take medication early in day to avoid diuretic effect at night.
- Tell patient to take drug with food or milk and to report GI symptoms.
- Advise patient to limit sodium intake for optimal drug effect.
- Advise patient to limit exposure to sun and to use sunscreen or wear protective clothing to avoid photosensitivity reaction.
- Instruct diabetic patients to report increased levels of blood glucose.
- Caution patient to avoid sudden position changes to prevent orthostatic hypotension.
- Tell patient to report these symptoms to physician: decrease in urinary output, jaundice, muscle cramps, weakness, nausea, blurred vision or dizziness.
- Instruct patient to drink 2-3 L/day of water unless contraindicated.
- Advise patient that drug may cause drowsiness and to use caution while driving or performing other tasks requiring mental alertness.

See Patient Guide, p. 293.

Hydrocodone Bitartrate/ Acetaminophen

(HIGH-droe-KOE-dohn by-TAR-trate/ass-eet-ah-MEE-noe-fen)

Amacodone, Anexsia, Anodynos DHC, Bancap-HC, Co-Gesic, Duocet, Dolacet, Duradyne DHC, Hydrocet, Hydrogesic, HY-PHEN, Margesic H, Lorcet-HD, Lortab, Norcet, Stagesic, T-Gesic, Vicodin, Vicodin ES, Zydone

Class: Narcotic analgesic

Action Inhibits synthesis of prostaglandins and binds to opiate receptors in CNS and peripherally blocks pain impulse generation; produces antipyresis by direct action on hypothalamic heat-regulating center; causes cough suppression by direct central action in medulla; may produce generalized CNS depression.

Indications Management of mild to moderate pain.

Contraindications Hypersensitivity to acetaminophen, hydrocodone or similar compounds.

Route/Dosage

Varies according to product and strength. ADULTS: **PO** 1-2 tablets or capsules (hydrocone 2.5-10 mg; acetaminophen 500-1000 mg) q 4-6 hr or 5-10 ml q 4-6 hr prn. CHILDREN < 12 YR: **PO** 10-15 mg acetaminophen/kg/dose q 4 hr to maximum of 2.6 g/24 hr.

Interactions

Anticholinergics: May produce paralytic ileus. *Carbamazepine, hydantoins, sulfinpyrazone:* May result in increased risk of hepatotoxicity from acetaminophen. *CNS depressants (eg, barbiturates, ethyl alcohol, other narcotics):* May cause CNS toxicity. *MAO inhibitors:* May cause additive CNS toxicity; may cause decreased BP. *Tricyclic antidepressants, phenzothiazines:* May cause additive CNS toxicity.

Lab Test Interferences

With Chemstrip bG, Dextrostix and Visidex II home blood glucose systems, may cause false decrease in mean glucose values. May give false-positive urinary 5-hydroxyindoleacetic acid test. Amylase or lipase may be increased for 24 hours due to narcotic-induced increase in biliary tract pressure.

Adverse Reactions

CV: Hypotension; bradycardia. *RESP:* Dyspnea; respiratory depression; irregular breathing. *CNS:* Lightheadedness; dizziness; sedation; drowsiness; weakness; anxiety; fear; fatigue; dysphoria; psychological dependence; confusion. *GI:* Nausea; vomiting; constipation. *GU:* Decreased urination; urethral spasm.

Precautions

Pregnancy: Category C. *Lactation:* Excreted in breast milk. *Special risk patients:* Closely monitor elderly, debilitated patients and those with conditions accompanied by hypoxia or hypercapnia to avoid decrease in pulmonary ventilation. Also use caution in patients sensitive to CNS depressants. Due to cough suppressant effects, exercise caution when using postoperatively or in patients with pulmonary disease. *Hepatic impairment:* Chronic alcoholics should limit acetaminophen intake to < 2 g/day. *Sulfite sensitivity:* Use caution in sulfite-sensitive individuals; some commercial preparations contain sodium bisulfite.

NURSING CONSIDERATIONS

Administration/Storage

- Administer before pain becomes severe.
- Give medication with food.
- Store at room temperature and protect from light.

Assessment/Interventions

- Obtain complete patient history, including drug history and any known allergies.
- Assess vital signs before and periodically after administration. If hypotension, bradycardia, bradypnea or difficulty in breathing occurs, notify physician.
- Monitor for orthostatic hypotension and supervise ambulation.
- Encourage coughing and deep breathing in patients with pulmonary problems.
- Monitor bowel and hepatic function. If decreased bowel sounds or abdominal distention, jaundice or dark urine occurs, notify physician.
- If confusion or blurred vision occur, institute safety measures and notify physician.
- Check for reduced dosage if another CNS depressant medication is being administered concurrently.

OVERDOSAGE: SIGNS & SYMPTOMS

Blood dyscrasias, respiratory depression and hepatic necrosis (all may occur up to several days after overdose); renal tubular necrosis, hypoglycemic coma, nausea, vomiting, diaphoresis, malaise, somnolence, skeletal muscle flaccidity, bradycardia, hypotension, apnea, cardiac arrest

Patient/Family Education

- Instruct patient to take before pain becomes severe.
- Advise patient to take with food or milk.
- When medication is being used for acute pain, advise patient of possible addiction and explain that drug should be used for short term only.
- Advise patient to change position slowly and to use caution when ambulating and performing other activities requiring mental alertness such as driving or operating machinery.
- Instruct patient to eat high-fiber diet, maintain adequate fluid intake and use stool softener or bulk laxative to prevent constipation.
- Advise patient to avoid alcohol and

any other drug that causes drowsiness such as sleeping aids and antihistamines.
- Instruct patient to discontinue drug and notify physician if blurred vision, rash, or yellowing of skin occurs.
- If lightheadedness, dizziness, drowsiness, nausea or vomiting occur, advise patient to lie down until symptoms subside and to notify physician if symptoms persist.

See Patient Guide, p. 294.

Hydrocortisone (Cortisol)

(HIGH-droe-CORE-tih-sone)

CaldeCort, Cortef Feminine Itch, Cortaid with Aloe, Corticaine, Dermol HC, Extra Strength Gynecort 10, Gynecort-5, Lanacort 5, Lanacort 10, Maximum Strength Lanacort 10, Proctocort, Westcort, U-Cort, ♣ *Barriere-HC, Cortoderm, Emo-Cort*

Hydrocortisone Acetate

Anugard, Anumed, Anusol, Anusol HC, Hemorrhoidal HC, Procto Cream, Proctofoam-HC, Rectocort, ♣ *Cortacet, Corticreme, Cortiment, Hyderm*

Hydrocortisone Cypionate

Cortef

Hydrocortisone Phosphate

Hydrocortone Phosphate

Hydrocortisone Sodium Succinate

A-Hydrocort, Solu-Cortef

Hydrocortisone Valerate

Westcort

Class: Corticosteroid

Action Short-acting glucocorticoid that depresses formation, release and activity of endogenous mediators of inflammation including prostaglandins, kinins, histamine, liposomal enzymes and complement system. Also modifies body's immune response.

Indications Treatment of primary or secondary adrenal cortex insufficiency, rheumatic disorders, collagen diseases, dermatologic diseases, allergic states, allergic and inflammatory ophthalmic processes, respiratory diseases, hematologic disorders (idiopathic thrombocytopenic purpura), neoplastic diseases, edematous states (resulting from nephrotic syndrome), GI diseases (ulcerative colitis and sprue), multiple sclerosis, tuberculous meningitis, trichinosis with neurologic or myocardial involvement. *Intra-articular or soft tissue administration:* Treatment of synovitis of osteoarthritis and symptoms of rheumatoid arthritis, bursitis, acute gouty arthritis, epicondylitis, acute nonspecific tenosynovitis and post-traumatic osteoarthritis. *Intralesional administration:* Treatment of keloids, lesions of lichen planus, psoriatic plaques, granuloma annulare, lichen simplex chronicus, discoid lupus erythematosus, necrobiosis lipoidica diabeticorum, alopecia areata, cystic tumors of aponeurosis or tendon. *Topical administration:* Treatment of inflammatory and pruritic manifestations of corticosteroid-responsive dermatoses. *Rectal administration:* Relief of discomfort associated with hemorrhoids, perianal itching or irritation.

STOP **Contraindications** Systemic fungal infections; IM use in idiopathic thrombocytopenic purpura; administration of live virus vaccines in patients receiving immunosuppressive corticosteroid doses.

Route/Dosage

Hydrocortisone and Hydrocortisone Cypionate

ADULTS & CHILDREN: **PO** 20-240 mg/day.

Hydrocortisone Sodium Phosphate

ADULTS & CHILDREN: **IV/IM/SC** 15-240 mg/day.

Hydrocortisone Sodium Succinate

ADULTS & CHILDREN: **IV/IM** 100-500 mg q 2-6 hr.

Hydrocortisone Acetate (Intralesional, Intra-Articular or Soft Tissue Injection Only)
LARGE JOINTS (KNEE) AND BURSAE: ADULTS & CHILDREN: 25-37.5 mg. SMALL JOINTS (INTERPHALANGEAL, TEMPOROMANDIBULAR) ADULTS & CHILDREN: 10-25 mg. TENDON SHEATHS ADULTS & CHILDREN: 5-12.5 mg. SOFT TISSUE INFILTRATION ADULTS & CHILDREN: 25-75 mg. GANGLIA ADULTS & CHILDREN: 12.5-25 mg. TOPICAL ADULTS & CHILDREN: Apply sparingly to affected areas bid-qid.

Interactions Oral administration of hydrocortisone: *Anticholinesterases:* May antagonize anticholinesterase effects in myasthenia gravis. *Anticoagulants, oral:* May alter anticoagulant dose requirements. *Barbiturates:* May decrease effect of hydrocortisone. *Cholestyramine:* May decrease hydrocortisone levels. *Contraceptives (oral) estrogens:* May decrease clearance of hydrocortisone. *Hydantoins, rifampin:* May increase clearance and decrease therapeutic efficacy of hydrocortisone. *Salicylates:* May reduce serum levels and efficacy of salicylates. *Troleandomycin:* May increase effects of hydrocortisone.

Lab Test Interferences
May cause increased urine glucose and serum cholesterol, decreased serum levels of potassium, T_3 and T_4, decreased uptake of Thyroid ^{131}I, false-negative nitroblue-tetrazolium test for bacterial infection, suppression of skin test reactions.

Adverse Reactions
CV: Thromboembolism or fat embolism; thrombophlebitis; necrotizing angiitis; cardiac arrhythmias or ECG changes; syncopal episodes; hypertension; myocardial rupture; CHF. *CNS:* Convulsions; increased intracranial pressure with papilledema (pseudotumor cerebri); vertigo; headache; neuritis; paresthesias; psychosis. *EENT:* Posterior subcapsular cataracts; increased IOP; glaucoma; exophthalmos. *GI:* Pancreatitis; abdominal distension; ulcerative esophagitis; nausea; vomiting; increased appetite and weight gain; peptic ulcer with perforation and hemorrhage; bowel perforation. *GU:* Increased or decreased motility and number of spermatozoa. *HEMA:* Leukocytosis. *DERM:* Impaired wound healing; thin, fragile skin; petechiae and ecchymoses; erythema; lupus erythematosus-like lesions; subcutaneous fat atrophy; striae; hirsutism; acneiform eruptions; allergic dermatitis; urticaria; angioneurotic edema; perineal irritation; hyperpigmentation or hypopigmentation. Topical application may cause burning; irritation; erythema; dryness; folliculitis; hypertrichosis; pruritus; perioral dermatitis; allergic contact dermatitis; stinging, cracking and tightening of skin; secondary infections; skin atrophy; striae; miliaria; telangiectasia. *META:* Sodium and fluid retention; hypokalemia; hypokalemic alkalosis; metabolic alkalosis; hypocalcemia. *OTHER:* Musculoskeletal effects (eg, weakness, myopathy, muscle mass loss, osteoporosis, spontaneous fractures); endocrine abnormalities (eg, menstrual irregularities, cushingoid state, growth suppression in children, sweating, decreased carbohydrate tolerance, hyperglycemia, glycosuria, increased insulin or sulfonylurea requirements in diabetics); anaphylactoid or hypersensitivity reactions; aggravation or masking of infections; malaise; fatigue; insomnia. Topical use may cause same adverse reactions seen with systemic use because of possibility of absorption.

Precautions
Pregnancy: Safety not established (systemic use); Category C (topical). *Lactation:* Excreted in breast milk. *Children:* Observe growth and development of infants and children on prolonged therapy. *Elderly:* May require lower doses. *Adrenal suppression:* Prolonged (daily systemic) therapy (> 7 days) may lead to hypothalamic-pituitary-adrenal suppression. *Fluid and electrolyte balance:* May cause elevation of blood pressure,

salt and water retention and increased excretion of potassium and calcium. Dietary salt restriction and potassium supplementation may be needed. *Hepatitis:* May be harmful in chronic active hepatitis positive for hepatitis B surface antigen. *Infections:* May mask signs of infection. May decrease host-defense mechanisms. *Ocular effects:* Use caution in patients with ocular herpes simplex because of possible corneal perforation. *Peptic ulcer:* May contribute to peptic ulceration, especially in large doses. *Renal impairment:* Use cautiously; monitor renal function. *Repository injections:* Do not inject SC; avoid injection into deltoid and repeated IM injection into the same site. *Stress:* Increased dosage of rapidly acting corticosteroid may be needed before, during and after stressful situations. *Withdrawal:* Abrupt discontinuation may result in adrenal insufficiency. Discontinue gradually; increase supplementation during times of stress.

NURSING CONSIDERATIONS

Administration/Storage

- Give medication with food.
- With large doses, administer antacids between meals.
- For intra-articular injection, local anesthetic may be administered prior to or mixed in same syringe and used immediately. Unused portions of mixture should be discarded.
- Shake optic solutions well prior to use.
- Apply topical doses sparingly.
- Topical absorption enhanced by heat, hydration, inflamed, denuded or thin skin surfaces or occlusive dressings.
- Avoid mixing topical preparations with other agents.
- Avoid abrupt discontinuation of systemic preparations used for > 7 days.

Assessment/Interventions

- Obtain patient history, including drug history and any known allergies. Note recent use of steroids.
- Monitor for covert infections.
- Monitor BP and body weight.
- Monitor routine laboratory studies including serum K^+ and Na^+.
- Monitor blood glucose.
- Monitor I&O for increased edema.
- Monitor growth and development in infants and children on prolonged therapy.
- Observe for signs of potassium depletion.
- Observe for signs of GI irritation.
- If local irritation occurs with topical use, discontinue and notify physician.
- Following dosage reduction or therapy withdrawal, monitor for signs of adrenal insufficiency, including fatigue, anorexia, nausea, vomiting, diarrhea, weight loss, weakness, dizziness or low blood sugar.
- Notify physician of weight gain, swelling, muscle weakness, black tarry stools, hematemesis, facial puffiness, menstrual irregularities, prolonged sore throat, fever, cold or signs of infection.

OVERDOSAGE: SIGNS & SYMPTOMS

Acute toxicity and death are rare. *Acute adrenal insufficiency (due to withdrawal after long-term use)*: fever, myalgia, arthralgia, malaise, anorexia, nausea, shedding of skin, orthostatic hypotension, dizziness, fainting, dyspnea, hypoglycemia *Cushingoid symptoms (due to chronic large doses)*: moonface, central obesity, striae, hirsutism, acne, ecchymoses, hypertension, osteoporosis, myopathy, sexual dysfunction, diabetes, hyperlipidemia, peptic ulcer, increased susceptibility to infection, electrolyte and fluid imbalance

Patient/Family Education

- Advise patient to take oral medication with food to minimize GI upset.
- Warn patient not to stop taking drug abruptly.
- Caution diabetic patients that insulin

or oral hypoglycemic agent needs may increase.

- Instruct elderly patient to have blood pressure, blood glucose and electrolytes monitored at least q 6 months.
- Advise patient that sunglasses may reduce sensitivity to sunlight that occurs with optic administration.
- Caution against eye contact with topical agents.
- Instruct patient that areas for topical administration should be washed or soaked prior to administration to increase absorption.
- Advise patient to apply topical agents sparingly, rubbing in lightly.
- Caution against covering topically treated areas unless specifically prescribed by physician.
- Advise against mixing topical agents with other products unless advised by physician.
- Instruct patient if topical dose is missed to apply as soon as remembered, but not to double doses.
- Teach patient using suppositories or other hemorrhoidal agents that appropriate diet, fluid intake and adequate exercise are useful treatment adjuncts.
- Remind patient to wear Medi-Alert identification while taking this medication.
- Advise that temporary burning is common after administration of optic preparations.
- Caution patient that systemic reactions may occur with topical applications.

See Patient Guide, pp. 295-297.

Hydromorphone HCl

(HIGH-droe-MORE-phone HIGH-droe-KLOR-ide)

Dilaudid, Dilaudid-HP

Class: Narcotic/analgesic

Action Relieves pain by stimulating opiate receptors in CNS; also causes respiratory depression, inhibition of cough reflex, peripheral vasodilation, inhibition of intestinal peristalsis, sphincter of Oddi spasm, stimulation of chemoreceptors that cause vomiting, and increased bladder tone.

Indications Relief of moderate to severe pain; control of persistent nonproductive cough.

Contraindications Hypersensitivity to similar compounds, depressed ventilatory function; acute asthma; diarrhea due to poisoning or toxins; patients not already receiving large amounts of parenteral narcotics; patients with respiratory depression without access to resuscitative equipment; labor.

Route/Dosage
ADULTS: **PO** 2 mg q 4-6 hr prn; ≥ 4 mg q 4-6 hr for more severe pain. **SC/IM** 1-2 mg q 4-6 hr prn; 3-4 mg q 4-6 hr for more severe pain. **IV** May give slowly over 2-5 min. Use high potency (10 mg/ml) only for patients tolerant to other opiates. **PR** 3 mg q 6-8 hr. *Antitussive:* **PO** 1 mg q 3-4 hr prn.

Interactions
CNS depressants (eg, tranquilizers, sedatives, alcohol): Additive CNS depression. *Barbiturate anesthetics:* May have additive effects.

Lab Test Interferences
Increased amylase and lipase may occur up to 24 hr after dose.

Adverse Reactions
CV: Hypotension; orthostatic hypotension; bradycardia; tachycardia. *RESP:* Respiratory depression; laryngospasm; depression of cough reflex. *CNS:* Lightheadedness; dizziness; sedation; disorientation; incoordination; lethargy; anxiety. *GI:* Nausea; vomiting; constipation; abdominal pain. *GU:* Urinary retention or hesitancy. *DERM:* Sweating; pruritus; urticaria. *OTHER:*

Tolerance; psychological and physical dependence with chronic use.

Precautions

Pregnancy: Category C. *Lactation:* Excreted in breast milk. *Children:* Safety and efficacy not established. *Special risk patients:* Use with caution in patients with myxedema, acute alcoholism, acute abdominal conditions, ulcerative colitis, decreased respiratory reserve, head injury or increased intracranial pressure, hypoxia, supraventricular tachycardia, depleted blood volume or circulatory shock. *Drug dependence:* Hydromorphone has abuse potential. *Hepatic or renal impairment:* May need to reduce dose.

NURSING CONSIDERATIONS

Administration/Storage

- Administer before pain becomes severe.
- Give medication with food.
- If vomiting occurs, administer with antiemetic.
- Store at room temperature and protect from light.

Assessment/Interventions

- Obtain complete patient history, including drug history and any known allergies.
- Assess vital signs before and periodically after administration. If hypotension, bradycardia, bradypnea, or difficulty in breathing occurs, notify physician.
- Monitor I&O and check for urinary retention.
- Monitor for orthostatic hypotension and supervise ambulation.
- Encourage coughing and deep breathing in patients with pulmonary problems.
- Monitor bowel function. If decreased bowel sounds or abdominal distention occur, notify physician.
- Check for reduced dosage in patients with impaired renal and liver function.

OVERDOSAGE: SIGNS & SYMPTOMS

Miosis, respiratory and CNS depression, apnea, bradycardia, hypotension, circulatory collapse, seizures, cardiopulmonary arrest, death

Patient/Family Education

- Instruct patient to take medication before pain becomes severe.
- Advise patient to take medication with food or milk to decrease stomach upset.
- Advise patient that drug may cause drowsiness and to use caution while driving or performing other tasks requiring mental alertness.
- Advise patient to eat high-fiber diet and to maintain adequate fluid intake. A stool softener or bulk laxative may be recommended to prevent constipation.
- Instruct patient to avoid intake of alcoholic beverages or other CNS depressants.
- Instruct patient to discontinue drug and notify physician if difficulty in breathing or persistent nausea, vomiting or constipation occurs.
- When medication is used for acute pain, caution patient about potential for addiction and explain that medication should be used for short term only.

See Patient Guide, p. 298.

Hydroxychloroquine Sulfate

(high-drox-ee-KLOR-oh-kwin SULL-fate)

Plaquenil Sulfate

Class: Anti-infective/antimalarial; antirheumatic

Action May interfere with parasitic nucleoprotein (DNA/RNA) synthesis and parasite growth or cause lysis of parasite or infected erythrocytes. In rheumatoid arthritis, may suppress formation of antigens responsible for symptom-producing hypersensitivity reactions.

Indications Prophylaxis and treatment of acute attacks of malaria due to *Plasmodium vivax, Plasmodium malariae, Plasmodium ovale* and susceptible strains of *Plasmodium falciparum*. Treatment of chronic discoid and systemic lupus erythematosus (SLE) and acute or chronic rheumatoid arthritis in patients not responding to other therapies.

Contraindications Retinal or visual field changes caused by any 4-aminoquinoline compound; hypersensitivity to 4-aminoquinoline compounds; long-term therapy in children.

Route/Dosage

Suppression of Malaria

ADULTS: **PO** 400 mg (310 mg of base) weekly on same day each week. CHILDREN: **PO** 5 mg/kg of base weekly on same day each week, up to maximum of 400 mg (310 mg of base). Begin 1-2 weeks prior to exposure; continue for 8 weeks after leaving area.

Acute Attack of Malaria

ADULTS: Initial dose **PO** 800 mg (620 mg of base). CHILDREN: Initial dose **PO** 10 mg/kg (base), up to adult dose; give half of initial dose 6 hours later and on days 2 and 3.

Rheumatoid Arthritis

ADULTS: Initially **PO** 400-600 mg/day (310-465 mg of base) with food or milk. Maintenance: After good response (usually 4-12 weeks), reduce dosage by 50% and continue at **PO** 200-400 mg/day (155-310 mg of base). CHILDREN: Although experience with hydroxychloroquine in children for rheumatoid arthritis or lupus erythematosus is limited, its use may be warrented in some cases. A dose of 3 to 5 mg/kg/day, up to a maximum of 400 mg/day (given once or twice daily) has been recommended. Do not exceed a dose of 7 mg/kg/day.

Lupus Erythematosus

ADULTS: Initially **PO** 400 mg/day or bid. For prolonged therapy, reduce to **PO** 200-400 mg/day (155-310 mg of base).

Interactions

Digoxin: May increase serum digoxin levels. *Hepatotoxic drugs:* May increase potential for hepatoxicity.

Lab Test Interferences

None well documented.

Adverse Reactions

CV: Hypotension; ECG changes. *CNS:* Headache; irritability; nervousness; emotional changes; nightmares; psychosis; dizziness; vertigo; nystagmus; nerve deafness; convulsions; ataxia. *EENT:* Disturbance of accommodation with blurred vision; transient corneal edema; corneal opacities; decreased corneal sensitivity; retinal edema; retinal atrophy; abnormal retinal pigmentation; loss of retinal reflexes; optic disc pallor and atrophy; scotoma; retinopathy; tinnitus. *GI:* Anorexia; nausea; vomiting; diarrhea; abdominal cramps. *HEMA:* Aplastic anemia; agranulocytosis; leukopenia; thrombocytopenia; hemolysis in G-6-PD deficiency; exacerbation of porphyria. *DERM:* Bleaching of hair; alopecia; pruritus; skin and mucosal pigmentation; skin eruptions; exacerbation of psoriasis. *META:* Weight loss. *OTHER:* Immunoblastic lymphadenopathy; extraocular muscle palsies; skeletal muscle weakness; absent or hypoactive deep tendon reflexes.

Precautions
Pregnancy: Category C. *Lactation:* Excreted in breast milk. *Children:* Deaths have occurred following accidental ingestion of relatively small doses. Do not exceed recommended doses for children with malaria. Not indicated for juvenile rheumatoid arthritis. *Special risk patients:* May exacerbate psoriasis, porphyria, or other dermatitis; may cause hemolysis in patients with G-6-PD deficiency. *Renal/hepatic disease or alcoholism:* May increase risk of hepatotoxicity in these conditions. *Muscular weakness:* If weakness occurs, discontinue. *Ophthalmic effects:* Irreversible retinal damage with long-term hydroxychloroquine therapy has been observed.

NURSING CONSIDERATIONS

Administration/Storage

- Give medication with food or milk.
- Store at room temperature in tightly closed container and protect from light.

Assessment/Interventions

- Obtain complete patient history, including drug history and any known allergies.
- Monitor periodic blood counts, and include eye examinations and knee and ankle reflex testing in assessments of patients on prolonged therapy.
- Monitor liver function throughout therapy.
- If unusual bleeding or bruising occurs, notify physician and withhold intramuscular injections.

OVERDOSAGE: SIGNS & SYMPTOMS

Headache, drowsiness, visual disturbances, cardiovascular collapse, convulsions, respiratory and cardiac arrest, bradycardia, ventricular fibrillation

Patient/Family Education

- Advise patient to take with food or milk and to discontinue drug and notify physician if severe stomach pain, loss of appetite, nausea, vomiting or diarrhea occurs.
- Explain that urine may be brown or rust color.
- If drug is being taken to prevent malaria, instruct patient to take each dose on same day each week.
- Advise patient to avoid alcohol during therapy.
- Instruct patient to have periodic eye examinations during long-term therapy.
- If drug is being taken for rheumatoid arthritis, explain to patient that it may take up to 6 months for drug to take effect and to notify physician if condition has not improved at this time.
- Advise patient to discontinue drug and notify physician if any of following occurs: fever, sore throat, unusual bleeding or bruising; changes in vision; ringing in ears or hearing loss; changes in color of skin or oral surfaces; skin rash or itching; muscle weakness; bleaching or loss of hair; mood or mental changes.
- If diarrhea, loss of appetite, nausea, vomiting, abdominal pain becomes persistent or bothersome, advise patient to notify physician.

See Patient Guide, p. 299.

Hydroxyurea

(high-DROX-ee-you-REE-uh)
Hydrea
Class: Antineoplastic

Action Inhibits DNA synthesis, thus interfering with normal cell repair process and decreasing cell survival rate.

Indications Treatment of melanoma; treatment of resistant chronic myelocytic leukemia; treatment of recurrent, metastatic or inoperable ovarian cancer; concomitant administration (with irradiation therapy) in treatment of primary squamous cell carcinomas of head and neck, excluding lip. *Orphan drug use:* Treatment of sickle cell anemia.

Contraindications Marked bone marrow depression; severe anemia.

Route/Dosage

Intermittent Therapy for Solid Tumors and Concomitant Therapy With Irradiation

ADULTS: **PO** 80 mg/kg as single dose every 3 days.

Continuous Therapy for Solid Tumors and for Resistant Chronic Myelocytic Leukemia

ADULTS: **PO** 20-30 mg/kg as single daily dose.

Interactions None well documented.

Lab Test Interferences

Serum uric acid, BUN and creatinine: Hydroxyurea may increase serum levels.

Adverse Reactions

GI: Stomatitis; gastric irritation; anorexia; nausea; vomiting; diarrhea; constipation; mucositis in combination with irradiation. *GU:* Renal tubular function impairment with elevated serum uric acid, BUN, creatinine levels. *HEMA:* Bone marrow depression; anemia; leukopenia; thrombocytopenia. *HEPA:* Elevation of hepatic enzymes. *DERM:* Maculopapular rash; facial erythema. *OTHER:* Fever; chills; malaise.

Precautions

Pregnancy: Not recommended in pregnancy. *Lactation:* Undetermined. *Children:* Safety and efficacy in children have not been established. *Elderly patients:* May be more sensitive to effects and need lower doses. *Bone marrow suppression:* Leukopenia is generally first manifestation. *Erythema:* Patients with prior irradiation therapy may have exacerbation of postirradiation erythema. *Erythrocytic abnormalities:* Self-limiting megaloblastic erythropoiesis is often seen early in therapy. *Renal impairment:* Use drug with caution.

NURSING CONSIDERATIONS

Administration/Storage

- If patient prefers or is unable to swallow capsule, empty contents of capsule into glass of water and have patient take immediately.
- Store away from excessive heat.

Assessment/Interventions

- Obtain patient history, including drug history and any known allergies.
- Monitor uric acid, CBC, BUN and serum creatinine levels and liver function tests throughout therapy.
- Monitor hydration if patient experiences nausea and vomiting.
- Observe patient's skin for changes.
- If WBC count falls, monitor patient for signs of infection.
- Take safety precautions if patient experiences drowsiness.
- Notify physician if signs of uric acid nephropathy occurs.
- Give extra fluids.
- If platelet count falls below 100,000/mm^3, notify physician.

Patient/Family Education

- Caution patient that this medication must not be taken during pregnancy or when pregnancy is possible. Advise patient to use reliable form of birth control while taking this drug.
- Instruct patient to drink at least 8 full glasses of fluid daily.
- Advise patient to avoid contact with people with contagious infections.

- Stress importance of returning for follow-up blood testing.
- Instruct patient to report these symptoms to physician: fever, chills, sore throat, nausea, vomiting, loss of appetite, diarrhea, sores in mouth and on lips or unusual bleeding or bruising.
- Inform patient of possibility of reversible hair loss.
- Advise patient that drug may cause drowsiness and to use caution while driving or performing other tasks requiring mental alertness.

See Patient Guide, p. 300.

Hydroxyzine HCl

(high-DROX-ih-zeen HIGH-droe-KLOR-ide)

Anxanil, Atarax, Atarax 100, E-Vista, Hydroxacen, Hyzine-50, Quiess, Vistacon, Vistaject-25, Vistaject-50, Vistaquel 50, Vistaril, Vistazine 50, ♣ *Multipax*

Class: Antipsychotic

Action May be due to suppression of activity in subcortical areas of CNS.

Indications Symptomatic relief of anxiety and tension associated with psychoneurosis; adjunct therapy in organic disease states with anxiety; management of pruritus due to allergic conditions; sedative before and after general anesthesia. *Intramuscular route only:* Relief of anxiety in acutely disturbed or hysterical patient; treatment of alcoholic delirium tremens or anxiety withdrawal symptoms; preoperative and postoperative and prepartum and postpartum adjunctive medication to permit reduction in narcotic dosage; alleviation of anxiety; control of emesis; adjunctive therapy in asthma.

Contraindications Standard considerations.

Route/Dosage

Anxiety

ADULTS: **PO** 50-100 mg qid. CHILDREN > 6 YR: **PO** 50-100 mg/day in divided doses. CHILDREN < 6 YR: **PO** 50 mg/day in divided doses.

Pruritus

ADULTS: **PO** 25 mg tid-qid. CHILDREN > 6 YR: **PO** 50-100 mg/day in divided doses. CHILDREN < 6 YR: **PO** 50 mg/day in divided doses.

Sedation

ADULTS: **PO** 50-100 mg. CHILDREN: **PO** 0.6 mg/kg.

Psychiatric and Emotional Emergencies (including acute alcoholism)

ADULTS: **IM** 50-100 mg stat and q 4-6 hr prn.

Nausea and Vomiting

ADULTS: **IM** 25-100 mg. CHILDREN: **IM** 1.1 mg/kg.

Preoperative and Postoperative Administration

ADULTS: **IM** 25-100 mg. CHILDREN: **IM** 1.1 mg/kg.

Prepartum and Postpartum Administration

ADULTS: **IM** 25-100 mg.

Interactions

Alcohol and CNS depressants: CNS depressant effects may be increased.

Lab Test Interferences

None well documented.

Adverse Reactions

CV: Chest tightness. *RESP:* Hypersensitivity reactions (eg, wheezing, shortness of breath). *CNS:* Transitory drowsiness; involuntary motor activity, including tremor and convulsions. *GI:* Dry mouth.

Precautions

Pregnancy: Safety not established; avoid use. *Lactation:* Undetermined.

NURSING CONSIDERATIONS

Administration/Storage

- Injectable form is for intramuscular use.
- Administer oral dose with meals to enhance absorption.
- Shake suspension well before administration.

Assessment/Interventions

- Obtain patient history, including drug history and any known allergies.
- Monitor lying and standing BP and pulse periodically throughout course of therapy.
- Assess degree of nausea and frequency and amount of emesis.
- Assist with ambulation during initial course of therapy.
- If CNS symptoms of dizziness or drowsiness occur, take safety precautions (side rails up, bed low, assist with ambulation).
- Notify physician if paradoxical CNS symptoms such as restlessness, insomnia, euphoria, tremors or seizures occur.

OVERDOSAGE: SIGNS & SYMPTOMS
Oversedation

Patient/Family Education

- Emphasize that drug is not to be used for everyday stress and should not be used for > 4 mo.
- Advise patient that drug may cause drowsiness and other CNS reactions and to use caution while driving or performing other tasks requiring mental alertness.
- Instruct patient to avoid intake of alcoholic beverages or any other CNS depressant drugs (eg, sleeping pills) while taking this drug.
- Advise patient to avoid sudden position changes to prevent orthostatic hypotension.
- Tell patient to avoid otc medications unless approved by physician.
- Instruct patient to report these symptoms to physician: tremor, seizures, dizziness, wheezing, difficulty breathing, chest tightness, involuntary movements or dry mouth.
- Instruct patient to take sips of water frequently, suck on ice chips or sugarless hard candy or chew sugarless gum if dry mouth occurs.
- Caution patient not to discontinue drug abruptly.

See Patient Guide, p. 301.

Ibuprofen

(eye-BYOO-pro-fen)

Advil, Arthritis Foundation, Children's Advil, Children's Motrin, Bayer Select, Genpril, Haltran, Ibu-Tab, Ibuprin, Menadol, Midol 220, Midol IB, Motrin, Motrin IB, Nuprin, Pamprin-IB, Rufen, Saleto-200, ♣ *Actiprofen, Novo-Profen.*
Class: Analgesic/NSAID

Action Decreases inflammation, pain and fever, probably through inhibition of cyclooxygenase activity and prostaglandin synthesis.

Indications Relief of symptoms of rheumatoid arthritis, osteoarthritis, mild to moderate pain, primary dysmenorrhea, reduction of fever. **Unlabeled uses:** Symptomatic treatment of juvenile rheumatoid arthritis, sunburn, resistant acne vulgaris.

Contraindications Hypersensitivity to aspirin, iodides or any other NSAID.

Route/Dosage

Rheumatoid Arthritis and Osteoarthritis

ADULTS: **PO** 300-800 mg tid-qid not to exceed 3.2 g/day.

Mild/Moderate Pain

ADULTS: **PO** 400 mg q 4-6 hr prn.

Primary Dysmenorrhea

ADULTS: **PO** 400 mg q 4 hr prn.

Juvenile Arthritis
CHILDREN: **PO** 30-40 mg/kg/day in 3-4 divided doses.

Fever Reduction
CHILDREN 1-12 YR: ≤ 39.2° C (102.5° F) recommended dose **PO** 5 mg/kg; > 39.2° C (102.5° F) recommended dose **PO** 10 mg/kg; maximum daily dose 40 mg/kg.

Interactions
Beta-blockers: Antihypertensive effect may be decreased. *Lithium:* May increase lithium levels. *Loop diuretics:* Diuretic effects may be decreased. *Methotrexate:* May increase methotrexate levels. *Warfarin:* May increase risk of gastric erosion and bleeding.

Lab Test Interferences
None well documented.

Adverse Reactions
CV: Peripheral edema; water retention; worsening or precipitation of CHF. *CNS:* Dizziness; lightheadedness; drowsiness; vertigo; headaches; aseptic meningitis. *EENT:* Visual disturbances; photophobia; tinnitus. *GI:* Gastric distress; occult blood loss; diarrhea; vomiting; nausea; heartburn; dyspepsia; anorexia. *GU:* Menometrorrhagia; hematuria; cystitis; acute renal insufficiency; interstitial nephritis; hyperkalemia; hyponatremia; renal papillary necrosis. *DERM:* Rash; pruritus; erythema. *OTHER:* Muscle cramps.

Precautions
Pregnancy: Pregnancy category undetermined. *Lactation:* Undetermined. *Children:* Safety and efficacy not established. *Elderly:* Increased risk of adverse reactions. *GI effects:* Serious GI toxicity (eg, bleeding, ulceration, perforation) can occur at any time, with and without warning symptoms. *Renal effects:* Increased risk of dysfunction in patients with preexisting renal disease.

NURSING CONSIDERATIONS

Administration/Storage
- Give medication soon after meals or with food, milk or antacids to minimize GI irritation.

Assessment/Interventions
- Obtain complete patient history, including drug history and any known allergies.
- Notify physician if visual changes or indications of GI distress or liver or renal impairment occur.
- Monitor patient's cardiac status: BP, pulse (quality and rhythm), edema, tachycardia, palpitations.
- Assess renal function before and during therapy. Serum creatinine, creatinine clearance and BUN should be monitored in patients with renal impairment.
- Document any changes in liver function (AST, ALT), eye examinations and Hgb and Hct in patients on long-term therapy.
- Notify physician if indigestion, epigastric pain, unusual bleeding or bruising or dark tarry stools occurs.

OVERDOSAGE: SIGNS & SYMPTOMS

Drowsiness, lethargy, GI irritation/bleeding, nausea, vomiting, tinnitus, sweating, acute renal failure, epigastric pain, metabolic acidosis

Patient/Family Education
- Tell patient to take medication soon after meals or with food, milk or antacids.
- Tell patient to avoid alcohol and medications containing aspirin, such as cold remedies.
- Advise patient to discontinue drug and notify physician if any of the following occur: persistent GI upset or headache, skin rash, itching, visual disturbances, black stools, weight gain or edema, changes in urine pattern, joint pain, fever, blood in urine.
- Instruct patient not to take otc preparation for more than 3 days for fever and 10 days for pain and to notify physician if condition does not improve.

- Advise patient that drug may cause drowsiness and to use caution while driving or performing other tasks requiring mental alertness.

See Patient Guide, p. 302.

Idarubicin HCl

(eye-DUH-RUE-bih-sin HIGH-droe-KLOR-ide)

Idamycin

Class: Antineoplastic/antibiotic

Action Interacts with enzyme topoisomerase II and binds DNA to inhibit nucleic acid synthesis.

Indications In combination therapy, treatment for acute myeloid leukemia in adults.

Contraindications Standard considerations.

Route/Dosage

Induction Therapy

ADULTS: **IV** 12 mg/m^2 daily by slow injection for 3 days. May give second course if needed. Reduce subsequent doses by 25% for patients experiencing severe mucositis. Dose may be reduced for patients with impaired renal or hepatic function.

Interactions None well documented. INCOMPATIBILITIES: Do not mix with other drugs unless specific data are available.

Lab Test Interferences None well documented.

Adverse Reactions *CV:* CHF; arrhythmia; chest pain; myocardial infarction. *CNS:* Mental status changes; fever; headache; seizure. *GI:* Nausea; vomiting; mucositis; abdominal pain; diarrhea; enterocolitis with perforation. *HEMA:* Hemorrhage; myelosuppression. *DERM:* Alopecia; extravasation; rash. *META:* Hyperuricemia. *OTHER:* Infection; hepatic and renal function impairment.

Precautions *Pregnancy:* Category D. *Lactation:* Undetermined. *Children:* Safety and efficacy not established. *Cardiac toxicity:* Potentially fatal congestive heart failure or arrhythmias may occur, particularly with high cumulative dosage or concurrent use of other potentially cardiotoxic drugs (eg, daunorubicin, cyclophosphamide), preexisting cardiac disease, prior radiation exposure to heart or in patients with anemia, infection, leukemic pericarditis or myocarditis. *Hepatic and renal function impairment:* May increase toxicity; dosage should be reduced. *Myelosuppression:* Severe myelosuppression will occur in all patients; may result in death from infection or hemorrhage. Avoid in patients with preexisting bone marrow suppression.

NURSING CONSIDERATIONS

Administration/Storage

- This medication should be administered under supervision of physician experienced in leukemia chemotherapy.
- Use of goggles, gloves and protective gown is recommended during preparation and administration of drug. If skin is exposed to drug, wash thoroughly with soap and water. If eyes are exposed, irrigate immediately.
- Reconstitute 5 and 10 mg vials with 5 and 10 ml, respectively, of 0.9% Sodium Chloride to yield final concentration of 1 mg/ml. Do not use bacteriostatic diluents.
- Use caution when inserting needle into vial since vial is under negative pressure.
- Administer IV slowly (over 10-15 min) into freely running IV infusion of 0.9% Sodium Chloride or D5W into large vein directed (tubing may

be attached to butterfly needle). Do not administer IM or SC.
- Reconstituted solution is stable for 72 hours at room temperature and for 7 days under refrigeration.

Assessment/Interventions
- Obtain patient history, including drug history and any known allergies.
- Frequently examine insertion site for pain, redness, edema. If extravasation occurs or is suspected, terminate infusion and notify physician. Treatment for extravasation includes intermittent ice packs (apply for 30 minutes immediately, then for 30 minutes qid for 3 days). Elevate extremity and frequently examine for pain, redness and edema.
- Assess hematology values, blood chemistry values and renal and hepatic function test results as available.
- Check for incompatibility before administering another drug.
- Keep patient well hydrated and monitor I&O.
- Monitor for signs and symptoms of myelosuppression, and notify physician if any of following occurs: fever, chills, sore throat; unusual bleeding (guiac, hematuria, hematemesis) or bruising.
- If nausea and diarrhea occur, give appropriate medication.
- Monitor for signs of cardiac toxicity: life threatening arrhythmias, cardiomyopathy and CHF (peripheral edema, dyspnea, rales/crackles, weight gain).

OVERDOSAGE: SIGNS & SYMPTOMS
Myelosuppression, GI toxicity

Patient/Family Education
- Advise patient to avoid crowds and persons with infections.
- Explain that hair loss may occur and suggest that patient may want to consider wearing wig.
- Instruct patient to notify physician immediately if any of these symptoms occur: irregular heartbeat, shortness of breath or swelling of lower extremities.
- Instruct patient to report these symptoms to physician: pain, redness or swelling at injection site; fever; chills; sore throat; unusual bleeding (gums, dark stools, blood in urine) or bruising.

See Patient Guide, p. 303.

Idoxuridine (IDU)

(EYE-dox-YOU-rih-deen)
Herplex
Class: Ophthalmic/antiviral

Action Blocks reproduction of herpes simplex virus by irreversibly inhibiting incorporation of thymidine into viral DNA.

Indication Treatment of herpes simplex keratitis.

Contraindications Standard considerations.

Route/Dosage
ADULTS: OPHTHALMIC SOLUTION: Instill 1 gtt into infected eye(s) q hr during day and q 2 hr during night. Alternate schedule: Instill 1 gtt q 1 min for 5 min; repeat q 4 hr night and day. OINTMENT: Apply ointment to infected conjunctival sac q 4 hr (5 applications daily).

Interactions
Boric acid-containing solution: May cause irritation; do not coadminister.

Lab Test Interferences
None well documented.

Adverse Reactions
EENT: Ocular irritation, pain, pruritus, inflammation or edema; photophobia; corneal clouding; stippling; punctate defects in corneal epithelium; follicular conjunctivitis; puncta occlusion; conjunctival scarring.

Precautions
Pregnancy: Category C. *Lactation:* Undetermined. *Children:* Safety and efficacy not established. *Carcinogenesis:* Based on animal studies, may be carcinogenic. *Recurrence:* Continue medication for 5-7 days after epithelial healing to avoid recurrence.

NURSING CONSIDERATIONS

Administration/Storage

- For patient convenience, drops may be prescribed for waking hours and ointment for nighttime.
- Wash hands before and after instillation of solution or ointment.
- Do not mix with other topical eye medications.
- Store at room temperature and protect from light.

Assessment/Interventions

- Obtain complete patient history, including drug history and any known allergies.
- Assess for allergy, itching, lacrimation, redness or swelling.
- Withhold drug and contact physician if unusual changes or inflammation of eye occurs.

Patient/Family Education

- Demonstrate proper technique for instillation of drops or ointment, emphasizing importance of handwashing and of not touching cap or tip of tube to eye, conjunctiva, fingers or any unsterile object.
- Inform patient that vision may be hazy for short time after instillation.
- Explain importance of continuing medication for prescribed time even after healing has occurred, to avoid recurrence.
- Advise patient to wear sunglasses and to avoid prolonged exposure to bright light.
- Instruct patient to notify physician if condition worsens or if no improvement is noted in 2 weeks. Physician should also be contacted if burning or stinging occurs.
- Caution patient not to use any other medications on eye such as boric acid.
- Warn patient not to use other persons' eye makeup, towels, washcloths or eye medications; reinfection may occur.
- Instruct patient to report these symptoms to physician: visual changes, pain, itching or swelling of eye.

See Patient Guide, p. 304.

Ifosfamide

(eye-FOSS-fuh-MIDE)
Ifex
Class: Antineoplastic/alkylating

Action Active metabolites interact with cellular DNA.

Indications In combination with other approved antineoplastic agents for third-line chemotherapy of germ-cell testicular cancer. **Unlabeled uses:** Also exhibits activity against lung, breast, ovarian, pancreatic and gastric cancers, sarcomas, acute leukemias (except acute monocytic leukemia) and malignant lymphomas.

Contraindications Severely depressed bone marrow function.

Route/Dosage
ADULTS: IV 1.2 g/m^2/day for 5 consecutive days. Give as slow infusion over at least 30 minutes. May repeat treatment q 3 weeks or after hematologic toxicity recovery.

Interactions None well documented.

Lab Test Interferences
None well documented.

Adverse Reactions
CNS: Somnolence; confusion; depressive psychosis; hallucinations; dizziness; disorientation; cranial nerve

dysfunction; seizures; coma. *GI:* Nausea; vomiting; anorexia; diarrhea. *GU:* Hematuria; renal impairment; hemorrhagic cystitis; dysuria; urinary frequency. *HEMA:* Myelosuppression; thrombocytopenia; leukopenia. *HEPA:* Liver dysfunction (increased liver enzymes or bilirubin). *DERM:* Alopecia. *OTHER:* Infection; phlebitis; fever; allergic reactions.

Precautions

Pregnancy: Category D. *Lactation:* Excreted in breast milk. *Children:* Safety and efficacy not established. *Compromised bone marrow reserve:* Administer cautiously in patients with leukopenia, granulocytopenia, extensive bone marrow metastases or prior radiation or cytotoxic therapy. *Neurologic manifestations:* Discontinue if CNS reactions occur. *Renal function impairment:* Use with caution. *Wound healing:* Ifosfamide may interfere with normal wound healing.

NURSING CONSIDERATIONS

Administration/Storage

- Reconstitute with Sterile Water for Injection or Bacteriostatic Water for Injection (preserved with benzylalcohol or paraben).
- Use strict aseptic technique in preparing drug.
- Do not allow drug to come in contact with skin, mucous membranes or eyes.
- Inspect parenteral solution for discoloration and precipitate.

Assessment/Interventions

- Obtain complete patient history, including drug history and any known allergies.
- Monitor BP, pulse, respiratory rate and body temperature during administration.
- Monitor I&O.
- Notify physician if any unusual bleeding, especially hematuria or bruising, fever, chills, sore throat, cough, shortness of breath or signs of infection occur.
- Closely monitor laboratory values for potential drug toxicities. Also check WBC and platelet count prior to each dose and at regular intervals throughout therapy. Drug should not be administered if WBC < 2000 or platelet count $< 50,000$.
- Obtain urinalysis prior to giving each dose. If microscopic hematuria is present, withhold dose until resolved.
- If nausea and vomiting occur, adjust diet accordingly and restrict activity.

Patient/Family Education

- Advise patient to avoid alcohol and medications containing aspirin such as medications for colds.
- Inform patient that hair loss may occur.
- Explain importance of using contraceptive measures during course of therapy.
- If nausea and vomiting occur, advise patient to adjust diet and restrict activity and to notify physician if symptoms persist.
- Instruct patient to avoid crowds and persons with infections.
- Emphasize importance of adequate fluid intake.
- Inform patient that drug may interfere with wound healing.
- Instruct patient to report these symptoms to physician: signs of superinfection (black "furry" tongue, vaginal itching or discharge, loose foul-smelling stools), any unusual bleeding or bruising, especially blood in urine, or fever, chills, sore throat, cough, shortness of breath.

See Patient Guide, p. 305.

Imipenem/Cilastatin

(ih-mih-PEN-em/SIGH-luh-STAT-in)
Primaxin IV, *Primaxin IM*
Class: Anti-infective/carbapenem

Action Imipenem inhibits bacterial cell wall synthesis. Cilastatin prevents metabolism of imipenem, resulting in increased urinary recovery and decreased renal toxicity.

Indications Treatment of serious infections of lower respiratory tract and urinary tract, intra-abdominal and gynecologic infections, bacterial septicemia, bone and joint infections, skin and skin structure infections, endocarditis, and polymicrobic infections due to susceptible microorganisms.

Contraindications IM use with hypersensitivity to local anesthetics of amide type or with severe shock or heart block.

Route/Dosage
ADULTS: **IV** 250-500 mg q 6-8 hr. Maximum: 50 mg/kg/day or 4 g/day, whichever is lower. ADULTS: **IM** 500-750 mg q 12 hr. Maximum: 1500 mg/day. CHILDREN < 40 KG: **IM** 60 mg/kg/day. CHILDREN ≥ 40 KG: **IM** Adult dose. PREMATURE INFANTS (≥ 36 WEEKS GESTATIONAL AGE): **IM** 20 mg/kg q 12 hr.

Interactions
Cyclosporine: CNS side effects (eg, myoclonia, seizures) may be increased. *Ganciclovir:* Generalized seizures may occur; avoid use. INCOMPATIBILITIES: Do not physically mix imipenem/cilastatin with other antibiotics.

Lab Test Interferences
May cause positive Coombs' test results.

Adverse Reactions
CV: Hypotension; palpitations; tachycardia; phlebitis; thrombophlebitis. *CNS:* Seizures. *GI:* Nausea; diarrhea; vomiting; pseudomembranous colitis; hemorrhagic colitis; hepatitis. *GU:* Presence of RBCs, WBCs, casts and bacteria in urine; increased BUN and creatinine. *HEMA:* Decreased Hgb and Hct; eosinophilia; increased or decreased WBCs and platelets; decreased erythrocytes. *HEPA:* Increased AST, ALT, alkaline phosphatase and bilirubin. *OTHER:* Pain at injection site.

Precautions
Pregnancy: Category C. *Lactation:* Undetermined. *Children:* Safety and efficacy in children < 12 yr not established. *CNS:* IV administration may result in myoclonic activity confusional states or seizures. *Hypersensitivity:* Administer drug with caution to penicillin-sensitive patients due to possible cross-activity. *Pseudomembranous colitis:* Consider possibility in patients with diarrhea. *Renal impairment:* Dosage reduction and/or alteration of dosage interval is required. *Superinfection:* May result in bacterial or fungal overgrowth of nonsusceptible organisms.

NURSING CONSIDERATIONS

Administration/Storage

- Do not inject by direct IV bolus.
- For IV administration, reconstitute with 100 ml of compatible diluent. Shake until suspension is clear; add suspension to 100 ml of appropriate infusion solution. Then add 10 ml of infusion to vial; shake well to ensure that all medication is used and transfer resulting suspension to infusion solution. Color of solution may range from colorless to yellow. Solution is stable for 4 hr at room temperature and for 24 hr when refrigerated. Do not administer if solution is cloudy.
- Do not use IM preparation for IV administration.
- For IM administration, prepare with 1% lidocaine hydrochloride solution (without epinephrine). Prepare 500 mg vial with 2 ml and 750 mg vial

with 3 ml of lidocaine. Agitate to form suspension. Color of solution may range from white to light tan. Withdraw and inject entire contents of vial intramuscularly. Use within 1 hr of preparation.

- Store unreconstituted powder at room temperature.

Assessment/Interventions

- Obtain complete patient history, including drug history and any known allergies, especially to penicillin and beta lactam antibiotics.
- Notify physician if signs of superinfection and/or resistance occur.
- Have epinephrine, antihistamines and resuscitation equipment available in case of anaphylaxis.
- If seizure occurs, withhold drug, institute safety measures and notify physician.
- If culture and sensitivity is ordered, obtain specimen prior to first dose.
- Withhold drug and notify physician if any of following occurs: fever, rash, hives, difficulty breathing, vaginitis, or severe diarrhea.
- Monitor vital signs, sputum, urine, stool and WBC at beginning of and throughout therapy.

OVERDOSAGE: SIGNS & SYMPTOMS

Seizures

Patient/Family Education

- Instruct patient to report to physician or nurse itching, rash, hives, difficulty breathing, diarrhea, black "furry" tongue, loose foul-smelling stool or vaginal itching or discharge.

See Patient Guide, pp. 307-308.

Imipramine

(im-IPP-ruh-meen)

Janimine, Tofranil, Tofranil-PM

Class: Tricyclic antidepressant

Action Inhibits reuptake of norepinephrine and, to a lesser degree, serotonin in CNS.

Indications Relief of symptoms of depression; treatment of enuresis in children ≥ 6 years. **Unlabeled uses:** Treatment of chronic pain, panic disorder and eating disorders (bulimia nervosa).

Contraindications Hypersensitivity to any tricyclic antidepressant. Generally, not to be given in combination with or within 14 days of treatment with MAO inhibitor or during acute recovery phase of MI.

Route/Dosage

Depression

Use parenterally only in patients who are not able or not willing to take oral medication. Give via IM route. Do not administer IV. Up to 100 mg/day in divided doses may be given IM. Switch to oral as soon as possible. ADULTS: **PO** 100-300 mg/day, in divided doses or once daily at bedtime. ELDERLY & ADOLESCENTS: **PO** 30-40 mg/day; may increase up to 100 mg/day. CHILDREN: **PO** 1.5 mg/kg/day in divided doses; up to maximum of 5 mg/kg/day. CHILDHOOD ENURESIS (6 YR): **PO** 25 mg/day given 1 hr before bedtime; if response unsatisfactory after 1 wk, may increase to 50 mg in children < 12 years. Children > 12 may receive 75 mg/night. Do not exceed 2.5 mg/kg/day.

Interactions

Carbamazepine: Carbamazepine levels may increase; imipramine levels may decrease. *Cimetidine, fluoxetine:* May cause increased imipramine blood levels and effects. *Clonidine:* May result in hypertensive crisis. *CNS depressants:* Depressant effects may be additive. *Dicumerol:* Anticoagulant actions may increase. *Guanethidine:* Hypotensive action may be inhibited. *MAO inhibitors:* May cause hyperpyretic crises, severe convulsions and death when given with imipramine. *Sympathomimetics:* Pressor response may be decreased by indirect-acting sympathomimetics and increased by direct-acting ones.

Lab Test Interferences
None well documented.

Adverse Reactions
CV: Orthostatic hypotension; hypertension; tachycardia; palpitations; arrhythmias; ECG changes; stroke; heartblock; CHF. *RESP:* Pharyngitis; rhinitis; sinusitis; laryngitis; coughing. *CNS:* Confusion; hallucinations; delusions; nervousness; restlessness; agitation; panic; insomnia; nightmares; mania; exacerbation of psychosis; drowsiness; dizziness; weakness; numbness; extrapyramidal symptoms; emotional lability; seizures; tremors. *EENT:* Nasal congestion; tinnitus; conjunctivitis; mydriasis; blurred vision; increased IOP. *GI:* Nausea; vomiting; anorexia; GI distress; diarrhea; flatulence; peculiar taste in mouth; dry mouth; constipation. *GU:* Impotence; sexual dysfunction; nocturia; urinary frequency; urinary tract infection; vaginitis; cystitis; dysmenorrhea; amenorrhea; urinary retention and hesitancy. *HEMA:* Bone marrow depression including agranulocytosis; eosinophilia; purpura; thrombocytopenia; leukopenia. *HEPA:* Hepatitis; jaundice. *DERM:* Rash; pruritis; photosensitivity reaction; dry skin; acne; itching. *META:* Elevation or depression of blood sugar. *OTHER:* Breast enlargement.

Precautions
Pregnancy: Category B. *Lactation:* Excreted in breast milk. *Children:* Do not exceed 2.5 mg/kg/day. *Special risk patients:* Use with caution in patients with history of seizures, urinary retention, ureteral spasm, angle-closure glaucoma or increased IOP, conduction disorders, hyperthyroid patients or those receiving thyroid medication, hepatic or renal impairment, schizophrenia or paranoia. *Hazardous tasks:* Patients should use caution while performing tasks requiring alertness.

NURSING CONSIDERATIONS

Administration/Storage

- Do not give via IV route.
- Use IM form only for patients unwilling or unable to take oral form.
- Give IM form in divided doses during day.
- Immerse ampules in hot tap water for 1 min if crystals have formed during storage.

Assessment/Interventions

- Obtain complete patient history, including drug history and any known allergies.
- Review ECG for prolongation of QT interval prior to starting large doses and periodically thereafter.
- Be alert for signs of orthostatic hypotension and take orthostatic BPs. Document and report significant changes to physician.
- Observe for onset of therapeutic effect in depressed patients in 7-21 days and full response in up to 6 wk.
- Assess patients receiving IM form for ability to switch to oral administration.
- Assess elderly patients for signs and symptoms of confusion.
- Report drowsiness, dry mouth, constipation or weight gain to physician.
- Watch for possible hypertension when coadministering clonidine.
- Be alert for possible drug interactions.

OVERDOSAGE: SIGNS & SYMPTOMS

Confusion, agitation, hallucinations, seizures, status epilepticus, clonus, choreoathetosis, hyperactive reflexes, positive Babinski's sign, coma, cardiac arrhythmias, renal failure, flushing, dry mouth, dilated pupils, hyperpyrexia

Patient/Family Education

- Tell patient to inform physician if she becomes pregnant or intends to become pregnant.
- Explain that it may be several weeks before a response is noticed.

- Instruct patient to avoid intake of alcoholic beverages or other CNS depressants.
- Advise patient that drug may cause drowsiness and to use caution while driving or performing other tasks requiring mental alertness.
- Caution patient to avoid exposure to sunlight and to use sunscreen or wear protective clothing to avoid photosensitivity reaction.
- Teach patient to avoid sudden position changes to prevent orthostatic hypertension.
- Inform patient that dizziness, dry mouth (suggest taking frequent sips of water, sucking on ice chips or sugarless hard candy or chewing sugarless gum), drowsiness, or constipation may occur, but that these side effects often subside with time.
- Instruct patient to report all problems to physician, including dizziness, drowsiness, dry mouth, constipation or weight gain.

See Patient Guide, p. 309.

Immune Globulin Intramuscular (IGIM; IG; Gamma Globulin; ISG)

(ih-MYOON GLAH-byoo-lin intramuscular)

Gamastan, Gammar

Class: Immune serum

Action Replaces normal human IgG antibodies.

Indications Passive immunization against or modification of hepatitis A. Prevention or modification of measles in susceptible persons exposed < 6 days previously. Passive immunization against varicella in immunocompromised patients if varicella-zoster immune globulin (VZIG) is not available and IGIM can be given promptly. IgG replacement therapy in certain persons with hypoglobulinemia or agammaglobulinemia.

Contraindications Immediate hypersensitivity to human antibody product or thimerosal; circulating anti-IgA antibodies; thrombocytopenia or any coagulation disorder.

Route/Dosage

Preexposure and Postexposure Hepatitis A Prophylaxis

ADULTS & CHILDREN: **IM** 0.02 ml/kg. Pre-exposure hepatitis A prophylaxis for travelers to developing countries who will stay < 3 mo. **IM** 0.06 mg/kg with booster doses q 4-6 mo throughout their stay.

Postexposure Measles Prophylaxis

ADULTS & CHILDREN: **IM** 0.25 ml/kg. SUSCEPTIBLE IMMUNOCOMPROMISED CHILDREN: **IM** 0.5 ml/kg (maximum 15 ml).

Postexposure Varicella Prophylaxis

ADULTS & CHILDREN: If VZIG is unavailable, **IM** 0.6-1.2 ml/kg.

Immunoglobulin Deficiency

ADULTS & CHILDREN: **IM** 0.66 ml/kg (100 mg/kg) q 3-4 wk. Larger initial dose (eg, 1.2 ml/kg) is often given at onset of therapy. Patients who rapidly metabolize may require more frequent or larger doses.

Interactions

Live vaccines: To avoid inactivating vaccines containing live viruses or bacteria, give live vaccines 2-4 wk before or 3-6 mo after IGIU, depending on dose.

Lab Test Interferences None well documented.

Adverse Reactions

OTHER: Local pain and tenderness at the injection site; urticaria; angioedema; anaphylactic reactions.

Precautions

Pregnancy: Category C. *Lactation:* Undetermined. *Special risk patients:* Give drug cautiously to persons receiving anticoagulant therapy because of IM administration. *Hypersensitivity:* Hypersensitivity, including anaphylaxis, may occur. Administer drug with caution in patients with prior systemic allergic reactions to human immunoglobulins.

NURSING CONSIDERATIONS

Administration/Storage

- Administer via IM injection only; do not give by IV route.
- In adults administer via IM injection, preferably in upper outer quadrant of gluteal region.
- In infants and children < 3 yr, administer intramuscularly in anterolateral thigh.
- Divide doses > 10 ml and inject into several muscle sites to reduce local pain and discomfort.
- It is better not to inject > 3 ml per injection site.
- Always record manufacturer's name and lot number of immune globulin in patient's permanent record file along with date of administration, name, address and title of person administering injection.
- Refrigerate vials. Do not freeze.

Assessment/Interventions

- Obtain patient history, including drug history and any known allergies.
- Monitor for hypersensitivity and/or anaphylaxis. Epinephrine should always be available to counteract any possible reactions.

Patient/Family Education

- Instruct patient to take analgesics (eg, acetaminophen) for local pain and tenderness at injection site if necessary.
- Provide patient or parent with immunization history record and record this injection in patient's medical records.

No patient monograph available.

Immune Globulin Intravenous (IGIV)

(ih-MYOON GLAH-byoo-lin intravenous)

Gamimune N, Gammagard SID, Gammar-P I.V., Iveegam, Polygam S/D, Sandoglobulin, Venoglobulin-I, Venoglobulin-S

Class: Immune serum

Action Replaces normal human IgG antibodies. Promotes opsonization, fixes complement, and neutralizes bacteria, viruses, fungi and parasites and their toxins.

Indications Treatment of primary immunodeficiency states in patients unable to produce sufficient amounts of IgG antibodies; prevention of bacterial infections in patients with hypogamma globulinemia, recurrent bacterial infections associated with B-cell chronic lymphocytic leukemia or Kawasaki syndrome, children with AIDS and bone-marrow transplant patients; treatment of immune thrombocytopenia purpura.

Contraindications Immediate hypersensitivity to human antibody product; circulating anti-IgA antibodies.

Route/Dosage

Immunodeficiency Syndrome

ADULTS & CHILDREN: *Gammagard:* **IV** 200-400 mg/kg initially; then monthly doses of at least 100 mg/kg are recommended. *Gammar S/D:* **IV** Initial dose of 0.5 ml/kg/hr; eventual—5%: 4 ml/kg/hr; 10%: 8 ml/kg/hr. *Gammar-P:* **IV** Initial dose—0.6 ml/kg/hr x 15-30 min; eventual—1.2-3.6 ml/kg/hr. *Gammar-IV:* **IV** Initial loading dose of at least 200 mg/kg; then 100-200 mg/kg q 3-4 wk. *Gamimune N:* **IV** 100-200 mg/kg monthly. If clinical response or level of IgG is insufficient, increase dose to 400 mg/kg or repeat infusion more frequently. *Iveegam:* **IV** 200 mg/kg monthly. If clinical response or level of IgG is insufficient, increase dose fourfold or repeat infusion more frequently. Doses up to 800 mg/kg monthly have been tolerated. *Polygam:* **IV** 200-400 mg/kg recommended initially; then 100 mg/kg monthly. Doses based on monitoring clinical response. *Polygam S/D:* **IV** Initial—0.5 ml/kg/hr; eventual—5%: 4 ml/kg/hr; 10%: 8 ml/kg/hr. *Sandoglobulin:* **IV** 200 mg/kg monthly. If clinical response or level of IgG is insufficient, increase dose to 300 mg/kg or repeat infusion more frequently. *Venoglobulin-I:* **IV** 200 mg/kg monthly. If clinical response or level of IgG is insufficient, increase dose to 300-400 mg/kg or repeat infusion more frequenly.

Immune Thrombocytopenic Purpura
ADULTS & CHILDREN: *Gammagard:* **IV** 1000 mg/kg. Give up to 3 doses on alternate days if required based on clinical response and platelet count. *Gammagard S/D:* **IV** Initial dose of 0.5 ml/kg/hr; eventual—5%: 4 ml/kg/hr; 10%: 8 ml/kg/hr. *Gamimune N:* **IV** 400 mg/kg for 5 consecutive days. *Polygam:* **IV** 1000 mg/kg recommended initially; then additional doses determined by clinical response and platelet count. Up to 3 doses may be given on alternate days if needed. *Polygam S/D:* **IV** Initial—0.5 ml/kg/hr; eventual—5%: 4 ml/kg/hr; 10%: 8 ml/kg/hr. *Sandoglobulin:* **IV** 400 mg/kg for 2-5 consecutive days. *Venoglobulin-I:* **IV** Induction: 500 mg/kg/day for 2-7 consecutive days. Patients responding to induction therapy by manifesting platelet count of 30,000-50,000/mm^3 may be discontinued after 2-7 daily doses. Maintenance: If platelet count falls below 30,000/mm^3 or patient manifests significant bleeding, infuse 500-2000 mg/kg as single dose q 2 wk or less as needed to maintain platelet count above 30,000/mm^3 in children and 20,000/mm^3 in adults.

B-Cell Chronic Lymphocytic Leukemia
ADULTS & CHILDREN: *Gammagard:* **IV** 400 mg/kg q 3-4 wk. *Polygam:* **IV** 400 mg/kg q 3-4 wk.

Interactions

Live vaccines: To avoid inactivating vaccines containing live viruses or bacteria, give live vaccines 2-4 wk before or 3-11 mo after IGIV depending on dose. INCOMPATIBILITIES: Admixture: Do not mix IGIV with other medications.

Lab Test Interferences

Blood type: Blood-group antibodies may be transferred to IGIV recipients, causing confusion regarding recipient's blood type.

Adverse Reactions

CV: Palpitations; hypotension; hypertension. *RESP:* Shortness of breath; wheezing. *CNS:* Anxiety; dizziness; headache. *GI:* Nausea; vomiting; abdominal cramps. *OTHER:* Pallor; cyanosis; immediate anaphylactic and hypersensitivity reactions; back pain; chills; muscle or joint pain; arthralgia; malaise; flushing; chest tightness.

Precautions

Pregnancy: Category C. *Lactation:* Undetermined. *Hypersensitivity:* Hypersensitivity, including anaphylaxis, may occur.

NURSING CONSIDERATIONS

Administration/Storage

- Administer via IV infusion only. Use separate IV line and electronic infusion device.
- Proceed with infusion only if reconstituted solution is clear and is at approximately body temperature.
- Store Gamimune N and Iveegam in refrigerator.
- Store Sandoglobulin, Gammagard S/D, Gammar-P, Polygam S/D and Venoglobulin-I at room temperature.
- Discard any unused solution.

- Avoid freezing. Do not use solution that has been frozen.

Assessment/Interventions

- Obtain patient history, including drug history and any known allergies.
- Keep epinephrine (1:1000) and resuscitation equipment readily available.
- Monitor vital signs continuously and observe for adverse symptoms (eg, anaphylaxis, fever, chills, nausea, vomiting) throughout infusion.
- If adverse reactions such as fever, chills, nausea or vomiting develop, slowing infusion rate will usually eliminate reaction.

Patient/Family Education

- Instruct patient to notify physician immediately of nausea, chills, shortness of breath, headache and chest tightness during infusion.

No patient monograph available.

Indapamide

(IN-DAP-uh-mide)

Lozol, ♣ *Lozide*

Class: Thiazide diuretic

Action Enhances excretion of sodium, chloride and water by interfering with transport of sodium ions across renal tubular epithelium.

Indications Treatment of edema associated with CHF, hepatic cirrhosis, renal dysfunction, and corticosteroid or estrogen therapy; management of hypertension. **Unlabeled uses:** Treatment of calcium nephrolithiasis, osteopororis or diabetes insipidus.

Contraindications Hypersensitivity to thiazides, related diuretics or sulfonamide-derived drugs; anuria.

Route/Dosage

ADULTS: **PO** 1.25-5 mg q AM. Maximum 5 mg/day.

Interactions

Bile acid sequestrants: May reduce thiazide absorption; give thiazide ≥ 2 hr before resin. *Diazoxide:* Hyperglycemia may occur. *Digitalis glycosides:* Diuretic-induced hypokalemia and hypomagnesemia may precipitate digitalis-induced arrhythmias. *Lithium:* May decrease renal excretion of lithium; monitor lithium levels. *Loop diuretics:* May result in synergistic effects and result in profound diuresis and serious electrolyte abnormalities. *Sulfonylureas, insulin:* May decrease hypoglycemic effect of sulfonylureas. May need to adjust dosage of sulfonylureas or insulin.

Lab Test Interferences

May decrease serum protein-bound iodine levels without signs of thyroid disturbance. May cause diagnostic interference of serum electrolyte levels, blood and urine glucose levels, serum bilirubin levels and serum uric acid levels. May increase serum magnesium levels in uremic patients.

Adverse Reactions

CV: Orthostatic hypotension; palpitations. *RESP:* Rhinorrhea. *CNS:* Dizziness; lightheadedness; vertigo; headache; weakness; restlessness; insomnia; drowsiness; fatigue; lethargy; anxiety; depression; nervousness. *EENT:* Blurred vision. *GI:* Anorexia; gastric irritation; epigastric distress; nausea; vomiting; abdominal pain/cramping/bloating; diarrhea; constipation; dry mouth. *GU:* Nocturia; impotence/reduced libido. *HEMA:* Neutropenia. *DERM:* Rash; necrotizing angiitis; vasculitis; cutaneous vasculitis; pruritus. *META:* Hyperglycemia; glycosuria; hyperuricemia. *OTHER:* Muscle cramp or spasm; acute gout.

Precautions

Pregnancy: Category B. *Lactation:* May be excreted in breast milk. *Hypersensitivity:* May occur in patients with or without history of allergy or bronchial asthma; cross-sensitivity with sulfonamides may also occur. *Electrolyte balance:* Severe hyponatremia and hypokalemia may infrequently occur with recommended doses; more common in elderly females. *Hepatic impairment:* Minor alterations of fluid and electrolyte balance may precipitate hepatic coma; use with caution. *Lipids:* May cause increased concentrations of total triglycerides and LDL in some patients. *Lupus erythematosus:* Exacerbation or activation may occur. *Postsympathectomy patients:* Antihypertensive effects may be enhanced. *Renal impairment:* May precipitate azotemia; use with caution.

NURSING CONSIDERATIONS

Administration/Storage

- Administer as morning dose to prevent nocturia.
- Give with food or milk if nausea occurs.
- Store in tightly closed, light-resistant container at room temperature.

Assessment/Interventions

- Obtain patient history, including drug history and any known allergies.
- Weigh patient daily.
- Assess feet, legs and sacral area for edema daily.
- Measure I&O throughout therapy.
- Monitor BP, with patient lying and standing.
- Monitor renal function (nonprotein nitrogen, BUN, creatinine, glomerular filtration) and serum potassium, sodium, calcium, magnesium, blood pH and uric acid as ordered.
- Assess for signs of metabolic alkalosis and hypokalemia.
- Report to physician signs of renal dysfunction (anuria, oliguria); liver dysfunction (dark urine, jaundice, pruritis); gout (rising serum uric acid, joint pain); muscle weakness, cramps, nausea, dizziness, numbness, irregular heartbeat and irritability.

OVERDOSAGE: SIGNS & SYMPTOMS

Orthostatic or general hypotension, syncope, electrolyte abnormalities, potassium deficiency, vomiting, respiratory depression, lethargy, shock, weakness, confusion, dizziness, cramps of calf muscles, thirst, polyuria, anuria

Patient/Family Education

- Tell patient to take medication early in day to prevent sleep problems.
- Instruct patient to take drug with food or milk to minimize GI irritation.
- Caution patient to avoid exposure to sunlight and to use sunscreen or wear protective clothing to avoid photosensitivity reaction.
- Instruct patients with diabetes to report increased blood glucose levels.
- Caution patients to avoid sudden position changes to prevent orthostatic hypotension.
- Advise patients to include in diet foods that are high in potassium (eg, bananas, broccoli, dried fruits, grapefruit, lima beans, nuts, oranges).
- Tell patient to report decrease in urinary output, jaundice, muscle cramps, weakness, nausea, blurred vision or dizziness.
- For patients being treated for hypertension, explain benefits of weight reduction, exercise, reduction of alcohol and sodium intake, cessation of smoking.

See Patient Guide, p. 310.

Indinavir Sulfate

(in-DIN-ah-veer SULL-fate)
Crixivan
Class: Antiviral

Action Inhibits human immunodeficiency virus (HIV) protease, the enzyme that cleaves viral polyprotein precursors into functional proteins in HIV-infected cells. Inhibition of this enzyme by indinavir results in formation of immature non-infectious viral particles.

Indications Treatment of HIV infection in adults when antiretroviral therapy is warranted.

Contraindications Standard considerations.

Route/Dosage
ADULTS: PO 800 mg (two 400-mg capsules) every 8 hrs.

Interactions
Rifabutin: Serum concentrations of rifabutin may be increased. A 50% reduction in rifabutin dosage is recommended by the manufacturer. *Ketoconazole:* Serum indinavir concentrations may be increased. Consider decreasing indinavir's dose. *Rifampin:* May induce enzymes that metabolize indinavir; concomitant use not recommended. *Didanosine:* Separate administration by at least 1 hr. The buffers in didanosine preparations may interfere with indinavir's absorption. *Astemizole, cisapride, midazolam, terfenadine, triazolam:* While not studied, metabolic enzyme inhibition by indinavir could lead to increases in the other drugs' levels and potentially serious reactions. Concomitant use is not recommended.

Lab Test Interferences
None well documented.

Adverse Reactions
CNS: Headache; insomnia; dizziness; somnolence; anxiety. *EENT:* Pharyngitis; altered taste; blurred vision. *CV:* Palpitation; syncope. *GI:* Nausea; vomiting; diarrhea; anorexia; acid reflux; dry mouth; abdominal pain; altered taste. *GU:* Nephrolithiasis; dysuria; hematuria. *HEPA:* Asymptomatic hyperbilirubinemia. *DERM:* Rash; dry skin; pruritus. *OTHER:* Asthenia; fatigue; flank pain; back pain; chest pain; malaise; fever; flu-like symptoms.

Precautions
Pregnancy: Category C. *Lactation:* Undetermined. *Children:* Safety and efficacy not established. *Hepatic insufficiency/cirrhosis:* Lower indinavir doses may be required since indinavir is hepatically metabolized.

NURSING CONSIDERATIONS

Administration/Storage

- Administer drug without food but with water 1 hour before or 2 hours after a meal; alternatively, administer with other liquids such as skim milk, juice, coffee or tea or a light meal (eg, dry toast with jelly, corn flakes with skim milk).
- The patient should drink 1.5 liters (48 ounces) of liquids in 24 hours.
- Store in a tightly closed container at room temperature, protected from moisture.

Assessment/Interventions

- Obtain patient history.
- Assess for evidence of hepatic insufficiency prior to starting therapy.
- Assess for nephrolithiasis during therapy.

Patient/Family Education

- Advise patient not to modify or discontinue treatment without first consulting the healthcare provider.
- Advise patient that this medicine must be taken at 8 hour intervals.
- If a dose is missed, the next dose should be taken as soon as possible but not doubled.

- If patient cannot take the drug with only water, the drug may be taken with other liquids or a light meal.
- Have patients store the drug in the original container to prevent moisture from affecting the drug.
- Advise patient that capsules should be used and stored in their original container.
- Inform patient that capsules are sensitive to moisture and the desiccant should remain in the bottle.
- Advise the patient that Indinavir is not a cure for H.I.V., and that its long-term effects are unknown.
- Advise patient to contact healthcare provider if any of the following occurs: back/flank pain; pink or red-colored urine, yellowing of skin or eyes.

See Patient Guide, p. 311.

Indomethacin

(in-doe-METH-uh-sin)

Indocin, Indocin SR, Indochron E-R, ♣ *Indocid, Indocid SR, Indocid Ophthalmic, NovoMethacin*

Indomethacin Sodium Trihydrate

Indocin IV

Class: Analgesic/NSAID

Action Decreases inflammation, pain and fever, probably through inhibition of cyclooxygenase activity and prostaglandin synthesis.

Indications *Indomethacin:* Symptomatic treatment of rheumatoid arthritis, osteoarthritis, ankylosing spondylitis, gouty arthritis, acute painful shoulder. *Indomethacin sodium trihydrate (IV):* Closure of patent ductus arteriosus. **Unlabeled uses:** Treatment of primary dysmenorrhea; migraine prophylaxis; treatment of cluster headache, polyhydramnios, sunburn; cystoid macular edema.

Contraindications Hypersensitivity to aspirin, iodides or any nonsteroidal anti-inflammatory agent. IV form is also contraindicated in these cases: proven or suspected untreated infection, bleeding, thrombocytopenia, coagulation defects, necrotizing enterocolitis, significant renal impairment, congenital heart disease when patency of ductus arteriosus is necessary for satisfactory blood flow. Suppositories contraindicated in recent bleeding or proctitis history.

Route/Dosage

Rheumatoid Arthritis, Osteoarthritis, Ankylosing Spondylitis

ADULTS: **PO** 25 mg bid or tid up to maximum of 200 mg/day (or 75 mg sustained release form 1-2 times daily)

Gouty Arthritis

ADULTS: **PO/PR** 50 mg tid; do not use sustained release form.

Acute Painful Shoulder

ADULTS: **PO** 75-150 mg/day in divided doses for 7-14 days.

Patent Ductus Arteriosus

IV 3 doses total. INFANTS < 2 DAYS OLD: **IV** 0.2 mg/kg followed by 2 doses of 0.1 mg/kg 12-24 hr apart. INFANTS 2-7 DAYS OLD: 3 doses of 0.2 mg/kg separated by 12-24 hr. INFANTS > 7 DAYS OLD: 0.2 mg/kg followed by 2 doses of 0.25 mg/kg separated by 12-24 hr.

Interactions *Anticoagulants:* May increase risk of gastric erosion and bleeding. *Beta-blockers, ACE inhibitors:* Antihypertensive effects may be decreased. *Digoxin:* May increase digoxin levels. *Lithium:* May decrease lithium clearance. *Loop diuretics:* May decrease diuretic effects. *Methotrexate:* May increase methotrexate levels.

Lab Test Interferences False-negative results may occur in dexamethasone suppression test.

Adverse Reactions

CV: Peripheral edema; water retention; worsening or precipitation of CHF. *CNS*: Dizziness; headache; drowsiness; confusion. *EENT*: Visual disturbances; tinnitus. *GI*: Gastric distress; occult blood loss; nausea; diarrhea; vomiting; ulceration; perforation. *GU*: Acute renal insufficiency; interstitial nephritis; hyponatremia; renal papillary necrosis. *META*: Hyperuricemia; hyperkalemia. *HEMA*: Leukopenia.

Precautions

Pregnancy: Safety not established. *Lactation*: Undetermined. *Children*: Safety and efficacy not established in children < 14 yr, except use of IV form in infants. *CNS effects*: May aggravate depression or other psychiatric disorders, epilepsy or Parkinsonism; use with caution. *Electrolyte imbalance*: IV indomethacin may suppress water excretion to greater extent than sodium excretion; monitor electrolytes and renal function. *GI effects*: Usually not given to patients with active GI lesions or history of recurrent GI lesions. *Renal impairment*: NSAIDs may worsen preexisting renal dysfunction.

NURSING CONSIDERATIONS

Administration/Storage

- Administer oral medication with food, milk or antacids to minimize GI upset.
- Do not crush, break or allow patient to chew sustained release capsules.
- Shake suspension before giving, do not mix with antacid or any other liquid.
- Rectal suppositories: Encourage patient to retain rectal suppositories for 1 hr.
- Refrigerate oral suspension and suppositories. Protect oral suspension from freezing.
- *IV for patent ductus*: Dilute 1 mg/ml or more with normal saline or Sterile Water for Injection without preservative. Administer over 5-10 sec. May also be given as retention enema or via orogastric tube.

Assessment/Interventions

- Obtain patient history, including drug history and any known allergies (especially allergy to aspirin).
- Observe for signs of rhinitis, asthma and urticaria.
- Assess patient with arthritis: Note type, location and intensity of limitation of movement and pain before and 1-2 hr after administration of standard release medication and 4-6 hr after sustained release form.
- Monitor BUN, creatinine, CBC, serum potassium, AST, and ALT prior to therapy and periodically during long-term therapy. Urine glucose and protein concentrations may be increased; leukocyte and platelet count may be decreased; bleeding time may be prolonged for 1 day after discontinuation.
- Assess for blurred vision, tinnitis, which could indicate toxicity.
- Observe for signs of GI bleeding (black stools, occult blood loss) throughout therapy.
- Assess for mood changes, depression, hallucinations, confusion.
- Report signs of adverse reactions to physician immediately, especially in elderly patients.

OVERDOSAGE: SIGNS & SYMPTOMS

Nausea, vomiting, headache, dizziness, mental confusion, disorientation, lethargy, paresthesias, numbness, convulsions, tinnitus

Patient/Family Education

- Tell patient to take medication with food, milk or antacids if GI upset occurs. Inform physician if stomach distress continues.
- Caution patient to avoid aspirin, alcohol and ibuprofen while taking this medication.
- Instruct patient to report these symptoms to physician: skin rash, itching,

black stools, unusual bruising or bleeding, visual disturbances, tinnitus, weight gain, edema or persistent headache.

- Advise patient that drug may cause drowsiness and to use caution while driving or performing other tasks requiring mental alertness.
- Explain that therapeutic effects for rheumatoid arthritis may not be seen for up to 1 mo of drug use.
- Explain purpose of medication and, for parents of infant with ductus arteriosus, emphasize need for frequent monitoring.

See Patient Guide, p. 312.

Influenza Virus Vaccine

(in-flew-EN-zuh virus vaccine)

Fluzone, Fluvirin, Fluogen, Flu-Shield

Class: Vaccine, inactivated virus

Action Induces formation of specific antibodies that protect against those strains of virus from which vaccine is prepared or closely related strains.

Indications Induction of active immunity against influenza A and B viruses corresponding to strains in current-year vaccine formula; prophylaxis for persons > 6 mo at increased risk of complications of or exposure to influenza.

Contraindications Immediate hypersensitivity to product or to thimerosal, neomycin or other components; immediate hypersensitivity (eg, hives, swelling of the mouth or throat, difficulty breathing, hypotension, shock) following ingestion of eggs. Delayed immunization is recommended for persons with active neurologic disorder characterized by changing neurologic findings; reconsider when disease process has stabilized. Defer immunization during acute respiratory disease or other active infection or during acute febrile illness.

Route/Dosage Both split-virus and whole-virus influenza vaccines are produced, with different viral strains included in each year's formula. CHILDREN ≤ 12 YR: Split-virus vaccine only. ADULTS & CHILDREN ≥ 13 YR: Use either vaccine. ADULTS & CHILDREN ≥ 9 YR: One 0.5 ml dose IM annually. PREVIOUSLY UNVACCINATED CHILDREN ≤ 8 YR: 2 doses IM at least 1 mo apart. Give second dose before December, if possible. CHILDREN 3-8 YR: 0.5 ml at each injection. CHILDREN 6-35 MO: 0.25 ml at each injection.

Interactions
Anticoagulants: As with other drugs given IM, give with caution to persons receiving anticoagulant therapy. *Immunosuppressant drugs (eg, high-dose corticosteroids), radiation therapy:* May result in inadequate response to immunization. *Pertussis vaccine:* In order to attribute causality of adverse reactions, do not give influenza vaccine within 3 days of pertussis vaccination.

Lab Test Interferences
None well documented.

Adverse Reactions Soreness at injection site; fever; malaise; myalgia; Guillain-Barré syndrome; immediate (probably allergic) reactions (eg, hives, angioedema, allergic asthma, systemic anaphylaxis) occur extremely rarely.

Precautions
Pregnancy: Category C. *Lactation:* Undetermined.

NURSING CONSIDERATIONS

Administration/Storage

- Agitate vial before administration.
- Use deltoid muscle for adults and older children.
- Use anterolateral aspect of thigh

for infants > 6 mo and for young children.
- Use only split vaccines in children < 13 yr.
- Have epinephrine 1:1000 readily available.
- Do not give intravenously.
- Do not give to infants < 6 mo.
- Do not give within 3 days of vaccination with pertussis vaccine.

Assessment/Interventions
- Obtain patient history, including drug history and any known allergies.
- Report skin reactions (erythema, rash, induration) or unusual neurological symptoms (paresthesias, paralysis, encephalopathies) to physician.
- Provide written record of immunization and any untoward effects.

Patient/Family Education
- Advise patient that soreness at injection site may occur for 1-2 days.
- Instruct patient to report fever, malaise, myalgia, weakness or headache to physician.
- Remind patient that vaccine needs to be given yearly.

See Patient Guide, p. 313.

Insulin

(IN-suh-lin)

Humulin 70/30, Humulin L, Humulin N, Humulin R, Humulin U, Iletin I Lente, Iletin I NPH, Iletin I Regular, Iletin II Lente (Pork), Iletin II NPH, Iletin II Regular, Iletin II Regular Concentrate, Lente Ilentin I, Lente L, Novolin 70/30, Novolin L, Novolin N, Novolin R, NPH Iletin I, NPH Insulin, NPH-N, Regular, Regular Iletin I, Regular Insulin, Ultralente U, Velosulin Human, ♣ Insulin-Toronto, Novolin Lente, Novolin-NPH, Novolin-Toronto (Regular), Novolin-Ultralente, Novolin 30/70, Protamine Zinc Iletin, Semilente, Semilente Iletin, Ultralente Iletin, Velosulin Human

Class: Antidiabetic

Action Regulates proper glucose use in normal metabolic processes.

Indications Management of diabetes mellitus type I (insulin-dependent) and diabetes mellitus type II (non-insulin-dependent) not properly controlled by diet, exercise and weight reduction. In hyperkalemia, infusions of glucose and insulin lower serum potassium levels. IV or IM regular insulin may be given for rapid effect in severe ketoacidosis or diabetic coma. Highly purified (single component) and human insulins are used for treatment of local insulin allergy, immunologic insulin resistance, lipodystrophy at injection site, temporary insulin administration and newly diagnosed diabetics.

Contraindications Hypersensitivity to pork or mixed beef/pork insulin unless successful desensitization has been accomplished.

Route/Dosage
Insulin preparations are classified into three groups based on promptness, duration and intensity of action following SC administration. These classifications are rapid-(Regular or Semilente), intermediate-(Lente or NPH) or long-(Ultralente) acting. Maintenance doses are given subcutaneously and must be individualized by monitoring patients closely. Consider following dosage guidelines. CHILDREN & ADULTS: 0.5 to 1 U/kg/day. ADOLESCENTS (DURING GROWTH SPURT): 0.8 to 1.2 U/kg/day. Adjust doses to achieve premeal and bedtime blood glucose levels of 80-140 mg/dl (children < 5 yr 100 to 200 mg/dl). Regular insulin is given IV or IM for severe ketoacidosis or diabetic coma.

Interactions Contraceptives (oral), corticosteroids, dextrothyroxine, diltiazem, dobutamine, epinephrine, smoking, thiazide diuretics, thyroid hormone: May decrease hypoglycemic effects of insulin. Alcohol, anabolic steroids, beta blockers, clofibrate, fenfluramine, guanthidine, MAO inhibitors, phenylbutazone, salicylates, sulfinpyrazone, tetracyclines: May increase hypoglycemic effects of insulin.

Lab Test Interferences

None well documented.

Adverse Reactions

DERM: Lipodystrophy (from repeated insulin injection into same site). *META:* Hypoglycemia. *OTHER:* Hypersensitivity reaction (eg, rash, shortness of breath, fast pulse, sweating, hypotension, anaphylaxis or angiodema); local reactions (eg, redness, swelling and itching at injection site).

Precautions

Pregnancy: Insulin is drug of choice for control of diabetes in pregnancy; supervise carefully. *Lactation:* Not excreted in breast milk. Breastfeeding may decrease insulin requirements despite increase in necessary caloric intake. *Changing insulin:* Changes in purity, strength, brand, type or species source of insulin may necessitate dosage adjustment. Make changes cautiously under medical supervision. *Diabetic ketoacidosis:* May result from stress, illness or insulin omission and may develop slowly after long period of poor insulin control. Condition is potentially life-threatening and requires prompt diagnosis and treatment. *Hypoglycemia:* May result from excessive insulin dose or increased work or exercise without eating or from illness with vomiting, fever or diarrhea. May also occur when insulin requirements decline. *Insulin resistance:* Requirements of > 200 units of insulin/day for > 2 days in absence of ketoacidosis or acute infection may occur, especially in obese patients, in patients with acanthosis nigricans, patients with insulin receptor defects or during infection.

NURSING CONSIDERATIONS

Administration/Storage

- For insulin suspension, ensure uniform dispersion by rolling vial gently between hands. Avoid vigorous shaking that may result in formation of air bubbles.
- When mixing insulins, draw regular insulin into syringe first.
- Use only insulin syringes.
- Select appropriate injection site according to patient history and needs; rotate administration sites to prevent lipodystrophy. (Subcutaneous insulin is absorbed most rapidly at abdominal injection sites, more slowly at sites on arms and slowest at sites on anterior thigh.)
- Administer insulin 30 min before meals.
- Store properly in accordance with patient's daily needs. (Insulin remains stable for 1 mo at room temperature or 3 mo under refrigeration.) Store extra bottle of insulin in refrigerator.
- Refrigerate prefilled plastic and glass syringes. (Can be stored under refrigeration for up to 14 days.)
- Do not freeze.
- Do not expose to extreme temperatures or sunlight.

Assessment/Interventions

- Obtain patient history, including drug history and any known allergies.
- Assess patient for signs of hypoglycemia (anxiety; chills; confusion; cool, pale skin; drowsiness; excessive hunger; headache; irritability; nausea; rapid pulse; tremors).
- Observe patient for signs of hyperglycemia (drowsiness; fruit-like breath odor; frequent urination; loss of appetite; thirst).
- Monitor blood glucose levels throughout course of therapy.
- Observe injection sites for signs of local hypersensitivity reaction, such as redness, itching or burning.
- Notify physician if hypoglycemia or adverse reactions occur.

- If lipoatrophy or lipohypertrophy develops at injection site, use alternate sites or use purified insulin.
- Document injection sites used.

OVERDOSAGE: SIGNS & SYMPTOMS

Fatigue, weakness, nervousness, confusion, headache, diplopia, convulsions, psychoses, dizziness, unconsciousness, rapid or shallow respiration, numb or tingling mouth, hunger, nausea, skin pallor, moist or dry skin

Patient/Family Education

- Teach name, dose, action and side effects of insulin.
- Tell patient not to change brand, strength, type or dose without physician's knowledge.
- Dosage adjustments may be necessary when type of insulin is changed.
- Tell patient to consult physician for dosage changes during illness.
- Instruct patient to use same type and brand of syringe each time to prevent dosage errors.
- Explain potential long-term complications of diabetes, and encourage regular, general physical and eye examinations.
- Tell patient to report redness, swelling or itching at injection site.
- Explain significance of and importance of reporting: visual changes; rash; infection that does not heal; increased thirst; increased urination; dry mouth; burning sensation in feet, legs or hands; pain in legs after exercise; and frequent episodes of very low or very high blood sugar levels.
- Show patient how to rotate injection sites to prevent scarring.
- Teach patient how to monitor blood glucose as directed.
- Identify source for obtaining medical ID (Medi-Alert) and explain importance of information.
- Teach patient and family how to draw up and administer insulin.
- Demonstrate self-care techniques for patient using insulin pump.
- Emphasize importance of compliance with diet and exchange system for meals.
- Emphasize importance of regular exercise.
- Tell patient to carry source of sugar (candy, sugar packets) to counteract hypoglycemia.

See Patient Guide, p. 314.

Interferon Alfa-2a (rIFN-A, IFLrA)

(IN-ter-FEER-ahn AL-fuh–2a)

Roferon-A

Class: Interferon/Immunomodulator

Action These small protein molecules bind to specific cell membranes and initiate complex sequence of intracellular events, including induction of certain enzymes; that may prevent proliferation of tumor cells.

Indications Treatment of hairy cell leukemia, AIDS-related Kaposi's sarcoma and chronic-phase, Philadelphia chromosome positive chronic myelogenous leukemia patients who are minimally pretreated (within 1 year of diagnosis). **Unlabeled uses:** Treatment of bladder tumors (locally for superficial tumors), carcinoid tumor, cutaneous T-cell lymphoma, certain leukemias, essential thrombocythemia, non-Hodgkin's lymphoma (low-grade), renal cell carcinoma, ovarian carcinoma, cervical carcinoma, malignant gliomas, Hodgkin's disease, melanoma, multiple myeloma, osteosarcoma, mycosis fungoides/Sezary syndrome, many viral infections, multiple sclerosis.

Contraindications Standard considerations.

Route/Dosage

Hairy Cell Leukemia

ADULTS: **SC/IM** Induction dose: 3 million IU daily for 16-24 wk. Maintenance: 3 million IU 3 times/wk for 6 mo;

evaluate benefit. Dosage reduction by one-half or withholding doses may become necessary with severe adverse reactions.

AIDS-Related Kaposi's Sarcoma
ADULTS: Induction dose: 36 million IU daily for 10-12 wk. Maintenance: 36 million IU 3 times/wk. Reduce to 50% if severe adverse effects occur.

Philadelphia Chromosome (Ph) Positive Chronic Myelogenous Leukemia ADULTS: **SC/TM:** Initial dose: 9 million IU daily. Short-term tolerance may be improved by gradually increasing the dose over the first week from 3 million IU daily for 3 days to 6 million IU daily for 3 days, then advancing to 9 million IU daily for the duration of the treatment period.

Interactions

Theophylline: Increased effects of theophylline.

Lab Test Interferences

None well documented.

Adverse Reactions

CV: Hypotension; edema; chest pain; hypertension; arrhythmias; palpitation; congestive heart failure; pulmonary edema; MI. *RESP:* Cough; chest congestion; dyspnea; chest pain; rhinorrhea; sinusitis. *CNS:* Headache; dizziness; anxiety; decreased mental status; depression; confusion; diaphoresis; paresthesias; numbness; lethargy; visual disturbances; sleep disturbances; nervousness; vertigo; forgetfulness; coma. *GI:* Anorexia; nausea; diarrhea; vomiting; abdominal pain; flatulence; constipation. *GU:* Transient impotence; BUN changes. *HEMA:* Leukopenia; neutropenia; thrombocytopenia; decreased Hgb; hypocalcemia; elevated fasting serum glucose and serum phosphorus; neutralizing antibodies to interferon. *HEPA:* Elevations in AST, alkaline phosphatase, LDH, bilirubin. *DERM:* Partial alopecia; rash; dryness or inflammation of oropharynx; pruritus; dry skin; urticaria reactivation of herpes labialis. *OTHER:* Flu-like symptoms (eg, fatigue, arthralgia, myalgia, chills); fever; weight loss; change in taste; night sweats.

Precautions

Pregnancy: Category C. *Lactation:* Undetermined. *Children:* Safety and efficacy in children < 18 yr not established. *Special risk patients:* Use caution in patients with severe renal or hepatic disease, seizure disorders or compromised CNS function; acute, self-limiting adverse effects may exacerbate these conditions. *CNS reactions:* Have occurred, including decreased mental status, exaggerated CNS function and dizziness. *Leukopenia and elevation of hepatic enzymes:* Occur frequently. *Platelet counts < 50,000:* Administer SC only.

NURSING CONSIDERATIONS

Administration/Storage

- Once powder is reconstituted, use within 30 days.
- Available IM or SC (SC administration is recommended for, but not limited to, patients who are thrombocytopenic [platelet count < 50,000/mm^3] or who are at risk for bleeding).
- Refrigerate; do not freeze; do not shake.

Assessment/Interventions

- Obtain patient history, including drug history and any known allergies.
- Assess patient for GI, CNS, respiratory, cardiovascular, hematological and dermatological side effects. If these effects are present, notify physician.
- Assess for flu-like symptoms (fever, headache, fatigue, myalgia, chills). If such symptoms occur, administer drug in evening, give acetaminophen as prescribed.
- Monitor hydration if patient experiences anorexia, nausea or diarrhea.

- Monitor results of patient's laboratory tests.
- If patient experiences adverse CNS symptoms, take safety precautions such as lowering bed, putting side rails up and supervising ambulation.
- Implement infection control precautions when WBC drops; implement bleeding precautions when platelet count drops.
- Discuss use of antiemetic with physician if nausea or vomiting develops.
- Maintain good hydration status.

Patient/Family Education

- Explain name, dose, action and side effects of drug. Emphasize that flu-like symptoms are most common.
- Assure male patient that impotence, when it occurs, is usually transient.
- Stress importance of follow-up blood tests.
- Teach infection control measures, bleeding precautions and energy conservation measures.
- Instruct patient to report swollen ankles, dyspnea, chest pain, noisy breathing.
- Caution patient if decreased mental status or dizziness occurs to take safety precautions and not to perform activities that require mental alertness such as operating machinery or driving.
- Advise patient to take medication at bedtime if flu-like symptoms occur.
- Tell patient to maintain a well-hydrated state.
- Teach patient or family how to reconstitute, administer and store SC or IM form of drug.
- Warn patient not to change brands of drug because of differences in manufacturing process, strength and product type.

See Patient Guide, p. 315.

Interferon Alfa-2b (IFN-alpha 2; rIFN-a2; a-2-interferon)

(IN-ter-FEER-ahn AL-fuh–2b)

Intron A

Class: Interferon/Immunomodulator

Action These small protein molecules bind to specific cell membranes and initiate complex sequence of intracellular events, including induction of certain enzymes.

Indications Treatment of hairy cell leukemia, condylomata acuminata, AIDS-related Kaposi's sarcoma, chronic hepatitis non-A, non-B/C, chronic hepatitis B and as an adjuvant treatment to surgery in adults at high risk for systemic recurrence of malignant melanoma. **Unlabeled uses:** Treatment of carcinoid tumor, cutaneous T-cell lymphoma, chronic myelogenous leukemia (CML), other leukemias, essential thrombocythemia, non-Hodgkin's lymphoma, primary malignant brain tumors, laryngeal papillomatosis, urinary bladder tumors, Hodgkin's disease, melanoma, multiple myeloma, osteosarcoma, many viral infections, multiple sclerosis.

Contraindications Standard considerations.

Route/Dosage

Hairy Cell Leukemia

ADULTS: **SC/IM** 2 million IU/m^2 3 times/wk; continue unless disease progresses rapidly or severe intolerance develops.

Condylomata Acuminata

ADULTS: **Intralesional** 1 million IU/lesion 3 times/wk for 3 wk.

AIDS-Related Kaposi's Sarcoma

ADULTS: **SC/IM** 30 million IU/m^2 3 times/wk. May reduce to 50% if severe adverse effects occur.

Chronic Hepatitis Non-A, Non-B/C

ADULTS: **SC/IM** 3 million IU 3 times/wk for 6 mo in patients with clinical response.

Chronic Hepatitis B

ADULTS: **SC/IM** 30-35 million IU/wk either as 5 million IU daily or 10 million IU 3 times/wk for 16 wk.

Malignant Melanoma

ADULTS: **IV** 20 million IU/m^2 5 consecutive days per week for 4 weeks. *Maintenance:* **SC** 10 million IU/m^2 3 times per week for 48 weeks.

Interactions

Zidovudine: May increase zidovudine serum levels and synergistic adverse effects, such as neutropenia.

Lab Test Interferences

None well documented.

Adverse Reactions

CV: Arrhythmia; atrial fibrillation; bradycardia; cardiac failure; cardiomyopathy; extrasystoles; hypertension; hypotension; palpitations; tachycardia. *RESP:* Pharyngitis; nasal congestion; cough; dry mouth; thirst; bronchospasm; cyanosis; epistaxis; pleural pain; pneumonia; rhinitis; rhinorrhea; sneezing. *CNS:* Headache; dizziness; paresthesia; depression; anxiety; confusion; hypoesthesia; amnesia; impaired concentration; irritability; somnolence; coma. *EENT:* Abnormal or blurred vision; conjunctivitis; diplopia; dry eyes; eye pain; periorbital edema; photophobia; hearing disorder; earache; lacrimal gland disorder; gingivitis; speech disorder; taste loss; tinnitus; vertigo; styes. *GI:* Nausea; diarrhea; vomiting; anorexia; dyspepsia; constipation; abdominal pain; abdominal distention; dysphagia; esophagitis; flatulence; gastric ulcer; gingival bleeding; increased appetite; increased saliva; melena; oral leukoplakia; rectal bleeding; stomatitis. *GU:* Amenorrhea; impotence; increased BUN; hematuria; keukorrhea; menorrhagia; micturition disorder; nocturia; polyuria; uterine bleeding. *HEMA:* Anemia; granulocytopenia; hemolytic anemia; leukopenia; thrombocytopenia; abnormal alkaline phosphatase, serum urea nitrogen. *HEPA:* Abnormal hepatic function test results; bilirubinemia; jaundice; hepatic encephalopathy; hepatic failure; abnormal AST, ALT. *DERM:* Rash; pruritus; dry skin; dermatitis; alopecia; facial edema; injection site reaction; abnormal hair texture; acne; epidermal necrolysis; photosensitivity; nonherpetic cold sores; peripheral ischemia; purpura; skin discoloration; urticaria; vitiligo. *META:* Aggravation of diabetes mellitus; gynecomastia; thyroid disorder; virilism. *OTHER:* Flu-like symptoms; fatigue; arthralgia; asthenia; rigors; chest or back pain; muscle pain or weakness; bone pain; leg cramps; increased sweating; malaise; taste alteration; insomnia; weight loss; hypercalcemia; lymphadenopathy; sepsis; weakness.

Precautions

Pregnancy: Category C. *Lactation:* Undetermined. *Children:* Safety and efficacy in children < 18 yr not established. *Fertility impairment:* May occur. Effective contraception use recommended. *Platelet counts < 50,000:* Administer SC only. *Pre-existing psychiatric condition:* Severe depression may occur; may need to discontinue. *Pre-existing thyroid abnormalities:* Do not use in patients whose thyroid function cannot be maintained in normal range by medication.

NURSING CONSIDERATIONS

Administration/Storage

- Once powder is reconstituted, use within 30 days.
- Use route of administration appropriate for patient (SC administration is recommended for, but not limited to, patients who are thrombocytopenic [platelet count less than 50,000/mm^3] or who are at risk for bleeding).
- Use only 10 million IU/vial strength for intralesional injections. Do not reconstitute with > 1 ml of diluent.
- Use only 50 million IU/vial strength for AIDS-related Kaposi's sarcoma.

- Use tuberculin syringe with 25- to 30-gauge needle for injection into condylomata acuminata lesions.
- If severe adverse reactions develop, dosage adjustment may be appropriate.
- Refrigerate medication. Do not freeze. Do not shake.

Assessment/Interventions

- Obtain patient history, including drug history and any known allergies.
- Assess patient for GI, CNS, respiratory, cardiovascular, hematological and dermatological side effects. If these effects occur, notify physician.
- Assess for flu-like symptoms (fever, headache, fatigue, myalgia, chills). If such symptoms occur, administer drug in evening, give acetaminophen as prescribed.
- Monitor hydration if patient experiences anorexia, nausea or diarrhea.
- Monitor results of patient's laboratory tests.
- If patient experiences adverse CNS symptoms, implement safety precautions such as lowering bed, putting side rails up and supervising ambulation.
- Implement infection control measures when WBC drops; implement bleeding precautions when platelet count drops.
- Discuss use of antiemetic with physician if patient develops nausea or vomiting.
- Maintain good hydration status.

Patient/Family Education

- Explain name, dose, action and potential side effects of drug. Emphasize that flu-like symptoms are most common.
- Advise patients that medication may impair fertility and to use effective contraception during therapy.
- Assure male patient that impotence, when it occurs, is usually transient.
- Stress importance of follow-up blood tests.
- Teach patient infection control measures, bleeding precautions and energy-conservation measures.
- Instruct patient to report swollen ankles, dyspnea, chest pain, noisy breathing.
- Caution patient if decreased mental status or dizziness occurs to take safety precautions and not to perform activities that require mental alertness such as operating machinery or driving.
- Advise patient to take medication at bedtime if flu-like symptoms occur and to use acetaminophen as prescribed.
- Tell patient to maintain a well-hydrated state.
- Teach patient or family how to reconstitute, administer and store SC or IM form of drug.
- Explain that skin changes such as rash, itching, dryness, alopecia, moniliasis, facial edema, and abnormal hair texture may occur.
- Warn patient not to change brands of drug because of differences in manufacturing process, strength and product type.
- Advise patient that this medication may cause photosensitivity and to use sunscreen or wear protective clothing until tolerance to sunlight is determined.

See Patient Guide, p. 316.

Interferon Alfa-n3

(IN-ter-FEER-ahn AL-fuh–n3)

Alferon N

Class: Interferon/Immunomodulator

Action These small proteins bind to specific cell membranes and initiate complex sequences of intracellular events, including induction of certain enzymes that produce antiproliferative action against tumor cells and inhibit viral replication in virus-infected cells.

Indications Treatment of condyloma acuminatum. **Unlabeled uses:** Treatment of bladder tumors, carcinoid tumors, certain leukemias, cutaneous T-cell lymphoma, essential thrombocythemia, non-Hodgkin's lymphoma, cervical carcinoma, Hodgkin's disease, malignant gliomas, melanoma, multiple myeloma, nasopharyngeal sarcoma, osteosarcoma, ovarian carcinoma, renal carcinoma, AIDS-related Kaposi's sarcoma and certain viral infections.

Contraindications None well documented.

Route/Dosage

Condyloma Acuminatum

ADULTS: **Intralesional** 250,000 IU (0.05 ml) (maximum recommended dose per treatment session) injected into base of each wart. Administer twice weekly for up to 8 wk.

Lab Test Interferences
None well documented.

Interactions None well documented.

Adverse Reactions
CV: Chest pain, hypotension; vasovagal response. *CNS:* Headache; depression; fatigue; malaise; dizziness; insomnia; sleepiness. *EENT:* Blurred vision; ocular rotation pain; sinus drainage; sore mouth; stomatitis; mucositis. *GI:* Nausea; vomiting; dyspepsia; diarrhea; anorexia; dry mouth. *HEMA:* Altered hemoglobin levels, WBC, platelet count, GGT. *HEPA:* Altered AST, alkaline phosphatase, total bilirubin. *DERM:* Soreness at injection site; generalized pruritus; sweating. *OTHER:* Fever; chills; myalgias; arthralgia; back pain; flu-like syndrome.

Precautions
Pregnancy: Category C. *Lactation:* Undetermined. *Children:* Safety and efficacy not established in children < 18 yr. *Debilitating medical conditions:* Fever and "flu-like" symptoms associated with drug may exacerbate medical conditions (eg, cardiovascular disease, pulmonary disease, diabetes mellitus with ketoacidosis, coagulation disorders, severe myelodepression, seizures). *Product interchange:* Interferon products are not interchangeable because of manufacturing processes, strength and type.

NURSING CONSIDERATIONS

Administration/Storage

- Do not shake solution.
- Inject into base of each wart, preferably with 30-gauge needle.
- Store in refrigerator. Do not freeze.

Assessment/Interventions

- Obtain patient history, including drug history and any allergies.
- Assess patient for GI, CNS, cardiovascular, respiratory, dermatological and hematological side effects. If present, notify physician.
- Monitor hydration if patient experiences anorexia, nausea or diarrhea. If vomiting and diarrhea occur frequently, increase patient's fluid intake to 2-3 L/day.
- Monitor results of laboratory tests.
- Assess patient for symptoms of infection because they may be masked by drug fever.
- If patient experiences adverse CNS symptoms (eg, LOC, mental status changes, dizziness, confusion), take safety precautions such as lowering bed, putting side rails up and supervising ambulation.
- Discuss need for antiemetic with physician if patient develops nausea or vomiting.
- If flu-like symptoms occur, administer drug in evening, and administer acetaminophen as prescribed for fever and headache.

Patient/Family Education

- Stress importance of returning for follow-up blood tests.
- Teach infection control measures, bleeding precautions and energy conservation measures.
- Emphasize importance of maintaining well-hydrated state.
- Caution patient not to change brand of drug because dosages vary among different forms.
- Advise patient to take medication at bedtime if flu-like symptoms occur and to use acetaminophen as needed.
- Instruct patient to report symptoms that may represent side effects: hives, swollen ankles, dyspnea, chest pain, noisy breathing.
- Caution patient that if decreased mental status or dizziness occurs to take safety precautions and not to perform activities that require mental alertness.

See Patient Guide, p. 317.

Interferon Beta-1b (rIFN-B)

(IN-ter-FEER-ahn BAY-tuh–1b)

Betaseron

Class: Interferon/immunomodulator

Action Has both antiviral and immunoregulatory activity. Decreases T-cell proliferation; blocks synthesis of interferon gamma; inhibits release of other cytokines that damage oligodendrocytes; increases T-suppressor cell activity.

Indications Reduction of frequency of clinical exacerbations in ambulatory patients with relapsing-remitting multiple sclerosis (RRMS). **Unlabeled uses:** Treatment of AIDS, AIDS-related Kaposi's sarcoma, metastatic renal-cell carcinoma, malignant melanoma, cutaneous T-cell lymphoma, and acute non-A/non-B hepatitis.

Contraindications Hypersensitivity to *E coli*–derived products or human albumin.

Route/Dosage

ADULTS: SC 0.25 mg (8 million IU) qod with 27-gauge needle into arm, abdomen, hip or thigh.

Interactions

Live virus vaccines (eg, measles, mumps, polio, rubella): May inhibit antibody response after immunization; avoid concurrent use.

Lab Test Interferences

None well documented.

Adverse Reactions

CV: Palpitation; hypertension; tachycardia; migraine; peripheral vascular disorders. *RESP*: Dyspnea. *CNS*: Asthenia; somnolence; dizziness; malaise. *EENT*: Laryngitis. *GI*: GI disorders; nausea; diarrhea; constipation. *GU*: Mild to moderate menstrual disorders; pelvic pain; cystitis. *HEPA*: Increased ALT, AST and total bilirubin. *OTHER*: Injection-site reactions; injection-site necrosis; sweating; breast pain; abdominal pain; "flu"-like symptoms (eg, myalgia, fever, chills); decreased absolute neutrophil count (ANC) and WBC.

Precautions

Pregnancy: Category C. *Lactation*: Undetermined. *Children*: Safety and efficacy in children < 18 yr not established. *Suicide/mental disorders*: Suicide attempts occurred in clinical trials. Depression and suicidal ideation should be reported immediately.

NURSING CONSIDERATIONS

Administration/Storage

- Reconstitute with supplied diluent.
- Do not shake solution.
- Discard solution if it contains particulate matter or is discolored.
- Administer SC with 27-gauge needle into arm, hip, abdomen or thigh.

- Do not inject into skin that is tender, red or hard.
- Rotate injection sites, not repeating same site more than once weekly.
- After reconstitution, refrigerate for no longer than 3 hours.
- Use product within 3 hr of reconstitution. Discard unused solution.
- Store drug in refrigerator before and after reconstitution.

Assessment/Interventions

- Obtain patient history, including drug history and any known allergies.
- Obtain baseline CBC with differential, platelets, LFTs, electrolytes. Monitor throughout therapy.
- Assess patient for GI, CNS, cardiovascular, respiratory, dermatological and hematological reactions. If present, notify physician.
- Monitor hydration if patient experiences anorexia, nausea or diarrhea.
- Monitor results of laboratory tests.
- Monitor I&O strictly. Increase fluid intake if patient becomes dehydrated. Weigh patient daily.
- Assess patient for depression and suicide potential.
- If patient experiences adverse CNS symptoms (LOC, mental status change, dizziness, confusion), take safety precautions such as lowering bed, putting side rails up and supervising ambulation.
- Implement infection control measures if WBC drops; implement bleeding precautions if platelet count drops.
- Discuss need for antiemetic with physician if nausea or vomiting develops.
- If flu-like symptoms occur, administer drug in evening and administer acetaminophen as prescribed for fever and headache.

Patient/Family Education

- Stress importance of returning for follow-up blood tests.
- Teach patient infection control measures, bleeding precautions and energy-conservation measures.
- Caution patient that if decreased mental status or dizziness occurs to use safety precautions and not to perform activities that require mental alertness.
- Advise patient to take medication at bedtime if flu-like symptoms occur and to use acetaminophen as needed.
- Explain importance of adequate hydration.
- Teach patient or family how to store, reconstitute and administer drug SC.
- Encourage patient to report depression or suicidal ideation immediately.
- Provide puncture-resistant container for disposal of used syringes and needles.
- Instruct patient to report symptoms that may represent side effects: swollen ankles, dyspnea, chest pain, noisy breathing.
- Instruct patient to report these symptoms to physician: flu-like symptoms; pain at injection site; headache; fever; fluid retention; pelvic pain; cysts; migraine headaches; pounding in chest; sleeplessness; menstrual problems; breast pain; frequent urination; hair loss, sweating; anxiety; confusion; joint and muscle aches; high blood pressure; sinus infection; difficulty breathing; laryngitis; convulsions.
- Caution patient to avoid exposure to sunlight and to use sunscreen or wear protective clothing to avoid photosensitivity reaction.

See Patient Guide, p. 318.

Interferon Gamma-1b

(IN-ter-FEER-ahn GAM-uh–1b)
Actimmune
Class: Interferon/immunomodulator

Action Produces potent phagocyte-activating effects, including generation of toxic oxygen metabolites within phagocytes, which mediate killing of microorganisms. Activities include enhancement of oxidative metabolism of tissue macrophages and enhancement of antibody-dependent cellular cytotoxicity and natural killer (NK) cell activity.

Indications Reduction of frequency and severity of serious infections associated with chronic granulomatous disease. **Unlabeled uses:** Treatment of small-cell lung cancer, atopic dermatitis, trauma-related infections, metastatic renal-cell carcinoma, cutaneous T-cell lymphoma, asthma and allergies, refractory leishmaniasis, chronic myelogenous leukemia and AIDS.

Contraindications Hypersensitivity to *E coli*–derived products.

Route/Dosage
ADULTS & CHILDREN: SC 50 mcg/m^2 (1.5 million U/m^2) if body surface area is > 0.5 m^2 or 1.5 mcg/kg/dose if body surface area is ≤ 0.5 m^2. Administer 3 times/wk (eg, Monday, Wednesday, Friday) into right or left deltoid or anterior thigh. If severe adverse reactions develop, reduced dosage or discontinuation of therapy may be necessary until those reactions subside.

Interactions
Live virus vaccines (eg, measles, mumps, polio, rubella): May inhibit antibody response after immunization; avoid concurrent use. *Myelosuppressive agents:* Additive neutropenic effects are possible.

Lab Test Interferences
None well documented.

Adverse Reactions
CNS: Decreased mental status; gait disturbance; dizziness; fatigue; headache. *GI:* Diarrhea; vomiting; nausea. *GU:* Proteinuria. *HEMA:* Thrombocytopenia. *OTHER:* Fever; chills; erythema or tenderness at injection site; myalgia; arthralgia.

Precautions
Pregnancy: Category C. *Lactation:* Undetermined. *Children:* Safety and efficacy in children < 1 yr not established. *Special risk patients:* Exercise caution in patients with seizure disorders, compromised CNS function, cardiac disease and myelosuppression.

NURSING CONSIDERATIONS

Administration/Storage

- Discard unused portion of any vial. Product contains no preservative, and vials are suitable for only single dose.
- Refrigerate; do not freeze. Any unopened vial should not be left at room temperature for more than 12 hr. Do not shake vial.
- Administer by SC route only in right or left deltoid and anterior thigh.
- Give at bedtime with acetaminophen for fever and headache.

Assessment/Interventions

- Obtain patient history, including drug history and any known allergies.
- Obtain baseline CBC with differential, platelets, renal and hepatic studies, BUN, creatinine, ALT and urinalysis. Monitor throughout therapy.
- Monitor results of laboratory tests.
- Assess patient for GI, CNS, cardiovascular, dermatological and hematological side effects. If present, notify physician.
- Monitor hydration if patient experiences anorexia, nausea or diarrhea.
- If patient experiences adverse CNS symptoms, implement safety precautions such as lowering bed, putting side rails up and supervising ambulation.
- Implement infection control measures if WBC drops; implement bleeding precautions if platelet count drops.
- Discuss need for antiemetic with physician if nausea or vomiting develops.

- If flu-like symptoms occur, administer drug in evening and give acetaminophen as prescribed.

Patient/Family Education

- Stress importance of returning for follow-up blood tests.
- Teach infection control measures, bleeding precautions and energy-conservation measures.
- Caution patient that if decreased mental status or dizziness occur to use safety precautions and not to perform activities that require mental alertness.
- Advise patient to take medication at bedtime if flu-like symptoms occur and to use acetaminophen as needed.
- Explain importance of adequate hydration.
- Teach patient or family to store, prepare and administer drug SC.
- Provide puncture-resistant container for disposal of used syringes and needles.
- Instruct patient to report these symptoms to physician: swollen ankles, dyspnea, chest pain, noisy breathing; flu-like symptoms; pain at injection site; headache; fever; fluid retention; pelvic pain; cysts; migraine headaches; pounding in chest; sleeplessness; menstrual problems; breast pain; frequent urination; hair loss; sweating; anxiety; confusion; joint and muscle aches; high blood pressure; sinus infection; difficulty breathing; laryngitis; convulsions.

See Patient Guide, p. 319.

Iodine

(EYE-uh-dine)

Iodine Tincture, Iodopen, Strong Iodine (Lugol's Solution), Thyro-Block

Potassium Iodide

Pima, SSKI

Class: Thyroid; trace metal; antiseptic; expectorant

Action

Antiseptic: Topical iodine possesses microbicidal properties. *Thyroid drug:* Large doses of iodides inhibit thyroid hormone production and release into bloodstream. Enhances secretion of respiratory fluids, thus decreasing mucus viscosity.

Indications

Antiseptic: Externally, to achieve broad microbicidal benefits. *Thyroid agent:* In adjunctive with antithyroid drug in hyperthyroid patients to prepare for thyroidectomy and to treat thyrotoxic crisis or neonatal thyrotoxicosis; thyroid blocking in radiation emergency. *Trace metal:* Supplement to IV solutions given for TPN. *Expectorant:* Treatment of chronic pulmonary diseases complicated by tenacious mucus, including bronchial asthma, chronic bronchitis, bronchiectasis and pulmonary emphysema; adjunctive treatment in respiratory conditions such as cystic fibrosis and chronic sinusitis and to prevent atelectasis after surgery.

Contraindications Hypersensitivity to iodides; impaired renal function; acute bronchitis; hyperthyroidism; Addison's disease; acute dehydration; heat cramps; hyperkalemia; iodism; tuberculosis.

Route/Dosage

Topical Antiseptic

Apply prn to intact skin.

Thyroid Agent Prior to Thyroidectomy

PO 2-6 drops of strong iodine solution (Lugol's solution) tid for 10 days prior to surgery.

For Thyroid Blocking in Radiation Emergency

Use at direction of state or local public health authorities.

Trace Metal for TPN (Supplied as Sodium Iodide)

FOR METABOLICALLY STABLE ADULTS: 1-2 mcg/kg/day (normal adults, 75-150 mcg/day). PREGNANT

AND LACTATING WOMEN, GROWING CHILDREN: 2-3 mcg/kg/day.

Expectorant

ADULTS: **PO** 300-1000 mg initially after meals. If tolerated, 1-1.5 g tid. CHILDREN: **PO** Half adult dose.

Interactions

Lithium: May have synergistic hypothyroid activity; may result in hypothyroidism. *Potassium-sparing diuretics:* Increase risk of hyperkalemia, cardiac arrhythmias and cardiac arrest.

Lab Test Interferences

Potassium iodide may alter thyroid function test results.

Adverse Reactions

CV: Irregular heart beat. *CNS:* Confusion; unusual tiredness. *EENT:* Swelling of neck, throat or salivary glands. *GI:* Bleeding. *DERM:* Rash; acne. *META:* Thyroid adenoma; goiter; myxedema; thyroid gland enlargement; acute parotitis. *OTHER:* Hypersensitivity manifested by angioneurotic edema, cutaneous and mucosal hemorrhages and symptoms resembling serum sickness (eg, fever, arthralgia, lymph node enlargement and eosinophilia); numbness; tingling; pain or weakness in hands or feet; unusual tiredness; weakness or heaviness of legs; fever; "iodism" (eg, metallic taste, burning mouth and throat, sore teeth and gums, symptoms of head cold and, sometimes, stomach upset and diarrhea).

Precautions

Pregnancy: Category C (trace metal); Category D (potassium iodide). *Lactation:* Excreted in breast milk. *Children:* Safety and efficacy not established. *Topical:* For external use only; highly toxic if ingested. Avoid contact with eyes and mucous membranes. Iodine preparations stain skin and clothing. *Oral: Hypothyroidism:* Prolonged use can lead to hypothyroidism. *Special risk patients:* Pulmonary tuberculosis is considered contraindication to use of iodides by some authorities; use with caution in such cases and in patients having cardiac disease, myotonia congenita or renal impairment. Cystic fibrosis patients may have increased susceptibility to adverse effects. *GI effects;* Nonspecific small bowel lesions have occurred with enteric-coated potassium salts.

NURSING CONSIDERATIONS

Administration/Storage

- Do not give trace metal undiluted by direct injection into peripheral vein.
- Measure solutions carefully with calibrated dropper.
- Dilute expectorant in 60 ml of flavored beverages (eg, chocolate or plain milk, orange juice) to minimize bitter taste.
- Mix solutions in full glass of fruit juice, water or milk.
- Administer after meals to minimize irritation.
- Have patient sip expectorant through straw to decrease burning sensation in mouth and to prevent discoloration of teeth.
- Store in airtight, light-resistant container at room temperature.

Assessment/Interventions

- Obtain patient history, including drug history and any known allergies.
- Assess for signs and symptoms of iodism (metallic taste, stomatitis, skin lesions, cold symptoms).
- Monitor thyroid function before and periodically during course of therapy.
- Notify physician of any signs of hyperthyroidism (tachycardia, palpitations, nervousness, insomnia, tremors, weight loss, diaphoresis).
- Report to physician any signs of iodism or sensitivity to drug.

OVERDOSAGE: SIGNS & SYMPTOMS

Iodine is corrosive; toxic symptoms are related primarily to local GI tract irritation. Gastroenteritis, abdominal pain and diarrhea (sometimes bloody) may be seen. Fatalities may occur from circulatory collapse, because of shock, corrosive gastritis or asphyxiation from swelling of glottis or larynx

Patient/Family Education

- Explain name, dose, action and side effects of iodine product.
- Tell patient to discontinue use and notify physician if fever, skin rash, metallic taste, swelling of throat, burning of mouth and throat, sore gums and teeth, head cold symptoms, severe GI distress or enlargement of thyroid gland (goiter) occurs.
- Inform patient if replacement therapy is to be taken for life.
- Explain that sudden discontinuation of drug should not be done without physician's guidance.
- Teach patient which foods are high in iodine (seafood, kale, turnips, and iodized salt).
- Explain that darkening of solution does not affect potency.

See Patient Guide, pp. 320-322.

Ipecac Syrup

(IPP-uh-kak syrup)

Available as generic only

Class: Antidote

Action Produces vomiting by local irritant effect and stimulation of chemoreceptor trigger zone.

Indications Treatment of drug overdose and certain poisonings.

Contraindications Do not use in semiconscious, unconscious, pregnant or lactating persons; do not use if strychnine, corrosives (eg, alkalis, strong acids) or petroleum distillates have been ingested.

Route/Dosage

ADULTS: **PO** 15-30 ml followed by 3-4 glasses of water. May repeat dose within 20 min if vomiting does not occur. CHILDREN < 1 YR: **PO** 5-10 ml followed by ½ glass of water. CHILDREN 1-12 YR: **PO** 15 ml followed by 1-2 glasses of water.

Interactions

Activated charcoal: Will absorb ipecac syrup. Give activated charcoal only after ipecac syrup has produced vomiting. *Milk or carbonated beverages:* Do not administer with ipecac syrup.

Lab Test Interferences

None well documented.

Adverse Reactions

CV: Heart conduction disturbances; atrial fibrillation; fatal myocarditis. *CNS:* Depression. *GI:* Diarrhea.

Precautions

Pregnancy: Category C. *Lactation:* Undetermined. *Abuse:* Severe cardiomyopathies and death may occur in bulimic and anorexic persons abusing ipecac syrup. *Syrup/fluid extract:* Do not confuse ipecac syrup with ipecac fluid extract, which is 14 times stronger and has caused some deaths.

NURSING CONSIDERATIONS

Administration/Storage

- Consult poison control center before administering, especially in children < 1 yr.
- Have patient sit upright with head forward before administering dose and for at least 30 min after administration.
- Follow administration with 3-4 glasses of water for adults and ½-2 glasses for children.
- If vomiting does not occur within 20 min, dose may be repeated.

- Do not administer with milk or carbonated beverages.
- Do not give to patient who is unconscious or convulsing.
- Do not give if patient has ingested caustic substances or oils.
- Administer activated charcoal only after vomiting has been induced and completed.

Assessment/Interventions

- Obtain patient history, including drug history and any known allergies. Determine what was ingested, paying particular attention to products for which ipecac is contraindicated (caustic substances, oils).
- Assess patient's level of consciousness.
- Assess for adverse reactions such as CNS stimulation or depression, respiratory depression, prolonged vomiting, lethargy or diarrhea.
- Assess effectiveness of drug shortly after administration.
- Assess respiratory rate and pattern, BP and heart rate.
- Monitor for cardiac arrhythmias in patient receiving high doses of ipecac syrup, particularly if patient is very young (< 1 yr) or elderly.
- Notify physician if adverse reactions occur.
- Take safety precautions if sedation occurs: place bed in low position with head of bed elevated, siderails up and assist patient with ambulation.
- Repeat initial dose of ipecac syrup in 20 min if first dose was not effective.
- Inform physician frequently about effectiveness of drug (frequency and amount of vomiting).
- Save all emesis for laboratory identification of ingested poison.
- If patient experiences extreme vomiting, take measures to maintain hydration such as IV fluid support including electrolytes.
- If vomiting does not occur within 30 min after second dose, perform gastric lavage.

OVERDOSAGE: SIGNS & SYMPTOMS

Cardiac conduction disturbances, bradycardia, atrial fibrillation, hypotension, fatal myocarditis

Patient/Family Education

- Caution parents not to induce vomiting if child has swallowed caustic substance or petroleum product or if child is unconscious, semiconscious or having convulsions.
- Instruct parents of children < 1 yr to keep small amount (one 30 ml bottle) on hand for emergencies.
- Instruct parents to always consult physician or poison control center before administration.
- Teach parents not to exceed recommended amounts.
- Teach families to give drug with adequate amounts of water—not milk or carbonated beverages.
- Advise parents that drug has shelf life of 1 yr and should be replaced yearly. Instruct parents to check expiration date before purchasing product.
- Do not give ipecac syrup to an unconscious or very drowsy child because vomited material may enter lungs and cause pneumonia.
- Teach parents to repeat dose if child does not vomit within 20 min and then to take child to emergency room, because gastric lavage may be necessary.

See Patient Guide, p. 323.

Ipratropium Bromide

(IH-pruh-TROE-pee-uhm BROE-mide)

Atrovent

Class: Respiratory inhalant/anticholinergic

Action Antagonizes action of acetylcholine on bronchial smooth muscle in lungs, causing bronchodilation.

Indications Maintenance treatment of bronchospasm associated with COPD, including chronic bronchitis and emphysema.

Contraindications Hypersensitivity to atropine or any anticholinergic derivatives.

Route/Dosage

ADULTS: **Inhalation:** 2 inhalations (36 mcg) qid (maximum 12 inhalations/24 hr). **Solution:** 500 mcg (1 unit dose vial) administered 3 to 4 times a day by oral nebulization, with doses 6 to 8 hours apart. The solution can be mixed in the nebulizer with albuterol if used within 1 hour.

Interactions None well documented.

Lab Test Interferences
None well documented.

Adverse Reactions
CV: Palpitations. *RESP:* Cough; exacerbation of symptoms. *CNS:* Nervousness; dizziness; headache. *EENT:* Blurred vision; local irritation. *GI:* Nausea; dry mouth; GI distress; constipation. *DERM:* Rash.

Precautions
Pregnancy: Category B. *Lactation:* Undetermined. *Children:* Safety and efficacy in children < 12 yr not established. *Special risk patients:* Use drug with caution in patients with narrow-angle glaucoma; prostatic hypertrophy, bladder neck obstruction due to increased risk for precipitation or worsening of underlying disease. *Acute bronchospasm:* Not indicated for initial treatment of acute episodes of bronchospasm in which rapid response is required.

NURSING CONSIDERATIONS

Administration/Storage

- If patient is also receiving an inhaled beta$_2$-agonist, give beta$_2$-agonist before administering ipratropium.
- Shake inhaler well before administration.
- Use spacing device (eg, Aerochamber) to facilitate intrapulmonary deposition.
- Allow 1-2 min between inhalations.
- Have patient rinse mouth with water or mouthwash after each use.
- **Inhalation:** Store at room temperature. Avoid excessive humidity. **Solution:** Store at room temperature. Protect from light. Store unused vials in the foil pouch.

Assessment/Interventions

- Obtain patient history, including drug history and any known allergies.
- Assess respiratory status before initiation of therapy and monitor after inhalation of ipratropium. Therapeutic response is demonstrated by patient's ability to breathe adequately.
- If exacerbation of symptoms occurs, notify physician.
- Give patient frequent sips of water and sugarless hard candy or gum to relieve dry mouth.
- Since drug tolerance may develop with long-term therapy, dosage may need to be increased.

Patient/Family Education

- Instruct patient on proper use of inhaler. Explain value of using spacing device.
- Instruct patient on proper sequencing

and timing if using more than one inhaled agent.
- Teach patient how to determine when canister is empty and needs to be replaced.
- Caution patient not to rely on ipratropium for acute bronchospasm.
- For relief of dry mouth, suggest use of saliva substitute, practice of good oral hygiene, rinsing of mouth after inhalation. Instruct patient to take sips of water frequently, suck on ice chips or sugarless hard candy or chew sugarless gum.
- Caution patient to avoid spraying aerosol in eyes; temporary blurred vision may result.
- Instruct patient to notify physician if condition worsens or the following symptoms occur: dizziness, nausea, headache, palpitations or cough.
- Advise patient that drug may cause dizziness and to use caution while driving or performing other tasks requiring mental alertness.

See Patient Guide, p. 324.

Iron Dextran

(iron DEX-tran)
InFeD
Class: Iron product

Action Replenishes Hgb and depleted iron stores.

Indications Treatment of iron deficiency anemia when oral administration of iron is unsatisfactory or impossible. **Unlabeled use:** Use with epoetin to ensure hematological response to epoetin.

Contraindications Anemia not associated with iron deficiency.

Route/Dosage
Prior to receiving the first **IV** or **IM** iron dextran injection, a 0.5 ml test dose should be given by the same route, respectively. Anaphylactic reactions occurring following iron dextran injection are usually evident within a few minutes or less; however, at least 1 hr should elapse before the remainder of the therapeutic dose is given.

Iron Deficiency Anemia
ADULTS & CHILDREN: **IM/IV** with dose based on formula to determine amount of iron required to restore hemoglobin to normal levels (maximum 2 ml/day undiluted iron dextran):

$$\text{Mg iron} = 0.3 \times \text{body weight in lb} \times \frac{(100 - \text{Hgb [g/dl]} \times 100)}{14.8}$$

Formula should not be used for patients weighing ≤ 30 lb.

Iron Replacement for Blood Loss
ADULTS & CHILDREN: Test dose: **IM/IV** with dose based on formula that 1 ml of normocytic, normochromic RBC cells contains 1 mg of elemental iron (maximum 2 ml/day undiluted iron dextran):

$$\text{Mg iron} = \text{blood loss (ml)} \times \text{Hct}$$

Each days' dose should not exceed 0.5 ml (25 mg iron) for infants < 10 lb or 1 ml (50 mg iron) for children < 20 lb (100 mg iron) for other patients.

Interactions
Chloramphenicol: May increase serum iron concentrations. INCOMPATIBILITIES: Do not mix with other medications or add to parenteral nutrition solutions for IV infusions.

Lab Test Interferences
Serum bilirubin: Drug may cause falsely elevated values. *Serum calcium:* Drug may cause falsely decreased values.

Adverse Reactions
CV: Hypotension; peripheral vascular flushing (IV). *CNS:* Headache; dizziness; malaise; transitory paresthesias. *GI:* Nausea. *HEMA:* Leukocytosis.

DERM: Brown skin discoloration at IM injection site. *OTHER:* Hypersensitivity (fatal anaphylaxis, shortness of breath, urticaria, itching, arthralgia, myalgia, fever); pain and inflammation at injection site; sterile abscesses (IM); phlebitis at IV injection site; reactivation of arthritis in patients with inactive rheumatoid arthritis; backache; shivering. Delayed reactions may occur 1-2 days after administration.

Precautions

Pregnancy: Safety not established. Based on animal studies, avoid if possible. *Lactation:* Undetermined. *Children:* Not recommended in children < 4 mo. *Allergies/asthma:* Use drug with caution in patients with history of significant allergies/asthma. *Arthritis:* Patients with iron deficiency anemia and rheumatoid arthritis may have acute exacerbation of joint pain and swelling after IV administration. *Hepatic impairment:* Use drug with extreme caution in severe hepatic impairment. *Hypersensitivity:* Hypersensitivity, including anaphylaxis, may occur. Have epinephrine immediately available.

NURSING CONSIDERATIONS

Administration/Storage

- Oral iron preparations should be discontinued before parenteral administration.
- Inject IM via/Z-track technique into upper outer quadrant of buttock; never inject iron dextran into arm or other exposed areas. Use 2- to 3-inch 19- or 20-gauge needle.
- If patient is standing, weight should be placed on leg opposite injection site. If in bed, patient should be in lateral position with injection site upper most.
- Change needles between withdrawal from container and injection to minimize staining of subcutaneous tissues. Stains are usually permanent.
- For IV administration, inject slowly at ≤ 1 ml/min.
- Store at room temperature.

Assessment/Interventions

- Obtain patient history, including drug history and any known allergies.
- Assess patient's nutritional status and dietary history to determine possible causes of anemia.
- Monitor Hgb, Hct and reticulocyte values; transferrin, ferritin, total iron-binding capacity; and plasma iron concentrations periodically during therapy.
- Assess patient for signs of anaphylaxis (rash, pruritus, laryngeal edema, wheezing).
- Monitor BP and heart rate frequently during IV administration.
- Assess patient for symptoms of GI distress and constipation regularly throughout therapy.
- Provide diet high in iron (organ meats; leafy, green vegetables; dried beans and peas; dried fruit; cereals).
- If constipation occurs, obtain order for laxative. Increase fiber and give additional fluids.

OVERDOSAGE: SIGNS & SYMPTOMS

Hemosiderosis

Patient/Family Education

- Teach family and patient the name, dose, action and side effects of iron.
- Advise patient to take additional fluids to prevent constipation.
- Teach patient that certain foods, such as coffee, tea, eggs and milk, interact with iron.
- Teach patient and family the daily iron requirements (children 6 mo-10 yr: 10 mg; adolescents 11-18 yr, male: 12 mg; adolescents 11-18 yr, female: 15 mg; adult women, pregnant: 30 mg; adult women, nonpregnant: 15 mg; adult men: 10 mg).

No patient monograph available.

Isoetharine

(EYE-so-ETH-uh-reen)

Isoetharine Hydrochloride

Arm-a-Med Isoetharine Hydrochloride, Bronkosol

Isoetharine Mesylate

Beta-2 Bronkometer

Class: Bronchodilator/ sympathomimetic

Action Produces bronchodilation by relaxing bronchial smooth muscle through beta-2 adrenergic receptor stimulation.

Indications Relief of bronchial asthma and reversible bronchospasm associated with bronchitis and emphysema.

Contraindications Hypersensitivity to any components; cardiac arrhythmias associated with tachycardia; tachycardia or heartblock caused by digitalis intoxication; narrow-angle glaucoma.

Route/Dosage Individualize dosage.

Aerosol Nebulizer/Metered Dose Inhaler

ADULTS & CHILDREN ≥ 12 YR: **Inhalation** 1-2 inhalations q 4 hr prn.

Hand Nebulizer

ADULTS & CHILDREN ≥ 12 YR: **Inhalation** 3-7 inhalations undiluted q 4 hr prn.

Intermittent Positive Pressure Breathing Administration

ADULTS & CHILDREN ≥ 12 YR: **Inhalation** 0.25-1 ml of 1% solution diluted 1:3 with saline.

Oxygen Aerosolization

ADULTS & CHILDREN ≥ 12 YR: **Inhalation** 0.25-0.5 ml of 1% solution diluted 1:3 with saline. Other solution strengths: Usual doses (volume) are based on equivalent 1% solution dose of 0.25-0.5 ml.

Interactions Epinephrine, other sympathomimetics: May cause excessive tachycardia.

Lab Test Interferences None well documented.

Adverse Reactions *CV:* Palpitations; elevated BP. *OTHER:* Anxiety.

Precautions *Pregnancy:* Category C. *Lactation:* Undetermined. *Children:* Safety and efficacy in children ≤ 12 yr not established. *Elderly patients:* Lower doses may be required. *Special risk patients:* Dosage needs to be carefully adjusted in patients with hyperthyroidism, hypertension, acute coronary disease and patients sensitive to sympathomimetic amine to prevent tachycardia, palpitations and headache. *Cardiovascular effects:* Toxic symptoms in patients with cardiovascular disorders may occur. *CNS effects:* CNS stimulation may occur; use drug with caution in patients with history of seizures or hyperthyroidism. *Diabetes mellitus:* Dosage adjustment of insulin or oral hypoglycemic agent may be required. *Excessive use:* Paradoxical bronchospasm and cardiac arrest have been associated with excessive inhalant use. *Sulfite sensitivity:* Some products contain sulfites that may cause allergic-type reactions including anaphylactic symptoms. *Tolerance:* If previously effective dose fails to provide relief, therapy may need to be reassessed.

NURSING CONSIDERATIONS

Administration/Storage

- Dilute 1% nebulizer/intermittent positive pressure breathing solution 1:3 with normal saline.
- Administer inhaled bronchodilator before giving other inhaled agents (eg, cromolyn, steroids).
- Initiate treatment on arising in morn-

ing and administer before meals to improve lung ventilation and reduce fatigue.

- Shake metered dose inhaler well before using.
- If using metered dose inhaler, use spacing device (eg, Aerochanger) to facilitate intrapulmonary deposition.
- Allow 5 min between metered dose inhalations in order to be certain whether another inhalation is necessary.
- Do not use if solution is discolored or contains precipitate.
- Store at room temperature and protect from light.

Assessment/Interventions

- Obtain patient history, including drug history and any known allergies.
- Monitor respiratory and cardiac status, including BP and pulse, before and after therapy.
- Observe for paresthesias and coldness of extremities and decreased peripheral blood flow.
- Notify physician of failure to respond to usual dosage and of dizziness and chest pain.
- Monitor respiratory functions: vital capacity, forced expiratory volume, arterial blood gases.
- Observe for therapeutic response as demonstrated by adequate breathing.

OVERDOSAGE: SIGNS & SYMPTOMS

Hypertension, tachycardia, palpitations, tremor, nausea, headache, anxiety, restlessness, insomnia, weakness, dizziness, excitation

Patient/Family Education

- Instruct patient on proper use of inhaler. Explain value of using spacing device.
- Instruct patient on proper method of determining when metered dose inhaler is empty and when it needs to be replaced.
- Advise patient to use bronchodilator before taking other inhaled agents (eg, cromolyn, steroids).
- Advise patient not to exceed or adjust recommended dosage and not to change brands without consulting physician.
- Caution patient to avoid spraying aerosol in eyes.
- Encourage patient to increase fluid intake, which helps in liquefying secretions.
- Instruct patient to withhold medication and notify physician if signs of paradoxical airway resistance (eg, sudden increase in shortness of breath) occur.
- Advise patient to notify physician of failure to respond to usual dosage and of dizziness and chest pain.
- Advise patient to avoid smoking, being in smoke-filled rooms and having contact with people who have respiratory infections.
- Instruct patient to wash inhaler with warm water daily.

See Patient Guide, p. 325.

Isometheptene Mucate/ Dichloralphenazone/ Acetaminophen

(eye-so-meth-EPP-teen MYOO-kate/die-klor-uhl-FEN-uh-zone/ASS-et-ah-MEE-noe-fen)

Isocom, Isopap, Midchlor, Midrin, Migratine

Class: Migraine

Action Isometheptene mucate acts as sympathomimetic to constrict dilated cranial and cerebral arterioles. Dichloralphenazone is mild sedative that reduces emotional reaction to pain of vascular and tension headaches. Acetaminophen is mild analgesic.

Indications Relief of tension and vascular headaches. FDA has classified drug as possibly effective in treatment of migraine headaches.

Contraindications Glaucoma; severe cases of renal disease; hypertension; organic heart disease; hepatic disease; MAO inhibitor therapy.

Route/Dosage

Migraine Headache

ADULTS: PO 2 capsules at once, followed by 1 capsule q hr until headache is relieved (maximum 5 capsules in 12 hr period).

Tension Headache

ADULTS: PO 1-2 capsules q 4 hr (maximum 8 capsules/day).

Interactions

MAO inhibitors: May result in severe headache, hypertension, hyperpyrexia and possible hypertensive crisis.

Lab Test Interferences

None well documented.

Adverse Reactions

CNS: Transient dizziness or drowsiness. *DERM:* Rash.

Precautions

Pregnancy: Pregnancy category undetermined. *Lactation:* Undetermined. *Children:* Safety and efficacy not established. *Special risk patients:* Observe caution in patients with hypertension or peripheral vascular disease and after recent CV attacks. *Hepatotoxicity:* Can occur with chronic ingestion of acetaminophen. Chronic alcohol abusers are especially at risk.

NURSING CONSIDERATIONS

Administration/Storage

- Administer at first sign of migraine headache.
- Administer with full glass of water.
- Store at room temperature in dry place in tightly closed container.

Assessment/Interventions

- Obtain patient history, including drug history and any known allergies.
- Assess frequency, duration, location and characteristics of chronic headaches.
- Monitor BP and pulse periodically during therapy.
- Notify physician if hypertension occurs.
- If relief from headache is not obtained, notify physician.

OVERDOSAGE: SIGNS & SYMPTOMS

Nausea, vomiting, drowsiness, confusion, liver tenderness, low or high BP, cardiac arrhythmias, jaundice, acute hepatic and renal failure

Patient/Family Education

- Instruct patient to take drug at first sign of impending headache.
- Encourage patient to rest in quiet, dark room after taking drug.
- Advise patient not to drink alcoholic beverages.

- Instruct patient to notify physician of dizziness or skin rash.
- Instruct patient to notify physician if headache persists.

See Patient Guide, p. 326.

Isoniazid (Isonicotinic Acid Hydrazide; INH)

(eye-so-NYE-uh-zid)
Laniazid, Nydrazid
Class: Anti-infective/antituberculer

Action Interferes with lipid and nucleic acid biosynthesis in actively growing tubercle bacilli.

Indications Treatment of all forms of tuberculosis. **Unlabeled use:** Improvement of severe tremor in multiple sclerosis.

Contraindications Previous isoniazid-associated hepatic injury, drug fever, chills or arthritis; acute liver disease.

Route/Dosage

Tuberculosis

Adults: **PO/IM** 5 mg/kg/day as single daily dose (maximum 300 mg/day). Infants & Children: **PO/IM** 10-20 mg/kg/day in single daily dose (maximum 300 mg/day).

Multiple Sclerosis

Adults: **PO/IM** 300-400 mg/day, increased over 2 wk to 20 mg/kg/day.

Interactions

Aluminum salts: May reduce oral absorption of isoniazid; give isoniazid 1-3 hr before aluminum salts. *Carbamazepine:* May result in carbamazepine toxicity or isoniazid hepatotoxicity. Monitor carbamazepine concentrations and liver function. *Disulfiram:* May result in increased incidence of CNS effects (coordination difficulties, confusion, irritability, aggressiveness). *Enflurane:* May result in high-output renal failure in rapid acetylators. Monitor renal function. *Hydantoins:* May increase serum hydantoin levels. *Rifampin:* May result in higher rate of hepatotoxicity.

Lab Test Interferences

None well documented.

Adverse Reactions

CNS: Peripheral neuropathy; convulsions; toxic encephalopathy; optic neuritis and atrophy; memory impairment; toxic psychosis. *GI:* Nausea; vomiting; epigastric distress. *HEMA:* Agranulocytosis; hemolytic, sideroblastic or aplastic anemia; thrombocytopenia; eosinophilia. *HEPA:* Hepatotoxicity including elevated serum transaminase levels, bilirubinemia, bilirubinuria, jaundice, severe and sometimes fatal hepatitis. *DERM:* Morbilliform, maculopapular, purpuric or exfoliative skin eruptions. *META:* Pyridoxine deficiency; pellagra; hyperglycemia; metabolic acidosis; hypocalcemia; hypophosphatemia. *OTHER:* Gynecomastia; rheumatic syndrome; systemic lupus erythematosus-like syndrome; local irritation at IM injection site.

Precautions

Pregnancy: Safety undetermined. *Lactation:* Excreted in breast milk. *Hepatic impairment:* Common prodromal symptoms of hepatotoxicity include anorexia, nausea, vomiting, fatigue, malaise and weakness. Patients with acute hepatic disease should have preventive tuberculosis treatment deferred. Incidence of hepatic reaction increases in patients over 50 yr. *Hypersensitivity:* Discontinue drug at first sign of hypersensitivity reaction. Restart only after symptoms have cleared. *Pyridoxine administration:* Prophylactic concomitant administration of pyridoxine (6-50 mg/day) is recommended in malnourished patients and those predisposed to neuropathy (eg, alcoholics, diabetics). *Renal impairment:* Monitor patients with severe renal dysfunction carefully.

NURSING CONSIDERATIONS

Administration/Storage

- Oral form available in tablet and syrup forms.
- Administer oral medication on empty stomach at least 1 hr before or 2 hr after meals.
- If GI irritation becomes problem, drug may be administered with food, although food decreases absorption of drug.
- Antacids may be administered 1 hr before administration.
- Store at room temperature and protect from moisture.

Assessment/Interventions

- Obtain patient history, including drug history and any known allergies.
- Assess mycobacterial studies and susceptibility tests before and periodically throughout therapy to detect possible resistance.
- Evaluate hepatic function studies before and monthly during therapy (SGOT [AST], SGPT [ALT]) and serum bilirubin.
- Assess patient for adverse reactions: GI distress, peripheral neuritis, optic neuritis or hypersensitivity reactions.
- If nausea, vomiting, anorexia or diarrhea develops, obtain order for antiemetic or antidiarrheal medication and assess for hepatotoxicity.
- Take safety precautions if patient experiences adverse CNS symptoms such as confusion or incoordination.

OVERDOSAGE: SIGNS & SYMPTOMS

Nausea, vomiting, dizziness, slurring of speech, blurring of vision, visual hallucinations, respiratory distress, CNS depression, stupor, coma, severe seizures

Patient/Family Education

- Teach patient and family the name, dose, action and side effects of isoniazid.
- Advise patient to minimize daily alcohol consumption while taking isoniazid due to the increased risk of hepatitis.
- Instruct patient to report these symptoms to physician: weakness, fatigue, loss of appetite, nausea and vomiting, yellowing of skin or eyes, darkening of urine, or numbness or tingling in hands or feet occurs.
- Emphasize to patient that treatment will be lengthy and that patient must complete entire course of therapy. Relapse of tuberculosis is higher if chemotherapy is discontinued prematurely.
- Advise patient to return for laboratory follow-up.
- Caution patient not to perform activities that require mental alertness if adverse CNS symptoms occur.

See Patient Guide, p. 327.

Isoproterenol

(eye-so-pro-TER-uh-nahl)

Isoproterenol Hydrochloride

Dispos-a-Med Isoproterenol HCl, *Isuprel*, *Isuprel Glossets*, *Isuprel Mistometer*

Isoproterenol Sulfate

Medihaler-ISO

Class: Bronchodilator/sympathomimetic

Action Produces bronchodilation by relaxing bronchial smooth muscle through beta-2 receptor stimulation; increases heart rate and myocardial contractility by stimulating cardiac beta-1 receptors, which increases cardiac output.

Indications

Inhalation: Treatment of bronchospasm associated with asthma, emphysema, bronchitis and bronchiectasis. *Injection:* Managment of bronchospasm during anesthesia; adjunctive treatment for shock. *Sublingual:* Management of bronchopulmonary disease, Adams-Stokes syndrome, atrioventricular heart block.

Contraindications Cardiac arrhythmias associated with tachycardia; tachycardia or heart block caused by digitalis intoxication; angina; ventricular arrhythmias requiring inotropic therapy.

Route/Dosage

Acute Bronchial Asthma

ADULTS & CHILDREN > 12 YR: **Inhalation** Hand bulb nebulizer: 5-15 inhalations of 1:200 (0.5%) solution. Adults may use 3-7 inhalations of 1:100 (1%) solution if needed. May repeat after 5-10 min; up to 5 times daily. Metered dose inhaler: 1-2 inhalations 4-6 times daily. Do not exceed 2 inhalations at one time, nor more than 6 inhalations/hr.

Bronchospasm in Chronic Obstructive Lung Disease

ADULTS: **Inhalation** Hand bulb nebulizer: 5-15 inhalations of 1:200 solution or 3-7 inhalations of 1:100 solution. May repeat at 3-4 hr intervals. Nebulization by compressed air or oxygen: 0.5 ml of 1:200 solution diluted to 2-2.5 ml with appropriate diluent. Deliver over 10-20 min. May repeat up to 5 times daily. Intermittent positive pressure breathing: 0.5 ml of 1:200 solution diluted to 2-2.5 ml with water or isotonic saline. Deliver over 15-20 min. May repeat up to 5 times daily. Metered dose inhaler: 1-2 inhalations 4-6 times daily. CHILDREN > 12 YR: Administration is similar to adults. For acute bronchospasm attack, 1:200 solution is recommended. Do not use more than 0.25 ml of 1:200 solution for each 10-15 min treatment. **IV** 0.01-0.02 mg. Repeat as necessary. Isoproterenol for shock is generally given IV (1:5000), starting at low dose and adjusting individually. ADULTS: **Sublingual** 10-20 mg. Do not exceed 60 mg/day. For shock, begin with 10 mg. CHILDREN: 5-10 mg. Do not exceed 30 mg/day. Do not repeat more often than every 3-4 hr or 3 times daily.

Interactions None well documented.

Lab Test Interferences

Bilirubin may be falsely elevated if measured by sequential multiple analyzer. Urinary epinephrine values may be elevated.

Adverse Reactions

CV: Palpitations; tachycardia; blood pressure changes; arrhythmias; Adams-Stokes attacks; cardiac arrest. *RESP:* Cough; throat irritation; bronchitis; sputum increase; pulmonary edema. *CNS:* Tremor; dizziness; nervousness; drowsiness; headache; insomnia. *GI:* Nausea; GI distress. *OTHER:* Parotid gland swelling with prolonged use; saliva discoloration; sweating; skin flushing.

Precautions

Pregnancy: Category C. *Lactation:* Undetermined. *Labor and delivery:* May inhibit uterine contractions and delay preterm labor. *Children:* Safety and efficacy of inhalation products in children ≤ 12 years not established. *Elderly patients:* Lower doses may be required. *Cardiovascular effects:* Toxic symptoms in patients with cardiovascular disorders may occur. *CNS effects:* Use cautiously in patients with history of seizures or hyperthyroidism. *Diabetes:* Dosage adjustment of insulin or oral hypoglycemic agent may be required. *Excessive use:* Paradoxical bronchospasm and cardiac arrest have been associated with excessive inhalant use. *Saliva discoloration:* Isoproterenol may cause saliva to turn pinkish-red.

NURSING CONSIDERATIONS

Administration/Storage

- IV injection: Dilute 1 ml of 1:5000 solution to 10 ml with sodium chloride or 5% dextrose injection to achieve 1:50,000 solution.
- IV infusion: Dilute 10 ml 1:5000 solution in 500 ml 5% dextrose to pro-

duce 1:250,000 solution. Use microdrip or continuous infusion pump to prevent sudden influx of large amount of drug.

- Metered dose inhaler: Shake container thoroughly to activate medication. Instruct patient in proper technique for use.
- IPPB: Position patient properly for treatment, either sitting or in semi-Fowler's. Have patient rinse mouth after each session.
- For sublingual administration, tell patient to allow tablet to disintegrate under tongue and not to crush, chew or suck tablet. Also tell patient not to swallow saliva until drug has been completely dissolved. Have patient rinse mouth after each sublingual dose.
- Discard solution if precipitate or discoloration is present.
- Store in tight, light-resistant container at room temperature.

Assessment/Interventions

- Obtain patient history, including drug history and any known allergies.
- Monitor heart rate, respirations, BP and urine output. Carefully monitor heart rate and rhythm and ECG pattern when used as treatment for shock.

OVERDOSAGE: SIGNS & SYMPTOMS

Tremor, palpitations, angina, arrhythmias, tachycardia, elevated or decreased blood pressure, seizures; nervousness, headache, dry mouth, nausea, dizziness, fatigue, malaise, insomnia

Patient/Family Education

- Use verbal instructions and demonstrations to teach technique for inhalation therapy and explain that if more than one inhalation is necessary, patient should wait 3-5 minutes between doses.
- Tell patient to notify physician if no response to usual dose.

See Patient Guide, p. 328.

Isosorbide Dinitrate

(EYE-sos-ORE-bide die-NYE-trate)

Dilatrate-SR, Iso-Bid, Isordil, Isordil Tembids, Isotrate Timecelles, Sorbitrate, Sorbitrate SA, ♣ *APO-ISDN, Cedocard-SR, Coradur, Coronex*

Class: Antianginal

Action Relaxation of smooth muscle of venous and arterial vasculature.

Indications Treatment and prevention of angina pectoris.

Contraindications Hypersensitivity to nitrates; severe anemia; closed-angle glaucoma; orthostatic hypotension; head trauma or cerebral hemorrhage.

Route/Dosage

Angina Pectoris

ADULTS: **SL** (sublingual tablets) 2.5-5 mg; **PO** (chewable tablets) 5 mg; **PO** (oral tablets) 5-40 mg q 6 hr; **PO** (sustained release tablets) 40-80 mg q 8-12 hr.

Acute Prophylaxis

ADULTS: **PO** (sublingual or chewable tablets) 5-10 mg q 2-3 hr.

Interactions

Alcohol: Severe hypotension and cardiovascular collapse. *Aspirin:* Increased nitrate concentration and actions. *Dihydroergotamine:* Increased systolic blood pressure and decreased antianginal effects.

Lab Test Interferences

May cause false report of reduced serum cholesterol with Zlatkis-Zak color reaction.

Adverse Reactions

CV: Tachycardia; palpitations; hypotension; syncope; arrhythmias. *RESP:* Bronchitis; pneumonia. CNS: Headache; apprehension; weakness;

vertigo; dizziness; agitation; insomnia. *EENT:* Blurred vision. *GI:* Nausea; vomiting; diarrhea; dyspepsia. *GU:* Dysuria; urinary frequency; impotence. *HEMA:* Methemoglobinemia; hemolytic anemia. *DERM:* Cutaneous vasodilation with flushing. *OTHER:* Arthralgia; perspiration; pallor; cold sweat; edema.

Precautions

Pregnancy: Category C. *Lactation:* Undetermined. *Children:* Safety and efficacy not established. *Special risk patients:* Use with caution in patients with acute MI or CHF. *Angina:* May aggravate angina caused by hypertrophic cardiomyopathy. *Orthostatic hypotension:* May occur even with small doses; alcohol accentuates this reaction. *Tolerance:* Tolerance to vascular and antianginal effects may develop.

NURSING CONSIDERATIONS

Administration/Storage

- Sublingual tablets should be placed under tongue to dissolve. Do not swallow.
- Chewable tablets should be chewed and swallowed. Do not crush before administering.
- Oral dosage forms should be taken on empty stomach with full glass of water.
- Store at room temperature.

Assessment/Interventions

- Obtain patient history, including drug history and any known allergies.
- Monitor for headache, hypotension, tachycardia, decreased pulse rate, heart block and decreased respiratory rate.
- Monitor hemoglobin levels.

OVERDOSAGE: SIGNS & SYMPTOMS

Hypotension, tachycardia, flushing, diaphoresis, headache, vertigo, palpitations, visual disturbances, nausea, vomiting, confusion, dyspnea

Patient/Family Education

- Instruct patient not to chew sublingual tablets. Emphasize need to hold chewable tablets in mouth for 1-2 min and then chew thoroughly before swallowing, to allow for absorption.
- Advise patient not to stop taking medication suddenly; withdrawal syndrome may occur.
- Instruct patient to notify physician immediately or go to nearest hospital emergency department if chest pain persists or worsens after taking prescribed dose.
- Advise patient to notify physician if effectiveness of therapy decreases over time; tolerance may develop.
- Instruct patient to report these symptoms to physician: severe or persistent headache, blurred vision, dry mouth, dizziness, flushing.
- Caution patient to avoid sudden position changes to prevent orthostatic hypotension.
- Instruct patient to avoid intake of alcoholic beverages or alcohol-containing products.

See Patient Guide, pp. 329-330.

Isosorbide Mononitrate

(EYE-sos-ORE-bide MAH-no-NYE-trate)

ISMO

Class: Antianginal

Action Relaxation of smooth muscle of venous and arterial vasculature.

Indications Prevention of angina pectoris.

Contraindications Hypersensitivity to nitrates; severe anemia; closed-angle glaucoma; orthostatic hypotension; head trauma or cerebral hemorrhage.

Route/Dosage
ADULTS: PO 20 mg bid, given 7 hr apart. Extended release tablets are given as 30 or 60 mg once daily.

Interactions
Alcohol: Severe hypotension and cardiovascular collapse may occur. *Aspirin:* Increased nitrate concentration and actions. *Calcium channel blockers:* Symptomatic orthostatic hypotension. *Dihydroergotamine:* Increased systolic BP and decreased antianginal effects may develop.

Lab Test Interferences
May cause false report of reduced serum cholesterol with Zlatkis-Zak color reaction.

Adverse Reactions
CV: Tachycardia; palpitations; hypotension; syncope; arrhythmias. *CNS:* Headache; apprehension; weakness; vertigo; dizziness; agitation; insomnia. *EENT:* Blurred vision. *GI:* Nausea; vomiting; diarrhea; dyspepsia. *GU:* Dysuria; urinary frequency; impotence. *HEMA:* Methemoglobinemia; hemolytic anemia. *DERM:* Cutaneous vasodilation with flushing. *OTHER:* Arthralgia; perspiration; pallor; cold sweat; edema.

Precautions
Pregnancy: Category C. *Lactation:* Undetermined. *Special risk patients:* Use with caution in patients with acute MI, CHF, glaucoma or angina caused by hypertrophic cardiomyopathy. *Acute angina:* Not indicated for treatment of acute anginal episodes. *Orthostatic hypotension:* May occur even with small doses; alcohol accentuates this reaction. *Tolerance:* Tolerance to vascular and antianginal effects may develop.

NURSING CONSIDERATIONS

Administration/Storage

- Administer first dose on awakening and second dose 7 hr later.
- Give on empty stomach with full glass of water.
- Store at cool temperature in tightly closed container.

Assessment/Interventions

- Obtain patient history, including drug history and any known allergies.
- Monitor for headache, hypotension and tachycardia.

OVERDOSAGE: SIGNS & SYMPTOMS

Hypotension, tachycardia, flushing, diaphoresis, headache, vertigo, palpitations, visual disturbances, nausea, vomiting, confusion, dyspnea

Patient/Family Education

- Instruct patient to take medication twice daily, with first dose in morning and second dose 7 hr later.
- Caution patient not to stop taking medication suddenly; withdrawal syndrome may occur.
- Advise patient to notify physician if effectiveness of therapy decreases over time; tolerance may develop.
- Instruct patient to report these symptoms to physician: nausea, vomiting, abdominal pain, appetite loss, persistent headache, faintness, apprehension, restlessness, chest pain, flushing, excessive sweating, cold sweat, visual disturbances, fever, involuntary passing of urine and feces.
- Caution patient to avoid sudden position changes to prevent orthostatic hypotension.
- Instruct patient to avoid intake of alcoholic beverages or alcohol-containing products.

See Patient Guide, p. 331.

Isotretinoin (13-*cis*-Retinoic Acid)

(EYE-so-TREH-tih-NO-in)

Accutane

Class: Acne

Action Reduces sebum secretion and sebaceous gland size, inhibits sebaceous gland differentiation and alters sebum lipid composition.

Indications Treatment of severe recalcitrant cystic acne. **Unlabeled uses:** Treatment of keratinization disorders, cutaneous T-cell lymphoma, leukoplakia; prevention of skin cancer in patients with xeroderma pigmentosum.

Contraindications Hypersensitivity to parabens; pregnancy.

Route/Dosage

ADULTS: **PO** 0.5-2 mg/kg/day divided into 2 doses for 15-20 wk.

Interactions

Sulfur, topical benzoyl peroxide, tretinoin: May potentiate drying effects of isotretinoin. *Vitamin A:* May increase toxic effects; do not take with isotretinoin.

Lab Test Interferences

None well documented.

Adverse Reactions

CV: Transient chest pain; vasculitis. *CNS:* Fatigue; headache; pseudotumor cerebri (benign intracranial hypertension with headache, visual disturbances and papilledema). *EENT:* Conjunctivitis; corneal opacities; cataracts; visual disturbances; dry eyes; contact lens intolerance; decreased night vision; epistaxis; dry nose. *GI:* Dry mouth; nausea; vomiting; abdominal pain; nonspecific GI symptoms; anorexia; inflammatory bowel disease. *GU:* WBC cells in urine; proteinuria; microscopic or gross hematuria; nonspecific urogenital findings. *HEMA:* Anemia; decreased RBC parameters and WBC counts; elevated platelet counts; elevated sedimentation rate. *HEPA:* Elevated liver enzymes; hepatitis. *DERM:* Cheilitis; skin fragility; dry skin; pruritus; facial skin desquamation; dry mucous membranes; nail brittleness; rash; thinning of hair; skin infections; photosensitivity; palmoplantar desquamation; exaggerated healing response manifested by exuberant granulation tissue with crusting; pyogenic granuloma; petechiae; bruising. *META:* Increased fasting serum glucose; hyperuricemia; elevated CPK levels after exercise. *OTHER:* Arthralgia; bone, joint and muscle pain and stiffness; flushing; reversibly elevated triglycerides; increased cholesterol level.

Precautions

Pregnancy: Category X. *Lactation:* Unknown. *Children:* Safety and efficacy not established. *Blood donation:* Patient should not donate blood for transfusion for 30 days after discontinuing therapy.

NURSING CONSIDERATIONS

Administration/Storage

- Instruct patient to swallow capsules whole. Do not open or crush capsules.
- Give medication with meals.
- Second course of therapy may be initiated if needed after 2 mo off therapy.
- Store in tightly-closed, light-resistant container at room temperature.

Assessment/Interventions

- Obtain patient history, including drug history and any known allergies. Note hypersensitivity to parabens.
- Obtain baseline lipid levels and then monitor q 2 wk for first month and then monitor monthly.
- Obtain liver function tests at 2- to

3-wk intervals for first 6 mo and then q mo throughout course of therapy.
- In diabetic patients, monitor glucose levels carefully.
- If increased triglyceride levels occur, discontinue drug immediately.
- Notify physician of signs and symptoms of decreased liver function (dark urine, jaundice, pruritus), visual disturbances, nausea, vomiting and headache.

OVERDOSAGE: SIGNS & SYMPTOMS

Transient headache, vomiting, facial flushing, cheilosis, abdominal pain, dizziness, ataxia

Patient/Family Education

- Because of teratogenic effects, instruct patient either to practice abstinence or to use reliable method of birth control during therapy and for 1 mo before and after therapy. Instruct patient to notify physician immediately if pregnancy is suspected. Pregnancy test given 2 wk before starting therapy is advised.
- Advise patient to take medication with meals.
- Instruct patient to discontinue any other acne medications (including otc topical preparations) before starting therapy.
- Advise patient to control weight, decrease dietary fat and restrict alcohol intake 36 hr before lipid determinations to avoid elevation in serum triglycerides.
- Caution patient against use of vitamin A, even in multivitamins, to avoid additive toxicity.
- Inform patient that contact lens tolerance may decrease.
- Suggest to patient to use lubricant (eg, petroleum jelly) on lips to prevent cheilitis.
- Advise patient not to donate blood for at least 30 days after discontinuing therapy.
- Inform patient that transient exacerbations of acne may be experienced during first few wk of therapy. Advise patient to continue drug therapy, because this may be normal response.
- Caution patient that decreased night vision can occur and onset can be sudden. Advise patient to be cautious when driving or operating any vehicle at night.
- Instruct patient to discontinue therapy and immediately notify physician if any of the following symptoms occur: abdominal pain, rectal bleeding, visual disturbances.
- Advise patient to take sips of water frequently, suck on ice chips or sugarless hard candy or chew sugarless gum if dry mouth occurs.
- Caution patient to avoid exposure to sunlight and to use sunscreen or wear protective clothing to avoid photosensitivity reactions.

See Patient Guide, p. 332.

Isoxsuprine HCl

(eye-SOX-you-preen HIGH-droe-KLOR-ide)

Vasodilan, Voxsuprine

Class: Peripheral vasodilator

Action Stimulates skeletal beta receptors to produce vasodilation; stimulates cardiac function (increased contractility, heart rate and cardiac output) and relaxes uterus. At higher doses, inhibits platelet aggregation and decreases blood viscosity.

Indications Possibly effective for treatment of cerebral vascular insufficiency, peripheral vascular disease caused by arteriosclerosis obliterans, thromboangiitis obliterans, Raynaud's disease. **Unlabeled uses:** Treatment of dysmenorrhea, premature labor.

Contraindications Arterial bleeding; use during immediate postpartum period.

Route/Dosage
ADULTS: PO 10-20 mg tid or qid.

Interactions None well documented.

Lab Test Interferences
None well documented.

Adverse Reactions
CV: Hypotension; tachycardia; chest pain. *CNS:* Dizziness; weakness. *GI:* Nausea; vomiting; abdominal distress. *DERM:* Severe rash.

Precautions
Pregnancy: Category C. *Lactation:* Undetermined.

NURSING CONSIDERATIONS

Administration/Storage

- Store at room temperature in tightly closed container.

Assessment/Interventions

- Obtain patient history, including drug history and any known allergies. Note cardiovascular disease.
- Monitor for hypotension, tachycardia and chest pain.
- If rash appears, withhold drug and notify physician.

Patient/Family Education

- Instruct patient to report these symptoms to physician: fast heart beat, chest pain, pounding in chest, severe rash, flushing, weakness, nausea, vomiting, stomach pain.
- Caution patient to avoid sudden position changes to prevent orthostatic hypotension.

See Patient Guide, p. 333.

Isradipine

(iss-RAHD-ih-peen)
DynaCirc
Class: Calcium channel blocker

Action Reduces systemic vascular resistance and BP by inhibiting movement of calcium ions across cell membrane in systemic and coronary vascular smooth muscle and myocardium.

Indications Treatment of hypertension.

Contraindications Standard considerations.

Route/Dosage
ADULTS: PO 2.5-10 mg/day in 2 divided doses (maximum dose 20 mg/day).

Interactions None well documented.

Lab Test Interferences
None well documented.

Adverse Reactions
CV: Peripheral edema; flushing; palpitations; angina; tachycardia; hypotension; syncope; CHF; MI; atrial or ventricular fibrillation. *RESP:* Shortness of breath; dyspnea; wheezing. *CNS:* Dizziness; lightheadedness; headache; fatigue; lethargy; weakness; shakiness; psychiatric disturbances. *GI:* Nausea; diarrhea; constipation; abdominal discomfort; cramps; dyspepsia; vomiting. *GU:* Urinary frequency; micturition disorders; sexual difficulties. *DERM:* Rash. *OTHER:* Transient ischemic attack; stroke.

Precautions
Pregnancy: Category C. *Lactation:* Undetermined. *Children:* Safety and efficacy not established. *CHF:* Use with caution in patients with CHF.

NURSING CONSIDERATIONS

Administration/Storage

- May administer with or without food.
- Store in tightly closed container at room temperature. Protect from light.

Assessment/Interventions

- Obtain patient history, including drug history and any known allergies. Note cardiovascular disease.
- Monitor BP, cardiac and respiratory function during therapy.
- Monitor for dizziness, headache and peripheral edema.
- Assist patient with ambulation if dizziness occurs.

OVERDOSAGE: SIGNS & SYMPTOMS

Hypotension, dizziness, slurred speech, nausea, weakness, drowsiness, confusion

Patient/Family Education

- Explain that dosage will be tapered slowly before stopping to avoid withdrawal symptoms. Warn patient that sudden discontinuation may cause serious chest pain.
- Tell patient to brush and floss teeth regularly to minimize gum changes (eg, overgrowth of gums).
- Instruct patient to report these symptoms to physician: irregular heart beat, shortness of breath, swelling of hands or feet, pronounced dizziness, constipation, nausea or hypotension.
- Advise patient that drug may cause dizziness and to use caution while driving or performing other tasks requiring mental alertness.

See Patient Guide, p. 334.

Itraconazole

(ih-truh-KAHN-uh-zole)

Sporanox

Class: Anti-infective/antifungal

Action Inhibits synthesis of ergosterol, which is a vital component of fungal cell membranes.

Indications Treatment of blastomycosis, aspergillosis, and histoplasmosis fungal infections. Treatment of ohychomycosis due to dermatophytes of the toenail with or without fungal involvement. **Unlabeled use:** Treatment of other fungal infections (eg, dermatophytoses, candidiasis, cryptococcus) and cutaneous Leishmaniasis.

Contraindications Coadministration with terfenadine, astemizole, cisapride, triazolam or oral midazolam; not for treatment of onychomycosis in pregnant women or women contemplating pregnancy.

Route/Dosage

Blastomycosis, Aspergillosis, Histoplasmosis

ADULTS: **PO** 200-400 mg/day. Give doses > 200 mg in 2 divided doses. LIFE-THREATENING SITUATIONS: Give loading dose of 200 mg tid for 3 days. Continue treatment for at least 3 mo and until clinical parameters and laboratory tests indicate active fungal infection has subsided. Inadequate period of treatment may lead to recurrence.

Onychomycosis

ADULTS: **PO** 200 mg/day for 12 consecutive weeks.

Interactions

Astemizole, cisapride, terfenadine: Increased terfenadine levels may result in life-threatening cardiac dysrhythmias and death. Do not use together. *Calcium blockers (eg, amlodipine, felodipine, nifedipine):* Edema has occurred with concomitant dihydropyridine calcium blockers. *Cyclosporine plus HMG-CoA reductase inhibitors:* There are rare reports of rhabdomyolysis in renal transplant patients receiving this drug combination. Increased cyclosporine levels may occur. Monitor cyclosporine levels; reduce cyclosporine dose by 50% when using itraconazole doses >100 mg/day. *Digoxin:* Increased digoxin levels. Monitor frequently. *H_2 antagonists:* Reduced plasma itraconazole levels. *Midazolam (oral), triazolam:* Elevated plasma levels of these drugs; may potentiate and prolong their hypnotic and sedative effects. Sedative effects of parenteral midazolam may be prolonged. *Phenytoin:* Reduced plasma intraconazole levels; altered phenytoin metabolism. *Rifampin:* Decreased itraconazole levels with decreased effectiveness. *Sulfonylurea:* Hypoglycemia may occur. *Tacrolimus:* Increased tacrolimus plasma concentrations. *Warfarin:* Increased warfarin levels with possible bleeding.

Lab Test Interferences

None well documented.

Adverse Reactions

CV: Hypertension; orthostatic hypotension; vasculitis. *CNS:* Headache; dizziness; decreased libido; somnolence; vertigo. *GI:* Nausea; vomiting; diarrhea; abdominal pain; anorexia; general GI disorders. *HEPA:* Abnormal liver function; elevated liver enzyme. *GU:* Impotence; albuminuria. *DERM:* Rash; pruritus. *META:* Hypokalemia. *OTHER:* Edema; fatigue; fever; malaise; myalgia.

Precautions

Pregnancy: Category C. *Lactation:* Excreted in breast milk. *Children:* Safety and efficacy not established. *Hepatitis:* Rare cases of hepatitis have been reported. *HIV-infected patients:* Absorption may be decreased in HIV-infected individuals with hypochlorhydria.

NURSING CONSIDERATIONS

Administration/Storage

- Administer after a full meal to increase absorption.
- Store at room temperature. Protect from light and moisture.

Assessment/Interventions

- Obtain patient history, including drug history (particularly use of terfenadine, astemizole or cisapride) and any allergies.
- Ensure that fungal cultures have been obtained before beginning therapy.
- Obtain baseline liver function test results. Ensure that liver function tests are performed 2 wk after initial administration. In patients receiving extended drug therapy, these tests should be repeated at routine intervals to monitor for signs of liver dysfunction.
- Monitor potassium levels after initial administration and repeat routinely with extended therapy.
- If loss of appetite, nausea, vomiting, sleeplessness, signs of liver dysfunction, dark urine, jaundice, or pruritus occurs, notify physician.
- Report decreased potassium levels to physician and give appropriate supplements as prescribed.

Patient/Family Education

- Instruct patient to take drug with food.
- Tell patient to report these symptoms to physician: nausea, vomiting, diarrhea, headache, rash, swelling, fever, itching, dizziness, inability to sleep, yellowing skin, pale stools, or dark urine.

See Patient Guide, p. 335.

Kanamycin Sulfate

(kan-uh-MY-sin SULL-fate)

Kantrex

Class: Antibiotic/aminoglycoside

Action Inhibits production of bacterial protein, causing cell death.

Indications

Parenteral: Short-term treatment of serious infections caused by susceptible strains of microorganisms, especially gram-negative bacteria. *Oral:* Short-term adjunctive therapy for suppression of intestinal bacteria; treatment of hepatic coma.

Contraindications

Hypersensitivity to aminoglycosides; intestinal obstruction (oral). Generally not indicated for long-term therapy (> 14 days) because of ototoxicity and nephrotoxicity.

Route/Dosage

Infection

ADULTS & CHILDREN: **IM/IV** 15 mg/kg/day in 2-4 divided doses. Do not exceed 1.5 g/day.

Suppression of Intestinal Bacteria

ADULTS: **PO** 1 g qh for 4 hr, then 1 g q 6 hr for 36-72 hr.

Hepatic Coma

ADULTS: **PO** 8-12 g/day in divided doses.

Interactions

Digoxin, methotrexate, vitamin A, vitamin K: Oral kanamycin may decrease absorption of these drugs. INCOMPATIBILITIES: *Beta-lactam antibiotics (eg, cephalosporins, penicillins):* Do not mix in IV solutions. *Drugs with nephrotoxic potential (eg, amphotericin, cephalosporins, enflurane, methoxyflurane, vancomycin):* Increased risk of nephrotoxicity. *Loop diuretics:* Increased auditory toxicity. *Neuromuscular blocking agents:* Enhanced effects of these agents. *Polypeptide antibiotics:* Increased risk of respiratory paralysis and renal dysfunction.

Lab Test Interferences

None well documented.

Adverse Reactions

RESP: Apnea. *CNS:* Neuromuscular blockade. *EENT:* Hearing loss, deafness, loss of balance. *GI:* Malabsorption syndrome (eg, increased fecal fat, decreased serum carotene, fall in xylose absorption), nausea, vomiting, diarrhea. *GU:* Oliguria, proteinuria, elevated serum creatinine and BUN, granular casts, red and white cells in urine, decreased creatinine clearance. *OTHER:* Pain and irritation at injection site, acute muscular paralysis; hypomagnesemia.

Precautions

Pregnancy: Category D. *Lactation:* Excreted in breast milk. *Children:* Use cautiously in premature infants and neonates because of renal immaturity. *Neuromuscular blockade:* Use with caution in patients with neuromuscular disorders, those receiving anesthesia or muscle relaxants, hypomagnesemia, hypocalcemia, hypokalemia or in neonates whose mothers received magnesium sulfate. *Oral absorption:* Increased absorption (and potential for toxicity) when intestinal mucosa is ulcerated or denuded. *Toxicity:* Can cause ototoxicity, both auditory and vestibular. Nephrotoxicity may occur; greater risk factors in the elderly, patients with renal impairment, high or frequent doses, long duration of therapy, other nephrotoxic drugs, potassium depletion and decreased intravascular volume.

NURSING CONSIDERATIONS

Administration/Storage

- Do not mix with other antibacterial agents; administer separately.
- For IV administration, dilute each 500 mg with at least 100-200 ml of 0.9% Sodium Chloride or D5W. Give slowly over 30-60 min.
- Give IM injection deeply into upper outer quadrant of gluteal muscle.
- Store at room temperature. Darkening of vials during shelf life does not indicate loss of potency.

Assessment/Interventions

- Obtain patient history, including drug history and any known aller-

gies. Note hypersensitivity to aminoglycosides.

- Ensure that culture and sensitivity, renal function tests and serum electrolytes have been performed before beginning therapy and repeat periodically.
- Assess for superinfection (bacterial or fungal overgrowth).
- Assess for allergic-type reactions including anaphylactic symptoms and life-threatening or less severe asthmatic episodes in susceptible persons (more frequent in asthmatic or atopic nonasthmatic persons).
- Keep patient well hydrated (especially important in elderly).
- Assess auditory function regularly.
- Monitor drug serum concentrations periodically.
- Monitor I&O.

OVERDOSAGE: SIGNS & SYMPTOMS

Nephrotoxicity, auditory toxicity, vestibular toxicity, neuromuscular blockade, respiratory paralysis

Patient/Family Education

- Advise patient that drug may cause nausea, vomiting or diarrhea.
- Instruct patient to drink plenty of fluids while taking medication.
- Emphasize importance of follow-up visits and serial audiograms, because ototoxicity may be asymptomatic.
- Instruct patient to report these symptoms to physician: ringing in ears, hearing impairment, rash, difficulty urinating or dizziness.

See Patient Guide, pp. 336-337.

Kaolin/Pectin

(KAY-oh-lin/PECK-tin)

Kao-Spen, Kapectolin

Class: Antidiarrheal combination

Action Absorbs fluid, binds and removes digestive tract irritants.

Indications Symptomatic treatment of diarrhea.

Contraindications Use in infants and children < 3 yr without physician guidance; use for > 2 days or in presence of high fever; intestinal obstruction; colitis.

Route/Dosage

All doses are given after each loose bowel movement. ADULTS: **PO** 60-120 ml (regular strength) or 45-90 ml (concentrate) after each loose bowel movement. CHILDREN 6-12 YR: **PO** 30-60 ml (regular strength) or 30 ml (concentrate) per dose. CHILDREN 3-5 YR: **PO** 15-30 ml (regular strength) or 15 ml (concentrate) per dose.

Interactions

Clindamycin, digoxin, lincomycin penicillamine (oral): Decreased absorption may occur; separate administration times by 2-4 hr.

Lab Test Interferences

None well documented.

Adverse Reactions

GI: Constipation; fecal impaction (especially infants and elderly).

Precautions

Pregnancy: Category B. *Lactation:* Kaolin and pectin are not absorbed from GI tract; transfer into breast milk is not expected.

NURSING CONSIDERATIONS

Administration/Storage

- Administer after each loose bowel movement.
- Shake suspension well before pouring.

Assessment/Interventions

- Obtain patient history, including drug history and any known allergies. Note usual bowel patterns and onset of recent condition.
- Conduct complete abdominal assess-

ment, including palpitation and auscultation.

- Assess for signs and symptoms of intestinal obstruction, fecal impaction or dehydration; notify physician if present.
- Assess vital signs, especially temperature. Notify physician if increased.

OVERDOSAGE: SIGNS & SYMPTOMS
Constipation

Patient/Family Education

- Instruct patient to take medication after each diarrheal or loose stool.
- Advise patient to notify physician if diarrhea persists for more than 48 hr or if fever develops.
- Caution patient not to exceed recommended dosage.

See Patient Guide, p. 338.

Ketamine HCl

(KEET-uh-MEEN HIGH-droe-KLOR-ide)

Ketalar

Class: General anesthetic

Action Produces rapid-acting anesthetic state with profound analgesia, normal pharyngeal-laryngeal reflexes, normal or slightly enhanced skeletal muscle tone, cardiovascular and respiratory stimulation and, occasionally, transient and minimal respiratory depression.

Indications Diagnostic and surgical procedures that do not require skeletal muscle relaxation; induction of anesthesia; supplementation of low-potency agents, such as nitrous oxide.

Contraindications Schizophrenia; acute psychoses; patients in whom significant BP elevation would be serious hazard.

Route/Dosage
ADULTS & CHILDREN: INDUCTION OF ANESTHESIA: Initial: **IV** 1-4.5 mg/kg via slow infusion (over 60 sec); usual dose for 5-10 min anesthesia: 2 mg/kg. **IM** Initial: 6.5-13 mg/kg. Maintenance: **IV/IM** One-half to full induction dose, repeated as needed. Alternatively **IV** 0.1-0.5 mg/min infusion, augmented with diazepam **IV** 2-5 mg.

Interactions
Halothane: Decreased cardiac output, BP and pulse. *Tubocurarine and other nondepolarizing muscle relaxants:* Increased neuromuscular effects, resulting in prolonged respiratory depression. INCOMPATIBILITIES: Ketamine is physically incompatible with diazepam and barbiturates.

Lab Test Interferences
None well documented.

Adverse Reactions
CV: Hypertension; tachycardia; hypotension; bradycardia; arrhythmia. *RESP:* Respiratory stimulation; severe respiratory depression; apnea after rapid injection; laryngospasm; other airway obstruction. *CNS:* Increased ICP. Emergence reaction: Vivid imagery; hallucinations; delirium; confusion; excitement; irrational behavior. *EENT:* Diplopia; nystagmus; increased intraocular pressure. *GI:* Anorexia; nausea; vomiting; hypersalivation. *DERM:* Transient erythema; morbilliform rash.

Precautions
Pregnancy: Pregnancy category undetermined. *Lactation:* Undetermined. *Hypertension or cardiac decompensation:* In patients with these conditions, monitor function continuously during procedure.

NURSING CONSIDERATIONS

Administration/Storage

- Premedicate patient with anticholinergic agent before giving anesthetic to prevent salivation.
- Administer slowly over 60 sec to prevent respiratory depression, unless otherwise indicated.

Assessment/Interventions

- Obtain patient history, including drug history and any known allergies. Note history of psychiatric disorders (schizophrenia or acute psychoses).
- Assess vital signs, especially BP, before administration.
- Place patient in quiet room with minimal stimulation to prevent recovery symptoms.
- Observe patient for signs of delirium and hallucinations during recovery period.
- Check patient's airway regularly to prevent aspiration caused by hypersalivation.
- If respiratory, neurologic or cardiovascular changes (hypertension, tachycardia, hypotension, bradycardia, arrhythmia) occur, notify physician. Be prepared to support patient physically.

OVERDOSAGE: SIGNS & SYMPTOMS

Respiratory depression

Patient/Family Education

- Advise patient that neurologic effects may persist for 24 hr after anesthesia. Advise patient to use caution during this period while driving or performing other tasks requiring mental alertness.

No patient monograph available.

Ketoconazole

(KEY-toe-KOE-nuh-zole)

Nizoral

Class: Anti-infective/antifungal

Action Impairs synthesis of ergosterol, allowing increased permeability in fungal cell membrane and leakage of cellular components.

Indications Treatment of susceptible systemic and cutaneous fungal infections. *Topical:* Seborrheic dermatitis; tinea corporis; tinea cruris; tinea pedis; tinea versicolor.

Contraindications Fungal meningitis.

Route/Dosage

ADULTS: **PO** 200-400 mg qd. CHILDREN > 2 YR: **PO** 3.3-6.6 mg/kg/day. Treatment may last from 1 wk-6 mo, depending on infection. ADULTS: **Topical** Apply to affected and immediate surrounding area qd for 2-4 wk.

Interactions

Antacids: Increased gastric pH may inhibit ketoconazole absorption; separate administration by at least 2 hr. *Antihistamines, nonsedating (eg, astemizole, terfenidine):* Increased levels of antihistamine may lead to serious adverse cardiovascular effects. *Corticosteroids:* Increased bioavailability and decreased clearance of corticosteroid. *Cyclosporine:* Increased cyclosporine concentrations. *H_2 receptor antagonists:* Increased gastric pH may inhibit ketoconazole absorption. *Rifampin:* Decreased serum levels of either drug; avoid concomitant use. *Theophylline:* Decreased theophylline serum concentrations. *Warfarin:* Increased anticoagulant effect.

Lab Test Interferences

None well documented.

Adverse Reactions

CNS: Headache; dizziness; somnolence. *GI:* Nausea; vomiting; abdominal pain. *GU:* Oligospermia (with high doses); impotence; gynecomastia. *HEPA:* Hepatitis. *DERM:* Pruritus; urticaria. *Topical use:* Severe irritation, stinging and itching.

Precautions

Pregnancy: Category C. *Lactation:* Undetermined. *Children:* PO Safety and efficacy in children < 2 yr not established. Topical: Safety and efficacy not established. *Anaphylaxis:* Has occurred after the first dose. *CNS infections:* Drug penetrates CSF poorly. Although high doses have sometimes been used in CNS fungal infections, this is not indicated use. *Gastric acidity.* Ketoconazole requires acid environment for dissolution and absorption. *Hepatotoxicity:* Hepatotoxicity, with rare fatalities, has occurred. Use with caution in patients receiving other potentially hepatotoxic drugs, those on long-term therapy and those with history of liver disease. *Hormone levels:* May lower serum testosterone or suppress adrenal corticosteroid secretion.

NURSING CONSIDERATIONS

Administration/Storage

- Give oral drug with food to minimize GI upset. Administer 2 hr before antacid is given.
- Tablets can be crushed and mixed with small amount of food or fluid.
- In achlorhydria, dissolve tablet in 4 ml of 0.2 Normal hydrochloride. Have patient use glass or plastic straw to avoid contact with teeth. Follow with glass of water.
- Apply topical medication once daily to cover affected and immediately surrounding area. Avoid contact with eyes.
- Store at room temperature in tightly closed container. Protect from light.

Assessment/Interventions

- Obtain patient history, including drug history and any known allergies. Note hepatic impairment and sensitivity to antifungal agents.
- Ensure that liver function tests have been obtained before beginning therapy and monitor regularly during treatment.
- Assess for jaundice, anorexia and hepatotoxicity. Notify physician immediately if these symptoms occur.
- Notify physician if severe irritation, itching or stinging occurs after topical application.

Patient/Family Education

- Instruct patient that if dose is missed, it should be taken as soon as possible. If several hours have passed or if close to time of next dose, do not double up. Notify physician if more than one dose is missed.
- Advise patient not to take medication with antacids. If antacids are required, ketoconazole should be taken 2 hr before antacid.
- Emphasize importance of completing full course of therapy, even if signs and symptoms resolve. Advise that maintenance therapy may be required for chronic infections.
- Instruct patient to notify physician if severe irritation, itching, or stinging occur after application.
- Instruct patient to report these symptoms to physician: fatigue, loss of appetite, nausea, vomiting, yellowing of skin, dark urine, pale stools, abdominal pain, fever or diarrhea.
- Advise patient that drug may cause drowsiness and to use caution while driving or performing other tasks requiring mental alertness.
- Instruct patient not to take otc medications, including antihistamine, without consulting physician.

See Patient Guide, pp. 339-341.

Ketoprofen

(KEY-toe-PRO-fen)

Fictron, Orudis, Orudis KT, Oruvail, ✤ *APO-Keto, APO-KETO-E, Novo-Keto-EC, Rhodis, Rhodis-EC*

Class: Analgesic/NSAID

Action Decreases inflammation, pain and fever, probably through inhibition of cyclooxygenase activity and prostaglandin synthesis.

Indications Treatment of rheumatoid arthritis, osteoarthritis, mild to moderate pain, primary dysmenorrhea. *Sustained-release form, only:* Treatment of rheumatoid arthritis and osteoarthritis. **Unlabeled uses:** Treatment of juvenile rheumatoid arthritis, sunburn, migraine prophylaxis.

Contraindications Patients in whom aspirin, iodides or any NSAID has caused allergic-type reactions.

Route/Dosage

Rheumatoid or Osteoarthritis

ADULTS: **PO** 75 mg tid or 50 mg qid; do not exceed 300 mg/day. Maintenance dose: Reduce initial dosage to 75-150 mg/day in elderly or disabled patients or patients with renal impairment. Sustained release capsule: 200 mg once daily can be used in patients already stabilized on that dose.

Mild to Moderate Pain, Primary Dysmenorrhea

ADULTS: **PO** 25-50 mg q 6-8 hr prn; do not exceed 300 mg/day.

Interactions *Anticoagulants:* Increased risk of gastric erosion and bleeding. *Aspirin:* Additive GI toxicity. *Cyclosporine:* Nephrotoxicity of both agents may be increased. *Lithium:* Serum lithium levels may be increased. *Methotrexate:* Increased methotrexate levels.

Lab Test Interferences May prolong bleeding time.

Adverse Reactions *CV:* Peripheral edema; fluid retention; CHF. *RESP:* Bronchospasm; laryngeal edema; rhinitis, dyspnea. *CNS:* Headache; dizziness; lightheadedness; drowsiness; vertigo. *EENT:* Visual disturbances; stomatitis. *GI:* Peptic ulcer; GI bleeding; dyspepsia; nausea; diarrhea; constipation; abdominal pain; flatulence; anorexia; vomiting. *GU:* Menorrhagia. *DERM:* Rash; pruritus.

Precautions *Pregnancy:* Category B. *Lactation:* Excreted in breast milk. *Children:* Safety and efficacy not established. *Elderly:* Increased risk of adverse reactions. *GI:* Bleeding, ulceration or perforation can occur at any time, with or without warning symptoms. *GU:* Acute renal insufficiency, interstitial nephritis, hyperkalemia, hyponatremia and renal papillary necrosis may occur. *Hepatic impairment:* Avoid sustained-release product. *Hypersensitivity:* May occur; use caution in aspirin-sensitive individuals because of possible cross-sensitivity. *Renal impairment:* Lower doses may be necessary.

NURSING CONSIDERATIONS

Administration/Storage

- Do not crush capsules.
- Administer with food, milk or antacids to minimize GI upset.
- Store at room temperature in tightly closed, light-resistant container.

Assessment/Interventions

- Obtain patient history, including drug history and any known allergies. Note renal or hepatic impairment or sensitivity to NSAIDs.
- Do not administer to patients in whom aspirin, iodides or other NSAIDs have induced symptoms of asthma, rhinitis, urticaria, nasal polyps, angioedema, bronchospasm and other symptoms of allergic or anaphylactoid reactions.
- Assess carefully for hypersensitivity (fever, rashes, abdominal pain, headache, nausea, vomiting, signs of liver damage) and for signs of infection (NSAIDs may mask the usual signs of infection).
- Monitor patients on long-term therapy for signs and symptoms of ulcera-

tion and bleeding of upper and lower GI tract.

- Monitor renal and hepatic function tests.
- If skin rash, diarrhea, weight gain, edema, black stools, constipation, persistent headache, blurred vision, dizziness, nervousness, ringing in the ears, taste changes or changes in vision occur or are reported, discontinue use and notify physician.

OVERDOSAGE: SIGNS & SYMPTOMS

Drowsiness, dizziness, confusion, disorientation, lethargy, numbness, vomiting, gastric irritation, nausea, abdominal pain, headache, tinnitus, convulsions, acute renal failure

Patient/Family Education

- Advise patient to take medication with food, milk or antacids. Capsule should be swallowed whole, not chewed or crushed.
- Warn patient not to take aspirin or other NSAIDs.
- Caution patient to report changes in stool (color, consistency, frequency), fluid retention and shortness of breath.
- Instruct patient to report these symptoms to physician: skin rash, itching, visual disturbances, weight gain, edema, black stools or persistent headache.
- Advise patient that drug may cause drowsiness and to use caution while driving or performing other tasks requiring mental alertness.
- Caution patient to avoid exposure to sunlight and other sources of ultraviolet light and to use sunscreen or wear protective clothing to avoid photosensitivity reaction.
- Instruct patient not to ingest alcohol or take otc medications without notifying physician.

See Patient Guide, pp. 342-343.

Ketorolac Tromethamine

(KEY-TOR-oh-lak tro-METH-uh-meen)

Acular, Toradol

Class: Analgesic/NSAID

Action Decreases inflammation, pain and fever, probably through inhibition of cyclooxygenase activity and prostaglandin synthesis.

Indications *Oral and intramuscular forms:* Short-term management of pain. *Ophthalmic form:* Relief of ocular itching caused by seasonal allergic conjunctivitis.

Contraindications Patients in whom aspirin, iodides or any NSAID has caused allergic-type reactions; active peptic ulcer disease, recent GI bleeding or perforation; advanced renal impairment and in patients at risk for renal failure due to volume depletion; suspected or confirmed cerebrovascular bleeding; hemorrhagic diathesis, incomplete hemostasis and those at high risk of bleeding; as prophylactic analgesia before any major surgery and intraoperatively when hemostasis is critical; for intrathecal or epidural administration due to its alcohol content; in labor and delivery; in lactation; in concomitant use with aspirin or other NSAIDSs. Ophthalmic use: Soft contact lens use.

Route/Dosage

Single dose

ADULTS: **IM** <65 years old-60 mg; >65 years old, renal impairment or weight <50 kg (110 lbs)—30 mg. **IV** <65 years old—30 mg; >65 years old, renal impairment or weight <50 kg (110 lbs)—15 mg.

Multiple dose

ADULTS: **IM** <65 years old—30 mg every 6 hours. Maximum daily dose should not exceed 120 mg; >65 years old, renal impairment or weight <50 kg (110 lbs)—15 mg every 6 hours. Maximum daily dose should not exceed 60 mg.

Transition from IV/IM to oral

ADULTS: <65 years old—20 mg as a first oral dose for patients who received 60 mg IM single dose, 30 mg IV single dose or 30 mg multiple dose IV/IM, followed by 10 mg every 4-6 hours, not to exceed 40 mg/24 hours. >65 years old, renal impairment or weight <50 kg (110 lbs)—10 mg as a first oral dose for patients who received a 30 mg IM single dose, 15 mg IV single dose or 15 mg multiple dose IV/IM, followed by 10 mg every 4-6 hours, not to exceed 40 mg/24 hours.

Ophthalmic

1 gtt qid.

Interactions

Anticoagulants: May increase risk of gastric erosion and bleeding. *Cyclosporine:* Nephrotoxicity of both agents may be increased. *Lithium:* Serum lithium levels may be increased. *Methotrexate:* May increase methotrexate levels. *Salicylates:* May cause additive GI toxicity.

Lab Test Interferences

Drug may prolong bleeding time.

Adverse Reactions

CV: Fluid retention; edema. *RESP:* Bronchospasm. *CNS:* Nervousness; abnormal thinking; depression; euphoria; headache; drowsiness; dizziness. *EENT:* Stomatitis. Ophthalmic use: Increased bleeding with ocular surgery; ocular irritation; allergic reactions; superficial keratitis. *GI:* Nausea; diarrhea; flatulence; GI fullness; abdominal distress; excessive thirst; GI toxicity. *HEPA:* Abnormal liver function test results. *DERM:* Rash. *OTHER:* Muscle cramps; aseptic meningitis.

Precautions

Pregnancy: Category C. *Lactation:* Excreted in breast milk. *Children:* Safety and efficacy have not been established. *Elderly patients:* Increased risk of adverse reactions. *Chronic use:* Intramuscular drug is not intended for long-term use. Limit to short-term therapy (not > 5 days). Oral drug is intended for limited duration of use. *GI effects:* Serious GI toxicity (eg, bleeding, ulceration, perforation) can occur at any time with or without warning symptoms. *Hypersensitivity:* May occur; use drug with caution in aspirin-sensitive individuals because of possible cross-sensitivity. *Photosensitivity:* Drug can cause photosensitization. *Renal effects:* Acute renal insufficiency, interstitial nephritis, hyperkalemia, hyponatremia and renal papillary necrosis may occur. *Renal impairment:* Assess function before and during therapy, because NSAID metabolites are eliminated renally. Dosage adjustments may be necessary.

NURSING CONSIDERATIONS

Administration/Storage

- The combined duration of ketorolac IV/IM and oral is not to exceed 5 days. Oral use is only indicated as continuation therapy to IV/IM.
- Do not mix IV/IM ketorolac in a small volume (eg, in a syringe) with morphine sulfate, meperidine HC1, promethazine HC1 or hydroxyzine HC1; this will result in precipitation of ketorolac from solution.
- When administering IM/IV, the IV bolus must be given over no less than 15 seconds. Give IM administration slowly and deeply into the muscle. The analgesic effect begins in 30 minutes with maximum effect in 1 to 2 hours after IV or IM dosing. Duration of the analgesic effect is usually 4 to 6 hours.
- If GI upset occurs, administer oral form with meals, milk or antacids to decrease GI irritation.
- With IM administration rotate injection sites.
- For ophthalmic administration, have patient tilt head back, instill drops

into conjunctival sac and close eyes. Apply light finger pressure to lacrimal sac for 1 min after instillation. Do not touch top of cap to eye, fingers or other surface.

- Wash hands before and after instillation.
- Lower doses may be necessary in patients with compromised renal or hepatic function.
- Store at room temperature. Protect from light.

Assessment/Interventions

- Obtain patient history, including drug history and any known allergies.
- Assess degree, location and type of pain before and after administration.
- With ophthalmic use, evaluate ocular itching before and after administration.
- Assess renal function before and during therapy. Monitor serum creatinine or creatinine clearance.
- Monitor for hematomas and bleeding, especially with perioperative intramuscular administration.
- Monitor liver function tests. Notify physician if abnormal liver function tests persist or worsen, if clinical signs and symptoms consistent with liver disease develop or if systemic manifestations (eg, eosinophilia, rash) occur.
- Monitor patients with compromised cardiac function and hypertension for signs of fluid retention (eg, peripheral edema).
- Observe for signs of GI toxicity, especially in elderly patients.
- Observe for signs of infection because ketorolac may mask usual signs.
- Hypersensitivity reactions, ranging from bronchospasm to anaphylactic shock, have occurred, and appropriate counteractive measures must be available when administering the first dose of ketorolac.

OVERDOSAGE: SIGNS & SYMPTOMS

Drowsiness, dizziness, mental confusion, disorientation, lethargy, paresthesia, numbness, vomiting, gastric irritation, nausea, abdominal pain, intense headache, tinnitus, sweating, convulsions, blurred vision, elevations in serum creatinine and BUN

Patient/Family Education

- Instruct patient to take drug with food, milk or antacid if GI upset occurs.
- Inform patient that drug is NSAID and can cause serious side effects such as GI bleeding.
- Instruct patient to avoid alcohol, aspirin and other NSAIDs.
- Advise patient to inform dentist and other physicians of drug therapy before any treatment or surgery.
- Instruct patient to report these symptoms to physician: skin rash, itching, visual disturbances, weight gain, edema, black stools or persistent headache.
- Inform patient using ophthalmic solution not to wear soft contact lenses during treatment; ocular irritation with redness and burning can occur.
- Caution patient to avoid exposure to sunlight and other sources of UV light and to use sunscreen or wear protective clothing to avoid photosensitivity reaction.
- Advise patient that drug may cause drowsiness or dizziness and to use caution while driving or performing other tasks requiring mental alertness.
- Instruct patient not to take any otc medications without consulting physician.

See Patient Guide, pp. 344-345.

Labetalol HCl

(la-BET-uh-lahl HIGH-droe-KLOR-ide)

Normodyne, Trandate

Class: Alpha-adrenergic blocker/beta-adrenergic blocker

Action Selectively blocks alpha-1 receptors and nonselectively blocks beta-receptors to decrease BP, heart rate and myocardial oxygen demand.

Indications Management of hypertension. **Unlabeled uses:** Treatment of pheochromocytoma; management of clonidine-withdrawal hypertension.

Contraindications Severe bradycardia; second- and third-degree heart block; heart failure; cardiogenic shock; bronchial asthma.

Route/Dosage

ADULTS: **PO** 100 mg bid initially; maintenance dose usually 200-400 mg bid. **IV** 20 mg over 2 min; then 40-80 mg q 10 min up to maximum of 300 mg. Infusions of 2 mg/min can be initiated and titrated to response.

Interactions

Beta-adrenergic agonists: Blunted bronchodilator effect. *Cimetidine:* Increased bioavailability of labetalol. *Indomethacin:* Impaired antihypertensive effect of labetalol. *Inhalation anesthetics:* May exaggerate hypotension. *Nitroglycerin:* Increased hypotension. INCOMPATIBILITIES: Injection not compatible with 5% sodium bicarbonate.

Lab Test Interferences

Drug may cause false-positive increases in levels of urinary catecholamines.

Adverse Reactions

CV: Orthostatic hypotension; edema; flushing; ventricular arrhythmias; atrioventricular block; bradycardia; heart failure; chest pain. *RESP:* Bronchospasm; shortness of breath; wheezing. *CNS:* Headache; fatigue; dizziness; depression; lethargy; drowsiness; forgetfulness; sleepiness; vertigo; paresthesias; nightmares. *EENT:* Dry eyes; visual disturbances; altered taste perception. *GI:* Nausea; vomiting; diarrhea; dyspepsia. *GU:* Impotence; urinary retention; difficulty with urination; failure to ejaculate; priapism; Peyronie's disease. *HEMA:* Leukopenia. *HEPA:* Elevated transaminases; jaundice; cholestasis. *DERM:* Tingling of scalp; rash; facial erythema; alopecia; urticaria; pruritus; increased sweating. *META:* Increases or decreases in serum glucose; increased creatinine and BUN. *OTHER:* Muscle cramps; systemic lupus erythematosus; increased hypoglycemic response to insulin; masking of hypoglycemic signs; asthenia.

Precautions

Pregnancy: Category C. *Lactation:* Excreted in breast milk. *Children:* Safety and efficacy not established. *Special risk patients:* Use drug with caution in patients with diabetes mellitus, CHF, respiratory difficulties or severely elevated BP. *Cardiac failure:* Has been observed in patients with or without history of cardiac failure. *Withdrawal:* Do not discontinue abruptly. Abrupt discontinuation may worsen angina and precipitate ischemic event in susceptible individuals.

NURSING CONSIDERATIONS

Administration/Storage

- Administer oral form with food. Tablets can be crushed.
- If nausea and dizziness occur with twice daily dosing of oral form, same total daily dose can be administered as divided doses 3 times/day.
- Keep patient supine during IV administration and for 3 hr afterward.
- For repeated IV injection, give 20 mg dose slowly over 2 min.

- For slow continuous infusion, dilute contents with compatible IV fluid and administer at rate of 2 mg/min. Use controlled administration device. Once satisfactory response is obtained, infusion can be discontinued and treatment with oral labetalol can be initiated.
- Labetalol is compatible with following parenteral solutions: Ringer's, lactated Ringer's 5% Dextrose and Ringer's, 5% lactated Ringer's and 5% Dextrose, 5% Dextrose, 0.9% Sodium Chloride, 5% Dextrose and 0.2% Sodium Chloride, 2.5% Dextrose and 0.45% Sodium Chloride, 5% Dextrose and 0.9% Sodium Chloride and 5% Dextrose and 0.33% Sodium Chloride.
- Store at room tempeature and protect from excessive moisture.
- Do not freeze injection vials. Protect from light. Parenteral solution is stable for 24 hr after dilution.

Assessment/Interventions

- Obtain patient history, including drug history and any known allergies.
- Measure vital signs and supine BP immediately before and at 5-10 min intervals after direct IV injection.
- Obtain renal and liver studies before therapy begins.
- Take safety precautions if orthostatic hypotension occurs.
- Closely monitor diabetic patients for signs of hypoglycemia.
- Assess skin turgor and dryness of mucous membranes for hydration status.

OVERDOSAGE: SIGNS & SYMPTOMS

Excessive orthostatic hypotension, excessive bradycardia, cardiac failure, bronchospasm, seizures

Patient/Family Education

- Caution patient to avoid sudden position changes to prevent orthostatic hypotension. Advise use of support hose.
- Advise patient to notify dentist and other physicians of drug therapy before treatment or surgery.
- Caution diabetic patient to monitor serum glucose carefully.
- Instruct patient not to discontinue drug abruptly.
- Advise patient to carry identification (eg, Medi-Alert) indicating medical condition and drug regimen.
- Instruct patient how to measure BP and pulse.
- Emphasize importance of other modalities on BP: weight control, regular exercise, smoking cessation and moderate intake of alcohol and salt.
- Inform patient that transient scalp tingling may occur, especially when treatment is initiated.
- Instruct patient to report these symptoms to physician: slow heart rate, dizziness, confusion, fever or depression, shortness of breath, fatigue, swelling of ankles and feet.
- Advise patient that drug causes dizziness and to use caution while driving or performing other tasks requiring mental alertness.
- Instruct patient not to take any otc medications without consulting physician.

See Patient Guide, p. 346.

Lactulose

(LAK-tyoo-lohs)

Cephulac, Cholac, Chronulac, Constilac, Constulose, Duphalac, Enulose, Evalose, Heptalac, ✤ *Alpha-Lac, Comalose-R, Gel-Ose, Lactulax, Rhodialax, Rhodialose*

Class: Laxative

Action Produces increased osmotic pressure within colon and acidifies its contents, resulting in increased stool water content and stool softening. Causes migration of ammonia from blood into colon where it is converted to ammonium ion and expelled through laxative action.

Indications Treatment of constipation; prevention and treatment of portal-systemic encephalopathy including stages of hepatic precoma and coma.

Contraindications Use in patients who require low-galactose diet.

Route/Dosage

Constipation (Chronulac, Constilac, Duphalac)

ADULTS: **PO** 15-30 ml (10-20 g lactulose) daily; may increase to 60 ml/day.

Portal-Systemic Encephalopathy (Cephulac, Cholac, Enulose)

ADULTS: **PO** 30-45 ml tid-qid. Adjust dosage to produce 2-3 soft stools/day. Hourly doses of 30-45 ml may be used for rapid laxation initially; once achieved, reduce to recommended daily dose. **PR** 300 ml with 700 ml water or physiologic saline solution via rectal balloon catheter; retain for 30-60 min. May repeat q 4-6 hr. OLDER CHILDREN AND ADOLESCENTS: **PO** 40-90 ml/day in divided doses to produce 2-3 soft stools/day. INFANTS: **PO** 2.5-10 ml/day in divided doses to produce 2-3 soft stools/day.

Interactions

Neomycin, other anti-infectives: May interfere with desired degradation of lactulose and prevent acidification of colonic contents. *Nonabsorbable antacids:* May inhibit colonic acidification.

Lab Test Interferences

None well documented.

Adverse Reactions

GI: Gaseous distention with flatulence or belching, abdominal discomfort and cramping; diarrhea; nausea; vomiting.

Precautions

Pregnancy: Category B. *Lactation:* Undetermined. *Children:* Safety and efficacy not established. Administer with caution. Infants receiving lactulose may develop hyponatremia and dehydration. *Elderly or debilitated patients:* With long-term therapy (> 6 mo) at increased risk of dehydration and electrolyte imbalance. *Concomitant laxative use:* Do not use other laxatives, especially during initial phase of therapy. Resultant loose stools may falsely suggest adequate lactulose dosage. *Diabetic patients:* Lactulose syrup contains galactose and lactose. Use drug with caution. *Electrocautery procedures:* Although not reported for lactulose, theoretical hazard exists for patients being treated with lactulose who may undergo electrocautery procedures during proctoscopy or colonoscopy. Accumulation of hydrogen gas in presence of electrical spark may result in explosion. Therefore patients should have thorough bowel cleansing with nonfermentable solution before undergoing such procedures.

NURSING CONSIDERATIONS

Administration/Storage

- Mix with fruit juice, water or milk to make more palatable.
- Administer with full glass of fruit juice, water or milk.
- May administer to adults during impending coma or coma stage of portal-systemic encephalopathy as retention enema via rectal balloon catheter when danger of aspiration exists or when endoscopic or intubation procedures interfere with oral administration. Do not use cleansing enemas containing soapsuds or other alkaline agents. If enema is inadvertently evacuated too promptly, may repeat it immediately.
- Store at room temperature; do not freeze.

Assessment/Interventions

- Obtain patient history, includ-

ing drug history and any known allergies.
- Assess for abdominal distention and discomfort.
- Evaluate bowel sounds and bowel function.
- Assess consistency and frequency of stool produced.
- Do not use other laxatives.
- Encourage fluid intake.
- Keep patient clean and dry. Assess skin integrity frequently.
- Monitor electrolyte balance and liver function.
- Monitor I&O.
- In elderly or debilitated patients who receive lactulose > 6 mo, measure serum electrolytes (potassium, chloride) and carbon dioxide periodically.
- Monitor mental status (eg, orientation, lethargy, irritability) in portal-systemic encephalopathy patients.
- If concomitant oral anti-infectives are given, monitor patient closely.
- If diarrhea, rectal bleeding, nausea, vomiting, abdominal cramps or distention occurs, discontinue medication and notify physician.

OVERDOSAGE: SIGNS & SYMPTOMS
Diarrhea, abdominal cramps

Patient/Family Education
- Advise patient that drug can be mixed with fruit juice, water or milk to make it more palatable.
- Inform patient that drug may cause belching, flatulence or abdominal cramps. Instruct patient to notify physician if these symptoms become bothersome or if diarrhea occurs.
- Instruct patient not to take other laxatives while receiving lactulose therapy.
- Encourage patient to increase dietary fiber and fluid intake and participate in regular exercise.

See Patient Guide, p. 347.

Lamivudine (3TC)

(la-MIH-view-deen)

Epivir

Class: Anti-infective/antiviral

Action Inhibits replication of HIV

Indications In combination with zidovudine when clinical or immunologic evidence demonstrates HIV progression.

Contraindications Standard considerations.

Route/Dosage
ADULTS: **PO** 150 mg bid in combination with zidovudine if weight > 50 kg; 2 mg/kg bid in combination with zidovudine if weight < 50 kg. ADOLESCENTS (12-16 YRS): **PO** 150 mg bid in combination with zidovudine if weight > 50 kg. CHILDREN 3 MO-12 YR: **PO** 4 mg/kg bid (maximum 150 mg bid) in combination with zidovudine. Dosage adjustment needed due to renal impairment. ADULTS: **PO** CrCl 30-49: 150 mg once/day; CrCl 15-29: 150 mg first dose then 100 mg once/day; CrCl 5-14: 150 mg first dose then 50 mg once/day; CrCl < 5: 50 mg first dose then 25 mg once/day.

Interactions
Trimethoprim-sulfamethoxazole: May decrease clearance of lamivudine, causing increase in its serum concentration. *Zidovudine:* Lamivudine may cause increase in zidovudine serum concentration.

Lab Test Interferences
None well documented.

Adverse Reactions
RESP: Nasal signs & symptoms; cough. *CNS:* Headache; neuropathy; dizziness; sleep disturbances; depression. *GI:* Nausea; vomiting; diarrhea; anorexia; abdominal pain/cramps; dyspepsia. *HEMA:* Anemia; neutropenia. *DERM:* Rash. *OTHER:* Malaise; fatigue; fever; chills; myalgia; arthralgia; pancreatitis; elevated liver enzymes.

Precautions

Pregnancy: Category C. *Lactation:* Undetermined. *Children:* Dosing regimen not determined for children < 3 mo. Use with extreme caution in children with history of pancreatitis or other risk factors for development of pancreatitis. *Renal impairment:* Dosage adjustment recommended.

NURSING CONSIDERATIONS

Administration/Storage

- Administer lamivudine in combination with zidovudine or alone for patients not responding to zidovudine as prescribed.
- Adhere strictly to the prescribed dosage and schedule.
- A reduced dosage is recommended for patients with impaired renal function.
- Store tablets at room temperature in a tight, dry container.
- Oral solution should be stored at room temperature in a tight container.

Assessment/Interventions

- There is no known antidote.
- Obtain patient history.
- Monitor for signs and symptoms of infection or neurological changes.
- Assess patient for change in severity of symptoms.
- Monitor patient for signs and symptoms of pancreatitis, especially pediatric patients.
- Monitor BUN, serum creatinine, liver function tests, amylase and CBC during the course of therapy.
- If any clinical signs, symptoms or laboratory tests suggest pancreatitis occurring, notify healthcare provider immediately.
- In patients receiving lamivudine with zidovudine (Retrovir), monitor patient for increased risk of adverse effects including headache, fatigue, nausea, neuropathy, nasal signs & symptoms, cough, skin rash and musculoskeletal pain.

OVERDOSAGE: SIGNS & SYMPTOMS

No signs or symptoms have been reported

Patient/Family Education

- Instruct patient that the lamivudine tablets and oral solution are for oral ingestion only and to take only as prescribed.
- Instruct patient to avoid over-the-counter medications unless prescribed by the healthcare provider.
- Instruct patient that lamivudine is not a cure for the HIV infection and opportunistic infections and other complications of HIV infection may continue to develop.
- Caution patient or guardian that long-term effects of lamivudine and results from controlled clinical trials evaluating therapeutic and adverse effects are unknown.
- Inform patient of the potential adverse effects.
- Instruct patient to notify the healthcare provider if signs of infection such as a sore throat, fever, cough and respiratory congestion occur.
- Instruct family to notify the healthcare provider of changes in neurological status such as memory loss or confusion.
- Advise patient that it may take 4 weeks or more for maximum effect.
- Warn patient that the risk of transmission of HIV to others through sexual contact or exposure to the patient's blood is still present. Instruct patient in methods and precautions to prevent transmission of the HIV virus.
- Instruct parents or guardians to monitor patients, especially pediatric patients, for signs and symptoms of pancreatitis.
- Caution mothers to discontinue nursing if they are receiving lamivudine due to the potential for adverse effects

from lamivudine in nursing infants as well as transmission of the HIV virus.
- Caution women to inform their healthcare provider if they are or become pregnant as lamivudine is transferred to the fetus through the placenta.
- Stress the importance of regular exams and laboratory work. Encourage patient to comply with the treatment regimen.

See Patient Guide, p. 348.

Lansoprazole

(lan-SO-pruh-zole)
Prevacid
Class: Gastrointestinal

Action Suppresses gastric acid secretion by blocking "acid (proton) pump" within gastric parietal cells.

Indications Short-term treatment of active duodenal ulcer; short-term treatment of all grades of erosive esophagitis; long-term treatment of pathological hypersecretory conditions, including Zollinger-Ellison syndrome.

Contraindications Standard considerations.

Route/Dosage
Duodenal Ulcer
ADULTS: **PO** 15 mg daily for 4 weeks.

Erosive Esophagitis
ADULTS: **PO** 30 mg daily for up to 8 weeks, an additional 8 weeks may be helpful for patients who do not heal.

Pathological Hypersecretory Conditions
ADULTS: **PO** Initial dose 60 mg once daily. Dosages up to 90 mg bid have been administered. Divide daily doses > 120 mg.

Interactions
Sucralfate: May delay and reduce absorption; give lansoprazole at least 30 minutes before sucralfate.

Lab Test Interferences
None well documented.

Adverse Reactions
CNS: Headache. *GI:* Diarrhea; abdominal pain; nausea.

Precautions
Pregnancy: Category B. *Lactation:* Undetermined. *Children:* Safety and efficacy not established. *Elderly:* Should not exceed 30 mg daily unless additional gastric acid suppression is necessary.

NURSING CONSIDERATIONS

Administration/Storage
- Take 30 min before meals for up to 8 weeks.
- Swallow each capsule whole. Do not open, crush or chew.
- Drink plenty of fluids as the capsules are swallowed.
- Store at room temperature, in tight container away from humidity.

Assessment/Interventions
- Obtain patient history.
- Assess for any symptoms of hyperacidity or acid-related disease (eg, dyspepsia, nausea, vomiting).
- Assess for coffee-ground or bloody emesis, tarry stools or constipation.
- Obtain baseline AST, ALT, alkaline phosphatase, electrolytes and liver function studies.

OVERDOSAGE: SIGNS & SYMPTOMS
None documented

Patient/Family Education
- Take with food.
- Instruct patient to follow bland diet per nutrition consultation/instruction.
- Stress importance of follow-up ap-

pointments with healthcare provider for laboratory tests and assessment of effectiveness.

- Inform patient that due to the long lasting effects of this medication on the reduction of gastric secretions, some medications that require an acid gastric pH (ketoconazole, ampicillin, iron preparations, digoxin) may not be well absorbed.
- Advise patient that antacids can be taken while taking lansoprazole.
- Instruct patient to avoid intake of alcoholic beverages while taking this medication.
- Inform patient to call the healthcare provider if they develop any severe side effects such as melena, rectal bleeding, difficulty breathing, hemoptysis or abnormal muscle movements.
- Instruct patient not to take any over-the-counter medications without checking with their healthcare provider first.

See Patient Guide, p. 349.

Leucovorin Calcium (Citrovorum Factor; Folinic Acid)

(loo-koe-VORE-in KAL-see-uhm)

Wellcovorin

Class: Folic acid derivative

Action Acts as antidote to drugs that antagonize folic acid, such as methotrexate.

Indications

Oral and parenteral: Treatment to diminish toxicity and counteract effect of overdosage of folic acid antagonists. *Parenteral:* Treatment of megaloblastic anemia due to folic acid deficiency when oral therapy is not feasible.

Contraindications Pernicious anemia and other megaloblastic anemias secondary to vitamin B_{12} deficiency.

Route/Dosage

Colorectal Cancer

ADULTS: **IV** Either 200 mg/m^2 followed by 5-fluorouracil (5-FU) 370 mg/m^2 or 20 mg/m^2 followed by 5-FU 425 mg/m^2 qd for 5 days.

Leucovorin Rescue

ADULTS: **PO/IV/IM** 10 mg/m^2 q 6 hr for 10 doses.

Megaloblastic Anemia Due to Folic Acid Deficiency

ADULTS: **IV/IM** 1 mg/day.

Interactions

Barbiturates, hydantoins (eg, phenytoin), primidone: May decrease anticonvulsant activity. *Fluorouracil:* Enhances toxicity of fluorouracil. *Methotrexate:* May decrease efficacy of intrathecal methotrexate.

Lab Test Interferences

None well documented.

Adverse Reactions

OTHER: Hypersensitivity, including anaphylaxis and urticaria. No other adverse reactions have been attributed to leucovorin alone.

Precautions

Pregnancy: Category C. *Lactation:* Undetermined. *Benzyl alcohol:* Present in 1 ml amp and some diluents. Benzyl alcohol has been associated with fatal "gasping syndrome" in premature infants. *5-FU toxicity:* Leucovorin enhances toxicity of 5-FU; dosage should be decreased. Administer only under supervision of physician experienced in use of antimetabolite cancer chemotherapy.

NURSING CONSIDERATIONS

Administration/Storage

- When drug is given for leucovorin rescue after high-dose methotrexate therapy, administer first dose 24 hr after beginning of methotrexate infusion.

- When drug is given as antidote for inadvertent overdosage of folic acid antagonists (eg, methotrexate), administer as soon as overdose is detected, preferably within first hour.
- Reconstitute parenteral solution using Bacteriostatic Water for Injection or Sterile Water for Injection. Bacteriostatic water mixtures must be used within 7 days; sterile water mixtures, immediately. If doses > 10 mg/m^2 are needed, reconstitute with Sterile Water for Injection.
- Administer IV solution slowly, at rate of < 160 mg/min, due to calcium content.
- If necessary, further dilution with 100-500 ml dextrose or saline solutions for intermittent infusion is possible.
- Tablets can be crushed if necessary.
- Store at room temperature and protect from light.

Assessment/Interventions

- Obtain patient history, including drug history and any known allergies.
- Ensure that baseline laboratory values, including liver and renal function tests, CBC and platelet count, have been obtained before beginning therapy and monitor during treatment.
- Ensure that daily methotrexate levels are obtained when leucovorin is used for high-dose methotrexate rescue.
- Keep patient well hydrated. Monitor I&O carefully during treatment.

Patient/Family Education

- Instruct patient not to double up doses, and to notify physician if dose is missed.
- Instruct patient to report these symptoms to physician: nausea, vomiting, diarrhea, sores in mouth, fatigue, difficulty breathing or skin disorders.
- Advise patient to notify physician if unable to keep dose down (ie, if vomiting occurs). Patient may need IM or IV therapy instead of oral medication.

See Patient Guide, p. 350.

Leuprolide Acetate

(loo-PRO-lide ASS-uh-TATE)

Lupron, Lupron Depot, Lupron Depot-Ped

Class: Gonadotropin-releasing hormone analog

Action A synthetic luteinizing hormone-releasing hormone (LHRH) agonist of greater potency than naturally occurring gonadotropin-releasing hormone (GnRH). Occupies pituitary GnRH receptors and thus desensitizes them, inhibiting gonadotropin secretion required for gonadal production of testosterone and estrogen.

Indications Palliative treatment of advanced prostatic cancer (alone or in combination with flutamide); management of endometriosis in women > 18 yr (depot preparation); treatment of children with central precocious puberty (CPP); uterine leiomyomata. **Unlabeled uses:** Breast, ovarian and endometrial carcinoma; leiomyoma uteri; infertility; prostatic hypertrophy.

Contraindications Pregnancy, lactation; hypersensitivity to GnRH, GnRH agonist analogs or product components; undiagnosed vaginal bleeding.

Route/Dosage

Advanced Prostate Cancer

ADULTS: **SC** 1 mg/day. **IM** 7.5 mg q mo (depot preparation).

Central Precocious Puberty (CPP)

Starting dose: **SC** 50 mcg/kg/day as single injection. Individualize dosage and titrate to response. Starting dose: **IM** 0.3 mg/kg q 4 wk (minimum 7.5 mg) as single injection (depot preparation). Must be administered by physician or designated health care provider.

Endometriosis

ADULTS: **IM** 3.75 mg as single monthly injection for 6 mo (depot preparation).

Uterine Leiomyomata

ADULTS: **IM** 3.75 mg as a single monthly injection for up to 3 months.

Interactions None well documented.

Lab Test Interferences

Diagnostic tests of pituitary gonadotropic and gonadal functions during treatment and up to 12 wk after discontinuing depot preparation may be misleading.

Adverse Reactions Incidence and type of reactions vary depending on usage and route of administration. *CV:* ECG changes; lethargy; ischemia; peripheral edema; hypertension; murmur; thrombosis; phlebitis; CHF. *RESP:* Dyspnea; sinus congestion. *CNS:* Depression; emotional lability; pain; insomnia; sleep disorders; headache; dizziness; lightheadedness; nervousness; parasthesias. *GI:* GI disturbances; anorexia; constipation; nausea; vomiting. *GU:* Vaginitis; bleeding; discharge; urinary frequency or urgency; hematuria; urinary tract infection. *DERM:* Dermatitis; acne. *META:* Androgen-like effects (in females); decreased testicular size; impotence; decreased libido; gynecomastia; breast tenderness (both sexes); hot flashes; sweats. *OTHER:* Weight gain or loss; anemia; asthenia; myalgia.

Precautions

Pregnancy: Category X (depot preparation). A non-hormonal method of contraception should be used. *Lactation:* Undetermined. *Children:* Safety and efficacy of injection not established; recommended depot preparation for CPP. *Bone density changes:* Use of depot preparation may result in decreased bone density. Decreased bone mineral content risk factors may cause additional bone loss with long-term use. *Hypersensitivity:* Injection contains benzyl alcohol, which can cause local hypersensitivity reactions. Depot preparation is preservative-free.

NURSING CONSIDERATIONS

Administration/Storage

- Use syringes included in the kit or low-dose insulin syringes (SC). Do not use needles smaller than 22-gauge (IM). Rotate injection sites.
- Reconstitute depot form only with diluent provided. Reconstituted suspension will appear milky. Suspension is stable for 24 hr after reconstitution.
- Store unreconstituted depot form at room temperature.
- Refrigerate injection (non-depot form) until used for first dose. May then be stored at room temperature until contents of vial have been administered. Protect from light.

Assessment/Interventions

- Obtain patient history, including drug history and any known allergies.
- Ensure that baseline laboratory tests (eg, testosterone, acid phosphase) have been obtained before beginning therapy and monitor periodically thereafter.
- Monitor I&O carefully and assess for bladder distention with prostate cancer. Transient exacerbation of symptoms (urinary obstruction, hematuria) occurs in many patients during first week of therapy.

Patient/Family Education

- Caution patient that depot preparation must not be taken during pregnancy or when pregnancy is possible. Advise patient to use reliable form of birth control while taking this drug.
- Advise patient/family to follow prescribed regimen. Do not alter dose or discontinue therapy without consulting physician.
- Instruct patient on proper injection

technique and have patient perform return demonstration.

- Advise patient to use nonhormonal forms of birth control because menstrual irregularities may occur.
- Inform patient that burning, itching or swelling may develop at injection site, and to notify physician if these symptoms worsen.
- Advise patient that increased bone pain and difficulty urinating may occur in early treatment of prostate cancer.
- With patients receiving drug for CPP, inform family that menses or spotting may occur initially but to notify physician if symptoms continue beyond second month.
- Inform patients receiving drug for endometriosis/uterine leiomyomata that menstruation should stop and to notify healthcare provider if it persists.

See Patient Guide, p. 351.

Levamisole HCl

(lev-AM-ih-sole HIGH-droe-KLOR-ide)

Ergamisol

Class: Antineoplastic

Action Restores depressed immune function by stimulating antibody formation to various antigens, enhancing T-cell responses and potentiating monocyte and macrophage functions including phagocytosis and chemotaxis. Inhibits alkaline phosphatase and has cholinergic activity.

Indications Adjuvant treatment (with fluorouracil [5-FU]) after surgical resection of Dukes' stage C colon cancer. **Unlabeled uses:** Treatment of bacterial and parasitic infections.

Contraindications Standard considerations.

Route/Dosage

ADULTS: Initial dose: **PO** 50 mg q 8 hr for 3 days. Maintenance: **PO** 50 mg q 8 hr for 3 days q 2 wk for 1 yr. Administer concomitantly with IV fluorouracil per protocol.

Interactions

Alcohol: Disulfuram-like reaction. *Phenytoin:* Increased phenytoin plasma levels.

Lab Test Interferences

None well documented.

Adverse Reactions

CNS: Dizziness; headache; paresthesia; somnolence; ataxia; depression; confusion; memory loss. *EENT:* Abnormal tearing; blurred vision; taste distortion. *GI:* Nausea; diarrhea; stomatitis; vomiting; anorexia; abdominal pain; constipation. *HEMA:* Agranulocytosis; leukopenia; thrombocytopenia; granulocytopenia; anemia; epistaxis. *DERM:* Dermatitis; rash; alopecia; pruritus. *OTHER:* Fatigue; fever; rigors; infection; arthralgia; myalgia; chills; edema.

Precautions

Pregnancy: Category C. *Lactation:* Undetermined. *Children:* Safety and efficacy in children not established. *Agranulocytosis:* Has occurred and been fatal. Often accompanied by flu-like symptoms. *Dosage adjustments:* Dosage of 5-FU and levamisole will need to be adjusted or discontinued in presence of neutropenia or thrombocytopenia.

NURSING CONSIDERATIONS

Administration/Storage

- Administer levamisole orally and fluorouracil by rapid push IV.
- Store in tightly closed, light-resistant container at room temperature.

Assessment/Interventions

- Obtain patient history, including drug history and any known allergies.
- Ensure that baseline CBC and plate-

let count, electrolytes and liver function tests have been performed before beginning therapy. Monitor CBC and platelets 1 wk before each 5-FU treatment. Electrolytes and liver function tests should be repeated every 3 mo for duration of treatment.

- Observe for fever or flu-like signs, signs of local infection, ecchymosis, oral ulcerations, neurologic deficits or edema. If present, notify physician.
- Monitor I&O during therapy.
- Weigh patient weekly.

OVERDOSAGE: SIGNS & SYMPTOMS

Leukopenia, thrombocytopenia, nausea, vomiting, stomatitis, infection

Patient/Family Education

- Instruct patient to check mucous membranes for signs of inflammation and ulceration. Discuss importance of oral hygiene in prevention of stomatitis.
- Advise patient to rinse mouth with water after eating and drinking, to avoid rigorous flossing, and to use soft toothbrush and electric razor.
- Instruct client to weigh self weekly and notify physician if weight gain > 2-3 lb or edema of ankles occurs.
- Advise patient to report any of these symptoms to physician: flu-like symptoms (fever, chills, fatigue); nausea; vomiting; increased bruising or bleeding; difficulty concentrating or lack of coordination; signs of infection (mouth sores, difficulty swallowing); dark stools.
- Warn patient to avoid contact with potentially infectious individuals and to avoid large groups.
- Tell patient to avoid any immunizations.
- Instruct patient to avoid intake of alcoholic beverages or alcohol-containing products. Caution patient to read *all* product labels carefully for hidden sources of alcohol (eg, mouthwash, cough medicine, sauces).
- Warn patient not to take otc medications (eg, aspirin, ibuprofen) without consulting physician.
- Advise patient to notify dentist or physician of drug regimen before surgical or dental procedures.
- Explain that routine laboratory tests will be scheduled to evaluate drug's effectiveness and to monitor for adverse reactions.
- Advise patient that drug may cause drowsiness and to use caution while driving or performing hazardous tasks.

See Patient Guide, p. 352.

Levobunolol

(LEE-voe-BYOO-no-lahl)

AK-Beta, Betagan Liquifilm

Class: Ophthalmic/glaucoma/beta-adrenergic blocker

Action Reduces IOP by reducing aqueous humor production.

Indications Treatment of IOP in chronic open-angle glaucoma or ocular hypertension.

Contraindications Bronchial asthma; severe chronic obstructive pulmonary disease; sinus bradycardia; second-degree and third-degree atrioventricular (AV) block; cardiac failure; cardiogenic shock.

Route/Dosage

ADULTS: **Topical** 1 drop in affected eye(s) qd or bid.

Interactions

Beta blockers, oral: Additive effects on systemic beta blockade. *Epinephrine, ophthalmic:* Hypertension due to unopposed alpha-adrenergic stimulation.

Lab Test Interferences

None well documented.

Adverse Reactions

CV: Arrhythmia; bradycardia; hypotension; syncope; heart block; cerebral vascular accident; cerebral ischemia; CHF; cardiac arrest. *RESP:* Bronchospasm. *CNS:* Headache; depression. *EENT:* Keratitis; blepharoptosis; visual disturbances; diplopia; ptosis; transient burning; stinging; blepharoconjunctivitis; decreased corneal sensitivity. *GI:* Nausea. *DERM:* Rash.

Precautions

Pregnancy: Category C. *Lactation:* Undetermined. *Children:* Safety and efficacy not established. *Special risk patients:* Use with caution in patients with cerebrovascular insufficiency and bronchial diseases. *Diabetes mellitus:* May mask hypoglycemic symptoms in patients with insulin-dependent diabetes. Use with caution. *Sulfite sensitivity:* Contains metabisulfite, which may cause allergic-type reactions in susceptible persons. *Systemic absorption:* Adverse effects like those seen with systemic beta-blockers may occur, due to absorption. *Thyroid disorders:* May mask clinical signs of hyperthyroidism.

NURSING CONSIDERATIONS

Administration/Storage

- Position patient with head tilted back. Instruct patient to look upward. Gently depress conjunctival sac to create small area for medication administration.
- Instill medication from ½ to 1 inch from eye. Instilling from greater distance may cause pain and injury.
- Avoid eyelash and eyelid contamination of medication dispenser.
- Compress lacrimal sac for at least 1 min after administration to delay drainage of medication into nasolacrimal duct and to prevent systemic absorption.
- Wait at least 5 min before administering other types of ophthalmic solution.
- Discard medication that has become contaminated by foreign material.
- Store at room temperature. Protect from light.

Assessment/Interventions

- Obtain patient history, including drug history and any known allergies. Note history of cerebrovascular accident, cardiac disease, chronic obstructive pulmonary disease or diabetes mellitus.
- Monitor BP and pulse throughout course of therapy.
- Monitor IOP periodically during therapy to determine effectiveness of therapy.
- Observe for loss of corneal sensitivity.
- Be alert for systemic effects, including bradycardia, CHF, cardiac arrhythmias, bronchospasm and dyspnea.

OVERDOSAGE: SIGNS & SYMPTOMS

Bradycardia, hypotension, bronchospasm, heart failure

Patient/Family Education

- Instruct patient in proper administration. Advise patient that if dose is missed, it should be administered as soon as possible unless close to time of next dose. Do not double up.
- Caution patient not to stop taking medication unless instructed to do so by physician.
- Emphasize importance of washing hands before drug administration and of not allowing dropper to come into contact with any surface including eyelashes.
- Instruct patient to report these symptoms to physician: eye infection, inflammation, rash, itching or decreased vision.
- Instruct patient to notify physician immediately if severe or sudden eye pain occurs.
- Advise diabetic patient that drug may mask signs of hypoglycemia and to monitor glucose levels carefully.
- Instruct patient not to take otc medications or allergy medications without consulting physician.
- Advise patient to inform physician or

dentist of medication regimen before surgical or dental procedures. Gradual withdrawal of medication may be necessary before procedure.

- Explain importance of scheduling regular follow-up examinations while taking medication.

See Patient Guide, p. 353.

Levodopa

(LEE-voe-DOE-puh)

Dopar

Class: Antiparkinson

Action Crosses the blood-brain barrier and is converted to dopamine in basal ganglia and periphery.

Indications Treatment of idiopathic, postencephalitic and symptomatic parkinsonism. **Unlabeled uses:** Relief of herpes zoster (shingles) pain and restless leg syndrome.

Contraindications Narrow-angle glaucoma; concomitant MAO inhibitor therapy (excluding MAO inhibitor–type B agents such as selegiline); history of or suspected melanoma.

Route/Dosage

ADULTS: **PO** 0.5-1 g/day in 2-4 divided doses initially. Increase dosage gradually in increments ≤ 0.75 g/day q 3-7 days as tolerated (maximum 8 g/day).

Interactions

Anticholinergics, benzodiazepines, hydantoins, methionine, papaverine, pyridoxine, tricyclic antidepressants: May reduce the effectiveness of levodopa. MAO *inhibitors* (except selegiline): Causes hypertensive reactions.

Lab Test Interferences

Antiglobulin Coombs' test: With extended therapy, drug may cause false-positive results. *Uric acid study:* May result in elevated values with colormetric method but not with uricase method.

Adverse Reactions

CV: Cardiac irregularity or palpitation; orthostatic hypotension; hypertension; phlebitis. *RESP:* Bizarre breathing patterns. *CNS:* Ataxia; headache; dizziness; numbness; weakness; faintness; confusion; insomnia; nightmares; mental changes (eg, psychosis, paranoia, depression, dementia, hallucinations, delusions); agitation; anxiety; fatigue; euphoria; psychopathology; adventitious movements (eg, choreiform or dystonic movements); increased hand tremor; muscle twitching; trismus; bradykinesia ("on-off" phenomenon). *EENT:* Blepharospasm; diplopia; blurred vision; dilated pupils; impaired taste perception; oculogyric crisis. *GI:* Anorexia; nausea; vomiting; abdominal pain; distress; dry mouth; dysphagia; excessive salivation; bruxism; GI bleeding; duodenal ulcer. *GU:* Urine retention; urinary incontinence; priapism. *HEMA:* Hemolytic anemia; anemia; agranulocytosis; leukopenia. *HEPA:* Elevated AST, ALT, LDH. *DERM:* Flushing; skin rash; sweating. *OTHER:* Malaise; hot flashes; weight gain or loss; dark sweat or urine; latent Horner's syndrome; elevated BUN, bilirubin, alkaline phosphatase and protein-bound iodine; activation of malignant melanoma.

Precautions

Pregnancy: Pregnancy category undetermined. *Lactation:* Undetermined. Do not use in nursing mothers. *Children:* Safety and efficacy in children < 12 yr not established. *Concomitant conditions:* Use cautiously in patients with severe cardiovascular or pulmonary disease; renal, hepatic or endocrine disease; affective disorder; major psychosis; and cardiac arrhythmias. *Dosage reduction:* Decrease levodopa dose by 75% to 80% when used in combination with carbidopa. *MI:* Administer cautiously to patients with history of MI who have residual arrhythmias. Administer drug in facility with coronary or intensive care unit. *Psychiatric patients:* Use cautiously. Observe all patients for development of depression or suicidal ideation. *Upper GI hemorrhage:* May occur in patients with prior history of peptic ulcer.

NURSING CONSIDERATIONS

Administration/Storage

- Give medication with food to reduce nausea.
- Tablets can be crushed and capsules opened for mixing with small amount of fruit juice for patients being given tube feedings.
- Store at room temperature in light-resistant container.

Assessment/Interventions

- Obtain patient history, including drug history and any known allergies.
- Assess for skin lesions or history of malignant melanoma.
- Determine if patient is receiving MAO inhibitor. MAO inhibitor therapy must be discontinued at least 3 wk before levodopa regimen is instituted.
- Perform complete baseline assessment of parkinsonian signs and symptoms before instituting therapy.
- Monitor BP closely for hypotension if patient is taking antihypertensives concurrently.
- Assist with ambulation during initial phase of therapy because of dizziness due to hypotension.
- Monitor protein intake because absorption of levodopa is decreased in the presence of high-protein foods.
- If uncontrollable movements, mental changes (eg, depression, paranoia), palpitations, difficult urination or severe or persistent nausea and vomiting occur, notify physician.
- Offer support to patient and family because relief of parkinsonian symptoms may take several weeks to months after therapy is initiated.

OVERDOSAGE: SIGNS & SYMPTOMS

Shock, coma, blepharospasm, arrhythmias, seizures, CNS depression, muscle twitching

Patient/Family Education

- Advise patient to take medication with food.
- Teach patient to avoid sudden position changes to avoid orthostatic hypotension.
- Inform patient that fluctuation in effectiveness of levodopa sometimes occurs with long-term therapy. Instruct patient to notify physician if fluctuation in effectiveness is experienced.
- Advise patient to avoid use of otc vitamins, fortified cereals and vitamin B_6, which reverse effects of levodopa.
- Warn patient not to increase dosage in an attempt to reduce parkinsonian symptoms more quickly. Noticeable lessening of symptoms may take more than 6 mo to occur.
- Advise patient to report these symptoms to physician: uncontrolled movements, mood or mental changes, irregular heartbeats, difficulty in urination, severe or persistent nausea or vomiting, worsening of parkinsonian symptoms.
- Advise patient that levodopa may cause urine and perspiration to become dark, which is a harmless side effect.
- Inform patient that drug may cause drowsiness and to use caution while driving or performing tasks that require mental alertness.
- Instruct patient to take sips of water frequently, suck on ice chips or sugarless hard candy or chew sugarless gum if dry mouth occurs.

See Patient Guide, p. 354.

Levodopa/Carbidopa

(LEE-voe-DOE-puh/CAR-bih-doe-puh)

Sinemet, Sinemet CR

Class: Antiparkinson

Action Levodopa is precursor of dopamine, which is deficient in parkinsonism patients. Carbidopa has no activity of its own but inhibits decarboxylation of levodopa, making it more available to brain.

Indications Treatment of symptoms of idiopathic Parkinson's disease (paralysis agitans), postencephalitic parkinsonism and symptomatic parkinsonism associated with carbon monoxide and manganese poisoning.

Contraindications Narrow-angle glaucoma; undiagnosed skin lesions or prior history of suspected melanoma; concurrent use of or within 2 wk of MAO inhibitors.

Route/Dosage

Individualize by careful titration. Combination tablets are available in ratios of carbidopa to levodopa of 1:4 (25 mg/100 mg) and 1:10 (10 mg/100 mg; 25 mg/250 mg). Tablets of the two ratios may be administered separately or combined prn to provide optimum dosage. Provide at least 70-100 mg/day of carbidopa to reduce side effects.

Immediate Release Tablets

ADULTS: Initial dose: **PO** 1 tablet of 25 mg carbidopa/100 mg levodopa tid or 10 mg carbidopa/100 mg levodopa tid-qid. Dosage may be increased by 1 tablet qd or qod prn (maximum 8 tablets/day).

Sustained Release Tablets (50 mg Carbidopa/200 mg Levodopa)

ADULTS: Initial dose: **PO** 1 tablet at intervals ≥ 6 hr. Adjust dosage based on response. Usual range is 2-8 tablets/day in divided doses 4-8 hr while awake. Allow at least 3-day interval between adjustments.

Interactions

Antihypertensive drugs: May cause symptomatic orthostatic hypotension. MAO *inhibitors:* May result in hypertensive crisis. Use is contraindicated. *Phenothiazines, butyrophenones, phenytoin and papaverine:* May reduce levodopa efficacy. *Tricyclic antidepressants:* Rare cases of hypertension and dyskinesia have occurred.

Lab Test Interferences

May cause false-positive reaction for urinary ketone bodies (Clinitest) and false-negative test results with glucose-oxidase methods of testing for glucosuria (Clinistix, Tes-tape).

Adverse Reactions

CV: Cardiac irregularities; palpitations; hypertension; phlebitis; orthostatic hypotension. *CNS:* Paranoid delusions; psychotic episodes; depression; suicidal ideation; dementia; convulsions; hallucinations; dizziness; choreiform; dystonic and other involuntary movements. *EENT:* Diplopia; blurred vision. *GI:* Nausea; anorexia; vomiting; GI distress; epigastric pain; GI bleeding; dry mouth; duodenal ulcer. *GU:* Dark urine; urinary retention; urinary incontinence; priapism. *HEMA:* Hemolytic and nonhemolytic anemia; thrombocytopenia; leukopenia; agranulocytosis. *HEPA:* Elevated liver function test results; hepatotoxicity. *OTHER:* Positive Coomb's test; flushing; malaise.

Precautions

Pregnancy: Safety and effects unknown. Sustained release: Category C. *Lactation:* Do not give to nursing mothers. *Special risk patients:* Use drug with caution in patients with severe cardiovascular or pulmonary disease, bronchial asthma, renal, hepatic or endocrine disease. *Abrupt withdrawal:* Rapid withdrawal of antiparkinson drugs may produce symptoms of neuroleptic malignant syndrome. *Dose conversion:* Patients previously given levodopa alone should discontinue levodopa use at least 8 hr before starting carbidopa/levodopa. Eventually substitute combination drug at dosage providing about 25% of previous levodopa dose. *GI hemorrhage:* Upper GI hemorrhage has been reported in patients with prior history of peptic ulcer. *MI:* Patients with previous history of MI who have residual arrhythmias should have their cardiac function closely monitored on initiating drug dosage adjustment in facility with provisions for intensive cardiac care. *Neurologic/psychiatric effects:* Levodopa may cause involuntary movement and mental disturbances. Use drug with caution in patients with psychosis. Dyskinesias may occur at lower doses and sooner than with levodopa alone. Dosages should be reduced if necessary.

NURSING CONSIDERATIONS

Administration/Storage

- Do not crush or allow patient to chew sustained release tablets; however, regular or sustained release tablet may be cut in half.
- Scored immediate release tablets may be crushed.
- Administer with food to reduce nausea.
- Do not administer with high-protein foods because they reduce absorption of medication.
- Discontinue levodopa at least 8 hr before initial dose of levodopa/carbidopa.
- Store at room temperature and protect from light.

Assessment/Interventions

- Obtain patient history, including drug history and any known allergies.
- Complete baseline assessment of parkinsonian symptoms before instituting therapy.
- Review baseline CBC and liver function test results.
- Determine if patient has taken MAO inhibitors within 3 wk of beginning levodopa/carbidopa therapy.
- Assess for adverse reactions and drug interactions throughout course of therapy.
- Observe for therapeutic effects. Parkinsonian movements are reduced for about 5 hr after administration of medication and then gradually increase in intensity.
- Assess for orthostatic hypotension, dizziness and mental changes during initial phase of therapy.
- Assist patient with position change and ambulation during initial therapy to prevent falling.
- Monitor BP and pulse routinely throughout therapy.
- Observe patients closely for possible depression or suicidal ideation.
- Monitor cardiac function closely, especially in patients with history of MI.
- Do not administer if significant changes in BP, pulse or mental status occur. Notify physician.

OVERDOSAGE: SIGNS & SYMPTOMS

Muscle twitching, blepharospasm

Patient/Family Education

- Teach patient and family how to administer tablets correctly; do not crush or chew sustained release tablets.
- Instruct patient to report these symptoms to physician: uncontrollable movements, mood or mental changes, irregular heartbeat, difficult urination, severe or persistent nausea or vomiting, appetite loss, dry mouth, difficulty swallowing or taste distortion.
- Instruct patient to avoid vitamin B_6 (pyridoxine), fortified cereals and otc vitamins because they reduce absorption of medication.
- Inform patient that drug may cause harmless darkening of sweat or urine.
- Advise patient that drug may cause drowsiness and to use caution while

driving or performing other tasks requiring mental alertness.

- Instruct patient and family about longer onset of action (about 1 hr) during initial phase of therapy. Reduction of parkinsonian symptoms may take several weeks to months to occur.
- Instruct patient to avoid sudden position changes to prevent orthostatic hypotension.

See Patient Guide, p. 355.

Levomethadyl Acetate HCl

(LEE-voe-METH-uh-dill ASS-uh-TATE HIGH-droe-KLOR-ide)

Orlaam

Class: Narcotic analgesic

Action Similar mechanism of action as other opiates; however, its slow onset and long duration of action make use as analgesic inappropriate.

Indications Management of opiate dependence.

Contraindications Standard considerations.

Route/Dosage

ADULTS: **PO** Induction: 20-40 mg 3 times/wk on Monday-Wednesday-Friday or Tuesday-Thursday-Saturday schedule. Higher dose may be needed at end of week to prevent withdrawal symptoms over 72-hour break. Dose can be increased in 5-10 mg increments until steady state is reached, usually in 1-2 wk. Never give on daily basis; if needed, give small doses of methadone on "off" day. For patients dependent on methadone, initial dose of levomethadyl is 1.2-1.3 times daily methadone dose. Maintenance: 60-90 mg 3 times/wk (range: 10-140 mg/dose); higher doses may be needed. Planned interruptions in therapy: Take-home doses of levomethadyl are not permitted; give methadone instead. Unplanned interruptions in therapy: After single missed dose, restart on every-other-day schedule. Wait until after weekend 72-hour break to reestablish prior schedule. If more than 1 dose is missed, restart at 50% to 75% of previous dose. After lapse of more than 1 wk, restart using induction schedule.

Interactions

Alcohol or drugs of abuse: Fatal overdose can occur; symptoms may be delayed. *Other CNS depressants (eg, tranquilizers, sedatives):* Additive CNS depression.

Lab Test Interferences

None well documented.

Adverse Reactions

CV: Hypertension; orthostatic hypotension; prolonged QT interval; nonspecific ST-T wave changes; peripheral edema. *RESP:* Cough. *CNS:* Drowsiness; insomnia; asthenia; nightmares; depression; euphoria; headache; nervousness. *GI:* Nausea; vomiting; dry mouth; constipation; abdominal pain. *GU:* Urinary retention. *DERM:* Sweating; pruritus; urticaria. *OTHER:* Tolerance; psychological and physical dependence with chronic use.

Precautions

Pregnancy: Category C. Infants may develop neonatal abstinence syndrome. Recommend switching to methadone during pregnancy. *Lactation:* Undetermined. *Special risk patients:* Use with caution in patients with myxedema, acute alcoholism, acute abdominal conditions, ulcerative colitis, decreased respiratory reserve, head injury or increased intracranial pressure, hypoxia, supraventricular tachycardia, depleted blood volume or circulatory shock. *Drug dependence:* Has abuse potential. *Renal or hepatic impairment:* Duration of action may be prolonged; may need to reduce dosage or convert to methadone.

NURSING CONSIDERATIONS

Administration/Storage

- Drug may not be dispensed for outpatient use. May be used only by treatment programs approved by FDA, DEA and designated state authorities.
- Administer in oral form only. Always dilute before administration.

Assessment/Interventions

- Obtain patient history, including drug history and any known allergies. Note renal or hepatic impairment or cardiac disease.
- Assess for hypertension or orthostatic hypotension, arrhythmias, peripheral edema and cough.
- Carefully monitor patients with cardiac disease or those receiving medications that affect cardiac conduction.
- Observe for withdrawal symptoms. Dosage may need to be adjusted to prevent unpleasant symptoms.
- Monitor I&O during therapy. Increasing fiber, fluids and exercise may help prevent constipation.
- Provide good oral hygiene.

OVERDOSAGE: SIGNS & SYMPTOMS

Miosis, respiratory and CNS depression, circulatory collapse, seizures, cardiopulmonary arrest, death

Patient/Family Education

- Advise patient that full effectiveness of drug may not occur for several days.
- Warn patient that drug may cause dependence and that detoxification/withdrawal program will be necessary if drug is discontinued.
- Advise patient that drug may cause drowsiness or impair judgment and to use caution while driving or performing other tasks requiring mental alertness.
- Remind patient to notify physicians, dentists and other health care providers of drug regimen.
- Instruct patient to avoid intake of alcoholic beverages or other CNS depressants.
- Instruct patient not to take otc medications without consulting physician.
- Encourage patient to wear identification bracelet or necklace and carry ID card.
- Emphasize importance of comprehensive treatment to include medical evaluation, planning and counseling.

See Patient Guide, p. 356.

Levonorgestrel (Levonorgestrel Implants)

(LEE-voe-nor-JESS-truhl)

Norplant System

Class: Hormone/contraceptive implant

Action Synthetic, biologically active progestin that transforms proliferative endometrium into secretory endometrium and inhibits secretion of pituitary gonadotropins, preventing follicular maturation and ovulation.

Indications Prevention of pregnancy.

Contraindications Active thrombophlebitis or thromboembolic disorders; undiagnosed abnormal genital bleeding; known or suspected pregnancy; acute liver disease; benign or malignant liver tumors; known or suspected carcinoma of breast.

Route/Dosage

ADULTS: **Subdermal** 6 capsules inserted in midportion of upper arm during first 7 days of onset of menses. Remove after 5 yr.

Interactions

Carbamazepine: Reduced contraceptive efficacy. *Phenytoin:* Reduced contraceptive efficacy. *Rifampin:* Possible reduced contraceptive efficacy.

Lab Test Interferences

Endocrine tests may be affected. Sex hormone-binding globulin concentrations may be decreased; thyroxine concentrations may be slightly decreased and triiodothyronine uptake may be increased.

Adverse Reactions

CNS: Headache; nervousness; dizziness. *GI:* Nausea; change in appetite; weight gain; abdominal discomfort. *GU:* Prolonged, irregular, frequent or scanty bleeding; spotting; amenorrhea; cervicitis; leukorrhea; vaginitis. *DERM:* Dermatitis; acne; hirsutism; hypertrichosis; scalp hair loss; pain, itching or infection near implant site. *OTHER:* Adnexal enlargement; mastalgia; breast discharge; implant removal difficulty; musculoskeletal pain.

Precautions

Pregnancy: Category X. *Lactation:* Excreted in breast milk. *Bleeding irregularities:* Most women can expect variation in menstrual bleeding patterns. *Delayed follicular atresia:* Follicle may grow beyond usual size and may resemble ovarian cyst. *Ectopic pregnancies:* Have occurred, although relationship to drug is not established. *Ocular lesions:* Retinal thrombosis has occurred with oral contraceptives; consider possibility in levonorgestrel users. *Thromboembolic disorders:* Remove capsules if thrombophlebitis or thromboembolic disease occurs. Consider removal in patients immobilized for prolonged periods.

NURSING CONSIDERATIONS

Administration/Storage

- Capsules must be inserted only by physician trained in procedure.

Assessment/Interventions

- Obtain patient history, including drug history and any known allergies. Note pregnancy and lactation status, current or past thrombophlebitis, abnormal menstrual or vaginal bleeding, cervical cytology, any degree of immobility, liver disease, breast abnormalities or hyperlipedemia.
- Ensure that complete physical examination is performed before insertion and repeated annually during use. Obtain baseline weight.
- After insertion, monitor site for healing and absence of infection.

OVERDOSAGE: SIGNS & SYMPTOMS

Fluid retention, uterine bleeding irregularities

Patient/Family Education

- Explain that contraceptive method will be effective for 5 yr; capsules should be removed after that period, but can be removed at any time; and that removal should be done by a physician trained in procedure.
- Encourage low-fat, low-cholesterol diet.
- Teach patient to identify and report signs of wound infection after insertion.
- Instruct patient to notify physician if capsule falls out.
- Instruct patient to report these symptoms to physician: jaundice, fluid retention, depression, vision changes, abnormal bleeding and weight gain.
- Emphasize that missed menstrual period is not accurate indicator of pregnancy.
- Explain that menstrual irregularities are common, especially during first year of therapy.
- Emphasize importance of keeping follow-up visits to evaluate effectiveness of contraceptive therapy.

See Patient Guide, p. 357.

Levothyroxine Sodium (T_4; L-thyroxine)

(lee-voe-thigh-ROX-een SO-dee-uhm)

Levothroid, Levoxyl, Synthroid, ♣ *Eltroxin*

Class: Thyroid hormone

Action Increases metabolic rate of body tissues; is needed for normal growth and maturation.

Indications Replacement or supplemental therapy in hypothyroidism; TSH suppression (in thyroid cancer, nodules, goiters and enlargement in chronic thyroiditis); diagnostic agent in suppression tests to differentiate suspected hyperthyroidism from euthyroidism.

Contraindications Acute MI and thyrotoxicocis uncomplicated by hypothyroidism; coexistence of hypothyroidism and hypoadrenalism (Addison's disease) unless treatment of hypoadrenalism with adrenocortical steroids precedes initiation of thyroid therapy.

Route/Dosage Individualize dosage.

Hypothyroidism

ADULTS: Initial dose: **PO** 0.05 mg/day, increased by 0.025 mg q 2-3 wk if needed.

Long-Standing Hypothyroidism

ADULTS: **PO** ≤ 0.025 mg/day, particularly if cardiovascular impairment is suspected. Reduce dosage if angina occurs. Maintenance: **PO** usually < 0.2 mg/day. **IV/IM** Half of previously established oral dosage initially. CHILDREN > 12 YR: **PO** > 150 mcg/day or 2-3 mcg/kg/day. **IV/IM** routes can be used for maintenance in children if child is unable to take medication orally. The initial parenteral dose should be approximately one-half the previously established oral dose. CHILDREN 6-12 YR: **PO** 100-150 mcg/day or 4-5 mcg/kg/day. CHILDREN 1-5 YR: **PO** 75-100 mcg/day or 5-6 mcg/kg/day. CHILDREN 6-12 MO: **PO** 50-75 mcg/day or 6-8 mcg/kg/day. CHILDREN 0-6 MO: **PO** 25-50 mcg/day or 8-10 mcg/kg/day.

Myxedema Coma

ADULTS: **IV/Nasogastric** 0.4 mg initially, followed by 0.1-0.2 mg/day until patient can take drug orally.

TSH Suppression

Requires larger amounts of thyroid hormone than those used for replacement therapy.

Thyroid Suppression Therapy

ADULTS: **PO** 2.6 mcg/kg/day for 7-10 days.

Interactions

Anticoagulants, oral: May increase anticoagulant effects. *Cholestyramine, cholestipol:* May decrease thyroid hormone efficacy. *Digitalis glycosides:* May reduce effects of glycosides. *Fasting:* Increases absorption from GI tract. *Iron salts:* May decrease efficacy of levothyroxine, resulting in hypothyroidism. *Theophyllines:* Hypothyroidism; may cause decreased theophylline clearance; clearance may return to normal when euthyroid state is achieved.

Lab Test Interferences

Consider changes in thyroxine-binding globulin concentration when interpreting thyroxine (T_4) and triiodothyronine (T_3) values; medicinal or dietary iodine interferes with all in vivo tests of radioiodine uptake, producing low uptakes that may not reflect true decrease in hormone synthesis.

Adverse Reactions

CV: Palpitations; tachycardia; cardiac arrhythmias; angina pectoris; cardiac arrest. *CNS:* Tremors; headache; nervousness; insomnia. *GI:* Diarrhea; vomiting. *OTHER:* Hypersensitivity; weight loss; menstrual irregularities; sweating; heat tolerance; fever; decreased bone density (in women using long term).

Precautions

Pregnancy: Category A. *Lactation:* Minimal amounts excreted in breast milk. *Children:* When drug is administered for congenital hypothyroidism, routine determinations of serum T_4 or TSH are strongly advised in neonates. In infants, excessive doses of thyroid hormone preparations may produce craniosynostosis. Children may experience transient partial hair loss in first few months of thyroid therapy. *Cardiovascular disease:* Use caution when integrity of cardiovascular system, particularly coronary arteries, is suspect (eg, angina, elderly). Development of chest pain or worsening cardiovascular disease requires decrease in dosage. *Endocrine disorders:* Therapy in patients with concomitant diabetes mellitus, diabetes insipidus or adrenal insufficiency (Addison's disease) exacerbates intensity of their symptoms. Therapy of myxedema coma requires simultaneous administration of glucocorticoids. In patients whose hypothyroidism is secondary to hypopituitarism, adrenal insufficiency, if present, should be corrected with corticosteroids. *Hyperthyroid effects:* Levothyroxine may rarely precipitate hyperthyroid state or may aggravate existing hyperthyroidism. *Infertility:* Drug is unjustified for treatment of male or female infertility unless condition is accompanied by hypothyroidism. *Morphologic hypogonadism and nephrosis:* Rule out before therapy. *Myxedema coma:* Patients are particularly sensitive to thyroid preparations. Sudden administration of large doses is not without cardiovascular risks. Small initial doses are indicated. *Obesity:* Drug should not be used for weight reduction; may produce serious or life-threatening toxicity in large doses, particularly when given with anorexiants.

NURSING CONSIDERATIONS

Administration/Storage

- Administer oral form once each day before breakfast. When given on empty stomach, absorption is increased. To maintain steady blood levels, be consistent in giving drug either with or without food.
- Do not give sooner than 4 hr after administration of cholestyramine or colestipol. Cholestyramine or colestipol reduces effectiveness of levothyroxine.
- Do not switch from one brand to another without comparison studies of bioavailability.
- For infants and children who cannot swallow intact tablets, crush proper dose tablet and suspend freshly crushed tablet in small amount of formula or water; give by spoon or dropper. Do not store suspension for any period of time. Crushed tablet may also be sprinkled over small amount of food (eg, cooked cereal, applesauce).
- Parenteral therapy may be used when oral form of medication cannot be tolerated.
- IV therapy is preferred in emergency treatment of myxedema coma. Can be administered via nasogastric tube. Give no faster than 100 mcg/min. Too rapid administration causes adverse cardiovascular reactions. Monitor closely during administration.
- Reconstitute injectable solution by adding 5 ml of 0.9% Sodium Chloride or Bacteriostatic Sodium Chloride (benzyl alcohol). Shake vial to ensure complete dissolution.
- Administer via Y-tubing or 3-way stopcock. Do not add to IV infusion.
- Use IV solution immediately after reconstitution. Discard any unused portion.
- Store in tightly closed, light-resistant container at room temperature.

Assessment/Interventions

- Obtain patient history, including drug history and any known allergies.

- Prior to initial administration, obtain baseline data of TSH and T_4 levels.
- Successful therapy achieves euthyroid state. Expect responses to initial therapy to be diuresis, weight loss, increased sense of well-being, increased appetite and activity, increased energy and return to normal texture of hair and skin.
- Monitor for signs and symptoms of thyroid deficit or excess.
- Do not give if pulse > 100 bpm.
- In infants, monitor for normal growth, development and intellectual functioning; monthly measurement of height is a good index.
- Compare laboratory tests of TSH and T_4 with baseline data; serum levels should return to normal. In some children TSH levels may remain abnormal.
- When given with oral anticoagulants, expect oral anticoagulant dosage to be reduced. Monitor for bleeding more closely.
- Give drug cautiously with catecholamines (eg, epinephrine, dopamine). When drug is given with catecholamines, monitor for cardiac arrhythmias.
- If patient is taking insulin, oral hypoglycemics or digitalis, monitor effectiveness of these agents. Dosages of these agents may need to be altered. Monitor serum glucose levels, ECG and pulse.
- Monitor thyroid function test results closely in patients over the age of 65 years; less levothyroxine is usually needed by elderly.

OVERDOSAGE: SIGNS & SYMPTOMS

Symptoms of hyperthyroidism: headache, irritability, nervousness, sweating, tachycardia, increased bowel motility, menstrual irregularities, palpitations, vomiting, psychosis, seizure, fever, angina pectoris, CHF, shock, arrhythmias, thyroid storm

Patient/Family Education

- Explain to patient that medication will probably need to be taken for life. Instruct patient not to discontinue taking medication or change dosage without consulting physician.
- Instruct patient to take levothyroxine at same time each day, preferably in morning before breakfast.
- Instruct patient not to switch from one brand of medication to another unless advised to do so by physician.
- Teach patient how to monitor for signs and symptoms of thyroid deficit or excess. Instruct patient to notify physician of following persistent signs and symptoms: headache, nervousness, diarrhea, excessive sweating, heat intolerance, chest pain, increased pulse rate and palpitations.
- Teach patient to keep a record of signs and symptoms for physician review.
- Advise patient of importance of keeping appointments with physician for regular checkups.
- Caution patient not to take otc or other prescribed medications without consulting physician.
- Advise patient to wear Medi-Alert bracelet or necklace and to carry Medi-Alert card in wallet.
- Caution patient not to take levothyroxine for weight control.
- Explain that partial hair loss may be experienced by child in first few months of therapy but that this side effect is transient.

See Patient Guide, p. 358.

Lidocaine HCl

(LIE-doe-cane HIGH-droe-KLOR-ide)

Anestacon, DermaFlex, Dilocaine, Duo-Trach Kit, L-Caine, Lidoject-1, Lidoject-2, LidoPen Auto-Injector, Nervocaine, Nulicaine, Octocaine, Solarcaine, Xylociane, Zilactin-L, ✤ *Xylocard*

Class: Antiarrhythmic/local anesthetic

Action Attenuates phase 4 diastolic depolarization, decreases automaticity, decreases action potential duration and raises ventricular fibrillation threshold; inhibits conduction of nerve impulses from sensory nerves.

Indications Acute management of ventricular arrhythmias; topical anesthesia in local skin disorders; local anesthesia of accessible mucous membranes. **Unlabeled use:** Intraosseous or endotracheal administration to pediatric patients with cardiac arrest.

Contraindications Hypersensitivity to amide local anesthetics; Stokes-Adams syndrome; Wolff-Parkinson-White syndrome; severe degrees of sinoatrial, atrioventricular (AV) or intraventricular block in absence of pacemaker; ophthalmic use.

Route/Dosage

ADULTS: **IM** 300 mg. May be repeated after 60-90 min. **IV Bolus** 50-100 mg at rate of 25-50 mg/min; may repeat, but do not exceed 200-300 mg/hr. Continuous infusion: 1-4 mg/min. CHILDREN: **IV bolus/intratracheal** 1 mg/kg/dose q 5-10 min (maximum dose: 5 mg/kg). Maintenance: 20-50 mcg/kg/min. **Topical:** Apply as needed to affected area; use lowest dose possible when applying to mucous membranes.

Interactions

Beta-adrenergic blockers: Increased lidocaine levels. *Cimetidine:* Decreased lidocaine clearance. *Class I antiarrhythmic agents (eg, tocainide, mexiletine):* Toxic effects are additive and potentially synergistic. *Procainamide:* Additive neurological and cardiac effects. *Succinylcholine:* Prolongation of neuromuscular blockade.

INCOMPATIBILITIES: Amphotericin B, parenteral cephalosporins, doxycycline, epinephrine, isoproterenol, methohexital, nitroprusside, norepinephrine, phenytoin, sodium bicarbonate, sulfadiazine.

Lab Test Interferences

IM administration may increase CPK levels.

Adverse Reactions

CV: Hypotension; bradycardia; cardiovascular collapse; cardiac arrest. *RESP:* Respiratory depression or arrest. *CNS:* Dizziness; lightheadedness; nervousness; drowsiness; apprehension; confusion; mood changes; hallucinations; tremors. *EENT:* Visual disturbances; diplopia; tinnitus. *GI:* Nausea; vomiting. *OTHER:* Hypersensitivity reactions. Local reactions, including soreness at IM injection site; venous thrombosis or phlebitis; extravasation; burning, stinging, sloughing, tenderness (with topical application). Difficulty in speaking, breathing and swallowing; numbness of lips or tongue and other paresthesias, including heat and cold.

Precautions

Pregnancy: Category B. *Lactation:* Excreted in breast milk. *Children:* Safety and efficacy not established. If used, reduce dose. IM autoinjector device not recommended in children < 50 kg. *Cardiac effects:* Use with caution and in lower doses in patients with CHF, reduced cardiac output, digitalis toxicity and in elderly. *Hypersensitivity reactions:* May occur. *IV use:* May result in excessive depression of cardiac conductivity. *Malignant hyperthermia:* Has been reported with administration of amide local anesthetics. *Methemoglobinemia:* Do not use in patients with congenital oridiopathic methomoglobinemia or in infants <12 months old who are receiving methemoglobin-inducing drugs.

Oral use: May impair swallowing and enhance danger of aspiration; avoid food for 1 hr if used in mouth or throat. *Renal or hepatic impairment:* Use caution with repeated doses or prolonged use in patients with renal or hepatic impairment. *Topical use:* Systemic effects can occur following topical use; use lowest possible dose to avoid serious toxicity, shock or heart block.

NURSING CONSIDERATIONS

Administration/Storage

- Use IM route for emergency situations (eg, no IV access, no ECG monitoring) only. Use 10% solution, only, for injection. Deltoid muscle is preferred IM site. Switch to IV route as soon as possible.
- When giving by IV route, use only 1-2% solutions of drug. Use only lidocaine specifically labeled for IV use (without preservatives or epinephrine). Do not administer with other agents.
- To initiate IV therapy, start IV of 5% Dextrose in Water at "keep vein open (KVO)" rate. Bolus loading dose of 50-100 mg may be given undiluted at rate of 25-50 mg/min. IV push is indicated for resuscitation situations.
- For continuous infusion, use prediluted solution or add 1 g of lidocaine to 500 ml of 5% Dextrose in Water to prepare 0.2% solution. Rate of administration should not exceed 1-4 mg/min. Adjust rate according to cardiac response.
- Use diluted solutions within 24 hr.
- When giving by topical route, apply thinly and to smallest area possible. Do not apply to abraded or otherwise injured areas of skin.
- Store all forms of drug at room temperature.
- For IV infusion, use microdropper and infusion pump or controller.

Assessment/Interventions

- Obtain patient history, including drug history and any known allergies. Note renal, cardiac or hepatic impairment and hypersensitivity to amide-type local anesthetics.
- Obtain baseline BP and ECG before administration.
- Monitor BP, ECG and respirations during IV administration. Continuous ECG monitoring is essential for proper administration. Have resuscitative equipment and medication immediately available.
- Monitor serum levels of drug if given via IV for more than 24 hr. Therapeutic serum levels range from 1.5-6 mcg/ml; toxic levels are > 6-10 mcg/ml.
- If serious adverse reactions occur, notify physician, but continue 5% dextrose IV. Continue to monitor patient closely.
- Keep bolus dose of 100 mcg of lidocaine available at all times.
- For topical use, apply thinly and to smallest area possible. Do not apply to abraded or otherwise injured areas of skin.
- Assess for systemic toxicity, which can result if excessive amounts of topical drug are absorbed. Risk of toxicity is greatest when large surface area, mucous membranes, and/or abraded or otherwise injured skin is involved.
- If topical preparation is used during labor and delivery, monitor vital signs and level of consciousness of newborn and mother.
- Monitor activity and position of patient post-anesthesia, until senses of pain, pressure, and temperature return.
- Monitor I&O and voiding.
- When topical drug is applied to pharynx, maintain npo status until gag reflex returns. If tongue and oral mucosa are numb, do not permit patient to eat food or chew gum until sensation returns.

OVERDOSAGE: SIGNS & SYMPTOMS

Confusion, drowsiness, unconsciousness, tremors, convulsions, hypotension, bradycardia, cardiovascular collapse, cardiac arrest, tinnitus, diplopia

Patient/Family Education

- Explain that adverse reactions related to central nervous system (drowsiness, confusion, paresthesias, convulsions, respiratory arrest) can occur and are related to CNS toxicity.
- Emphasize importance of not allowing topical solution to come in contact with eyes or broken skin.
- Advise patient not to chew gum or eat food until 60 min after oral anesthetic has been administered.
- Advise patient that drug may cause dizziness or drowsiness and to avoid getting out of bed or walking without assistance.

See Patient Guide, pp. 359-360.

Liothyronine Sodium (T3; triiodothyronine)

(lie-oh-THIGH-row-neen SO-dee-uhm)

Cytomel, Triostat

Class: Thyroid hormone

Action Increases metabolic rate of body tissues; is needed for normal growth and maturation.

Indications Replacement or supplemental therapy in hypothyroidism; TSH suppression for treatment or prevention of euthyroid goiters (eg, thyroid nodules, multinodular goiters and enlargement in chronic thyroiditis); diagnostic agent in suppression tests to differentiate suspected hyperthyroidism from euthyroidism.

Contraindications Acute MI and thyrotoxicosis uncomplicated by hypothyroidism; coexistence of hypothyroidism and hypoadrenalism (Addison's disease), unless treatment of hypoadrenalism with adrenocortical steroids precedes initiation of thyroid therapy.

Route/Dosage

Individualize dosage

Hypothyroidism

ADULTS: **PO** 25 mcg/day initially, increase by 12.5-25 mcg q 1-2 wk, if needed. CHILDREN: **PO** 5 mcg/day initially, increase by 5 mcg q 1-2 wk, if needed.

Congenital hypothyroidism

CHILDREN: **PO** 5 mcg/day initially: **PO** 5 mcg/day, increase by 5 mcg q 3-4 d until desired response achieved.

Simple (nontoxic) goiter

ADULTS: **PO** 5 mcg/day initially, increase by 5-10 mcg q 1-2 wk. When 25 mcg/day is reached, increase by 12.5-25 mcg q 1-2 wk, if needed. CHILDREN: **PO** 5 mcg/day initially, increase by 5 mcg q 1-2 wk, if needed.

Myxedema

ADULTS: **PO** 5 mcg/day initially, increase by 5-10 mcg q 1-2 wk. When 25 mcg/day is reached, increase by 12.5-25 mcg q 1-2 wk, if needed. CHILDREN: **PO** 5 mcg/day initially, increase by 5 mcg q 1-2 wk, if needed.

Myxedema coma/precoma

ADULTS: **IV** 25-50 mcg initially; additional doses administered q 4-12 hr, as needed.

TSH suppression test

ADULTS: **PO** 75-100 mcg/day for 7 days.

Interactions

Anticoagulants, oral: May increase anticoagulant effects. *Beta-blockers:* May reduce effects of beta-blockers. *Cholestyramine, colestipol:* May decrease thyroid hormone efficacy. *Digitalis glycosides:* May reduce effects of glycosides. *Theophyllines:* Hypothyroidism; may cause decreased theophylline clearance;

clearance may return to normal when euthyroid state is achieved.

Lab Test Interferences

Consider changes in thyroxine-binding globulin concentration when interpreting thyroxine (T4) and triiodothyronine (T3) values; medicinal or dietary iodine interferes with all *in vivo* tests of radioiodine uptake, producing low uptakes that may not reflect true decrease in hormone synthesis.

Adverse Reactions

CV: Palpitations; tachycardia; cardiac arrhythmias; angina pectoris; cardiac arrest. *CNS:* Tremors; headache; nervousness; insomnia. *GI:* Diarrhea; vomiting. *OTHER:* Hypersensitivity; weight loss; menstrual irregularities; sweating; heat intolerance; fever; decreased bone density (in women using long term).

Precautions

Pregnancy: Category A. *Lactation:* Minimal amounts excreted in breast milk. *Children:* When drug is administered for congenital hypothyroidism, routine determinations of serum T4 or TSH are strongly advised in neonates. In infants, excessive doses of thyroid hormone preparations may produce craniosynostosis. Children may experience transient partial hair loss in first few months of thyroid therapy. *Elderly:* Therapy should be started with 5 mcg q day and increased by 5 mcg increments at recommended intervals. *Cardiovascular disease:* Use caution when integrity of cardiovascular system, particularly coronary arteries, is suspect (eg, angina, elderly). Development of chest pain or worsening cardiovascular disease requires decrease in dosage. *Endocrine disorders:* Therapy in patients with concomitant diabetes mellitus, diabetes insipidus or adrenal insufficiency (Addison's disease) exacerbates intensity of their symptoms. Therapy of myxedema coma requires simultaneous administration of glucocorticoids. Corticosteroids should be used to correct adrenal insufficiency in patients whose hypothyroidism is secondary to hypopituitarism. *Hyperthyroid effects:* Liothyronine may rarely precipitate hyperthyroid state or may aggravate existing hyperthyroidism. *Infertility:* Drug is unjustified for treatment of male or female infertility unless condition is accompanied by hypothyroidism. *Morphologic hypogonadism and nephrosis:* Rule out before therapy. *Myxedema coma:* Patients are particularly sensitive to thyroid preparations. Sudden administration of large doses is not without cardiovascular risks. Small initial doses are indicated. *Obesity:* Drug should not be used for weight reduction; may produce serious or life-threatening toxicity in large doses, particularly when given with anorexiants.

NURSING CONSIDERATIONS

Administration/Storage

- Administer once a day in the early morning to prevent sleep disturbances.
- Administer liothyronine injection IV only, do not give IM or SC.
- Administer with caution to patients with known cardiovascular disease.
- Administer cautiously to patients with possible thyroid gland autonomy as there is danger of an additive effect between the exogenous and endogenous sources.
- Administer only by injection to patients in Myxedema coma and with precoma diagnoses.
- Ensure oral therapy is resumed as soon as patient is stabilized.
- Discontinue IV injection therapy gradually when switching to tablets. Expect a low dosage that will be increased gradually according to response.
- Administer cautiously to elderly patients and patients with known or suspected cardiovascular disease. Note contraindications in some serious cardiovascular conditions and thyrotoxicosis.

- Do not administer large doses of liothyronine with sympathomimetic amines as serious and even life threatening results can occur.
- Administer cholestyramine and thyroid hormones 4 to 5 hours apart.
- Store tablets in tightly closed container at room temperature; store injectable under refrigeration.

Assessment/Interventions

- Obtain patient history.
- Prior to initial administration, obtain baseline data of TSH and T4 levels.
- Monitor for signs and symptoms of thyroid deficit or excess.
- Periodically assess thyroid status by using the TSH suppression test.
- Monitor patients on anticoagulants for signs of bleeding.
- Monitor patients on insulin or oral hypoglycemics closely during initiation of thyroid replacement therapy. Increase in insulin or oral hypoglycemic dosage may be required.
- If patient is switching therapies, be aware that liothyronine has a rapid onset of action, but residual effects of other thyroid preparations may persist for the first several weeks of therapy.
- Inform laboratory if patient is pregnant or taking androgens, corticosteroids, estrogens, oral contraceptives, iodine-containing preparations, preparations containing salicylates, or medicinal or dietary iodine as these drugs are known to interfere with tests of patients on liothyronine therapy. Interacting medications may need to be held or discontinued prior to the test.
- Assess for side effects that can occur more rapidly with liothyronine because of its rapid onset.
- Monitor patient on digoxin for signs and symptoms of potential digitalis toxicity as thyroid hormone increases metabolic rate which requires an increased digitalis dosage.

OVERDOSAGE: SIGNS & SYMPTOMS

Symptoms of hyperthyroidism: Headache, irritability, nervousness, sweating, tachycardia, increased bowel motility, menstrual irregularities, palpitations, vomiting, psychosis, seizure, fever, angina pectoris, CHF, shock, arrhythmias, thyroid storm

Patient/Family Education

- Instruct patient to take liothyronine as directed. Do not change or discontinue dosage without consulting healthcare provider. Explain that liothyronine does not cure hypothyroidism and that therapy will continue for the rest of his or her life.
- Instruct patient with diabetes mellitus to closely monitor urinary glucose levels. The daily dosage of antidiabetic medication may need readjustment as thyroid hormone replacement is achieved or if thyroid medication is stopped.
- Explain that partial hair loss may be experienced by children in first few months of therapy, but that this side effect is transient.
- Advise patient to wear Medi-Alert bracelet or necklace and to carry Medi-Alert card in wallet.
- Inform patient that liothyronine's effects are more rapid than levothyroxine, which requires several days before onset of action.
- Teach patient to take their pulse and inform the healthcare provider if signs of tachycardia or dysrhythmias occur.
- Instruct patient to call the healthcare provider immediately if any adverse symptoms such as chest pain, palpitations, headaches, irritability, increased nervousness, diaphoresis, tachycardia, dysrhythmias or heat intolerance occur.
- Inform patient of possible adverse reactions with other drugs or foods they may be taking. Caution them to inform their healthcare provider of any

drugs, including over-the-counter drugs, they may be taking or plan to take.

- Emphasize the importance of follow-up examinations and periodic laboratory tests.

See Patient Guide, p. 361.

Lisinopril

(lie-SIN-oh-prill)

Prinivil, Zestril

Class: Antihypertensive/ACE inhibitor

Action Competitively inhibits angiotensin I–converting enzyme, prevention of angiotensin I conversion to angiotensin II, a potent vasoconstrictor that also stimulates aldosterone secretion. Results in decrease in sodium and fluid retention, decrease in BP and increase in diuresis.

Indications Treatment of hypertension; treatment of heart failure not responding to diuretics and digitalis.

Contraindications Hypersensitivity to ACE inhibitors.

Route/Dosage

Hypertension

ADULTS: **PO** Initial dose: 10 mg qd. Maintenance: 20-40 mg/day; may add diuretic if needed and decrease dose.

CHF

ADULTS: **PO** Initial dose: 5 mg qd with diuretics and digitalis; reduce concomitant diuretic dose, if possible, to minimize hypovolemia. In patients with hyponatremia, initiate with 2.5 mg qd. Usual dose: 5-20 mg/day.

Interactions

Allopurinol: Greater risk of hypersensitivity possible with coadministration. *Antacids:* Lisinopril bioavailability may be decreased. Separate administration times by 1 to 2 hrs. *Capsaicin:* Cough may be exacerbated. *Digoxin:* May increase plasma digoxin levels. *Indomethacin:* Reduced hypotensive effects, especially in low-renin or volume-dependent hypertensive patients. *Lithium:* Increased lithium levels and symptoms of lithium toxicity. *Potassium-sparing diuretics, potassium preparations:* May increase serum potassium levels. *Phenothiazines:* May increase pharmacological effect of phenothiazines.

Lab Test Interferences

False elevation of liver enzymes, serum bilirubin, uric acid or blood glucose may occur.

Adverse Reactions

CV: Chest pain; hypotension; orthostatic hypotension. *RESP:* Cough (especially in females); upper respiratory symptoms; dyspnea. *CNS:* Headache; dizziness; fatigue. *GI:* Nausea; vomiting; diarrhea. *HEMA:* Small decreases in hemoglobin and hematocrit; neutropenia; bone marrow depression; eosinophilia. *DERM:* Rash; pruritus. *META:* Hyperkalemia; hyponatremia. *OTHER:* Asthenia; angioedema.

Precautions

Pregnancy: Category D (second and third trimester); Category C (first trimester). Can cause injury or death to fetus if used during second or third trimester. *Lactation:* Undetermined. Avoid use in nursing women if possible. *Children:* Safety and efficacy not established. *Elderly:* Reduced dosage may be necessary. *Angioedema:* Use with extreme caution in patients with hereditary angioedema. *Hypotension/first-dose effect:* Significant decreases in BP may occur after first dose, especially in severely salt- or volume-depleted patients or those with heart failure. Minimize risk by discontinuing diuretics, decreasing dose or increasing salt intake approximately 1 wk prior to initiating drug. *Neutropenia and agranulocytosis:* May occur; risk appears greater in patients with renal dysfunction, heart failure or immunosuppression. *Renal impairment:* Reduce dose and give less frequently. In renal insufficiency, stable elevations in BUN and serum creatinine may occur due to inadequate renal perfusion; monitor renal function during first few weeks of therapy and adjust dosage carefully, especially if glomerular filtration rate < 30 ml/min.

NURSING CONSIDERATIONS

Administration/Storage

- May be administered with or without food.
- Store at room temperature in tightly closed, light-resistant container.

Assessment/Interventions

- Obtain patient history, including drug history and any known allergies. Note history of angioedema, hypersensitivity to ACE inhibitors, renal disease, CHF and use of diuretics/dialysis.
- Ensure that baseline blood, renal and thyroid function studies have been obtained before administration and monitor during treatment.
- Obtain baseline BP and pulse and monitor closely for at least 2 hr after initial dose and during first 2 wk of therapy. If systolic BP is < 90 mm Hg, withhold medication and notify physician.
- If patient develops sudden severe dyspnea, swelling of lips or eyes or edema of hands and feet, withhold medication and notify physician.
- Monitor for hyperkalemia in patients with impaired renal function or diabetes mellitus and in patients receiving potassium supplements or potassium-sparing diuretics.
- Assist patient with position changes and ambulation during initial phase of therapy. Orthostatic hypotension is common.
- Keep side rails raised if hypotension or dizziness occur.

OVERDOSAGE: SIGNS & SYMPTOMS

Hypotension

Patient/Family Education

- Instruct patient not to discontinue medication suddenly. Tell patient that missed doses should be taken as soon as possible unless close to time of next dose. Do not double up doses.
- Explain that chronic cough may occur. Instruct patient to avoid cough, cold or allergy medications and to notify physician.
- Instruct patient not to use potassium-containing salt substitute without consulting physician.
- Tell patient to avoid sudden position changes to prevent orthostatic hypotension.
- Instruct patient to report these symptoms to physician: dyspnea, loss of taste; swelling of eyes, face, lip, tongue or throat; difficulty breathing, speaking or swallowing.
- Advise patient to use caution while driving or performing other tasks requiring mental alertness until response to medication is known.
- Instruct patient to avoid intake of alcoholic beverages and not to take otc medications without consulting physician.
- Emphasize importance of follow-up visits and frequent assessment of BP while taking drug.
- Advise patient and family that life-style changes (exercise, salt restriction, weight loss) will enhance effectiveness of medication and may facilitate lower medication doses.

See Patient Guide, p. 362.

Lithium

(LITH-ee-uhm)

Cibalith-S, Eskalith, Eskalith CR, Lithane, Lithobid, Lithonate, Lithotabs, ♣ *Carbolith, Duralith*

Class: Antipsychotic/antimanic

Action Specific mechanism unknown; alters sodium transport in nerve and muscle cells and effects shift toward intraneuronal metabolism of catecholamines.

Indications Management of bipolar disorder and manic episodes of manic-depressive illness. **Unlabeled uses:** Treatment of neutropenia; unipolar depression; schizoaffective disorder; prophylaxis of cluster headaches; premenstrual tension; tardive dyskinesia; hyperthyroidism; syndrome of inappropriate secretion of antidiuretic hormone, postpartum affective psychosis; corticosteroid-induced psychosis.

Contraindications History of leukemia.

Route/Dosage

ADULTS: **PO** 900-1800 mg/day in 2-4 divided doses. Give regular capsules tid or qid; slow-release tablets bid or tid. Maximum dose: 2400 mg/day. CHILDREN ≥ 12 YR: 15-20 mg/kg/day in 2-3 divided doses.

Interactions

Acetazolamide, osmotic diuretics, theophyllines, urinary alkalinizers: Increased renal excretion of lithium. *ACE inhibitors, fluoxetine, loop diuretics, NSAIDs, thiazide diuretics:* Increased lithium serum levels. *Carbamazepine, haloperidol, methyldopa:* Increased neurotoxic effects despite therapeutic serum levels and normal dosage range. *Iodide salts:* Increased risk of hypothyroidism. *Neuromuscular blocking agents, tricyclic antidepressants:* Increased pharmacological effects of additive drug. *Phenothiazines:* Neurotoxicity; decreased phenothiazine concentrations or increased lithium concentrations may occur. *Verapamil:* Reductions in lithium levels and lithium toxicity have occurred.

Lab Test Interferences

None well documented.

Adverse Reactions

CV: Arrhythmias; hypotension; bradycardia; peripheral circulatory collapse. *CNS:* Tremor; muscle hyperirritability; headache; fatigue; ataxia; dizziness; pychomotor retardation; confusion; dystonia; hallucinations; blackouts; seizures; pseudotumor cerebri; drowsiness; poor memory and intellectual function; muscular weakness; slurred speech. *EENT:* Blurred vision; tinnitus. *GI:* Anorexia; nausea; vomiting; diarrhea; sialorrhea; dry mouth; parotitis. *GU:* Urinary urgency; stress incontinence; polyuria; albuminuria; sexual dysfunction; symptoms of nephrogenic diabetes; decreased creatinine clearance. *HEMA:* Leukocytosis; leukemia. *DERM:* Drying or thinning hair; dry skin; pruritis; exacerbation of psoriasis; acne. *META:* Hypothyroidism; hypercalcemia; hyperparathyroidism; hyponatremia; dehydration; weight gain. *OTHER:* Tast distortion; thirst; fever; swollen joints.

Precautions

Pregnancy: Category D. *Lactation:* Excreted in breast milk. *Children:* Safety and efficacy not established in children < 12 yr. *Encephalopathic syndrome:* Has occurred in patients also taking neuroleptic, and may cause irreversible brain damage. Characterized by weakness, lethargy, fever, tremors, confusion, extrapyramidal symptoms, leukocytosis, and elevated serum enzymes, BUN and fasting blood sugar. *Hypothyroidism:* Has occurred with chronic use. Thyroid hormone replacement therapy may be required. *Infections:* Reduction in dose or discontinuation may be required if patient has infection with fever, especially if accompanied by protracted sweating, vomiting or diarrhea. *Renal function:* Chronic use may lead to nephrogenic diabetes insipidus. Patients, including elderly, who have reduced renal function, should take lower doses. *Sodium/volume depletion:* Because drug decreases renal sodium absorption, patients must maintain adequate salt and fluid intake. *Tartrazine sensitivity:* Some products contain tartrazine, which may cause allergic-type reactions in susceptible individuals. *Toxicity:* Toxicity can occur even at therapeutic doses. Toxicity risk is greater in patients with renal or cardiovascular disease, debilitation, dehydration or sodium depletion.

NURSING CONSIDERATIONS

Administration/Storage

- Administer with meals to minimize GI upset.
- Do not crush, chew or break extended release capsules or coated tablets.
- Observe carefully during administration to make such patient swallows medication.
- Store at room temperature. Protect capsules from moisture.

Assessment/Interventions

- Obtain patient history, including drug history and any known allergies.
- Ensure that baseline renal and thyroid function studies and ECG have been obtained before beginning therapy.
- Assess mood and behavior before beginning medication and frequently, thereafter. Note particularly: flight of ideas, elation, grandiosity, aggressiveness and hyperactivity.
- Assess for lithium toxicity: persistent nausea/vomiting, diarrhea, ataxia, blurred vision, tinnitus.
- Periodically assess thyroid and renal function.
- Ensure that weekly lithium blood levels are obtained until therapeutic level has been reached; monthly levels should be obtained thereafter.
- Monitor lithium level frequently while titrating, then periodically once dose is stable. Therapeutic doses are 1-1.5 mEq/L during acute manic attacks and 0.6-1.2 mEq/L for maintenance. Lithium serum testing should be performed as close as possible to 12 hr after last dose. Withhold dose and consult physician if blood level is > 1.5 mEq/L.
- Record I&O and weight daily. Report sudden changes to physician.
- Provide diet matching patient's normal sodium intake. Do not dramatically alter sodium intake from patient's usual amount.
- Encourage intake of 2500-3000 ml of fluids daily.
- If signs of neurological toxicity occur, withhold drug and notify physician.

OVERDOSAGE: SIGNS & SYMPTOMS

ECG changes, slurred speech, seizures, acute renal failure, coma, diarrhea, vomiting, drowsiness, muscle weakness, ataxia

Patient/Family Education

- Explain that therapeutic improvement will be noted in 1-3 wk.
- Instruct patient to take medication regularly even if feeling well. Symptoms may return if medication is discontinued.
- Advise patient not to decrease or increase dietary sodium intake.
- Tell patient to drink 8-10 glasses of water or other caffeine-free liquids daily.
- Caution patient to avoid excessive caffeine intake, as caffeine may increase urinary excretion of drug.
- Advise patient that thirst, frequent polyuria, taste distortion and fine hand tremors are common side effects.
- Instruct patient to report these symptoms to physician immediately: nausea, vomiting, diarrhea, muscular weakness, ataxia, blurred vision or tinnitus.
- Advise patient that drug may cause drowsiness and to use caution while

driving or performing other tasks requiring mental alertness.

- Emphasize need for serum lithium level monitoring every 1 or 2 mo or as advised by physician.
- Encourage patient to wear a Medi-Alert tag at all times stating medication name and dosage.

See Patient Guide, p. 363.

Lomefloxacin HCl

(low-MUH-FLOX-uh-sin HIGH-droe-KLOR-ide)

Maxaquin

Class: Antibiotic/fluoroquinolone

Action Interferes with microbial DNA synthesis.

Indications Treatment of infections of the lower respiratory tract and urinary tract caused by susceptible organisms; prevention of urinary tract infections in patients undergoing transurethral procedures.

Contraindications Hypersensitivity to fluoroquinolones or quinolone antibiotics.

Route/Dosage

ADULTS: **PO** 400 mg qd for 10-14 days.

Surgical Prophylaxis

PO 400 mg 2-6 hr preoperatively.

Interactions

Antacids, iron salts, zinc salts, sucralfate, didanosine: Decreased oral absorption of lomefloxacin. Stagger administration times. *Antineoplastic agents:* Decreased lomefloxacin serum levels. *Probenecid:* Decreased renal elimination of lomefloxacin.

Lab Test Interferences

None well documented.

Adverse Reactions

CNS: Headache; dizziness. *GI:* Diarrhea; nausea. *DERM:* Photosensitivity.

Precautions

Pregnancy: Category C. *Lactation:* Excreted in breast milk. *Children:* Do not use in children < 18 yr. *Elderly:* Clearance may be decreased. *Chronic bronchitis:* Lomefloxacin is not indicated for empiric treatment of acute bacterial exacerbation of chronic bronchitis when *Streptococcus pneumoniae* is probable pathogen. *Convulsions:* CNS stimulation can occur; use with caution in patients with known or suspected CNS disorders. *Hypersensitivity reactions:* Serious and potentially fatal reactions have occurred. Discontinue if allergic reaction occurs. *Pseudomembranous colitis:* Should be considered in patients who develop diarrhea. *Renal impairment:* Reduced clearance may occur; adjust dose accordingly. *Superinfection:* Use may result in bacterial or fungal overgrowth.

NURSING CONSIDERATIONS

Administration/Storage

- May be administered with or without food; however, absorption is more rapid on empty stomach.
- Do not give antacids, sucralfate, iron or zinc-containing products within 2 hr before or after medication.
- Store at room temperature in tightly closed light-resistant container.

Assessment/Interventions

- Obtain patient history, including drug history and any known allergies, especially to fluoroquinolones or quinolone antibiotics. Note renal impairment.
- Assess patient for signs of infection before beginning treatment.
- Obtain specimens for culture and sensitivity before beginning treatment.
- Take baseline vital signs and reassess at least bid.
- Monitor I&O.

- Assess for symptoms of superinfection, such as vaginitis or stomatitis.

> **OVERDOSAGE: SIGNS & SYMPTOMS**
>
> Renal failure (severely decreased urine output, weight gain, confusion, dry flaky skin), tremor, seizures

Patient/Family Education

- Instruct patient to continue taking medication until completed, even if signs and symptoms of infection abate.
- Warn patient not to take antacids or vitamins less than 4 hr before or 2 hr after taking medication.
- Encourage patient to drink plenty of fluids, especially citrus fruit juices and cranberry juice.
- Advise patient that drug may cause dizziness and to use caution while driving or performing other tasks requiring mental alertness.
- Caution patient to avoid prolonged exposure to sunlight even when using sunscreens or sunblocks and to wear protective clothing to avoid photosensitivity reaction.

See Patient Guide, p. 364.

Lomustine

(LOW-muss-teen)

CCNU

Class: Antineoplastic/alkylator

Action Acts as alkylating agent but may also inhibit cellular enzymes.

Indications As single agent or in combination chemotherapy for treatment of primary and metastatic brain tumors (post surgical or radiotherapy) and in combination as secondary therapy for relapsing or non-responsive Hodgkin's disease.

Contraindications Standard considerations.

Route/Dosage

ADULTS & CHILDREN: **PO** Initial dose: 130 mg/m^2 as single dose q 6 wk. In compromised bone marrow function, reduce dose to 100 mg/m^2 q 6 wk. Do not repeat dose until blood counts return to acceptable levels (platelets > 100,000/mm^3; leukocytes > 4000/mm^3). Subsequent doses: Adjust to lower dose if nadir of leukocytes was < 3000/mm^3 or platelets were < 75,000/mm^3.

Interactions None well documented.

Lab Test Interferences

None well documented.

Adverse Reactions

RESP: Pulmonary toxicity with infiltrates or fibrosis. *CNS:* Disorientation; lethargy; ataxia; dysarthria. *GI:* Nausea; vomiting; stomatitis. *GU:* Decreased kidney size; progressive azotemia; renal failure. *HEMA:* Delayed myelosuppression (usually occurs 4-6 wk post administration and is dose related); thrombocytopenia and leukopenia (may persist for 1-2 wk); anemia. *HEPA:* Reversible liver toxicity with increased transaminase, alkaline phosphatase and bilirubin levels. *OTHER:* Secondary malignancies (ie, acute leukemia, bone marrow dysplasia); alopecia and stomatitis (infrequent).

Precautions

Pregnancy: Category D. *Lactation:* Undetermined. *Bone marrow suppression:* Most common and severe toxic effect of lomustine. Because bone marrow suppression may be delayed, blood counts should be monitored weekly for at least 6 wk after each dose. *Concomitant therapy:* Adjust dose if given with other myelosuppressive drugs.

NURSING CONSIDERATIONS

Administration/Storage

- Administer on empty stomach to minimize GI upset.
- Store at room temperature in tightly closed light-resistant container.

Assessment/Interventions

- Obtain patient history, including drug history and any known allergies.
- Ensure that baseline CBC, blood chemistry, platelets, liver, renal and urinalysis studies have been performed before administration and monitor regularly during therapy.
- Monitor for fever, signs of local infection, ecchymosis, tarry stools, hematuria or edema.
- Assess for signs of systemic infection, such as fever or chills.
- Assess for signs of superimposed infection, such as vaginitis or stomatitis.

> **OVERDOSAGE: SIGNS & SYMPTOMS**
>
> Liver and lymph node enlargement, bone marrow depression, epistaxis

Patient/Family Education

- Advise patient that nausea and vomiting are common side effects. Fasting before taking medication may help decrease nausea. Explain that antiemetics also may be used to minimize GI upset.
- Explain that temporary hair loss may occur rarely. Discuss possible coping strategies and use of scarves or wigs.
- Instruct patient to check mucous membranes for signs of inflammation and ulceration. Discuss importance of oral hygiene in prevention of stomatitis.
- Advise patient to use soft toothbrush and electric razor, and to avoid vigorous flossing.
- Instruct patient to report these symptoms to physician: fever, chills, sore throat, unusual bleeding or bruising, shortness of breath, dry cough, edema, yellowing of skin or eyes, confusion, mouth sores and unusual lethargy.
- Warn patient to avoid contact with potentially infectious individuals and to avoid large groups.
- Tell patient to avoid any immunizations.
- Instruct patient not to take otc medications (eg, aspirin, ibuprofen) without consulting physician.
- Advise patient to notify dentist or physician of drug regimen before surgical or dental procedures.
- Explain that follow-up blood tests will be scheduled q 6 wk to evaluate drug effects.

See Patient Guide, p. 365.

Loperamide HCl

(low-PEHR-uh-mide HIGH-droe-KLOR-ide)

Imodium, Imodium A-D, Kaopectate, Maalox Anti-Diarrheal, Pepto Diarrhea Control

Class: Antidiarrheal

Action Slows intestinal motility, affects water and electrolyte movement through intestine, inhibits peristalsis, reduces daily fecal volume, increases viscosity and bulk density of stool, diminishes loss of fluid and electrolytes.

Indications Control and symptomatic relief of acute nonspecific or chronic diarrhea; reduction in volume of ileostomy output.

Contraindications Pseudomembranous colitis due to antibiotic use; acute diarrhea associated with organisms that penetrate intestinal wall (eg, toxigenic *Escherichia coli*, *Salmonella*, and *Shigella*); conditions in which constipation should be avoided;

bloody diarrhea; fever; acute ulcerative colitis (potential for toxic megacolon).

Route/Dosage

Acute Diarrhea

ADULTS: **PO** 4 mg followed by 2 mg after each unformed stool; not to exceed 16 mg/24 hr. CHILDREN 8-12 YR (> 30 KG): 2 mg tid. 6-8 YR (20-30 KG): 2 mg bid. 2-5 YR (13-20 KG): First day: 1 mg tid. May decrease to adjust for nutritional and hydration status after 24 hr; usually 0.1 mg/kg after each loose stool but do not exceed total first day dosing recommendations on any day.

Chronic Diarrhea

ADULTS: **PO** 4-8 mg qd or bid.

Interactions None well documented.

Lab Test Interferences
None well documented.

Adverse Reactions
CNS: Fatigue; drowsiness; dizziness. *GI:* Abdominal pain; distention or discomfort; constipation; nausea; vomiting; dry mouth. *DERM:* Rash.

Precautions
Pregnancy: Category B. *Lactation:* Undetermined. *Children:* Not recommended for children < 2 yr. Use with caution in young children. *Acute ulcerative colitis:* Agents that inhibit intestinal motility or delay intestinal transit time may induce toxic megacolon. Discontinue if abdominal distention or other untoward symptoms occur. *Hepatic impairment:* Hepatic coma may be precipitated in patients with advanced hepatorenal disease or hepatic dysfunction.

NURSING CONSIDERATIONS

Administration/Storage

- Administer as ordered, usually after each unformed stool.
- Store at room temperature.

Assessment/Interventions

- Obtain patient history, including drug history and any known allergies.
- Assess frequency and consistency of stools.
- Assess bowel sounds before and throughout course of therapy.
- Monitor I&O, fluid and electrolyte balance and skin turgor for signs of dehydration.

OVERDOSAGE: SIGNS & SYMPTOMS

Constipation, CNS depression, GI irritation

Patient/Family Education

- Instruct patient to record number and consistency of stools.
- Inform patient that medication may cause dry mouth. Encourage patient to drink plenty of clear fluids to help prevent dehydration that may accompany diarrhea.
- Advise patient to notify physician if diarrhea persists more than 48 hr or if fever develops.
- Inform patient that drug may cause drowsiness or dizziness and to use caution while driving or performing other tasks requiring mental alertness.

See Patient Guide, p. 366.

Loratadine

(lore-AT-uh-DEEN)

Claritin

Class: Antihistamine

Action Competitively antagonizes histamine at the H_1 receptor site.

Indications Symptomatic relief (nasal and nonnasal) of symptoms associated with perennial and seasonal allergic rhinitis. **Unlabeled uses:** Treatment of allergic and nonallergic pruritic symptoms; treatment of mild, uncomplicated urticaria.

Contraindications Hypersensitivity to antihistamines; use in nursing women.

Route/Dosage

ADULTS & CHILDREN ≥ 12 YR: **PO** 10 mg qd.

Hepatic Impairment

ADULTS & CHILDREN ≥ 12 YR: **PO** 10 mg qod.

Interactions

Alcohol, CNS depressants: Additive CNS depressant effects. *Azole antifungals (eg, ketoconazole, itraconazole):* Use of these agents with similar antihistamines has resulted in serious cardiac toxicity, including death. *Food:* May increase absorption of loratadine. *MAO inhibitors:* Concomitant use may prolong and intensify anticholinergic effects of loratadine and may result in hypotensive episodes.

Lab Test Interferences

May prevent or diminish otherwise positive reactions to dermal reactivity indicators.

Adverse Reactions

CV: Hypotension; hypertension; palpitations; tachycardia. *RESP:* Nasal dryness; pharyngitis; epistaxis; nasal congestion; dyspnea; coughing; rhinitis; hemoptysis; sinusitis; sneezing; bronchospasm; bronchitis; laryngitis. *CNS:* Hyperkinesia; paresthesia; dizziness; migraine; tremor; vertigo; headache; somnolence; fatigue. *EENT:* Conjunctivitis; blurred vision; earache; eye pain; blepharospasm; dysphonia; altered taste. *GI:* Anorexia; increased appetite and weight gain; nausea; vomiting; diarrhea; constipation; flatulence; gastritis; dyspepsia; dry mouth. *GU:* Urinary discoloration; altered micturation; menstrual irregularities. *DERM:* Dermatitis; dry hair; dry skin; urticaria; rash; pruritus; purpura; photosensitivity. *OTHER:* Breast pain; arthralgia; myalgia.

Precautions

Pregnancy: Category B. *Lactation:* Excreted in breast milk. *Children:* Safety and efficacy not established in children < 12 yr. *Hepatic impairment:* Use drug with caution in patients with hepatic impairment. *Hypersensitivity:* May occur.

NURSING CONSIDERATIONS

Administration/Storage

- Administer on empty stomach 1 hr before or 2 hr after eating.
- Store at room temperature.

Assessment/Interventions

- Obtain patient history, including drug history and any known allergies, especially to antihistamines.
- Obtain baseline BP, respirations and pulse before beginning therapy.
- Monitor closely for signs of hypersensitivity if patient has history of allergic reactions to other antihistamines.
- Observe for dizziness, excessive sedation, syncope, confusion and hypotension, especially in elderly patients.

OVERDOSAGE: SIGNS & SYMPTOMS

Somnolence, tachycardia, headache

Patient/Family Education

- Warn patient not to increase dose to obtain quicker relief of symptoms.
- If patient is to have allergy skin testing, advise to avoid taking medication for 4 days before test.
- Tell patient that drug may be used alone for symptoms of sneezing and runny nose with slight nasal congestion.
- Advise patient not to take any otc medications without consulting physician.
- Instruct patient to maintain fluid in-

take of 1½ to 2 quarts/day to decrease viscosity of secretions.

- Caution patient to avoid exposure to sunlight and to use sunscreen or wear protective clothing to avoid photosensitivity reaction.
- Instruct patient to avoid intake of alcoholic beverages or other CNS depressants (sedatives, hypnotics, tranquilizers).
- Advise patient that drug may cause drowsiness and to use caution while driving or performing other tasks requiring mental alertness until response to medication is known.

See Patient Guide, p. 367.

Lorazepam

(lore-AZE-uh-pam)

Ativan, ♣ *Nu-Loraz*

Class: Antianxiety/benzodiazepine

Action Potentiates action of GABA, resulting in increased neuronal inhibition and CNS depression, especially in limbic system and reticular formation.

Indications Treatment of anxiety, anxiety associated with depression; preanesthetic medication for sedation/anxiety and decreased recall (IV). **Unlabeled uses:** Treatment of status epilepticus; relief of chemotherapy-induced nausea and vomiting; acute alcohol withdrawal; psychogenic catatonia.

Contraindications Psychoses; acute narrow-angle glaucoma intra-arterial administration (injection); hypersensitivity to benzodiazepines.

Route/Dosage

Antianxiety

ADULTS: **PO** Usual dose: 2-6 mg/day (range 1-10 mg/day) in divided doses; largest dose at bedtime. ELDERLY/DEBILITATED PATIENTS: Initial dose: 1-2 mg/day in divided doses; increase gradually.

Preanesthesia

ADULTS: **IM** 0.05 mg/kg at least 2 hr before procedure; up to 4 mg maximum. **IV** Initial dose: 2 mg total or 0.044 mg/kg, whichever is smaller. Do not exceed in patients > 50 yr. For increased lack of recall: 0.05 mg/kg, up to 4 mg maximum, 15-20 min before procedure.

Interactions *Alcohol/CNS depressants:* Additive CNS depressant effects. *Digoxin:* Increased serum digoxin concentrations. *Theophyllines:* May antagonize sedative effects.

Lab Test Interferences None well documented.

Adverse Reactions *CV:* Cardiovascular collapse; hypotension; phlebitis or thrombosis at IV sites. *RESP:* Partial airway obstruction (injection). *CNS:* Drowsiness; confusion; ataxia; dizziness; lethargy; fatigue; apathy; memory impairment; disorientation; anterograde amnesia, restlessness; headache; slurred speech; aphonia; stupor; coma; euphoria; irritability; vivid dreams; psychomotor retardation; paradoxical reactions (eg, anger, hostility, mania, insomnia). *EENT:* Visual or auditory disturbances; depressed hearing. *GI:* Constipation; diarrhea; dry mouth; coated tongue; nausea; anorexia; vomiting. *DERM:* Rash. *HEMA:* Leukopenia. *HEPA:* Elevated LDH, ALT, AST and alkaline phosphatase; hepatic dysfunction, including hepatitis and jaundice. *OTHER:* Dependence/withdrawal syndrome (eg, confusion, abnormal perception of movement, depersonalization, muscle twitching, psychosis, paranoid delusions, seizures); pain, burning, redness at IM injection site.

Precautions *Pregnancy:* Category D. Avoid use, especially during first trimester, due to possible increased risk of congenital malformations. Advise women of childbearing age to use effective contraceptive method. Not recommended during labor and delivery. *Lactation:* Undetermined. *Children:* Do not use in patients < 18 yr (IM/IV); safety and efficacy in patients < 12 yr (oral) not established. *Dependence:* Prolonged use can lead to dependence. *Parenteral administration:* Primarily for acute states. Keep patients under observation for up to 3 hr. Use with extreme care in elderly, very ill patients or those with limited pulmonary reserve due to possibility of apnea or cardiac arrest. Do not give to patients in shock, coma or those with acute alcohol intoxication. *Psychiatric disorders:* Not intended for use in patients with primary depressive disorder, psychosis or disorders in which anxiety is not prominent. *Renal or hepatic impairment:* Injection is not recommended in these patients. Use oral form with caution. *Suicide:* Use with caution in patients with suicidal tendencies; do not allow access to large quantities.

NURSING CONSIDERATIONS

Administration/Storage

- Oral form may be given with food to minimize GI upset. Drug may be crushed and mixed with food or juice if patient has difficulty swallowing.
- When giving by IM route, inject undiluted, deep into muscle mass.
- Prepare IV solution immediately before administration. Dilute drug with equal volume of 5% Dextrose in Water, sterile water or saline.
- When giving by IV route, inject into large veins to minimize risk of thrombophlebitis. Administer IV push at rate not to exceed 2 mg/min.
- Direct IV push injection should be made with repeated aspiration to prevent intra-arterial administration, which may produce arteriospasm leading to gangrene.
- Do not administer IV or IM solution if discolored or if precipitate has formed.
- Oral form should be stored at controlled room temperature in tightly closed container.
- IM and IV forms should be refrigerated and protected from light.

Assessment/Interventions

- Obtain patient history, including drug history and any known allergies. Note glaucoma, renal or hepatic impairment, suicidal tendencies and use of nicotine (smoking may decrease drug effectiveness).
- Assess patient's anxiety level before beginning therapy and reassess daily.
- Assess for suicidal ideation as CNS depressants may aggravate symptoms of depression.
- Assess respiratory function carefully, particularly in elderly, very ill patients or those with compromised pulmonary reserve. Apnea or cardiac arrest may occur when drug is given parenterally. Have resuscitation equipment available.
- Monitor vital signs twice daily throughout therapy and every 10 min during IV administration.
- Ensure bedrest for 3 hr after IV administration. Supervise ambulation for up to 8 hr after IV administration.
- Offer sugarless hard candy, gum or frequent sips of water if dry mouth occurs.
- Monitor for symptoms of withdrawal syndrome, which may occur within 4-6 wk of treatment with therapeutic doses.

> **OVERDOSAGE: SIGNS & SYMPTOMS**
>
> Ataxia, lethargy, slurred speech, hypotension, respiratory depression, coma, CNS depression

Patient/Family Education

- Advise women of childbearing potential to use effective contraceptive method while taking lorazepam.
- Instruct patients who have used lorazepam regularly for more than a few weeks not to stop taking drug

abruptly as serious withdrawal symptoms may occur. Advise that prolonged use may result in dependence.
- Advise patient to avoid sudden position changes to prevent orthostatic hypotension.
- Instruct patient to report these symptoms to physician: sedation, dizziness, weakness, unsteadiness, disorientation, depression or paradoxical reactions such as anger, mania or insomnia.
- Explain that amnesia may occur, especially if drug is given via IV route.
- Advise patient that drug will cause drowsiness and to avoid driving or performing other tasks requiring mental alertness for at least 24-48 hr after administration of IM form.
- Instruct patient to avoid alcohol and other CNS depressants and otc medications while taking this drug.

See Patient Guide, p. 368.

Losartan Potassium

(low-SAHR-tan poe-TASS-ee-uhm)

Cozaar

Class: Antihypertensive/Angiotensin II antagonist

Action Antagonizes the effect of angiotension II (vasoconstriction and aldosterone secretion) by blocking the angiotensin II receptor (AT1 receptor) in vascular smooth muscle and the adrenal gland, producing decreased BP.

Indications Treatment of hypertension.

Contraindications Standard considerations.

Route/Dosage
ADULTS: PO Initial dose 50 mg once/day; 25 mg once/day if volume depleted or history of hepatic impairment. Maintenance: 25-100 mg/day.

Interactions None well documented.

Lab Test Interferences
None well documented.

Adverse Reactions
RESP: Cough; sinusitis. *CNS:* Dizziness; insomnia. *EENT:* Nasal congestion. *GI:* Diarrhea; dyspepsia. *OTHER:* Muscle cramps; myalgia; back pain; leg pain.

Precautions
Pregnancy: Category D (second and third trimester); Category C (first trimester). Can cause injury or death to fetus if used during second or third trimester. *Lactation:* Undetermined. *Children:* Safety and efficacy in children < 18 yr not established. *Hypotension/volume-depleted patients:* Symptomatic hypotension may occur after initiation of losartan in patients who are intravascularly volume depleted (eg, those treated with diuretics). Correct these conditions prior to administration of losartan or use a lower starting dose. *African-Americans:* Losartan may not be as effective as in non-African-Americans. *Renal impairment:* Use caution in treating patients whose renal function may depend on the activity of the renin-angiotension-aldosterone system (eg, patients with severe CHF). *Hepatic impairment:* Losartan total plasma clearance is lower (50%) and total bioavailability is higher (2-fold) in patients with hepatic insufficiency as compared to healthy subjects. A lower initial dose is recommended for patients with a history of hepatic impairment.

NURSING CONSIDERATIONS

Administration/Storage
- Administer alone or in combination with other antihypertensives.
- Administer with caution and reduce dosage in patients with possible depletion of intravascular volume or a history of hepatic impairment.

- Can be administered with or without food.
- Do not administer to pregnant women as fetal and neonatal morbidity and death can occur.
- Safety has not been established for nursing infants and children.
- Store in tightly closed, light-resistant container at room temperature.

Assessment/Interventions

- Obtain patient history.
- Monitor blood pressure and pulse. Should hypotension, tachycardia or bradycardia result, hold the medication and notify the physician.
- Monitor for signs of hypersensitivity including angioedema involving swelling of the face, lips and tongue.

OVERDOSAGE: SIGNS & SYMPTOMS

Hypotension, tachycardia

Patient/Family Education

- Instruct patient to take the medication as prescribed at the same time each day.
- Inform patient that losartan controls, but does not cure, hypertension.
- Caution patient to take the dose exactly as prescribed and not to stop taking the medication even if they feel better. Instruct patient not to decrease or increase the dosage.
- Instruct patient in blood pressure and pulse measurement skills. Caution patient to call their healthcare provider should abnormal measurements occur.
- Instruct patient in methods of fall prevention including rising slowly and sitting on the side of the bed before standing, especially early in therapy.
- Inform patient of the importance of adjunct therapies such as dietary planning, regular exercise program, weight reduction, low sodium diet, smoking cessation program, alcohol reduction and stress management.
- Instruct patient to report symptoms of weakness, fatigue, dizziness or lightheadedness to their healthcare provider.
- Caution patient to notify healthcare provider or dentist prior to surgery or treatment.
- Caution female patients to notify their healthcare provider at once should they become or plan to become pregnant.

See Patient Guide, p. 369.

Lovastatin (Mevinolin)

(LOW-vuh-STAT-in)

Mevacor, Mevinolin

Class: Antihyperlipidemic/HMG-coenzyme A reductase inhibitor

Action Increases rate at which body removes cholesterol from blood and reduces production of cholesterol in body by inhibiting enzyme that catalyzes early rate-limiting step in cholesterol synthesis; increases HDL; reduces LDL, VLDL and triglycerides.

Indications Reduction of elevated cholesterol and LDL cholesterol levels in patients with primary hypercholesterolemia (types IIa and IIb). **Unlabeled uses:** Treatment of diabetic dyslipidemia, nephrotic hyperlipidemia, familial dysbetalipoproteinemia, familial combined hyperlipidemia.

STOP **Contraindications** Active liver disease or unexplained persistent elevations of liver function tests; pregnancy; lactation.

Route/Dosage

ADULTS: **PO** 20-80 mg/day in single or divided doses with meals.

Interactions

Cyclosporine, erythromycin, gemfibrozil, niacin: Severe myopathy or rhabdomyolysis may occur with coadministration. *Warfarin:* Enhanced anticoagulant effect.

Lab Test Interferences

None well documented.

Adverse Reactions

CNS: Headache; dizziness; paresthesia; insomnia. *EENT:* Blurred vision; dysfunction of certain cranial nerves (including alteration of taste, impairment of extraocular movement, facial paresis). *GI:* Nausea; vomiting; diarrhea; abdominal pain; constipation; flatulence; heartburn; dyspepsia; pancreatitis. *HEPA:* Hepatitis; cholestatic jaundice; fatty change in liver; cirrhosis; fulminant hepatic necrosis; hepatoma. *DERM:* Rash; pruritus. *OTHER:* Myalgia; muscle cramps; myopathy; rhabdomyolysis with increased CPK; arthralgias; hypersensitivity syndrome (eg, anaphylaxis, angioedema, lupus erythematosus–like syndrome, polymyalgia rheumatica, vasculitis, purpura, thrombocytopenia, leukopenia, hemolytic anemia, arthritis, arthralgia, urticaria, fever, chills, dyspnea, toxic epidermal necrolysis, erythema multiforme.)

Precautions

Pregnancy: Category X. *Lactation:* Undetermined. *Children:* Safety and efficacy not established in children < 18 yr. *Liver dysfunction:* Use with caution in patients who consume substantial quantities of alcohol or those with liver disease. Marked, persistent increases in serum transaminases have occurred during lovastatin therapy. *Skeletal muscle effects:* Rhabdomyolysis with renal dysfunction secondary to myoglobinuria has been reported, mostly in those taking lovastatin concomitantly with cyclosporine, erythromycin, gemfibrozil or nicotinic acid. Immunosuppressants may increase active lovastatin metabolites, which are associated with myopathy, myalgia and muscle weakness associated with markedly increased CPK levels.

NURSING CONSIDERATIONS

Administration/Storage

- Administer with meals. If given as a single dose, administer with evening meal.
- Store at room temperature in tightly closed, light resistant container.

Assessment/Interventions

- Obtain patient history, including drug history and any known allergies. Note hepatic impairment, alcohol consumption and other medications that may increase risk of myopathy.
- Ensure that blood cholesterol and triglyceride levels are assessed before beginning therapy and repeated periodically during treatment.
- Place patient on standard cholesterol-lowering diet before beginning therapy and continue diet during treatment.
- Ensure that liver function tests are performed q 4-6 wk during first 3 mo of therapy, q 6-8 wk during next 18 mo and q 6 mo thereafter.
- If elevated serum transaminase levels develop during treatment, repeat tests more frequently.
- If transaminase levels rise to 3 times upper limit of normal and are persistent, notify physician. Drug may be discontinued.
- If muscle tenderness or weakness develops during therapy, monitor CPK levels. Notify physician if CPK levels are markedly increased or if symptoms continue.

OVERDOSAGE: SIGNS & SYMPTOMS

No specific symptoms with overdose of up to 6 g

Patient/Family Education

- Caution patient that this medication must not be taken during pregnancy or when pregnancy is possible. Advise patient to use reliable form of birth control while taking this drug.

- Advise patient to take medication with evening meal if possible.
- Explain importance of adhering to low-cholesterol, low-fat diet during treatment. Suggest consultation with nutritionist as needed.
- Instruct patient to report these symptoms to physician: unexplained muscle pain, tenderness or weakness, especially if accompanied by fever or malaise.
- Caution patient to avoid or decrease alcohol intake.
- Advise patient not to take any additional medications or supplementation without approval by physician.
- Emphasize importance of returning for follow-up liver function and blood cholesterol tests as instructed.
- Explain that this treatment must be continued over years.

See Patient Guide, p. 370.

Magaldrate (Hydroxymagnesium Aluminate)

(MAG-al-drate)

Isopan, Riopan, ♣ *Riopan Extra Strength*

Class: Antacid

Action Neutralizes gastric acid, thereby increasing pH of stomach and duodenal bulb. Increases lower esophageal sphincter tone and inhibits smooth muscle contraction and gastric emptying.

Indications Symptomatic relief of upset stomach associated with hyperacidity, including heartburn, gastroesophageal reflux, acid indigestion and sour stomach; relief of hyperacidity associated with peptic ulcer, gastritis, peptic esophagitis, gastric hyperacidity and hiatal hernia.

Contraindications Severe renal dysfunction; hypophosphatemia; nausea; vomiting; severe abdominal pain; acute surgical abdomen; impaction; intestinal obstruction.

Route/Dosage

ADULTS: PO 480-1080 mg qid prn or to aid in peptic ulcer healing or chronic reflux, give 1 hr and 3 hr after meals and at bedtime (7 doses/day). CHILDREN: PO 5-10 mg/dose q 3-6 hr or 1 hr and 3 hr after meals and at bedtime for peptic ulcer.

Interactions

Iron: Decreased pharmacologic effect of iron. *Ketoconazole:* Decreased pharmacologic effect of ketoconazole. *Nitrofurantoin:* Decreased effects of nitrofurantoin. *Penicillamine:* Decreased pharmacologic effect of penicillamine. *Quinidine:* Increased pharmacologic effect of quinidine. *Quinolones:* Decreased pharmacologic effect of quinolones. *Salicylates:* Decreased pharmacologic effect of salicylates. *Sodium polystyrene sulfonate:* Concomitant use may cause metabolic alkalosis in patients with renal failure. *Tetracyclines:* Decreased pharmacologic effect of tetracyclines.

Lab Test Interferences

None well documented.

Adverse Reactions

CNS: Neurotoxicity; encephalopathy. *GI:* Diarrhea; constipation; intestinal obstruction; rebound hyperacidity. *META:* Hypophosphatemia; hypermagnesemia. *OTHER:* Osteomalacia; bone pain; muscular weakness; malaise; decreased fluoride absorption; aluminum accumulation in serum, bone and CNS; milk-alkali syndrome.

Precautions

Pregnancy: Pregnancy category undetermined. *Lactation:* Undetermined. *GI hemorrhage:* Use with care in patients with recent massive upper GI hemorrhage. *Renal insufficiency:* Use with caution in patients with renal impairment to avoid hypermagnesemia and toxicity.

NURSING CONSIDERATIONS

Administration/Storage

- Administer 1 hr and 3 hr after meals and at bedtime when ordered for treatment of ulcers or 4 times/day when ordered as necessary for relief of symptoms.
- If possible, administer antacid 1-2 hr before or after other medications.
- Shake suspension vigorously before pouring. Administer with sufficient water (approximately 4 oz) to ensure that drug reaches stomach.
- Chewable tablet should be chewed thoroughly before swallowing, followed by half a glass of water.
- Store at room temperature.

Assessment/Interventions

- Obtain patient history, including drug history and any allergies.
- Assess for heartburn and indigestion, noting location, duration, character and precipitating factors of GI pain.
- Monitor serum magnesium level in patients with renal impairment.
- Monitor level of relief obtained by patient following medication.

OVERDOSAGE: SIGNS & SYMPTOMS

Nausea, vomiting, diarrhea, constipation, hypermagnesemia, hypophosphatemia

Patient/Family Education

- Instruct patient to take medication 1 and 3 hr after meals and at bedtime.
- Warn patient not to take other medications within 2 hr of antacid.
- Review proper use of suspension or tablet form.
- Advise patient to consult physician if problem recurs, if any symptoms that suggest bleeding occur (eg, black tarry stools) or if patient has taken antacids for more than 2 wk.

See Patient Guide, p. 371.

Magnesium Citrate

(mag-NEE-zee-uhm SIH-trate)

Citrate of Magnesia, Citro-Nesia,
♣ *Citro-Mag*

Class: Laxative

Action Attracts and retains water in intestinal lumen, thereby increasing intraluminal pressure and inducing urge to defecate.

Indications Short-term treatment of constipation; evacuation of colon for rectal and bowel evaluations.

Contraindications Hypersensitivity to any ingredient; nausea, vomiting or other symptoms of appendicitis; acute surgical abdomen; fecal impaction; intestinal obstruction; undiagnosed abdominal pain; intestinal bleeding; renal disease.

Route/Dosage
ADULTS: PO 1 glassful (approximately 240 ml) prn. CHILDREN 2-6 YR: PO 4-12 ml. CHILDREN 6-12 YR: PO 50-100 ml. Repeat if necessary.

Interactions
Nitrofurantoin: Reduced anti-infective action. *Penicillamine:* Reduced action of penicillamine. *Tetracyclines:* Impaired absorption of tetracyclines.

Lab Test Interferences
None well documented.

Adverse Reactions
CV: Palpitations. *CNS:* Dizziness; fainting. *GI:* Excessive bowel activity (eg, cramping, diarrhea, nausea, vomiting); perianal irritation; bloating; flatulence; abdominal cramping. *OTHER:* Sweating; weakness; fluid and electrolyte imbalance.

Precautions
Pregnancy: Pregnancy category undetermined. *Lactation:* Undetermined. *Children:* Exercise caution; consult physician. One 6-wk-old infant de-

veloped magnesium poisoning after several doses for constipation. *Abuse/dependency:* Chronic use of laxatives may lead to laxative dependency, which may result in fluid and electrolyte imbalances, steatorrhea, osteomalacia and vitamin and mineral deficiencies. *Fluid and electrolyte imbalance:* Excessive laxative use may lead to significant fluid and electrolyte imbalance. *Rectal bleeding or failure to respond:* May indicate serious condition requiring further attention. *Renal impairment:* Avoid in patients with renal dysfunction. Hypermagnesemia and toxicity may occur due to decreased clearance of magnesium ion.

NURSING CONSIDERATIONS

Administration/Storage

- Chilling medication or giving with ice may improve palatability.
- Administer on empty stomach and give with full glass of water to increase effectiveness of medication.
- Store in tightly closed container in cool dry place.

Assessment/Interventions

- Obtain patient history, including drug history and any known allergies. Note symptoms of appendicitis, fecal impaction, renal disease or small bowel obstruction.
- Observe for distended abdomen and auscultate for presence of bowel sounds.
- Monitor for electrolyte imbalances and dehydration.
- If nausea, diarrhea, abdominal distention, increased abdominal pain or rectal bleeding occur, notify physician.

OVERDOSAGE: SIGNS & SYMPTOMS

Severe/protracted diarrhea, fluid and electrolyte disturbances, hypermagnesemia

Patient/Family Education

- Explain that drug should not be used routinely for constipation; dependence can result.
- Instruct patient to report any of these symptoms to physician: unrelieved constipation, vomiting, diarrhea, abdominal fullness, rectal bleeding, dizziness and muscle cramps.
- Review information on proper use and storage of medication.

See Patient Guide, p. 372.

Magnesium Oxide

(mag-NEE-zee-uhm OX-ide)

Mag-Ox 400, Maox, Uro-Mag

Class: Antacid

Action Neutralizes gastric acid, thereby increases pH of stomach and duodenal bulb; also increases lower esophageal sphincter tone.

Indications Symptomatic relief of upset stomach associated with hyperacidity, including heartburn, gastroesophageal reflux, acid indigestion and sour stomach; relief of hyperacidity associated with peptic ulcer, gastritis, peptic esophagitis, gastric hyperacidity and hiatal hernia. Also used for treatment of hypomagnesemia, or magnesium depletion resulting from malnutrition, restricted diet, alcoholism or magnesium-depleting drugs.

Contraindications Standard considerations.

Route/Dosage

ADULTS: **PO** 140 mg (caps) 3-4 times/day or 400-840 mg/day (tabs).

Interactions

Iron: Decreased pharmacological effect of iron. *Nitrofurantoin:* Decreased pharmacological effect of nitrofurantoin. *Penicillamine:* Decreased pharmacological effect of penicillamine. *Tetracyclines:* Decreased pharmacological effect of tetracyclines.

Lab Test Interferences None well documented.

Adverse Reactions *GI:* Laxative effect (diarrhea); rebound hyperacidity. *META:* Hypermagnesemia. *OTHER:* Milk-alkali syndrome.

Precautions *Pregnancy:* Category B. *Lactation:* Undetermined. *Renal insufficiency:* Caution with renal impairment to avoid hypermagnesemia and toxicity.

NURSING CONSIDERATIONS

Administration/Storage

- Administer caps or tabs with full glass of water or other liquid.
- Give 1-2 hr before or after other medications if possible.
- Store in airtight container in cool location unless otherwise specified by manufacturer.

Assessment/Interventions

- Obtain patient history, including drug history and any known allergies. Note renal disease.
- Monitor for symptoms of renal insufficiency (elevated BUN and creatinine, decreased urine output).
- Encourage patient to increase fluid intake.
- Monitor serum magnesium levels in patients being treated for hypomagnesemia and in patients with impaired renal function.
- Assess for heartburn and indigestion. Note location, duration, character and precipitating factors.

OVERDOSAGE: SIGNS & SYMPTOMS

Diarrhea, fluid and electrolyte abnormalities, hypermagnesemia

Patient/Family Education

- Advise patient that drug may be laxative and cause diarrhea.
- If being used for antacid effect, instruct patient to notify physician if symptoms are not relieved or if black, tarry stools or "coffee-ground" vomitus occurs. These symptoms can indicate bleeding.
- Explain that drug should not be used routinely for laxative effect. Advise patient to use other forms of bowel regulation such as increasing fluid intake, mobility and bulk in diet.
- Warn patient not to take other medications within 2 hr of antacids.

See Patient Guide, p. 373.

Magnesium Sulfate

(mag-NEE-zee-uhm SULL-fate)

Epsom Salt

Class: Anticonvulsant; electrolyte; laxative

Action Magnesium has CNS-depressant effect; prevents/controls seizures by blocking neuromuscular transmission and decreasing amount of acetylcholine liberated at end plate by motor nerve impulse. Orally it attracts/retains water in intestinal lumen, thereby increasing intraluminal pressure and inducing urge to defecate.

Indications *Parenteral:* Seizure prevention and control in severe pre-eclampsia or eclampsia without deleterious CNS depression in mother, fetus or neonate, and in convulsions associated with hypomagnesemia. **Unlabeled uses:** Control of hypertension, encephalopathy and convulsions in children with acute nephritis; inhibition of premature labor; treatment of life-threatening ventricular arrhythmias; prevention and treatment of nutritional magnesium deficiency. *Oral:* Laxative.

Contraindications Toxemia of pregnancy during 2 hr preceding delivery; MI; myocardial damage; heartblock.

Route/Dosage

Severe Hypomagnesemia

ADULTS & OLDER CHILDREN: **IM** 1-5 g (2-10 ml of 50% solution)/day in divided doses until correction of serum magnesium. ADULTS & OLDER CHILDREN: **IV** Must be given very carefully due to risk of cardiac arrest. **IV** 1-4 g diluted to 10% or 20% solution at rate not to exceed 1.5 ml (of 10% solution) or its equivalent per minute.

Milder Hypomagnesemia and Electrolyte Supplement

ADULTS: **IM** 1-2 g of 50% solution qd-qid. CHILDREN: **IM** 20-40 mg/kg of 20% solution.

Eclampsia

ADULTS: **IM** 1-2 g (as 25% or 50% solution) followed by **IM** 1 g q 30 min until relaxation is obtained. IV infusion may be given as **IV** 4-5 g in 250 ml D5W not to exceed 3 ml/min.

Anticonvulsant

ADULTS: **IM** 1-5 g as 25% or 50% solution. May be repeated up to 6 times/day prn. CHILDREN: **IM** 20-40 mg/kg as 20% solution.

Laxative

Usually one-time dose. ADULTS: **PO** 10-15 g. CHILDREN: **PO** 5-10 g.

Interactions

Neuromuscular blocking agents: Potentiation of neuromuscular blockade. *Nitrofurantoin:* Decreased absorption of nitrofurantoin (oral magnesium). *Penicillamine:* Reduced penicillamine effects (oral magnesium). *Tetracyclines:* Decreased absorption of tetracyclines (oral magnesium). INCOMPATIBILITIES: Amphotericin B, calcium salts, clindamycin, dobutamine, doxycycline, hydrocortisone sodium succinate, nafcillin, sodium bicarbonate, tetracycline, thiopental, vasopressin.

Lab Test Interferences

None well documented.

Adverse Reactions

CV: Cardiac depression; circulatory collapse; hypotension; cardiac arrest. *RESP:* Respiratory paralysis. *CNS:* CNS depression; depressed reflexes; muscle weakness; flaccid paralysis. *META:* Hypocalcemia. *OTHER:* Flushing; sweating; hypothermia; hypomagnesemia.

Precautions

Pregnancy: Category A. *Lactation:* Excreted in breast milk during parenteral use. *Eclampsia:* Use IV form only for immediate control of life-threatening convulsions. *Renal impairment:* Use with caution; renal insufficiency may lead to magnesium intoxication.

NURSING CONSIDERATIONS

Administration/Storage

- When giving by IV route, use infusion pump. Deliver in separate line and do not mix with other IV drugs unless compatibility has been established.
- Administer loading dose followed by drip titrated to maintain therapeutic serum level with minimal side effects.
- When giving by IM route, use deep, slow injection. Rotate sites to prevent tissue irritation.
- Administer oral drug early in day on empty stomach.
- Dilute oral drug in glass of water containing ice chips or flavored with lemon or orange juice. Follow with full glass of water.

Assessment/Interventions

- Obtain patient history, including any drug history and any known allergies. Note kidney impairment and hydration status.
- Ensure that baseline ECG, calcium, phosphorus, magnesium, BUN and creatinine levels have been obtained before beginning parenteral magnesium administration and monitor regularly. Serum magnesium levels

should be obtained q 6 hr or when toxicity is suspected and as necessary when using for therapeutic benefit (eg, eclampia, hypomagnesia). Notify physician if deviations from normal laboratory values occur.

- Obtain baseline vital signs, patellar reflex and neurologic assessment. Continue to assess throughout parenteral magnesium administration.
- Assess vital signs q 5-15 min while infusing IV loading dose, then q ½-1 hr.
- Assess bowel sounds, abdominal distention and bowel patterns when using oral magnesium as laxative.
- If drug is being given for prevention of preterm labor, assess fetal heart rate and uterine contractions prior to first dose and continuously during administration.
- If patient experiences symptoms of parenteral magnesium toxicity (including sweating, flushing, hypotension, respiratory depression, diminished reflexes, oliguria or depressed CNS function), notify physician and discontinue drug.
- Maintain safety precautions such as keeping bed in low position with side rails up and instructing patient not to rise without assistance after receiving parenteral magnesium.
- Maintain strict, hourly I&O and keep patient well hydrated. Urine output should be at least 100 ml q 4 hr when giving parenteral magnesium.
- Keep 10% calcium chloride at bedside for adult patients (calcium gluconate for neonates and pediatric patients).
- Keep resuscitation equipment readily available.
- If drug is being given for pre-eclampsia, eclampsia or convulsions, maintain seizure precautions. Provide a quiet, nonstimulating environment.
- If drug was administered during labor, prepare for neonatal resuscitation. Monitor neonate for magnesium toxicity and administer IV calcium if hypermagnesemia is present. Observe for uterine atony following delivery.
- If used as laxative, utilize additional measures to prevent constipation including increased dietary fiber and fluids.

OVERDOSAGE: SIGNS & SYMPTOMS

Early signs: sweating, flushing, thirst, decreased deep tendon reflexes, weakness. Later signs: sedation, loss of deep tendon reflexes, hypothermia, hypotension, heart block and respiratory paralysis.

Patient/Family Education

- Instruct patient to take oral drug with full glass of water and emphasize importance of maintaining sufficient fluid intake.
- If drug is prescribed for home laxative use, advise patient about correct administration, side effects and other measures to prevent constipation.
- Caution that drug is for short-term laxative use only. Explain that prolonged use can lead to dehydration and electrolyte imbalance.
- After parenteral administration, instruct patient to report any of these symptoms to physician: tremors, tetany, muscle cramps, thirst, sedation, confusion, muscle weakness, inability to urinate.

See Patient Guide, pp. 374-375.

Maprotiline HCl

(ma-PRO-tih-leen HIGH-droe-KLOR-ide)

Ludiomil

Class: Tetracyclic antidepressant

Action Inhibits norepinephrine (but not serotonin) reuptake.

Indications Depression; anxiety associated with depression. **Unlabeled use:** Relief of chronic neurogenic pain.

Contraindications Hypersensitivity to tricyclic antidepressants; MI acute recovery period; seizure disorder; concomitant use with MAO inhibitors.

Route/Dosage

ADULTS: Initial dose: **PO** 25-75 mg/day as single dose or divided doses. May be increased to 150 mg/day (outpatient) or 225 mg/day (inpatient).

Interactions

Alcohol, CNS depressants: Additive CNS effects possible. MAO *inhibitors:* May precipitate hypertensive crisis and convulsions with possibly fatal results. Discontinue at least 14 days before starting maprotiline.

Lab Test Interferences

None well documented.

Adverse Reactions

CV: Syncope; tachycardia; palpitations; orthostatic hypotension; hypertension; MI; arrhythmias; heart block. *CNS:* Drowsiness; dizziness; hallucinations; disorientation; mania; exacerbation of psychosis; nervousness; fatigue; headache; anxiety; tremor; insomnia; agitation; seizures. *EENT:* Blurred vision; mydriasis. *GI:* Dry mouth; constipation; nausea; diarrhea. *GU:* Impotence; urinary retention. *HEMA:* Bone marrow depression, including agranulocytosis; eosinophilia; purpura; thrombocytopenia; leukopenia. *HEPA:* Increased bilirubin and alkaline phosphatase. *META:* Altered blood glucose levels. *OTHER:* Hypersensitivity (eg, rash, itching, photosensitivity, petechiae, edema, drug fever).

Precautions

Pregnancy: Category B. *Lactation:* Excreted in breast milk. *Children:* Safety and efficacy not established. *Elderly:* Use lower doses. *Special risk patients:* Use with caution in patients with history of seizures, urinary retention, urethral or ureteral spasm, angle-closure glaucoma or increased IOP, cardiovascular disorders, hyperthyroid patients or those receiving thyroid medication, hepatic or renal impairment, schizophrenic or paranoid patients. *Severe depression:* Do not allow patient to possess more than small quantities of drug. *Seizures:* May occur in therapeutic dose or overdose.

NURSING CONSIDERATIONS

Administration/Storage

- Administer at bedtime to reduce side effects.
- Store in cool, dry place.

Assessment/Interventions

- Obtain patient history, including drug history and any known allergies. Note MI, seizure disorder, hypersensitivity to drug and concomitant use of MAO inhibitors.
- Ensure that CBC with differential is obtained prior to initial dose and monitored routinely throughout therapy.
- Take baseline vital signs with postural BP and pulse on initiation and reassess routinely.
- Monitor blood glucose closely in diabetic patients.
- Monitor patient's mood and affect closely. If mood changes or suicidal tendencies develop, notify physician and take suicide precautions.
- Assess patient's level of sedation. If patient becomes too lethargic or becomes restless and agitated, notify physician.
- Observe for signs of dizziness, palpitations, orthostatic hypotension, drowsiness, chest pain, tremors or seizures. Notify physician if these symptoms occur.
- If constipation occurs, increase fiber and fluid intake and mobility.
- Observe for inability to urinate or bladder fullness. If these symptoms occur, notify physician.

OVERDOSAGE: SIGNS & SYMPTOMS
Hypotension, tachycardia, ventricular arrhythmias, CNS depression, seizures, respiratory depression, coma

Patient/Family Education
- Explain that full effectiveness of drug may not occur until after several doses.
- Instruct patient that if dose is missed, it should be taken as soon as possible unless close to time of next dose. Warn patient not to double up doses and to notify physician if more than one dose is missed.
- Explain that drug may cause dry mouth and constipation. Advise patient about measures to manage these side effects.
- Advise diabetic patient that drug may alter blood glucose level.
- Instruct patient not to take otc medications without consulting physician.
- Instruct patient to avoid intake of alcoholic beverages or other CNS depressants.
- Instruct patient to report these symptoms to physician: difficult or infrequent voiding, dizziness, chest pain, palpitations, anxiety, depression, blurred vision, excessive dry mouth, mouth sores, severe constipation.
- Advise patient that drug may cause drowsiness and to use caution while driving or performing other tasks requiring mental alertness.

See Patient Guide, p. 376.

Masoprocol

(mass-OH-prah-KOLE)

Actinex

Class: Topical; antiproliferative

Action Thought to have antiproliferative activity against keratinocytes.

Indications Topical treatment of actinic (solar) keratoses.

Contraindications Standard considerations.

Route/Dosage
ADULTS: **Topical** Massage evenly into area containing actinic keratoses each morning and evening for 28 days.

Interactions None well documented.

Lab Test Interferences
None well documented.

Adverse Reactions
EENT: Eye irritation. *DERM:* Erythema; flaking; itching; dryness; edema; burning; soreness; bleeding; crusting; oozing; rash; skin irritation; stinging; tightness; tingling.

Precautions
Pregnancy: Category B. *Lactation:* Undetermined. *Children:* Safety and efficacy not established. *Application:* Occlusive dressings should not be used with this product. *External use:* This product is for external use only. Avoid contact with eyes and mucous membranes. *Sulfite sensitivity:* Use caution in sulfite-sensitive individuals; preparation contains bisulfites.

NURSING CONSIDERATIONS

Administration/Storage
- Before application, wash, rinse and dry affected area.
- Apply each morning and evening for 28 days. Gently and evenly massage into affected area.
- Wash hands immediately after application.
- Avoid contact with eyes or mucous membranes. If contact occurs, promptly flush eye or mucous membranes with water.
- Do not cover with occlusive dressing.
- Store at room temperature.

Assessment/Interventions
- Obtain patient history, includ-

ing drug history and any known allergies.

- Assess number and severity of lesions before beginning therapy and throughout use of medication.
- Assess area after administration for local reactions such as redness, flaking, itching, dryness, swelling, continued burning, oozing, blistering or bleeding.
- If adverse reactions occur, notify physician immediately.

Patient/Family Education

- Explain proper method of administration. Tell patient that temporary stinging or burning sensation is common but should disappear quickly.
- Warn patient that medication may stain clothing or other fabrics.
- Advise patient not to use makeup or other skin products without consulting physician.
- Caution patient to avoid excessive exposure to sun.
- Instruct patient to avoid taking any other medications unless prescribed by physician.

See Patient Guide, p. 377.

Measles, Mumps and Rubella Vaccine, Live

(MEE-zuhls, mumps and roo-BELL-uh vaccine, live)

M-M-R-II

Class: Vaccine, live virus

Action Induces protective antibodies against measles, mumps and rubella viruses.

Indications Vaccination of individuals known to be susceptible to measles, mumps or rubella; prevention of occurrence of congenital rubella syndrome (CRS) among offspring of women who contract rubella during pregnancy. Preferred immunizing agent for most children and many adults.

Contraindications Pregnancy; moderate to severe hypersensitivity reaction to eggs; immunosuppressive therapy; blood dyscrasia, leukemia, lymphoma of any type or other malignant neoplasms affecting the bone marrow or lymphatic systems; primary or acquired immunodeficiency; active untreated tuberculosis; family history of congenital or hereditary immunodeficiency, until immune competence of potential vaccine recipient is demonstrated. (*Exception:* Vaccinate asymptomatic children with HIV infection.)

Route/Dosage

ADULTS & CHILDREN: SC 0.5 ml. Optimal schedule: Give first dose at 12-15 mo; revaccinate routinely at 5-6 yr or 11-12 yr.

Interactions

Human antibody products: To avoid inactivating vaccine, give MMR 2-4 wk before or 3-11 mo after AGIV, depending on dose. Susceptible postpartum women who received blood products or Rho(D) immune globulin may receive rubella vaccine prior to discharge, provided that rubella titer is measured 6-8 wk after vaccination to ensure seroconversion. *Immunosuppressants, interferon, meningococcal vaccine:* May inhibit response to MMR vaccine.

Lab Test Interferences

May cause delayed hypersensitivity skin tests (eg, tuberculin, histoplasmin) to appear falsely negative. Effect may persist for several weeks after vaccination. Methacoline inhalation challenge may be falsely positive for a few days.

Adverse Reactions

CNS: Fever; headache; encephalitis; dizziness; polyneuritis; arthralgia; arthritis (rarely chronic); convulsions or seizures. *EENT:* Sore throat; optic neuritis. *GI:* Nausea; vomiting; diarrhea. *HEMA:* Thrombocytopenia; purpura. *DERM:* Urticaria; rash; erythema multiforme. *OTHER*: Local pain, induration, erythema or allergic reaction at injection site; mild regional lymphadenopathy; malaise.

Precautions

Pregnancy: Category C (contraindicated). *Lactation*: Excreted in breast milk (vaccine-strain rubella). *Acute febrile illness*: Defer immunization during course of any acute febrile illness.

NURSING CONSIDERATIONS

Administration/Storage

- If patient is febrile, delay administration if possible.
- Reconstitute using supplied diluent.
- With 25-gauge ⅝-inch needle, inject total volume of reconstituted vaccine SC, preferably into outer aspect of upper arm.
- Refrigerate before and after reconstitution and protect from light.
- Discard unused reconstituted vaccine if not used within 8 hr.

Assessment/Interventions

- Obtain patient history, including drug history and any known allergies. Note untreated tuberculosis, history of immunocompromised disease, immunosuppressive therapy, or hypersensitivity to eggs, egg products or neomycin.
- Ensure that pregnancy test has been performed on sexually active women.
- Observe for local redness and warmth at injection site.
- Monitor for fever, dizziness, arthritis or rash. Notify physician if these symptoms occur.
- Record immunization in patient's record.

Patient/Family Education

- Advise patient that tenderness, redness, swelling and warmth at site of injection may occur.
- Applying warm compress to site will decrease these symptoms.
- Instruct patient to notify physician if local symptoms persist.
- Caution sexually active women to avoid pregnancy for 3 mo after vaccination.

No patient monograph available.

Mebendazole

(meh-BEND-uh-zole)

Vermox

Class: Antihelmintic

Action Kills parasitic worms by blocking glucose uptake, thus depleting stored glycogen. Without glycogen, parasite cannot reproduce or survive.

Indications Treatment of pinworm (*Enterobius vermicularis*), round worm (*Ascaris lumbricoides*), common hookworm (*Ancylostoma duodenale*), American hookworm (*Necator americanus*) and whipworm (*Trichuris trichiura*) in single or mixed parasitic infections.

Contraindications Standard considerations.

Route/Dosage

Trichuriasis, Ascariasis and Hookworm Infection

ADULTS & CHILDREN: **PO** 100 mg tablet AM and PM on 3 consecutive days.

Ascaris Infection

ADULTS & CHILDREN: Alternative dose: **PO** 500 mg as single dose.

Enterobiasis

ADULTS & CHILDREN: **PO** 100 mg as single dose.

Interactions

Carbamazepine; hydantoins (eg, phenytoin): Pharmacological effects of mebendazole may be decreased.

Lab Test Interferences
None well documented.

Adverse Reactions
GI: Transient abdominal pain and diarrhea. *OTHER:* Fever.

Precautions
Pregnancy: Category C. *Lactation:* Undetermined. *Children:* Safety and efficacy in children < 2 yr not established.

NURSING CONSIDERATIONS

Administration/Storage

- Give with food; crush or allow patient to chew tablets if patient has difficulty tolerating ingestion.
- Store in tightly closed container.

Assessment/Interventions

- Obtain patient history, including drug history and any known allergies.
- Monitor results of stool testing prior to and 3 wk after treatment is initiated.
- Obtain baseline vital signs and monitor throughout therapy.
- Notify physician of new-onset fever after initiation of therapy and diarrhea during expulsion of worms.
- Report to physician any signs of abdominal pain with diarrhea.
- Disinfect toilet facilities, towels, bed linens, and clothing daily.
- Avoid self-contamination. Practice thorough hand washing.
- Check for infection in other family members.

OVERDOSAGE: SIGNS & SYMPTOMS
GI complaints

Patient/Family Education

- Advise patient to chew tablet or to crush tablet and mix with food.
- Instruct patient to wash clothing, bed linens and towels daily and to disinfect bathroom facilities daily.
- Advise that infected person sleep alone.
- Caution patient not to put fingers in mouth.
- Emphasize importance of thorough hand washing, especially after toileting, to avoid reinfecting self.
- Explain that all family members should be treated to eradicate infestation.
- Tell patient that second treatment is sometimes necessary.
- Instruct family/patient to call physician if fever, abdominal pain or diarrhea develops.

See Patient Guide, p. 378.

Meclizine

(MEK-lih-zeen)
Antivert, Antrizine, Bonine, Dizmiss, Dramamine II, Meni-D, Ru-Vert-M Vergon, ✤ *Bonamine*
Class: Antiemetic and antivertigo/anticholinergic

Action Acts on CNS to decrease vestibular stimulation and depress labyrinthine activity.

Indications Prevention and treatment of nausea, vomiting and dizziness of motion sickness; possibly effective treatment for vertigo of vestibular dysfunction origin.

Contraindications Hypersensitivity to cyclizine; asthma; glaucoma; emphysema; chronic pulmonary disease; shortness of breath; difficulty breathing; urinary retention caused by enlarged prostate.

Route/Dosage
Motion Sickness
ADULTS: **PO** 25-50 mg 1 hr before travel; may repeat q 24 hr during travel.

Vertigo
ADULTS: **PO** 25-100 mg/day in divided doses.

Interactions
Alcohol, CNS depressants: Additive CNS effects.

Lab Test Interferences
False-negative result in allergy skin testing.

Adverse Reactions
CV: Hypotension; tachycardia; palpitations. *CNS:* Drowsiness; excitation; nervousness; restlessness; insomnia; euphoria; vertigo; hallucinations. *EENT:* Dry nose and throat; visual disturbances; tinnitus. *GI:* Nausea; vomiting; dry mouth; diarrhea; constipation; anorexia. *GU:* Urinary frequency; urinary retention; difficulty urinating. *DERM:* Rash; urticaria.

Precautions
Pregnancy: Category B. *Lactation:* Undetermined. *Children:* Safety and efficacy not established. Not recommended in children < 12 yr.

NURSING CONSIDERATIONS

Administration/Storage
- Tablets may be chewed, swallowed whole or allowed to dissolve in water.
- Store at room temperature.

Assessment/Interventions
- Obtain patient history, including drug history and any known allergies. Note glaucoma and prostatic hypertrophy.
- Monitor for side effects, especially sedation, hypotension, tachycardia and urinary retention.
- Implement safety precautions (eg, keep bed in low position and instruct patient to call for assistance when rising) if patient is experiencing sedation or vertigo.

OVERDOSAGE: SIGNS & SYMPTOMS
Hyperexcitability, drowsiness, hallucinations, convulsions

Patient/Family Education
- When given for motion sickness, inform patient that first dose should be taken 1 hr before exposure to motion.
- Instruct patient to take sips of water frequently, suck on ice chips or sugarless hard candy or chew sugarless gum if dry mouth occurs.
- Explain that high-fiber diet and drinking plenty of fluids may help to prevent constipation, which is common side effect.
- Instruct patient to report these symptoms to physician: sedation, dizziness, palpitations, difficulty urinating or urinary retention.
- Instruct patient to notify physician if vomiting increases or becomes severe.
- Advise patient that drug may cause drowsiness and to use caution while driving or performing other tasks requiring mental alertness.
- Instruct patient to avoid intake of alcoholic beverages or other CNS depressants.
- Advise patient not to take otc medications or other prescription medications without consulting physician.

See Patient Guide, p. 379.

Meclofenamate Sodium

(mek-loe-FEN-uh-mate SO-dee-uhm)
Meclomen
Class: Analgesic/NSAID

Action Decreases inflammation, pain and fever, probably through inhibition of cyclooxygenase activity and prostaglandin synthesis.

Indications Treatment of rheumatoid and osteoarthritis; treatment of primary dysmenorrhea; relief of mild to moderate pain; idiopathic heavy menstrual blood loss. **Unlabeled**

uses: Relief of sunburn; pain; migraine (abort acute attacks).

Contraindications Patients in whom aspirin, iodides or any NSAID has caused allergic-type reactions.

Route/Dosage

Osteoarthritis or Rheumatoid Arthritis; Mild to Moderate Pain

ADULTS: PO 200-400 mg/day in 3-4 equally divided doses.

Excessive Menstrual Blood Loss; Primary Dysmenorrhea

ADULTS: PO 100 mg tid for up to 6 days.

Interactions

Anticoagulants: Increased risk of gastric erosion and bleeding. *Cyclosporine:* Nephrotoxicity of both agents may be increased. *Lithium:* Serum lithium levels may be increased. *Methotrexate:* Increased methotrexate levels. *Salicylates:* Additive GI toxicity.

Lab Test Interferences

May prolong bleeding time.

Adverse Reactions

CV: Edema. *RESP:* Breathing difficulties in aspirin-sensitive individuals. *CNS:* Headache; vertigo; drowsiness; dizziness; tinnitus. *GI:* Diarrhea; vomiting; nausea; abdominal pain; dyspepsia; peptic ulcer; GI bleeding. *GU:* Acute renal failure; nephrotic syndrome. *HEMA:* Fall in hemoglobin; positive Coombs' test; bruising; prolonged bleeding time; thrombocytopenia purpura; anemia. *HEPA:* Abnormal liver function test results. *DERM:* Rash; urticaria; fasciitis. *META:* Porphyria; hyponatremia.

Precautions

Pregnancy: Safety not established; avoid use, especially during first and last trimester. *Lactation:* Undetermined. *Children:* Not recommended for children < 14 yr. *Elderly patients:* Increased risk of adverse reactions. *Diarrhea:* If diarrhea occurs, reduce dosage or temporarily discontinue. *GI toxicity:* Bleeding, ulceration or perforation can occur at any time, with or without warning symptoms. *Hypersensitivity:* May occur; use with caution in aspirin-sensitive individuals due to possible cross-sensitivity. *Renal effects:* Acute renal insufficiency, interstitial nephritis, hyperkalemia, hyponatremia and renal papillary necrosis may occur. *Renal impairment:* Lower doses may be necessary.

NURSING CONSIDERATIONS

Administration/Storage

- Administer with meals, followed by full glass of water or milk to reduce GI or esophageal irritation. May be given with antacids if stomach upset occurs.
- Store at room temperature in tightly closed, light-resistant container.

Assessment/Interventions

- Obtain patient history, including drug history and any known allergies. Note chronic alcohol use, fluid retention, nasal polyps, bronchospastic disease or hypersensitivity to aspirin or NSAIDs.
- Monitor carefully for hypersensitivity. Note any ecchymosis or rash.
- Notify physician if stomach pain develops or continues.
- Monitor renal and liver function and blood studies throughout treatment.
- Monitor for diarrhea or blood in stools. If diarrhea occurs, notify physician. Dosage may need to be reduced or drug temporarily withheld.
- Weigh patient daily if fluid retention is a concern.

OVERDOSAGE: SIGNS & SYMPTOMS

Sweating, disorientation, vomiting, convulsions, electrolyte imbalance, metabolic acidosis

Patient/Family Education

- Explain that therapeutic effects may take up to 1 mo to be noticed.

- Instruct patient to report these symptoms to physician: rash, dark stools, persistent headache or stomach pain, unusual bruising or bleeding, decreased urinary output.
- Advise patient to avoid intake of alcoholic beverages.
- Caution patient to avoid exposure to sunlight and to use sunscreen or wear protective clothing to avoid photosensitivity reaction.
- Instruct patient that drug may cause dizziness and to use caution while driving or performing other activities requiring mental alertness until effects of drug are known.
- Tell patient to notify physician if diarrhea occurs. Review symptoms of dehydration. Explain that if diarrhea becomes severe or nausea and vomiting are severe, patient should stop taking medication and contact physician.
- Instruct patient to weigh self twice weekly and to notify physician if weight gain of > 3-4 lb/wk occurs.
- Instruct patient not to take otc medications, including aspirin and ibuprofen, or other prescription medications, without consulting physician.
- Warn patient about potential for bleeding and advise to notify other health care professionals that drug is being taken.

See Patient Guide, p. 380.

Medroxyprogesterone Acetate

(meh-DROX-ee-pro-JESS-tuh-rone ASS-uh-TATE)

Amen, Curretab, Cycrin, Depo-Provera, Provera

Class: Progestin

Action Inhibits secretion of pituitary gonadotropins, thereby preventing follicular maturation and ovulation (contraceptive effect); inhibits spontaneous uterine contraction; transforms proliferative endometrium into secretory endometrium; produces antineoplastic effect in advanced endometrial or renal carcinoma.

Indications *Oral form:* Treatment of secondary amenorrhea and abnormal uterine bleeding due to hormonal imbalance. *Parenteral form:* Prevention of pregnancy; adjunctive and palliative treatment of inoperable, recurrent and metastatic endometrial or renal carcinoma. **Unlabeled uses:** Treatment of menopausal symptoms; stimulation of respiration in obstructive sleep apnea.

Contraindications Hypersensitivity to progestins; current or past history of thrombophlebitis, thromboembolic disorders, cerebrovascular disease or cerebral hemorrhage; impaired liver function; breast cancer; undiagnosed vaginal bleeding; missed abortion; diagnostic test for pregnancy.

Route/Dosage

Secondary Amenorrhea

ADULTS: **PO** 5-10 mg/day for 5-10 days.

Abnormal Uterine Bleeding

ADULTS: **PO** 5-10 mg/day for 5-10 days beginning on 16th or 21st day of menstrual cycle.

Contraceptive

ADULTS: **IM** 150 mg q 3 mo.

Endometrial or Renal Carcinoma

ADULTS: **IM** 400-1000 mg weekly initially; maintenance: 400 mg/mo.

Interactions *Aminoglutethamide:* May increase metabolism and decrease effect of medroxyprogesterone.

Lab Test Interferences Endocrine, coagulation (increased amounts of some clotting factors), thyroid and liver function test results may be affected by progestins;

may alter metyrapone test results; may decrease glucose tolerance.

Adverse Reactions

CV: Thrombophlebitis; edema. *RESP:* Pulmonary embolism. *CNS:* Depression; headache; nervousness; dizziness; insomnia; fatigue; somnolence. *GI:* Abdominal pain or discomfort; nausea. *GU:* Breakthrough bleeding; spotting; change in menstrual flow; amenorrhea; decrease in libido; changes in cervical erosion and secretions. *HEPA:* Cholestatic jaundice. *DERM:* Rash; acne; melasma; chloasma; alopecia; hirsutism; photosensitivity. *OTHER:* Breast tenderness; masculinization of female fetus; edema; weight changes, especially weight gain; anaphylactoid reactions; bone mineral density changes, increasing risk of osteoporosis; hyperglycemia.

Precautions

Pregnancy: Category X. *Lactation:* Excreted in breast milk. *Conception:* Has prolonged contraceptive effect, which may delay time to potential conception once therapy is discontinued. *Contraception:* If period between injections is > 14 days determine that patient is not pregnant before administering drug. *Fluid retention:* Use with careful observation when conditions that might be affected by this factor are present (eg, asthma, cardiac or renal dysfunction, epilepsy). *Mental depression:* Carefully observe patients with history of depression. *Ophthalmic effects:* Discontinue medication if there are any sudden changes in vision, sudden onset of proptosis, diplopia, migraine, papilledema or retinal vascular lesions.

NURSING CONSIDERATIONS

Administration/Storage

- Administer oral dose on same days of month as prescribed.
- Give medication with food if GI upset occurs.
- Parenteral dosage form is for IM administration only. Inject deeply into large muscle.
- Shake vial vigorously prior to IM administration.
- Rotate site of IM administration and observe for redness and warmth at injection site.
- When using contraceptive injection, give during first 5 days after onset of normal menstrual period or within 5 days postpartum if not breastfeeding or at 6 weeks postpartum if breast feeding.
- Store at room temperature.

Assessment/Interventions

- Obtain patient history, including drug history and any known allergies.
- Monitor serum glucose in patients with diabetes.
- Monitor results of liver function tests throughout therapy.
- Assess patient's weight daily. Notify physician of > 5 lb gain.
- Include breast and pelvic examination and Papanicolaou smear in pretherapy physical assessment.
- Assess BP at beginning of therapy and periodically during treatment.
- Assess fluid and respiratory status and notify physician of any changes.
- Notify physician of pain in calves accompanied by swelling, warmth and redness; sudden severe headache; visual disturbances; numbness in extremities; signs of depression; signs of liver dysfunction (eg, dark urine, jaundice).
- Monitor mental status: affect, mood, depression, behavioral changes.
- Monitor I&O.

Patient/Family Education

- Caution patient that this medication must not be taken during pregnancy or when pregnancy is possible. Advise patient to use reliable form of birth control while taking this drug.
- Advise patient to take tablets with food if GI upset occurs.

- Explain significance of irregular menstrual cycles, breakthrough bleeding or change in menstrual flow, and tell patient to notify physician of heavy or continuous menstrual flow.
- Caution patient to avoid prolonged exposure to sunlight and other sources of ultraviolet light and to use sunscreen and wear protective clothing to avoid photosensitivity reaction.
- Encourage patients with diabetes to monitor blood glucose more frequently until effect on diabetes control is determined.
- Tell patient to notify physician of pain in calves with swelling, warmth or redness; sudden severe headache; visual disturbances; numbness in extremities.
- Instruct patient to report these symptoms to physician: breast abnormalities, vaginal bleeding, edema, jaundice, dark urine, clay-colored stools, dyspnea, chest pain or suspected pregnancy.
- Remind patient using agent for contraception that doses must be administered every 3 mo to ensure effectiveness.

See Patient Guide, p. 381.

Mefenamic Acid

(MEH-fen-AM-ik acid)

Ponstel, ♣ *Ponstan*

Class: Analgesic/NSAID

Action Decreases inflammation, pain and fever, probably through inhibition of cyclooxygenase activity and prostaglandin synthesis.

Indications Relief of moderate pain lasting < 1 wk; treatment of primary dysmenorrhea. **Unlabeled uses:** Treatment of sunburn, migraine (acute attack), PMS.

Contraindications Patients in whom aspirin, iodides or any NSAID has caused allergic-type reactions; preexisting renal disease; active ulceration or chronic inflammation of GI tract.

Route/Dosage

Acute Pain

ADULTS & CHILDREN > 14 YR: **PO** 500 mg, followed by 250 mg q 6 hr prn. Usually not used longer than 1 wk.

Primary Dysmennorhea

ADULTS & CHILDREN > 14 YR: **PO** 500 mg, followed by 250 mg q 6 hr starting with onset of bleeding and associated symptoms.

Interactions

Anticoagulants: Increased risk of gastric erosion and bleeding. *Cyclosporine:* Nephrotoxicity of both agents may be increased. *Lithium:* Serum lithium levels may be increased. *Methotrexate:* Increased methotrexate levels. *Salicylates:* Additive GI toxicity.

Lab Test Interferences

May cause prolonged bleeding time or false-positive reaction for urinary bile using diazo tablet test.

Adverse Reactions

CV: Edema; weight gain; CHF; altered BP; palpitations; chest pain; bradycardia; tachycardia. *RESP:* Bronchospasm; laryngeal edema; rhinitis; dyspnea; pharyngitis; hemoptysis; shortness of breath. *CNS:* Headache; vertigo; drowsiness; dizziness; insomnia. *EENT:* Blurred vision; tinnitus; salivation; glossitis. *GI:* Diarrhea; dry mouth; vomiting; abdominal pain; dyspepsia; GI bleeding. *GU:* Hematuria; proteinuria; dysuria; renal failure. *HEMA:* Decreased hematocrit; bleeding; neutropenia; leukopenia; pancytopenia; eosinophilia; thrombocytopenia. *HEPA:* Mild elevations in liver function test results. *DERM:* Rash; urticaria; purpura. *OTHER:* Autoimmune hemolytic anemia may occur if used long term.

Precautions

Pregnancy: Category C. *Lactation:* Undetermined. *Children:* Not recommended for children < 14 yr. *Elderly:* Increased risk of adverse reactions. *Diarrhea:* If diarrhea occurs, reduce dosage or temporarily discontinue. *GI toxicity:* Bleeding, ulceration, or perforation can occur at any time, with or without warning symptoms. *Hypersensitivity:* May occur; use with caution in aspirin-sensitive individuals because of possible cross-sensitivity. *Rash:* Promptly discontinue if rash develops. *Renal effects:* Acute renal insufficiency, interstitial nephritis, hyperkalemia, hyponatremia and renal papillary necrosis may occur. *Renal impairment:* Lower doses may be necessary.

NURSING CONSIDERATIONS

Administration/Storage

- Administer with meals, followed by full glass of water or milk to avoid GI and esophageal irritation. May be given with antacids if stomach upset occurs.
- Store at room temperature in tightly closed, light-resistant container.

Assessment/Interventions

- Obtain patient history, including drug history and any known allergies. Note chronic alcohol use, fluid retention, nasal polyps, bronchospastic disease or hypersensitivity to aspirin or NSAIDs.
- Weigh patient daily if fluid retention is a concern.
- Monitor carefully for hypersensitivity. Note any ecchymosis or rash.
- Monitor renal and liver function and blood studies throughout treatment.
- Monitor for diarrhea or blood in stools. If diarrhea occurs, notify physician. Dosage may need to be reduced or drug temporarily withheld.
- Notify physician if stomach pain develops or continues.

OVERDOSAGE: SIGNS & SYMPTOMS

Acute renal failure, coma, grand mal seizures, muscle twitching

Patient/Family Education

- Inform patient not to use drug for more than 1 wk. If given for dysmenorrhea, instruct patient to begin taking drug with onset of bleeding and associated symptoms.
- Warn patient about potential for bleeding and advise to notify other health care professionals that drug is being taken.
- Advise patient to discontinue medication if rash develops and to contact physician.
- Instruct patient to report these symptoms to physician: rash, visual problems, dark stools, decreased urinary output, persistent headache or stomach pain and unusual bruising or bleeding.
- Advise patient to avoid intake of alcoholic beverages.
- Instruct patient that drug may cause drowsiness and to use caution while driving or performing other activities requiring mental alertness.
- Caution patient to avoid prolonged exposure to sunlight and to use sunscreen or wear protective clothing to avoid photosensitivity reaction.
- Instruct patient not to take otc medications, including aspirin and ibuprofen or other prescription drugs, without consulting physician.

See Patient Guide, p. 382.

Megestrol Acetate

(meh-JESS-trole ASS-uh-TATE)

Megace

Class: Progestin

Action Inhibits secretion of pituitary gonadotropins, thereby preventing follicular maturation and ovulation (contraceptive effect); inhibits spontaneous uterine contraction; transforms proliferative endometrium into secretory endometrium.

Indications Palliative treatment of advanced inoperable, recurrent or metastatic carcinoma of breast or endometrium. **Unlabeled use:** Appetite stimulation in HIV-related cachexia.

Contraindications Hypersensitivity to progestins; as diagnostic test for pregnancy.

Route/Dosage

Breast Cancer

ADULTS: **PO** 40 mg qid.

Endometrial Cancer

ADULTS: **PO** 40-320 mg/day in divided doses.

Cachexia

ADULTS: **PO** Usual dose: 160-320 mg/day. Up to 800 mg/day *or* 20 ml/day of suspension has been given.

Interactions None well documented.

Lab Test Interferences

Endocrine, coagulation (increased amounts of coagulation factors), thyroid and liver function test results may be affected by progestins; may alter metyrapone test results; may decrease glucose tolerance.

Adverse Reactions

CV: Hypertension; thromboembolic phenomena, including thrombophlebitis and pulmonary embolism. *RESP:* Dyspnea. *CNS:* Insomnia; fatigue. *GI:* Abdominal pain or discomfort; nausea; vomiting. *GU:* Breakthrough bleeding; change in menstrual flow; changes in cervical erosion and secretions; impotence. *HEPA:* Cholestatic jaundice. *DERM:* Rash; alopecia. *OTHER:* Breast tenderness; masculinization of female fetus; edema; weight changes; decreased libido; tumor flare; carpal tunnel syndrome.

Precautions

Pregnancy: Category X. *Lactation:* Excreted in breast milk. *Children:* Safety and efficacy not established. *Fluid retention:* Use with careful observation when conditions that might be affected by this factor are present (eg, asthma, cardiac or renal dysfunction, epilepsy). *Hepatic impairment:* Use drug with caution and with close monitoring in patients with liver dysfunction. *Mental depression:* Carefully observe patients with history of depression. *Ophthalmic effects:* Discontinue medication if there are any sudden changes in vision, sudden onset of proptosis, diplopia, migraine, papilledema or retinal vascular lesions. *Thromboembolic disease:* Use drug with caution in patients with history of thromboembolic disease.

NURSING CONSIDERATIONS

Administration/Storage

- Store in dry, cool place at room temperature.

Assessment/Interventions

- Obtain complete patient history, including drug history and any known allergies. Note history of thromboembolic disease.
- Assess results of baseline liver and thyroid tests and coagulation tests prior to initiation of therapy and routinely during therapy.
- Monitor blood glucose in patients with diabetes.
- Monitor patient's mental status: affect, mood, depression, behavioral changes.
- Notify physician if any of these symp-

toms occur: pain in calves accompanied by swelling, warmth and redness; severe sudden headache; visual disturbances; numbness in extremities; signs of depression; signs of liver dysfunction (eg, dark urine, jaundice); breakthrough bleeding.

Patient/Family Education

- Caution patient that this medication must not be taken during pregnancy or when pregnancy is possible. Advise patient to use reliable form of birth control while taking this drug.
- Explain potential significance of breakthrough bleeding, irregular menstrual cycles and possible lack of menstrual cycle. Tell patient to notify physician of heavy or continuous menstrual flow.
- Encourage patients with diabetes to monitor blood glucose more frequently until effect on diabetes control has been determined.
- Instruct patient to report these symptoms to physician: pain in calves of legs with redness, warmth and swelling; sudden severe headache; visual disturbances; numbness in extremities; dyspnea; chest pain; edema; jaundice; dark urine; clay-colored stools.
- Caution patient to avoid exposure to sunlight and other sources of ultraviolet light and to use sunscreen or wear protective clothing to avoid photosensitivity reaction.

See Patient Guide, p. 383.

Melphalan (L-PAM, Phenylalanine Mustard, L-Sarcolysin)

(MELL-fuh-lan)

Alkeran

Class: Antineoplastic/alkylating agent

Action Phenylalanine derivative of nitrogen mustard that acts as alkylating agent by cross-linking DNA and RNA strands and by protein synthesis inhibition.

Indications Palliative treatment of multiple myeloma; Hodgkin's lymphoma and nonresectable epithelial ovarian carcinoma. **Unlabeled uses:** Treatment of polycythemia vera, breast carcinoma, chronic myelogenous leukemia, testicular seminoma, osteogenic sarcoma, amyloidosis.

Contraindications Prior resistance to this drug.

Route/Dosage

Multiple Myeloma

ADULTS: **PO** 6 mg/day for 2-3 wk; discontinue drug for up to 4 wk, then institute maintenance dose of 2 mg/day on the basis of blood counts. **IV** 16 mg/m^2.

Ovarian Cancer

ADULTS: **PO** 0.2 mg/kg/day for 5 days. May repeat as infusion q 2 wk for 4 doses, then q 4 wk.

Interactions

Carmustine: Threshold for lung toxicity may be reduced. *Cyclosporine:* Severe renal failure may develop when high doses of melphalan and cyclosporine are used. *Nalidixic acid:* Increased incidence of hemorrhagic necrotic enterocolitis. INCOMPATIBILITIES: Amphotericin B, chlorpromazine.

Lab Test Interferences

None well documented.

Adverse Reactions

RESP: Pulmonary fibrosis; interstitial pneumonitis. *EENT:* Stomatitis. *GI:* Nausea; vomiting; diarrhea. *HEMA:* Bone marrow suppression; hemolytic anemia. *DERM:* Skin hypersensitivity; alopecia; ulcerative at injection site. *OTHER:* Vasculitis; allergic reaction; amenorrhea.

Precautions

Pregnancy: Category D. *Lacta-*

tion: Undetermined. *Children:* Safety and efficacy not established. *Special risk patients:* Use with caution in patients with prior radiation or chemotherapy or in renal impairment. Reduce dose up to 50% in renal impairment. *Bone marrow depression:* Most significant toxicity. Frequent blood counts are essential to determine optimum dosage and to avoid toxicity. *Carcinogenesis/mutagenesis:* Probably leukemogenic in humans. Secondary malignancies have occurred. *Hypersensitivity reactions:* Have occurred with IV form; may cause anaphylaxis. Usually occurs after multiple treatments.

NURSING CONSIDERATIONS

Administration/Storage

- Administer oral form with food to reduce nausea and vomiting.
- Administer under supervision of health care professional experienced in use of chemotherapeutic agents. Use caution when administering (eg, wear gloves when handling injectable form to prevent contact with drug).
- Reconstitute IV solution according to manufacturer's instructions with supplied diluent. Shake vigorously until solution is clear. Administer within 60 min of reconstitution.
- Administer IV solution as single infusion over 15-20 min.
- Dispense medication to patient in glass container.
- Store at room temperature and protect from light. Do not refrigerate reconstituted product.

Assessment/Interventions

- Obtain patient history, including drug history and any known allergies. Note any infectious processes.
- Ensure that baseline CBC and renal studies have been obtained before beginning therapy and monitor weekly.
- Monitor for fever, signs of local infection, ecchymosis, tarry stools, hematuria and unusual lumps or masses.
- Monitor serum uric acid levels.
- If IV solution comes in contact with skin or mucosa, wash immediately and thoroughly with soap and water.

OVERDOSAGE: SIGNS & SYMPTOMS

Immediate signs: vomiting, mouth ulcerations, diarrhea and GI hemorrhage. Major effect involves bone marrow suppression.

Patient/Family Education

- Advise patient to take oral form with food to reduce nausea and vomiting.
- Encourage patient to increase fluid intake, if not contraindicated.
- Instruct patient to use soft toothbrush and electric razor and to avoid vigorous flossing.
- Caution patient to avoid crowds and potentially infectious individuals if WBC decreases.
- Instruct patient to consult with physician before receiving immunizations.
- Advise patient to notify dentist or physician of drug regimen before surgical or dental procedures.
- Explain that follow-up blood tests will be scheduled to monitor drug effects.
- Advise patient that temporary hair loss or changes in hair texture or color may occur. Discuss possible coping strategies and use of scarves or wigs.
- Inform female patient that menstrual periods may cease or become irregular.
- Instruct patient to check mucous membranes for signs of inflammation and ulceration. Discuss importance of oral hygiene in prevention of stomatitis.
- Advise patient to report these symptoms to physician: sore throat; chills; nausea; vomiting; increased bruising or bleeding; dark stools or urine; flank, abdominal or joint pain; weight loss; skin rash; presence of unusual lumps or masses.
- Instruct patient not to take otc medications (eg, aspirin, ibuprofen) without consulting physician.

See Patient Guide, p. 384.

Meperidine HCl

(meh-PEHR-ih-deen HIGH-droe-KLOR-ide)
Demerol HCl
Class: Narcotic analgesic

Action Relieves pain by stimulating opiate receptors in CNS; also causes respiratory depression, peripheral vasodilation, inhibition of intestinal peristalsis, sphincter of Oddi spasm, stimulation of chemoreceptors that cause vomiting and increased bladder tone.

Indications
Oral and parenteral: Relief of moderate to severe pain. *Parenteral:* Preoperative sedation; support of anesthesia; obstetrical analgesia.

Contraindications Upper airway obstruction; acute asthma; diarrhea due to poisoning or toxins; patients who are receiving or have received MAO inhibitor within last 14 days.

Route/Dosage
Pain
ADULTS: **IM/SC/PO** 50-150 mg q 3-4 hr prn. If IV administration is required, reduce dose and administer slowly. CHILDREN: **IM/SC/PO** 1-1.8 mg/kg (up to adult dose) q 3-4 hr prn.

Preoperative Sedation
ADULTS: **IM/SC** 50-100 mg 30-90 min before anesthetic.

Support of Anesthesia
ADULTS: **IV** Repeated doses diluted to 10 mg/ml by slow injection or by continuous infusion diluted to 1 mg/ml.

Obstetrical Analgesia
ADULTS: **IM/SC** 50-100 mg q 1-3 hr prn when pains become regular.

Interactions
CNS depressants (eg, tranquilizers, sedatives, alcohol): Additive CNS depression. *MAO inhibitors, furazolidone:* Potentially fatal reactions can occur if meperidine is used in patients within 14 days of receiving MAO inhibitor or furazolidone. *Phenothiazines:* Excessive sedation and hypotension. INCOMPATIBILITIES: Do not co-infuse with solutions of soluble barbiturates, aminophylline, heparin, morphine, methicillin, phenytoin, sodium bicarbonate, iodine, sulfadiazine and sulfisoxazole.

Lab Test Interferences
Increased amylase and lipase may occur up to 24 hr after dose.

Adverse Reactions
CV: Hypotension; orthostatic hypotension; bradycardia; tachycardia. *RESP:* Respiratory depression; laryngospasm; depression of cough reflex. *CNS:* Lightheadedness; dizziness; sedation; disorientation; incoordination; seizures. *GI:* Nausea; vomiting; constipation; abdominal pain. *GU:* Urinary retention or hesitancy. *DERM:* Sweating; pruritus; urticaria.

Precautions
Pregnancy: Pregnancy category undetermined. Safety not established. *Lactation:* Excreted in breast milk. *Special risk patients:* Use with caution in patients with myxedema, acute alcoholism, acute abdominal conditions, ulcerative colitis, decreased respiratory reserve, head injury or increased intracranial pressure, hypoxia, supraventricular tachycardia, depleted blood volume, circulatory shock or renal dysfunction. *Drug dependence.* Tolerance and psychological and physical dependence may occur with chronic use. *Hepatic or renal impairment:* Dosage reduction may be necessary. *Neurotoxicity:* Can cause dysphoria, hallucinations and seizures in patients with renal impairment or with chronic high-dose therapy. *Sulfite sensitivity:* Some parenteral products contain sulfites; may

cause allergic-type reactions in susceptible individuals.

NURSING CONSIDERATIONS

Administration/Storage

- Administer as soon as pain occurs or prophylactically 30 min before painful procedures. Effect is reduced as pain severity increases.
- Administer meperidine syrup with half glass of water to avoid anesthetizing oral mucous membranes.
- Give oral preparations with food if stomach upset occurs.
- IM administration is preferred for repeated doses.
- Prepare IV injection or solution by diluting in 5% Dextrose and Lactated Ringer's; Dextrose-Saline combinations; 2.5%, 5%, or 10% Dextrose in Water; Lactated Ringer's or Ringer's; 0.45% or 0.9% Sodium Chloride; or ⅙ Molar Sodium Lactate.
- Administer direct IV over at least 3 min.
- Place patient in reclining position and institute safety measures before administering parenteral medication.
- Do not administer if solution is cloudy or if precipitate is present.
- Do not administer IV solution if antidote is not readily available.
- Store at room temperature in tightly closed, light-resistant container.

Assessment/Interventions

- Obtain patient history, including drug history and any known allergies.
- Reduce environmental stimuli and provide maximum comfort measures before administration.
- Obtain vital signs before administration. If respirations are diminished (or 12 breaths/min), withhold medication and notify physician.
- Reassess vital signs 30 min after administration (5-10 min after direct IV administration).
- Assess bowel and bladder function regularly in patients receiving repeated dosages.
- Encourage coughing and deep breathing exercises q 2 hr while awake.

OVERDOSAGE: SIGNS & SYMPTOMS

Miosis, respiratory and CNS depression, circulatory collapse, seizures, cardiopulmonary arrest, death

Patient/Family Education

- Instruct patient that if dose is missed, it should be taken as soon as possible unless close to time of next dose. Do not double up doses.
- If medication is given long term, explain that dosage will be tapered gradually before stopping to prevent withdrawal symptoms.
- Instruct patient not to wait until pain level is high to self-medicate, because drug will not be as effective.
- Encourage increased fluid intake and moderate exercise to prevent constipation. Stool softeners or fiber laxative may also be used.
- Advise patient to use humidifier to liquefy secretions. Teach deep breathing exercises.
- Instruct patient to avoid sudden position changes to avoid orthostatic hypotension.
- Tell patient to avoid intake of alcoholic beverages or other CNS depressants (eg, sleeping pills, antihistamines).
- Advise patient that drug may cause drowsiness and to use caution while driving or performing other tasks requiring mental alertness.

See Patient Guide, p. 385.

Mephentermine Sulfate

(meh-FEN-ter-meen SULL-fate)

Wyamine Sulfate

Class: Vasopressor

Action Acts directly and indirectly (via release of norepinephrine) on beta and alpha receptors, causing increase in cardiac contraction and, to lesser degree, increase in peripheral vasoconstriction.

Indications Treatment of hypotension secondary to ganglionic blockade and to spinal anesthesia; maintenance of blood pressure until blood or blood substitutes may be administered during hypovolemic shock.

Contraindications Hypotension induced by chlorpromazine; use of MAO inhibitors.

Route/Dosage

Shock and Hypotension

ADULTS: **IM** 0.5 mg/kg undiluted. **IV** 1 mg/ml solution in D5W titrated to clinical response.

Hypotension Following Spinal Anesthesia

ADULTS: **IV** 30-45 mg; repeat doses of 30 mg prn; or give as 1 mg/ml infusion in D5W titrated to clinical response.

Prevention of Hypotension Following Spinal Anesthesia

ADULTS: **IM** 30-45 mg 10-20 min prior to anesthesia, operation or termination of operative procedure.

Hypotension Secondary to Spinal Anesthesia During Cesarean Section

ADULTS: **IV** 15 mg; repeat prn.

Hemorrhagic Shock

ADULTS: **IV** Continuous infusion of 1 mg/ml solution in D5W until whole blood replacement can be accomplished.

Interactions

Guanethidine: Antihypertensive effects of guanethidine may be negated. *Halogenated hydrocarbon anesthetics:* May sensitize myocardium to arrhythmogenic effects of catecholamines. MAO *inhibitors, furazolidone, rauwolfia alkaloids, methyldopa:* May significantly increase pressor response, possibly resulting in hypertensive crisis and intracranial hemorrhage. *Oxytoxic drugs:* Synergistic or additive vasoconstrictive effects may occur, resulting in hypertension and possible gangrene in the extremities. *Tricyclic antidepressants:* May decrease pressor response.

Lab Test Interferences

None well documented.

Adverse Reactions

CV: Cardiac arrhythmias; excessive hypertension, especially in patients with heart disease. *CNS:* Anxiety; seizures.

Precautions

Pregnancy: Category C. *Lactation:* Undetermined. *Cardiovascular effects:* May be profound. Use with caution in chronically ill patients and patients with known cardiovascular disease or hyperthyroidism. *Hypovolemia:* Avoid in patients with uncorrected hypovolemia. Persistent hypotension may indicate hypovolemia.

NURSING CONSIDERATIONS

Administration/Storage

- If solution is discolored, do not use; discard.
- IV solution can be prepared by adding 10 or 20 ml of 30 mg/ml mephentermine to 250 ml or 500 ml of D5W, respectively.
- Store reconstituted solution no longer than 24 hr.

Assessment/Interventions

- Obtain patient history, including drug history and any known allergies.
- Use electronic infusion device for IV administration.

- Monitor I&O. If urinary output is < 30 ml/hr, notify physician.
- Monitor BP during IV administration and every 5 min after IM administration.

OVERDOSAGE: SIGNS & SYMPTOMS

Hypertension, cardiac arrhythmias, seizures

Patient/Family Education

- Instruct patient and family to notify physician if any otc cold or allergy preparation has been used within 3 days of surgery.
- Inform physician of use of MAO inhibitors or tricyclic antidepressants within 1 mo of surgery.

No patient monograph available.

Meprobamate

(meh-pro-BAM-ate)

Equanil, Meprospan, Miltown

Class: Antianxiety

Action Produces CNS depressant action at multiple sites, including thalamic and limbic systems.

Indications Management of anxiety. **Unlabeled use:** Sedative-hypnotic.

Contraindications Hypersensitivity to meprobamate or related compounds, such as carisoprodol; acute intermittent porphyria.

Route/Dosage

ADULTS: Tablets: **PO** 1.2-1.6 g/day in 3-4 divided doses. Sustained release capsules: **PO** 400-800 mg bid. CHILDREN 6-12 YR: Tablets: **PO** 100-200 mg bid-tid. Sustained release capsules: **PO** 200 mg bid.

Interactions

Alcohol, CNS depressants: May produce additive CNS depression.

Lab Test Interferences

None well documented.

Adverse Reactions

CV: Palpitations; tachycardia; syncope; hypertension; hypotensive crisis; arrhythmias. *CNS:* Drowsiness; ataxia; euphoria; slurred speech; dizziness; headache; paradoxical excitement. *GI:* Nausea; vomiting; diarrhea. *HEMA:* Leukopenia; thrombocytopenia; agranulocytosis; aplastic anemia. *OTHER:* Hypersensitivity (eg, rash, itching, fever, chills, edema, bronchospasm, anaphylaxis, erythema multiforme, exfoliative dermatitis, Stevens-Johnson syndrome, bullous dermatitis); exacerbation of porphyria symptoms.

Precautions

Pregnancy: Category D. Use with extreme caution, if at all. *Lactation:* Excreted in breast milk. *Children:* Do not give to children < 6 yr; safety and efficacy not established. Do not give 600 mg tablet to children. *Dependence:* Physical and psychological dependence and abuse may occur. Avoid prolonged use, especially in patients prone to addiction. Abrupt discontinuation after prolonged or excessive use may precipitate withdrawal symptoms with risk of seizures. *Elderly or debilitated patients:* Use lowest effective dose to avoid oversedation. *Hypersensitivity:* Usually seen between first and fourth dose in patients without previous exposure. *Renal or hepatic impairment:* Use drug with caution to avoid accumulation.

NURSING CONSIDERATIONS

Administration/Storage

- Do not alter medication form prior to administration.
- Store in dry, cool place.

Assessment/Interventions

- Obtain patient history, including drug history and any known allergies.
- Monitor results of liver and renal function tests throughout therapy.

- Watch patient take medication to ensure that it is swallowed.
- Notify physician if tachycardia, syncope or palpitations occur.
- Monitor blood studies and CBC during long-term therapy.
- Notify physician if patient experiences signs of hypersensitivity and withhold drug.
- Assess for signs of drowsiness, ataxia, lethargy, itching, rash or stupor and report findings to physician.
- Assist patient with ambulation during beginning of therapy.
- Institute safety measures (eg, siderails).
- Monitor mental status: mood, sensorium, affect, sleeping patterns.
- Monitor pulse and lying and standing BP; if BP is < 20 mm Hg, withhold drug and notify physician.

OVERDOSAGE: SIGNS & SYMPTOMS

Drowsiness, lethargy, stupor, ataxia, coma, shock, vasomotor and respiratory collapse, death

Patient/Family Education

- Instruct patient not to crush or chew tablets or capsules.
- Advise patient that drug may cause drowsiness and to use caution while driving or performing other tasks requiring mental alertness.
- Instruct patient to avoid intake of alcoholic beverages or other CNS depressants.
- Explain potential side effects, and encourage patient to notify physician if signs of itching, rash, fever, drowsiness, dizziness, difficulty walking, nausea, vomiting, diarrhea, palpitations, shortness of breath or sore throat occur.
- Caution patient to change position slowly to minimize orthostatic hypotension.
- Caution patient not to discontinue taking drug abruptly since doing so may precipitate pre-existing symptoms or withdrawal reactions.
- Advise female patients that if they become pregnant or intend to become pregnant to consult their physician about continued use of this drug.

See Patient Guide, p. 386.

Mercaptopurine (6-Mercaptopurine; 6-MP)

(mer-cap-toe-PURE-een)

Purinethol

Class: Antineoplastic/antimetabolite

Action Mercaptopurine (6-MP) competes directly with hydroxyxanthine and guanine for enzyme hypoxanthine-guanine phosphoribosyltransferase and is converted into active metabolites, which inhibit inosinic acid and de novo ribonucleoside synthesis.

Indications Remission induction and maintenance therapy of acute lymphatic (lymphocytic, lymphoblastic) leukemia in children and adults; induction of remission in acute myelogenous (and acute myelomonocytic) leukemia.

Contraindications Prior resistance to this drug or thioguanine. 6-MP is not effective for prophylaxis or treatment of CNS leukemia, chronic lymphatic leukemia, lymphomas (including Hodgkin's disease) or solid tumors.

Route/Dosage

Induction Therapy

ADULTS & CHILDREN: PO 2.5 mg/kg/day for several wk. May increase to 5 mg/kg/day after 4 wk. Maintenance: PO 1.5-2.5 mg/kg/day.

Interactions

Allopurinol: Enhanced toxicity of mercaptopurine. Dose of mercaptopurine must be reduced to 25%-33% of usual dose. *Nondepolarizing muscle relaxants:* Effects of these agents may be reduced or reversed.

Lab Test Interferences

None well documented.

Adverse Reactions

GI: Ulceration; nausea; vomiting; anorexia; diarrhea; stomatitis; sprue-like symptoms. *HEMA:* Bone marrow suppression; marrow hypoplasia; leukopenia; granulocytopenia; thrombocytopenia; anemia. *HEPA:* Hepatomegaly; jaundice; ascites; toxic hepatitis; cholestasis; biliary stasis; hepatic necrosis. *DERM:* Skin rash; hyperpigmentation. *OTHER:* Hyperuricemia; drug fever; weakness; oral thrush-like lesions.

Precautions

Pregnancy: Category D. *Lactation:* Undetermined. *Bone marrow depression:* Most consistent dose-related toxicity. *Crohn's disease:* Pancreatitis may occur when drug is used in treatment of Crohn's disease. *Hepatotoxicity:* Usually occurs when recommended doses are exceeded. Deaths have occurred from hepatic necrosis. Use drug with caution in patients given other hepatotoxic drugs (eg, doxorubicin) or those with known preexisting liver disease. Withhold drug if liver toxicity is suspected. *Immunosuppression:* May be manifested by decreased cellular hypersensitivities, impaired allograph rejection or lower immunity to infection or vaccine response. *Renal impairment:* Start with lower doses.

NURSING CONSIDERATIONS

Administration/Storage

- Total daily dose may be given at one time.
- Reduce dose by 66%-75% when given together with allopurinol.
- Store at room temperature in tightly closed light-resistant container.

Assessment/Interventions

- Obtain patient history, including drug history and any known allergies. Note hepatic impairment or use of other hepatotoxic drugs.
- Ensure that baseline CBC, chemistry, platelets, liver, renal and urinalysis studies have been performed before beginning therapy and monitor weekly.
- If abnormally large or rapid decrease in leukocyte or platelet count occurs, withhold drug, notify physician and protect patient from exposure to infection, stress and trauma.
- Monitor for fever, signs of local infection, ecchymosis, tarry stools, hematuria, edema, bleeding gums and petechiae.
- Monitor I&O and daily weight.
- Observe for jaundice, which indicates hepatotoxicity. Monitor liver function test results weekly when initiating treatment and monthly thereafter.

OVERDOSAGE: SIGNS & SYMPTOMS

Anorexia, nausea, vomiting, diarrhea (may be immediate), myelosuppression, liver or GI disturbance (may be delayed)

Patient/Family Education

- Encourage patient to increase fluid intake, if not contraindicated, to limit hyperuricemia.
- Instruct patient to check mucous membranes for signs of inflammation and ulceration. Discuss importance of oral hygiene in prevention of stomatitis.
- Instruct patient to use soft toothbrush and electric razor and to avoid vigorous flossing.
- Explain that diarrhea, fever and weakness are common side effects, but to notify physician if these become persistent problems.
- Instruct patient to report these symptoms to physician: sore throat; chills; nausea; vomiting; increased bruising or bleeding; dark stools or urine; flank, abdominal or joint pain; and yellow discoloration of skin or eyes.

- Caution patient to avoid crowds and potentially infectious individuals.
- Tell patient to avoid any immunizations.
- Instruct patient to notify dentist or physician of drug regimen before surgical or dental procedures.
- Instruct patient not to take otc medications (eg, aspirin, ibuprofen) without consulting physician.
- Explain that follow-up blood tests will be scheduled to monitor drug effects.

See Patient Guide, p. 387.

Mesalamine (5-aminosalicylic acid, 5-ASA)

(me-SAL-uh-MEEN)

Asacol, Pentasa, Rowasa

Class: Intestinal anti-inflammatory/aminosalicylic acid derivative

Action Reduces inflammation of colon topically by preventing production of substances involved in inflammatory process such as arachidonic acid.

Indications Treatment of active, mild to moderate distal ulcerative colitis, proctosigmoiditis or proctitis. **Unlabeled use:** Treatment of Crohn's disease.

Contraindications Hypersensitivity to salicylates.

Route/Dosage

ADULTS: Controlled release tablets or capsules: **PO** 800 mg tid for total of 2.4 g/day for 6 wk. Suppositories: **PR** 500 mg suppository bid for up to 6 wk. Retain suppository in rectum for 1-3 hr or more to achieve maximum benefit. Suspension enema: **PR** 4 g in 60 ml as rectal instillation q day for up to 6 wk, preferably at bedtime, retained for 8 hr.

Interactions None well documented.

Lab Test Interferences

May cause transient asymptomatic elevations in liver function test results (AST, ALT, alkaline phosphatase) and serum creatinine. Hepatitis is rare.

Adverse Reactions

CV: Chest pain. *RESP:* Cough. *CNS:* Headache; asthenia; chills; dizziness; fever; sweating; malaise. *EENT:* Rhinitis; sore throat; pharyngitis. *GI:* Abdominal pain; cramps; discomfort; colitis exacerbation; constipation; diarrhea; dyspepsia; vomiting; flatulence; nausea; eructation; rectal pain; soreness; burning. *DERM:* Acne; itching; rash. *OTHER:* Arthralgia; back pain; hypertonia; myalgia; dysmenorrhea; edema; flu syndrome; pain.

Precautions

Pregnancy: Category B. *Lactation:* Excreted in breast milk. *Children:* Safety and efficacy not established. *Intolerance and colitis exacerbation:* Some patients develop acute intolerance syndrome or exacerbation of colitis characterized by cramping, acute abdominal pain and bloody diarrhea, and occasionally fever, headache, malaise, pruritus, conjunctivitis and rash. Symptoms generally abate when mesalamine is discontinued. *Pericarditis:* Rarely, pericarditis has been reported. Observe for chest pain or dyspnea. *Pyloric stenosis:* Gastric retention of oral mesalamine may occur in patients with pyloric stenosis. *Renal impairment:* Patients with history of renal disease or dysfunction may have worsening of renal function. *Sulfite sensitivity:* Some products may contain sulfites, which may cause allergic reactions in susceptible individuals.

NURSING CONSIDERATIONS

Administration/Storage

- Instruct patient to swallow tablets or capsules whole.
- Do not alter form of medication prior to administration.
- Shake suspension well and position patient in knee-chest position or on left side with lower leg extended and upper right leg flexed for administration.
- Be certain that suppositories are retained for 1-3 hr and enemas retained for about 8 hr (preferably at bedtime) to achieve maximum effectiveness.
- Full course of therapy may last up to 6 wk and patient response may occur within 3-12 days.
- Store at room temperature.

Assessment/Interventions

- Obtain patient history, including drug history and any known allergies.
- Monitor results of renal function tests throughout therapy.
- Assess for increased abdominal pain, nausea, diarrhea and vomiting and notify physician of any problems.
- Document character and frequency of stools.

Patient/Family Education

- Tell patient to swallow capsules or tablets whole. Explain that outer coating must be intact to pass through stomach and travel to sigmoid colon.
- Tell patient to notify physician if any remnant of capsule or tablet is seen in stool.
- Tell patient to retain suppository 1-3 hr or to retain enema for 8 hr.
- Teach patient proper positioning and technique for self-administering enema. Include knee-chest and left side positions to promote medication advancement to sigmoid colon.
- Tell patient to report these symptoms to physician: increase in abdominal pain, diarrhea or vomiting.
- Instruct patient to notify physician of hives, itching, wheezing, rash or fever.

See Patient Guide, p. 388.

Metaproterenol Sulfate

(MEH-tuh-pro-TEHR-uh-nahl SULL-fate)

Alupent, Arm-a-Med Metaproterenol, Metaprel

Class: Bronchodilator/sympathomimetic

Action Relaxes bronchial smooth muscle through beta-2 receptor stimulation.

Indications Treatment of bronchial asthma and reversible bronchospasm associated with bronchitis and emphysema; control of acute asthma attacks in children ≥ 6 yr (inhalation solution only).

Contraindications Cardiac arrhythmias associated with tachycardia.

Route/Dosage

ADULTS & CHILDREN ≥ 12 YR: Metered dose inhaler: **Inhalation** 2-3 inhalations q 3-4 hr, not to exceed 12 inhalations/day. Hand nebulizer: **Inhalation** 5-15 inhalations q 4 hr prn. Intermittent positive pressure breathing apparatus: **Inhalation** 0.2-0.3 ml of 5% solution in 2.5 ml of diluent q 4 hrs prn. ADULTS & CHILDREN > 9 YR OR > 60 LB: **PO** 20 mg tid-qid. CHILDREN 6-9 YR OR < 60 LB: **PO** 10 mg tid-qid. CHILDREN < 6 YR: **PO** 1.3-2.6 mg/kg/day of syrup in divided doses.

Interactions

MAO inhibitors, tricyclic antidepressants: Pressor effects may be potentiated.

Lab Test Interferences

None well documented.

Adverse Reactions

CV: Palpitations; hypertension; tachycardia; cardiac arrest. *RESP:* Cough; asthma exacerbation. *CNS:* Tremor; dizziness; nervousness; weakness; headache. *EENT:* Throat irritation. *GI:* GI distress; nausea; vomiting. *DERM:* Rash.

Precautions

Pregnancy: Category C. *Lactation:* Undetermined. *Elderly patients:* Lower doses may be required. *CNS effects:* CNS stimulation may occur; use drug with caution in patients with history of seizures or hyperthyroidism. *Cardiovascular disorders:* Toxic symptoms may occur. *Diabetes mellitus:* Dosage adjustment of insulin or oral hypoglycemic agent may be required. *Excessive use:* Paradoxical bronchospasm and cardiac arrest have been associated with excessive inhalant use. *Labor and delivery:* May inhibit uterine contractions and delay preterm labor. *Tolerance:* May occur.

NURSING CONSIDERATIONS

Administration/Storage

- Oral form may be given with food to minimize GI upset.
- Shake metered-dose inhaler prior to administration. To administer, instruct patient to exhale through nose as completely as possible; tilt head back, and put inhaler mouthpiece between lips or 2 inches from open mouth. Tell patient to inhale slowly, press down on cannister, hold breath at least 10 sec or as long as comfortable, then exhale slowly.
- Pressurized inhalation should be administered during second half of inspiration to achieve better distribution of medication. Instruct patient to wait at least 1 full min between inhalations and to give second inhalation at 10 min.
- Store metered-dose inhaler in pressurized container at room temperature; do not freeze. Keep away from extreme heat. Do not use near open flame or discard in incinerator.
- Refrigerate unit dose nebulizer vials at 35 to 46°F. Protect from excessive heat and light.

Assessment/Interventions

- Obtain patient history, including drug history and any known allergies.
- Review baseline ECG for cardiac dyrhythmias associated with tachycardia.
- Obtain baseline blood values and monitor during therapy. Notify physician of abnormal results.
- Take vital signs before, during and after treatment, noting elevations in BP and pulse. If tachycardia, cardiac arrhythmia or chest pain are present, withhold medication and notify physician immediately.
- Assess baseline respiratory function, vital capacity and forced expiratory volume.
- Auscultate lung sounds before and after treatment. If increase in extra sounds, notify physician.
- Observe for signs of tremors and anxiety. If present, discontinue therapy and notify physician.
- Have epinephrine 1:1000 available for immediate or delayed hypersensitivity reaction.

OVERDOSAGE: SIGNS & SYMPTOMS

Tremor, palpitations, angina, arrhythmias, tachycardia, elevated or decreased BP, seizures, nervousness, headache, dry mouth, nausea, dizziness, fatigue, malaise, insomnia

Patient/Family Education

- Ask patient to demonstrate correct use of inhaler. It may be necessary to repeat instructions and demonstrations more than once.
- Instruct patient that if more than 1 inhalation is necessary, to wait 10 min between doses.

- Instruct patient to wash and dry inhaler every day in warm water.
- Explain that tolerance may occur with prolonged use, but temporary cessation of drug usually restores its original effectiveness. Instruct patient to notify physician if medication is ineffective.
- Warn patient to avoid excessive use (not more than q 4 hr), which can lead to side effects or loss of effectiveness.
- Advise patient to increase fluid intake to liquefy secretions.
- Instruct patient to report these symptoms to physician: palpitations, nervousness, dizziness, shortness of breath, rash, or asthma exacerbation.
- Caution patient to avoid getting aerosol medication in eyes.
- Advise patient to avoid smoke-filled rooms and smoking.
- Instruct patient not to take otc medications without consulting physician.

See Patient Guide, p. 389.

Metaraminol

(met-uh-RAM-in-ole)
Aramine
Class: Vasopressor

Action Acts directly on alpha receptors, causing peripheral vasoconstriction. Increase in systolic, diastolic blood and pulmonary pressure results, as does increase in cardiac output.

Indications Prevention and treatment of acute hypotensive state occurring with spinal anesthesia; adjunctive treatment of hypotension due to hemorrhage, reactions to medications, surgical complications and shock associated with brain damage due to trauma or tumor. Probably effective as adjunct in hypotension due to cardiogenic shock or septicemia.

Contraindications Use with cyclopropane or halothane anesthesia unless essential.

Route/Dosage

Prevention of Hypotension

ADULTS: **SC/IM** 2-10 mg; wait at least 10 min before readministering. CHILDREN: **SC/IM** 0.1 mg/kg.

Treatment of Hypotension

ADULTS: **IV** 15-100 mg in 250-500 ml of normal saline or D5W; adjust rate to response; may concentrate further in fluid-restricted states. CHILDREN: **SC/IM** 0.1 mg/kg.

Treatment of Severe Shock

ADULTS: **IV push** 0.5-5 mg followed by infusion of 15-100 mg in 500 ml of normal saline or D5W. CHILDREN: **IV** 0.01 mg/kg as single dose or via infusion of 1 mg/25 ml in normal saline or D5W.

Interactions *Guanethidine:* Antihypertensive effects of guanethidine may be negated. *MAO inhibitors, furazolidone, rauwolfia alkaloids, methyldopa:* May significantly increase pressor response, possibly resulting in hypertensive crisis and intracranial hemorrhage. *Tricyclic antidepressants:* May decrease pressor response. INCOMPATIBILITIES: Metaraminol is incompatible with many drugs; consult reference prior to admixture.

Lab Test Interferences None well documented.

Adverse Reactions *CV:* Sinus or ventricular tachycardia or other arrhythmias, especially in predisposed patients; hypertension or hypotension following cessation of drug; cardiac arrest; palpitations; flushing. *CNS:* Headaches; dizziness; apprehension. *GI:* Nausea. *OTHER:* Sweating; abscess formation; tissue necrosis; sloughing at injection site.

Precautions *Pregnancy:* Category C. *Lactation:* Undetermined. *Extravasation:* Avoid by infusing into large vein and monitoring carefully. *Sulfite sensitivity:* Use caution in sulfite-sensitive individuals; some preparations contain sodium bisulfite.

NURSING CONSIDERATIONS

Administration/Storage

- Dilute in normal saline or D5W. Use large veins to decrease irritation and/or tissue necrosis at parenteral administration sites. If given directly IV, follow with infusion to decrease possibility of necrosis.
- After administration, observe patient for effects before repeating dose. Pressor effects occur 1-2 min after IV dose, 10 min after IM dose, and 5-20 min after SC dose.
- Avoid IM injection to prevent tissue sloughing at injection site.
- Use infusion solutions within 24 hrs of mixing.
- Avoid exposing drug to excessive heat. Protect from light.

Assessment/Interventions

- Obtain patient history, including drug history and any known allergies.
- Monitor cardiac status, BP, pulse and respiration rate frequently, especially with IV administration. Fall in BP may occur with repeated use of metaraminol. Check BP every 5 min until stabilized and then check every 5 min throughout therapy.
- Notify physician if significant changes or arrhythmias occur.
- Monitor I&O.
- Monitor patient for sympathomimetic side effects such as: dizziness, headaches, restlessness, faintness, anxiety, flushing and apprehension.
- Monitor for hypertensive crisis and intracranial hemorrhage if given with MAO inhibitors, furazolidone, rauwolfia alkaloids and methyldopa.
- Observe for metabolic acidosis with prolonged use.
- When infusion is to be discontinued, gradually reduce flow rate.
- Document any side effects or adverse reactions, including arrhythmias, hypertension or hypotension after stopping drug, cardiac arrest and nausea.

OVERDOSAGE: SIGNS & SYMPTOMS

Convulsions, severe hypertension, cerebral hemorrhage, cardiac arrhythmias, headache, constricting sensation in chest, nausea, vomiting, euphoria, sweating, pulmonary edema, MI, cardiac arrest, convulsions

Patient/Family Education

- Alert patient to the possible problems of extravasation. Instruct patient to report symptoms such as paresthesia, respiratory distress, chest pain, palpitations or irritation or pain at injection site.
- Educate patient and family regarding sympathomimetic side effects.

No patient monograph available.

Metformin Hydrochloride

(met-FORE-min HIGH-droe-KLOR-ide)

Glucophage

Class: Antidiabetic/biguanide

Action Decreases blood glucose by decreasing hepatic glucose production. May also decrease intestinal absorption of glucose and increase response to insulin.

Indications Adjunct to diet to lower blood glucose in patients with noninsulin-dependent diabetes mellitus (type II) whose hyperglycemia cannot be controlled by diet alone.

Contraindications Renal disease or dysfunction as suggested by serum creatinine > 1.5 mg/dl in males or > 1.4 mg/dl in females or abnormal creatinine clearance; conditions which predispose to renal dysfunction (eg, cardiovascular collapse, acute MI or septicemia); in patients undergoing radiologic studies involving parenteral administration of iodinated contrast material (potential to acutely alter renal function); acute or chronic metabolic acidosis, including diabetic ketoacidosis.

Route/Dosage

Metformin 500 mg

ADULTS: **PO** 500 mg bid initially, increase by 500 mg q wk (maximum 2500 mg/day in divided doses).

Metformin 850 mg

ADULTS: **PO** 850 mg qd initially, increase by 850 mg q 2 weeks (maximum 2550 mg/day in divided doses).

Interactions

Alcohol: Potentiates effect of metformin on lactate metabolism. *Cationic drugs (eg, amiloride, digoxin, quinidine, etc):* May increase metformin serum concentration by competing for tubular secretion. *Cimetidine:* Increases metformin serum concentration. *Furosemide:* May increase metformin serum concentration; metformin may reduce furosemide serum concentration. *Iodinated contrast material:* May cause acute renal failure and has been associated with lactic acidosis in patients receiving metformin. *Nifedipine:* Increases metformin serum concentration.

Lab Test Interferences

None well documented.

Adverse Reactions

EENT: Unpleasant/metallic taste. *GI:* Diarrhea; nausea; vomiting; abdominal bloating; flatulence; anorexia. *META:* Lactic acidosis. *OTHER:* Subnormal vitamin B_{12} levels.

Precautions

Pregnancy: Category B. Insulin is recommended to maintain blood glucose levels during pregnancy. *Lactation:* Undetermined. *Children:* Safety and efficacy not established. *Elderly:* Use with caution. Maximum doses are generally not used because of age-related decreases in renal function. *Lactic acidosis:* Can occur as a result of metformin accumulation (eg, renal impairment) or in association with pathophysiologic conditions associated with tissue hypoperfusion and hypoxia. The risk of lactic acidosis increases with the degree of renal dysfunction and the patient's age. *Renal impairment:* Decreased renal function results in decreased renal clearance and prolongation of the metformin half-life. Concomitant medications that affect renal function, result in significant hemodynamic changes or interfere with disposition of metformin (eg, cationic drugs eliminated by renal tubular secretion) should be used with caution. *Hepatic disease:* Avoid metformin in patients with clinical or laboratory evidence of hepatic disease. *GI symptoms:* GI symptoms occurring after a patient is stabilized on metformin are unlikely to be drug related but could be due to lactic acidosis or other serious disease. *Iodinated contrast material:* Withhold metformin for at least 48 hours before parenteral contrast studies with iodinated materials. Reinstitute therapy 48 hours after the study and after renal function has been determined to be normal.

NURSING CONSIDERATIONS

Administration/Storage

- Administer in divided doses with meals starting with a low dose with gradual escalation of dose.
- Dosage of metformin should be individualized on basis of effectiveness and tolerance.
- Ensure determination of fasting plasma level prior to initial dose to ascertain therapeutic response to metformin.
- Metformin can be administered alone or in combination with a sulfonylurea.
- Monitor for possible hypoglycemic effects.

- A reduced dose may be needed in elderly and debilitated or malnourished patients.
- Monitor blood glucose as indicated to ensure blood sugar control; measure glycosylated hemoglobin at intervals of about 3 months.
- Do not administer during pregnancy; insulin is usually given.

Assessment/Interventions

- Obtain patient history.
- Monitor patient for signs and symptoms of hypoglycemia.
- Assess for potential drug-drug interactions. A patient receiving hyperglycemic agents should be closely monitored to maintain adequate glycemic control.
- Assess patient for factors that put them at high risk for lactic acidosis.
- Hold metformin if patient is to have an X-ray procedure with contrast dyes or surgery.
- Should the patient become ill, review laboratory studies as indicated for abnormalities in serum electrolytes, CBC and blood glucose levels for signs of acidosis and dehydration.
- Assess for gastrointestional symptoms, especially with higher doses.
- When transferring from standard oral hypoglycemic agents, other than chlorpropamide, no transition period is usually necessary; however, when transferring from chlorpropamide, care should be exercised during the first 2 weeks due to the long retention of chlorpropamide in the body, leading to overlapping drug effects and possible hypoglycemia.
- Determine possible pregnancy or lactation as safety for these conditions has not been established.
- Administer with caution to elderly patients.
- Store in a tightly closed container at room temperature.

OVERDOSAGE: SIGNS & SYMPTOMS

Lactic acidosis: Malaise, myalgia, respiratory distress, increasing somnolence, abdominal distress

Patient/Family Education

- Emphasize the importance of taking this medication exactly as prescribed and not double dosing.
- Caution patient to inform the healthcare provider of over-the-counter drugs or other prescription drugs they may be taking.
- Evaluate the patient's knowledge about diabetes type II and its relationship to metformin therapy.
- Explain the difference between metformin and other glucose-control medications.
- Inform patient of the importance of following dietary instructions, of a regular exercise program and of regular testing of blood glucose, glycosylated hemoglobin, renal function and hematologic parameters.
- Instruct patient to take the medication as prescribed at the same time each day.
- Instruct patient in the proper techniques of glucose monitoring.
- Explain metallic or unpleasant taste is sometimes present at the start of therapy and should be temporary.
- Caution patient to inform the healthcare provider immediately if GI discomfort is severe. If symptoms do not go away within the first few weeks, or if symptoms come back after or start later on during the therapy, the patient should inform the healthcare provider so that the dosage can be adjusted.
- Caution patient to be aware of signs and symptoms of hypoglycemia.
- Caution patient to be aware of the signs and symptoms of lactic acidosis.
- Caution patient that they should not take metformin if they have chronic liver or kidney problems; drink alcohol excessively; are severely dehydrated; are having a diagnostic procedure with contrast agents; are having

surgery or develop a serious condition such as a myocardial infarction, severe infection or a stroke.

- Caution patient to inform the healthcare provider if they have an illness that results in severe vomiting, diarrhea or fever.
- Instruct female patients to inform the healthcare provider if they are or plan to become pregnant, as metformin should not be taken during pregnancy.

See Patient Guide, p. 390.

Methadone HCl

(METH-uh-dohn HIGH-droe-KLOR-ide)

Dolophine HCl

Class: Narcotic analgesic

Action Relieves pain by stimulating opiate receptors in CNS; also causes respiratory depression, peripheral vasodilation, inhibition of intestinal peristalsis, sphincter of Oddi spasm, stimulation of chemoreceptors that cause vomiting and increased bladder tone.

Indications Management of severe pain; detoxification and temporary maintenance treatment of narcotic addiction.

Contraindications Standard considerations.

Route/Dosage

Pain

ADULTS: **IM/SC/PO** 2.5-10 mg q 3-4 hr prn. May need higher doses in patients with severe pain or tolerance.

Detoxification

ADULTS: **PO** 15-20 mg initially to suppress withdrawal symptoms. Additional doses may be needed. PATIENTS PHYSICALLY DEPENDENT ON HIGH DOSES OF NARCOTICS: **PO** 40 mg/day may be given for 2-3 days; decrease dose q 1-2 days. Maintenance: **PO** 20-40 mg initially to suppress withdrawal symptoms in patients who are heavy heroin users. Additional 10 mg doses can be given prn. Adjust dose as tolerated and required, up to 120 mg/day.

Interactions

Barbiturate anesthetics: Drug actions may be additive. *CNS depressants (eg, tranquilizers, sedatives, alcohol):* Additive CNS depression. *Hydantoins, rifampin, barbiturates:* May decrease effectiveness of methadone. *Urinary acidifiers:* May increase renal clearance of methadone.

Lab Test Interferences

Increased amylase and lipase may occur up to 24 hr after dose.

Adverse Reactions

CV: Hypotension; palpitations; bradycardia; tachycardia. *RESP:* Laryngospasm; depression of cough reflex. *CNS:* Lightheadedness; euphoria; dysphoria; headache; insomnia; dizziness; sedation; disorientation; incoordination. *GI:* Nausea; vomiting; constipation; abdominal pain; dry mouth. *GU:* Urinary retention or hesitancy. *HEMA:* Thrombocytopenia. *DERM:* Sweating; pruritus; urticaria. *OTHER:* Tolerance; psychological and physical dependence with chronic use.

Precautions

Pregnancy: Pregnancy category undetermined. *Lactation:* Excreted in breast milk. *Children:* Not recommended for children; dosage is not well defined. *Special risk patients:* Use drug with caution in patients with myxedema, acute alcoholism, acute abdominal conditions, ulcerative colitis, decreased respiratory reserve, head injury or increased intracranial pressure, hypoxia, supraventricular tachycardia, depleted blood volume or circulatory shock. *Drug dependence:* Methadone has abuse potential. *Hepatic or renal impairment:* May need to decrease dose. *Treatment of drug addiction:* Methadone for detoxification should not be given for > 21 days and treatment should not be repeated within 4 wk. More than 3 wk in methadone treatment of narcotic dependence is considered maintenance therapy; only approved programs can provide this therapy.

NURSING CONSIDERATIONS

Administration/Storage

- If GI upset occurs, give with food.
- Adjust dose as tolerated and required (up to 120 mg/day) for adequate pain relief. When withdrawing methadone, decrease by 10% every 1-2 days.
- Use reduced dose in elderly or debilitated patients.
- IM administration is preferred over SC injection, which can cause local irritation.
- Rotate injection sites.
- Store at room temperature in light-resistant container.

Assessment/Interventions

- Obtain patient history, including drug history and any known allergies.
- Monitor vital signs, especially respirations.
- Monitor bowel function and treat constipation as indicated.
- Monitor I&O. Observe for urinary retention.
- Assess for pain relief.
- Have patient turn, cough and deep breathe every 2 hr.
- Watch for additive CNS effects when used with other CNS depressants.
- Carefully monitor patients with acute abdominal problems, acute alcoholism, myxedema, respiratory disease, supraventricular tachycardia or shock.
- Document and notify physician of any side effects, including hypotension, bradycardia, tachycardia, laryngospasm, decreased cough reflex, dizziness, disorientation, nausea and vomiting, constipation, urinary retention, sweating, pruritus, physical and psychological dependence with long-term use.

OVERDOSAGE: SIGNS & SYMPTOMS

Miosis, respiratory and CNS depression, cool/clammy skin, skeletal muscle flaccidity, circulatory collapse, seizures, cardiopulmonary arrest, apnea, hypotension, coma, death

Patient/Family Education

- Tell patient to take methadone regularly, as prescribed. If dose is missed, tell patient to take as soon as possible. If close to next dose, wait and take next regularly scheduled dose.
- Advise patient that drug may cause dizziness, drowsiness, or blurred vision and to use caution while driving or performing other hazardous tasks.
- Caution patient to avoid intake of alcoholic beverages or other CNS depressants.
- If constipation occurs, tell patient to increase fluids and fiber or to use fiber laxative.
- Explain that use of methadone before pain becomes acute will allow it to alleviate pain better.
- Caution patient to avoid sudden position changes to prevent orthostatic hypotension.
- Explain types and potential significance of sympathomimetic side effects.

See Patient Guide, p. 391.

Methamphetamine HCl (Desoxyephedrine HCl)

(meth-am-FET-uh-meen HIGH-droe-KLOR-ide)

Desoxyn, Desoxyn Gradumets

Class: CNS stimulant/amphetamine

Action Activates noradrenergic neurons causing CNS and respiratory stimulation; stimulates the satiety center in the brain causing appetite suppression.

Indications Treatment of attention deficit disorder in children; short-term exogenous obesity adjunct.

Contraindications Advanced arteriosclerosis; symptomatic cardiovascular disease; moderate to severe hypertension; hyperthyroidism; hypersensitivity to sympathomimetic amines; glaucoma; agitated states; history of drug abuse. Drug should not be used concomitantly with or within 14 days of MAO inhibitor use.

Route/Dosage

Attention Deficit Disorder

CHILDREN: PO 5 mg 1-2 times/day; may be increased weekly by 5 mg to maximum of 20-25 mg/day in divided doses. Long-acting form: Once daily.

Exogenous Obesity

ADULTS & CHILDREN > 12 YR: PO 5 mg 1-3 times/day 30 min before meals. Long-acting form: 10-15 mg in AM. Not to be used beyond a few weeks.

Interactions *Guanethidine:* Amphetamines may decrease effectiveness. *MAO inhibitors, furazolidone:* Hypertensive crisis and intracranial hemorrhage may occur. *Tricyclic antidepressants:* Decreased amphetamine effect. *Urinary acidifiers:* Decreased amphetamine levels. *Urinary alkalinizers:* Increased amphetamine levels.

Lab Test Interferences Plasma and urinary steroid levels may be altered.

Adverse Reactions *CV:* Palpitations; tachycardia; hypertension; arrhythmias. *CNS:* Hyperactivity; dizziness; insomnia; euphoria; restlessness; tremors; headache. *GI:* Dry mouth; unpleasant taste; diarrhea; constipation; anorexia. *GU:* Impotence. *DERM:* Urticaria.

Precautions *Pregnancy:* Category C. *Lactation:* Excreted in breast milk. *Children:* Not recommended as anorectic agent in children < 12 yr. *Drug dependence:* Has high potential for dependence and abuse. Tolerance may occur; recommended dose should not be exceeded. *Tartrazine sensitivity:* Some products contain tartrazine, which may cause allergic reactions in susceptible individuals.

NURSING CONSIDERATIONS

Administration/Storage

- Administer last dose several hours before bedtime.
- Store in tightly closed container at room temperature.

Assessment/Interventions

- Obtain patient history, including drug history and any known allergies. Note cardiovascular disease, hyperthyroidism, glaucoma or sensitivity to sympathomimetic drugs.
- Take vital signs and auscultate heart and lungs before administration; monitor closely during treatment.
- Assess mental status: mood, sensorium, affect, stimulation, insomnia, aggressiveness. Depressed patients are more likely to misuse drug to induce euphoria and mood elevation.
- Monitor renal function.
- Monitor blood glucose level closely in diabetic patient. Changes in appetite and food intake will occur.

- Monitor for weight loss (may be desired effect).
- If hypertension, dysrhythmias, marked agitation, restlessness or confusion occur, withhold medication and notify physician.

OVERDOSAGE: SIGNS & SYMPTOMS

Restlessness, tremor, hyperreflexia, rapid respiration, confusion, assaultiveness, hallucinations, panic attack, hyperpyrexia

Patient/Family Education

- Instruct patient to take medication exactly as ordered and not to increase dosage unless advised by physician.
- Advise patient to take sips of water frequently, suck on ice chips or sugarless hard candy, or chew sugarless gum if dry mouth occurs.
- Instruct patient to report excessive dryness of mouth, constipation or prolonged insomnia as dosage may need to be adjusted.
- Tell patient to avoid caffeine, which increases drug effect.
- Advise patient that drug may cause dizziness and to use caution while driving or performing other tasks requiring mental alertness or coordination.
- Instruct patient not to take otc medications without consulting physician.
- Tell parents to report decreased appetite to pediatrician.

See Patient Guide, p. 392.

Methenamine and Methenamine Salts

(meh-THEN-uh-meen and meh-THEN-uh-meen salts)

Methenamine Hippurate

Hiprex, Urex

Methenamine Mandelate

Mandameth, Mandelamine

Class: Urinary anti-infective

Action In acidic urine, methenamine is hydrolyzed to ammonia and formaldehyde, which is bactericidal to certain bacteria in urine. Acid salts (methenamine mandelate and hippurate) have some nonspecific bacteriostatic activity and help to maintain low urine pH.

Indications Suppression or elimination of bacteriuria associated with pyelonephritis, cystitis and other chronic urinary tract infections; treatment of infected residual urine, sometimes accompanying neurologic disease or diabetes.

Contraindications Renal insufficiency; severe dehydration; severe hepatic insufficiency with hyperammonemia; acute urinary tract infections involving renal parenchyma.

Route/Dosage

Methenamine Hippurate

ADULTS & CHILDREN > 12 YR: **PO** 1 g bid. CHILDREN 6-12 YR: **PO** 500 mg-1 g bid.

Methenamine Mandelate

ADULTS: **PO** 1 g qid after meals and at bedtime. CHILDREN 6-12 YR: **PO** 500 mg qid. CHILDREN < 6 YR: **PO** 250 mg for q 30 lb body weight qid (18.4 mg/kg qid).

Interactions

Sulfonamides: May increase chance of crystalluria. *Urine alkalizers (acetazolamide, sodium bicarbonate or carbonate):* Prevents hydrolysis of methenamine to formaldehyde with possible decrease in antimicrobial action.

Lab Test Interferences

Methenamine may interfere with laboratory urine determinations of 17-hydroxycorticosteroids, catecholamines and vanillylmandelic acid (false increases) and 5-hydroxyindoleacetic acid (false decrease). Taken during pregnancy, can interfere with laboratory tests for urine estriol (false decrease) when acid hydrolysis procedure is used; use enzymatic hydrolysis procedure.

Adverse Reactions

RESP: Dyspnea. *CNS*: Headache. *GI*: Nausea; vomiting; cramps; diarrhea; stomatitis; anorexia. *GU*: Bladder irritation; dysuria; proteinuria; hematuria; frequency; urgency; crystalluria. *HEMA*: Serum transaminase elevation. *DERM*: Pruritus; urticaria; erythematous eruptions; rash. *OTHER*: Generalized edema.

Precautions

Pregnancy: Category C. *Lactation*: Undetermined. *Debilitated patients and patients with swallowing difficulty*: Use with caution to avoid inducing lipoid pneumonia. *Acid urine*: If acidification of urine cannot be obtained or is contraindicated, drug is not recommended. *Gout*: May cause precipitation of urate crystals in urine. *Lipoid pneumonia*: Methenamine mandelate oral suspension is vegetable oil–based; aspiration could result in lipoid pneumonitis. *Tartrazine sensitivity*: Some products contain tartrazine, which may cause rash or bronchial asthma in susceptible patients.

NURSING CONSIDERATIONS

Administration/Storage

- Administer after meals and at bedtime to minimize GI distress.
- Reconstitute granules by dissolving 1 packet (500 mg-1 g) in 60-120 ml of water immediately before use. Solution may be cloudy.
- Urinary acidification using ascorbic acid to maintain low pH may be necessary.
- Store at room temperature in tightly closed container. Protect from excessive heat.

Assessment/Interventions

- Obtain patient history, including drug history and any known allergies.
- Obtain clean-catch urine specimen for culture and sensitivity before beginning therapy.
- Monitor I&O, and watch for bladder irritation (painful/frequent urination, proteinuria, hematuria); dose may need to be decreased if these symptoms occur. Fluid intake should be maintained at 1500-2000 ml/day (if medically acceptable).
- Monitor liver function test results for transient increase in enzymes.
- Avoid concurrent use of sulfonamides (may cause precipitates), or any drugs that will alkalize urine.

Patient/Family Education

- Explain significance of adequate hydration.
- Tell patient to report these symptoms to physician: painful urination, skin rash, headache, swelling or severe stomach upset.
- Instruct patient to avoid use of milk products and antacids while taking drug to help keep urine acidic and allow drug to work better. Instruct patient to take vitamin C and drink cranberry or prune juice to acidify urine.
- Caution patient not to self-medicate with otc medications containing sodium bicarbonate or sodium carbonate.
- Teach patient how to read dipstick tests for urine pH and specific gravity and to report to physician if required values are not attained.

See Patient Guide, p. 393.

Methicillin Sodium

(meth-ih-SILL-in SO-dee-uhm)
Staphcillin
Class: Antibiotic/penicillin

Action Inhibits bacterial cell wall mucopeptide synthesis.

Indications Treatment of infections caused by penicillinase-producing staphylococci; initial therapy of suspected staphylococcal infection.

Contraindications Hypersensitivity to penicillins.

Route/Dosage
ADULTS: **IM/IV** 4-12 g/day in divided doses q 4-6 hr. ADULTS WITH RENAL FAILURE: **IM/IV** 1 g q 8-12 hr when creatinine clearance is ≤ 10 ml/min. CHILDREN: **IM/IV** 100-300 mg/kg/day in divided doses q 4-6 hr. INFANTS: **IM/IV** 50-100 mg/kg/day in divided doses q 6-12 hr.

Interactions
Aminoglycosides, parenteral: May inactivate aminoglycosides in vitro; do not mix in same IV solution. *Contraceptives, oral:* May reduce efficacy of oral contraceptives. *Probenecid:* May increase serum concentrations of methicillin by slowing rate of renal tubular secretion. *Tetracyclines:* May impair bactericidal effects of methicillin. INCOMPATIBILITIES: Do not mix with other agents; administer separately.

Lab Test Interferences
Antiglobulin Coombs' test: Drug may cause false-positive results in certain patient groups. *Urinary steroid test:* May cause false increase in 17-hydroxycorticosteroids using Porter-Silber method. *Urine glucose test:* Drug may cause false-positive results with copper sulfate tests (Benedict's test, Fehling's test, or Clinitest tablets); enzyme-based tests (eg, Clinistix, Tes-tape) are not affected. *Urine protein determinations:* Drug may cause false-positive reactions with turbidimetric method using sulfosalicylic acid and trichloroacetic acid; bromphenol blue test (Multi-Stix) is not affected.

Adverse Reactions
CNS: Neurotoxicity (lethargy, neuromuscular irritability, hallucinations, convulsions, seizures); dizziness; fatigue; insomnia; reversible hyperactivity; prolonged muscle relaxation. *EENT:* Itchy eyes. *GI:* Nausea; vomiting; abdominal pain or cramps; diarrhea or bloody diarrhea; rectal bleeding; flatulence; enterocolitis; pseudomembranous colitis; anorexia. *GU:* Interstitial nephritis (oliguria, proteinuria, hematuria, hyaline casts, pyuria); nephropathy; elevated creatinine or BUN. *HEPA:* Transient hepatitis; cholestatic jaundice. *HEMA:* Anemias; thrombocytopenia; eosinophilia; leukopenia; granulocytopenia; neutropenia; bone marrow depression; agranulocytosis; reduced hemoglobin or hematocrit; prolongation of bleeding time and PT; altered blood cell counts. *DERM:* Ecchymosis. *META:* Elevated serum alkaline phosphatase; hypernatremia; reduced serum potassium, albumin, total proteins and uric acid. *OTHER:* Hypersensitivity reactions that may lead to death; vaginitis; hyperthermia; pain at site of injection; deep vein thrombosis; hematomas; vein irritation; phlebitis; sciatic neuritis.

Precautions
Pregnancy: Category B. *Lactation:* Excreted in breast milk. *Hypersensitivity:* Reactions range from mild to life threatening. Administer cautiously to cephalosporin-sensitive patients because of possible cross-reactivity. *Pseudomembranous colitis:* Consider possibility in patients with diarrhea. *Superinfection:* May result in bacterial or fungal overgrowth of nonsusceptible organisms.

NURSING CONSIDERATIONS

Administration/Storage

- Dilute methicillin with Sterile Water for Injection or Sodium Chloride for Injection. Shake vigorously.
- Use preparation on mixing; do not allow to stand more than 8 hr at concentrations 10-30 mg/ml to prevent significant loss of potency.
- Carefully infuse intravenous medication to prevent thrombophlebitis, especially in elderly.
- IM medication should be well diluted to avoid causing tissue atrophy, and caution must be taken during injection to avoid sciatic nerve injury. Inject deep intragluteally. Rotate injection sites.
- Administer after culture and sensitivity results are obtained.
- Discard any unused portion.

Assessment/Interventions

- Obtain patient history, including drug history and any known allergies. Note hepatic or renal disease and sensitivity to penicillins, cephalosporins or imipenem.
- Be aware of amount of sodium in methicillin for patients on restricted sodium diets.
- Isolate patient with methicillin-resistant *Staphylococcus aureus* (MRSA) until appropriate antibiotic therapy can be instituted.
- Monitor vital signs and signs and symptoms of superinfection (sore mouth, foul-smelling stools, vaginal discharge, fever, cough) and inflammation.
- Monitor I&O, observing for hematuria or oliguria resulting from nephrotoxicity. This is more likely to occur in those patients with decreased renal function.
- Monitor patient for signs and symptoms of interstitial nephritis.
- If diarrhea occurs, increase fluid intake.

OVERDOSAGE: SIGNS & SYMPTOMS

Neuromuscular hyperexcitability, convulsive seizures, agitation, confusion, asterixis, hallucinations, stupor, coma, multifocal myoclonus, encephalopathy

Patient/Family Education

- Instruct patient to drink plenty of fluids.
- Inform patient that methicillin may decrease efficacy of birth control pills. Suggest use of alternate method of birth control while taking this medication.
- Instruct patient to report these symptoms to physician: signs of superinfection (fever, vaginitis, oral candidiasis, fatigue, foul-smelling stools, black "furry" tongue, cough), severe diarrhea.

See Patient Guide, p. 394.

Methimazole

(meth-IMM-uh-zole)

Tapazole

Class: Antithyroid

Action Inhibits synthesis of thyroid hormones.

Indications Long-term therapy of hyperthyroidism; amelioration of hyperthyroidism in preparation for subtotal thyroidectomy or radioactive iodine therapy.

Contraindications Use in nursing women.

Route/Dosage

ADULTS: Initial dose: PO 15-60 mg/day in 3 equal doses at approximately 8-hr intervals. Maintenance: PO 5-15 mg/day. CHILDREN: Initial dose: PO 0.4 mg/kg/day. Maintenance: PO Approximately ½ initial dose. Alternately, children may be given 0.5-0.7 mg/kg/day in 3 divided doses as initial therapy and ⅓-⅔ of initial dose for maintenance.

Interactions

Anticoagulants: May decrease or increase anticoagulant action. *Beta blockers:* May increase effects of beta blockers, resulting in toxicity. *Digoxin:* May cause increase in effects of digitalis glycosides, including toxicity. *Theophyllines:* May alter theophylline clearance in hyperthyroid or hypothyroid patients.

Lab Test Interferences

None well documented.

Adverse Reactions

CNS: Paresthesias; neuritis; headache; vertigo; drowsiness; neuropathies; CNS stimulation; depression. *EENT:* Loss of taste; sialadenopathy. *GI:* Nausea; vomiting; epigastric distress. *GU:* Nephritis. *HEPA:* Jaundice; hepatitis. *HEMA:* Inhibition of myelopoiesis (eg, agranulocytosis, granulocytopenia, thrombocytopenia); aplastic anemia; hypoprothrombinemia; periarteritis. *DERM:* Rash; urticaria; pruritus; erythema nodosum; skin pigmentation; exfoliative dermatitis; lupus-like syndrome including splenomegaly, hepatitis, periarteritis, hypoprothrombinemia and bleeding. *OTHER:* Abnormal hair loss; arthralgia; myalgia; edema; lymphadenopathy; drug fever; interstitial pneumonitis; insulin autoimmune syndrome.

Precautions

Pregnancy: Category D. *Lactation:* Avoid nursing. *Agranulocytosis:* Potentially most serious side effect. Discontinue drug in presence of agranulocytosis, aplastic anemia, hepatitis, fever or exfoliative dermatitis. *Hemorrhage:* May cause hypoprothrombinemia and bleeding. Monitor PT.

NURSING CONSIDERATIONS

Administration/Storage

- Administer around clock in 3 equal doses (ie, q 8 hr).
- Administer each dose with same amount of food to facilitate uniform absorption.
- Store in light-resistant container at room temperature.

Assessment/Interventions

- Obtain patient history, including drug history and any known allergies.
- Assess for history of liver disease.
- Assess symptoms of hyperthyroidism that patient is experiencing.
- Obtain baseline vital signs and monitor during treatment.
- Obtain baseline hepatic blood work including bilirubin and liver enzymes.
- Obtain baseline CBC and monitor carefully during first 2 months of treatment.
- Obtain baseline thyroid levels and monitor monthly initially and q 2-3 mo for long-term therapy.
- Monitor drug's effects on hyperthyroid symptoms.
- Monitor PT, especially before surgery, to assess increased risk of bleeding.
- Observe for potential adverse reactions including rash or fever, and notify physician if any occur.

OVERDOSAGE: SIGNS & SYMPTOMS

Nausea, vomiting, epigastric distress, headache, fever, arthralgia, pruritus, edema, pancytopenia, agranulocytosis, exfoliative dermatitis, hepatitis, neuropathies, CNS stimulation or depression

Patient/Family Education

- Instruct patient in importance of taking proper dose exactly as scheduled.
- Advise patient not to stop, start or adjust dose of any medications, including otc, without discussing with physician.
- Explain to patient the importance of complying with follow-up appointments and lab work.
- Instruct patient to check pulse daily.
- Advise patient that iodine-restrictive diet may be necessary.

- Inform patient that response to therapy may take months.
- Instruct patient to report these symptoms to physician: rash, fever, sore throat, bruising or signs of infection or jaundice.
- Advise patient that drug may cause drowsiness and to use caution while driving or performing other tasks requiring mental alertness.

See Patient Guide, p. 395.

Methocarbamol

(meth-oh-CAR-buh-mahl)

Robaxin, Robaxin-750

Class: Skeletal muscle relaxant/centrally acting

Action May cause relaxation of skeletal muscle via general CNS depression. Does not directly relax tense skeletal muscles.

Indications Adjunctive therapy for relief of painful, acute musculoskeletal conditions; control of neuromuscular manifestations of tetanus.

Contraindications Renal pathologic disorders (parenteral form).

Route/Dosage

Skeletal Muscle Relaxation

ADULTS: Initial dose: **IV/IM** 3 g over ≤ 3 consecutive days. Repeat course after 48 hr lapse if condition persists. **PO** 1.5 g qid. Maintenance: **PO** 1 g qid or 750 mg q 4 hr, or 1.5 g tid. For first 48-72 hr, 6-8 g/day is recommended; then reduce to 4 g/day.

Tetanus

ADULTS: **IV** 1-2 g; additional 1-2 g may be added to infusion up to 3 g total. Repeat q 6 hr until oral form may be administered. CHILDREN: **IV/IV infusion** 15 mg/kg initially; then 15 mg/kg q 6 hr.

Interactions None well documented.

Lab Test Interferences

Screening tests for 5-hydroxyindoleacetic acid or vanillylmandelic acid: Drug may cause color interference.

Adverse Reactions

CV: Syncope; hypotension; bradycardia. *CNS:* Dizziness; lightheadedness; vertigo; headache; drowsiness; fainting; mild muscular incoordination; convulsions in epileptic patients. *EENT:* Blurred vision; conjunctivitis with nasal congestion; nystagmus; diplopia; metallic taste. *GI:* GI upset; nausea. *DERM:* Urticaria; pruritus; rash; flushing. *OTHER:* Thrombophlebitis; pain or sloughing at injection site; anaphylactic reaction; fever.

Precautions

Pregnancy: Safety not established. Avoid use, if possible. *Lactation:* Undetermined. *Children:* Safety and efficacy in children < 12 yr not established, except for management of tetanus.

NURSING CONSIDERATIONS

Administration/Storage

- Administer parenteral form for no more than 3 days.
- Wait 48 hr before repeating with additional course if needed.
- For parenteral administration, do not administer SC; drug should be given IV or IM.
- Assess patency of IV site prior to administration; if patency is in doubt, start new IV to avoid extravasation.
- Administer via slow IV push or as infusion.
- Infuse in solution of D5W or saline solution ≤ 1 vial/250 ml.
- Keep prepared infusion at room temperature.
- For IV administration, place patient in recumbent position; have patient

remain recumbent for 10-15 min after administration to prevent orthostatic hypotension.
- Monitor vital signs and IV flow rate.
- For IM administration, inject deeply and do not exceed 5 ml in each gluteal area. Rotate injection sites.
- For oral administration, administer loading dose followed by maintenance dose.
- May crush tablets if necessary.
- Administer with food to decrease stomach upset.
- Store at room temperature.

Assessment/Interventions
- Obtain patient history, including drug history and any known allergies. Note epilepsy and renal pathologic conditions.
- Perform physical assessment noting muscle tone, range of motion, pain, CNS function, mentation and vital signs.
- Observe IV site for phlebitis.
- Provide safe environment (eg, keep bed in low position with side rails up, instruct patient to call for assistance when rising).
- Move patient slowly from recumbent to sitting or standing position.
- Keep oxygen and epinephrine available in event of anaphylaxis.
- Monitor for effectiveness of drug and side effects, especially dizziness, drowsiness, rash, pruritus, fever and congestion.
- If patient experiences syncope, place in reverse Trendelenburg's position and monitor vital signs.
- Notify physician if patient does not spontaneously recover.
- Notify physician if extravasation occurs.

OVERDOSAGE: SIGNS & SYMPTOMS
Coma, CNS depression

Patient/Family Education
- Instruct patient regarding additional therapy recommended to treat muscle spasm such as activity restrictions or physical therapy.
- Advise patient that drug may cause drowsiness, dizziness and lightheadedness and to use caution while driving or performing other tasks requiring mental alertness.
- Caution patient not to discontinue medication abruptly without consulting physician.
- Inform patient that urine may become different or darker color.
- Instruct patient to report these symptoms to physician: skin rash, itching, fever or nasal congestion.
- Caution patient to avoid sudden changes in position to prevent orthostatic hypotension.
- Instruct patient to avoid intake of alcoholic beverages or other CNS depressants.
- Advise patient not to take otc medications without consulting physician.

See Patient Guide, p. 396.

Methotrexate (Amethopterin; MTX)

(meth-oh-TREK-sate)

Folex, Folex PFS, Rheumatrex Dose Pack, Rheumatrex Tablets

Class: Antineoplastic/antimetabolite; antipsoriatic; antiarthritic

Action Competitively inhibits dihydrofolic acid reductase and thereby inhibits DNA synthesis and cellular replication. In rheumatoid arthritis, believed to reduce immune function.

Indications Antineoplastic chemotherapy for treatment of gestational choriocarcinoma, chorioadenoma destruens, hydatidiform mole; treatment and prophylaxis of acute (meningeal) lymphocytic leukemia; treatment of breast cancer, epidermoid cancers of head and neck, advanced mycosis fungoides and lung cancer; in combination therapy in advancedstage non-Hodgkin's lymphoma; as adjunct in high doses followed by leucovorin rescue in nonmetastatic osteosarcoma (postsurgically); symptomatic control of severe psoriasis and severe rheumatoid arthritis. **Unlabeled use:** Reduction of corticosteroid requirements in patients with severe corticosteroid-dependent asthma.

Contraindications Use in nursing mothers. In patients with psoriasis or rheumatoid arthritis, methotrexate is contraindicated in pregnancy, alcoholism, alcoholic liver disease, chronic liver disease, overt or laboratory evidence of immunodeficiency syndrome and preexisting blood dyscrasias (eg, leukopenia, thrombocytopenia).

Route/Dosage

Choriocarcinoma and Thromboblastic Diseases

ADULTS: **PO/IM** 15-30 mg for 5 days. Repeat courses 3-5 times as required, with rest periods of > 1 wk between courses.

Leukemia

ADULTS & CHILDREN: INDUCTION: 3.3 mg/m^2/day in combination with prednisone 60 mg/m^2/day usually for 4 to 6 wk. POSTREMISSION MAINTENANCE THERAPY (USUALLY IN COMBINATION WITH OTHER DRUGS): **PO/IM** 2 times weekly in total weekly doses of 30 mg/m^2 or **IV** 2.5 mg/kg q 14 days.

Meningeal Leukemia

ADULTS: **Intrathecal** 12 mg/m^2 or empirical dose of 15 mg. Administer q 2-5 days until cell count of CSF returns to normal; then give one additional dose. Dose reduction may be required in elderly patients because of differences in CSF volume. CHILDREN ≥ 3 YR: 12 mg. Administer q 2-5 days until CSF cell count returns to normal. CHILDREN 2 YR: 10 mg. CHILDREN 1 YR: 8 mg. CHILDREN < 1 YR: 6 mg.

Lymphoma: Burkitt's Lmphoma, Stages 1 & 2

ADULTS: **PO** 10-25 mg/day for 4-8 days. Provide 7- to 10-day rest period between courses.

Stage 3 Lymphosarcoma as Part of Combination Therapy

ADULTS: **PO** 0.625-2.5 mg/kg/day.

Mycosis Fungoides

ADULTS: **PO** 2.5-10 mg/day for weeks to months (based on clinical response or hematologic function). **IM** 25 mg twice weekly or 50 mg weekly.

Osteosarcoma

Complex high dose with leucovorin rescue and other chemotherapeutic agents. Starting dose for high-dose methotrexate is 12 gm/m^2.

Rheumatoid Arthritis

ADULTS: Initial therapy: **PO** 7.5 mg/week in single dose or 2.5 mg q 12 hr for 3 doses each wk. Gradually adjust dosage to maximal response; do not exceed 20 mg/wk.

Psoriasis

Individualize dosage. Administer 5-10 mg parenteral test dose 1 wk prior to therapy. ADULTS: **IM/IV** 10-25 mg/wk (maximum 50 mg/wk). ADULTS: **PO** 2.5 mg q 12 hr for 3 doses or at 8 hr intervals for 4 doses q wk (maximum 30 mg/wk). ALTERNATIVE SCHEDULE: **PO** 2.5 mg qd for 5 days followed by 2-day rest period (maximum 6.25 mg qd). This schedule may pose increased risk of liver toxicity.

Interactions

Charcoal, folic acid: May reduce methotrexate efficacy. *Digoxin:* May reduce serum digoxin levels and actions. *Hydantoins:* May reduce plasma levels. *Etretinate, NSAIDs, penicillins, probenecid, salicylates, sulfonamides:* May increase methotrexate blood levels and toxicity.

Lab Test Interferences

None well documented.

Adverse Reactions

RESP: Deaths from interstitial pneumonitis; chronic interstitial obstructive pulmonary disease. *CNS:* Dizziness; fatigue; headache; aphasia;

hemiparesis; paresis; convulsions; leukoencephalopathy (IV after craniospinal irradiation); chemical arachnoiditis; transient paresis; neurotoxicity. *EENT:* Blurred vision; ulcerative stomatitis; gingivitis; pharyngitis. *GI:* Nausea; abdominal distress (common); anorexia; vomiting; diarrhea; hematemesis; melena; GI ulceration and bleeding; enteritis. *GU:* Renal failure; azotemia; cystitis; hematuria; severe nephropathy; reproductive disorders; infertility; abortion; fetal defects. *HEMA:* Leukopenia; bone marrow depression; thrombocytopenia; anemia; hypogammaglobulinemia; hemorrhage; septicemia. *HEPA:* Hepatotoxicity; hepatic cirrhosis and fibrosis. *DERM:* Erythematous rashes; pruritus; urticaria; photosensitivity; pigmentary changes; alopecia; ecchymosis; telangiectasia; acne; furunculosis; aggravation of psoriasis by ultraviolet light. *OTHER:* Malaise; chills; fever; lower resistance to infections; arthralgia; myalgia; diabetes; osteoporosis; anaphylactoid reaction; sudden death.

Precautions

Pregnancy: Category X (for rheumatoid arthritis and psoriasis); Category D (other uses). *Lactation:* Contraindicated in nursing mothers. *Children:* Safety and efficacy not established other than for cancer treatment. *Elderly patients:* Closely monitor for early signs of toxicity. May require dose reduction. *Infection:* Severe reactions may occur if live vaccines are administered. *Intrathecal therapy:* Large doses may cause convulsions and systemic toxicity. Dosage regimens based on age may be more effective and associated with fewer neurotoxic side effects. Do not use formulations or diluents containing preservatives. *Renal impairment:* Use drug with extreme caution. Determine renal status before and during therapy. *Severe effects:* Use of high-dose methotrexate regimens (ie, to treat osteosarcoma) require meticulous care. Deaths have occurred after use of methotrexate for any condition. Potential toxicities include bone marrow depression; hepatotoxicity; lung disease (suggested by symptoms of dry, nonproductive cough); nephrotoxicity and GI toxicity.

NURSING CONSIDERATIONS

Administration/Storage

- Ensure that leucovorin is available from pharmacy before beginning high-dose administration of methotrexate. Leucovorin diminishes methotrexate toxicity.
- Oral administration is often preferred. Give medication 1-2 hr before meals.
- Preservative-free methotrexate may be given IM, IV, intra-arterially or intrathecally.
- For intrathecal use, reconstitute immediately prior to use with preservative-free medium such as 0.9% Sodium Chloride for Injection.
- Follow procedures for proper handling and disposal of anticancer drugs. Wear gloves and avoid skin exposure and inhalation of fumes.
- Store medication in tightly closed, light-resistant container.

Assessment/Interventions

- Obtain patient history, including drug history and any known allergies.
- Before beginning therapy, check that serum creatinine is normal and creatinine clearance is > 60 ml/min.
- Assess for alcoholism, alcoholic liver disease or other chronic liver disease.
- Determine whether patient has any evidence of immunodeficiency syndromes, active infection, preexisting blood dyscrasias (eg, bone marrow hypoplasia, leukopenia, thrombocytopenia or significant anemia).
- Assess pulmonary function; note especially presence of any pulmonary

effusion. Establish baseline pulmonary function measurements.

- Maintain adequate hydration and urine alkalinization during therapy. Monitor I&O.
- Avoid IM injections and taking temperatures rectally during methotrexate therapy; apply pressure to venipuncture sites for at least 10 min.
- Determine renal status before therapy and monitor during therapy.
- During therapy monitor periodically for toxicity. Mandatory monitoring includes CBC with differential and platelet counts and liver and renal function tests. Periodic liver biopsies may be indicated in some situations.
- Assess frequently for pulmonary symptoms, especially dry, nonproductive cough or nonspecific pneumonitis.
- Monitor closely for any symptoms of diarrhea and ulcerative stomatitis.
- Inspect patient's mouth daily. Report any patchy necrotic areas, bleeding and discomfort or black/"furry" tongue.
- Inform physician if diarrhea or ulcerative stomatitis occur during treatment; therapy must be interrupted.
- Inform physician of development of pulmonary symptoms (dry, nonproductive cough, fever, shortness of breath, hypoxemia or presence of infiltrate on chest x-ray film) during therapy. Methotrexate must be discontinued and symptoms investigated and treated.

OVERDOSAGE: SIGNS & SYMPTOMS

Hepatotoxicity, nephrotoxicity, GI toxicity, bone marrow toxicity, pulmonary toxicity

Patient/Family Education

- Advise patient to contact physician if vomiting occurs after medication is taken.
- Inform patient that pregnancy should be avoided during therapy if either partner is receiving methotrexate and for minimum of 3 mo after therapy for men and during and for at least one ovulatory cycle after therapy for women.
- Advise patient and parents that immunization with live virus vaccines is generally not recommended during methotrexate therapy.
- Instruct patient to avoid crowds and persons with known infections.
- Emphasize importance of lab tests during therapy and encourage patient to keep all scheduled appointments.
- Stress importance of strict oral hygiene to prevent infection.
- Inform patient of possibility of hair loss and reassure patient that hair will regrow following discontinuation of therapy.
- Instruct patient to report these symptoms to physician immediately: any symptoms of pulmonary infection (cough, shortness of breath, fever) or GI complications (diarrhea, abdominal pain, black tarry stools) occur. Instruct patient to report these symptoms to physician: presence of chills and fever, unusual bleeding or bruising, jaundice, dark or bloody urine, swelling of feet or legs and joint pain.
- Advise patient to avoid intake of alcoholic beverages, salicylates and NSAIDs.
- Caution patient to avoid exposure to sunlight or sunlamps and to wear protective clothing to avoid photosensitivity reaction.
- Instruct patient not to take otc preparations (including vitamins) without notifying physician. Folic acid, an ingredient in some otc products, reduces methotrexate efficacy.

See Patient Guide, p. 397.

Methyldopa and Methyldopate HCl

(meth-ill-DOE-puh and meth-ill-DOE-pate HIGH-droe-KLOR-ide)

Aldomet, Amodopa, ♣ *Novo-Medopa, Nu-Medopa*

Class: Antihypertensive/antiadrenergic, centrally acting

Action Causes central alpha-adrenergic stimulation, which inhibits sympathetic cardioaccelerator and vasoconstrictor centers; reduces plasma renin activity; reduces standing and supine BP.

Indications Treatment of hypertension.

Contraindications Active hepatic disease or previous hepatic disease associated with methyldopa therapy.

Route/Dosage

ADULTS: **PO** 250 mg bid-tid initially, then 500 mg-3 g/day in 2-4 divided doses. Adjust doses at intervals ≥ 2 days. **IV** 250-500 mg q 6 hr prn (maximum 1 g q 6 hr). CHILDREN: **PO** 10 mg/kg/day in 2-4 doses (maximum 65 mg/kg/day or 3 g/day, whichever is less). **IV** 20-40 mg/kg/day in 4 divided doses (maximum 65 mg/kg/day or 3 g/day, whichever is less).

Interactions

Haloperidol: May result in dementia and/or sedation. *Lithium:* May precipitate lithium toxicity. *Sympathomimetics:* May potentiate pressor effects of sympathomimetics and lead to hypertension.

Lab Test Interferences

May interfere with tests for urinary uric acid, serum creatinine, AST; may give falsely high levels of urinary catecholamines, abnormal liver function test results, positive Coombs' test or rise in BUN.

Adverse Reactions

CV: Bradycardia; aggravation of angina pectoris; pericarditis; myocarditis; orthostatic hypotension; edema. *CNS:* Drowsiness; dizziness; sedation; nightmares; headache; paresthesias; parkinsonism; Bell's palsy; decreased mental acuity; verbal memory impairment. *EENT:* Sore or "black" tongue; nasal stuffiness. *GI:* Constipation; dry mouth; nausea; vomiting; distention; flatus; diarrhea. *GU:* Impotence; decreased libido; failure to ejaculate; rise in BUN. *HEPA:* Abnormal liver function tests; jaundice; hepatitis or liver disorders. *HEMA:* Hemolytic anemia; bone marrow depression; leukopenia; granulocytopenia; thrombocytopenia; reduced WBC count. *DERM:* Rash; toxic epidermal necrolysis. *META:* Gynecomastia; lactation; amenorrhea; galactorrhea. *OTHER:* Fever; lupus-like syndrome; mild arthralgia or myalgia; septic shock-like syndrome.

Precautions

Pregnancy: Category B (methyldopa); Category C (methyldopate hydrochloride). *Lactation:* Excreted in breast milk. *Hepatic and renal dysfunction:* Use with caution in patients with hepatic or renal dysfunction. *IV use:* Paradoxical pressor response has been reported. *Liver disorders:* Jaundice, with or without fever, may occur. Fatal hepatic necrosis has been reported rarely. If symptoms or tests indicate liver effects, may need to discontinue drug. *Positive Coombs' test, hemolytic anemia, and liver disorders:* May occur; monitor patient closely because of potentially fatal complications.

►

NURSING CONSIDERATIONS

Administration/Storage

- Add 100 ml of D5W to dose and infuse intravenous medication slowly over 30-60 min.
- Shake oral suspension well prior to administration.
- Make dosage increases with evening dose to avoid daytime drowsiness.
- Methyldopa: Protect oral suspension from light. Avoid freezing.
- Methyldopate hydrochloride: Refrigerate. Do not freeze.

Assessment/Interventions

- Obtain patient history, including drug history and any known allergies. Determine whether patient has active hepatic or renal disease.
- Prior to therapy perform baseline blood counts (hematocrit and hemoglobin or RBC count) and BP readings.
- During therapy monitor carefully for hemolytic anemia and liver disorders (fever, jaundice).
- Monitor for paradoxical pressor response after IV administration of methyldopa or methyldopate hydrochloride.
- Monitor I&O and weight.
- Monitor renal studies: BUN, creatinine, protein.
- If Coombs' test–positive hemolytic anemia occurs, discontinue methyldopa and notify physician.

OVERDOSAGE: SIGNS & SYMPTOMS

Sedation, coma, acute hypotension, weakness, bradycardia, dizziness, lightheadedness, constipation, distention, flatus, diarrhea, nausea, vomiting, impaired atrioventricular conduction

Patient/Family Education

- Encourage patient's compliance with physician recommendations of weight reduction, sodium and alcohol restriction, cessation of smoking, regular exercise, stress reduction and other methods of BP control.
- Teach patient or family proper technique for BP monitoring at home.
- Prepare schedule for return visits to physician for additional monitoring of BP and hepatic function. Emphasize importance of return visits.
- Caution patient not to stop taking drug abruptly.
- Warn patient that dizziness may occur and that hot baths or showers may aggravate dizziness.
- Inform patient that nausea, vomiting or diarrhea may cause increase in hypotensive effect due to dehydration. If this occurs the patient should contact physician for dosage adjustment.
- Advise patient that urine may darken when exposed to air after voiding and assure patient that this is not a problem.
- Instruct patient to report these symptoms to physician: fever, muscle aches, jaundice or flu-like symptoms.
- Advise patient to take sips of water frequently, suck on ice chips or sugarless hard candy or chew sugarless gum if dry mouth occurs. Dry mouth usually does not continue for more than 2 wk; if it does, patient should report to physician.
- Caution patient to avoid sudden position changes to avoid orthostatic hypotension.
- Instruct patient to avoid intake of alcoholic beverages.
- Advise patient that drug may cause drowsiness, especially during first days of therapy or when dose is increased, and to use care while driving or performing other activities requiring mental alertness.
- Caution patient to avoid exposure to sunlight and to use sunscreen or wear protective clothing to avoid photosensitivity reaction.
- Instruct patient not to take otc medications without consulting physician.

See Patient Guide, p. 398.

Methylphenidate HCl

(meth-ill-FEN-ih-date HIGH-droe-KLOR-ide)

Ritalin, Ritalin-SR

Class: Psychotherapeutic/CNS stimulant

Action Acts as mild cortical stimulant with CNS action; exact mechanism of action unknown.

Indications Treatment of attention-deficit hyperactivity disorder; treatment of narcolepsy.

Contraindications Marked anxiety, agitation and tension; glaucoma; motor tics; family history or diagnosis of Tourette's syndrome.

Route/Dosage

ADULTS: PO 10-60 mg/day in 2-3 divided doses. CHILDREN > 6 YR: PO 5 mg before breakfast and lunch initially; increase by increments of 5-10 mg weekly up to 60 mg/day. Give sustained-release tablets at 8 hr intervals.

Interactions None well documented.

Lab Test Interferences

None well documented.

Adverse Reactions

CV: Changes in pulse and BP; tachycardia; angina; cardiac arrhythmias; palpitations. *CNS:* Nervousness; insomnia; dizziness; headache; dyskinesias; drowsiness; convulsions; toxic psychosis. *EENT:* Blurred vision. *GI:* Anorexia; nausea; abdominal pain; weight loss during prolonged therapy. *HEMA:* Leukopenia; anemia. *OTHER:* Hypersensitivity reactions (eg, rash, itching, fever, joint pain, exfoliative dermatitis, erythema multiforme, thrombocytopenia purpura).

Precautions

Pregnancy: Safety not established. *Lactation:* Undetermined. *Children:* Do not give to children < 6 yr because safety and efficacy have not been established. Children on long-term therapy should be monitored carefully, especially for height growth and weight gain. *Dependence:* Chronic use may lead to tolerance, psychological dependence and abnormal behavior. Use with caution in patients with history of drug abuse. Monitor withdrawal from drug therapy, symptoms of which can include severe depression. *Hypertension:* Use drug with caution; monitor BP. *Seizure disorders:* Drug may lower seizure threshold in susceptible patients. Safe concomitant use with anticonvulsants is not established. If seizures occur, notify physician and consider withholding drug. *Uses:* Do not use to treat severe depression or normal fatigue.

NURSING CONSIDERATIONS

Administration/Storage

- Discontinue MAO inhibitors at least 14 days before initiating treatment.
- Administer last daily dose 6 hr before bedtime to avoid sleeplessness.
- Do not crush or allow patient to chew sustained-release tablet. Instruct patient to swallow sustained-release tablet whole.
- Store at room temperature.

Assessment/Interventions

- Obtain patient history, including drug history and any known allergies. Note history of drug abuse, alcoholism, hypertension, liver disease, glaucoma, motor tics, seizures, Tourette's syndrome and family history of Tourette's syndrome.
- Obtain psychological history noting anxiety, agitation or tension.
- With parental permission, consult with school personnel regarding drug effectiveness.
- Discontinue drug periodically to assess behavior and determine need to continue drug.
- Evaluate ability of family to comply

with regimen and follow-up. Assist with problem-solving barriers that inhibit compliance.

- Promote holistic team approach to management of attention-deficit hyperactivity disorder including parents, day care providers, school personnel and health care providers.
- Monitor height and weight in children.
- Monitor vital signs, noting increase in BP.
- Monitor for drug effectiveness, hypersensitivity and side effects, especially insomnia, tremors, restlessness, anorexia and tachycardia.
- Monitor for depression of psychotic reaction when drug is discontinued after long-term use.
- Monitor CBC, differential and platelet counts if patient is undergoing long-term treatment.
- Monitor sleep habits in adults.

OVERDOSAGE: SIGNS & SYMPTOMS
Vomiting, agitation, tremors, hyperreflexia, muscle twitching, convulsions, euphoria, confusion, hallucinations, delirium, sweating, flushing, headache, hyperpyrexia, tachycardia, palpitations, cardiac arrhythmias, hypertension, mydriasis, dry mucous membranes

Patient/Family Education

- Instruct patient to take last daily dose 6 hr before bedtime to avoid insomnia.
- Stress importance of complying with follow-up appointments and lab work.
- Instruct patient to measure weight 2-3 times/wk and report weight loss to physician.
- Advise parents regarding behavior management of children and coping strategies.
- Instruct parent to provide relaxing environment at bedtime with sleep rituals to promote sleep and prevent insomnia.
- Advise parents to alert school or day care personnel about drug use and administration.
- Refer parents to attention-deficit hyperactivity disorder support group.
- Instruct patient to report these symptoms to physician: nervousness, insomnia, palpitations, vomiting, fever or rash.
- Suggest that patient take sips of water frequently, suck on ice chips or sugarless hard candy or chew sugarless gum if dry mouth occurs.
- Instruct patient to avoid intake of caffeine and alcoholic beverages.
- Advise patient that drug may cause drowsiness and to use caution while driving or performing other tasks requiring mental alertness.
- Instruct patient not to take otc medications without consulting physician.

See Patient Guide, p. 399.

Methylprednisolone

(METH-ill-pred-NIH-suh-lone)

Medrol, ✤ *Medrol Veriderm*

Methylprednisolone Sodium Succinate

A-Methapred, Solu-Medrol

Methylprednisolone Acetate

Adlone, depMedalone 40, depMedalone 80, Depoject, Depo-Medrol, Depopred-40, D-Med 80, Duralone-40, Duralone-80, Medralone-40, Medralone-80, Medrol Acetate Topical, M-Prednisol-40, M-Prednisol-80, Rep-Pred 40, Rep-Pred 80

Class: Corticosteroid

Action Depresses formation, release and activity of endogenous mediators of inflammation including prostaglandins, kinins, histamine, liposomal enzymes and complement system. Modifies body's immune response.

Indications Replacement therapy in primary or secondary adrenal cortex insufficiency; adjunctive therapy for short-term administration in rheumatic disorders; exacerbation or maintenance therapy in collagen diseases; treatment of dermatologic diseases; control of allergic states or allergic and inflammatory ophthalmic processes; management of respiratory diseases; treatment of hematologic disorders; palliative management of neoplastic diseases; management of cerebral edema associated with primary or metastatic brain tumor, craniotomy or head injury; induction of diuresis in edematous states (from nephrotic syndrome); management of critical exacerbations of GI diseases; management of acute exacerbations of multiple sclerosis; treatment of tuberculous meningitis; management of trichinosis with neurologic or myocardial involvement. *Intra-articular or soft tissue administration:* Adjunctive therapy for short-term administration in synovitis of osteoarthritis, rheumatoid arthritis, bursitis, acute gouty arthritis, epicondylitis, acute nonspecific tenosynovitis and posttraumatic osteoarthritis. *Intralesional administration:* Management of keloids; treatment of localized hypertrophic, infiltrated, inflammatory lesions of lichen planus, psoriatic plaques, granuloma annulare, lichen simplex chronicus; treatment of discoid lupus erythematosus, necrobiosis lipoidica diabeticorum, alopecia areata and cystic tumors of aponeurosis or tendon. *Topical administration:* Treatment of inflammatory and pruritic manifestations of corticosteroid-responsive dermatoses. **Unlabeled uses:** Reduction of mortality in severe alcoholic hepatitis; prevention of respiratory distress syndrome; treatment of septic shock; improvement of neurologic function in acute spinal cord injury.

Contraindications Systemic fungal infections; idiopathic thrombocytopenic purpura (IM administration); administration of live virus vaccines; topical monotherapy in primary bacterial infections; topical use on face, groin or axilla; use in premature infants (sodium succinate salt).

Route/Dosage

Methylprednisolone

ADULTS: **PO** 4-48 mg/day.

Methylprednisolone Sodium Succinate

ADULTS: **IV/IM** 10-40 mg administered over 1 to several min. In severe condition, 30 mg/kg infused over 30 min; may repeat q 4-6 hr for 48-72 hr. INFANTS & CHILDREN: **IV/IM** Not less than 0.5 mg/kg/24 hr.

Methylprednisolone Acetate

ADULTS: **IM** 40-120 mg q wk for 1-4 wk. **Intra-articular/intralesional** 4-80 mg into joints or lesions. **Topical** Apply sparingly to affected areas 2-4 times daily.

Interactions

Anticholinesterases: May antagonize anticholinesterase effects in myasthenia gravis. *Barbiturates:* May decrease pharmacologic effect of methylprednisolone. *Hydantoins, rifampin:* May increase clearance and decrease efficacy of methylprednisolone. *Ketoconazole:* May decrease clearance of methylprednisolone. *Macrolide antibiotics:* Significantly decreases methylprednisolone clearance; may need to decrease dose. *Salicylates:* May reduce serum levels and efficacy of salicylates.

Lab Test Interferences

Drug may cause increased levels of urine glucose and serum cholesterol, decreased serum levels of potassium, T_3 and T_4, decreased uptake of thyroid I^{131}, false-negative result in nitroblue-tetrazolium test for systemic bacterial infection and suppression of skin-test reactions.

Adverse Reactions

CV: Thromboembolism or fat embolism; thrombophlebitis; necrotizing angiitis; cardiac arrhythmias or ECG changes; syncopal episodes; hypertension; myocardial rupture; fatal arrest; circulatory collapse; CHF. *CNS:* Convulsions; pseudotumor cerebri (increased intracranial pressure with papilledema); vertigo; headache; neuritis; paresthesias; psychosis. *EENT:* Posterior subcapsular cataracts; increased intraocular pressure; glaucoma; exophthalmos. *GI:* Pancreatitis; abdominal distention; ulcerative esophagitis; nausea; vomiting; increased appetite and weight gain; peptic ulcer with perforation and hemorrhage; bowel perforation. *GU:* Increased or decreased motility and number of spermatozoa. *HEMA:* Leukocytosis. *DERM:* Impaired wound healing; thin, fragile skin; petechiae and ecchymoses; erythema; lupus erythematosus–like lesions; subcutaneous fat atrophy; striae; hirsutism; acneiform eruptions; allergic dermatitis; urticaria; angioneurotic edema; perineal irritation; hyperpigmentation or hypopigmentation. Topical application: burning; itching; irritation; erythema; dryness; folliculitis; hypertrichosis; pruritus; perioral dermatitis; allergic contact dermatitis; stinging, cracking and tightening of skin; secondary infections; skin atrophy; striae; miliaria; telangiectasia. *META:* Sodium and fluid retention; hypokalemia; hypokalemic alkalosis; metabolic alkalosis; hypocalcemia. *OTHER:* Musculoskeletal effects (eg, weakness, myopathy, muscle mass loss, osteoporosis, spontaneous fractures); endocrine abnormalities (eg, menstrual irregularities, cushingoid state, growth suppression in children, sweating, decreased carbohydrate tolerance, hyperglycemia, glycosuria, increased insulin or sulfonylurea requirements in diabetic patients, hirsutism); anaphylactoid or hypersensitivity reactions; aggravation or masking of infections; fatigue; insomnia. Intra-articular administration: Osteonecrosis; tendon rupture; infection; skin atrophy; postinjection flare; hypersensitivity; facial flushing. Topical application may produce adverse reactions seen with systemic use because of absorption.

Precautions

Pregnancy: Pregnancy category undetermined (systemic use); Category C (topical use). *Lactation:* Excreted in breast milk. *Children:* May be more susceptible to adverse effects from topical use. Benzyl alcohol/gasping syndrome may occur with use of methylprednisolone sodium succinate. *Elderly patients:* May require lower doses. *Adrenal suppression:* Prolonged therapy may lead to hypothalmic-pituitary-adrenal suppression. *Hepatitis:* Drug may be harmful in chronic active hepatitis positive for hepatitis B surface antigen. *Hypersensitivity:* Reactions, including anaphylaxis, may occur rarely. *Immunosuppression:* Because drug causes immunosuppressed state, do not administer live virus vaccines during treatment. *Infections:* May mask signs of infection. May decrease host-defense mechanisms to prevent dissemination of infection. *Ocular effects:* Use drug systemically with caution in ocular herpes simplex because of risk of possible corneal perforation. *Peptic ulcer:* Drug may contribute to peptic ulceration, especially in large doses. *Repository injections:* Do not inject subcutaneously. Avoid injection into deltoid muscle and repeated intramuscular injection into same site. *Stress:* Increased dosage of rapidly acting corticosteroid may be needed before, during and after stressful situations. *Tartrazine sensitivity:* May contain tartrazine, which may cause allergic-type reactions in susceptible individuals.

NURSING CONSIDERATIONS

Administration/Storage

- When initiating or discontinuing drug therapy, taper dose.
- With oral administration, give with food. Tablets can be crushed and given with fluid.
- Administer once-daily dose or alternate-day dosing in morning before 9 AM.
- Administer multiple doses at evenly spaced intervals throughout day. When large doses are given, administer antacids between meals to help to prevent peptic ulcers. For long-term

use, alternate-day regimen may be used.

- With intra-articular injection, inject into synovial space. Do not inject unstable joints.
- When treating conditions such as tendinitis or tenosynovitis, inject into tendon sheath rather than into substance of tendon.
- When treating conditions such as epicondylitis, outline area of greatest tenderness and infiltrate drug into area.
- When treating ganglia of tendon sheaths, inject drug directly into cyst.
- When treating dermatologic conditions, avoid injection of sufficient material to cause blanching, which may cause small slough.
- Do not inject into deltoid muscle. IM injection should be administered deeply into gluteal muscle.
- If giving as injection, rotate sites.
- Although methylprednisolone sodium succinate can be given both IM and IV, methylprednisolone acetate can only be administered IM; it *cannot* be administered IV.
- With topical application, once ointment is applied, plastic wrap can be used over area to increase absorption. To avoid skin irritation, do not leave plastic wrap in place > 12 hr. Wash hands before and after application.
- Do not use topically on face, groin or axilla.
- Use solution within 48 hr of mixing.
- Store at room temperature.

Assessment/Interventions

- Obtain patient history, including drug history and any known allergies. Note renal and liver function; state of mental health; hemologic, cardiac, vision and skin problems; and history of frequent fungal infections.
- Assess baseline renal function (ie, creatinine, electrolytes, frequency, 24-hr urine output).
- Check for history of hepatitis B.
- Assess for signs of adrenal insufficiency: low blood glucose, nausea, anorexia, weakness, dizziness, weight loss and diarrhea.
- Obtain baseline vital signs, weight and lab test results (ie, electrolytes, CBC, T_3, T_4, cholesterol, urine glucose).
- Observe growth and development of infants and children on prolonged therapy.
- Monitor renal function, especially in patients with renal impairment.
- If skin irritation occurs, withhold medication and notify physician.
- If signs of infection, renal or liver dysfunction, bleeding, circulatory problems, edema, weight gain or respiratory changes occur, notify physician.
- If difficulties with GI tract or vision changes occur, notify physician.
- If patient is having difficulty with weight control, obtain dietary counseling.
- If patient is diabetic, monitor closely for possible increased requirements for insulin or sulfonylurea.

> **OVERDOSAGE: SIGNS & SYMPTOMS**
>
> Cushingoid changes, moonface, central obesity, striae, hirsutism, acne, ecchymoses, hypertension, osteoporosis, myopathy, sexual dysfunction, diabetes mellitus, hyperlipidemia, peptic ulcer, increased susceptibility to infection, electrolyte and fluid imbalance

Patient/Family Education

- Instruct patient to take medication at same time each day and with food if taking orally.
- With cream or ointment application, instruct patient to soak area of skin before gently applying light film of medication, to increase absorption. Caution patient to wash hands before and after application.
- Encourage patient to eat low-sodium, low-fat foods.
- Advise patient to practice frequent, thorough handwashing to help to prevent infections.
- Advise patient on chronic steroid

therapy to wear or carry identification (eg, Medi-Alert) indicating condition and medication regimen.
- Inform patient of potential for mood swings.
- Warn patient regarding increasing appetite and consequent weight gain. Instruct patient to weigh self daily.
- Inform patient of moonface, which often occurs with this medication.
- Advise patient of acne and skin flushing, which are often associated with this medication. Instruct patient in proper skin care practices to help to prevent irritation and/or acne.
- Instruct patient to report these symptoms to physician: swelling in feet and ankles, signs of infection (fever, overgrowth in mouth, vaginal yeast, wound not healing or with drainage), diarrhea, nausea, vomiting, weight loss, discolored or painful urine, vision changes, menstrual irregularity and fatigue.

See Patient Guide, p. 400.

Methysergide Maleate

(METH-ih-SIR-jide MAL-ee-ate)

Sansert

Class: Analgesic/migraine

Action Semisynthetic ergot derivative possessing no intrinsic vasoconstrictor activity; believed to work by antagonizing effects of serotonin in lowering pain threshold.

Indications Prevention or reduction of intensity of severe and frequent (once weekly or more) vascular headaches; prophylaxis of vascular headache. Not for management of acute attack.

Contraindications Pregnancy; peripheral vascular disease; severe arteriosclerosis; severe hypertension; coronary artery disease; phlebitis or cellulitis in lower limbs; pulmonary disease; collagen disease or fibrotic processes; impaired liver or renal function; valvular heart disease; debilitated states; serious infections.

Route/Dosage

ADULTS: **PO** 4-8 mg daily with meals. There must be drug-free interval of 3-4 wk after 6 mo of treatment.

Interactions

Beta blockers: May result in peripheral ischemia, manifested by cold extremities with possible peripheral gangrene.

Lab Test Interferences

None well documented.

Adverse Reactions

CV: Encroachment of retroperitoneal fibrosis on aorta, inferior vena cava and common iliac branches may cause vascular insufficiency of lower limbs; fibrotic thickening of cardiac valves; murmurs; bruits; arterial vasoconstriction causing chest pain; coldness, numbness or pain in extremities; diminished or absent pulse; ischemic tissue damage; orthostatic hypotension; tachycardia; peripheral edema. *RESP:* Pleuropulmonary fibrosis. *CNS:* Insomnia; drowsiness; mild euphoria; dizziness; ataxia; weakness; lightheadedness; hyperesthesia; hallucinatory dissociation; parasthesias. *GI:* Nausea; vomiting; diarrhea; heartburn; abdominal pain; constipation. *DERM:* Facial flush; telangiectasia; rash; initial increased hair loss. *HEMA:* Neutropenia; eosinophilia. *OTHER:* Arthralgia; myalgia; weight loss.

Precautions

Pregnancy: Contraindicated in pregnancy due to oxytocic properties. *Lactation:* Excreted in breast milk. *Children:* Not recommended for children. *Fibrosis:* Long-term methylsergide therapy may cause retroperitoneal fibrosis, pleuropulmonary fibrosis and fibrotic complications within cardiovascular system. These may be reversible. This drug should be reserved for prophylaxis of frequent, severe or uncontrollable vascular headaches under close supervision. To reduce fibrotic risks, continuous use should not exceed 6 mo. Reduce dosage gradually over 2-3 wk to avoid "rebound headache." Provide 3-4 wk drug-free interval between each 6-mo course of therapy. *Tartrazine sensitivity:* Contains tartrazine, which may cause allergic reactions in susceptible people.

NURSING CONSIDERATIONS

Administration/Storage

- Administer as supplied; do not crush.
- Give with meals.

Assessment/Interventions

- Obtain patient history, including drug history and any known allergies. Note tartrazine sensitivity.
- Obtain cardiac and renal function studies, blood count and sedimentation rate before administration and monitor throughout therapy.
- Palpate for diminished or absent peripheral pulses, changes in extremity color/temperature or peripheral edema throughout prolonged therapy.
- Implement appropriate safety precautions, as patient may be at risk for falls due to insomnia, lightheadedness, hyperesthesia or hallucinatory experiences.
- Notify physician of orthostatic hypotension or tachycardia, chest or flank pain, leg cramps or shortness of breath.

OVERDOSAGE: SIGNS & SYMPTOMS

Peripheral vasospasm, cyanotic extremities, coldness of extremities

Patient/Family Education

- Caution patient that this medication must not be taken during pregnancy or when pregnancy is possible. Advise patient to use reliable form of birth control while taking this drug.
- Explain that medication can be taken with food or milk if GI upset occurs.
- Tell patient that medication may cause drowsiness and to use caution while driving or performing other tasks requiring mental alertness, coordination, dexterity.
- Instruct patient or family member to check regularly for cold or numb extremities.
- Advise patient to report these symptoms to physician immediately: leg cramps, chest pain, flank pain, shortness of breath or painful urination.
- Caution patient to avoid sudden position changes to prevent orthostatic hypotension.
- Tell patient to consult physician after 6 mo of therapy regarding tapering of regimen.
- Explain that medication should not be discontinued abruptly; which may cause rebound headache.
- Educate patient to report rapid weight gain and to check for peripheral edema. Explain benefits of low salt, reduced calorie diet if necessary.

See Patient Guide, p. 401.

Metoclopramide

(MET-oh-kloe-PRA-mide)

Maxolon, Octamide PFS, Reglan, ✤ *APO-Metoclop, Maxeran*

Class: GI stimulant

Action Stimulates upper GI tract motility, resulting in accelerated gastric emptying and intestinal transit and increased resting tone of lower esophageal sphincter. Exerts antiemetic properties through antagonism of central and peripheral dopamine receptors.

Indications *Oral form:* Relief of symptoms associated with acute and recurrent diabetic gastroparesis; short-term therapy of symptomatic, documented gastroesophageal reflux disease in adults who fail to respond to conventional therapy. *Parenteral form:* Prevention of nausea and vomiting associated with emetogenic cancer chemotherapy; prophylaxis of postoperative nausea and vomiting when nasogastric suction is undesirable; facilitation of small bowel intubation when tube does not pass pylorus with conventional maneuvers. **Unlabeled uses:** Treatment of hiccoughs, migraines, postoperative gastric bezoars, improvement in lactation.

Contraindications Patients in whom increase in GI motility could be harmful (eg, in presence of GI hemorrhage, mechanical obstruction, perforation); pheochromocytoma; epilepsy; patients receiving drugs likely to cause extrapyramidal reactions.

Route/Dosage

Diabetic Gastroparesis

ADULTS: **PO/IV** 10 mg 30 min before meals and at bedtime for 2-8 wk.

Symptomatic Gastroesophageal Reflux Disease

ADULTS: **PO** 10-15 mg up to qid, 30 min before meals and at bedtime. For intermittent symptoms or those occurring at specific times, single doses up to 20 mg prior to provoking situations may be preferred. Patients sensitive to therapeutic or adverse effects (eg, elderly) require only 5 mg per dose. Maximum duration of therapy: 12 wk.

Postoperative Nausea and Vomiting

ADULTS: **IM** 10 mg near end of surgery (20 mg may be used).

Chemotherapy-Induced Emesis

ADULTS: **IV** 1-2 mg/kg 30 min before cancer chemotherapy; infuse slowly over not less than 15 min. Repeat q 2 hr for 2 doses, then q 3 hr for 3 doses.

Small Bowel Intubation

ADULTS: **IV** 10 mg (2 ml) as single undiluted dose infused slowly over 1-2 min. CHILDREN 6-14 YR: 2.5-5 mg (0.5-1 ml) as single undiluted dose infused slowly over 1-2 min. CHILDREN < 6 YR: 0.1 mg/kg as single undiluted dose infused slowly over 1-2 min.

Interactions

Cyclosporine: May increase cyclosporine absorption. *Digoxin:* May reduce digoxin absorption. *Succinylcholine:* May increase neuromuscular blocking effects. INCOMPATIBILITIES: Cephalothin, chloramphenicol, sodium bicarbonate.

Lab Test Interferences

None well documented.

Adverse Reactions

CV: Hypotension; hypertension; supraventricular tachycardia; bradycardia. *CNS:* Extrapyramidal symptoms, including acute dystonic reactions; Parkinson-like symptoms (eg, bradykinesia, tremor, cogwheel rigidity, masklike facies); tardive dyskinesia; akathesia; restlessness; drowsiness; fatigue; lassitude; dizziness; anxiety; dystonia; insomnia; headache; myoclonus; confusion; mental depression with suicidal ideation; convulsive seizures; hallucinations. *EENT:* Visual disturbances. *GI:* Nausea and bowel disturbances, primarily diarrhea. *GU:* Urinary frequency; incontinence. *HEPA:* Hepatotoxicity, characterized by jaundice and altered liver function tests. *HEMA:* Neutropenia; leukopenia; agranulocytosis; methemoglobinemia. *OTHER:* Galactorrhea; amenorrhea; gynecomastia; impotence; fluid retention; neuroleptic malignant syndrome; transient flushing of face and upper body (after high IV doses).

Precautions

Pregnancy: Category B. *Lactation:* Excreted in breast milk. *Children:* Some efficacy has been demonstrated. However, methemoglobinemia has occurred in neonates. *Anastomosis or closure of gut:* Drug could theoretically put increased pressure on suture lines after gut anastomosis or closure. *Carcinogenesis:* Because drug elevates serum prolactin concentration, use caution if administration of metoclopramide is considered in patient with previously detected breast cancer. *Depression:* Has occurred with or without prior history of depression. Symptoms have ranged from mild to severe and have included suicidal ideation and suicide. *Extrapyramidal symptoms:* Manifest primarily as acute dystonic reactions, occurring usually during first 24 to 48 hr and more frequently in children and young adults or at higher doses. *Hypertension:* Use drug with caution in hypertensive patients. *Parkinson-like symptoms:* Occur more commonly within first 6 mo of treatment but also can occur after longer periods. Symptoms generally subside within 2-3 mo after drug discontinuation. Give drug cautiously, if at all, to patients with preexisting Parkinson's disease. *Renal impairment:* Initiate therapy at approximately ½ normal dosage in patients whose creatinine clearance is < 40 ml/min. *Tardive dyskinesia:* May develop, especially in elderly and elderly women. Risk of development and likelihood of irreversibility increases with treatment duration and total cumulative dose.

NURSING CONSIDERATIONS

Administration/Storage

- Administer oral form 30 min before meals and at bedtime.
- For IV admixture, when diluted in parenteral solution, administer slowly over no less than 15 min.
- For IV bolus, inject slowly over 1-2 min.
- For parenteral doses > 10 mg, dilute in 50 ml Sodium Chloride Injection.
- May be stored unprotected from light for 24 hr after preparation.

Assessment/Interventions

- Obtain patient history, including drug history and any known allergies. Note history of epilepsy, seizures, hypertension, Parkinson disease, GI bleeding or bowel obstruction.
- Take safety precautions because of high risk for falls because of drowsiness and decreased dexterity.
- Evaluate digoxin level routinely during therapy.
- Check BP and pulse q 8 hr.
- Patients at high risk for arrhythmia should be monitored with telemetry monitoring system.
- In diabetic patients, monitor blood glucose level closely.
- Notify physician of acute CNS reactions, arrhythmias, hypotension, hypertension and suicidal ideations.

OVERDOSAGE: SIGNS & SYMPTOMS

Drowsiness, disorientation, extrapyramidal reactions, muscle hypertonia, irritability, agitation

Patient/Family Education

- Instruct patient to take medication 30 min before meals.
- Instruct patient to report these symptoms to physician: involuntary movement of eyes, face or limbs.
- Caution patient to avoid intake of alcoholic beverages.
- Advise patient that drug may cause drowsiness and to use caution while driving or performing other tasks requiring mental alertness.

See Patient Guide, p. 402.

Metolazone

(meh-TOLE-uh-ZONE)

Zaroxolyn, Mykrox

Class: Thiazide-like diuretic

Action Increases urinary excretion of sodium and chloride by inhibiting reabsorption in ascending limb of loop of Henle and early distal tubules.

Indications Treatment of edema and hypertension. **Unlabeled uses:** Prevention of calcium nephrolithiasis; reduction of postmenopausal osteoporosis; reduction of urine volume in diabetes insipidus.

Contraindications Anuria; renal decompensation; hepatic coma or precoma.

Route/Dosage

ADULTS: PO 0.5-1 mg/day (*Mykrox*) or 2.5-20 mg/day (*Zaroxolyn*). Do not interchange *Mykrox* with *Zaroxolyn*. *Mykrox* is absorbed more rapidly and more completely than *Zaroxolyn*.

Interactions

Cholestyramine, colestipol: May decrease effects of metolazone by decreasing absorption. *Diazoxide:* Concurrent use may produce severe hyperglycemia. *Digitalis glycosides (eg, digoxin):* Urinary loss of potassium and magnesium may predispose patient to digitalis-induced arrhythmia. *Lithium:* Metolazone may decrease renal elimination of lithium, resulting in toxicity. *Loop diuretics (eg, furosemide):* Concurrent use may produce profound diuresis and electrolyte abnormalities. *Sulfonylureas (eg, tolbutamide):* Metolazone may decrease hypoglycemic effect of sulfonylureas by increasing blood glucose.

Lab Test Interferences

None well documented.

Adverse Reactions

CV: Rapid-acting formulation: Orthostatic hypotension; palpitations; chest pain; cold extremities; edema. Slow-acting formulation: Venous thrombosis, palpitations; chest pain; excessive volume depletion; hemoconcentration. *RESP:* Rapid-acting formulation: Cough; epistaxis; sinus congestion; sore throat. *CNS:* Rapid-acting formulation: Dizziness; headache; weakness; "weird" feeling; neuropathy; fatigue; lethargy; lassitude; depression. Slow-acting formulation: Dizziness; syncope; neuropathy; vertigo; headache; weakness; fatigue; lethargy; lassitude; anxiety; depression; nervousness. *EENT:* Bitter taste. *GI:* Rapid-acting formulation: Nausea. Slow-acting formulation: Nausea; anorexia; pancreatitis. *GU:* Slow-acting formulation: Impotence. *HEMA:* Slow-acting formulation: Leukopenia; agranulocytosis; aplastic anemia. *HEPA:* Slow-acting formulation: Jaundice; hepatitis. *DERM:* Rapid-acting formulation: Necrotizing angiitis; vasculitis; cutaneous vasculitis; dry skin. Slow-acting formulation: Photosensitivity; necrotizing angiitis; vasculitis; cutaneous vasculitis. *META:* Hypokalemia; hyperuricemia; hyponatremia; hypochloremia; hypochloremic alkalosis. *OTHER:* Rapid-acting formulation: Impotence; joint pain; back pain; itching eyes; tinnitus; muscle cramps and spasms. Slow-acting formulation: Swelling; chills; acute gouty attack; hypergylcemia; glucosuria; muscle cramps and spasms.

Precautions

Pregnancy: Category B. *Lactation:* Undetermined. *Children:* Not recommended for children. *Fluid and electrolytes:* May be altered; periodic determinations of serum electrolytes, BUN, uric acid and glucose are indicated. *Hepatic impairment:* May precipitate hepatic coma; use drug with caution. *Hypersensitivity:* May occur; cross-sensitivity to sulfonamides or thiazides possible. *Hyperuricemia:* May increase serum uric acid and precipitate gout. *Lipids:* May cause increases in total serum cholesterol, triglycerides and LDL. *Lupus erythematosus:* May be activated or exacerbated. *Post-sympathectomy patients:* Antihypertensive effects may be increased. *Renal impairment:* May precipitate azotemia; use drug with caution. *Tartrazine-sensitivity:* Some products contain tartrazine, which may cause allergic-type reactions (eg, bronchial asthma).

NURSING CONSIDERATIONS

Administration/Storage

- For treatment of edema, establish schedule for intermittent therapy every other day or 3-5 days/wk schedule to reduce potential for electrolyte imbalance.
- For treatment of hypertension, check orders for dosage adjustments of other agents to prevent hypotension.
- Do not interchange product with other brand or generic forms because some formulations are more rapidly bioavailable and not therapeutically equivalent at same doses of other thiazides.
- Administer medication in morning to prevent nocturia.
- Store at room temperature in tight, light-resistant container.

Assessment/Interventions

- Obtain patient history, including drug history and any known allergies.
- Assess for signs of fluid or electrolyte imbalance (dry mouth, thirst, confusion, muscle fatigue, hypotension, tachycardia).
- Maintain accurate I&O records.
- Monitor blood sugar closely for diabetic patients.
- Monitor serum uric acid levels periodically.
- Assess initial and periodic determinations of serum electrolytes and uric acid levels.
- For treatment of diabetic patients, monitor output. If output increases, dosage may need to be increased.

OVERDOSAGE: SIGNS & SYMPTOMS

Orthostatic hypotension, syncope, lethargy, GI hypermotility, dizziness, electrolyte abnormalities, CNS depression, drowsiness, hemoconcentration, GI irritation

Patient/Family Education

- Advise patient to take early in day to avoid sleep disruption.
- Tell patient to take with food if stomach upset occurs.
- Explain significance of potential potassium loss, and identify appropriate supplemental food sources (eg, bananas, orange juice, dates, citrus fruits, apricots). Teach patient signs and symptoms of hypokalemia (muscle weakness, cramping).
- Explain that dizziness or lightheadedness may occur if patient stands up too fast.
- Tell patient to avoid exposure to sunlight and to use sunscreen or wear protective clothing until tolerance to sunlight can be established.
- Explain that BP should be checked periodically by patient or family member.
- Review signs and symptoms of fluid imbalance.

See Patient Guide, p. 403.

Metoprolol

(meh-TOE-pro-lahl)

Lopressor, Toprol XL, ♣ *Betaloc, Betaloc Durules, Novo-Metoprol, Nu-Metoap*

Class: Beta-adrenergic blocker

Action Blocks beta receptors, primarily affecting cardiovascular system (decreases heart rate, decreases contractility, decreases BP) and lungs (promotes bronchospasm).

Indications Used alone or in combination with other antihypertensive agents, for management of hypertension, long-term management of angina pectoris, myocardial infarction (immediate-release tablets and injection).

Contraindications Greater than first-degree heart block; congestive heart failure unless secondary to tachyarrhythmia treatable with beta-blockers; overt or moderate to severe cardiac failure; sinus bradycardia; cardiogenic shock; hypersensitivity to beta-blockers; systolic blood pressure < 100 mm Hg; MI in patients with heart rate < 45 beats/min.

Route/Dosage

Hypertension

ADULTS: **PO** 100 mg/day in single or divided doses initially; maintenance: 100-450 mg/day.

Angina

ADULTS: **PO** 100 mg/day in 2 divided doses initially; maintenance: 100-400 mg/day.

Myocardial Infarction

ADULTS: **IV bolus injection** 5 mg slowly; may repeat every 2 min up to total of 15 mg. If tolerated, give **PO** 50 mg q 6 hr beginning 15 min after last IV dose; continue for 48 hr followed by **PO** 100 mg bid for 1-3 mo. If patient is intolerant of full IV dose, give **PO** 25-50 mg q 6 hr starting 15 min after last IV dose.

Interactions

Barbiturates: Bioavailability of metoprolol may decrease. *Cimetidine:* May increase metoprolol levels. *Clonidine.* May enhance or reverse antihypertensive effect; potentially life-threatening situations may occur, especially on abrupt withdrawal of clonidine. *Hydralazine:* Serum levels of both drugs may increase. *Lidocaine:* Lidocaine levels may increase, leading to toxicity. *NSAIDs:* Some agents may impair antihypertensive effect. *Prazosin:* Orthostatic hypotension may increase. *Propafenone, quinidine, thioamines:* Effects of metoprolol may increase. *Rifampin:* May decrease effects of metoprolol. *Verapamil:* Effects of both drugs may be increased.

Lab Test Interferences

Antinuclear antibodies may develop but are usually reversible on discontinuation.

Adverse Reactions

CV: Hypotension; edema; flushing; bradycardia. *RESP:* Bronchospasm; dyspnea; wheezing. *CNS:* Headache; fatigue; dizziness; depression; lethargy; drowsiness; forgetfulness; sleepiness; vertigo; paresthesias. *EENT:* Dry eyes; visual disturbances. *GI:* Nausea; vomiting; diarrhea. *GU:* Impotence; urinary retention; difficulty with urination. *DERM:* Rash; facial erythema; alopecia; urticaria; pruritus. *OTHER:* Increased hypoglycemic response to insulin; may mask hypoglycemic signs; muscle cramps; asthenia; systemic lupus erythematosus.

Precautions

Pregnancy: Category C. *Lactation:* Excreted in breast milk. *Children:* Safety and efficacy not established. *Anaphylaxis:* Deaths have occurred; aggressive therapy may be required. *AV block:* Slows AV conduction and may cause heart block. *Bradycardia:* Metoprolol decreases heart rate in most patients. *Congestive heart failure:* Administer cautiously in CHF patients controlled by digitalis and diuretics. Notify physician at first sign or symptom of CHF or of unexplained respiratory symptoms in any patient. *Peripheral vascular disease:* May precipitate or aggravate symptoms of atrial insufficiency. *Renal/hepatic function impairment:* Reduced daily dose advised. *Thyrotoxicosis:* May mask clinical signs (eg, tachycardia) of developing or continuing hyperthyroidism. Abrupt withdrawal may exacerbate symptoms of hyperthyroidism, including thyroid storm.

NURSING CONSIDERATIONS

Administration/Storage

- Tablets (immediate release) and injection: Give at same time every day.
- When switching from immediate-release tablets, give same total daily dose.
- Give drug at same time consistently with or without meals. Food slightly enhances drug's bioavailability.

- Store at room temperature and protect from light.

Assessment/Interventions

- Obtain patient history, including drug history and any known allergies.
- Implement periodic ECG or telemetry monitoring, as ordered, if bradyarrhythmias occur.
- Check BP and pulse every 8 hours.
- Monitor levels of BUN, LDH and uric acid and glucose tolerance.
- In diabetic patients, monitor blood sugar closely.
- Notify physician of CNS changes, unstable diabetes, rash, pruritus, visual disturbance or eye irritation, dyspnea, bronchospasm, asthma, arthralgia, muscle cramps.
- Avoid abrupt withdrawal of therapy, which may precipitate ventricular arrhythmia, angina, MI, death.
- Assess peripheral pulses for evidence of arterial occlusion.

OVERDOSAGE: SIGNS & SYMPTOMS

Bradycardia, hypotension, bronchospasm, cardiac failure

Patient/Family Education

- Teach patient how to check pulse and BP.
- Advise patient to contact physician if pulse is < 50 bpm.
- Explain why medication should not be discontinued abruptly.
- Tell patient to check blood sugar regularly and consult physician if levels are unstable.
- Explain that adverse effects are usually mild and transient and will generally subside with continued therapy.
- Instruct patient to report these symptoms to physician: difficulty breathing, night cough or edema.
- Advise patient that drug may cause drowsiness and to use caution while driving or performing tasks requiring mental alertness.
- Instruct patient not to take otc cold preparations without consulting physician.

See Patient Guide, p. 404.

Metronidazole

(meh-troe-NID-uh-zole)

Flagyl, Flagyl I.V., Flagyl I.V. RTU, MetroGel, MetroGel-Vaginal, Metro I.V., Protostat, ♣ *Novo-Nidazol, Trikacide*

Class: Anti-infective

Action Enters bacterial or protozoal cell and impairs synthesis of DNA, resulting in cell death.

Indications Treatment of serious infections caused by susceptible anaerobic bacteria; prophylaxis of postoperative infection in patients undergoing colorectal surgery; treatment of amebiasis; treatment of trichomoniasis and asymptomatic partners of infected patients. *Topical:* Treatment of inflammatory papules, pustules and erythema of acne rosacea. *Vaginal:* Treatment of bacterial vaginosis. **Unlabeled uses:** Prophylaxis of postoperative infection in gynecologic and abdominal surgery; treatment of hepatic encephalopathy, Crohn's disease, antibiotic-associated pseudomembranous colitis, *Helicobacter pylori* infections, giardiasis and *Gardnerella vaginalis* infections.

Contraindications Hypersensitivity to nitroimidazole derivatives; first trimester of pregnancy in patients with trichomoniasis.

Route/Dosage

Anaerobic Bacterial Infections

ADULTS: **IV** 15 mg/kg loading dose infused over 1 hr; then 7.5 mg/kg infused over 1 hr q 6 hr. Do not exceed 4 g in 24 hr. May follow with similar oral dose. For prophylaxis, loading dose is to be completed 1 hr before surgery, followed by maintenance dose 6 and 12 hrs later.

Amebiasis

ADULTS: **PO** 500-750 mg tid for 5-10 days. CHILDREN: 35-50 mg/kg/24 hr in 3 divided doses.

Trichomoniasis

ADULTS: **PO** 2 g in 1 or 2 doses in 1 day or 250 mg tid for 7 days. *Topical:* Apply and rub in thin film twice daily to affected area. *Vaginal:* 1 applicatorful (approximately 37.5 mg metronidazole) intravaginally bid for 5 days.

Interactions

Anticoagulants: Anticoagulant effect may be increased. *Barbiturates:* Therapeutic failure of metronidazole may occur. *Disulfiram:* Concurrent use may result in acute psychosis or confusional state. Metronidazole should not be given to patients who have taken disulfiram within last 2 wk. *Ethanol:* Disulfiram-like reaction including flushing, palpitations, tachycardia, nausea and vomiting may occur with concurrent use. INCOMPATIBILITIES: Do not use aluminum-containing equipment with metronidazole, because solution will turn orange/rust color.

Lab Test Interferences

May interfere with chemical analyses for AST, ALT, LDH, triglycerides and hexokinase glucose; zero values may occur.

Adverse Reactions

CV: Flattening of T-wave. *CNS:* Seizures; peripheral neuropathy; dizziness; vertigo; incoordination; ataxia; confusion; depression; insomnia; syncope. *EENT:* Metallic taste; glossitis; stomatitis. *GI:* Nausea; anorexia; vomiting; diarrhea; epigastric distress; cramps; proctitis; pseudomembranous colitis. *GU:* Darkening of urine; dysuria; cystitis; polyuria; incontinence; vaginal *Candida* proliferation; decreased libido. *HEMA:* Mild leukopenia. *DERM:* Thrombophlebitis; urticaria; erythematous rash; flushing. *OTHER:* Hypersensitivity reactions including dermatologic reactions, nasal congestion, dry mouth or vagina, and fever; fleeting joint pains; pancreatitis. Topical or vaginal use may cause similar adverse effects. After prolonged IV use, thrombophlebitis may occur.

Precautions

Pregnancy: Category B. *Lactation:* Excreted in breast milk. *Children:* Safety and efficacy not established, except for amebiasis. *Elderly:* Monitoring serum levels may be necessary for proper dosing. *Hepatic impairment:* Patients with severe hepatic disease metabolize drug slowly; use caution and lower dose. *Neurologic effects:* Seizures and peripheral neuropathy have occurred. Use extra caution with prolonged use, high doses or history of CNS disease.

NURSING CONSIDERATIONS

Administration/Storage

- Add 4.4 ml of Sterile Water for Injection, bacteriostatic water or sterile saline solution to vial to reconstitute medication.
- Add solution to either D5W, 0.9% normal saline or Lactated Ringer's solution; do not exceed concentration of 8 mg/ml.
- Neutralize IV solution with 5 mEq sodium bicarbonate for each 500 ml of solution.
- Monitor IV infusion for slow continuous or intermittent drip only. If administered by intermittent infusion, discontinue primary fluid during infusion.
- Use IV metronidazole cautiously in patients on sodium-restricted diet. Each gram contains 28 mEq of sodium.
- Do not use equipment containing aluminum.
- Clean treatment area prior to topical applications.
- Apply topical applications in thin film each morning and evening for 9 wk course of therapy. Wash hands

before and after application. Avoid contact with eyes.

- Store at 30°F in room light; reconstituted solutions are stable for 96 hours.
- Use neutralized solutions within 24 hr.
- Prior to reconstitution, store below 86°F. Protect from light.

Assessment/Interventions

- Obtain patient history, including drug history and any known allergies.
- Assess blood levels of medication when used in pediatric and geriatric patients.
- Observe for therapeutic results, which may take 3 wk to occur.
- Notify physician if patient experiences numbness or paresthesia of extremities, seizures or GI distress.
- Observe for psychotic reactions in alcoholic patients.

OVERDOSAGE: SIGNS & SYMPTOMS

Nausea, vomiting, ataxia, seizures, peripheral neuropathy

Patient/Family Education

- Instruct patient to crush tablet if difficult to swallow whole.
- Tell patient not to engage in vaginal intercourse during treatment with vaginal cream.
- Discuss current drug therapies (anticoagulants, disulfiram) with physician, and explain any specific precautions.
- Tell patient to wash hands before and after application of topical or vaginal creams and to avoid eye contact.
- Explain that cosmetics may be applied over topical metronidazole.
- Advise patient that oral medications can be taken with food to decrease GI upset.
- Inform patient that medication may cause darkening of urine or metallic taste in mouth.
- Instruct patient to refrain from sexual intercourse during treatment for trichomoniasis.
- Explain that sexual partner should undergo evaluation and treatment by physician.
- Tell patient that mineral oil base in vaginal cream may weaken latex or rubber products such as condom or diaphragm and should not be used for 72 hours after treatment is completed.
- Explain that vaginal cream should be inserted high in vagina.
- Instruct patient to avoid intake of alcoholic beverages for at least 1 full day after therapy is stopped.

See Patient Guide, pp. 405-407.

Mexiletine HCl

(MEX-ih-leh-teen HIGH-droe-KLOR-ide)

Mexitil

Class: Antiarrhythmic

Action Reduces rate of rise of action potential; decreases effective refractory period in Purkinje fibers; has local anesthetic actions.

Indications Treatment of documented life-threatening ventricular arrhythmias such as sustained ventricular arrhythmias. **Unlabeled uses:** Prevention of ventricular arrhythmias in acute phase of MI; reduction of pain, dysesthesia and paresthesia associated with diabetic neuropathy.

Contraindications Preexisting second- or third-degree atrioventricular block (if pacemaker is not present); cardiogenic shock.

Route/Dosage

Ventricular Arrhythmias

ADULTS: **PO** 200 mg q 8 hr initially, increasing up to 400 mg q 8 hr if necessary (maximum 1200 mg/day). Adjust dose by 50-100 mg increments q 2-3 days. For rapid control of ventricular arrhythmias, give loading dose of 400 mg followed by 200 mg in 8 hr. With dose ≤ 300 mg q 8 hr, may give total daily dose q 12 hr (maximum 450 mg q 12 hr).

Interactions

Hydantoins, rifampin: May increase mexiletine clearance. *Theophylline:* May increase serum theophylline levels.

Lab Test Interferences

May result in abnormal liver function tests, positive ANA titer or thrombocytopenia.

Adverse Reactions

CV: Palpitations; chest pain; increased ventricular arrhythmias or premature ventricular contractions; angina or angina-like pain; CHF. *RESP:* Shortness of breath. *CNS:* Dizziness; lightheadedness; tremor; nervousness; coordination difficulties; changes in sleep habits; headache; paresthesias or numbness; weakness; fatigue; speech difficulties; confusion; depression. *EENT:* Blurred vision; tinnitus. *GI:* Nausea; constipation; abdominal pain; vomiting; diarrhea; anorexia; heartburn; dry mouth; changes in appetite. *HEPA:* Hepatitis; hepatic necrosis. *OTHER:* Fever; rash; nonspecific edema; arthralgias.

Precautions

Pregnancy: Category C. *Lactation:* Excreted in breast milk. *Children:* Safety and efficacy not established. *Cardiovascular effects:* Has proarrhythmic effect; therapy should be initiated in hospital. *Convulsions:* Have occurred; use drug with caution in patients with known seizure disorder. *Hepatic impairment:* Use drug with caution in patients with hepatic impairment. Reduce dosage in patients with severe liver disease. *Urinary pH:* Marked alterations in urinary pH may alter mexiletine elimination; avoid drugs or diets that alter pH.

NURSING CONSIDERATIONS

Administration/Storage

- Administer with food or antacids to reduce GI distress.
- When transferring from lidocaine, stop lidocaine when first oral dose is administered.
- Store at room temperature.

Assessment/Interventions

- Obtain patient history, including drug history and any known allergies. Note history of blood dyscrasias and second- or third-degree heart block without pacemaker.
- Maintain IV during conversion from lidocaine until suppression of arrhythmia appears satisfactory.
- Perform continuous ECG monitoring. Evaluate when desired antiarrhythmic effect has been obtained.
- Monitor BP continuously throughout therapy.
- Monitor I&O.
- Monitor drug serum levels to evaluate for toxic or subtherapeutic dosage regimens.
- Monitor serum electrolytes and liver enzymes periodically throughout therapy.
- If worsening of arrhythmia or CNS symptoms occurs, notify physician.

OVERDOSAGE: SIGNS & SYMPTOMS

CNS symptoms, coma, respiratory arrest, dizziness, drowsiness, nausea, hypotension, sinus bradycardia, paresthesia, seizures

Patient/Family Education

- Instruct patient to take medication with food or antacid.
- Teach patient to monitor pulse rate. Advise patient to notify physician if pulse rate is < 50 bpm or becomes irregular.
- Explain that medication may cause dizziness and lightheadedness. Caution patient to take appropriate safety precautions.
- Remind patient to carry identification describing cardiac disease and medication regimen.
- Instruct patient to report these symptoms to physician: unexplained gen-

eral tiredness, jaundice, fever, sore throat, bruising or bleeding.

See Patient Guide, p. 408.

Mezlocillin Sodium

(MEZZ-low-SILL-in SO-dee-uhm)
Mezlin
Class: Antibiotic/penicillin

Action Inhibits biosynthesis of bacterial cell wall mucopeptide.

Indications Treatment of infections of lower respiratory tract, urinary tract, skin or skin structure, intra-abdominal infections, uncomplicated gonorrhea, gynecological infections and septicemia caused by susceptible strains of specific microorganisms.

Contraindications Hypersensitivity to penicillins.

Route/Dosage
ADULTS: **IM/IV** 200-300 mg/kg/day in 4-6 divided doses. Usual doses are 3 g q 4 hr or 4 g q 6 hr. IM doses should not exceed 2 g/injection. CHILDREN 1 MO-12 YR: **IM/IV** 50 mg/kg q 4 hr. NEONATES: **IV** 75 mg/kg q 6-12 hr.

Interactions
Contraceptives, oral: May reduce efficacy of oral contraceptives. *Tetracyclines:* May impair bactericidal effects of mezlocillin. INCOMPATIBILITIES: Parenteral aminoglycosides may inactivate aminoglycosides in vitro; do not mix in same IV solution.

Lab Test Interferences
Antiglobulin (Coombs') test: Drug may cause false-positive results in certain patient groups. *Urine glucose test:* Drug may cause false-positive results with copper sulfate tests (Benedict's test, Fehling's test or Clinitest tablets); enzyme-based tests (eg, Clinistix, Tes-tape) are not affected. *Urine protein determinations:* Drug may cause false-positives with sulfosalicylic acid and boiling test, acetic acid test, biuret reaction and nitric acid test; bromphenol blue test (Multi-Stix) not affected.

Adverse Reactions
CNS: Neurotoxicity (lethargy, neuromuscular irritability, hallucinations, convulsions and seizures); dizziness; fatigue; insomnia; reversible hyperactivity; prolonged muscle relaxation. *EENT:* Itchy eyes. *GI:* Nausea; vomiting; abdominal pain or cramp; diarrhea or bloody diarrhea; rectal bleeding; flatulence; enterocolitis; pseudomembranous colitis; anorexia. *GU:* Interstitial nephritis (oliguria, proteinuria, hematuria, hyaline casts, pyuria); nephropathy; elevated creatinine or BUN. *HEPA:* Transient hepatitis; cholestatic jaundice. *HEMA:* Anemias; thrombocytopenia; eosinophilia; leukopenia; granulocytopenia; neutropenia; bone marrow depression; agranulocytosis; reduced hemoglobin or hematocrit; prolongation of bleeding time and PT; altered blood cell counts. *DERM:* Ecchymosis. *META:* Elevated serum alkaline phosphatase; hypernatremia; reduced serum potassium, albumin, total proteins and uric acid. *OTHER:* Hypersensitivity reactions that may lead to death; vaginitis; hyperthermia; pain at site of injection; deep vein thrombosis; hematomas; vein irritation; phlebitis; hyperthermia; sciatic neuritis.

Precautions
Pregnancy: Category B. *Lactation:* Excreted in breast milk. *Bleeding abnormalities:* Hemorrhagic manifestations associated with abnormalities of coagulation tests (bleeding time, PT, platelet aggregation) may occur. Abnormalities should revert to normal once drug is discontinued. *Hypersensitivity:* Reactions range from mild to life threatening. Administer cautiously to cephalosporin-sensitive patients because of possible cross reactivity. *Pseudomembranous colitis:* Consider in patients with diarrhea. *Sodium content:* 1.85 mEq sodium/g. *Superinfection:* May

result in bacterial or fungal overgrowth of nonsusceptible organisms.

NURSING CONSIDERATIONS

Administration/Storage

- For IV administration reconstitute each gram of mezlocillin sodium with 9-10 ml of sterile water, D5W, or 0.9% Sodium Chloride Injection; shake vigorously.
- Temporarily discontinue administration of any other solution during infusion.
- May inject reconstituted solution ≥ 10% into vein or IV tubing; infuse slowly over 3-5 min.
- For IM administration reconstitute each gram of mezlocillin sodium with 3-4 ml of 0.5%-1% lidocaine HCl without epinephrine. Inject into large muscle slowly (12-15 sec) to minimize discomfort.
- Store unreconstituted mezlocillin at room temperature.

Assessment/Interventions

- Obtain patient history, including drug history and any allergies.
- Monitor I&O throughout therapy.
- Monitor liver function, hematology (WBC, RBC, hgb, hct, bleeding time) and renal function.
- Assess bowel function.
- Assess respiratory status.
- Observe IV site for thrombophlebitis.
- Notify physician of hemorrhagic manifestations associated with abnormalities in coagulation time.

OVERDOSAGE: SIGNS & SYMPTOMS

Neuromuscular hyperexcitability, seizures, convulsive seizures, agitation, confusion, asterixis, hallucinations, stupor, coma, multifocal myoclonus, encephalopathy, hyperkalemia

Patient/Family Education

- Instruct patient to report these symptoms to physician: skin rash, itching, hives, severe diarrhea, shortness of breath, wheezing, black tongue, sore throat, nausea, vomiting, fever, swollen joints or any unusual bleeding or bruising.

See Patient Guide, p. 409.

Miconazole

(my-KAHN-uh-zole)

Breezee Mist Antifungal, Fungoid Tincture, Maximum Strength Desenex Antifungal, Micatin, Monistat, Monistat 3, Monistat 5, Monistat 7, Monistat 7 Combination Pack, Monistat-Derm, Monistat Dual-Pak, Monistat i.v., Zeasorb-AF

Class: Anti-infective/antifungal

Action Alters permeability of fungal cell membrane, leading to cell death.

Indications

Parenteral form: Treatment of severe systemic fungal infections. *Vaginal form:* Local treatment of vulvovaginal candidiasis (moniliasis). *Topical form:* Treatment of topical fungal infections, including tinea infections and candidiasis.

Contraindications Hypersensitivity to imidazoles.

Route/Dosage

Systemic Infections

ADULTS: **IV** 200-3600 mg/day. May divide into 3 doses. Treatment of meningitis is supplemented by intrathecal injections of 20 mg/dose. Treatment of bladder infections is supplemented by bladder instillations of 200 mg per dose. CHILDREN 1-12 YR: **IV** 20-40 mg/kg/day (maximum 15 mg/kg/dose). CHILDREN < 1 YR: **IV** 15-30 mg/kg/day (maximum 15 mg/kg/dose).

Vaginal Infections

ADULTS: **Intravaginal** 1 suppository (200 mg) at bedtime for 3 days or 1 suppository (100 mg) for 7 days *or* 1 applicatorful at bedtime for 7 days.

Topical Infections

ADULTS: **Topical** Apply to infected area bid.

Interactions

Anticoagulants, oral: May cause increased anticoagulant effect. *Antihistamines, nonsedating type (eg, astemizole, terfenadine):* Cardiotoxicity, including arrhythmias and death, has occurred when agents of this type were used together with azole-type antifungals.

Lab Test Interferences

None well documented.

Adverse Reactions

CV: Tachycardia; arrhythmia; cardiorespiratory arrest. *GI:* Nausea; vomiting; diarrhea; anorexia. *HEMA:* Transient decreases in hematocrit; thrombocytopenia. *DERM:* Phlebitis at infusion site; pruritus; rash; skin irritation, sensitization and burning from topical preparations. *META:* Hyperlipemia possibly caused by vehicle. *OTHER:* Anaphylaxis; fever; chills. Topical or vaginal forms may cause similar reactions.

Precautions

Pregnancy: Category C. *Lactation:* Undetermined. *Children:* Safety and efficacy in children < 1 yr not studied sufficiently. *Cardiac effects:* Have occurred, possibly because of too-rapid administration. *Cremophor-type vehicle:* Present in IV formulation; may cause electrophoretic abnormalities of lipoprotein; usually reversible.

NURSING CONSIDERATIONS

Administration/Storage

- Dilute IV admixture in 200 ml of 0.9% Sodium Chloride Injection or D5W. Infuse at rate of 2 hr/amp.
- Continue treatment until clinical and lab tests indicate absence of fungal infection.
- Topical lotion is preferred in intertriginous areas. If cream is used, use sparingly to avoid maceration effects.
- Spray or sprinkle powder liberally over affected area bid.

Assessment/Interventions

- Obtain patient history, including drug history and any known allergies. Note history of blood dyscrasias and hyperlipidemia.
- Monitor hemoglobin, hematocrit, electrolytes and lipids.
- Avoid having topical products come into contact with eyes.
- Refrigerate suppositories.

Patient/Family Education

- With topical therapy, instruct patient to use for full treatment time, even if symptoms improve. Advise patient to notify physician if there is no improvement in 2 wk.
- With topical therapy, if condition worsens or if burning, itching or redness occurs, instruct patient to discontinue use and notify physician.
- With vaginal therapy, instruct patient to refrain from sexual intercourse or to have partner use condom for protection and to prevent reinfection. Advise patient to apply medication at bedtime.
- Suggest patient use sanitary pad to prevent staining of clothing.
- With vaginal therapy, instruct patient not to discontinue use during menstruation.

See Patient Guide, p. 410.

Midazolam HCl

(meh-DAZE-oh-lam HIGH-droe-KLOR-ide)

Versed

Class: General anesthetic/benzodiazepine

Action Depresses all levels of CNS, including limbic and reticular formation, probably through increased action of GABA, which is major inhibitory neurotransmitter in brain.

Indications Preoperative sedative; conscious sedation prior to diagnostic or endoscopic procedures; induction of general anesthesia; supplement to nitrous oxide and oxygen for short surgical procedures.

Contraindications Hypersensitivity to benzodiazepines; uncontrolled pain; existing CNS depression; shock; acute narrow-angle glaucoma; acute alcohol intoxication; coma.

Route/Dosage

Preoperative Sedative

ADULTS: **IM** 0.07-0.08 mg/kg approximately 1 hr before surgery.

Conscious Sedation

ADULTS: **IV** 1-2.5 mg as 1 mg/ml dilution over 2 min. Increase by small increments to total dose of ≤ 5 mg at no less than 2 min intervals; use less if patient is premedicated with other CNS depressants.

Induction of General Anesthesia

UNPREMEDICATED ADULT PATIENTS: **IV** 0.3-0.35 mg/kg as 1 mg/ml dilution over 20-30 sec, allowing 2 min for effect; may use increments of approximately 25% of initial dose. PREMEDICATED ADULT PATIENTS: **IV** 0.15-0.35 mg/kg over 20-30 sec.

Interactions

Barbiturates, alcohol, other CNS depressants: May prolong effect and increase risk of underventilation or apnea. *Cimetidine:* May increase midazolam levels. *Droperidol, narcotics, secobarbital:* May accentuate hypnotic effect of midazolam. INCOMPATIBILITIES: Dimenhydrinate, pentobarbital, perphenazine, prochlorperazine, ranitidine.

Lab Test Interferences

None well documented.

Adverse Reactions

CV: Hypotension; PVCs; tachycardia; cardiac arrest. *RESP:* Respiratory depression or arrest; decreased tidal volume, decreased respiratory rate; apnea, coughing. *CNS:* Headache; oversedation; retrograde amnesia; euphoria or dysphoria; confusion; argumentativeness; anxiety; emergence delirium and dreaming; nightmares; tonic/clonic movements; tremor; athetoid movements; ataxia; dizziness; slurred speech; paresthesia; weakness; loss of balance. *EENT:* Vision disturbances; nystagmus; pinpoint pupils; cyclic eyelid movements; blocked ears. *GI:* Nausea; vomiting; acid taste; excessive salivation; retching. *DERM:* Hives; burning, coldness at injection site; rash; pruritus. *OTHER:* Pain, tenderness and induration at injection site; hiccoughs; yawning; chills.

Precautions

Pregnancy: Category D. *Labor and delivery:* Drug not recommended because of transplacental transfer. *Lactation:* Undetermined. *Children:* Safety and efficacy not established in children < 18 yr. *Elderly or debilitated patients:* May need to decrease dosage. Titration should be more gradual. *Special risk patients:* High-risk surgical patients require lower doses. Patients with COPD are unusually sensitive to respiratory depressant effects. In renal or heart failure patients, give less frequently. Exercise care when administering to patients with uncompensated acute illness (eg, severe fluid or electrolyte disturbances). *Serious cardiorespiratory events:* Have occurred, including respiratory depression, apnea, respiratory arrest or cardiac arrest, sometimes resulting in death.

NURSING CONSIDERATIONS

Administration/Storage

- For IM administration, inject deeply in large muscle mass.
- Prior to intravenous administration, ensure availability of resuscitative equipment.
- For IV administration, titrate slowly to achieve desired effect (initiation of slurred speech).
- Give no more than 2.5 mg over at least 2 min; wait additional 2 min to fully evaluate the sedative effect.
- Continuously monitor patients for hypoventilation or apnea.
- Do not administer IV medication as rapid or bolus dose. Excessive or rapid IV dosing may result in respiratory arrest.
- Avoid intra-arterial injection.
- Avoid extravasation.
- May mix midazolam in same syringe as morphine, meperidine, atropine or scopolamine.
- Midazolam is compatible with Sodium Chloride for Injection, D5W, Ringer's Lactate Solution for 24 hr.
- Store at room temperature.

Assessment/Interventions

- Obtain patient history, including drug history and any known allergies. Note history of glaucoma, hypersensitivity to benzodiazepines and existing CNS depression.
- Continuously monitor patient for hypoventilation or apnea.
- Assist with ambulation after procedure until drowsiness resolves.
- Because serious life-threatening cardiorespiratory events have been reported, make provision for monitoring, detection and correction of these reactions for every patient regardless of health status.

OVERDOSAGE: SIGNS & SYMPTOMS

Sedation, impaired coordination and reflexes, hypotension, hypoventilation, solomnolence, coma, confusion

Patient/Family Education

- Inform patient and family preoperatively about possibility of temporary postoperative amnesia.
- Advise patient that drug may cause drowsiness and to use caution while driving or performing other tasks requiring mental alertness until drowsiness has subsided or until day after administration, whichever is longer.
- Advise patient to avoid alcohol and other CNS depressants for 24 hr following administration.

No patient monograph available.

Milk of Magnesia (Magnesium Hydroxide)

(milk of mag-NEE-zhuh)

Phillips' Milk of Magnesia

Class: Laxative; antacid

Action As antacid, neutralizes gastric acidity, resulting in increased gastric pH. As laxative, attracts and retains water in intestinal lumen, thereby increasing intraluminal pressure and inducing urge to defecate.

Indications Symptomatic relief of upset stomach associated with hyperacidity; short-term treatment of constipation.

Contraindications Nausea, vomiting or other symptoms of appendicitis; acute surgical abdomen; fecal impaction; intestinal obstruction; undiagnosed abdominal pain.

Route/Dosage

Antacid

ADULTS & CHILDREN > 12 YR: PO 5-15 ml (liquid) or 2.5-7.5 ml (liquid concentrate) or 650 mg-1.3 g (tablets) qid.

Laxative

ADULTS: PO 30-60 ml/day. CHILDREN ≥ 2 YR: PO 5-30 ml depending on age.

Interactions

Iron salts: May reduce absorption of iron. *Penicillamine:* May reduce penicillamine absorption. *Nitrofurantoin, quinolone antibiotics (ie, ciprofloxacin), tetracyclines:* Decreases absorption of anti-infectives and thus action. *Quinidine:* May increase effects of quinidine. *Salicylates:* May reduce serum salicylates levels. *Sodium polystyrene sulfonate:* May cause metabolic alkalosis in patients with renal failure.

Lab Test Interferences

None well documented.

Adverse Reactions

CV: Palpitations. CNS: Dizziness; fainting. *GI:* Excessive bowel activity (eg, griping, diarrhea, nausea, vomiting); perianal irritation; bloating; flatulence; abdominal cramping. *OTHER:* Hypermagnesemia in renal failure patients; sweating; weakness.

Precautions

Pregnancy: Pregnancy category undetermined. *Lactation:* Undetermined. *Children:* Consult physician and exercise caution. Magnesium poisoning developed in a 6-wk-old infant after several doses given for constipation. *Abuse/dependency:* Chronic use of laxatives may lead to laxative dependency, which may result in fluid and electrolyte imbalances, steatorrhea, osteomalacia and vitamin and mineral deficiencies. *Fluid and electrolyte imbalance:* Excessive laxative use may lead to significant fluid and electrolyte imbalance. *Rectal bleeding or failure of drug to produce desired response:* May indicate serious condition requiring further attention. *Renal impairment:* Avoid drug in renal dysfunction. Hypermagnesemia and toxicity may occur because of decreased clearance of magnesium ion.

NURSING CONSIDERATIONS

Administration/Storage

- Administer 1-3 hr after meals or at bedtime with full glass of water.
- May give via nasogastric tube.
- Store in original container at room temperature.

Assessment/Interventions

- Obtain patient history, including drug history and any known allergies. Note history of renal insufficiency and sodium restriction.
- Record bowel activity and bowel sounds.
- Encourage patients to drink 8-10 oz of water daily.
- Monitor I&O throughout therapy.

OVERDOSAGE: SIGNS & SYMPTOMS

Severe/protracted diarrhea, hypermagnesemia, fluid and electrolyte disturbances

Patient/Family Education

- If patient is taking chewable tablets, instruct patient to thoroughly chew before swallowing and then drink full glass of water.
- Because antacids may impair absorption of other drugs, instruct patient not to take oral medications within 1-2 hr of antacid administration.
- Instruct patient not to use maximum dose of antacid for more than 2 wk except under supervision of physician.

See Patient Guide, p. 411.

Milrinone Lactate

(MILL-rih-nohn LAK-tate)

Primacor

Class: Cardiovascular

Action Has direct arterial vasodilator activity and positive inotropic effect; increases myocardial contractility.

Indications Short-term treatment of CHF.

Contraindications Standard considerations.

Route/Dosage

ADULTS: **IV** Loading dose: 50 mcg/kg over 10 min; adjust infusion rate according to hemodynamic and clinical response.

Interactions None well documented. INCOMPATIBILITIES: Precipitate forms if furosemide is injected into same IV line as milrinone; do not administer both in same IV line.

Lab Test Interferences

None well documented.

Adverse Reactions

CV: Ventricular arrhythmia (eg, ventricular ectopic activity, nonsustained ventricular tachycardia, sustained ventricular tachycardia, ventricular fibrillation); supraventricular arrhythmia; hypotension; angina. *CNS:* Headaches; tremor. *HEMA:* Thrombocytopenia. *OTHER:* Hypokalemia.

Precautions

Pregnancy: Category C. *Lactation:* Undetermined. *Children:* Safety and efficacy not established. *Cardiovascular effects:* Do not use in patients with severe obstructive aortic or pulmonic valvular disease; may exacerbate hypertrophic subaortic stenosis; may cause supraventricular and ventricular arrhythmias; may shorten atrioventricular node conduction. *Renal impairment:* Use drug with caution; monitor renal function. Dosage reduction, based on creatinine clearance, may be needed.

NURSING CONSIDERATIONS

Administration/Storage

- For short-term (up to 5 days) IV use only.
- Prepare drug for IV infusion by diluting with 0.45% or 0.9% Sodium Chloride Injection D5W.
- Use infusion pump for administration.
- Adjust maintenance infusion rate on the basis of hemodynamic and clinical response (maximum rate is 0.75 mcg/kg/min or 1.13 mg/kg/day).
- Store at room temperature and protect from light.

Assessment/Interventions

- Obtain patient history, including drug history and any known allergies.
- Evaluate renal function and identify whether patient has severe obstructive aortic or pulmonic valvular disease.
- Provide close cardiac and BP monitoring.
- Be especially observant for supraventricular and ventricular arrhythmias and excessive decreases in BP and report to physician.
- Carefully monitor fluid and electrolyte changes as well as renal function during therapy.
- Observe IV site for signs of irritation. Rotate injection site every 48 hr.
- Correct hypokalemia by potassium supplementation prior to and during use of drug.
- Observe for other common side effects (headaches, hypokalemia, tremor and thrombocytopenia) and report to physician.

OVERDOSAGE: SIGNS & SYMPTOMS

Hypotension

Patient/Family Education

- Explain what medication does.
- Inform patient that treatment with this drug usually does not exceed 5 days.
- Instruct patient to report these symptoms to physician: headache or tremors.

No patient monograph available.

Minocycline

(min-oh-SIGH-kleen)

Minocin, Minocin IV

Class: Antibiotic/tetracycline

Action Inhibits bacterial protein synthesis.

Indications Treatment of infections caused by susceptible strains of gram-positive and gram-negative bacteria, *Rickettsia* and *Mycoplasma* pneumonia, and trachoma; treatment for susceptible infections when penicillins are contraindicated; adjunctive treatment of acute intestinal amebiasis; treatment of asymptomatic carriers of *Neisseria meningitidis* to eliminate meningococci from nasopharynx, chlamydia, inflammatory acne, syphilis, gonorrhea, and lymphogranuloma nervosum. **Unlabeled uses:** Alternative to sulfonamides in treatment of nocardiosis; sclerosing agent to control malignant pleural effusion.

Contraindications Hypersensitivity to tetracyclines.

Route/Dosage

Susceptible Infections

ADULTS: **PO/IV** 200 mg initially, then **PO/IV** 100 mg q 12 hr or **PO** 50 mg qid. CHILDREN > 8 YR: **PO/IV** 4 mg/kg initially, then 2 mg/kg q 12 hr.

Gonococcal Infection

ADULTS: **PO** 200 mg initially, then 100 mg bid for minimum of 4 days; 100 mg bid for 5 days.

Inflammatory Acne

ADULTS: **PO** 50 mg 1-3 times daily.

Primary/Secondary Syphilis

ADULTS: **PO** 200 mg initially then 100 mg q 12 hr for 10-15 days.

Chlamydia

ADULTS: **PO** 100 mg bid for at least 7 days.

Meningococcal Carrier State

ADULTS: **PO** 100 mg q 12 hr for 5 days.

Interactions

Antacids (containing aluminum, calcium, magnesium, zinc), bismuth salts, divalent or trivalent cations: May decrease oral absorption of minocycline. *Digoxin:* May increase digoxin serum levels. *Insulin:* Increases hypoglycemic potential. *Iron salts:* May decrease absorption of minocycline. *Methoxyflurane:* Increased potential for nephrotoxicity exists; do not use together. *Oral anticoagulants:* Increased anticoagulant activity. *Oral contraceptives:* May reduce effect of oral contraceptives. *Penicillins:* May interfere with bactericidal action of penicillins. *Urinary alkalinizers, zinc salts:* May decrease serum minocycline levels. INCOMPATIBILITIES: Calcium-containing solutions other than Ringer's Injection and Ringer's Injection Lactate.

Lab Test Interferences

May increase liver function test

values and BUN. False-negative results in urine glucose testing with glucose oxidase (eg, Clinistix, Tes-tape). False increase in urinary catecholamines with fluorometric method.

Adverse Reactions

CNS: Lightheadedness; dizziness; vertigo. *EENT:* Glossitis, black hairy tongue, dysphagia, sore throat; hoarseness. *GI:* Diarrhea; nausea; vomiting; abdominal pain or discomfort; esophageal ulcers; anorexia; bulky, loose stools. *GU:* Increased BUN. *HEMA:* Hemolytic anemia; thrombocytopenia; neutropenia. *HEPA:* Hepatitis; increased liver enzymes. *DERM:* Urticaria; rash; photosensitivity; blue-gray pigmentation of skin and mucous membranes. *OTHER:* Hypersensitivity, including anaphylaxis; pseudotumor cerebri.

Precautions

Pregnancy: Category D. *Lactation:* Excreted in breast milk. Advise against nursing. *Children:* Avoid in children < 8 yr because abnormal bone formation and discoloration of teeth may occur unless other appropriate drugs are ineffective or contraindicated. *Esophageal irritation/ulceration:* May result from tablet or capsule lodging in esophagus. Greater risk in patients with esophageal obstructive disease or hiatal hernia. *Expiration:* Outdated product should not be used because degraded product is highly nephrotoxic. *Hepatic effects:* Large IV doses can be dangerous, leading to liver failure. *Parenteral therapy:* Prolonged periods of parenteral use may result in thrombophlebitis. *Pseudotumor cerebri (benign intracranial hypertension):* Has been reported in adults. Usual manifestations are headache and blurred vision. *Superinfection:* Prolonged use may result in bacterial or fungal overgrowth.

NURSING CONSIDERATIONS

Administration/Storage

- Do not use outdated drug; degraded product is highly nephrotoxic.
- Administer tablets or capsules with full glass of water. If possible, have patient in standing position for 90 sec after ingestion.
- Administer evening dose at least 1 hr before bedtime.
- Administer oral form at least 2 hr before or after ingesting antacids containing aluminum, calcium, zinc or magnesium; bismuth salts; ferrous salts or other divalent or trivalent cations.
- Reserve parenteral therapy for situations when oral therapy is not indicated; switch to oral therapy as soon as possible.
- Initially dissolve powder for injection with Sodium Chloride Injection, Dextrose Injection, Dextrose and Sodium Chloride Injection, Ringer's Injection or Lactated Ringer's Injection. Do not use any solution containing calcium (a precipitate may form).
- Store prepared solution for up to 24 hr at room temperature; discard if stored longer.
- Immediately before use further dilute prepared solution to 500-1000 ml with one of solutions listed for initial preparation.
- Store suspension at room temperature. Do not freeze.

Assessment/Interventions

- Obtain patient history, including drug history and any known allergies. Note renal insufficiency or liver impairment.
- In long-term therapy perform hematopoietic, renal and hepatic studies.
- Observe for common side effects of nausea, diarrhea, vomiting, rash, blue-gray pigmentation of skin and mucous membranes, lightheadedness, dizziness or vertigo and report to physician.
- Report headache and blurred vision, symptoms of pseudotumor cerebri (benign intracranial hypertension), to physician.

- Be alert for possible thrombophlebitis with prolonged parenteral therapy.
- Be alert for superinfection; prolonged use of drug may result in bacterial or fungal overgrowth. Superinfection of bowel with staphylocci may be life threatening.

Patient/Family Education

- Instruct patient to avoid simultaneous ingestion of drug and antacids, oral iron supplements and vitamins with iron.
- Advise patient to take every 12 hr.
- Instruct patient that if antacid is needed or if iron supplement or vitamin with iron is being taken, to take it at least 2 hr before or 2 hr after drug.
- Advise patients using suspension to store it in refrigerator and to shake well before use.
- Warn patient that using expired drug is dangerous.
- Encourage patients with gonococcal or chlamydia infections to keep follow-up visits.
- Inform patient that drug may interfere with effectiveness of birth control pills and advise use of alternative or additional nonhormonal birth control methods while patient is taking drug.
- Instruct patient to report these symptoms to physician: nausea, diarrhea, vomiting, headache, lightheadedness, dizziness, vertigo, rash, blue-gray pigmentation of the skin and mucous membranes, visual disturbances or other bothersome physical complaints.
- Caution patient to avoid exposure to sunlight and to use sunscreen or wear protective clothing to avoid photosensitivity reaction.
- Advise patient that drug may cause dizziness and lightheadedness and to use caution while driving or performing other tasks requiring mental alertness.

See Patient Guide, p. 412.

Minoxidil

(min-OX-ih-dill)

Loniten, Rogaine, ♣ *APO-Gain Topical Solution*

Class: Antihypertensive; topical hair growth

Action Directly dilates vascular smooth muscle by mechanism possibly related to blockade of calcium uptake or stimulation of catecholamine release; reduces elevated systolic and diastolic BP by decreasing peripheral arteriolar resistance; triggers sympathetic, vagal inhibitory and renal homeostatic mechanisms including increased renin release, which results in increased cardiac rate and output and fluid retention; stimulates hair growth by unknown mechanism but likely is related to its arterial vasodilating action.

Indications *Oral form:* Management of severe hypertension associated with target organ damage in patients who have failed to respond to maximum doses of other antihypertensive agents. *Topical form:* Treatment of androgenic alopecia. **Unlabeled use:** *Topical form:* Treatment of alopecia areata.

Contraindications Pheochromocytoma; acute MI; dissecting aortic aneurysm.

Route/Dosage

ADULTS & CHILDREN > 12 YR: **PO** 5 mg/day initially. If necessary, can increase to 10-40 mg/day in single or divided doses (maximum 100 mg/day). CHILDREN < 12 YR: **PO** 0.2 mg/kg/day as single dose initially. May increase in 50%-100% increments until optimal BP control is achieved (usually 0.25-1 mg/kg/day; maximum 50 mg/day). ADULTS: **Topical** Apply 1 ml to affected scalp areas morning and evening (maximum 2 ml/day).

Interactions

Guanethidine: May result in

profound orthostatic hypotensive effects; discontinue guanethidine before minoxidil therapy. *Topical corticosteroids or retinoids, petrolatum:* May enhance cutaneous drug absorption of topically applied minoxidil.

Lab Test Interferences

None well documented.

Adverse Reactions

CV: Topical form: Edema; chest pain; BP changes; palpitations; heart rate changes. Systemic form: Tachycardia; edema; pericardial effusion leading to tamponade; angina; changes in T waves; rebound hypertension following withdrawal. *CNS:* Systemic form: Headache; fatigue. *CNS:* Topical form: Headache; dizziness; faintness. *GI:* Diarrhea; nausea; vomiting. *HEMA:* Systemic form: Hct, Hgb and RBC counts may fall but return to normal. *DERM:* Topical form: Irritant or allergic dermatitis; eczema; local erythema; pruritus; dry scalp; exacerbation of hair loss; alopecia. Systemic and topical forms: Hypertrichosis. *OTHER:* Systemic form: Darkening of skin.

Precautions

Pregnancy: Category C. *Lactation:* Excreted in breast milk. In general, nursing should not be undertaken. *Children:* Safety and efficacy not established. *Abnormal scalp:* Use of topical form of drug may result in increased absorption and systemic effects; avoid use on scalps with decreased integrity. *ECG changes:* T wave changes may occur; significance unknown. *Fluid/electrolytes imbalance:* Sodium and water retention occur, leading to edema and possible CHF. *Heart disease:* Patients may be predisposed to cardiovascular side effects. *Hypersensitivity:* Can occur and is manifested by rash. *Pericardial effusion:* Has occurred rarely, sometimes with tamponade. *Renal impairment:* Dosage reduction required; pericardial effusion more likely. *Severe hypertension:* Avoid too rapid BP correction. Patients should be hospitalized to monitor carefully. *Tachycardia:* Can be prevented by concomitant use of beta-blocker or other agent.

NURSING CONSIDERATIONS

Administration/Storage

- Dry hair and scalp before topical administration.
- Wear gloves to apply topical form.
- Wash hands after topical administration.
- Administer oral form with diuretic to counteract fluid retention and with beta-blocker to counteract tachycardia.
- Give oral medication with meals to minimize GI symptoms.
- Store tablets at room temperature in tightly closed container.
- Store topical solution at room temperature.

Assessment/Interventions

- Obtain patient history, including drug history and any known allergies. Note renal insufficiency or cardiac disease.
- Perform urinalysis, renal function tests, ECG, chest x-ray and echocardiogram at initiation of therapy. Repeat any tests with abnormal results q 1-3 mo. After stabilization occurs, repeat tests at 6-12 mo intervals.
- Monitor fluid and electrolyte balance and body weight.
- Avoid too rapid control of very severe high BP; syncope, cerebrovascular accidents, MI and ischemia of special sense organs, decreasing hearing and vision, may result.
- Closely supervise patients with renal impairment to prevent cardiac failure or exacerbation of renal failure.
- Observe for tachycardia or angina and report to physician.
- Report patient complaints of nausea, vomiting, diarrhea, dizziness, lightheadedness, rash or skin irritation to physician.
- Observe patients, especially those

with renal impairment, closely for signs of pericardial effusion. If condition is suspected, notify physician; ECG must be performed.

- Monitor patients receiving topical therapy for possible systemic effects after 1 mo of therapy and every 6 mo thereafter.
- If systemic effects appear in patients using drug topically, discontinue drug and notify physician.

OVERDOSAGE: SIGNS & SYMPTOMS

Exaggerated hypotension, fluid retention, tachycardia

Patient/Family Education

- Advise patient not to change dose without physician direction.
- Tell patient that diuretic and beta-blocker are necessary to enhance effectiveness and to decrease side effects of minoxidil.
- Instruct patient to notify physician of heart rate ≥ 20 beats/min over normal, rapid weight gain of > 5 lb, unusual swelling, breathing difficulty, angina symptoms, dizziness or lightheadedness.
- Tell patient to report these symptoms to physician: skin irritation, diarrhea, vomiting, rash or other bothersome physical complaints.
- Warn patient taking oral form that enhanced growth and darkening of fine body hair may occur. It may take 1-6 mo to return to pretreatment appearance.
- Inform patient using topical form that 4 mo of continuous use is required before hair growth is seen and that stopping treatment will lead to hair loss within few mo.
- Advise patient using topical form that more frequent applications or use of larger doses will not enhance hair growth and may lead to side effects.
- Inform patient using topical form to expect initial hair growth to be soft, downy, colorless and barely visible and that after further treament new hair should match other scalp hair.
- Tell patient using topical form not to use it in conjunction with other topical scalp medications, to apply drug only to healthy areas of scalp, not to use if scalp becomes irritated or sunburned and not to use it on other parts of body.
- For topical application, instruct patient to dry head and scalp before application and to wash hands after application.
- Explain that product contains significant amount of alcohol as base. Caution patient to avoid having topical form coming into contact with eyes, mucous membranes or sensitive skin areas. If accidental contact occurs, instruct patient to rinse area with large amounts of cool tap water and to notify physician.

See Patient Guide, pp. 413-414.

Misoprostol

(MY-so-PRAHST-ole)

Cytotec

Class: Prostaglandin

Action Synthetic prostaglandin E_1 analog that inhibits gastric acid secretion and exerts mucosal-protective properties.

Indications Prevention of gastric ulcers in high-risk patients who are taking nonsteroidal anti-inflammatory drugs (NSAIDs). **Unlabeled uses:** Treatment of duodenal ulcers and duodenal ulcers unresponsive to H_2 receptor antagonists.

Contraindications History of allergy to prostaglandins; pregnancy.

Route/Dosage

ADULTS: PO 100-200 mcg qid, in conjunction with NSAID therapy.

Interactions None well documented.

Lab Test Interferences

None well documented.

Adverse Reactions

CNS: Headache. *GI:* Diarrhea (dose-related, developing usually early in course of therapy and self-limiting; may require discontinuation in some patients); abdominal pain; nausea; flatulence; dyspepsia; vomiting; constipation. *GI:* Menstrual disorders.

Precautions

Pregnancy: Category X. *Lactation:* Undetermined. *Children:* Safety and efficacy not established in children < 18 yr. *Elderly:* Reduce dosage if usual dose is not tolerated. *Fertility impairment:* May adversely affect fertility. *Renal impairment:* May reduce clearance of drug; routine dosage adjustment is not recommended unless usual dose is not tolerated. *Duodenal ulcers:* Not for prevention of duodenal ulcers in patients on NSAIDs. *Women of childbearing potential:* Contraindicated in pregnant women because of its abortifacient property. Avoid in women of childbearing potential unless patient requires NSAIDs and is at high risk of complications from gastric ulcers associated with use of NSAIDs. If used in woman of childbearing potential, patient should be capable of complying with effective contraceptive measures; have received oral and written warnings of the hazards of misoprostol, risk of possible contraception failure and danger to other women of childbearing potential should drug be taken by mistake; and have negative serum pregnancy test within 2 wk prior to starting therapy.

NURSING CONSIDERATIONS

Administration/Storage

- If used in woman of childbearing potential, begin therapy on second or third day of menstrual cycle.
- Administer with food and at bedtime to reduce incidence of diarrhea.
- Store in tight container in dry cool place.

Assessment/Interventions

- Obtain patient history, including drug history and any known allergies. Note history of headaches, types of contraception, renal function.
- Monitor patient for signs and symptoms of gastric irritation and ulcers.
- Ensure that pregnancy test has been performed within 2 wk prior to initiation of therapy. Make sure that test result is negative before beginning therapy.
- If headaches, GI distress, menstrual irregularities, or signs of renal dysfunction occur, notify physician.
- Ensure that female patients of childbearing potential have received both oral and written warning regarding hazards of misoprostol in pregnancy.

OVERDOSAGE: SIGNS & SYMPTOMS

Sedation, tremor, seizure, dyspnea, abdominal pain, diarrhea, fever, palpitations, hypotension, bradycardia

Patient/Family Education

- If patient is woman of childbearing potential, review the following: medication may adversely affect pregnancy, causing miscarriage; need for effective contraception; need to stop medication and notify physician immediately if pregnancy is suspected.
- Advise patient to take with food to reduce incidence of diarrhea.
- Instruct patient not to give this medication to anyone else.
- Inform patient not to discontinue or alter dose unless directed by physician.
- Advise patient to avoid magnesium-containing antacids because of risk of diarrhea.
- Advise patient to avoid alcohol and foods that may increase GI irritation.
- Instruct patient to notify physician

if increasing or persistent headache occurs.

- Teach patient to report these symptoms to physician: diarrhea, constipation, nausea, vomiting, menstrual changes.

See Patient Guide, p. 415.

Mitomycin (Mitomycin-C; MTC)

(MY-toe-MY-sin)

Mutamycin

Class: Antineoplastic/antibiotic

Action Suppresses cellular division by selectively inhibiting DNA and RNA synthesis.

Indications In combination therapy for treatment of disseminated adenocarcinoma of stomach or pancreas and palliative treatment when other modalities fail. **Unlabeled uses:** Superficial bladder cancer by intravesical route; as an ophthalmic solution for treating pterygia.

Contraindications Thrombocytopenia, coagulation disorders or increased bleeding tendency.

Route/Dosage

ADULTS: **IV** 10-20 mg/m^2 as single dose q 6-8 wk. Adjust based on patient response (leukocyte/platelet counts) and use of other myelosuppressive agents.

Interactions

Vinca alkaloids: Acute shortness of breath or severe bronchospasm with previous or concurrent use of mitomycin.

Lab Test Interferences

None well documented.

Adverse Reactions

RESP: Dyspnea with nonproductive cough; pulmonary infiltrates; adult respiratory distress syndrome (ARDS). *CNS:* Headache; confusion; drowsiness; fatigue. *GI:* Stomatitis; anorexia; nausea; vomiting; diarrhea. *GU:* Increased serum creatinine; renal failure. *HEMA:* Thrombocytopenia; leukopenia; anemia. *DERM:* Necrosis/tissue sloughing with extravasation; alopecia; cellulitis at injection site. *OTHER:* Fever; hemolytic uremic syndrome.

Precautions

Pregnancy: Pregnancy category undetermined. *Lactation:* Undetermined. *ARDS:* Has occurred in some patients receiving combination chemotherapy and maintained at FIO_2 concentrations > 50% perioperatively. *Bone marrow suppression:* Thrombocytopenia and leukopenia may contribute to overwhelming infection. Myelosuppression is cumulative and is most common and severe toxic drug effect. *Renal toxicity:* Hemolytic uremic syndrome (eg, microangiopathic hemolytic anemia, thrombocytopenia and irreversible renal failure) has occurred.

NURSING CONSIDERATIONS

Administration/Storage

- Administer only under supervision of physician certified in cancer chemotherapy.
- Administer antiemetic 30-60 min prior to giving medication.
- Reconstitute with Sterile Water for Injection. If drug does not dissolve immediately, allow to stand at room temperature until solution is obtained.
- Dilute with IV fluids to a concentration of 20-40 mcg/ml.
- Administer by IV route only via slow infusion. Extravasation may result in tissue damage that may not become apparent for weeks to months after use.
- Do not administer to patient with platelet count < 100,000/mm^3 or WBC < 4000/mm^3 or with progressive decline in either blood value.

- Do not administer to patient with serum creatinine > 1.7 mg/dl.
- Reconstituted drug (in Sterile Water) may be stored for up to 7 days at room temperature and up to 14 days under refrigeration. Use solution within 3 hr when diluted with 5% Dextrose Injection; use within 12 hr when diluted with 0.9% Sodium Chloride for Injection; use within 24 hr when diluted with Sodium Lactate Injection.
- Combination of 5-15 mg of drug and 1000-10,000 U of heparin in 30 ml of 0.9% Sodium Chloride for Injection is stable for 48 hr at room temperature.
- Store powder for injection at room tempeature. Protect from light. Avoid excessive heat.

Assessment/Interventions

- Obtain patient history, including drug history and any known allergies. Note renal impairment, bone marrow suppression, coagulation disorders or increased bleeding tendency.
- Ensure that baseline CBC counts have been obtained before starting therapy and continue for at least 8 wk following completion of therapy.
- Assess renal function periodically, especially serum creatinine.
- Monitor I&O throughout therapy.
- Monitor for possible pulmonary toxicity (dyspnea with nonproductive cough and radiographic evidence of pulmonary infiltrates) or adult respiratory distress. Notify physician immediately if these symptoms occur.
- Be alert for possible hemolytic uremic syndrome (microangiopathic hemolytic anemia and irreversble renal failure). Closely monitor patients receiving ≥ 60 mg for unexplained anemia with fragmented cells on peripheral blood smear, thrombocytopenia and decreased renal function.
- Observe for fever, stomatitis, nausea, vomiting, anorexia, alopecia, extravasation or cellulitis at injection site and report to physician.
- Be alert for possible drug interaction with vinca alkaloids. Acute shortness of breath and severe bronchospasm may occur in patients who are currently or who have previously received mitomycin.

Patient/Family Education

- Explain that temporary hair loss or changes in hair texture or color may occur. Discuss coping strategies and possible use of scarves or wigs.
- Instruct patient to examine mouth daily to check mucous membranes for signs of inflammation and ulceration. Discuss importance of oral hygiene in prevention of stomatitis.
- Advise patient to use soft toothbrush and electric razor and to avoid vigorous flossing.
- Instruct patient to report these symptoms to physician: fever, nausea, vomiting, anorexia, alopecia and extravasation or cellulitis at injection site.
- Advise patient to notify physician immedaitely if the following symptoms occur: dyspnea with nonproductive cough, other respiratory distress, evidence of a bleeding problem (black tarry stools, bloody stools, unusual bleeding or bruising) or decreased urinary output.
- Caution patient to avoid crowds and potentially infectious individuals.
- Tell patient to avoid immunizations.
- Instruct patient to notify dentist or physician of drug regimen before surgical or dental procedures.
- Instruct patient not to take otc medications without consulting physician.
- Explain that follow-up blood tests will be scheduled to monitor drug effects.

See Patient Guide, p. 416.

Mitotane (o,p′-DDD)

(MY-toe-TANE)
Lysodren
Class: Antineoplastic

Action Adrenal cytotoxic agent with primary action on adrenal cortex. Reduces production of adrenal steroids and modifies peripheral metabolism of steroids.

Indications Treatment of inoperable adrenal cortical carcinoma (functional and nonfunctional).

Contraindications Standard considerations.

Route/Dosage
ADULTS: PO 2-6 g divided into 3-4 doses/day. Increase dose incrementally; reduce to maximum tolerated dose (2-19 g/day).

Interactions
Spironolactone: May decrease therapeutic effects of mitotane. *Warfarin:* May decrease therapeutic effects of warfarin.

Lab Test Interferences
None well documented.

Adverse Reactions
CNS: Depression; lethargy; somnolence; dizziness; vertigo. *GI:* Anorexia; nausea; vomiting; diarrhea. *DERM:* Transient skin rash.

Precautions
Pregnancy: Category C. *Lactation:* Undetermined. *Adrenal insufficiency:* May develop; patients may need adrenal steroid replacement. *Hepatic impairment:* Drug accumulation can occur in patients with hepatic insufficiency due to decreased metabolism. *Long-term therapy:* Continuous long-term administration of high doses may lead to brain damage and impairment of function. Behavioral and neurologic assessment are indicated when treatment exceeds 2 yr. *Shock or severe trauma:* If these occur during therapy, temporarily discontinue drug and use exogenous steroids to supplement adrenal function.

NURSING CONSIDERATIONS

Administration/Storage
- Administer only under the supervision of physician certified in cancer chemotherapy.
- Wear goggles, gloves and gown while preparing and administering drug.
- Give antiemetic 30-60 min prior to giving drug.
- Administer drug after evening meal but before bedtime.
- Treatment should be initiated and continued in hospital until dosage regimen is stable.
- Store at room temperature in tight, light-resistant container.

Assessment/Interventions
- Obtain patient history, including drug history and any known allergies. Note hepatic impairment.
- Ensure that behavioral and neurologic assessments are performed on patients receiving long-term therapy (eg, > 2 yr).
- If aching muscles, muscle twitching or fever persist or increase in severity, notify physician.
- Monitor I&O throughout therapy.
- Increase patient's fluid intake unless contraindicated.
- If shock or severe trauma occurs during therapy, temporarily discontinue drug and use exogenous steroids to supplement adrenal function.
- Observe for possible adrenal insufficiency. Adrenal steroid replacement may be needed.
- If no clinical benefits are noted after 3 mo at maximum tolerated dose, consider case a failure.

Patient/Family Education
- Instruct patient to report these symptoms to physician: aching mus-

cles, muscle twitching, fever, depression, lethargy, somnolence, dizziness, vertigo, diarrhea, nausea, vomiting, anorexia or skin rash.

- Advise patient that drug may cause drowsiness and to use caution while driving or performing other tasks requiring mental alertness.
- Advise patient to carry identification describing medication regimen.
- Explain need for continuing medical follow-up, including neurologic examination, to assess effectiveness and possible side effects of medication.

See Patient Guide, p. 417.

Mitoxantrone HCl

(MY-toe-ZAN-trone HIGH-droe-KLOR-ide)

Novantrone

Class: Antineoplastic/antibiotic

Action Suppresses cellular division by inhibiting DNA synthesis throughout cell cycle.

Indications Combination therapy for acute nonlymphocytic leukemia (ANLL) in adults, including myelogenous, promyelocytic, monocytic and erythroid acute leukemias. **Unlabeled uses:** Treatment of breast cancer, refractory lymphomas; non-Hodgkin's lymphoma.

Contraindications Standard considerations.

Route/Dosage

Combination Therapy for ANLL

ADULTS: **IV** Initial induction: 12 mg/m^2/day on days 1-3. Second induction (if needed): 12 mg/m^2/day for 2 days.

Consolidation Therapy

12 mg/m^2/day on days 1 and 2 approximately 6 wk after final induction course. Second consolidation course is generally given 4 wk after first.

Interactions None well documented. INCOMPATIBILITIES: *Heparin:* Precipitate may form if mixed together in same infusion. Do not mix mitoxantrone with other drugs unless specific data are available.

Lab Test Interferences None well documented.

Adverse Reactions *CV:* CHF; arrhythmias: *RESP:* Dyspnea; cough. *CNS:* Seizures; headache. *EENT:* Conjunctivitis. *GI:* Nausea; vomiting; diarrhea; GI pain; stomatitis. *GU:* Renal failure. *HEMA:* Myelosuppression; bleeding; petechiae. *DERM:* Alopecia; rash. *HEPA:* Hepatotoxicity; jaundice. *META:* Hyperuricemia. *OTHER:* Infections; transient discoloration of urine (blue-green) and sclera (blue); fever; tissue necrosis following extravasation; phlebitis.

Precautions *Pregnancy:* Category D. *Lactation:* Undetermined. *Children:* Safety and efficacy not established. *Cardiac toxicity:* CHF and decreased left ventricular ejection fraction may occur; patients with pre-existing cardiac disease are at greatest risk. *Hepatotoxicity:* Transient elevations of AST and ALT have occurred. *Hyperuricemia:* May occur due to rapid tumor cell lysis. *Myelosuppression:* Severe bone marrow depression will occur; risk of infection and bleeding is increased. Blood and blood products must be available.

NURSING CONSIDERATIONS

Administration/Storage

- For IV administration only.
- Administer only under supervision of physician certified in cancer chemotherapy.
- Wear goggles, gloves and gown while preparing and administering drug.

- Dilute solution to at least 50 ml with either 0.9% Sodium Chloride for Injection or 5% Dextrose Injection.
- Administer antiemetic 30 min before drug.
- Introduce solution slowly into tubing as freely running IV infusion of 0.9% Sodium Chloride for Injefction or 5% Dextrose Injection over not < 3 min.
- Minimize risk of extravasation by avoiding areas of previous irradiation and extremities with poor venous circulation.
- Avoid contact with skin or eyes. Rinse copiously with warm water if exposure occurs.
- Do not freeze.

Assessment/Interventions

- Obtain patient history, including drug history and any known allergies. Note cardiac disease or prior mediastinal radiotherapy.
- Ensure that baseline ECG, CBC with differential and liver function tests have been performed and monitor throughout therapy.
- If risk of hyperuricemia is high, monitor serum uric acid levels and institute hypouricemic therapy prior to initiation of antileukemic therapy.
- If risk of severe bone marrow depression is high, have blood and blood products available to support patient, perform serial blood count and be alert for increased risk of infection.
- If extravasation occurs, stop administration immediately and restart in another vein.

OVERDOSAGE: SIGNS & SYMPTOMS
Leukopenia, infection

Patient/Family Education

- Explain that temporary hair loss or changes in hair texture or color may occur. Discuss coping strategies and possible use of scarves or wigs.
- Instruct patient to report these symptoms to physician: black tarry stools, unusual bleeding or bruising, shortness of breath, cough, swelling or fast or irregular heartbeat.
- Advise patient that diarrhea, nausea and vomiting are common side effects, but that patient should notify physician if symptoms persist or become bothersome.
- Tell patient that blue-green urine color is expected for 24 hr after administration and that sclera may have bluish discoloration.
- Instruct patient to monitor mouth daily, checking mucous membranes for signs of inflammation and ulceration.
- Discuss importance of oral hygiene in prevention of stomatitis.
- Instruct patient to use soft toothbrush and electric razor and to avoid vigorous flossing.
- Instruct patient not to take any otc products without consulting physician.
- Caution patient to avoid crowds and potentially infectious individuals.
- Tell patient to avoid immunizations.
- Instruct patient to notify dentist or physician of drug regimen before surgical or dental procedures.

See Patient Guide, p. 418.

Mivacurium Chloride

(mih-vuh-CURE-ee-uhm KLOR-ide)

Mivacron

Class: Muscle relaxant/nondepolarizing neuromuscular blocker

Action Binds competitively to cholinergic receptors on motor end-plate to antagonize action of acetylcholine, resulting in block of neuromuscular transmission.

Indications Adjunct to general anesthesia; facilitation of mechanical ventilation; facilitation of tracheal intubation.

Contraindications Hypersensitivity to mivacurium or similar agents; use of multidose vials in benzyl alcohol–sensitive patients.

Route/Dosage
ADULTS: **IV** Initial dose: 0.15 mg/kg over 5-15 sec. Maintenance: 0.1 mg/kg q 15 min prn or 9-10 mcg/kg/min infusion initially followed by titration (range 1-15 mg/kg/min). CHILDREN 2-12 YR: **IV** Initial dose: 0.2 mg/kg over 5-15 sec. Maintenance: 14 mcg/kg/min infusion initially followed by titration (range 5-31 mcg/kg/min).

Interactions
Aminoglycosides, clindamycin, inhalation anesthetics ketamine, parenteral magnesium salts, polypeptide antibiotics, quinidine, quinine, trimethaphan, verapamil: Action of mivacurium potentiated. *Azathioprine:* Action of mivacurium may be decreased or reversed. *Carbamazepine:* Shortened action of mivacurium and decreased effectiveness. *Theophyllines:* Dose-dependent reversal of neuromuscular blockade. *Trimethaphan:* Prolonged apnea. *Verapamil:* Enhanced action of mivacurium (eg, respiratory depression). INCOMPATIBILITIES: Alkaline solutions (pH > 8.5).

Lab Test Interferences
None well documented.

Adverse Reactions
CV: Flushing; hypotension; tachycardia; bradycardia; arrhythmia; plebitis. *RESP:* Bronchospasm; wheezing; hypoxemia. *DERM:* Rash; urticaria; erythema; injection site reaction. *OTHER:* Dizziness; muscle spasms.

Precautions
Pregnancy: Category C. *Lactation:* Undetermined. *Children:* Safety and efficacy in children < 2 yr not established. *Elderly patients:* Neuromuscular blockade may be longer. *Cachectic or debilitated patients, patients with neuromuscular disease, burns:* Use test dose of ≤ 0.015-0.02 mg/kg. *Cardiovascular disease or allergy/sensitivity (eg, asthma):* Administer initial dose of ≤ 0.15 mg/kg over 60 sec. *Obese patients:* Use ideal body weight to determine initial dose. *Reduced plasma cholinesterase activity:* Use drug with great caution, if at all. *Renal and hepatic impairment:* Duration of action is longer; use lower maintenance doses.

NURSING CONSIDERATIONS

Administration/Storage

- Administer via IV route only.
- Administer only under supervision of health care provider familiar with drug actions and possible complications.
- Ensure that personnel and facilities for resuscitation and life support (tracheal intubation, artificial ventilation, oxygen therapy) are available and have antagonist of drug (anticholinesterase) immediately available.
- Administer to unconscious patients only.
- Prepared drug dilutions in compatible solutions may be stored at room temperature for up to 24 hr when protected from ultraviolet light and from temperature extremes.
- Do not introduce additives into infusion solution.
- Discard unused portion of diluted drug after each use.

Assessment/Interventions

- Obtain patient history, including drug history and any known allergies. Note cardiovascular disease, asthma or other conditions resulting in sensitivity to release of histamine or related mediators; neuromuscular disease; carcinomatosis; renal or hepatic impairment; history of reduced plasma cholinesterase activity.
- Observe for flushing, hypotension, increases or decreases in heart rate, dizziness or muscle spasms and report to physician.

- Use nerve stimulator to assess neuromuscular blockade.
- Maintain adequate hydration and monitor hemodynamic status in patients with clinically significant cardiovascular disease and with asthma or other conditions resulting in sensitivity to release of histamine or related mediators.
- Perform eye care (eg, artificial tears, covering eye) frequently to prevent corneal drying.

OVERDOSAGE: SIGNS & SYMPTOMS
Flaccid paralysis, apnea, hypotension

Patient/Family Education

- Explain that drug will be administered while patient is unconscious.
- Advise patient that dizziness or muscle spasms sometimes occur during recovery.

No patient monograph available.

Moexipril Hydrochloride

(moe-EX-ah-pril HIGH-droe-KLOR-ide)

Univasc

Class: Antihypertensive/ACE inhibitor

Action Competitively inhibits angiotensin I-converting enzyme, preventing conversion of angiotensin I to angiotensin II, which is a potent vasoconstrictor and also stimulates aldosterone secretion from the adrenal cortex. This results in a decrease in BP.

Indications Treatment of hypertension.

Contraindications Hypersensitivity to ACE inhibitors.

Route/Dosage

ADULTS: Initial dose: **PO** 7.5 mg qd. Maintenance: 7.5-30 mg/day; may add diuretic if needed and decrease dose.

Interactions

Diuretics: Excessive reductions in blood pressure may occur. *Indomethacin:* Reduced hypotensive effects, especially in low-renin or volume-dependent hypertensive patients. *Lithium:* Increased lithium levels and symptoms of lithium toxicity. *Potassium-sparing diuretics, potassium preparations:* May increase serum potassium levels.

Lab Test Interferences

False elevation of liver enzymes and uric acid may occur.

Adverse Reactions

CV: Chest pain; peripheral edema. *RESP:* Cough. *CNS:* Dizziness; fatigue; headache. *EENT:* Pharyngitis. *GI:* Nausea; diarrhea; dyspepsia. *DERM:* Flushing; rash. *META:* Hyperkalemia. *OTHER:* Myalgia; flu syndrome; angioedema.

Precautions

Pregnancy: Category D (second and third trimester); Category C (first trimester). Can cause injury or death to fetus if used during second or third trimester. *Lactation:* Undetermined. *Children:* Safety and efficacy not established. *Elderly:* Use reduced dosage. *Angioedema:* Use with extreme caution in patients with hereditary angioedema. *Hypotension/first dose effect:* Significant decreases in blood pressure may occur after the first dose, especially in severely salt- or volume-depleted patients or in those with heart failure. Minimize risk by discontinuing diuretics, decreasing dose or increasing salt intake approximately 2-3 days prior to initiating drug. *Neutropenia/agranulocytosis:* Has been reported with other ACE inhibitors. Risk appears greater in patients with renal dysfunction, heart failure or immunosuppression. *Hepatic failure:* Has been associated with other ACE inhibitors. Patients who develop jaundice or marked elevations of liver enzymes should discontinue drug and receive medical follow-up. *Renal impairment:* In renal insufficiency, stable elevations in

BUN and serum creatinine may occur due to inadequate renal perfusion; monitor renal function during first few weeks of therapy and adjust dosage carefully; for patients with CrCl < 40 ml/1.73 m^2, an initial dose of 3.75 mg should be given. Doses may be carefully titrated to maximum of 15 mg/day.

NURSING CONSIDERATIONS

Administration/Storage

- Administer 1 hour before meal.
- Store in a tightly closed container. Protect from excessive moisture.

Assessment/Interventions

- Obtain patient history.
- Monitor patient for orthostatic hypotension and tachycardia.
- If patient is using diuretics, inform the prescriber as diuretics should be either discontinued 2 to 3 days prior to beginning therapy or the dose reduced until blood pressure is stabilized.
- Monitor blood pressure closely for at least 2 hours after initial dose during the first several days of therapy.
- Observe for sudden, exaggerated hypotension response.
- Monitor blood studies, electrolytes, and renal and hepatic functions throughout therapy.
- Report increased serum potassium and decreased sodium levels to physician.
- Report signs of hyperkalemia or hyponatremia to physician.
- Notify physician if patient develops hypotension, nausea, vomiting, headache, dizziness, fatigue, angioedema, fever, infection or mouth sores.

OVERDOSAGE: SIGNS & SYMPTOMS

Hypotension

Patient/Family Education

- Instruct patient to take as prescribed.
- Advise patient that chronic, dry cough may develop and to notify healthcare provider if this occurs.
- Advise patient to consult the healthcare provider before taking any over-the-counter medications. Excessive amounts of tea, coffee, cola or other drinks that could create a diuretic effect leading to volume depletion or electrolyte imbalance should be avoided.
- Explain that this medicine controls, but does not cure, hypertension and do not discontinue drug unless directed by healthcare provider.
- Teach patient and family to monitor blood pressure, keep a written record and report abnormal readings to the healthcare provider.
- Instruct patient to change positions slowly, especially after the initial dose, to decrease hypotensive effects.
- If dizziness is present, instruct patient not to drive or operate machinery or perform any tasks that require mental alertness.
- Encourage patient to comply with additional interventions for hypertension such as regular exercise, weight control, smoking cessation, sodium and alcohol restriction, diet and stress reduction.
- Instruct patient to notify healthcare provider of persistent rash, sore throat, heart palpitations, chest pain, abdominal pain, difficulty breathing, fever, excessive fatigue or angioedema.
- Caution female patients to inform healthcare provider immediately if she becomes pregnant or is planning to become pregnant.

See Patient Guide, p. 419.

Mometasone Furoate

(moe-MET-uh-SONE FYU-roh-ate)

Elocon, ✤ *Elocom*

Class: Topical corticosteroid

Action Medium-potency topical corticosteroid that depresses formation, release and activity of endogenous mediators of inflammation including prostaglandins, kinins, histamine, liposomal enzymes and complement system; modifies body's immune response.

Indications Relief of inflammatory and pruritic manifestations of corticosteroid-responsive dermatoses.

Contraindications Hypersensitivity to other corticosteroids; monotherapy in primary bacterial infections; ophthalmic use.

Route/Dosage

ADULTS: **Topical** Apply sparingly to affected areas once daily.

Interactions None well documented.

Lab Test Interferences

None well documented.

Adverse Reactions

EENT: Cataracts; glaucoma. *DERM:* Burning; itching; irritation; erythema; dryness; folliculitis; hypertrichosis; acneiform eruptions; hypopigmentation; perioral dermatitis; allergic contract dermatitis; numbness of fingers; stinging; cracking and tightening of skin; skin maceration; secondary infection; skin atrophy; striae; miliaria; telangiectasis. *OTHER:* Systemic absorption may produce reversible hypothalamic pituitary adrenal (HPA) axis suppression, manifestations of Cushing's syndrome, hyperglycemia and glycosuria.

Precautions

Pregnancy: Category C. *Lactation:* May be excreted in breast milk. *Children:* May be more susceptible to topical corticosteroid–induced HPA axis suppression and Cushing's syndrome. *Occulsive therapy:* Should not be used with mometasone treatment regimens.

NURSING CONSIDERATIONS

Administration/Storage

- For topical use only.
- Apply as thin film, rubbing in lightly (washing or soaking area before application may enhance drug penetration).
- Avoid prolonged use near eyes, on face, on genital and rectal areas and in skinfolds.
- Do not use with occlusive dressings.
- When applied in diaper area, avoid using tight-fitting diapers or plastic pants.
- Store at room temperature.

Assessment/Interventions

- Obtain patient history, including drug history and any known allergies. Note liver failure, diabetes, Cushing's disease or HPA axis suppression.
- Observe for local irritation. If redness, itching or other skin changes occur, notify physician.
- Observe for signs of systemic absorption (HPA axis suppression, manifestations of Cushing's syndrome, hyperglycemia and glycosuria), particularly in children, in patients with liver failure and in those receiving high doses of drug.
- If systemic absorption is suspected, ensure that appropriate tests (morning plasma cortisol, urinary free cortisol, ACTH stimulation) are performed.

OVERDOSAGE: SIGNS & SYMPTOMS

Hypothalamic-pituitary-adrenal suppression, Cushing's syndrome

Patient/Family Education

- Explain that product is for topical use only.
- Tell patient to not put other skin products, cosmetics, bandages or dressings over affected area.
- Remind patient to wash hands before and after application of drug.
- Warn patient to avoid contact with eyes and prolonged use around eyes.
- Instruct patient in proper application (apply sparingly once daily; washing or soaking area before application will increase effectiveness).
- Instruct patient to notify physician if condition worsens or if local irritation occurs.

See Patient Guide, p. 420.

Monoctanoin

(MAHN-ahk-tuh-NO-in)

Moctanin

Class: Gallstone solubilizer

Action Dissolves cholesterol gallstones via perfusion of common bile duct.

Indications Solubilizing agent for cholesterol (radiolucent) gallstones retained in biliary tract after cholecystectomy, via perfusion of common bile duct, when other means of removing them have failed or cannot be undertaken.

Contraindications Impaired hepatic function, significant biliary tract infection or history of recent duodenal ulcer or jejunitis; portosystemic shunting, so that there is saturation of hepatic uptake and metabolism of material absorbed from gut lumen; acute pancreatitis; any active life-threatening problems that would be complicated by perfusion into biliary tract.

Route/Dosage

ADULTS: **Biliary/nasobiliary:** 3-5 ml/hr continuous perfusion for 2-10 days.

Interactions None well documented.

Lab Test Interferences
None well documented.

Adverse Reactions
CNS: Fatigue; lethargy; depression; headache. *GI:* Abdominal pain or discomfort; nausea; vomiting; diarrhea; loose stools; anorexia; indigestion; burning; increased fistula drainage; irritation of duodenal mucosa. *HEMA:* Leukopenia. *HEPA:* Increased serum amylase; bile shock. *DERM:* Pruritus. *META:* Hypokalemia. *OTHER:* Fever; chills; diaphoresis; allergic reaction.

Precautions
Pregnancy: Category C. *Lactation:* Undetermined. *Children:* Safety and efficacy not established. *Hepatic impairment:* Patients with impaired hepatic function may experience metabolic acidosis during drug perfusion.

NURSING CONSIDERATIONS

Administration/Storage

- Use caution in patients with obstructive jaundice due to stones.
- Not for parenteral (IM/IV) use.
- Prepare vials by adding 13 ml of Sterile Water for Injection.
- Continuously perfuse on a 24-hour basis at a rate of 3 to 5 ml/hr. Continuous perfusion usually requires 2 to 10 days for elimination or size reduction of stones. If, after 10 days, cholangiography shows neither elimination nor reduction in size or density of stones, an endoscopy should be performed to determine advisability of additional perfusion based on friability, softness or reduction of stone density.
- Maximize benefits of therapy by administering drug at 37°C (98.6°F).

- Perfuse into biliary tract either directly via catheter inserted through T-tube or via catheter inserted through mature sinus tract through nasobiliary tube placed endoscopically.
- Place tip of catheter as close to stone as possible. Drug is effective only when in direct contact with stone.
- Store at room temperature. If stored below 59°F (15°C), drug may form semisolid, which will reliquefy on rewarming.

Assessment/Interventions

- Obtain patient history, including drug history and any known allergies. Note impaired hepatic function, significant biliary tract infection, acute pancreatitis, recent duodenal ulcer, recent jejunitis, portosystemic shunting or active life-threatening problems that would be complicated by perfusion into biliary tract.
- Ensure that liver function tests are performed routinely in patients with impaired liver function.
- Monitor flow rate and pressure carefully. Irritation to GI and biliary tracts is related to perfusion pressure and rate of administration.
- Monitor for intolerable abdominal pain, nausea, diarrhea or emesis. If symptoms occur, stop perfusion for 1 hr, aspirate duct, then restart. If symptoms persist, stop perfusion for 1 hr, aspirate duct, then restart at reduced rate of 3 ml/hr. If symptoms still persist, temporarily discontinue perfusion during mealtimes.
- Observe for fever, anorexia, chills, severe right upper quadrant abdominal pain or jaundice. If these symptoms occur, discontinue drug and notify physician.

OVERDOSAGE: SIGNS & SYMPTOMS

Abdominal pain

Patient/Family Education

- Instruct patient to report these symptoms to physician: fever, chills, anorexia, severe right upper quadrant abdominal pain, jaundice, fatigue, lethargy, abdominal pain or discomfort, nausea, vomiting, diarrhea, anorexia, depression or any other problem.

No patient monograph available.

Morphine Sulfate

(MORE-feen SULL-fate)

Astramorph PF, Duramorph, MS Contin, MSIR, RMS, Roxanol, Roxanol SR, Roxanol 100, Roxanol UD,
Epimorph, M.O.S., *Statex*

Class: Narcotic analgesic

Action Relieves pain by stimulating opiate receptors in CNS; also causes respiratory depression, peripheral vasodilation, inhibition of intestinal peristalsis, sphincter of Oddi spasm, stimulation of chemoreceptors that cause vomiting and increased bladder tone.

Indications Relief of moderate to severe acute and chronic pain; preoperative sedation and adjunct to anesthesia. **Unlabeled use:** Management of dyspnea associated with left ventricular failure and pulmonary edema.

Contraindications Hypersensitivity to opiates; upper airway obstruction; acute asthma; diarrhea caused by poisoning or toxins. *Intrathecal/epidural:* Infection at injection site; anticoagulation; bleeding condition; parenteral corticosteroids within past 2 wk; any other drug or condition that would contraindicate intrathecal/epidural therapy.

Route/Dosage

ADULTS: **PO** 10-30 mg q 4 hr prn. **SC/IM** 5-20 mg/70 kg q 4 hr prn. **IV** 2.5-15 mg/70 kg in 4-5 ml Water for Injection over 5 min prn. **PR** 10-20 mg q 4 hr prn. **Epidural** Initial injection: 5 mg may provide pain relief for up to 24 hr; if pain is not controlled within 1 hr, give incremental doses of 1-2 mg. Do not exceed 10 mg/24 hr. **Intrathecal** Usual dose is 10% of epidural dose. Single injection of 0.2-1 mg may provide pain relief for 24 hr. Do not inject more than 2 ml of 5 mg/10 ml ampul or 1 ml of 10 mg/10 ml ampul. Repeat injections not recommended. CHILDREN: **SC/IM** 0.1-0.2 mg/kg q 4 hr. Maximum dose: 15 mg.

Interactions

CNS depressants (eg, alcohol, sedatives, tranquilizers): Additive CNS depression. INCOMPATIBILITIES: *Acyclovir, barbiturates, furosemides, heparin, sargramostim, sodium bicarbonate*: Precipitation of IV solutions.

Lab Test Interferences

Increased amylase and lipase may occur up to 24 hr after dose.

Adverse Reactions

CV: Hypotension; orthostatic hypotension; bradycardia; tachycardia; palpitations. *RESP*: Respiratory depression; apnea; respiratory arrest; laryngospasm; depression of cough reflex. *CNS*: Lighheadedness; dizziness; drowsiness; sedation; euphoria; dysphoria; delerium; disorientation; incoordination. *EENT*: Blurred vision; miosis. *GI*: Nausea; vomiting; constipation; abdominal pain. *GU*: Urinary retention or hesitancy. *DERM*: Sweating; pruritus; urticaria. *OTHER*: Tolerance; psychological and physical dependence with chronic use; pain at injection site; local irritation and induration following SC use.

Precautions

Pregnancy: Category C. *Lactation*: Excreted in breast milk. *Elderly patients*: Dosage reduction may be necessary. *Special risk patients*: Use drug with caution in patients with myxedema, acute alcoholism, acute abdominal conditions, ulcerative colitis, decreased respiratory reserve, head injury or increased intracranial pressure, hypoxia, supraventricular tachycardia, depleted blood volume or circulatory shock. *Drug dependence*: Has abuse potential. *Hepatic or renal impairment*: May need to reduce dose.

NURSING CONSIDERATIONS

Administration/Storage

- Administer medication as soon as pain occurs. Effect is reduced as pain increases.
- Give oral form with food to decrease GI upset.
- Administer antiemetic for nausea and vomiting, if ordered.
- Controlled-release tablets should not be chewed or crushed.
- Prepare IV solution by diluting in 4-5 ml of Water for Injection. Administer over 4-5 min.
- For continuous IV infusion, add drug to prepare solution of 0.1-1 mg/ml in D5W. Control infusion with electronic infusion device.
- Do not administer IV solution if cloudy, precipitate is present or antidote is not readily available.
- Intrathecal and epidural injection should be administered only in lumbar region.
- To reduce chance of adverse effects with intrathecal administration, constant IV infusion of naloxone (0.6 mg/hr for 24 hr after intrathecal injection) is recommended.
- Subcutaneous injection can irritate tissues; use IM injection for repeated doses.
- Store at room temperature.

Assessment/Interventions

- Obtain patient history, including drug history and any known allergies.
- Assess type, location and intensity of pain before and 30-60 min after administration.
- Assess vital signs before and periodically during therapy.

- Assess bowel and bladder function regularly in patients receiving repeated doses.
- Assist patient with ambulation. Keep siderails up and call bell within reach.
- Evaluate therapeutic response. Prolonged use may lead to physical dependence and tolerance. Progressively higher doses may be necessary to control pain in patients receiving long-term therapy.
- With continuous infusion, titrate dose to ensure adequate pain relief without excessive sedation, respiratory depression or hypotension.
- Monitor for CNS changes: dizziness, drowsiness, hallucinations, euphoria, level of consciousness, pupil reaction.

OVERDOSAGE: SIGNS & SYMPTOMS

Miosis, respiratory and CNS depression, circulatory collapse, seizures, cardiopulmonary arrest, death

Patient/Family Education

- Instruct patient to take oral preparations with food or juice if GI upset occurs.
- Tell patient not to crush or chew controlled-release tablets.
- Explain that full effectiveness of drug may not occur for 30-60 min after administration. Emphasize that drug is more effective if taken regularly to prevent pain rather than to treat pain after it occurs.
- If patient is to receive patient-controlled analgesia (PCA), instruct on use of PCA pump.
- Explain that physical dependency may occur with long-term therapy and that dosage will be tapered slowly before stopping to prevent withdrawal symptoms (nausea, vomiting, cramps, fever, faintness, anorexia).
- Encourage patient to turn, cough and breathe deeply every 2 hr to prevent atelectasis.
- Advise patient to consult with physician if excessive sedation occurs or if pain relief is inadequate.
- Inform patient that drug may cause constipation. Stool softener, fiber laxative, increased fluid intake and bulk in diet may help alleviate problem.
- Caution patient to avoid sudden position changes to prevent orthostatic hypotension.
- Instruct patient to avoid intake of alcoholic beverages and other CNS depressants.
- Advise patient that drug may cause drowsiness, dizziness or blurred vision and to use caution while driving or performing other tasks requiring mental alertness.
- Instruct patient not to take otc medications without consulting physician.

See Patient Guide, p. 421.

Mupirocin (Pseudomonic Acid A)

(myoo-PIHR-oh-sin)

Bactroban

Class: Topical/anti-infective

Action Inhibits bacterial protein synthesis.

Indications Topical treatment of impetigo caused by *Staphylococcus aureus*, *Staphylococcus pyogenes*, *Streptococci*, and *Bacillus hemolyticus*.

Contraindications Standard considerations.

Route/Dosage

ADULTS: **Topical** Apply tid for 3-5 days.

Interactions None well documented.

Lab Test Interferences

None well documented.

Adverse Reactions

DERM: Burning; stinging; pain; rash; itching; contact dermatitis.

Precautions

Pregnancy: Category B. *Lacta-*

tion: Undetermined. *Hypersensitivity:* Chemical irritation may occur.

NURSING CONSIDERATIONS

Administration/Storage

- Apply topically only; avoid contact with eyes and mucous membranes. Treated area may be covered with gauze dressing.
- Wash hands before and after application.

Assessment/Interventions

- Obtain patient history, including drug history and any known allergies.
- Assess for signs of superinfection (bacterial or fungal overgrowth of nonsusceptible organisms).
- Assess for therapeutic response: decrease in size and number of lesions.
- If a skin reaction develops, discontinue therapy, wash affected area and notify physician.

Patient/Family Education

- Warn the patient to avoid contact of drug with eyes and mucous membranes.
- Instruct patient to wash hands before and after application.
- Tell patient to inform physician if no improvement is seen within 3-5 days or if condition worsens.
- Advise patient to keep fingernails well trimmed to prevent scratching.
- Review with patient and family appropriate hygiene measures to prevent spread of impetigo.
- Instruct patient to report these symptoms to physician: burning, stinging, pain, nausea, tenderness, swelling, rash, dry skin or increased exudate.

See Patient Guide, p. 422.

Muromonab–CD3

(MYOO-row-MOE-nab–CD3)

Orthoclone OKT3

Class: Immunosuppressive

Action Blocks T cell function, which plays major role in graft rejection, by reacting with and blocking T3(CD3) molecule on membrane of human T cells associated with antigen recognition.

Indications Treatment of renal, cardiac or hepatic allograft rejection.

Contraindications Hypersensitivity to any product of murine origin; antimouse antibody titers ≥ 1:1000; fluid overload or uncompensated heart failure; seizures or predisposition to seizures; pregnancy; breastfeeding.

Route/Dosage

ADULTS: **IV** 5 mg/day as bolus over < 1 min for 10-14 days.

Interactions

Immunosuppressants (eg, azathioprine, corticosteroids, cyclosporine): Psychosis, infections, malignancies, seizures, encephalopathy and thrombotic events have occurred with immunosuppressants alone and in conjunction with muromonab-CD3. *Indomethacin:* Encephalopathy and other CNS effects. INCOMPATIBILITIES: Do not administer in conjunction with other drug solutions.

Lab Test Interferences

None well documented.

Adverse Reactions

CV: Cardiac arrest; hypotension; shock; cardiovascular collapse; MI; tachycardia; bradycardia; hypertension; left ventricular dysfunction; arrhythmias; chest pain/tightness; hemodynamic instability. *RESP:* Respiratory arrest; cardiogenic and noncardiogenic pulmonary edema; apnea; dyspnea; wheezing; bronchospasm; shortness of breath; hypoxemia; hyperventilation; pneumonia. *CNS:* Seizures;

encephalopathy; cerebral edema; aseptic meningitis; headache; paresis; cerebrovascular accident; subarachnoid hemorrhage; aphasia; transient ischemic attack; hearing loss; nerve palsy. *EENT:* Blindness; photophobia; vision disturbances; conjunctivitis; hearing loss; otitis media; tinnitus; vertigo; nasal and ear stuffiness. *HEPA:* Increases in liver function tests; hepatomegaly; hepatitis. *GI:* Diarrhea; nausea; vomiting; abdominal pain; anorexia; bowel infarction; splenomegaly. *GU:* Anuria; oliguria; increases in BUN and serum creatinine; abnormal urinary cytologic results. *HEMA:* Pancytopenia; aplastic anemia; neutropenia; leukopenia; thrombocytopenia; lymphopenia; leukocytosis; lymphadenopathy; thrombosis; disturbances in coagulation. *DERM:* Rash; urticaria; pruritus; erythema; flushing; diaphoresis. *OTHER:* Fever; chills; tremor; rigor; malaise; weakness; arthralgia; arthritis; muscle stiffness; aches, and pains; infections; neoplasias; cytokine release syndrome.

Precautions

Pregnancy: Category C. *Lactation:* Undetermined. *Children:* Safety and efficacy not established. *Cytokine release syndrome (CRS):* Temporally associated with administration of first few doses of drug and linked to release of cytokines. Reactions range from mild flu-like illness to more rare and serious shock-like cardiovascular and CNS manifestations. Common reactions include high, spiking fever; chills; rigors; headache; tremor; nausea; vomiting; diarrhea; abdominal pain; malaise; muscle and joint aches; weakness. Cardiorespiratory findings include dyspnea, shortness of breath, bronchospasm, tachypnea, respiratory arrest, cardiovascular collapse, cardiac arrest, angina, MI, chest pain, tachycardia, hypertension, hemodynamic instability, hypotension, adult respiratory distress syndrome, pulmonary edema, hypoxemia, apnea, arrhythmias. Decreased urine output may occur. *Hypersensitivity:* Anaphylactic or anaphylactoid reactions may occur after administration of any dose or course of drug. Serious and occasionally life-threatening systemic, cardiovascular and CNS reactions have been reported, including pulmonary edema (especially in patients with volume overload), shock, cardiovascular collapse, cardiac or respiratory arrest, seizures and coma. *Immunosuppression:* Increases risk, severity and morbidity from infectious complications. *Intravascular thrombosis:* Arterial or venous thromboses of allografts and other vascular beds have been reported. *Neoplasia:* Immunosuppression can increase risk of malignancies developing. *Neuropsychiatric events:* Have occurred even after first dose and include seizures, encephalopathy, cerebral edema, aseptic meningitis syndrome, headache.

NURSING CONSIDERATIONS

Administration/Storage

- Administer under supervision of physician knowledgeable about immunosuppressive agents. Patient must be hospitalized during administration.
- Withdraw medication through 0.2-0.22 mcg filter into syringe. Replace filter with needle.
- Do not mix other medications in same IV line. If IV line must be used for other medications, flush line with saline before and after use.
- Administer as IV bolus.
- Be prepared to respond to life-threatening reactions (anaphylaxis, CRS).
- Methylprednisolone sodium succinate and hydrocortisone sodium succinate given prior to medication administration may reduce incidence of first-dose reactions. Acetaminophen and antihistamines given prior to drug administration may also reduce early reactions.
- Use immediately after opening am-

pule (contains no preservative). Discard any unused portion.
- Store in refrigerator. Do not freeze or shake.

Assessment/Interventions
- Obtain patient history, including drug history and any known allergies.
- Take baseline vital signs and assess fluid balance and level of consciousness.
- Ensure that chest x-ray is ordered within 24 hr before initiating treatment.
- Reassess for signs and symptoms of fluid overload, fever, chills, malaise, dyspnea and neuropsychiatric events immediately after administration and for up to 6 hr after first dose.
- Ensure availability of resuscitative equipment.
- Monitor renal, hepatic, and blood count values before and during therapy.
- Monitor I&O and weigh daily.
- Monitor patient closely for 48 hr after first dose. Notify physician of any spiking fever or other adverse effects.

Patient/Family Education
- Advise patient about first-dose adverse effects. Explain that these effects will become less severe as treatment progresses.
- Explain that it will be necessary to resume lifelong therapy with other immunosuppressive drugs after completing course of muromonab.
- Instruct patient to report these symptoms to physician: chest pain, difficulty breathing, nausea, vomiting, fever, chills, sore throat.

See Patient Guide, p. 423.

Mycophenolate Mofetil

(my-koe-FEN-oh-late MOE-feh-till)
CellCept
Class: Immunosuppressive

Action Inhibits immune-mediated inflammatory responses, but exact mechanism not known.

Indications In combination with cyclosporine and corticosteroids for prophylaxis of organ rejection in patients receiving allogenic renal transplants.

Contraindications Standard considerations.

Route/Dosage
ADULTS: **PO** 1 g administered within 72 hours following transplantation; then 1 g twice daily in combination with corticosteroids and cyclosporine.

Interactions
Acyclovir: Possible increased plasma concentrations of both drugs. *Antacids containing magnesium and aluminum hydroxides:* Decreased absorption of mycophenolate; do not administer simultaneously. *Azathioprine:* Avoid use due to lack of clinical studies. *Cholestyramine:* Decreased mycophenolate plasma concentrations; do not give mycophenolate with cholestyramine or other agents that may interfere with enterohepatic recirculation. *Ganciclovir:* Possible increased plasma concentrations of both drugs. *Probenecid:* May increase plasma concentrations of mycophenolate.

Lab Test Interferences
None well documented.

Adverse Reactions
CV: Hypertension; hypotension; orthostatic hypotension; peripheral edema; tachycardia; chest pain; palpitations. *RESP:* Infection; dyspnea; cough; bronchitis; asthma; pulmonary edema; pleural effusion. *CNS:* Headache; tremor; insomnia; dizziness; anxiety; depression; somnolence; paresthesia. *EENT:* Amblyopia; cataracts; conjunctivitis; rhinitis; sinusitis; pharyngitis. *GI:* Diarrhea; constipation; nausea; abdominal pain; dyspepsia; vomiting; oral moniliasis; anorexia; esophagitis; flatu-

lence; gastritis; GI hemorrhage; gingivitis; gingival hyperplasia; ileus. *GU:* Urinary tract infection; hematuria; kidney tubular necrosis; dysuria; impotence; pyelonephritis; urinary frequency. *HEMA:* Anemia; hypochromic anemia; leukopenia; thrombocytopenia; leukocytosis. *HEPA:* Elevated liver function tests. *DERM:* Acne; rash; alopecia; pruritis; sweating. *META:* Hypercholesterolemia; hypophosphatemia; hypokalemia; hyperkalemia; hyperglycemia. *OTHER:* Body/back pain; fever; chills; infection; sepsis; asthenia; arthralgia; myalgia; leg cramps; myasthenia; lymphoma/lymphoproliferative disease; nonmelanoma skin carcinoma.

Precautions

Pregnancy: Category C. *Lactation:* Undetermined. *Children:* Safety and efficacy not established. *Women of childbearing potential:* Should have a negative serum or urine pregnancy test within 1 week of beginning therapy; effective contraception (abstinence or two reliable methods) must be used before, during and for 6 weeks following discontinuation of therapy. *Lymphomas/malignancies:* Patients receiving immunosuppressive regimens involving combinations of drugs are at increased risk of developing lymphomas and other malignancies, particularly of the skin. Risk appears to be related to intensity and duration of immunosuppression rather than to any specific agent. *Infection:* Suppression of the immune system increases susceptibility to infection. *Neutropenia:* Monitor patients for neutropenia; dosage changes may be indicated. *Monitoring:* Complete blood counts should be performed weekly during the first month, twice monthly during the second and third months, then monthly through the first year. *GI hemorrhage:* GI tract hemorrhage has been observed; administer with caution to patients with active serious digestive system disease. *Impaired renal function:* Do not exceed 2 g per day doses in patients with GFR < 25 ml/min/1.73 m^2; carefully monitor these patients.

NURSING CONSIDERATIONS

Administration/Storage

- Initial oral dose should be administered within 72 hours after transplantation.
- Oral medication is most effective on an empty stomach.
- Medication should be used concurrently with cyclosporine and corticosteroids.
- Do not open or crush capsules. Avoid inhalation or direct contact with skin or mucous membranes of the capsule powder. If contact occurs, wash thoroughly with soap and water; rinse eyes with plain water.
- Store at room temperature.

Assessment/Interventions

- Obtain patient history.
- Obtain baseline laboratory tests, including BUN, creatinine, lipid levels, potassium, WBC with diff and CBC. Perform and evaluate these tests periodically during treatment.
- Assess for any signs of infection, bleeding or bruising.
- Maintain medical asepsis and eliminate any potential sources of environmental contamination.
- Monitor for signs and symptoms of organ rejection.

OVERDOSAGE: SIGNS & SYMPTOMS

Nausea, vomiting, diarrhea, neutropenia

Patient/Family Education

- Instruct patient not to change dose or discontinue medication without consulting healthcare provider.
- Instruct patient to check with healthcare provider before taking any over-the-counter or prescription medications, and vaccinations.
- Instruct patient to report any serious

side effects to healthcare provider, including: tremors, headaches, diarrhea, hypertension, nausea and low urine output.

- Inform patient of need for frequent laboratory tests while taking this medication. Be sure to keep appointments.
- Instruct patient to avoid contact with others who may have infections.
- Instruct patient to use a soft toothbrush and to practice frequent oral hygiene.
- Instruct patient to take medication 30 minutes before or 2 hours after meals. If medication causes GI upset, take with a full glass of water. May be taken with food, but is less effective.
- Instruct women of childbearing potential to use effective contraception before beginning therapy, during therapy and for 6 weeks after stopping therapy.

See Patient Guide, p. 424.

Nabumetone

(nab-YOU-meh-TONE)
Relafen
Class: Analgesic/NSAID

Action Decreases inflammation, pain and fever, probably through inhibition of cyclooxygenase activity and prostaglandin synthesis.

Indications Relief of symptoms of chronic and acute rheumatoid arthritis and osteoarthritis.

Contraindications Hypersensitivity to aspirin, iodides or any NSAID.

Route/Dosage
Osteoarthritis/Rheumatoid Arthritis
ADULTS: **PO** 1000 mg initially; may increase to 1500-2000 mg daily in 1-2 divided doses.

Interactions
Anticoagulants: May increase effect of anticoagulants. May increase risk of gastric erosion and bleeding. *Cyclosporine:* Neurotoxicity of both agents may be increased. *Lithium:* May increase lithium levels. *Methotrexate:* Increased risk of methotrexate toxicity. *Salicylates:* Additive GI toxicity.

Lab Test Interferences
May prolong bleeding time.

Adverse Reactions
CV: Edema; weight gain; congestive heart failure; alterations in blood pressure; vasodilation; palpitations; tachycardia; chest pain; bradycardia. *CNS:* Dizziness; lightheadedness; drowsiness; confusion; increased sweating; vertigo; headaches; nervousness; migraine; anxiety; aggravated Parkinson's or epilepsy; paresthesia; peripheral neuropathy; myalgia; tremors; fatigue. *RESP:* Bronchospasm; laryngeal edema; dyspnea; hemoptysis; shortness of breath. *EENT:* Blurred vision; tinnitus; rhinitis; salivation; glossitis; pharyngitis. *GI:* Diarrhea; ulceration; dry mouth; heartburn; dyspepsia; nausea; vomiting; anorexia; diarrhea; constipation; flatulence; indigestion; appetite changes; abdominal cramps; epigastric pain; hematemesis. *GU:* Acute renal insufficiency; interstitial nephritis; hyperkalemia; hyponatremia; papillary necrosis; melena; menometrorrhagia; impotence; menstrual disorders; hematuria; cystitis; nocturia; proteinuria. *HEPA:* Hepatitis. *HEMA:* Increased prothrombin time; bleeding; anemia; neutropenia; leukopenia; pancytopenia; eosinophilia; thrombocytopenia. *DERM:* Rash; urticaria; purpura. *OTHER:* Photosensitivity.

Precautions
Pregnancy: Category C. *Lactation:* Undetermined. *Children:* Safety and efficacy not established. *Elderly patients:* Increased risk of adverse reactions. *GI effects:* Serious GI toxicity (eg, bleeding, ulceration, perforation) can

occur at any time, with or without warning symptoms. *Hypersensitivity:* May occur; use drug with caution in aspirin-sensitive patients because of possible cross-sensitivity. *Renal impairment:* Lower doses may be necessary.

NURSING CONSIDERATIONS

Administration/Storage

- Give medication with full glass of water, either with or without food.
- Store in tightly-closed, light-resistant container at room temperature.

Assessment/Interventions

- Obtain patient history, including drug history and any known allergies. Note fluid retention, nasal polyps, bronchospastic disease and hypersensitivity to aspirin or other NSAIDs.
- Obtain baseline assessments of pain and ability to perform activities of daily living.
- For patients undergoing long-term therapy or with history of GI or renal disease, monitor for abnormalities/trends in liver/kidney function test results, hematocrit, hemoglobin and platelets.
- Use caution if patient is also receiving anticoagulants or thrombolytics.
- Monitor for signs and symptoms of GI distress or bleeding.

OVERDOSAGE: SIGNS & SYMPTOMS

Drowsiness, dizziness, confusion, disorientation, lethargy, numbness, vomiting, gastric irritation, nausea, abdominal pain, headache, tinnitus, sweating, convulsions, blurred vision, renal failure, coma

Patient/Family Education

- Remind patient to take medication with full glass of water, either with or without food.
- Explain that therapeutic effects may take up to 1 mo to be noted.
- Instruct patient to report these symptoms to physician: rash, visual disturbance, ringing in ears, dark stools, persistent headache or abdominal pain, unusual bleeding or bruising, decreased urinary output, weight gain, edema. Caution patient to avoid intake of alcoholic beverages and to avoid smoking.
- Advise patient that drug may cause drowsiness and to use cauton while driving or performing other tasks requiring mental alertness.
- Caution patient to avoid exposure to sunlight and to use sunscreen or wear protective clothing to avoid photosensitvity reaction.

See Patient Guide, p. 425.

Nadolol

(nay-DOE-lahl)

Corgard, ✤ *APO-Nadol*

Class: Beta-adrenergic blocker

Action Blocks beta-receptors, which primarily affect cardiovascular system (decreases heart rate, contractility and BP) and lungs (promotes broncho-spasm).

Indications Management of hypertension and angina pectoris.

Contraindications Hypersensitivity to beta blockers; greater than first-degree heart block; CHF unless secondary to tachyarrhythmia treatable with beta-blockers or untreated hypotension; overt cardiac failure; sinus bradycardia; cardiogenic shock; bronchial asthma or bronchospasm, including severe COPD.

Route/Dosage

Hypertension

ADULTS: **PO** Initiate with 40 mg/day; titrate in 40-80 mg increments to desired response. Maintenance: 40-320 mg/day.

Angina

ADULTS: **PO** Initiate with 40 mg/day; titrate in 40-80 mg increments at 3-7 day intervals to desired response. Maintenance: 40-240 mg/day. Dosage intervals may need to be altered in patients with decreased renal function.

Interactions

Clonidine: May enhance or reverse antihypertensive effect; potentially life-threatening situations may occur, especially on withdrawal. *Epinephrine:* Initial hypertensive episode followed by bradycardia may occur. *Ergot alkaloids:* Peripheral ischemia, manifested by cold extremities and possible gangrene, may occur. *Insulin:* Prolonged hypoglycemia with masking of symptoms may occur. *Lidocaine:* Lidocaine levels may increase, leading to toxicity. *NSAIDs:* Some agents may impair antihypertensive effect. *Prazosin:* Orthostatic hypotension may be increased. *Verapamil:* Effects of both drugs may be increased.

Lab Test Interferences

Serum glucose may decrease; may interfere with glucose or insulin intolerance tests.

Adverse Reactions

CV: Bradycardia; hypotension; CHF; cold extremities; heart block; worsening angina; edema. *RESP:* Wheezing; bronchospasm; difficulty breathing. *CNS:* Depression; fatigue; lethargy; drowsiness; short-term memory loss; headache; dizziness. *EENT:* Dry eyes; visual disturbances. *GI:* Nausea; vomiting; diarrhea. *GU:* Impotence; urinary retention; difficulty with urination. *HEMA:* Agranulocytosis. *DERM:* Alopecia; rash. *META:* May increase or decrease blood glucose; elevated triglycerides and total cholesterol; decreased HDL cholesterol. *OTHER:* Increased sensitivity to cold.

Precautions

Pregnancy: Category C. *Lactation:* Excreted in breast milk. *Children:* Safety and efficacy not established. *Abrupt withdrawal:* Beta-blocker withdrawal syndrome (hypertension, tachycardia, anxiety, angina, MI) may occur 1-2 wk following sudden discontinuation of systemic beta-blocker therapy. Treatment should be withdrawn gradually over 1-2 wk. *Anaphylaxis:* Deaths have occurred; aggressive therapy may be required. *CHF:* Administer cautiously in CHF patients controlled by digitalis and diuretics. Notify physician at first sign or symptom of CHF or unexplained respiratory symptoms in any patient. *Diabetics:* May mask signs and symptoms of hypoglycemia, eg, tachycardia, blood pressure changes. May potentiate insulin-induced hypoglycemia. *Nonallergic bronchospasm:* Give drug with caution in patients with bronchospastic disease. *Peripheral vascular disease:* May precipitate or aggravate symptoms of arterial insufficiency. *Renal/hepatic impairment:* Reduced dosage advised. *Thyrotoxicosis:* May mask clinical signs (eg, tachycardia) of developing or continuing hyperthyroidism. Abrupt withdrawal may exacerbate symptoms of hyperthyroidism, including thyroid storm.

NURSING CONSIDERATIONS

Administration/Storage

- Assess heart rate and BP before administering medication.
- Administer on regular schedule.
- Give medication with full glass of water, either with or without food.
- Discontinue drug gradually over 1-2 wk.
- Store in tightly closed, light-resistant container at room temperature.

Assessment/Interventions

- Obtain patient history, includ-

ing drug history and any known allergies. Note CHF, asthma, diabetes mellitus or hyperthyroidism.

- Obtain baseline cardiac assessment including heart rate, BP, capillary refill, pulse rhythm, presence of angina. Monitor BP and pulse frequently during initial phase of therapy and when changing dosage.
- If patient is scheduled for surgery, confer with physician regarding use of medication prior to surgery.
- For postoperative patients, monitor for trends in heart rate and blood pressure.
- Monitor I&O and weigh patient daily.
- Withhold medication and notify physician if heart rate is < 60 bpm or systolic BP < 90 mm Hg. Atropine may be needed for treatment of persistent bradycardia.
- For diabetic patients receiving hypoglycemic agents, monitor blood glucose test results. Signs and symptoms of hypoglycemia may be masked with nadolol.
- For patients discontinuing medication, monitor for signs or symptoms of thyroid storm. Abrupt withdrawal may precipitate thyrotoxicosis.
- Observe for signs of beta-blocker withdrawal syndrome (hypotension, tachycardia, anxiety, angina, MI) if medication is discontinued suddenly.
- Use caution in patients with CHF, COPD or asthma. Monitor cardiovascular and respiratory status carefully and frequently.

OVERDOSAGE: SIGNS & SYMPTOMS

Bradycardia, cardiogenic shock, intraventricular conduction disturbances, hypotension, AV block, depressed consciousness, CHF, asystole, coma

Patient/Family Education

- Teach patient how to measure pulse rate before taking medication. Explain that if pulse rate is < 50 bpm, patient needs to discontinue taking medication immediately and notify physician.
- Ensure that patient has independently demonstrated how to measure pulse rate.
- Show patient how to monitor blood sugar levels, and explain that signs and symptoms of low blood sugar levels may be masked.
- Caution patient not to stop taking medication abruptly but to consult physician for instructions on safest way to discontinue medication.
- Instruct patient to report these symptoms to physician: bradycardia, palpitations, dizziness, fatigue, insomnia or sleep disturbances, altered sensorium, GI symptoms, changes in blood sugar levels.
- Advise patient that drug may cause drowsiness and to use caution while driving or performing other tasks requiring mental alertness.
- Instruct patient not to take otc medications without consulting physician.

See Patient Guide, p. 426.

Nafarelin Acetate

(NAFF-uh-RELL-in ASS-uh-TATE)

Synarel

Class: Gonadotropin-releasing hormone

Action Initially causes synthesis and release of luteinizing hormone (LH) and follicle-stimulating hormone (FSH). With continued use (> 4 wk) suppresses secretion of LH and FSH.

Indications Treatment of endometriosis, central precocious puberty in children of both sexes.

Contraindications Hypersensitivity to gonadotropin-releasing hormone (GnRH); or GnRH-agonist analogs; undiagnosed abnormal vaginal bleeding; pregnancy; lactation.

Route/Dosage

Endometriosis

ADULTS: **Intranasal** 400 mcg/day (200 mcg [1 spray] in 1 nostril in morning and 200 mcg [1 spray] in other nostril in evening. For long-term suppression, 800 mcg/day (1 spray in each nostril bid) may be necessary.

Central Precocious Puberty

CHILDREN: **Intranasal** 1600 mcg/day (400 mcg [2 sprays] in each nostril in morning and 400 mcg [2 sprays] in each nostril in evening). In some patients 1800 mcg/day (3 sprays in alternating nostrils tid) may be necessary.

Interactions

None well documented.

Lab Test Interferences

Diagnostic tests of pituitary gonadotropic and gonadal function during treatment and 4-8 wk after discontinuation of treatment may be misleading.

Adverse Reactions

CNS: Headaches; insomnia; depression. *EENT:* Nasal irritation. *DERM:* Acne; seborrhea. *GU:* Vaginal dryness. *OTHER:* Hot flushes; decreased libido; emotional lability; myalgia; reduced breast size; edema; weight gain; hirsutism; decreased bone density.

Precautions

Pregnancy: Category X. *Lactation:* Do not use in lactating women. *Bone density loss:* May be small loss in bone density during therapy, some of which may not be reversible. Risk is greater in patients who smoke or have osteoporosis and in alcoholics. *Intercurrent rhinitis:* If patient must use topical nasal decongestant during nafarelin therapy, should be used at least 2 hr after nafarelin dosing to decrease possibility of reduced absorption. *Menstruation:* Should stop with effective doses. *Noncompliance:* Irregular or incomplete doses may result in stimulation of pituitary-gonadal axis. *Ovarian cysts:* Have occurred in first 2 mo of therapy.

NURSING CONSIDERATIONS

Administration/Storage

- When treating endometriosis, begin treatment between days 2 and 4 of menstrual cycle.
- Administer intranasally with metered-spray pump. Patient's head should be tilted back slightly.
- If administering > 1 spray per nostril, wait 30 sec between sprays.
- Store container upright at room temperature.
- Protect from light.

Assessment/Interventions

- Obtain patient history, including drug history and any known allergies.
- Obtain baseline assessments of last menstrual period, pregnancy status in patients with endometriosis, height and weight in patients with central precocious puberty.
- Monitor menstrual cycles.
- Monitor for drug-related hypoestrogenism. Note patient complaints of hot flushes, libido decrease, vaginal dryness, headaches, emotional lability.
- Monitor for signs of androgenism, including acne, myalgia, breast size reduction, edema, weight gain.

Patient/Family Education

- Caution patient that this medication must not be taken during pregnancy or when pregnancy is possible. Advise patient to use nonhormonal form of birth control while taking this drug.
- Advise patient regarding proper administration techniques and storage information.
- Tell patient to begin treatment between days 2 and 4 of menstrual cycle if being treated for endometriosis.
- Instruct patient not to blow nose and to avoid sneezing immediately after administration.
- Tell patient using topical nasal

decongestant to use 2 hr after nafarelin has been administered.

- Advise patient that each bottle contains approximately 60 sprays and plan refills accordingly.
- Explain side effects of medication and instruct patient to report these symptoms to physician: bleeding/menses continues, breakthrough bleeding or adverse/side effects.

See Patient Guide, p. 427.

Nalbuphine HCl

(NAL-byoo-FEEN HIGH-droe-KLOR-ide)

Nubain

Class: Narcotic agonist-antagonist analgesic

Action An opiate analgesic with both narcotic agonist and antagonist actions. Analgesic potency is about equal to that of morphine, and antagonist potency is about 1/25 that of naloxone. May cause sphincter of Oddi spasm. Does not increase pulmonary artery pressure, systemic vascular resistance or myocardial work load.

Indications Management of moderate to severe pain; preoperative and postoperative analgesia; supplement to balanced anesthesia; obstetrical analgesia during labor and delivery.

Contraindications Standard considerations.

Route/Dosage
ADULTS: **SC/IM/IV** 10 mg/70 kg q 3-6 hr prn. Individualize dosage. In nontolerant patients, do not exceed 20 mg/dose or 160 mg/day.

Interactions
CNS depressants, including barbiturate anesthetics: Increased respiratory and CNS depression. INCOMPATIBILITIES: Diazepam, pentobarbital, promethazine.

Lab Test Interferences
None well documented.

Adverse Reactions
CV: Hypertension; hypotension; bradycardia; tachycardia; pulmonary edema. *RESP:* Respiratory depression. *CNS:* Sedation; dizziness; vertigo; headache. *EENT:* Miosis. *GI:* Nausea; vomiting; constipation; dry mouth. *DERM:* Urticaria. *OTHER:* Sweaty or clammy feeling.

Precautions
Pregnancy: Pregnancy category undetermined. Safety (except during labor) is unknown. May cause respiratory depression in neonate; use drug with caution in women delivered of premature infants. *Lactation:* Undetermined. *Children:* Not recommended in patients < 18 yr. *Special risk patients:* Use drug with caution in patients with impaired respiration, head injury, increased intracranial pressure, or MI with nausea or vomiting and in patients about to undergo biliary tract surgery. *Dependence:* Low abuse potential; however, withdrawal symptoms can occur after long-term use. Use drug with caution in patients who are emotionally unstable or have history of narcotic abuse. *Opiate-dependent patients:* Nalbuphine can precipitate withdrawal; small doses of morphine can be given to relieve discomfort. If patient has received morphine, meperidine, codeine or other opiate of similar duration, give 25% of normal nalbuphine dose first. Observe for signs of withdrawal and increase nalbuphine dose slowly. *Renal or hepatic impairment:* Duration of action may be prolonged; may need to reduce dose. *Sulfite sensitivity:* Contains sodium metabisulfite, which may cause allergic-type reactions including anaphylactic symptoms and life-threatening asthma.

NURSING CONSIDERATIONS

Administration/Storage

- Administer via parenteral route only.
- Store in light-resistant container at room temperature.

Assessment/Interventions

- Obtain patient history, including drug history and any known allergies.
- Obtain baseline assessments of pain, respiratory rate and level of consciousness. Withhold medication and notify physician if respiratory rate < 10/min.
- For patients receiving opiate agonists (eg, morphine, codeine), assess for signs and symptoms of withdrawal, which may include restlessness, abdominal cramps, nausea, vomiting, lacrimation, piloerection, increased temperature. Check physician's orders for notes on use of morphine sulfate to relieve withdrawal symptoms.
- Monitor effectiveness of medication by evaluating patient's pain perception.
- Monitor for sedation. May need to take precautions against falling to ensure patient safety.
- Carefully monitor patients with neurologic injury.
- Monitor for constipation and urinary retention.

OVERDOSAGE: SIGNS & SYMPTOMS

Respiratory depression, hypoxemia, sedation

Patient/Family Education

- Explain importance of communicating effectiveness of pain relief.
- Tell patient to inform nurse if difficulty breathing, dizziness, drowsiness or lethargy occurs.
- Explain importance of fall precautions and of asking for assistance with ambulation.
- Emphasize importance of informing caregivers of potential problems, including sedation, dizziness, headache, vertigo, nausea, vomiting, dry mouth, itching, shortness of breath, blurred vision, flushing.
- Instruct patient to avoid intake of alcoholic beverages or other CNS depressants.
- Advise patient that drug may cause drowsiness and to use caution while driving or performing other tasks requiring mental alertness.

See Patient Guide, p. 428.

Nalidixic Acid

(nal-ih-DIK-sik acid)

NegGram

Class: Urinary anti-infective

Action Interferes with DNA formation of certain bacteria.

Indications Treatment of UTIs caused by susceptible gram-negative bacteria, including most *Proteus* strains, *Klebsiella* and *Enterobacter* species and *E coli*.

Contraindications History of seizures.

Route/Dosage

ADULTS: PO Initial therapy: 1 g qid for 1 or 2 wk. PROLONGED THERAPY: 1 g bid after initial therapy. CHILDREN 3 MO-12 YR: PO Initial therapy: 55 mg/kg/day divided into 4 equal doses. PROLONGED THERAPY: 33 mg/kg/day in 4 divided doses after initial therapy.

Interactions

Oral anticoagulants: May enhance anticoagulant effect.

Lab Test Interferences

False-positive urinary glucose results with Benedict's or Fehling's solutions or Clinitest reagent tablets; use Clinistix or Tes-tape. Urinary 17-keto and ketogenic steroids may be falsely elevated; Porter-Silber method should be used.

Adverse Reactions

CNS: Drowsiness; weakness; headache; dizziness; vertigo; seizures; intracranial hypertension; increased intracranial pressure; sixth cranial nerve palsy in children and infants. *EENT:* Visual disturbances. *GI:* Abdominal pain; nausea; vomiting; diarrhea. *HEMA:* Thrombocytopenia; leukopenia, eosinophilia or hemolytic anemia (associated with G-6-PD deficiency or acute immune reaction). *HEPA:* Cholestatic jaundice; cholestasis. *DERM:* Rash; pruritus; urticaria; angioedema; photosensitivity. *META:* Metabolic acidosis.

Precautions

Pregnancy: Pregnancy category undetermined. Do not use during first trimester. *Lactation:* Excreted in breast milk. *Children:* Use drug with caution in prepubertal children; may affect cartilage and joints. *CNS effects:* Convulsions, increased intracranial pressure and toxic psychosis may occur with overdose or predisposing factors (eg, epilepsy, cerebral arteriosclerosis). *Hematologic:* Can produce clinically significant hemolysis in patients with G-6-PD deficiency. *Renal failure:* Patients with compromised renal function may fail to accumulate nalidixic acid, decreasing its effectiveness.

NURSING CONSIDERATIONS

Administration/Storage

- Give medication at least 1 hr before meals.
- Shake suspension well before use.
- Store in tightly closed container at room temperature. Do not freeze.

Assessment/Interventions

- Obtain patient history, including drug history and any known allergies.
- Obtain baseline assessments of burning/pain with urination, urinary urgency or frequency, level of consciousness.
- Assess for adverse reactions, primarily with CNS and GI systems.
- Obtain urine specimens as needed for culture and sensitivity.
- Monitor blood counts, liver and renal function test values if treatment is continued longer than 2 wk.
- Re-evaluate patient for improvement of symptoms.

OVERDOSAGE: SIGNS & SYMPTOMS

Increased intracranial pressure, metabolic acidosis, lethargy, psychosis, nausea, hyperglycemia, convulsions, vomiting

Patient/Family Education

- Tell patient to take with food or milk.
- Explain importance of adequate hydration and encourage intake of 1500-3000 ml fluids/day, unless otherwise specified by physician.
- Instruct patient to report these symptoms to physician: if no improvement of UTI discomfort, signs or symptoms 48 hours after initiation of treatment and if adverse effects occur.
- Advise patient that drug may cause drowsiness or dizziness and to use caution while driving or performing other tasks requiring mental alertness.
- Caution patient to avoid exposure to ultraviolet light and sunlight and to use sunscreen or wear protective clothing and to use sunglasses when outdoors. Explain that photosensitivity may last up to 3 mo after last dose.

See Patient Guide, p. 429.

Naproxen

(nay-PROX-ehn)

EC Naprosyn, Naprosyn, ✤ Naxen, Novo-Naprox

Naproxen Sodium

Aleve, Anaprox, Anaprox DS, ✤ Novo-Naprox Sodium, Nu-Naprox, Synflex, Synflex DS

Class: Analgesic/NSAID

Action Decreases inflammation, pain and fever, probably through inhibition of cyclooxygenase activity and prostaglandin synthesis.

Indications Management of mild to moderate pain, symptoms of rheumatoid or osteoarthritis, bursitis, tendinitis, ankylosing spondylitis, primary dysmenorrhea, acute gout. Naproxen (not naproxen sodium) also indicated for treatment of juvenile rheumatoid arthritis. Delayed-release naproxen is not recommended for initial treatment of acute pain because absorption is delayed compared to other naproxen formulations. **Unlabeled uses:** Relief of fever, sunburn, migraine, PMS.

Contraindications Allergy to aspirin, iodides or any NSAID; patients in whom aspirin or other NSAIDs induce symptoms of asthma, rhinitis or nasal polyps.

Route/Dosage

Naproxen

Rheumatoid Arthritis, Osteoarthritis, Ankylosing Spondylitis ADULTS: PO 250-500 mg bid; maximum dose of 1.5 g/day should be used short term only. **Delayed release naproxen:** PO 375 to 500 mg twice/day.

Pain, Dysmenorrhea, Bursitis, Tendinitis

ADULTS: PO 500 mg initially, then 250 mg q 6-8 hr. Do not exceed 1250 mg/day.

Juvenile Rheumatoid Arthritis

CHILDREN: PO 10 mg/kg/day in 2 divided doses. For children requiring suspension, 2.5 ml bid can be given for weights of ≥ 13 kg; 5 ml bid for weights of ≥ 25 kg, or 7.5 ml bid for weights of ≥ 38 kg.

Naproxen Sodium

Rheumatoid Arthritis, Osteoarthritis, Ankylosing Spondylitis ADULTS: PO 275 mg bid.

Acute Gout

ADULTS: 825 mg initially, then 275 mg q 8 hr prn.

Pain, Dysmenorrhea, Tendinitis, Bursitis

ADULTS: PO 500 mg initially, then 275 mg q 6-8 hr prn. Do not exceed 1375 mg/day.

Interactions

Anticoagulants: May increase effect of anticoagulants because of decreased plasma protein binding. May increase risk of gastric erosion and bleeding. *Lithium:* May decrease lithium clearance. *Methotrexate:* May increase methotrexate levels.

Lab Test Interferences

May falsely increase urinary 17-ketosteroid values; may interfere with urinary assays for 5-hydroxyindoleacetic acid.

Adverse Reactions

CV: Edema; weight gain; congestive heart failure; alterations in blood pressure; vasodilation; palpitations; tachycardia; chest pain; bradycardia. *RESP:* Bronchospasm; laryngeal edema; dyspnea; shortness of breath. *CNS:* Headache; dizziness; drowsiness; vertigo; lightheadedness; mental depression; nervousness; irritability; fatigue; malaise; insomnia; sleep disorders; dream abnormalities; aseptic meningitis. *EENT:* Visual changes; tinnitus; rhinitis; pharyngitis, stomatitis. *GI:* Constipation; heartburn; abdominal pain; peptic ulceration and bleeding; nausea; dyspepsia; diarrhea; vomiting; anorexia; colitis; flatulence. *GU:* Glomerulonephritis; interstitial nephritis; nephrotic syndrome; acute renal insufficiency and renal failure; dysuria; hyperkalemia; hyponatremia; renal papillary necrosis. *HEPA:* Increased liver function test results. *HEMA:* Increased bleeding time; leukopenia; thrombocytopenia; granulocytopenia; eosinophilia. *DERM:* Rash; urticaria; purpura.

Precautions

Pregnancy: Category B. *Lactation:* Excreted in breast milk. *Elderly patients:* Increased risk of adverse reactions. *Cardiovascular disease:* Drug may worsen CHF and may decrease hypertension control. *GI effects:* Serious GI toxicity (eg, bleeding, ulceration, perforation) can occur at any time, with or without warning symptoms. *Hepatic impairment:* May need to reduce dose. *Renal impairment:* Assess function before and during therapy because NSAID metabolites are eliminated renally.

NURSING CONSIDERATIONS

Administration/Storage

- Give with meals, milk or antacids.
- To facilitate dosing accuracy, for juvenile rheumatoid arthritis use suspension only.
- Store in tightly closed, light-resistant container at room temperature.

Assessment/Interventions

- Obtain patient history, including drug history and any known allergies.
- Obtain baseline assessments of pain and ability to perform activities of daily living.
- Review baseline CBC, renal and hepatic studies and coagulation studies.
- For patients on long-term therapy, history of GI or renal disease, monitor liver function test results, serum creatinine, hematocrit, hemoglobin and platelets.
- Carefully monitor patients also receiving anticoagulants or thrombolytics. Be alert for GI bleeding.

OVERDOSAGE: SIGNS & SYMPTOMS

Drowsiness, nausea, heartburn, vomiting, indigestion, seizures

Patient/Family Education

- Tell patient to take with milk, meals or antacids; follow with ½-1 glass of water to reduce GI upset.
- Advise patient to shake oral suspension before measuring.
- Explain that it may take 2-4 wk with naproxen and 1-2 days with naproxen sodium for anti-inflammatory effects to occur. Peak analgesic effect may occur in 1-2 hr.
- Caution patient that use with aspirin, alcohol, steroids and other GI irritants may cause increased GI upset.
- Instruct patient to report these symptoms to physician: visual problems, abdominal pain, symptoms of gastric bleeding.
- Caution patient to avoid intake of alcoholic beverages and smoking.
- Advise patient to use caution while driving or performing other activities that require coordinated motor movements and mental alertness.

See Patient Guide, p. 430.

Natamycin

(NAT-uh-MY-sin)

Natacyn

Class: Ophthalmic/anti-infective

Action Binds to fungal cell membrane, altering membrane permeability and depleting essential cellular constituents.

Indications Treatment of fungal blepharitis, conjunctivitis and keratitis caused by susceptible organisms.

Contraindications Standard considerations.

Route/Dosage
ADULTS: **Ophthalmic** 1 gtt in conjunctival sac q 1-2 hr initially; after 3-4 days, frequency of instillation usually reduced to 1 gtt 6-8 times daily. Continue for 14-21 days or until there is resolution of active fungal keratitis.

Interactions None well documented.

Lab Test Interferences
None well documented.

Adverse Reactions
EENT: Conjunctival chemosis; hyperemia.

Precautions
Pregnancy: Category C. *Lactation:* Undetermined. *Children:* Safety and efficacy not established. *Keratitis:* Continue medication for 14-21 days or until active fungal keratitis has resolved, to avoid recurrence.

NURSING CONSIDERATIONS

Administration/Storage

- Administer as topical ophthalmic suspension.
- Shake well before administering medication.
- To administer, wash hands thoroughly. Have patient tilt head back. Pull lower eyelid down to create pocket. Place prescribed number of drops in pocket, taking care not to touch eye or allow dropper to touch eye, eyelid or other surfaces. Wash hands again after instillation.
- Store at room temperature or refrigerate. Do not freeze. Protect from light and excessive heat.

Assessment/Interventions

- Obtain patient history, including drug history and any known allergies.
- Obtain baseline ophthalmic assessment: presence of pain, visual changes, signs and symptoms that prompted patient to seek treatment.
- Assess for ocular inflammation or irritation. Note presence of discharge, including amount and characteristics.
- Re-evaluate patient regularly for effectiveness of therapy.

Patient/Family Education

- Review proper method of instillation of medication. Instruct patient to clean excessive exudate before instilling drops and to apply light pressure to lacrimal sac for 1 min after drops are instilled.
- Emphasize importance of thorough handwashing before and after instillation and need to avoid touching eye or allowing dropper to touch eye, lids or other surfaces, to prevent spread of infection to unaffected eye or others.
- Warn patient to avoid scratching, rubbing or touching eyes.
- Instruct patient to consult physician before applying medication while wearing contact lenses.
- Advise patient to notify physician if no improvement in 7-10 days.
- Instruct patient to report this symptom to physician: conjunctivitis (ie, pain, itching, changes in vision and sense of foreign body in eye).

See Patient Guide, p. 431.

Nedocromil Sodium

(NEH-doe-KROE-mill SO-dee-uhm)
Tilade
Class: Respiratory inhalant

Action Inhibits release of mediators from inflammatory cell types associated with asthma, including histamine from mast cells and beta-glucuronidase from macrophages. May also suppress local production of leukotrines and prostaglandins. Inhibits development of bronchoconstriction responses to inhaled antigen and other challenges such as cold air.

Indications Maintenance of mild to moderate bronchial asthma.

Contraindications Standard considerations.

Route/Dosage

SYMPTOMATIC ADULTS & CHILDREN > 12 YR: **Aerosol inhalation** 2 inhalations qid at regular intervals to provide 14 mg/day. May attempt lower frequency of doses (bid-tid) over several wk in well-controlled patients.

Interactions None well documented.

Lab Test Interferences

None well documented.

Adverse Reactions

RESP: Rhinitis; upper respiratory tract infection. *GI*: Nausea; vomiting; dyspepsia; abdominal pain. *OTHER*: Unpleasant taste.

Precautions

Pregnancy: Category B. *Lactation*: Undetermined. *Children*: Safety and efficacy in children < 12 yr not established. *Acute bronchospasm*: Should not be used for reversal of acute bronchospasm, particularly status asthmaticus. However, continue to administer during acute exacerbations, unless patient becomes intolerant to inhaled dosage forms. *Cough/bronchospasm*: If cough or bronchospasm follows inhalation, may need to discontinue. *Dosing interval*: Optimal effect depends on administration at regular intervals, even during symptom-free periods.

NURSING CONSIDERATIONS

Administration/Storage

- Shake container well and invert before activation.
- Clean inhaler at least twice/wk.
- Store in light-resistant container at room temperature.
- Protect from heat and moisture.

Assessment/Interventions

- Obtain patient history, including drug history and any known allergies.
- Obtain baseline respiratory assessment, carefully documenting any shortness of breath, presence of mucus and breath sounds.

Patient/Family Education

- Ensure appropriate demonstration of how to connect medication and inhalant cartridge. Supply adequate information for home use.
- Provide appropriate demonstration of how to administer inhalant dose.
- Advise patient to increase fluid intake (if not contraindicated) to promote flow of nasal secretions.
- Caution patient to avoid exhaling into mouthpiece to avoid moisture accumulation.
- Tell patient to notify physician if coughing and bronchospasm occur with inhalation therapy. Alternative therapy may be needed.
- Explain that therapeutic effect may take approximately 2 wk.
- Tell patient that nedocromil sodium cannot be substituted for bronchodilator (for acute attacks) or steroids.
- If patient being tapered from steroids, explain that increased asthmatic symptoms may occur and to notify physician if this occurs.
- Demonstrate proper method of cleaning inhaler and remind patient that cleaning should be done at least twice/wk.
- Tell patient to report any adverse effects.

See Patient Guide, p. 432.

Nefazodone Hydrochloride

(neff-AZE-oh-dohn HIGH-droe-KLOR-ide)

Serzone

Class: Antidepressant

Action Undetermined; inhibits neuronal uptake of serotonin and norepinephrine; antagonizes alpha$_1$-adrenergic receptors.

Indications Treatment of depression.

Contraindications Coadministration with terfenadine or astemizole; hypersensitivity to nefazodone or other phenylpiperazine antidepressants (eg, trazodone).

Route/Dosage

ADULTS: **PO** 100 mg bid initially, increase by 100-200 mg increments q wk (maximum 600 mg/day). ELDERLY/DEBILITATED PATIENTS: **PO** 50 mg bid initially, increase by 100 mg increments q wk (maximum 600 mg/day).

Interactions

Antihistamines, nonsedating: Increased plasma levels and cardiac effects of astemizole and terfenadine; do not use concurrently. *Benzodiazepines:* Increased plasma concentrations and effects of alprazolam and triazolam. *Digoxin:* Increased plasma levels of digoxin. *Haloperidol:* Decreased haloperidol clearance; may need to adjust haloperidol dose. MAO *inhibitors:* Do not use nefazodone concurrently or within 14 days of discontinuing a MAO inhibitor; do not start MAO inhibitors within 1 week of stopping nefazodone. *Propranolol:* Nefazodone may decrease propranolol serum concentration; propranolol may interfere with nefazodone metabolism.

Lab Test Interferences

None well documented.

Adverse Reactions

CV: Hypotension; orthostatic hypotension; peripheral edema; sinus bradycardia. *RESP:* Pharyngitis; cough. *CNS:* Headache; somnolence; dizziness; insomnia; lightheadedness; confusion; memory impairment; paresthesia; abnormal dreams; decreased concentration; ataxia; incoordination; psychomotor retardation; tremor; hypertonia; decreased libido. *EENT:* Blurred vision; abnormal vision; visual field defects; eye pain; tinnitus; abnormal taste. *GI:* Dry mouth; nausea; constipation; dyspepsia; diarrhea; increased appetite; vomiting. *GU:* Urinary frequency; urinary tract infection; urinary retention; vaginitis; breast pain; impotence. *HEMA:* Decreased hematocrit. *DERM:* Pruritus; rash. *OTHER:* Asthenia; flu syndrome; chills; fever; neck rigidity; arthralgia.

Precautions

Pregnancy: Category C. *Lactation:* Undetermined. *Children:* Safety and efficacy in children < 18 yr not established. *Elderly patients:* Initiate treatment at half the usual dose. Dosage range same as younger patients. *Bradycardia:* Sinus bradycardia reported in 1.5% of patients; use with caution in patients with recent MI or unstable heart disease. *Hepatic cirrhosis:* Use with caution; may need smaller doses. *Postural hypotension:* Use with caution in patients with known cardiovascular or cerebrovascular disease that could be exacerbated by hypotension (eg, history of MI, angina, ischemic stroke) and conditions that would predispose to hypotension (eg, dehydration, hypovolemia, treatment with antihypertensive medications). *Mania/hypomania:* May activate mania/hypomania; use with caution in patients with history of mania. *Suicide:* Patients at risk should be closely monitored and not be given access to excessive quantities. *Priapism:* Priapism (prolonged, painful, inappropriate penile erection) has been reported with closely related antidepressants. Discontinuation of therapy is necessary.

NURSING CONSIDERATIONS

Administration/Storage

- Cautiously administer to elderly patients; patients with suicidal behavior, mania, heart disease or dysrhythmias.
- Administer with caution to patients with known cardiac conditions that could be exacerbated by hypotension (eg, history of MI, angina, ischemic stroke).
- Store at room temperature in a tightly closed container.

Assessment/Interventions

- Obtain patient history.
- Advise patient to avoid use of alcohol and OTC medications without consulting healthcare provider.
- Evaluate mental and neurological status, mood changes and suicidal tendencies.
- Assess debilitated or elderly patients for signs of overdose or adverse reactions.
- Determine whether suicide precautions are advisable and implement them as necessary.
- Monitor patient for postural hypotension and cardiac dysrhythmias. Blood pressure and pulse should be monitored at periodic intervals throughout therapy.

OVERDOSAGE: SIGNS & SYMPTOMS

Nausea, vomiting, somnolence

Patient/Family Education

- Instruct patient to take exactly as directed by healthcare provider.
- Inform patient or family that several weeks of treatment may be required to obtain the full therapeutic antidepressant effect.
- Instruct patient to inform healthcare provider of all prescription and over-the-counter drugs they are presently taking or plan to take.
- Instruct patient to avoid alcohol or other CNS depressant drugs during therapy.
- Caution patient not to drive or operate hazardous machinery until certain that therapy does not adversely affect ability to perform these activities.
- Instruct patient to notify healthcare provider if they develop a rash, hives or any signs of an allergic reaction.
- Instruct female patients to notify healthcare provider if they are pregnant, plan to become pregnant or are nursing an infant.
- Advise patient to take sips of water frequently or to suck on ice chips, sugarless hard candy or chew sugarless gum if dry mouth occurs.
- Instruct male patients to immediately notify healthcare provider should symptoms of priapism occur.
- Reinforce the necessity of follow-up examinations and continued therapy.

See Patient Guide, p. 433.

Neostigmine

(nee-oh-STIGG-meen)

Prostigimin

Class: Cholinergic muscle stimulant/anticholinesterase

Action Facilitates myoneural junction impulse transmission by inhibiting acetylcholine destruction by cholinesterase.

Indications

Neostigmine bromide (oral) and methylsulfate (injection): Diagnosis of myasthenia gravis; symptomatic control of myasthenia gravis; antidote for nondepolarizing neuromuscular blocking agents after surgery. *Neostigmine methylsulfate*: Prevention and treatment of postoperative distention and urinary retention.

Contraindications Hypersensitivity to anticholinesterases and bromides; mechanical intestinal or urinary obstruction; peritonitis.

Route/Dosage

Diagnosis of Myasthenia Gravis

ADULTS: **IM** 0.022 mg/kg. CHILDREN: **IM** 0.04 mg/kg.

Control of Myasthenia Gravis

ADULTS: **PO** 15-375 mg/day; **SC/IM** 1 ml of 1:2000 solution (0.5 mg); individualize subsequent doses. CHILDREN: **IM/IV/SC** 0.01-0.04 mg/kg dose q 2-3 hr prn.

Antidote

ADULTS: **IV** 0.5-2 mg by slow infusion repeated as needed, preceded by 0.6-1.2 mg of atropine sulfate. May be repeated prn up to total dose of 5 mg. CHILDREN: **IV** 0.07-0.08 mg/kg/dose preceded by 0.008-0.025 mg/kg/dose atropine sulfate.

Prevention of Postoperative Urinary Distention and Retention

ADULTS: **SC/IM** 1 ml of 1:4000 solution (0.25 mg) after surgery; repeat q 4-6 hr for 2 or 3 days.

Treatment of Postoperative Distention

ADULTS: **SC/IM** 1 ml of 1:2000 solution (0.5 mg), as required.

Treatment of Urinary Retention

ADULTS: **SC/IM** 1 ml of 1:2000 solution (0.5 mg) after bladder is emptied; continue 0.5 mg injection every 3 h for at least 5 injections.

Interactions

Corticosteroids: May antagonize anticholinesterases in myasthenia gravis, producing profound muscular depression. *Succinylcholine:* Neuromuscular blockade produced by succinylcholine may be either prolonged or antagonized.

Lab Test Interferences

None well documented.

Adverse Reactions

CV: Arrhythmia (bradycardia; tachycardia; atrioventricular block; nodal rhythm); nonspecific ECG changes; cardiac arrest; hypotension; syncope. *RESP:* Increased tracheobronchial secretions; laryngospasm; bronchiolar constriction; respiratory paralysis; dyspnea; respiratory depression; respiratory arrest; bronchospasm. *CNS:* Convulsions; dysarthria; dysphonia; dizziness; loss of consciousness; drowsiness; headache. *EENT:* Lacrimation; miosis; spasm of accommodation; diplopia; conjunctival hyperemia; visual changes. *GI:* Increased salivary, gastric and intestional secretions; nausea; vomiting; dysphagia; increased peristalsis; diarrhea; abdominal cramps; flatulence. *GU:* Urinary urgency; frequency and incontinence. *DERM:* Rash; urticaria; flushing. *OTHER:* Allergy and anaphylaxis; weakness; fasciculations; muscle cramps and spasms; arthralgia; diaphoresis.

Precautions

Pregnancy: Category C. *Lactation:* Undetermined. *Children:* Safety and efficacy in urinary tract indications not established. *Special risk patients:* Use with caution in patients with epilepsy, bronchial asthma, bradycardia, recent coronary occlusion, vagotonia, hyperthyroidism, cardiac arrhythmias or peptic ulcer. *Anticholinesterase insensitivity:* May develop. *Hypersensitivity:* Anaphylaxis may occur. Have atropine and antishock meds available.

NURSING CONSIDERATIONS

Administration/Storage

- Give with food or milk to reduce adverse effects. Tablet is poorly absorbed via GI tract and requires considerably larger dose than parenteral form.
- If administering IV, push at rate of 0.5 mg/min.
- Store tablets in tightly closed containers.
- Protect injectable product from light.

Assessment/Interventions

- Obtain patient history, including drug history and any known allergies.
- Obtain baseline assessment of pulse rate, respiratory rate, blood pressure.
- Provide oxygen and oxygen delivery system set-up at bedside.
- Continuously reassess for respiratory depression.
- Ensure availability of atropine to prevent or reduce adverse effects. When administering atropine and neostigmine, use separate syringes.
- If used for urinary retention, consult with physician to catheterize patient if no effects noted after 1 hr of administration.
- Notify physician if heart rate is < 80/min. Atropine may be needed to restore heart rate.
- If patient becomes hypotensive, place in supine position until BP has stabilized.

OVERDOSAGE: SIGNS & SYMPTOMS

Abdominal cramps, miosis, diarrhea, sweating, excessive salivation, panic attacks, progressive muscle weakness leading to paralysis and death, urinary urgency, anxiety

Patient/Family Education

- Identify potential adverse effects and tell patient to inform physician if any occur. Tell patient to report time effects occur, length of time since last dose and type of adverse effects.
- Explain that long-term use may induce drug tolerance and dosage adjustment may be necessary.
- When drug is used for myasthenia gravis, advise patient to keep diary to record time at which muscle weakness and other symptoms occur. This log will enable dosage adjustment. Timing of dose is very important and schedule must be adhered to.

See Patient Guide, p. 434.

Niacin (B_3; nicotinic acid)

(NYE-uh-sin)

Nia-Bid, Niac, Niacels, Niacor, Nico-400, Nicobid, Nicolar, Nicotinex, Slo-Niacin

Class: Vitamin/antihyperlipidemic

Action Necessary for lipid metabolism, tissue respiration and glycogenolysis. At pharmacologic doses, it reduces total cholesterol, LDL cholesterol and triglycerides while increasing HDL cholesterol. Also causes peripheral vasodilation, especially cutaneous vessels.

Indications Prevention and treatment of niacin deficiency or pellagra; treatment of hyperlipidemia. **Unlabeled uses:** Treatment of peripheral vascular disease, vascular spasm, migraine, headache, Menière's disease.

Contraindications Significant liver disease; active peptic ulcer; severe hypotension; arterial hemorrhaging.

Route/Dosage

Pellagra

ADULTS: **PO** Up to 500 mg daily in divided doses. **Slow IV/SC/IM** When oral route is not possible.

Dietary Supplementation

ADULTS: **PO** RDA is 15-20 mg/day for adult males and 13-15 mg/day for adult females. Niacin needs increase to 17-20 mg/day during pregnancy and lactation. CHILDREN: **PO** RDA is 5-20 mg/day.

Hyperlipidemia

ADULTS: **PO** 1-2 g tid, with or after meals. Titrate doses gradually. Lower doses may be effective if using sustained-release products.

Interactions

Adrenergic blocking agent: May potentiate hypotensive effect. *Lovastatin:* Increased risk of myopathy.

Lab Test Interferences

May produce fluorescent substances, which may cause false elevation in some fluorometric measurements of urinary catecholamines. May produce false-positive reaction with cupric sulfate solution used for urinary glucose determination.

Adverse Reactions

CV: Hypotension; tachycardia. *CNS:* Dizziness; syncope; headache. *EENT:* Blurred vision; xerostomia. *GI:* Nausea; bloating; flatulence; hunger; vomiting; heartburn; diarrhea; activation of peptic ulcer. *HEPA:* Jaundice; liver damage; abnormal liver function test results. *DERM:* Flushing; pruritus; burning or tingling sensation; rash; hyperpigmentation (acanthosis nigricans); dry skin. *OTHER:* Hyperuricemia; hyperglycemia; decreased glucose tolerance test results.

Precautions

Pregnancy: Category C if used in doses above RDA. *Lactation:* Undetermined. *Children:* Safety and efficacy not established for doses exceeding nutritional requirements. Extended-release preparations not recommended for children. *Special risk patients:* Use drug with caution when administering to patients with gallbladder disease, history of jaundice, diabetes mellitus, gout, peptic ulcer or allergy. Also, patients allergic to aspirin may be allergic to this product. *Flushing:* Commonly appears with oral therapy. Aspirin (325 mg) 30 min-1 hr before niacin may decrease flushing. *Long-acting dosage form:* Increases risk of jaundice and hepatitis. Avoid use if possible. *Tartrazine sensitivity:* Nicolar contains FD&C yellow #5, which may cause asthma in susceptible patients.

NURSING CONSIDERATIONS

Administration/Storage

- When giving orally, start with small doses, then increase gradually.
- Administer with food.
- Do not crush or break oral medication.

Assessment/Interventions

- Obtain patient history, including drug history and any known allergies.
- If giving for hyperlipidemia, check baseline and monitor cholesterol level.
- Check blood glucose, liver function tests and uric acid level as ordered.
- Monitor vital signs.
- Assess for signs of jaundice, light-colored stools, dizziness or faint feeling.
- Notify physician of changes from baseline assessment.

OVERDOSAGE: SIGNS & SYMPTOMS

Nausea, dizziness, pruritus, vomiting, tachycardia, GI distress, hypotension, flushing

Patient/Family Education

- Tell patient not to break up medication if taking orally.
- Explain that flushing may appear 2 hours after taking medication but should dissipate with continued therapy.
- Tell patient to take medication with food.
- Identify specific elements of well-balanced, low-fat diet.
- Instruct patient to report these symptoms to physician: jaundice, light-colored stools, excessive thirst, urinary frequency, dizziness or faint feeling.
- Caution patient to avoid sudden position changes, especially lying to sitting, to prevent dizziness.
- Advise patient to avoid intake of alcoholic beverages and large doses of medication (> 500 mg) at one time to minimize flushing and warmth sensation.

See Patient Guide, p. 435.

Nicardipine HCl

(NYE-CAR-dih-peen HIGH-droe-KLOR-ide)

Cardene, Cardene I.V., Cardene SR

Class: Calcium channel blocker

Action Inhibits movement of calcium ions across cell membrane in systemic and coronary vascular smooth muscle and myocardium.

Indications Treatment of chronic stable (effort-associated) angina (immediate-release capsules); management of hypertension (immediate- and sustained-release capsules). **Unlabeled use:** Treatment of CHF.

Contraindications Sick sinus syndrome; second- or third-degree atrioventricular (AV) block except with functioning pacemaker; advanced aortic stenosis.

Route/Dosage

ADULTS: **PO** 20-40 mg tid (immediate-release capsules) *or* 30-60 mg bid (sustained-release capsules).

Interactions

Cyclosporine: May cause increased cyclosporine levels with possible toxicity. *Other hypertensive agents:* May have additive effects.

Lab Test Interferences

None well documented.

Adverse Reactions

CV: Peripheral edema; palpitations; AV block; MI; angina; tachycardia; abnormal ECG. *CNS:* Dizziness; lightheadedness; asthenia; psychiatric disturbances; headache; paresthesia; somnolence; weakness. *GI:* Nausea; abdominal discomfort; cramps; dyspepsia; dry mouth; thirst. *DERM:* Rash. *OTHER:* Flushing; allergic reaction; myalgia.

Precautions

Pregnancy: Category C. *Lactation:* Undetermined. *Children:* Safety and efficacy not established. *Antiplatelet effects:* Calcium channel blockers may inhibit platelet function. *Beta-blocker withdrawal:* Patients withdrawn from beta-blockers while taking nicardipine may experience increased angina. Gradually taper beta-blocker dose. *CHF:* Use drug with caution in patients with CHF. *Hepatic impairment:* Adjust dosage and use drug with caution in patients with impaired hepatic function or reduced hepatic blood flow. *Increased angina:* Occasionally patients have increased frequency, duration or severity of angina on starting or increasing dose. *Renal impairment:* Adjust dose in patients with renal dysfunction. *Withdrawal:* Abrupt withdrawal may cause increased frequency and duration of angina.

NURSING CONSIDERATIONS

Administration/Storage

- Administer without regard to meals. Avoid giving with high-fat meals.
- If patient is taking sustained-released capsules, instruct patient to swallow capsule whole and not to chew, divide or crush.
- If stopping medication, taper dose slowly. Stopping drug quickly could result in immediate angina.
- If patient has history of liver or renal disease, start with low doses and titrate.
- Do not increase dose for minimum of 3 days after starting medication or dose changes.
- When converting from immediate-release form to sustained-release form, note that dosage may differ.
- Store at room temperature in tight, light-resistant container.

Assessment/Interventions

- Obtain patient history, including drug history and any known allergies.
- Evaluate cardiac, hepatic, renal and thyroid function.

- Obtain baseline vital signs and monitor 1-2 hr and 8 hr after administration of immediate-release product and 2-4 hr and at end of dosing interval if sustained-release product is used.
- Obtain baseline ECG and any follow-up ECGs as ordered by physician.
- Assess for edema, dizziness, headache, sore throat, renal changes, palpitations, liver dysfunction or flushing.
- If patient has history of liver, renal or cardiac dysfunction, monitor patient closely for changes from baseline.
- If there are any changes from baseline assessment, notify physician.
- If drug used to treat angina, monitor frequency of anginal episodes and consumption of sublingual nitroglycerin.

OVERDOSAGE: SIGNS & SYMPTOMS

Nausea, weakness, dizziness, drowsiness, confusion, slurred speech, marked and prolonged hypotension, bradycardia, functional rhythms, second- or third-degree AV block, palpitations, flushing, nervousness, vomiting

Patient/Family Education

- Instruct patient to swallow sustained-release capsules whole and not to crush or chew.
- Caution patient that increased angina may occur initially when starting, changing dose or stopping medication.
- Advise patient not to stop taking drug abruptly.
- Instruct patient to report these symptoms to physician: any unusual bleeding, bruising, rash, palpitations, irregular heartbeat, shortness of breath, nausea, change in angina, constipation, changes in gums, dizziness or swelling in hands or feet.
- Advise patient that drug may cause dizziness or drowsiness and to use caution while driving or performing other tasks requiring mental alertness.

See Patient Guide, pp. 436-437.

Nicotine

(NIK-oh-TEEN)

Habitrol, Nicoderm, Nicorette, Nicorette DS, Nicotrol, Polacrilex, ProStep

Class: Smoking deterrent

Action Reduces nicotine withdrawal symptoms by providing nicotine levels lower than those associated with smoking.

Indications Aid to smoking cessation. Part of comprehensive behavioral smoking-cessation program.

Contraindications Nonsmokers; during immediate post-MI period; life-threatening arrhythmias; severe or worsening angina pectoris; active temporomandibular joint disease (nicotine Polacrilex [gum]).

Route/Dosage

Transdermal Patches

ADULTS: **Topical** Apply one patch daily. Start with 14-22 mg/day patches. Gradually decrease dose by using smaller dose patches over 2-5 mo.

Nicotine Polacrilex (Nicotine Gum)

ADULTS: **PO** 4 mg pieces (maximum 20 pieces/day) for highly dependent patients. For others, 2 mg pieces (maximum 30 pieces/day). Chew 1 piece prn or on fixed schedule of 1 piece q 1-2 hr initially. Initiate gradual weaning from treatment after 2-3 mo and complete withdrawal by 4-6 mo.

Interactions

Acetaminophen, caffeine, imipramine, oxazepam, pentazocine, propanolol, theophylline: Smoking tends to increase metabolism and may lower blood levels of these drugs or others. Smoking cessation, with or without nicotine medication, may reverse these effects. *Food:* Effective absorption of nicotine Polacrilex (gum) depends on mildly alkaline saliva. Coffee, cola and other drinks or food may reduce salivary pH and should probably be avoided 15 min before and during chewing of gum.

Lab Test Interferences

None well documented.

Adverse Reactions

CV: Edema; flushing; hypertension; palpitations; tachyarrhythmias; tachycardia; MI; CHF; cardiac arrest; cerebrovascular accident. *RESP:* Increased cough; pharyngitis; sinusitis; difficulty breathing; hoarseness; sneezing. *CNS:* Insomnia; dizziness; lightheadedness; irritability; headache; impaired concentration; confusion; convulsions; depression; paresthesia; abnormal dreams. *EENT:* Buccal cavity irritation; mouth or throat soreness or dryness. With gum chewing: traumatic injury to oral mucosa or teeth; jaw ache; changes in taste perception. *GI:* GI distress; belching; indigestion; nausea; vomiting; excess salivation; hiccoughs; anorexia; constipation; diarrhea. *HEPA:* Alterations of liver function tests. *DERM:* Erythema; rash; itching; urticaria. *OTHER:* Pain; myalgia; arthralgia; dysmenorrhea.

Precautions

Pregnancy: Category C (nicotine polacrilex); Category D (transdermal nicotine). *Lactation:* Excreted in breast milk. *Children:* Safety and efficacy not established. *Elderly or debilitated patients:* May be more susceptible to adverse effects. *Abuse/dependence:* Transference of nicotine dependence from smoking to deterrent product exists. If patient continues to smoke while on nicotine therapy, patient may experience severe effects because of higher nicotine levels. *Cardiovascular effects:* Patients with coronary heart disease, serious cardiac arrhythmias, systemic hypertension or vasospastic disease need to be carefully evaluated and monitored closely because of cardiac effects. *Dental problems:* Might be exacerbated by chewing nicotine gum. *Endocrine effects:* Use with caution in patients with hyperthyroidism, pheochromocytoma or insulin-dependent diabetes because of action of nicotine on adrenal medulla. *GI effects:* May delay healing in patients with peptic ulcer disease. *Hepatic impairment:* May reduce nicotine clearance.

NURSING CONSIDERATIONS

Administration/Storage

Transdermal System

- Apply patch promptly on removal from pouch.
- Apply patch once daily to nonhairy, clean, dry skin site on upper body or upper outer arm.
- After patch has been on for 24 hr, remove and apply new patch to alternate skin site. Skin sites should not be reused for at least 1 wk (exception is Nicotrol, which is applied on awakening and removed at bedtime).
- After handling active patch, wash hands with water alone, because soap may increase nicotine absorption. Do not touch eyes.
- After removing used patch from skin, fold over, place in protective pouch and immediately dispose of it so that it is inaccessible to children and pets.
- Store in cool location. Do not store out of pouch.

Nicotine Chewing Gum

- Instruct patient to chew gum 1 piece at a time.
- Tell patient to chew intermittently for about 30 min. Proper chewing technique is slow-paced chewing and intermittent "parking".
- If gum is chewed fast, increased side effects will result.
- Do not allow patient to eat or drink for 15 min before chewing and during chewing.

Assessment/Interventions

- Obtain patient history, including drug history and any known allergies.
- Assess for edema, cardiac irregularities or changes, headache, dizziness, inability to sleep, GI distress or signs of liver dysfunction.
- Assess for history or signs of depression. If present, notify physician.
- If patient is diabetic, monitor blood sugar closely.
- Monitor oral mucosa and teeth for traumatic injury related to medicated gum.
- Report cardiac, hepatic or CNS changes from baseline assessment to physician.

OVERDOSAGE: SIGNS & SYMPTOMS

Nausea, salivation, abdominal pain, vomiting, diarrhea, cold sweat, headache, dizziness, disturbed hearing and vision, mental confusion, marked weakness, faintness, prostration, hypotension, difficult breathing, rapid, weak, irregular pulse, respiratory collapse

Patient/Family Education

- Review package insert information with patient.
- Inform patient of serious effects if he/she continues to smoke while chewing gum or using patch. Instruct patient not to smoke anymore. Encourage patient to participate in comprehensive smoking cessation program.
- Warn patient that he/she could become dependent on medication.
- Tell patient that gum or patch is not for long-term use and that dose will be gradually tapered off over course of few wk to months.
- Inform patient it will take a few days to adjust to taste of gum.
- Instruct patient to avoid drinking or eating 15 min before and during chewing of gum.
- Advise patient to chew gum slowly 1 piece at a time when urge to start smoking is felt.
- Instruct patient regarding proper use of gum (intermittent technique of slow-paced chewing and "parking").
- Advise patient not to exceed 30 pieces of gum/day (2 mg size) or 20 pieces/day (4 mg size) and to decrease this number gradually over first mo.
- Tell patient to inspect mouth daily (if chewing gum) for signs of irritation.
- Instruct patient in proper use and disposal of patch. Tell patient to always remove old patch before applying new one and to wash hands after applying patch.
- Advise patient regarding proper storage of patch (heat sensitive, rapid evaporation once opened).
- Instruct patient to report these symptoms to physician: GI distress (ie, constipation, diarrhea, nausea), headache, depression, dizziness, hiccups, sore throat, pain or mouth discomfort.

See Patient Guide, pp. 438-439.

Nifedipine

(nye-FED-ih-peen)

Adalat, Adalat CC, Procardia, Procardia XL, ♣ *Adalat PA 10, Adalat PA 20, Adalat XL, APO-Nifed, Nu-Nifed*

Class: Calcium channel blocker

Action Inhibits movement of calcium ions across cell membrane in systemic and coronary vascular smooth muscle and myocardium. Increases CO and decreases peripheral vascular resistance. Minimal effect on sinoatrial and atrioventricular (AV) nodal conduction. Reduces myocardial oxygen demand; relaxes and prevents coronary artery spasm.

Indications Treatment of vasospastic (Prinzmetal's or variant) angina, chronic stable angina, hypertension (sustained-release tablets only). **Unlabeled uses:** Management of hypertensive emergencies; treatment of Raynaud's phenomenon; control of primary pulmonary hypertension.

Contraindications Sick sinus syndrome; second- or third-degree AV block, except with functioning pacemaker.

Route/Dosage

Angina

ADULTS: **PO** 10-30 mg tid (immediate-release capsules) (maximum 120 mg/day).

Angina or Hypertension

ADULTS: **PO** 30-90 mg qd (sustained-release tablets) (maximum 120 mg/day).

Hypertensive Emergency

ADULTS: **PO/SL** 10-20 mg (immediate-release capsule that has been punctured). Allow up to 20-30 min for full onset of effects. May be repeated according to BP readings.

Interactions

Barbiturates: May reduce nifedipine concentrations. *Cimetidine:* May increase bioavailability of nifedipine. *Diltiazem:* May increase nifedipine levels and effects. *Fentanyl, parenteral magnesium:* Hypotension may occur. *Other hypertensive agents:* May have additive effects.

Lab Test Interferences

None well documented.

Adverse Reactions

CV: Peripheral edema; hypotension; palpitations; syncope; CHF; MI; arrhythmia; pulmonary edema; angina; tachycardia. *RESP:* Nasal or chest congestion; shortness of breath; wheezing; cough; respiratory infection. *CNS:* Dizziness; lightheadedness; giddiness; nervousness; headache; sleep disturbances; insomnia; abnormal dreams; blurred vision; equilibrium disturbances; weakness; jitteriness; paresthesia; somnolence; malaise; anxiety. *EENT:* Tinnitus; sinusitis; rhinitis. *GI:* Nausea; diarrhea; constipation; abdominal discomfort; cramps; dyspepsia; dry mouth; flatulence. *GU:* Micturition disorders; sexual difficulties. *HEPA:* Hepatitis; hepatotoxicity; elevations of liver function test enzymes. *HEMA:* Anemia; leukopenia; thrombocytopenia; bruising; positive Coombs' test with or without hemolytic anemia. *DERM:* Dermatitis; rash; pruritus; urticaria; Stevens-Johnson syndrome. *OTHER:* Flushing; gingival hyperplasia; sweating; muscle cramps, pain and inflammation; joint stiffness, pain, or arthritis; chills; fever; thirst.

Precautions

Pregnancy: Category C. *Lactation:* Excreted in breast milk in small amounts. *Children:* Safety and efficacy not established. *Elderly patients:* May experience greater hypotensive effects. *Acute hepatic injury:* In rare instances nifedipine has been associated with significant elevations in liver enzymes, symptoms consistent with acute hepatic injury, cholestasis with or without jaundice and allergic hepatitis. *Antiplatelet effects:* Nifedipine decreases platelet aggregation and can increase bleeding time in some patients. *Beta-blocker withdrawal:* Patients withdrawn from beta-blockers while taking nifedipine may experience increased angina. *CHF:* Use drug with caution in patients with CHF. *Edema:* Nifedipine has been associated with edema in some cases and should be distinguished from fluid retention secondary to heart failure. *Hepatic impairment:* Use drug with caution in patients with impaired hepatic function, reduced hepatic blood flow or hepatic cirrhosis. *Increased angina:* Occasional patients may have increased frequency, duration or severity of angina at start of therapy or when dose is increased. *Withdrawal:* Abrupt withdrawal may cause increased frequency and duration of angina.

NURSING CONSIDERATIONS

Administration/Storage

- Initiation and discontinuation of drug should be tapered over 7-14 days.
- May be administered without regard to meals.
- Have patient swallow sustained-release tablets whole; do not allow patient to chew, divide or crush.
- Procardia XL and Adalat CC are not rated as generic equivalents and should not be interchanged without physician authorization.
- If beta-blockers are being withdrawn while patient is taking nifedipine, beta-blocker dose should be gradually tapered.
- Patients with impaired hepatic function should start with low doses.
- When using immediate-release capsules for treatment of hypertensive emergencies, puncture capsules and squeeze liquid contents under tongue or puncture capsule several times and have patient chew.
- Store capsules at room temperature and protect from light and moisture.

Assessment/Interventions

- Obtain history, including drug history and any known allergies. Evaluate cardiac, endocrine, respiratory, hepatic, CNS, renal and GI systems.
- Obtain baseline and follow-up vital signs; assess for chest pain.
- If drug is used as antihypertensive, routinely monitor BP and note any orthostatic hypotension.
- Inspect skin for rashes.
- Assess for any unusual bruising or bleeding.
- Check BP at least once daily when patient is taking both nifedipine and cimetidine. If possible, another H_2 antagonist may be prescribed instead of cimetidine.
- Administer sublingual nitroglycerin if breakthrough chest pain occurs. Record frequency and duration of anginal attacks and use of sublingual nitroglycerin.
- If any changes from baseline vital signs occur, notify physician.

OVERDOSAGE: SIGNS & SYMPTOMS

Hypotension, nausea, weakness, dizziness, drowsiness, confusion, slurred speech, second- or third-degree AV block, marked and prolonged hypotension and bradycardia, decreased cardiac output, functional rhythms

Patient/Family Education

- Remind patient that sustained-release capsules must be swallowed whole, not chewed, divided or crushed.
- Teach patient the importance of good dental care and advise that patient visit dentist on routine basis because gum swelling may occur.
- Instruct patient to maintain increased fluid intake (if not contraindicated) to avoid constipation.
- Instruct patient that medication must be used chronically to obtain benefit and to notify physician if ≥ 2 doses are missed.
- Teach patient/family to notify physician of any changes from baseline evaluation (ie, chest pain, shortness of breath).
- Inform patient that there may be increased chest pain at start of medication and with dose changes but that this effect is transient. If it persists, notify physician.
- If physician prescribes concomitant administration of sublingual nitroglycerin, teach patient how to take nitroglycerin sublingually.
- Explain that when sustained-release form is used, partially undigested tablet may appear in feces but that this effect is no cause for concern.
- Instruct patient to report these symptoms to physician: ringing in ears, swollen gums, respiratory changes, inability to sleep, fever or chills.

- Advise patient that drug may cause dizziness, lightheadedness and blurred vision and to use caution while driving or performing other tasks requiring mental alertness.

See Patient Guide, pp. 440-441.

Nimodipine

(NYE-MOE-dih-peen)

Nimotop

Class: Calcium channel blocker

Action Inhibits movement of calcium ions across cell membrane in systemic and coronary vascular smooth muscle and myocardium. Has greater effect on cerebral arteries than on other arteries.

Indications Improvement of neurologic deficits caused by vasospasm after subarachnoid hemorrhage from ruptured congenital intracranial aneurysms. **Unlabeled uses:** Treatment of common and classic migraine and chronic cluster headache.

Contraindications Standard considerations.

Route/Dosage

Subarachnoid Hemorrhage

ADULTS: **PO/Nasogastric** 60 mg q 4 hr for 21 consecutive days. Initiate therapy within 96 hr of subarachnoid hemorrhage.

Headaches

ADULTS: **PO** 30 mg tid.

Interactions

Beta-blockers: May cause increased adverse effects because of myocardial contractility or atrioventricular (AV) conduction depression. *Fentanyl:* May cause severe hypotension or increased fluid requirements. *Other hypertensive agents:* May have additive effects.

Lab Test Interferences

None well documented.

Adverse Reactions

CV: Peripheral edema; hypotension; hypertension; bradycardia; CHF; tachycardia; abnormal ECG. *RESP:* Shortness of breath; wheezing. *CNS:* Rebound vasospasm; headache; dizziness; psychiatric disturbances. *GI:* Nausea; diarrhea; abdominal discomfort; cramps; dyspepsia; GI hemorrhage. *HEPA:* Hepatitis; hepatotoxicity; elevated LDH, alkaline phosphatase and ALT levels. *HEMA:* Disseminated intravascular coagulation; thrombocytopenia; deep vein thrombosis. *DERM:* Rash; acne. *OTHER:* Flushing; muscle cramps, pain, and inflammation.

Precautions

Pregnancy: Category C. *Lactation:* Undetermined. *Children:* Safety and efficacy not established. *Antiplatelet effects:* Calcium channel blockers may inhibit platelet function. *Hepatic impairment:* Use drug with caution in patients with impaired hepatic function or reduced hepatic blood flow.

NURSING CONSIDERATIONS

Administration/Storage

- If capsule cannot be swallowed, make hole in both ends of capsule with 18-gauge needle and extract contents into syringe. Empty contents into patient's nasogastric tube and wash down tube with 30 ml of normal saline solution.
- Patient may require decreased dose if liver dysfunction is present.
- Administer drug around the clock.
- Do not abruptly withdraw drug; dosage must be tapered.
- Store at room temperature in original foil packaging.

Assessment/Interventions

- Obtain patient history, including drug history and any known allergies. Note liver dysfunction, respiratory difficulties, unusual bruising or bleeding, GI problems, rashes, acne, joint pain, deep vein thrombosis or muscle cramping.

- Obtain baseline vital signs.
- Assess patient's neurological status and document any deficits.
- If patient has history of liver, renal or cardiac dysfunction, monitor closely for change from baseline.
- If patient is hypotensive or bradycardic or has respiratory difficulties, notify physician.
- If nausea, vomiting, diarrhea, abdominal cramping or increased bruising or bleeding occurs, notify physician.

OVERDOSAGE: SIGNS & SYMPTOMS

Nausea, weakness, dizziness, drowsiness, confusion, slurred speech, marked and prolonged hypotension, bradycardia, decreased cardiac output, junctional rhythms, second- or third-degree AV block, palpitations, flushing, nervousness, loss of consciousness, vomiting, generalized edema

Patient/Family Education

- Explain that medication needs to be taken around the clock for 21 days.
- Instruct patient to report these symptoms to physician: shortness of breath, nausea, abdominal cramping, diarrhea, unusual bruising or bleeding, palpitations, dizziness, faint feeling or swelling of hands or feet.

See Patient Guide, p. 442.

Nitrofurantoin

(nye-troe-FYOOR-an-toyn)

Furadantin, Macrobid, Macrodantin

Class: Urinary anti-infective

Action May interfere with bacterial cell wall formation and bacterial duplication. Inhibits bacterial carbohydrate metabolism. Bacteriostatic in low concentrations; bactericidal at higher concentrations.

Indications Treatment of urinary tract infections caused by susceptible strains of *E coli*, enterococci, *Staphylococcus aureus*, certain strains of *Klebsiella*, *Enterobacter* and *Proteus* species.

Contraindications Renal impairment (creatinine clearance < 40 ml/min); anuria or oliguria; pregnant women at term; infants < 1 mo.

Route/Dosage

ADULTS & CHILDREN > 12 YR: PO 50-100 mg qid with meals for minimum of 7 days and for at least 3 days after sterile urine is obtained. CHILDREN > 1 MO: PO 5-7 mg/kg/24 hr in 4 divided doses with meals and at bedtime for minimum of 7 days and for at least 3 days after sterile urine is obtained.

Long-Term Suppressive Therapy

ADULTS: PO 50-100 mg at bedtime. CHILDREN: PO 1 mg/kg/24 hr as single or 2 divided doses.

Interactions

Anticholinergic drugs and food: Increased absorption of nitrofurantoin. *Magnesium salts:* May reduce anti-infective action by decreasing absorption. *Probenicid:* May increase nitrofurantoin serum levels by reducing renal elimination.

Lab Test Interferences

Urinary creatinine elevation and false-positive urine glucose determination with Benedict's reagent (copper sulfate solution) may occur.

Adverse Reactions

RESP: Acute, subacute or chronic pulmonary reaction (eg, shortness of breath, chest pain, cough, fever, chills); permanent pulmonary impairment. *CNS:* Peripheral neuropathy; headache; dizziness; nystagmus; drowsiness. *GI:* Anorexia; nausea; emesis; abdominal pain; diarrhea; parotiditis; pancreatitis. *GU:* Superinfection. *HEPA:* Hepatitis; hepatotoxicity; jaundice; increased bilirubin and alkaline phosphatase; permanent liver dysfunction. *HEMA:* Hemolytic anemia from G-6-PD deficiency; granulocytopenia; agranulocytosis; leukopenia; thrombocytopenia; eosinophilia; megaloblastic anemia; aplastic anemia. *DERM:* Exfoliative dermatitis; erythema multiforme; maculopapular, erythematous or eczematous eruption; pruritus; urticaria; angioedema; alopecia; photosensitivity. *OTHER:* Anaphylaxis; asthmatic attack in patient with history of asthma; drug fever; arthralgia; sialadenitis; muscular aches.

Precautions

Pregnancy: Category B. Contraindicated in women at term. Do not give to pregnant patient with G-6-PD deficiency. *Lactation:* Excreted in breast milk. *Children:* Contraindicated in infants < 1 mo. *Hemolysis:* Hemolytic anemia has occurred, apparently linked to G-6-PD deficiencies. Discontinue at any sign of hemolysis. *Peripheral neuropathy:* May become severe or irreversible; fatalities have been reported. Predisposing conditions such as renal impairment, anemia, diabetes, electrolyte imbalance, vitamin B deficiency and debilitating diseases may increase risk. *Pulmonary reactions:* Acute and chronic reactions, including interstitial pneumonia, respiratory failure and death, have occurred. Do not give to any patient who has had pulmonary reaction to drug. *Superinfection:* Prolonged or repeated therapy with antibiotics may result in overgrowth of nonsusceptible bacteria or fungi.

NURSING CONSIDERATIONS

Administration/Storage

- Administer with food or milk.
- Oral suspension can be mixed with water, juice or formula.
- Have patient rinse mouth after administration to avoid staining teeth.
- Have patient swallow tablets or capsules whole. Instruct patient not to open capsule or crush tablets.
- Nitrofurantoin and nitrofurantoin macrocrystalline are not interchangeable because of differences in absorption. *Macrobid* brand is formulated for every 12-hr administration.
- Store at room temperature in tightly closed container. Protect from light.

Assessment/Interventions

- Obtain patient history, including drug history and any known allergies.
- Obtain urine for culture and sensitivity prior to starting drug.
- Obtain results of CBC and other lab tests ordered by physician (ie, creatinine, electrolytes, alkaline phosphatase, bilirubin).
- Obtain vital signs. Monitor weight and I&O.
- Evaluate for signs of infection (ie, fever, chills, drainage, burning, frequency or hesitancy).
- Evaluate for dizziness, headaches, GI upset, skin changes, hearing or vision changes.
- If patient exhibits shortness of breath, chest pain, continued fever, numbness, tingling, headache, dizziness, drowsiness, nystagmus, blood in urine or signs of hemolysis, notify physician.

OVERDOSAGE: SIGNS & SYMPTOMS

Nausea, anorexia, vomiting, diarrhea

Patient/Family Education

- Remind patient to shake nitrofurantoin suspension before measuring dose.
- Instruct patient to take medication with food or milk.
- Inform patient to expect urine to be

orange or brown in color while taking medication.

- Teach patient importance of completing full course of antibiotic to avoid recurrent infection.
- Instruct patient to report these symptoms to physician: shortness of breath, difficulty breathing, changes in urination (other than orange discoloration), nausea, vomiting, diarrhea, cramping, skin changes, chest pain, cough, fever, headache, dizziness, vision changes, unusual bleeding (ie, red or black urine or stool), yellowing of skin, light-colored stools or edema.
- Caution patient to avoid exposure to sunlight and to use sunscreen or wear protective clothing to avoid photosensitivity reaction.

See Patient Guide, p. 443.

Nitroglycerin

(nye-troe-GLIH-suh-rin)

Deponit, Minitran, Nitro-Bid Plateau Caps, Nitrocine, Nitrocine Timecaps, Nitrodisc, Nitrogard, Nitroglyn, Nitrolingual, Nitrong, Nitrostat, Nitro-Dur, Nitrol, Transderm-Nitro, Tridil

Class: Antianginal

Action Relaxation of smooth muscle of venous and arterial vasculature.

Indications Treatment of acute angina (SL, translingual, IV, transmucosal); prophylaxis of angina (SL, transmucosal, translingual, sustained release, transdermal, topical); control of blood pressure in perioperative or intraoperative hypertension (IV); CHF associated with MI (IV). **Unlabeled uses:** Reduce cardiac workload in patients with MI and in refractory CHF (SL, topical, oral, IV); adjunctive treatment of Raynaud's disease (topical); treatment of hypertensive crisis (IV).

Contraindications Hypersensitivity to nitrates; severe anemia; closed-angle glaucoma; orthostatic hypotension; early MI; pericarditis or pericardial tamponade; head trauma or cerebral hemorrhage; allergy to adhesives (transdermal); hypotension or uncorrected hypovolemia (IV); increased intracranial pressure or decreased cerebral perfusion (IV).

Route/Dosage

Perioperative Hypertension

ADULTS: **IV** 5 mcg/min using non–peripheral vein catheter (PVC) IV administration set initially; titrate to response.

Angina

ADULTS: **SL** 0.15-0.6 mg dissolved under tongue or in buccal pouch at first sign of acute angina attack; repeat q 5 min (do not exceed 3 tablets in 15 min). **Translingual** 1-2 sprays onto or under tongue at onset of attack. **Transmucosal** 1 mg every 3-5 hr during waking hours; tablet placed between lip or cheek and gum. **PO** 2.5 or 2.6 mg (sustained-release form) tid-qid initially; titrate to response. **Transdermal** 0.2-0.4 mg/hr patch initially applied once daily; titrate dose to response. **Topical** 1-2 inches q 8 hr up to 4-5 inches spread over 3 x 4 inch area and cover with plastic wrap to prevent staining of clothes or application q 4 hr prn. Allow a nitrate-free period of 10-12 hr/day.

Refractory Angina, CHF Secondary to Acute MI:

ADULTS: **IV** 5 mcg/min initially; titrate according to hemodynamic readings (BP, heart rate, pulmonary capillary wedge pressure).

Interactions

Alcohol: Severe hypotension and cardiovascular collapse may occur. *Calcium channel blockers:* Symptomatic orthostatic hypotension may occur. *Dihydroergotamine:* May increase systolic blood pressure and decrease antianginal effects. *Heparin:* May decrease anticoagulation effect when used in conjunction with IV nitroglycerin.

Lab Test Interferences

May cause false report of reduced serum cholesterol with Zlatkis-Zak color reaction. May cause false-positive results in urinary catecholamines and VMA determinations.

Adverse Reactions

CV: Tachycardia; palpitations; hypotension; syncope; arrhythmias. *RESP:* Bronchitis; pneumonia. *CNS:* Headache; apprehension; weakness; vertigo; dizziness; agitation; insomnia. *EENT:* Blurred vision. *GI:* Nausea; vomiting; diarrhea; dyspepsia. *GU:* Dysuria; urinary frequency; impotence. *HEMA:* Methemoglobinemia; hemolytic anemia. *DERM:* Cutaneous vasodilation with flushing; contact dermatitis (transdermal); topical allergic reactions (ointment); local burning or tingling sensation in oral cavity (sublingual). *OTHER:* Arthralgia; perspiration; pallor; cold sweat; edema.

Precautions

Pregnancy: Category C. *Lactation:* Undetermined. *Children:* Safety and efficacy not established. *Alcohol intoxication:* Has occurred in patients receiving high doses of IV nitroglycerin. *Angina:* May aggravate angina caused by hypertrophic cardiomyopathy. *Defibrillation:* Do not discharge cardioverter/defibrillator through paddle electrode overlying transdermal system. Arcing may occur and burn patient. *Glaucoma:* May increase intraocular pressure; administer with caution in patients with glaucoma. *Hepatic and renal impairment:* Use IV product with caution. *Hypotension:* Avoid excessive, prolonged hypotension with IV product because of possible harmful effects on brain, heart, liver and kidneys. *MI:* Safety of oral or sublingual products in acute MI not established; use only with close observation and monitoring. However, IV nitroglycerin is drug of choice in acute MI. *Orthostatic hypotension:* May occur even with small doses; alcohol accentuates this reaction. *Sublingual administration:* Absorption is dependent on salivary secretion; dry mouth decreases absorption. *Tolerance:* Tolerance to vascular and antianginal effects may occur. *Transdermal nitroglycerin:* Not for immediate relief of anginal attacks.

NURSING CONSIDERATIONS

Administration/Storage

- IV: Dilute in D5W or 0.9% Sodium Chloride injection prior to infusion. Do not mix with any other infusions. Use glass bottles only and non-PVC tubing provided. Use with infusion pump. Do not use IV filter. Store premixed IV solution in dark. Do not freeze.
- Topical: Apply uniform layer with applicator or on dose-measuring paper. Apply in thin, uniform layer on nonhairy area on upper arm or upper torso. After spreading measured dose, cover skin with plastic wrap to prevent staining of clothes. Wash hands after application. Store in original tube. Do not freeze.
- Sublingual: Give while patient is lying or sitting. Place in buccal pouch to decrease stinging. Do not swallow. Store at room temperature in original, brown glass container. If cotton is in bottle, remove and discard after opening. Do not place cotton or other materials within bottle because they may absorb nitroglycerin. Protect from moisture. Discard unused amounts after 6 months.
- PO: Sustained release—Tell patient not to chew or dissolve capsule in mouth. Store at room temperature.
- Transdermal: Apply patch to nonhairy area on upper arm or torso. Do not apply over cuts or abrasions. Remove old patch prior to applying new patch. Store at room temperature. Do not open until ready to use.

- Translingual: Do not shake canister prior to using. Patient should release spray under tongue. Do not inhale spray.

Assessment/Interventions

- Obtain patient history, including drug history and any known allergies.
- Assess baseline vital signs, ECG, lung and heart sounds.
- IV: Monitor vital signs frequently while patient is receiving infusion, and titrate dosage to systolic BP or pain relief as prescribed.
- IV: Monitor LOC. Notify physician of any significant hypotension, bradycardia, headache or no reduction of anginal pain. Keep patient on bedrest.
- IV: Monitor pulmonary capillary wedge pressure and I&O.
- All other forms: monitor vital signs, I&O. Assess for tolerance of drug effects.
- Monitor for nausea, diarrhea, incontinence, abdominal pain, chest pain, bradycardia, flushing, pruritus, rash or contact dermatitis.
- Assess lung and heart sounds regularly during IV therapy.
- Notify physician of any muscle twitching, diaphoresis, pallor, edema, blurred vision, wheezes, hypotension or chest pain.

OVERDOSAGE: SIGNS & SYMPTOMS

Hypotension, tachycardia, flushing, perspiring skin, headache, vertigo, palpitations, visual disturbances, nausea, vomiting, confusion, and dyspnea may occur as a result of vasodilation and methemoglobinemia

Patient/Family Education

- Review with patient and family the signs and symptoms of angina: pressure-like chest pain of acute onset, often associated with physical activity, that may radiate down to left arm or up to neck and jaw.

Sublingual

- Advise patient to dissolve tablet under tongue and not to swallow. If pain remains, the dose may be repeated every 5 min until 3 tablets are taken. If pain still persists or becomes more intense, patient should be taught to call 911 or appropriate local number to obtain emergency services.
- Tell patient to place tablet between gum and cheek if stinging sensation occurs.
- Caution patient to sit or lie down while taking and for 20 minutes after initial dose. If dizziness occurs, instruct patient to lie down.
- Teach patient storage instructions (per Administration/Storage information).
- Advise patient to discard 6 mo after opening package.
- Instruct patient to report these symptoms to physician: severe headache, blurred vision, dry mouth, dizziness or flushing.

Ointment, Spray, Sustained-Release, Transdermal

- Advise patient to wear gloves or use dose-determining applicator when applying ointment.
- Teach patient to leave a 10-12 hr nitrate-free period at night to decrease likelihood of developing tolerance.
- For transdermal form, tell patient to change site of application to avoid skin sensitization.
- Explain that swimming or bathing does not affect effectiveness of drug.
- Advise patient to notify physician of any decrease in effectiveness of medication.
- Caution patient to avoid sudden position changes to prevent orthostatic hypotension.
- Instruct patient to avoid intake of alcoholic beverages.

See Patient Guide, pp. 444-445.

Nitroprusside Sodium

(nye-troe-PRUSS-ide SO-dee-uhm)
Nipride, Nitropress
Class: Agent for hypertensive emergencies

Action Relaxes vascular smooth muscle and dilates peripheral veins and arteries.

Indications Immediate reduction of blood pressure in hypertensive crisis; production of controlled hypotension to reduce bleeding during surgery. **Unlabeled uses:** Has been used alone or with dopamine in severe refractory congestive heart failure and acute myocardial infarction.

Contraindications Treatment of compensatory hypertension, in which primary hemodynamic lesion is aortic coarctation or arteriovenous shunting; to produce hypotension during surgery in patients with known inadequate cerebral circulation or in moribund patients (A.S.A. Class 5E) coming to emergency surgery; patients with congenital (Leber's) optic atrophy or with tobacco amblyopia.

Route/Dosage
Give by IV infusion using infusion pump, preferably volmetric pump. ADULTS & CHILDREN: **IV** 0.3 mcg/kg/min initially; titrate upward gradually every few minutes to desired effect. Do not exceed 10 mcg/kg/min. Do not use maximum rate for more than 10 min. Average rate of infusion is 3 mcg/kg/min; some patients require much lower doses, especially if other hypotensive agents are used.

Interactions
Antihypertensives, ganglionic blocking agents, volatile anesthetics (eg, enflurane, halothane): Additive hypotensive effects.

Lab Test Interferences
None well documented.

Adverse Reactions
CV: Evidence of rapid blood pressure reduction (eg, abdominal pain; apprehension; diaphoresis; dizziness; headache; muscle twitching; nausea; palpitations; restlessness; retching; retrosternal discomfort); bradycardia; ECG changes; tachycardia. *GI*: Ileus. *HEMA*: Methemoglobinemia; decreased platelet aggregation. *DERM*: Flushing; venous streaking; irritation at infusion site; rash. *META*: Hypothyroidism. *OTHER*: Thiocyanate toxicity; cyanide toxicity; increased intracranial pressure.

Precautions
Pregnancy: Category C. *Lactation*: Undetermined. *Elderly patients*: May be more sensitive to hypotensive effects. *Anesthesia*: Patient's ability to compensate for anemia and hypovolemia may be diminished during anesthesia. *Cyanide toxicity*: Infusions faster than 2 mcg/kg/min generate cyanide faster than body can dispose of it. Symptoms of cyanide toxicity include venous hyperoxemia with bright red venous blood, metabolic (lactic) acidosis, air hunger, confusion and death. *Excessive hypotension*: Precipitous drops in BP can occur. If not properly monitored, decreases can lead to irreversible ischemic injuries or death. *Hepatic impairment*: Cyanide may accumulate. *Intracranial pressure*: Use with extreme caution in patients with elevated intracranial pressure; nitroprusside can increase intracranial pressure. *Methemoglobinemia*: Clinically significant methemoglobinemia is seen rarely, but suspect condition in patients who have received more than 10 mg/kg of nitroprusside and who have signs of impaired oxygen delivery despite adequate cardiac output and arterial Po_2. Blood may be chocolate brown. *Severe renal disease, anuria*: Thiocynate may accumulate. *Thiocyanate toxicity*: Cyanide is eliminated in form of thiocyanate. When cyanide elimination is accelerated by infusion of thiosulfate or when

prolonged infusions are used, thiocyanate levels may increase. Thiocyanate is neurotoxic (tinnitus, miosis, hyperreflexia) and toxicity may be life threatening.

NURSING CONSIDERATIONS

Administration/Storage

- Dilute 50 mg in 2 ml D5W. Add to 250-500 ml D5W. Resulting solution is 200 mcg/ml or 100 mcg/ml. Use only D5W; no other diluent should be used. No other medication should be infused with nitroprusside medication. Protect solution from light, usually by wrapping with aluminum foil. However, it is not necessary to protect drip chamber or tubing.
- Do not use if solution is discolored or if particulate matter is seen.
- Store diluted solution at room temperature for no longer than 24 hr and protect from light.
- Do not give by bolus infusion; infuse slowly using pump or controller to regulate rate.

Assessment/Interventions

- Obtain patient history, including drug history and any known allergies.
- Assess baseline vital signs, ECG, heart sounds and lung sounds.
- Assess baseline neurological status.
- Place patient in Trendelenburg position to increase venous return.
- Perform continuous ECG monitoring.
- Monitor vital signs every 15 min while on drip and every 5 min while infusion is being titrated.
- Monitor I&O throughout therapy.
- Monitor plasma cyanogen level if used for > 48 hr or with hepatic impairment.
- Monitor thiocynate level (< 10 mg/dl) if used for > 48 hr or in severe renal dysfunction.
- Monitor for chest pain or flushing.
- Notify physician of severe hypotension, abdominal pain, apprehension, dizziness, headache, vomiting, bradycardia or tachycardia, ECG changes or syncope.
- Notify physician of signs of cyanide toxicity such as bright red venous blood, metabolic acidosis, air hunger and mental confusion.
- Monitor for and notify physician of signs of thiocyanate toxicity (ie, tinnitus, miosis, hyperreflexia).

OVERDOSAGE: SIGNS & SYMPTOMS

Severe hypotension, dyspnea, loss of consciousness, metabolic acidosis, headache, death

Patient/Family Education

- Instruct patient to report these symptoms to physician: dizziness; retching, nausea, abdominal pain, chest pain, palpitations, tinnitus or flushing.
- Caution patient to avoid sudden position changes to prevent orthostatic hypotension.

No patient monograph available.

Nizatidine

(nye-ZAT-ih-deen)

Axid Pulvules

Class: Histamine H_2 antagonist

Action Reversibly and competitively blocks histamine at H_2 receptors, particularly those in gastric parietal cells, leading to inhibition of gastric acid secretion.

Indications Treatment and maintenance of duodenal ulcer, gastroesophageal reflux disease (GERD, including erosive or ulcerative disease) and benign gastric ulcer.

Contraindications Hypersensitivity to H_2 antagonists.

Route/Dosage

Duodenal Ulcer (Active)

ADULTS: PO 300 mg at bedtime *or* 150 mg bid for up to 8 wk; maintenance: 150 mg at bedtime.

Benign Gastric Ulcer (Acute)

ADULTS: PO 300 mg at bedtime *or* 150 mg bid.

GERD

ADULTS: PO 150 mg bid.

Moderate to Severe Renal Insufficiency

Dosage adjustment recommended.

Interactions

Aspirin: Increased salicylate levels in patients taking very high doses of aspirin (3.9 gm/day). *Ketoconazole:* Effects of ketoconazole may be reduced.

Lab Test Interferences

False-positive tests for urobilinogen with Multistix may occur.

Adverse Reactions

CV: Cardiac arrhythmias. *CNS:* Headache; somnolence; fatigue; dizziness. *GI:* Diarrhea; constipation; nausea; vomiting; abdominal discomfort; anorexia; cholestatic or hepatocellular effects. *GU:* Hyperuricemia unassociated w/gout or nephrolithiasis. *HEMA:* Thrombocytopenia; eosinophilia. *HEPA:* Hepatocellular injury; elevated AST, ALT and alkaline phosphatase concentrations. *DERM:* Exfoliative dermatitis; erythroderma; rash; pruritus; urticaria. *OTHER:* Gynecomastia; sweating; fever.

Precautions

Pregnancy: Category C. *Lactation:* Excreted in breast milk. *Children:* Safety and efficacy not established. *Elderly patients:* May have reduced renal function; decreased clearance may be more common. *Hepatic impairment:* Use drug with caution; decreased clearance may occur. In patients with normal renal function and uncomplicated hepatic dysfunction, nizatidine disposition is generally normal. *Hepatocellular injury:* Abnormalities appear to be reversible after discontinuation of drug. *Renal function impairment:* Decreased clearance may occur; reduced dosage may be needed.

NURSING CONSIDERATIONS

Administration/Storage

- Give twice daily after breakfast and at bedtime, or if once daily, give at bedtime.
- Do not administer within 1 hr of antacids.
- Store at room temperature.

Assessment/Interventions

- Obtain patient history, including drug history and any known allergies.
- Assess baseline AST, ALT and alkaline phosphatase levels.
- Monitor liver function test results, CBC, BUN and creatinine levels.
- Assess for constipation and encourage increased fluid intake.
- Assess for fatigue, somnolence, skin rashes and diaphoresis.

Patient/Family Education

- Advise patient to take medication after breakfast and at bedtime if prescribed for twice-daily regimen or at bedtime if prescribed for once-daily dosage.
- Caution patient to stay active and to increase fluid and roughage in diet to prevent constipation.
- Instruct patient to take missed dose as soon as possible, and caution not to double doses.
- Advise patient to avoid cigarette smoking, which increases gastric acid secretions and therefore decreases effectiveness of nizatidine therapy.
- Instruct patient to report these symptoms to physician: abdominal pain, coffee-ground emesis, tarry stools, extreme fatigue or weakness.

See Patient Guide, p. 446.

Norepinephrine (Levarterenol)

(NOR-eh-pih-NEFF-reen)
Levophed
Class: Vasopressor

Action Stimulates alpha-receptors in arterial and venous beds and $beta_1$ receptors of heart, resulting in peripheral vasoconstriction and stimulation of heart rate and contractility. Coronary vasodilation occurs secondary to enhanced myocardial contractility.

Indications Restoration of blood pressure in certain acute hypotensive states; adjunct in treatment of cardiac arrest and profound hypotension.

Contraindications Hypovolemic states, except temporarily until blood volume replacement is accomplished; mesenteric or peripheral vascular thrombosis, unless essential; generally contraindicated during cyclopropane and halothane anesthesia; profound hypoxia or hypercarbia.

Route/Dosage

Acute Hypotensive States

ADULTS: **IV** 2-3 ml/min of 4 mcg base/ml solution (8-12 mcg/min); adjust to response. Higher concentration (up to 16 mcg/ml) may be used in fluid-restricted patients. Usual maintenance dose is 2-4 mcg/min, but higher doses and prolonged therapy may be needed.

Interactions

Blood or plasma: Chemically incompatible with norepinephrine. *Furazolidone, guanethidine, MAO inhibitors, methyldopa, rauwolfia alkaloids:* May increase pressor response, resulting in severe hypertension. *Normal saline:* Norepinephrine may lose potency in normal saline solution. *Oxytocic drugs:* May cause severe, persistent hypertension. *Phenothiazines (eg, chlorpromazine):* May decrease pressor effect. *Tricyclic antidepressants:* May increase pressor response.

Lab Test Interferences

None well documented.

Adverse Reactions

CV: Hypotension; increased peripheral vascular resistance; decreased carbon monoxide; precordial pain; ventricular arrhythmias; reflex bradycardia. *RESP:* Respiratory difficulties. *CNS:* Headache; dizziness; tremor; insomnia; anxiety. *META:* Metabolic acidosis; hyperglycemia. *OTHER:* Gangrene (when infused into small vein); thyroid enlargement; irritation from extravasation; decreased urinary output.

Precautions

Pregnancy: Category D. *Lactation:* Undetermined. *Children:* Safety and efficacy not established. *Extravasation:* Avoid by infusing into large vein and monitoring carefully. *Sulfite sensitivity:* Use caution in sulfite-sensitive individuals; some preparations contain sodium bisulfite.

NURSING CONSIDERATIONS

Administration/Storage

- Administer in D5W or 5% dextrose in saline. Do not prepare infusion with normal saline alone because doing so may cause degradation.
- Use infusion pump and plastic catheter. Enter antecubital or other large vein.
- Do not discontinue therapy abruptly.
- Discard solution after 24 hr.
- Store undiluted solution at room temperature. Protect from light.

Assessment/Interventions

- Obtain patient history, including drug history and any known allergies.
- Obtain baseline vital signs, neurological assessment, urinary output and ECG.
- Monitor vital signs, ECG, I&O and

neurological status regularly during therapy.

- Monitor for cyanosis: bluish skin color and cold extremities.
- Assess for signs of extravasation (blanching and coolness of skin over vein) at infusion site. If this occurs, notify physician immediately and change infusion site as soon as possible. Have phentolamine readily available for local infiltration in case extravasation occurs.

OVERDOSAGE: SIGNS & SYMPTOMS

Severe hypertension, reflex bradycardia, decreased cardiac output, increased peripheral vascular resistance, ventricular arrhythmias, tissue hypoxia and ischemic injury

Patient/Family Education

- Advise patient to notify nurse if IV site feels cool or painful.
- Instruct patient to report these symptoms to physician: dizziness, nausea, syncope, abdominal pain, chest pain or confusion.
- Caution patient to avoid sudden position changes to prevent orthostatic hypotension.

No patient monograph available.

Norfloxacin

(nor-FLOX-uh-SIN)

Chibroxin, Noroxin, Ocuflox

Class: Antibiotic/fluoroquinolone

Action Interferes with microbial DNA synthesis.

Indications Oral treatment of urinary tract infections caused by susceptible organisms; treatment of sexually transmitted diseases caused by *Neisseria gonorrheae*; ocular solution for treatment of superficial ocular infections due to strains of susceptible organisms; prostatitis due to *E. coli*.

Contraindications Hypersensitivity to fluoroquinolones, quinolones or any component. *Ophthalmic use:* Epithelial herpes simplex keratitis; fungal disease of ocular structure; mycobacterial infections of eye; vaccinia; varicella.

Route/Dosage

Urinary Tract Infections

ADULTS: **PO** 400 mg q 12 hr for 3-21 days.

Sexually Transmitted Diseases

ADULTS: **PO** 800 mg as single dose.

Ocular Infections

ADULTS & CHILDREN: **Topical** Acute infection: 1-2 gtt q 15-30 min; moderate infections: 1-2 gtt 4-6 times daily.

Prostatitis due to E. Coli

ADULTS: **PO** 400 mg q 12h for 28 days.

Interactions

Antacids, iron salts, zinc salts, sucralfate, didanosine: May decrease oral absorption of norfloxacin. *Antineoplastic agents:* Serum norfloxacin levels may be decreased. *Cyclosporine:* Elevated serum cyclosporine levels. *Theophylline:* Decreased clearance and increased plasma levels of theophylline may result in toxicity.

Lab Test Interferences

None well documented.

Adverse Reactions

CNS: Headache; dizziness; fatigue; drowsiness. *EENT:* Ophthalmic use: Conjunctival hyperemia; chemosis; photophobia; transient burning, itching or stinging. *GI:* Diarrhea; nausea; vomiting; abdominal pain/discomfort. *GU:* Increased serum creatinine and BUN. *HEMA:* Eosinophilia; leukopenia; neutropenia. *HEPA:* Increased ALT, AST, LDH. *DERM:* Rash.

Precautions

Pregnancy: Category C. *Lactation:* Undetermined. *Children:* Safety and efficacy not established (oral form). *Convulsions:* CNS stimulation can occur; use drug with caution in patients with known or suspected CNS disorders. *Photosensitivity:* Moderate to severe reactions have occurred; avoid excessive sunlight and ultraviolet light. *Pseudomembranous colitis:* Consider possibility in patients who develop diarrhea. *Renal impairment:* Reduced clearance may occur; adjust dose accordingly. *Superinfection:* Use of antibiotics may result in bacterial or fungal overgrowth.

NURSING CONSIDERATIONS

Administration/Storage

Ophthalmic

- Store at room temperature in original container.

Tablets

- Store at room temperature.
- Give 1 hr before or 2 hr after meals with full glass of water.
- Do not administer antacids within 2 hr of dose.

Assessment/Interventions

- Obtain patient history, including drug history and any known allergies.
- Assess baseline CBC, taste alterations, conjunctivitis or mycobacterial infections.
- Review baseline BUN, creatinine, ALT, AST and LDH.
- Monitor vital signs, elimination patterns, food intolerance, sedation and sleep patterns.
- Monitor conjunctival color and edema if using eyedrop preparation.
- Encourage fluid intake, full glass with each dose and full glass between each dose if not medically contraindicated.
- Notify physician of any nausea, rashes, diarrhea, shortness of breath, dizziness, extreme headache or lethargy.

OVERDOSAGE: SIGNS & SYMPTOMS

Nausea, headache, dizziness, crystalluria, vomiting, drowsiness, seizures

Patient/Family Education

- For ophthalmic use, demonstrate and observe return demonstration of correct technique for instillation of drops.
- Advise patient to take medication on empty stomach with full glass of water.
- Caution patient to avoid exposure to sunlight and to use sunscreen or wear protective clothing to avoid photosensitivity reaction.
- Advise patient not to double dose if one dose is missed and to notify physician if more than one dose is missed.
- Advise patient to notify physician of any nausea, rashes, diarrhea, shortness of breath, dizziness, unusual headache or lethargy.
- Instruct patient to maintain increased fluid intake (if not contraindicated) while taking this medication.
- Advise patient to use caution when driving or performing tasks that require mental alertness until effects of medication are determined.
- Remind patient to complete full course of therapy, even if symptoms of urinary tract or eye infection have resolved.

See Patient Guide, p. 447.

Nortriptyline HCl

(nor-TRIP-tih-leen HIGH-droe-KLOR-ide)

Aventyl, Aventyl HCl, Pamelor

Class: Tricyclic antidepressant

Action Inhibits reuptake of norepinephrine and serotonin in CNS.

Indications Relief of symptoms of depression. **Unlabeled uses:** Treatment of panic disorder, premenstrual depression, dermatologic disorders (eg, chronic urticaria, angioedema, nocturnal pruritis in atopic eczema).

Contraindications Hypersensitivity to any tricyclic antidepressant. Generally, not to be given in combination with or within 14 days of treatment with MAO inhibitor or during acute recovery phases of MI.

Route/Dosage

ADULTS: **PO** 25 mg tid-qid. Doses > 150 mg/day are not recommended. ELDERLY & ADOLESCENTS: **PO** 30-50 mg/day in divided doses.

Interactions

Anticoagulants: Dicumaral actions may increase. *Carbamazepine:* Carbamazepine levels may increase; nortriptyline levels may decrease. *Cimetidine, fluoxetine:* Concomitant administration may increase nortriptyline blood levels and effects. *CNS depressants:* Depressant effects may be additive. *Clonidine:* May result in hypertensive crisis. *Guanethidine:* Hypotensive action may be inhibited. *MAO Inhibitors:* Hyperpyretic crisis, convulsions and death may occur. *Sympathomimetics:* Pressor response may decrease.

Lab Test Interferences

None well documented.

Adverse Reactions

CV: Orthostatic hypotension; hypertension; tachycardia; palpitations; arrhythmias; ECG changes; stroke; heart block; CHF. *RESP:* Pharyngitis; rhinitis; sinusitis; laryngitis; coughing. *CNS:* Confusion; hallucinations; delusions; nervousness; restlessness; agitation; panic; insomnia; nightmares; mania; exacerbation of psychosis; drowsiness; dizziness; weakness; fatigue; emotional lability; seizures; tremors; extrapyramidal symptoms (eg, pseudoparkinsonism, movement disorders, akathesia). *EENT:* Nasal congestion; tinnitus; conjunctivitis; mydriasis; blurred vision; increased IOP; peculiar taste in mouth. *GI:* Nausea; vomiting; anorexia; GI distress; diarrhea; flatulence; dry mouth; constipation. *GU:* Impotence; sexual dysfunction; nocturia; urinary frequency; urinary tract infection; vaginitis; cystitis; dysmenorrhea; amenorrhea; urinary retention and hesitancy. *HEMA:* Bone marrow depression including agranulocytosis; eosinophilia; purpura; thrombocytopenia; leukopenia. *DERM:* Rash; pruritus; photosensitivity reaction; dry skin; acne. *HEPA:* Hepatitis; jaundice. *META:* Elevation or depression of blood sugar. *OTHER:* Numbness; breast enlargement.

Precautions

Pregnancy: Safety not established. *Lactation:* Excreted in breast milk. *Children:* Safety and efficacy not established. *Special risk patients:* Use drug with caution in patients with history of seizures, urinary retention, urethral or ureteral spasm, angle-closure glaucoma or increased IOP, cardiovascular disorders, hyperthyroid patients or those receiving thyroid medication, patients with hepatic or renal impairment, schizophrenia or paranoia.

NURSING CONSIDERATIONS

Administration/Storage

- Give with food or milk.
- Store at room temperature in tight container.
- If prescribed as single daily dose, give at bedtime to reduce side effects.

Assessment/Interventions

- Obtain patient history, including drug history and any known allergies.
- Obtain baseline renal function tests, liver function tests, CBC and ECG and monitor throughout therapy.
- Drug levels may be obtained to determine if patient is in optimal range (50-150 ng/ml).
- Assess emotional status (appearance, speech patterns, mood, level of interest), and monitor level of consciousness and suicidal ideation.
- Monitor daily elimination pattern, BP and pulse, and notify physician of potential problems.
- Assess for bladder distention and constipation.

> **OVERDOSAGE: SIGNS & SYMPTOMS**
>
> Confusion, vomiting, muscle rigidity, ECG abnormalities, seizures, agitation, fever, hyperactive reflexes, CHF, coma, respiratory depression, death

Patient/Family Education

- Advise patient to avoid sudden position changes to prevent orthostatic hypotension.
- Explain that it may take up to 2 wk for therapeutic effects to become evident.
- Caution patient to avoid exposure to sunlight and to use sunscreen or wear protective clothing to avoid photosensitivity reaction.
- Instruct patient to notify physician of visual disturbances.
- Advise patient to take sips of water frequently, suck on ice chips or sugarless hard candy or chew sugarless gum if dry mouth occurs.
- Caution patient that drug may cause drowsiness and to use caution while driving or performing other tasks requiring mental alertness.
- Instruct patient not to double dose if one is missed and to notify physician if more than one dose is missed.
- Advise that side effects will be decreased if taken at bedtime if prescribed as once-daily dose.

See Patient Guide, p. 448.

Nystatin

(nye-STAT-in)

Mycostatin, Nilstat, Nystex, Mycostatin Pastilles, ♣ *Nadostine, Nyaderm*

Class: Anti-infective/antifungal

Action Binds to fungal cell membrane, changing membrane permeability and allowing leakage of intracellular components.

Indications Treatment of intestinal, oral, vulvovaginal, cutaneous or mucocutaneous candidiasis.

Contraindications Standard considerations.

Route/Dosage

Intestinal Candidiasis

ADULTS & CHILDREN: **PO** 500,000-1,000,000 U tid. Continue treatment for at least 48 hr after clinical cure.

Oral or Mucocutaneous Candidiasis

ADULTS & CHILDREN: **PO** (suspension) 200,000-600,000 U qid; swish and swallow, *or* **PO** (oral pastilles) 1-2 pastilles (200,000-400,000 U) dissolved in mouth 4-5 times/day. INFANTS: **PO** 200,000 units qid.

Vaginal Candidiasis

ADULTS: **Intravaginal** 100,000 U qd for 2 wk.

Cutaneous Candidiasis
ADULTS & CHILDREN: **Topical** Apply to affected areas bid-tid.

Interactions None well documented.

Lab Test Interferences
None well documented.

Adverse Reactions
GI: Diarrhea; GI distress; nausea; vomiting (with large oral doses). *DERM:* Irritation (with topical use).

Precautions
Pregnancy: Category C (oral); Category A (vaginal). *Lactation:* Undetermined. *Effectiveness:* Has no activity against bacteria or trichomonads. Not indicated for systemic mycoses. *Topical preparations:* Not for ophthalmic use.

NURSING CONSIDERATIONS

Administration/Storage

- For troche/pastilles administration, have patient dissolve troche in mouth. Instruct patient not to chew or swallow troche whole. Have patient retain troche in mouth as long as possible before swallowing.
- For administration of oral suspension, place half of dose in each side of mouth. Have patient swish thoroughly around in mouth and retain in mouth as long as possible before swallowing. Shake suspension well. Use calibrated dropper provided.
- Do not mix oral suspension in foods.
- To use powder for extemporaneous compounding, reconstitute ⅛ tsp (500,000 U) in half glass of water and stir well. Use immediately; do not store. Can be administered in form of flavored frozen popsicle.
- Cream or ointment is preferred for affected intertriginous areas. Wash and dry affected area before application. Use gloves or swabs to apply enough medication to cover lesion completely.
- To use powder, clean and dry affected area before application. Dust powder on feet and in socks and shoes for infection of feet. Very moist lesions are best treated with powder.
- For vaginal use, insert 1 tablet high into vagina with applicator.
- Refrigerate vaginal tablets.
- Avoid contact with eyes.
- Store oral suspension in refrigerator. Protect from heat, light, moisture and air.

Assessment/Interventions

- Obtain patient history, including drug history and any known allergies.
- Although allergic reactions are rare, assess for rash, urticaria, burning, stinging, redness and swelling.
- Assess for factors predisposing to infection: pregnancy, antibiotic therapy, diabetes, sexual partner infections (vaginal infections). However, vaginal yeast infections are very common and may not be associated with any of these factors.
- Inspect mucous membranes before and frequently throughout course of therapy.

OVERDOSAGE: SIGNS & SYMPTOMS
Nausea, diarrhea, vomiting

Patient/Family Education

- Instruct patient that long-term therapy may be needed to clear infection and that patient should complete entire course of medication. Take drug for 2 days after symptoms have disappeared or as directed.
- Advise patient using vaginal preparations to wear light-day pad; drug may stain clothing and linens.
- Advise patient to notify physician if irritation occurs.
- Assure patient that relief from itching may occur after 24-72 hr.
- Instruct patient to practice good hand washing before and after each application of topical or vaginal medication. Remind patient to wash applicator after each use.

- Advise patient with oral candidiasis not to use mouthwash, which may alter normal flora and promote infections.
- Teach patient to continue using vaginal tablets even when menstruating because treatment should be continued for 2 wk. Instruct patient to avoid using tampons.
- Advise patient to prevent reinfection (ie, avoid intercourse during therapy or use condoms).
- Instruct patient to discontinue drug and notify physician if vaginal tablets cause irritation, redness or swelling.

See Patient Guide, pp. 449-452.

Octreotide Acetate

(ock-TREE-oh-tide ASS-uh-TATE)
Sandostatin
Class: Hormone

Action Actions mimic those of natural hormone somatostatin. Suppresses secretion of serotonin and gastroenteropancreatic peptides (gastrin, insulin, glucagon, secretin, motilin). Also suppresses growth hormone.

Indications Symptomatic treatment of diarrhea associated with carcinoid tumors; treatment of profuse watery diarrhea associated with vasoactive intestinal peptide tumors (VIPoma); to reduce blood levels of growth hormone and IGF-1 in acromegaly patients who have had inadequate response to or cannot be treated with resection, pituitary irradiation and bromocriptine at maximally tolerated doses. **Unlabeled uses:** To reduce output from GI fistulas; for variceal bleeding; for relief of diarrhea associated with a variety of conditions; to reduce output from pancreatic fistulas; to treat irritable bowel syndrome; to treat dumping syndrome; to treat the following conditions: enteric fistula; pancreatitis; pancreatic surgery; glucagonoma; insulinoma; gastrinoma (Zollinger-Ellison syndrome); intestinal obstruction; local radiotherapy; chronic pain management; antineoplastic therapy; decrease insulin requirements in diabetes mellitus; thryotropin- and TSH-secreting tumors.

Contraindications Standard considerations.

Route/Dosage

Carcinoid Tumors

ADULTS: **SC** 100-600 mcg/day in 2-4 divided doses, adjusting to response.

VIPoma

ADULTS: **SC** 200-300 mcg/day in 2-4 divided doses, adjusting to response.

Acromegaly

ADULTS: **SC** 50 mcg-500 mcg/tid. Most common dose is 100 mcg/tid; doses >300 mcg/day seldom result in additional benefit.

Interactions *Cyclosporine:* May decrease plasma levels of cyclosporine. INCOMPATIBILITIES: Parenteral nutrition solutions.

Lab Test Interferences None well documented.

Adverse Reactions *CNS:* Headache; dizziness; lightheadedness; fatigue; sinus bradycardia; conduction abnormalities; arrhythmias. *GI:* Nausea; constipation; flatuence; diarrhea; abdominal pain or discomfort; loose stools; vomiting; fat malabsorption. *HEPA:* Increased liver transaminase. *META:* Hyperglycemia; hypoglycemia. *OTHER:* Injection site pain; flushing; asthenia; weakness.

Precautions *Pregnancy:* Category B. *Lactation:* Undetermined. *Children:* Has been used in children as young as 1 mo. *Elderly:* Dose adjustments may be necessary due to significant increases in half-life and significant decrease in the clearance of octreotide. *Cardiac effects:* In acromegalics, bradycardia, conduction abnormalities and arrhythmias have occurred. Other ECG changes observed include QT prolongation, axis shifts, early repolarization, low voltage, R/S transition and early wave progression. Dose adjustments in drugs such as beta blockers that have bradycardia effects may be necessary. Pancreatitis: Several cases have occurred in patients receiving octreotide. *Cholelithiasis:* Cholelithiasis may occur; periodically monitor gallbladder function. *Hypoglycemia or hyperglycemia:* Serum glucose control may be altered; carefully monitor patient and adjust insulin requirements accordingly. *Renal impairment:* Dosage reduction may be necessary.

NURSING CONSIDERATIONS

Administration/Storage

- Do not administer if particulate matter or discoloration is observed.
- Rotate sites for subcutaneous injection.
- Store ampules at room temperature for day of use.
- Refrigerate for prolonged storage.

Assessment/Interventions

- Obtain patient history, including drug history and any known allergies.
- Monitor glucose, CBC, T_3, T_4, TSH, renal function tests, BUN, creatinine, and electrolytes and obtain baseline weight and BP.
- Assess for nausea, headache, shortness of breath, hyperglycemia/hypoglycemia or abdominal pain.
- Monitor I&O and daily weight.
- Monitor BP, pulse and respiration weekly during treatment.
- Assess frequency and consistency of stools.
- Assess lung sounds, and report any edema or decrease in urine output.
- Diatary fat absorption may be altered in some patients. Periodic quantitative 72-hour fecal fat and serum carotene determination should be performed to aid in assessment of possible drug-induced aggravation of fat malabsorption.

OVERDOSAGE: SIGNS & SYMPTOMS

Possible hyperglycemia and hypoglycemia

Patient/Family Education

- Instruct and observe return demonstration of correct technique for subcutaneous injection. Explain that preferred sites for injection are abdomen, thigh and hip.
- Advise patient of importance of regular follow-up with physician.
- Caution patient to report these symptoms to physician: icterus, jaundice, dark urine or clay-colored stools.
- Advise patient to notify physician of abdominal pain, edema, chest pain, fainting, dry mouth or shortness of breath.
- Advise patient that various laboratory tests may be required during therapy.

See Patient Guide, p. 453.

Ofloxacin

(oh-FLOX-uh-SIN)

Floxin, Ocuflox

Class: Antibiotic/fluoroquinolone

Action Interferes with microbial DNA synthesis.

Indications Treatment of infections of lower respiratory tract, skin and skin structure and urinary tract caused by susceptible organisms; treatment of sexually transmitted diseases; treatment of prostatitis caused by *Escherichia coli*. *Ophthalmic:* Treatment of superficial ocular infections due to susceptible organisms.

Contraindications Hypersensitivity to fluoroquinolones, quinolone antibiotics or any product component. *Ophthalmic:* Epithelial herpes simplex keratitis; vaccinia; varicella; fungal disease of ocular structure; mycobacterial infections of the eye.

Route/Dosage

UTIs

ADULTS: **PO/IV** 200 mg q 12 hr.

Prostatitis

ADULTS: **PO/IV** 300 mg q 12 hr for 6 wk.

Infections of Respiratory Tract, Skin and Skin Structure

ADULTS: **PO/IV** 400 mg q 12 hr.

Acute, Uncomplicated Gonorrhea

ADULTS: **PO/IV** 400 mg as single dose.

Cervicitis/Urethritis

ADULTS: **PO/IV** 300 mg q 12 hr.

Ocular Infection

ADULTS: **Ophthalmic** 1-2 gtt as directed.

Interactions

Antacids, iron salts, zinc salts, sucralfate, didanosine: May decrease oral absorption of ofloxacin. *Antineoplastic agents:* Serum ofloxacin levels may be decreased. *Theophylline:* Decreased clearance and increased plasma levels of theophylline may result in toxicity.

Lab Test Interferences

None well documented.

Adverse Reactions

CNS: Headache; dizziness; fatigue; lethargy; drowsiness; insomnia. *EENT:* Visual disturbances. Ophthalmic use: Transient burning, itching, stinging, inflammation, angioneurotic edema, urticaria and dermatitis. *GI:* Diarrhea; nausea; vomiting; abdominal pain or discomfort; dry or painful mouth; flatulence. *HEPA:* Increased ALT, AST. *HEMA:* Eosinophilia; lymphocytopenia. *DERM:* Rash; pruritus. *OTHER:* Vaginitis; fever; decreased appetite. Ophthalmic use may possibly cause same adverse reactions seen with systemic use, due to absorption.

Precautions

Pregnancy: Category C. *Lactation:* Excreted in breast milk. *Children:* Do not use in children < 18 yr. *Elderly patients:* Half-life may increase. *Convulsions:* CNS stimulation can occur; use drug with caution in patients with known or suspected CNS disorders. *Photosensitivity:* Moderate to severe reactions may occur; avoid excessive sunlight and ultraviolet light. *Pseudomembranous colitis:* Consider possibility in patients who develop diarrhea. *Renal impairment:* Reduced creatinine clearance may occur; decrease dose accordingly. *Syphilis:* Not effective for treating syphilis.

NURSING CONSIDERATIONS

Administration/Storage

- Store all forms at room temperature. IV solution is stable after dilution for 72 hr at room temperature and 2 wk if refrigerated.
- Discard unused portion of IV preparation.

Oral Form

- Administer 1 hr before or 2 hr after meals.
- Do not administer concurrently with antacids.
- Administer with full glass of water.

IV Solution

- Do not give as IV push or bolus. To reduce likelihood of hypotension, infuse over 60 min.
- Dilute to concentration of 4 mg/ml.
- Do not infuse in IV line with any other drug.

Assessment/Interventions

- Obtain patient history, including drug history and any known allergies.
- Obtain baseline CBC, renal and liver function tests and electrolytes.
- Assess for any skin rashes. Notify physician if skin rash occurs.
- Obtain baseline vital signs. Monitor

vital signs at least bid while administering medication.
- Monitor patterns of elimination and stool consistency.
- Monitor for signs of superinfection.
- Encourage fluid intake.
- Notify physician if vomiting, fatigue, lymphocytopenia, increased liver function test results, seizures or visual disturbances occur.
- Notify physician if extreme burning, angioneurotic edema or dermatitis occurs with ophthalmic use.

OVERDOSAGE: SIGNS & SYMPTOMS

Nausea, headache, dizziness, crystalluria, vomiting, drowsiness, seizures

Patient/Family Education

- Advise patient to take on empty stomach 1 hr before or 2 hr after meals.
- Instruct patient not to take antacids within 4 hr before or 2 hr after dose.
- Caution to avoid exposure to sunlight and to use sunscreen or wear protective clothing to avoid photosensitivity reaction.
- Advise patient to notify physician of signs of superinfection.
- Caution patient to report these symptoms to physician: seizures, nausea, rash, itching, diarrhea, shortness of breath, dizziness or headache.
- Demonstrate and observe return demonstration of correct technique for instillation of ophthalmic drops.
- Advise patient using ophthalmic solution to discontinue medication and notify physician of rash or allergic reaction.
- Instruct patient to complete full course of therapy, even if symptoms have resolved.

See Patient Guide, pp. 454-455.

Olsalazine Sodium

(OLE-SAL-uh-zeen SO-dee-uhm)

Dipentum

Class: Intestinal anti-inflammatory/aminosalicylic acid derivative

Action Bioconverted to 5-aminosalicylic acid (mesalamine) in colon. Although mechanism of action is unknown, it probably reduces inflammation of colon topically by preventing production of substances involved in inflammatory process such as arachidonic acid.

Indications Maintenance of remission of ulcerative colitis in patients intolerant of sulfasalazine.

Contraindications Hypersensitivity to salicylates or any product component.

Route/Dosage

ADULTS: **PO** 500 mg bid (2 capsules) (total of 1 g/day).

Interactions None well documented.

Lab Test Interferences

None well documented.

Adverse Reactions

CNS: Headache; fatigue; drowsiness; lethargy; depression. *GI:* Diarrhea; abdominal pain, cramps; nausea; dyspepsia; bloating; anorexia. *DERM:* Rash; itching. *OTHER:* Arthralgia; upper respiratory infection.

Precautions

Pregnancy: Category C. *Lactation:* Undetermined. *Children:* Safety and efficacy not established. *Renal impairment:* Patients with history of renal disease or dysfunction may have worsening of renal function.

NURSING CONSIDERATIONS

Administration/Storage

- Administer with meals.
- Store at room temperature.

Assessment/Interventions

- Obtain patient history, including drug history and any known allergies.
- Assess baseline vital signs, weight, BUN, creatinine, ALT and AST.
- Monitor elimination patterns, color and consistency of stools.
- Assess for rashes, respiratory difficulty, abdominal pain, vomiting, diarrhea, abdominal distention or lethargy and notify physician of any problems.

Patient/Family Education

- Caution patient to notify physician of rashes, respiratory difficulty, lethargy, muscle weakness, vomiting, diarrhea or abdominal distention or worsening of abdominal pain.
- Advise patient not to double doses if one is missed. If more than one dose is missed, tell patient to notify physician.

See Patient Guide, p. 456.

Omeprazole

(oh-MEH-pray-ZAHL)

Prilosec, *Losec*

Class: Gastrointestinal

Action Suppresses gastric acid secretion by blocking "acid (proton) pump" within gastric parietal cell.

Indications Short-term treatment of active duodenal ulcer, gastroesophageal reflux disease (GERD), including severe erosive esophagitis and symptomatic GERD poorly responsive to customary medical treatment; long-term treatment of pathologic hypersecretory conditions (eg, Zollinger-Ellison syndrome, multiple endocrine adenomas, systemic mastocytosis); to maintain healing of erosive esophagitis. **Unlabeled uses:** Treatment of gastric ulcers; healing of gastric ulcers in patients receiving NSAIDs; in combination with other drugs for eradication of *Helicobacter pylori* gastric infection.

Contraindications Standard considerations.

Route/Dosage

Active Duodenal Ulcer

ADULTS: **PO** 20 mg/day for 4-8 wk.

Severe Erosive Esophagitis or Poorly Responsive GERD

ADULTS: **PO** 20 mg/day for 4-8 wk.

Pathologic Hypersecretory Conditions

ADULTS: **PO** Initial dose: 60 mg/day. Doses up to 120 mg tid have been given. Divide daily doses > 80 mg.

Maintenance of Healing Erosive Esophagitis

ADULTS: **PO** 20 mg daily.

Interactions

Benzodiazepines: Clearance of benzodiazepines may be decreased. *Drugs depending on gastric pH for bioavailability (eg, ketoconazole, iron salts, ampicillin):* Absorption of these drugs may be affected. *Phenytoin:* Decreased plasma clearance and increased half-life phenytoin. *Warfarin:* Prolonged warfarin elimination.

Lab Test Interferences

None well documented.

Adverse Reactions

CV: Angina; tachycardia; bradycardia; palpitation. *RESP:* Cough; upper respiratory infection. *CNS:* Headache; dizziness. *GI:* Diarrhea; abdominal pain; acid regurgitation; nausea; vomiting; constipation; flatulence. *DERM:* Rash. *OTHER:* Asthenia; back pain.

Precautions

Pregnancy: Category C. *Lacta-*

tion: Undetermined. *Children:* Safety and efficacy in children not established.

NURSING CONSIDERATIONS

Administration/Storage

- Do not open, chew or crush capsule. Instruct patient to swallow capsule whole.
- Daily doses > 80 mg should be divided.
- Give before meals or as one-time daily dose. If medication is administered once daily, give before dinner.
- Store at room temperature in original container tightly closed and protected from light.

Assessment/Interventions

- Obtain patient history, including drug history and any known allergies.
- Review baseline CBC and liver function test results and monitor as indicated.
- Assess for coffee ground emesis, tarry stools or constipation.
- Assess for any symptoms of hyperacidity (dyspepsia, nausea or vomiting).
- Monitor elimination patterns and document any problems such as constipation.
- Assess skin for rashes or hives.
- Encourage adequate fluid intake and roughage in diet.

Patient/Family Education

- Advise patient not to chew or crush medication and to swallow whole.
- Remind patient to take medication before meals.
- Inform patient that antacids may be taken concurrently with omeprazole.
- Advise patient to avoid tasks requiring alertness until response to medication is established.
- Caution patient to report these symptoms to physician: cramping, diarrhea, rash or hives.

See Patient Guide, p. 457.

Ondansetron HCl

(ahn-DAN-SEH-trahn HIGH-droe-KLOR-ide)

Zofran

Class: Antiemetic/antivertigo

Action Selective serotonin (5-HT_3) receptor antagonist that inhibits serotonin receptors in GI tract or chemoreceptor trigger zone.

Indications *Parenteral or oral:* Prevention of nausea and vomiting associated with emetogenic chemotherapy. *Parenteral only:* Prevention of postoperative nausea and vomiting in patients at risk.

Contraindications Standard considerations.

Route/Dosage

Prevention of Chemotherapy-Induced Nausea and Vomiting

ADULTS: **IV** 0.15 mg/kg infused over 15 min beginning 30 min before chemotherapy with 2 additional doses 4 and 8 hr after chemotherapy. Alternatively give 32 mg over 15 min, 30 min before chemotherapy. ADULTS & CHILDREN > 12 YR: **PO** 8 mg tid; give first dose 30 min before chemotherapy with 2 additional doses 4 and 8 hr after chemotherapy. Can give 8 mg q 8 hr for 1-2 days after chemotherapy. CHILDREN 4-18 YR: **IV** 0.15 mg/kg infused over 15 min beginning 30 min before chemotherapy with 2 additional doses 4 and 8 hr after chemotherapy. CHILDREN 4-12 YR: **PO** 4 mg tid.

Postoperative Nausea and Vomiting

ADULTS: **IV** 4 mg undiluted over 2-5

min ideally at induction of anesthesia or shortly after surgery is completed.

Interactions None well documented. INCOMPATIBILITIES: Alkaline solutions.

Lab Test Interferences
None well documented.

Adverse Reactions
CV: Chest pain; tachycardia. *RESP:* Bronchospasm. *CNS:* Headache; seizures. *GI:* Dry mouth; constipation; abdominal pain. *META:* Hypokalemia. *DERM:* Rash. *OTHER:* Fever; anaphylaxis; weakness.

Precautions
Pregnancy: Category B. *Lactation:* Undetermined. *Children:* Dosing in children < 4 yr is not well defined. *Hepatic impairment:* In patients with severe hepatic impairment, do not exceed 8 mg daily oral dose. For IV use, give single 8 mg daily dose over 15 min beginning 30 min before chemotherapy. *Peristalsis:* Ondansetron does not stimulate gastric or intestinal peristalsis; may mask progressive ileus or gastric distention.

NURSING CONSIDERATIONS

Administration/Storage

- Dilute solution in 50 ml of 5% Dextrose in Water or 0.9% Sodium Chloride for Injection.
- Do not mix with solutions for which compatibility has not been established.
- Preparation is stable for 48 hr at room temperature following dilution.

Assessment/Interventions

- Obtain patient history, including drug history and any known allergies. Note hepatic impairment.
- Ensure that baseline hepatic studies have been performed before beginning therapy.
- Assess patient for nausea, vomiting and bowel sounds.
- Monitor I&O carefully.
- Be prepared to give additional IV fluids to patient who is vomiting, but do not overhydrate.
- Discontinue IV infusion if signs of hypersensitivity develop.

OVERDOSAGE: SIGNS & SYMPTOMS

Hypotension, constipation

Patient/Family Education

- Advise patient that headache is common side effect.
- Advise patient that medication will greatly reduce likelihood of nausea and vomiting but that these are still possible.

See Patient Guide, p. 458.

Oral Contraceptives, Combination Products

Brevicon, Demulen 1/35, Demulen 1/50, Desogen, Genora 0.5/35, Genora 1/35, Genora 1/50, Jenest-28, Levlen, Levora, Loestrin 21 1/20, Loestrin 21 1.5/30, Loestrin Fe 1/20, Loestrin Fe 1.5/30, Lo/Ovral, ModiCon, N.E.E., Nelova 0.5/35 E, Nelova 1/35 E, Nelova 1/50 M, Nelova 10/11, Nordette, Norethin 1/35 E, Norethin 1/50 M, Norinyl 1 + 35, Norinyl 1 + 50, Ortho-Cept, Ortho-Cyclen, Ortho-Novum 1/50, Ortho-Novum 1/35, Ortho-Novum 10/11, Ortho Tri-Cyclen, Ovcon-35, Ovcon-50, Ovral, Tri-Levelen, Tri-Norinyl, Triphasil
Class: Hormone/contraceptive

Action Inhibits ovulation by suppressing gonadotropins, follicle-stimulating hormone and luteinizing hormone.

Indications Prevention of pregnancy. **Unlabeled use:** Postcoital contraceptive.

Contraindications Thrombophlebitis; thromboembolic disorders; history of deep vein thrombophlebitis; cerebral vascular disease; MI; coronary artery disease; known or suspected breast carcinoma or estrogen-dependent neoplasia; past or present benign or malignant liver tumors that developed during use of estrogen-containing products; past or present angina pectoris; undiagnosed abnormal genital bleeding; known or suspected pregnancy; cholestatic jaundice of pregnancy or jaundice with prior pill use.

Route/Dosage

Sunday-Start Packaging

ADULTS: **PO** 1 tablet daily beginning on first Sunday after menstruation begins. If menstruation begins on Sunday, take first tablet on that day.

21-day Regimen

ADULTS: **PO** 1 tablet daily for 21 days, beginning on day 5 of cycle. Take no tablets for 7 days; then start new course of 21-day regimen.

28-day Regimen

ADULTS: **PO** 1 tablet daily.

Interactions *Barbiturates, hydantoins, rifampin, griseofulvin, penicillin, tetracyclines:* Decreased effectiveness of oral contraceptive. Use additional form of birth control during concomitant therapy. *Benzodiazepines:* Increased benzodiazepine therapeutic effect or toxicity. *Caffeine:* Increased caffeine therapeutic effect or toxicity. *Corticosteroids:* Increased corticosteroid effect or toxicity. *Metoprolol:* Increased metoprolol effect or toxicity. *Theophyllines:* Increased theophylline effect or toxicity. *Tricyclic antidepressants:* Increased tricyclic antidepressant effect or toxicity. *Troleandomycin:* Increased frequency of cholestatic jaundice.

Lab Test Interferences

May cause increases in sulfobromophthalein retention; factors II, VII, VIII, IX, X; plasminogen, fibrinogen; norepinephrine-induced platelet aggregation; thyroid-binding globulin, leading to increased total thyroid hormone measurements; transcortin; corticosteroid levels; triglycerides and phospholipids; ceruloplasmin; aldosterone; amylase; gamma-glutamyl transpeptidase; iron-binding capacity; transferrin; prolactin; renin activity; vitamin A. May cause decreases in anti-thrombin III; free T_3 resin uptake; pregnanediol excretion; response to metyrapone test; folate; glucose tolerance; albumin; cholinesterase; haptoglobin; zinc; vitamin B_{12}.

Adverse Reactions

CV: Coronary thrombosis; MI; hypertension. *RESP:* Pulmonary embolism. *CNS:* Cerebral thrombosis; cerebral hemorrhage; migraine; mental depression. *EENT:* Steepening of corneal curvature; contact lens intolerance. *GI:* Nausea and vomiting; abdominal cramps; bloating; mesenteric thrombosis. *GU:* Renal artery thrombosis; breakthrough bleeding; spotting; change in menstrual flow; dysmenorrhea; amenorrhea; temporary infertility after discontinuation; change in cervical erosion and cervical secretions; endocervical hyperplasia; increase in size of uterine leiomyomata; vaginal candidiasis. *HEMA:* Thrombophlebitis and thrombosis; arterial thromboembolism. *HEPA:* Cholestatic jaundice; gallbladder disease. *DERM:* Melasma; rash; photosensitivity. *OTHER:* Raynaud's disease; congenital anomalies; liver tumors; hepatocellular carcinoma; breast tenderness, enlargment, secretion, diminished lactation; edema; weight change; reduced carbohydrate tolerance; prolactin-secreting pituitary tumors; increased prevalence of cervical chlamydia trachomatous.

Precautions

Pregnancy: Category X. *Lactation:* Excreted in breast milk. Defer use until infant weaned. *Acute intermittent porphyria:* May be precipitated by estrogen therapy in susceptible individuals. *Carbohydrate and lipid metabolism:* Glucose tolerance may decrease; triglycerides and total phospholipids may increase. Progestins may elevate LDL levels. *Depression:* Use drug with caution in patients with history of depression. *Fibroids:* Oral contraceptives may cause an increase in size of pre-existing uterine leiomyomata (fibroids). *Fluid retention:* Use drug with caution in patients with hypertension, convulsive disorders, migraines, asthma, cardiac, hepatic or renal dysfunction. *Liver dysfunction:* May impair metabolism of oral contraceptives. *Pyridoxine deficiency:* May occur due to disturbance in normal tryptophan metabolism. *Serum folate:* May be depressed by oral contaceptive therapy. *Tartrazine sensitivity:* Some products may contain tartrazine, which may cause allergic-type reaction in susceptible individuals.

NURSING CONSIDERATIONS

Administration/Storage

- Give at same time each day. Efficacy depends on strict adherence to dosage schedule.
- May be given with or without food.

Assessment/Interventions

- Obtain patient medical history, including drug history and any known allergies.
- Monitor blood glucose levels in patients with diabetes.
- If spotting or breakthrough bleeding continues past second month, notify physician.
- Do not administer oral contraceptives to induce withdrawal bleeding as test for pregnancy.

OVERDOSAGE: SIGNS & SYMPTOMS

Withdrawal bleeding

Patient/Family Education

- Advise patient to use additional method of birth control until after first week of administration in initial cycle.
- Advise patient what to do if dose is missed: (1) if you miss 1, take when you remember or take 2 the next day; (2) if you miss 2, take 2 on 2 consecutive days; (3) if you miss ≥ 3, stop pills; (4) use alternative form of birth control in all cases.
- Advise patient to take multiple daily vitamin.
- Encourage patient who smokes to stop. Cardiovascular dysfunction and thromboembolic disease have been associated with use of oral contraceptives in patients who smoke.
- Advise patient that oral contraceptives may change the fit of rigid contact lenses.
- Caution patient to avoid prolonged exposure to sunlight and to use sunscreen or wear protective clothing to avoid photosensitivity reaction.
- Advise patient to wait at least 3 mo after discontinuing oral contraceptives to try to become pregnant.
- Caution patient that antibiotics may decrease effectiveness of oral contraceptives and to use a nonhormonal form of contraception while taking antibiotics and for 7 days after stopping antibiotics.
- Instruct patient to report symptoms of blood clots (eg, pain, numbness, shortness of breath, visual disturbances).
- Teach patient routine breast self-examination technique.
- Warn patient that side effects such as nausea and breakthrough bleeding are common at first.

See Patient Guide, p. 459.

Oral Contraceptives, Progestin-only Products

Micronor, Nor-Q.D., Orvette
Class: Hormone/contraceptive

Action Alters cervical mucus, interferes with implantation and may suppress ovulation.

Indications Prevention of pregnancy.

Contraindications Thrombophlebitis; thromboembolic disorders; history of deep vein thrombophlebitis; cerebral vascular disease; MI; coronary artery disease; known or suspected breast carcinoma; impaired liver function or disease; undiagnosed abnormal genital bleeding; known or suspected pregnancy; as diagnostic test for pregnancy.

Route/Dosage
ADULTS: PO 1 tablet daily, starting on first day of menstruation.

Interactions
Rifampin: Reduced plasma levels and pharmacologic effects of norethindrone.

Lab Test Interferences
Results of liver function tests, coagulation tests (increased prothrombin, factors VII, VIII, IX and X), thyroid function tests, metyrapone test and endocrine function tests may be altered. Pregnanediol determination may be altered.

Adverse Reactions
CV: Thrombophlebitis; cerebrovascular disorders. *RESP:* Pulmonary embolism. *CNS:* Depression; tiredness; fatigue. *EENT:* Retinal thrombosis. *GU:* Breakthrough bleeding; spotting; hypomenorrhea; amenorrhea; changes in cervical erosion and cervical secretions. *HEPA:* Cholestatic jaundice. *DERM:* Rash with and without pruritus; acne; melasma or chloasma; photosensitivity. *OTHER:* Breast changes; masculinization of female fetus; edema; weight change.

Precautions
Pregnancy: Category X. *Lactation:* Excreted in breast milk. *Depression:* Use drug with caution in patients with history of depression. *Fluid retention:* Use with caution in patients with hypertension, convulsive disorders, migraines, asthma, cardiac, hepatic or renal dysfunction. *Lipid disorders:* Progestins may elevate LDL levels. *Tartrazine sensitivity:* Some products may contain tartrazine, which may cause allergic-type reaction in susceptible individuals.

NURSING CONSIDERATIONS

Administration/Storage
- Administer at same time each day.
- Start on first day of menstruation.
- If GI upset occurs, administer with food.
- Do not administer oral contraceptives to induce withdrawal bleeding as test for pregnancy.

OVERDOSAGE: SIGNS & SYMPTOMS
Nausea

Assessment/Interventions
- Obtain patient history, including drug history and any known allergies.
- Perform baseline physical examination before beginning therapy.
- If spotting or breakthrough bleeding continues past second month, notify physician.

Patient/Family Education
- Advise patient to use additional method of birth control until after first wk of administration in initial cycle.
- Teach patient what to do if dose is missed. If 1 tablet is missed, take as soon as remembered and then take

next tablet at regular time. If 2 consecutive tablets are missed, do not take missed tablets; discard and take next tablet at regular time. Use additional form of contraception until pregnancy is ruled out or menses occurs. If 3 consecutive tablets are missed, discontinue drug immediately. Use additional form of contraception until pregnancy is ruled out or menses occurs.

- Encourage patient who smokes to stop. Cardiovascular dysfunction and thromboembolic disease have been associated with use of oral contraceptives in patients who smoke.
- Advise patient that oral contraceptives may change fit of rigid contact lenses.
- Caution patient to avoid prolonged exposure to sunlight and to use sunscreen or wear protective clothing to avoid photosensitivity reaction.
- Advise patient to wait at least 3 mo after discontinuing oral contraceptives before trying to become pregnant.
- Instruct patient to report symptoms of blood clots (eg, pain, numbness, shortness of breath, visual disturbances).

See Patient Guide, p. 460.

Orphenadrine Citrate

(ore-FEN-uh-dreen SIH-trate)

Banflex, Flexoject, Flexon, Myolin, Norflex, Norgesic, Norgesic Forte

Class: Skeletal muscle relaxant/centrally acting

Action Unknown; may be related to analgesic properties since drug acts on brain stem and does not act directly on muscles; possesses anticholinergic actions.

Indications Adjunctive treatment for acute, painful musculoskeletal conditions. **Unlabeled use:** Treatment of quinine-resistant leg cramps.

Contraindications Glaucoma; pyloric or duodenal obstruction; stenosing peptic ulcers; prostatic hypertrophy; obstruction of bladder neck; esophageal achalasia; myasthenia gravis.

Route/Dosage
ADULTS: **IV/IM** 60 mg q 12 hr prn. **PO** 100 mg bid.

Interactions
Alcohol, other CNS depressants: Increased CNS depression. *Haloperidol:* Worsening schizophrenic symptoms, decreased haloperidol levels, tardive dyskinesia. *Phenothiazines:* Decreased effects of phenothiazines.

Lab Test Interferences
None well documented.

Adverse Reactions
CV: Tachycardia; palpitations; transient syncope. *CNS:* Weakness; headache; dizziness; lightheadedness; confusion (especially in elderly); hallucinations; agitation; tremor; drowsiness. *EENT:* Blurred vision; pupil dilation; increased ocular tension. *GI:* Dry mouth; vomiting; nausea; constipation; gastric irritation. *GU:* Urinary hesitancy and retention. *DERM:* Hypersensitivity reactions (eg, rashes).

Precautions
Pregnancy: Category C. *Lactation:* Undetermined. *Children:* Safety and efficacy not established. *Elderly patients:* May be more sensitive to anticholinergic effects. *Cardiac disease:* Use drug with caution in patients with cardiac decompensation, coronary insufficiency, cardiac arrhythmias or tachycardia. *Heat prostration:* Can occur in presence of high environmental temperature. *Hypersensitivity reactions:* May occur. *Sulfite sensitivity:* Some products contain bisulfites, which may cause allergic-type reactions in certain persons.

NURSING CONSIDERATIONS

Administration/Storage

- Do not crush or have patient chew sustained release preparations.
- Give IV solution over 5 min with patient in supine position. Administer carefully; intoxication is very rapid and can be lethal.
- Store at room temperature.

Assessment/Interventions

- Obtain patient history, including drug history and any known allergies.
- Monitor patient's vital signs.
- Monitor blood, urine, and liver function values during long-term therapy.
- Assess degree of pain relief obtained.
- Implement safety precautions if patient becomes drowsy or dizzy.
- Notify physician if rapid heart rate, palpitations or mental confusion occurs.
- Carefully document voiding.

OVERDOSAGE: SIGNS & SYMPTOMS

Cardiac arrhythmias, seizures, coma, shock

Patient/Family Education

- Tell patient not to increase dosage of medication. Even slight overdose may be highly toxic.
- Instruct patient to take sips of water frequently, suck on ice chips or sugarless hard candy, or chew sugarless gum if dry mouth occurs.
- Advise patient that drug may cause drowsiness or dizziness and to use caution while driving or performing other tasks requiring mental alertness.
- Instruct patient to report these symptoms to physician: urinary retention, constipation, palpitations or tremors.
- Instruct patient to avoid alcohol or other CNS depressants.

See Patient Guide, p. 461.

Oxacillin Sodium

(ox-uh-SILL-in SO-dee-uhm)

Bactocill, Prostaphlin

Class: Antibiotic/penicillin

Action Inhibits mucopeptide synthesis in bacterial cell wall.

Indications Treatment of infections caused by penicillinase-producing staphylococci; initial therapy of suspected staphylococcal infection.

Contraindications Hypersensitivity to penicillins. Do not treat severe pneumonia, empyema, bacteremia, pericarditis, meningitis and purulent or septic arthritis with oral oxacillin during acute state.

Route/Dosage

ADULTS: **PO/IV/IM** 250 mg-1 g q 4-6 hr. CHILDREN: **PO/IV/IM** 50-100 mg/kg/day in divided doses q 4-6 hr.

Interactions

Contraceptives, oral: Reduced efficacy of oral contraceptives. *Probenecid:* Increased oxacillin levels. *Tetracyclines:* Impaired bactericidal effects of oxacillin. INCOMPATIBILITIES: Aminoglycosides.

Lab Test Interferences

Urine glucose test: May cause false-positive urine glucose test result with Benedict's solution, Fehling's solution or Clinitest tablets but not with enzyme-based tests (eg, Clinistix, Tes-tape). *Antiglobulin (Coombs') test:* Drug may cause false-positive results. *Urine and serum protein determinations:* Drug may cause false-positive reactions with sulfosalicylic acid and boiling test, acetic acid test, biuret reaction, and nitric acid test but not with brompheol blue test (Multi-Stix).

Adverse Reactions

CNS: Neurotoxicity (lethargy, neuromuscular irritability, hallucinations, convulsions and seizures); dizziness; fatigue; insomnia; reversible hyperactivity; prolonged muscle relaxation. *EENT:* Itchy eyes; abnormal taste perception. *GI:* Glossitis; stomatitis; gastritis; sore mouth or tongue; dry mouth; furry tongue; black "hairy" tongue; nausea; anorexia; vomiting; abdominal pain or cramp; diarrhea or bloody diarrhea; rectal bleeding; flatulence; enterocolitis; pseudomembranous colitis; anorexia. *GU:* Interstitial nephritis (oliguria, proteinuria, hematuria, hyaline casts, pyuria); nephropathy; increased creatinine and BUN; vaginitis. *HEMA:* Deep vein thrombosis; hematomas; phlebitis; anemias; thrombocytopenia; eosinophilia; leukopenia; granulocytopenia; neutropenia; bone marrow depression; agranulocytosis; reduced Hgb or Hct; prolongation of bleeding and prothrombin time. *HEPA:* Transient hepatitis; cholestatic jaundice; increased liver function test results. *DERM:* Ecchymosis. *META:* Elevated serum alkaline phosphatase, AST, ALT, bilirubin and LDH; hypernatremia; hypokalemia; reduced albumin, total proteins and uric acid. *OTHER:* Hypersensitivity reactions that may lead to death; hyperthermia; pain at site of injection; hyperthermia; sciatic neuritis.

Precautions

Pregnancy: Category B. *Lactation:* Excreted in breast milk. *Hypersensitivity:* Reactions range from mild to life-threatening. Administer cautiously to cephalosporin-sensitive or imipenem-sensitive patients due to possible cross-reactivity. *Pseudomembranous colitis:* Should be considered in patients who develop diarrhea. *Sodium content:* Contains 2.5-3.1 mEq sodium per gram. *Superinfection:* May result in bacterial or fungal overgrowth of nonsusceptible organisms.

NURSING CONSIDERATIONS

Administration/Storage

- Administer at regular intervals around the clock.
- Administer oral doses on empty stomach at least 1 hr before or 2 hr after meals.
- Reconstitute IM preparation to dilution of 250 mg/1.5 ml. Use deep, slow injection. Rotate sites to prevent tissue irritation.
- Reconstitute IV preparation with Sterile Water for Injection or Sodium Chloride for Injection. Administer slowly over approximately 10 min to prevent vein irritation.
- IM solution is stable for up to 3 days at room temperature or 7 days under refrigeration.
- IV solutions are stable for at least 6 hr at room temperature.
- Reconstituted oral solution is stable for 14 days if refrigerated.

Assessment/Interventions

- Obtain patient history, including drug history and any known allergies.
- Ensure that specimens for culture and sensitivity have been obtained before starting therapy.
- Assess for infection at beginning and throughout course of therapy (fever, appearance of wound, increased WBC).
- Observe patient for signs and symptoms of anaphylaxis (rash, pruritis, laryngeal edema, wheezing). Discontinue drug if these symptoms occur.
- Keep resuscitation equipment, adrenaline and antihistamines available.
- Notify physician if unusual bleeding or bruising occurs.

OVERDOSAGE: SIGNS & SYMPTOMS

Neuromuscular hyperexcitability, stupor, agitation, confusion, asterixis, hallucinations, coma, multifocal myoclonus, seizures, encephalopathy

Patient/Family Education

- Advise patient to complete full course of therapy even if symptoms abate to prevent reoccurrence of infection.

- Instruct patient to discard any liquid forms of medication after 7 days if stored at room temperature; after 14 days if refrigerated.
- Instruct patient to notify physician if symptoms of infection do not improve.
- Advise patient to report puritus and rash immediately.
- Instruct patient to report signs of superinfection: black, "furry" tongue, loose or foul-smelling stools, vaginal itching or discharge.

See Patient Guide, p. 462.

Oxaprozin

(ox-uh-PRO-zin)

DayPro

Class: Analgesic/NSAID

Action Decreases inflammation, pain and fever, probably through inhibition of cyclooxygenase activity and prostaglandin synthesis.

Indications Relief of symptoms of rheumatoid arthritis and osteoarthritis.

Contraindications Hypersensitivity to aspirin, iodides or any other NSAID.

Route/Dosage

ADULTS: **PO** 1200 mg once a day (maximum 1800 mg/day or 26 mg/kg, whichever is lower).

Interactions

Beta-blockers: Antihypertensive effects may be decreased. *Lithium:* May increase lithium levels. *Loop diuretics:* Diuretic effects may be decreased. *Methotrexate:* May increase methotrexate levels. *Warfarin:* May increase risk of gastric erosion and bleeding.

Lab Test Interferences

None well documented.

Adverse Reactions

CV: Edema; blood pressure changes; worsening or precipitation of CHF. *CNS:* Depression; sedation; somnolence; confusion; disturbed sleep. *EENT:* Visual disturbances; tinnitus. *GI:* Gastric distress; peptic ulcers; occult blood loss; diarrhea; constipation; vomiting; nausea; dyspepsia; flatuence; anorexia. *GU:* Difficult or painful urination; urinary frequency; decreased menstrual flow. *HEMA:* Anemia; neutropenia; thrombocytopenia; leukopenia. *HEPA:* Hepatitis. *DERM:* Rash; pruritus; erythema; photosensitivity; ecchymosis.

Precautions

Pregnancy: Category C. *Lactation:* Undetermined. *Children:* Safety and efficacy not established. *GI effects:* Serious GI toxicity (eg, bleeding, ulceration, perforation) can occur at any time, with or without warning symptoms. *Elderly:* Increased risk of adverse reactions. *Hepatic function impairment:* Exercise caution when administering to patients with impaired hepatic function or history of liver disease. *Platelet aggregation:* Can inhibit platelet aggregation; use with caution in patients with intrinsic coagulation defects or those on anticoagulant therapy. *Renal impairment:* May need to reduce dose.

NURSING CONSIDERATIONS

Administration/Storage

- Foods may reduce the rate of absorption but not the extent. Antacids have no effect on rate or extent of absorption.
- Not recommended for patients with renal or hepatic disease, low body weight, advanced age, a known ulcer susceptibility or known sensitivity to other NSAIDs.
- Store below 86°F in a tight, light-resistant container.

Assessment/Interventions

- Obtain patient history.
- Closely monitor patients at risk for peptic ulcer disease such as those with a history of serious GI problems, alcoholism, smoking or other ulcer-associated factors.
- Determine if patient is taking aspirin, oral anticoagulants, H_2-receptor antagonists, beta-blockers, iodides or other NSAIDs as drug interactions can occur and discontinuation or adjustment in therapy would be indicated.
- Assess for adverse reactions. Notify physician if adverse reactions are noted; the most common include abdominal pain, anorexia, dyspepsia, flatulence, nausea, vomiting, depression, sedation, somnolence, confusion, sleep disturbances, rash, tinnitus and dysuria or frequency of urination.
- Ensure dosage is individualized to the lowest effective dose to minimize adverse effects.
- Anticipate a greater risk of reactions from patients on higher dosages or elderly patients.
- Monitor renal function tests (creatinine, BUN).
- Monitor CBC, especially hemoglobin, hematocrit and platelets.
- If patient is taking beta-blockers, monitor blood pressure when starting therapy for increases in sitting and standing blood pressure.

OVERDOSAGE: SIGNS & SYMPTOMS

Drowsiness, nausea, heartburn, vomiting, indigestion, seizures

Patient/Family Education

- Instruct patient to take medication as prescribed and not to make up missed doses.
- Inform patient that analgesic effects are usually achieved after a single dose, but that it requires several days of dosing to reach the maximum effect.
- Inform patient concerning the expected therapeutic effects of the medication which include analgesic, antipyretic and anti-inflammatory benefits.
- Instruct patient to inform the healthcare provider of symptom relief so that the dosage is individualized to the lowest effective dose to minimize adverse effects.
- Instruct patient to take the dose exactly as prescribed about the same time each day with a full glass of water.
- Caution patient to avoid taking other NSAIDs, aspirin, alcohol or other over-the-counter medications unless advised to do so by the healthcare provider.
- Instruct patient concerning drug/drug interactions as applicable to their situation.
- Advise patient to discontinue drug and notify healthcare provider if any of the following occurs: persistent GI upset or headache, skin rash, itching, visual disturbances, black stools, weight gain or edema, changes in urine pattern, joint pain, fever or blood in urine.
- Caution patient regarding the serious gastrointestinal, renal, hepatic, hematologic and dermatologic adverse effects that can occur at any time, with or without warning symptoms.
- Advise patients on long-term therapy that lab tests may be required and to keep appointments.
- Caution patients to inform their dentist or surgeon prior to any procedure that they are taking oxaprozin.
- Advise elderly or debilitated patients regarding their increased risk of adverse reactions.
- Caution patient regarding possibility of photosensitivity and to use protective measures until tolerance is determined.
- Advise patient that medication may cause drowsiness and to use caution while driving or performing other tasks requiring mental alertness.

See Patient Guide, p. 463.

Oxazepam

(ox-AZE-uh-pam)
Serax
Class: Antianxiety/benzodiazepine

Action Potentiates action of GABA (gamma-aminobutyric acid), an inhibitory neurotransmitter, resulting in increased neuronal inhibition and CNS depression, especially in limbic system and reticular formation.

Indications Control of anxiety, anxiety associated with depression; control of anxiety, tension, agitation and irritability in elderly; treatment of alcoholics with acute tremulousness, inebriation or anxiety; treatment and prevention of alcohol withdrawal.

Contraindications Hypersensitivity to benzodiazepines; psychoses.

Route/Dosage

Mild to Moderate Anxiety

ADULTS: PO 10-15 mg tid-qid.

Severe Anxiety Syndromes, Anxiety Associated with Depression, Alcoholics

ADULTS: PO 15-30 mg tid-qid. ELDERLY: PO 10 mg tid; increase cautiously up to 15 mg tid-qid.

Interactions

Alcohol, CNS depressants: Additive CNS depressant effects. *Digoxin:* Increased serum digoxin concentrations. *Theophyllines:* May antagonize sedative effects.

Lab Test Interferences

None well documented.

Adverse Reactions

CV: Cardiovascular collapse; hypotension. *CNS:* Drowsiness; confusion; dizziness; lethargy; fatigue; apathy; memory impairment; disorientation; anterograde amnesia; restlessness; headache; slurred speech; aphonia; stupor; coma; euphoria; irritability; vivid dreams; psychomotor retardation; paradoxical reactions (eg, anger, hostility, mania, insomnia). *EENT:* Visual or auditory disturbances; depressed hearing. *GI:* Constipation; diarrhea; dry mouth; coated tongue; nausea; anorexia; vomiting. *HEMA:* Blood dyscrasias including agranulocytosis; anemia; thrombocytopenia; leukopenia; neutropenia; decreased Hct. *HEPA:* Hepatic dysfunction including hepatitis and jaundice; elevated LDH, ALT, AST and alkaline phosphatase. *DERM:* Rash. *OTHER:* Dependence/withdrawal syndrome (eg, confusion, abnormal perception of movement, depersonalization, muscle twitching, psychosis, paranoid delusions, seizures).

Precautions

Pregnancy: Category D. *Lactation:* Excreted in breast milk. *Children:* Dosage and efficacy not established. *Elderly/debilitated patients:* Initial dose should be small; increase gradually. *Dependence:* Prolonged use may lead to dependence. Withdrawal syndrome has occurred within 4-6 wk of treatment with therapeutic doses, especially if abruptly discontinued. Use caution and taper dosage. *Long-term use (> 4 mo):* Effectiveness has not been assessed. *Psychiatric disorders:* Not intended for use in patients with primary depressive disorder, psychosis or disorders in which anxiety is not prominent. *Suicide:* Use drug with caution in patients with suicidal tendencies; do not allow access to large quantities of drug.

NURSING CONSIDERATIONS

Administration/Storage

- Administer with food if GI irritation occurs.
- Store at room temperature in tight container.

Assessment/Interventions

- Obtain patient history, including drug history and any known allergies.
- Assess BP while patient is lying down and standing. If systolic BP falls 20 mm Hg, withhold dose and notify physician.
- Assess patient's level of anxiety and level of sedation before administration and periodically throughout therapy.
- Take safety precautions (keep siderails up; assist with ambulation) to prevent falls caused by sedation.
- If drug is being given for alcohol withdrawal, assess tremulousness, anxiety level. Take seizure precautions.
- If serum bilirubin, ALT and AST levels rise, notify physician.
- If signs of drug dependence develop, notify physician. Do not discontinue therapy abruptly. Oxazepam is more commonly habit forming. Observe for excessive use and drug-seeking behavior.

OVERDOSAGE: SIGNS & SYMPTOMS

Slurred speech, sedation, respiratory depression, ataxia, hypotension

Patient/Family Education

- Emphasize importance of not exceeding recommended dosage. If symptoms do not improve within 2-3 days of beginning therapy or if tolerance develops, notify physician.
- If patient has been taking drug for weeks to months, tell patient not to stop taking drug abruptly to avoid withdrawal symptoms.
- Caution patient to avoid sudden position changes to prevent orthostatic hypotension.
- Instruct patient not to take otc medications without consulting physician.
- Instruct patient to use safety precautions if dizziness or sedation occurs.
- Advise patient to avoid intake of alcoholic beverages or other CNS depressants without consulting physician.
- Instruct patient to notify physician if dizziness or excessive drowsiness occurs.
- Advise patient that drug may cause drowsiness and to avoid driving or performing other tasks requiring mental alertness after taking drug.

See Patient Guide, p. 464.

Oxybutynin Chloride

(OX-ee-BYOO-tih-nin KLOR-ide)

Ditropan

Class: Urinary tract product/antispasmodic

Action Increases bladder capacity, diminishes frequency of uninhibited contractions of detrusor muscle and delays initial desire to void.

Indications Treatment of symptoms of bladder instability associated with voiding in patients with uninhibited and reflex neurogenic bladder (eg, urinary leakage, dysuria).

Contraindications Untreated angle-closure glaucoma; untreated narrow anterior chamber angles; GI obstruction; paralytic ileus; intestinal atony of elderly or debilitated patients; toxic megacolon complicating ulcerative colitis; severe colitis; obstructive uropathy; myasthenia gravis; unstable cardiovascular status in acute hemorrhage.

Route/Dosage

ADULTS: PO 5 mg bid-tid (maximum: 5 mg qid). CHILDREN > 5 YR: PO 5 mg bid (maximum: 5 mg tid).

Interactions

Haloperidol: Worsening of schizophrenic symptoms; tardive dyskinesia; decreased serum haloperidol concentrations, reducing therapeutic effect. *Phenothiazines:* Decreased therapeutic effects of phenothiazines; increased incidence of anticholinergic side effects.

Lab Test Interferences
None well documented.

Adverse Reactions
CV: Tachycardia; palpitations; vasodilatation. *CNS:* Drowsiness; dizziness; hallucinations; insomnia; restlessness. *EENT:* Decreased lacrimation; mydriasis; amblyopia; cycloplegia. *GI:* Nausea; vomiting; constipation; decreased GI motility; dry mouth. *GU:* Urinary hesitancy and retention; impotence. *DERM:* Rash. *OTHER:* Decreased sweating; asthenia; suppression of lactation.

Precautions
Pregnancy: Category B. *Lactation:* Undetermined. *Children:* Safety and efficacy in children < 5 yr not established. *Anticholinergic effects:* Use cautiously with phenothiazines or other drugs with anticholinergic properties because side effects will be additive. *Diarrhea:* May be early symptom of intestinal obstruction in which oxybutinin is contraindicated. *Heat prostration:* May occur when exposed to high environmental temperature.

NURSING CONSIDERATIONS

Administration/Storage
- If patient experiences nausea, administer with food.
- Store in tightly closed container at room temperature.

Assessment/Interventions
- Obtain patient history, including drug history and any known allergies.
- Assess patient for urinary retention before administrating drug and periodically during treatment. If symptoms of urinary retention (suprapubic pain in conjunction with urgency and frequency with voiding of small amounts) occur, notify physician.
- If signs of heat stroke develop (elevation in body temperature, dehydration, mental changes), move patient to a cooler area; cover torso with wet towels; use fans or air conditioners. Give extra fluids.
- If patient has difficulty voiding, use bladder massage.
- If passing urinary catheter becomes difficult, use extra lubricant and inflexible catheter, allow time for spasms to diminish.
- If diarrhea occurs, discontinue use and notify physician.

OVERDOSAGE: SIGNS & SYMPTOMS
CNS excitation, flushing, fever, tachycardia, nausea, respiratory depression, coma

Patient/Family Education
- Instruct patient to take sips of water frequently, suck on ice chips or sugarless hard candy or chew sugarless gum if dry mouth occurs.
- Teach patient to use bladder massage to empty bladder.
- Advise patient to use caution in hot weather to reduce risk of heat stroke.
- Advise patient that drug may cause drowsiness or dizziness and to use caution while driving or performing other tasks requiring mental alertness.

See Patient Guide, p. 465.

Oxycodone HCl

(OX-ee-KOE-dohn HIGH-droe-KLOR-ide)

OxyContin, Roxicodone, Roxicodone Intensol, ♣ *Supeudol*

Class: Narcotic analgesic

Action Relieves pain by stimulating opiate receptors in CNS; as side effects, may cause respiratory depression, peripheral vasodilation, inhibition of intestinal peristalsis, sphincter of Oddi spasm, stimulation of chemoreceptors that cause vomiting and increased bladder tone.

Indications Relief of moderate to moderately severe pain.

Contraindications Hypersensitivity to opiates; upper airway obstruction; acute asthma; diarrhea due to poisoning or toxins.

Route/Dosage
ADULTS: PO 5 mg q 6 hr prn. CHILDREN > 12 YR: PO 1.25 mg q 6 hr prn. CHILDREN 6-12 YR: PO 0.62 mg q 6 hr prn.

Interactions
CNS depressants (eg, alcohol, barbiturate anesthetics, phenothiazines, sedatives, tricyclic antidepressants, other narcotics): Additive CNS depression.

Lab Test Interferences
Increased amylase and lipase may occur up to 24 hr after administration.

Adverse Reactions
CV: Hypotension; orthostatic hypotension; bradycardia; tachycardia. *RESP*: Respiratory depression; laryngospasm; depression of cough reflex. *CNS*: Lightheadedness; dizziness; sedation; disorientation; incoordination. *GI*: Nausea; vomiting; constipation; abdominal pain. *GU*: Urinary retention or hesitancy. *DERM*: Sweating; pruritus; urticaria. *OTHER*: Tolerance; psychologic and physical dependence with chronic use.

Precautions
Pregnancy: Category C. *Lactation*: Excreted in breast milk. *Children*: Not recommended for children. *Special risk patients*: Use with caution in elderly and debilitated patients and patients with myxedema, acute alcoholism, acute abdominal conditions, ulcerative colitis, decreased respiratory reserve, head injury or increased intracranial pressure, hypoxia, supraventricular tachycardia, depleted blood volume or circulatory shock. *Drug dependence*: Has abuse potential. *Hepatic or renal impairment*: Dosage reduction may be necessary.

NURSING CONSIDERATIONS

Administration/Storage
- Administer with food or milk to minimize GI irritation.
- Store at room temperature in tightly closed container and protect from light.

Assessment/Interventions
- Obtain patient history, including drug history and any known allergies.
- Assess type, location and intensity of pain before administration and frequently during treatment.
- Assess vital signs before administration and periodically during treatment.
- Assess for signs of narcotic dependence.
- Assess bowel function routinely. If constipation develops, provide additional fluids, high-fiber foods or stool softeners. Administer laxative if indicated.
- If respiratory depression develops, notify physician immediately and prepare emergency equipment.
- If sedation or confusion develops, take safety precautions (keep side rails up; assist with ambulation).
- Evaluate patient's continuing need for therapy since psychological and physical dependence and tolerance may develop.

OVERDOSAGE: SIGNS & SYMPTOMS

Miosis, respiratory depression, CNS depression (somnolence progressing to stupor or coma), circulatory collapse, seizures, cardiopulmonary arrest, death

Patient/Family Education
- Instruct patient to take medi-

cation before pain becomes severe for greatest effectiveness.

- Teach patient methods to prevent constipation.
- Instruct patient to make position changes slowly if lightheadedness or sedation occur.
- Advise patient to avoid intake of alcoholic beverages or products containing alcohol while using this medication.
- Advise patient that drug may cause drowsiness and to use caution while driving or performing other tasks requiring mental alertness.
- Instruct patient not to take any otc medications without consulting physician.
- Explain that physical dependency may occur and that withdrawal symptoms may be noted on discontinuation after long-term therapy.

See Patient Guide, p. 466.

Oxycodone/ Acetaminophen

(OX-ee-KOE-dohn/ass-cet-ah-MEE-noe-fen)

Percocet, Roxicet Tablets, Roxicet Oral Solution, Roxicet 5/500, Roxilox, Tylox

Class: Narcotic analgesic combination

Action Acetaminophen inhibits its synthesis of prostaglandins and peripherally blocks pain impulse generation, whereas, oxycodone binds to opiate receptors in CNS. Combination has synergistic effect on alleviating pain.

Indications Relief of moderate to moderately severe pain.

Contraindications Hypersensitivity to acetaminophen, oxycodone or similar compounds.

Route/Dosage
ADULTS: **PO** 5 mg (1 tablet, caplet, or teaspoonful) q 6 hr prn.

Interactions
Anesthetics: Additive CNS depression. *Carbamazepine, hydantoins, sulfinpyrazone:* Increased risk of hepatotoxicity. *CNS depressants (eg, barbiturates, tricyclic antidepressants, phenothiazines, sedatives, hypnotics, alcohol, other narcotics):* Additive CNS depression.

Lab Test Interferences
With Chemstrip bG, Dextrostix and Visidex II home blood glucose systems, may cause false decrease in mean glucose values.

Adverse Reactions
CV: Hypotension; bradycardia; tachycardia. *RESP:* Dyspnea; respiratory depression. *CNS:* Lightheadedness; dizziness; weakness; fatigue; sedation; euphoria; dysphoria; nervousness; headache; confusion. *GI:* Nausea; vomiting; constipation; abdominal pain; anorexia; biliary spasm; dry mouth. *GU:* Urinary retention or hesitancy. *DERM:* Pruritus; rash. *OTHER:* Malaise; tolerance; psychological and physical dependence with chronic use.

Precautions
Pregnancy: Category C. *Lactation:* Undetermined. *Children:* Safety and efficacy not established. *Special risk patients:* Use with caution in elderly, debilitated patients and those with hepatic or kidney failure or conditions accompanied by hypoxia or hypercapnia; monitor carefully to avoid decrease in pulmonary ventilation. Also use cautiously in patients sensitive to CNS depressants, postoperatively and in patients with pulmonary disease. *Acute abdominal conditions:* Diagnosis may be obscured; use with caution. *Dependence:* Can produce drug dependence; has abuse potential. *Head injury:* Respiratory depression and elevation of CSF pressure may be exacerbated. *Hepatic impairment:* Chronic alcoholics should limit acetaminophen intake to < 2 g/day. *Sulfite sensitivity:* Use with caution in patients known to be sensitive, as some products contain bisulfites.

NURSING CONSIDERATIONS

Administration/Storage

- Administer with food or milk to minimize GI irritation.
- Store at room temperature in tightly closed container.

Assessment/Interventions

- Obtain patient history, including drug history and any known allergies.
- Assess type, location and intensity of pain before administration and frequently during treatment.
- Assess vital signs before administration and periodically during treatment.
- Assess for signs of narcotic dependence.
- Assess bowel function routinely. If constipation develops, provide additional fluids, high-fiber foods or stool softeners.
- If respiratory depression develops, notify physician immediately and prepare emergency equipment.
- If sedation or confusion develops, take safety precautions (keep side rails up; assist with ambulation).
- Evaluate patient's continuing need for therapy since psychological and physical dependence and tolerance may develop.

OVERDOSAGE: SIGNS & SYMPTOMS

Miosis, respiratory depression, CNS depression (somnolence progressing to stupor or coma), hepatic damage, circulatory collapse, cardiopulmonary arrest, death

Patient/Family Education

- Instruct patient to take medication before pain becomes severe for greatest effectiveness.
- Teach patient methods to prevent constipation.
- Instruct patient to make position changes slowly if lightheadedness or sedation occurs.
- Advise patient to avoid intake of alcoholic beverages or products containing alcohol while using this medication.
- Advise patient that drug may cause drowsiness and to use caution while driving or performing other tasks requiring mental alertness.
- Caution patient that physical dependency and withdrawal symptoms may occur following discontinuation of long-term therapy.
- Instruct patient not to take any otc medications without consulting physician.

See Patient Guide, p. 467.

Oxytocin

(ox-ih-TOE-sin)

Pitocin, Syntocinon, ♣ *Toesen*

Class: Oxytocic hormone

Action Endogenous hormone with uterine stimulant properties and vasopressive and antidiuretic effects.

Indications Initiation or improvement of uterine contractions to achieve early vaginal delivery for maternal or fetal reasons (IV); management of inevitable or incomplete abortion (IV); stimulation of uterine contractions during third stage of labor (IV); stimulation reinforcement of labor, as in selected cases of uterine inertia (IV). Control of postpartum bleeding or hemorrhage (IV, IM); initiation of milk let-down (nasal). **Unlabeled uses:** Antepartum fetal heart rate testing; relief of breast engorgement.

Contraindications Significant cephalopelvic disproportion; inadequate, undeliverable fetal position; obstetric emergencies in which surgical intervention is preferred; cases of fetal distress in which delivery is not imminent; prolonged use in uterine inertia or severe toxemia; hypertonic or hyperactive uterine patterns; when adequate uterine activity fails to achieve satisfactory response; induction or augmentation of labor when vaginal delivery is not indicated (eg, prolapse); pregnancy (nasal product only).

Route/Dosage

Induction or Stimulation of Labor

ADULTS: **IV** 1-2 mU/min; adjust by no more than 1-2 mU/min at 15-30 min intervals until contraction pattern similar to normal labor is obtained.

Control of Postpartum Uterine Bleeding

IV infusion 10-40 U in 1000 mL diluent to run as infusion at rate necessary to control uterine atony. **IM** 10 U (1 ml) after delivery of placenta.

Treatment of Incomplete or Inevitable Abortion

IV infusion 10-20 mU/min.

Initial Milk Let-Down

Nasal 1 spray into one or both nostrils 2-3 min before nursing or pumping of breasts.

Interactions

Cyclopropane anesthesia: May cause maternal hypotension, bradycardia and abnormal atrioventricular rhythms. *Parenteral sympathomimetics (eg, methoxamine, dopamine):* Increased pressor effect, possibly resulting in postpartum hypertension. INCOMPATIBILITIES: Sodium bicarbonate. Oxytocin is rapidly decomposed in the presence of sodium bisulfite.

Lab Test Interferences

None well documented.

Adverse Reactions

CV: Cardiac arrhythmias; fetal reactions include bradycardia, premature ventricular contractions, death, jaundice, low Apgar scores, retinal hemorrhage and other arrythmias. *RESP:* Hypoxia. *CNS:* Neurologic damage; convulsions. *GI:* Nausea; vomiting. *GU:* Postpartum hemorrhage; cervical/vaginal lacerations; uterine hypertoxicity; uterine rupture; tetanic contractions; decreased uterine blood flow; pelvic hematoma. *OTHER:* Maternal reactions include anaphylaxis; death; increased blood loss.

Precautions

Pregnancy: No indication for use in first trimester unless related to spontaneous or induced abortion. *Lactation:* Excreted in breast milk. If used post partum to control bleeding, patient should not nurse for 24 hr after last dose. *Children:* Contraindicated in children. *Special risk patients:* Not recommended in prematurity, borderline cephalopelvic disproportion, previous major surgery on cervix or uterus (including cesarean section), uterine overdistention, grand multiparity, history of uterine sepsis, traumatic delivery, fetal distress, partial placenta previa or invasive cervical carcinoma, except in unusual circumstances. *Mortality:* Hypertensive episodes, subarachnoid hemorrhage and rupture of uterus have resulted in maternal deaths. Fetal deaths and infant brain damage have been reported with IV use during first and second stages of labor. *Overstimulation of uterus:* Can occur and can be hazardous to mother and fetus. *Water intoxication:* Consider possibility when patient is receiving oxytocin by IV infusion and fluids by mouth.

NURSING CONSIDERATIONS

Administration/Storage

- Add 1 ml (10 U) to 500-1000 ml normal saline or 5% Dextrose in Water to prepare infusion solution. Final concentration will be 20 mU/ml and 10 mU/ml, respectively.
- Always use infusion pump to control IV oxytocin administration.
- When administering by IV infusion, rotate solution gently to distribute drug throughout solution.
- When administering drug by nasal

spray, ensure that patient is seated (patient should not lie down); hold squeeze bottle upright (do not tilt hand); spray into one or both nostrils 2-3 min before nursing or pumping breasts.

Assessment/Interventions

- Obtain patient history, including drug history and any allergies. Note hypersensitivity to drug, epilepsy, nephritis, placenta previa, umbilical cord prolapse or other potential contraindications.
- Have emergency resuscitation equipment readily available.
- Assess cardiovascular function before administration and frequently during IV therapy.
- Assess fetal maturity, presentation and pelvic adequacy before administration.
- Monitor vital signs, I&O and strength, duration and frequency of contractions throughout infusion.
- If contractions occur < 2 min apart, last 60-90 sec or longer, or if significant change in fetal heart rate develops, stop infusion and turn patient on left side. Notify physician.
- If maternal heartbeat becomes irregular, BP rises, skin color changes or if patient develops chest discomfort, notify physician at once.
- Monitor patient for signs of water intoxication. If signs of water intoxication occur (drowsiness, listlessness, confusion, headache, anuria), notify physician.
- Check fundus frequently during first few hours postpartum.
- Inspect nasal passages frequently when given nasally and look for irritation, ulcerations and rhinorrhea.

OVERDOSAGE: SIGNS & SYMPTOMS

Uterine hyperactivity (hyperstimulation with hypertonic or tetonic contractions) uterine rupture, cervical and vaginal lacerations, postpartum hemorrhage, fetal complications, water intoxication with seizures

Patient/Family Education

- Teach patient how to administer nasal spray (clear nasal passages first; sit; do not lie down or tilt head back; hold bottle upright into vertical nares).
- Explain purpose of IV oxytocin to patient and family.
- Tell patient that early contractions will feel like strong menstrual cramps.

See Patient Guide, p. 468.

Paclitaxel

(pak-lih-TAX-uhl)

Taxol

Class: Antineoplastic

Action Exhibits antitumor activity by stabilizing microtubule network of cells, inhibiting normal cell division.

Indications Management of metastatic ovarian carcinoma and of metastatic breast cancer. **Unlabeled uses:** Treatment of advanced head and neck cancer, untreated small-cell lung cancer, adenocarcinoma of upper GI tract, hormone-refractory prostate cancer, advanced non-small cell lung cancer and leukemias.

Contraindications Hypersensitivity to paclitaxel or other drugs formulated in Cremophor EL (polyoxyethylated castor oil); patients with baseline neutropenia of < 1500 cells/mm^3.

Route/Dosage

Ovarian Cancer

ADULTS: IV 135 mg/m^2 through microporous 0.22-micron filter over 24 hr q 3 wk.

Breast Cancer

ADULTS: IV 175 mg/m^2 through microporous 0.22-micron filter over 3 hr q 3 wk.

Interactions

Cisplatin: Increased risk of myelosuppression of paclitaxel given after cisplatin. *Ketoconazole:* Inhibition of paclitaxel elimination.

Lab Test Interferences

None well documented.

Adverse Reactions

CV: Bradycardia or hypotension; abnormal ECG; atrioventricular block requiring treatment or pacemaker. *CNS:* Peripheral neuropathy. *GI:* Nausea; vomiting; diarrhea; mucositis. *HEMA:* Neutropenia; leukopenia; thrombocytopenia; anemia; bleeding; infections; need for transfusions of packed cells and platelets. *HEPA:* Elevations in serum bilirubin; alkaline phosphatase, AST. *DERM:* Alopecia. *OTHER:* Hypersensitivity reaction (shortness of breath; hypotension; urticaria; angioedema); myalgia; arthralgia.

Precautions

Pregnancy: Category D. *Lactation:* Undetermined. Avoid nursing. *Children:* Safety and efficacy have not been established. *Bone marrow suppression:* Major dose-limiting toxicity. *Cardiac effects:* Severe conduction abnormalities have occurred rarely. *Hepatic impairment:* Use drug with caution. *Peripheral neuropathy:* If condition is severe, patient will require 20% reduction in dose.

NURSING CONSIDERATIONS

Administration/Storage

- Administer only intravenously through polyethylene-lined administration set containing 0.22-micron microporous filter.
- Dilute concentrate just before infusion with 0.9% Sodium Chloride for Injection, 5% Dextrose in Water, 5% Dextrose and 0.9% Sodium Chloride for Injection, 5% Dextrose in Ringer's Injection to achieve final concentration of 0.3-1.2 mg/ml.
- Exercise caution in handling drug. Use gloves during preparation and administration of drug.
- If paclitaxel comes into contact with skin, wash immediately with soap and water. If paclitaxel comes into contact with mucous membranes, thoroughly flush membranes with water.
- Administer paclitaxel carefully via IV infusion to prevent extravasation. Avoid areas of previous irradiation and extremities with poor circulation.
- If extravasation occurs, discontinue infusion and contact physician regarding treatment.
- Prepared solution is stable at room temperature for 24 hr. Store in non-PVC bottles or plastic bags.
- Store unopened vials in refrigerator. Retain in original package to protect from light.
- Patient should be pretreated with corticosteroids, diphenhydramine and/or H_2 antagonists to reduce risk of severe allergic reaction.

Assessment/Interventions

- Obtain patient history, including drug history and any known allergies.
- Monitor vital signs frequently during first 3 hr of infusion.
- Assess lab values before and during therapy (leukocytes, thrombocytes, hemoglobin, bleeding studies, bilirubin, alkaline phosphatase, AST, neutrophils).
- Assess for infection (elevated WBC, fever, redness, drainage) before and during therapy.
- If anemia develops, packed cells should be administered as ordered.
- If thrombocytopenia develops, platelets should be administered as ordered.
- If cardiac conduction abnormalities develop during treatment, notify physician immediately. During subsequent infusions, monitor cardiac status continuously.

OVERDOSAGE: SIGNS & SYMPTOMS
Bone marrow suppression, peripheral neurotoxicity, mucositis

Patient/Family Education

- Instruct patient to notify physician of any signs of infection (sore throat, fever, rash or chills).
- Caution patient to avoid crowds and persons with known infections.
- Inform patient of possibility of hair loss.
- Instruct patient to notify physician if muscle and joint pain occurs.
- Advise patient to notify physician if symptoms of infection or excessive bruising or bleeding occur.
- Instruct patient to notify physician if paresthesia of extremities occurs. Explain that diarrhea and nausea also may be noted.

See Patient Guide, p. 469.

Pamidronate Disodium

(pam-IH-DROE-nate die-SO-dee-uhm)

Aredia

Class: Hormone/biphosphonate

Action Inhibits normal and abnormal bone resorption.

Indications Treatment of moderate to severe hypercalcemia associated with malignancy with or without bone metastases; treatment of Paget's disease of bone; treatment of osteolytic bone lesions of multiple myelma in conjunction with standard antimyeloma chemotherapy. **Unlabeled uses:** Treatment of postmenopausal osteoporosis; control of bone metastases from breast cancer; treatment of hyperparathyroidism; prevention of glucocorticoid-induced osteoporosis; management of immobilization-related hypercalcemia.

Contraindications Hypersensitivity to biphosphonates.

Route/Dosage

Moderate to Severe Hypercalcemia of Malignancy

ADULTS: **IV** 60 mg as an initial single-dose infusion over at least 4 hrs. For more severe condition, 90 mg as an initial single-dose infusion over 24 hours. Retreatment: Same as initial therapy, on or after 7 days.

Paget's Disease

ADULTS: **IV** 30 mg/day as a 4 hour infusion on 3 consecutive days for a total dose of 90 mg. Retreatment: Same as initial therapy, when clinically indicated.

Osteolytic Bone Lesions

ADULTS: **IV** 90 mg as a 4 hour infusion on a monthy basis.

Interactions None well documented. INCOMPATIBILITIES: Calcium-containing infusion solutions (eg, Ringer's solution). Do not mix.

Lab Test Interferences None well documented.

Adverse Reactions *CV:* Hypertension; atrial fibrillation; syncope; tachycardia. *CNS:* Fatigue; headache; insomnia; psychosis; drowsiness. *EENT:* Uveitis; iritis. *GI:* Abdominal pain; anorexia; constipation; diarrhea; GI hemorrhage; stomatitis; dyspepsia; nausea; vomiting. *GU:* Urinary tract infection; uremia. *HEMA:* Anemia; leukopenia; neutropenia; thrombocytopenia. *META:* Hypophosphatemia; hypomagnesemia; hypothyroidism; hypokalemia; hypocalcemia. *RESP:* Upper respiratory infection; rales/rhinitis. *OTHER:* Infusion site reaction (eg, redness, swelling or induration, pain on palpation); transient mild elevation of temperature 24-48 hr after administration; bone pain; fluid overload; generalized pain; back pain; arthrosis; myalgias; arthralgias; moniliasis; edema.

Precautions

Pregnancy: Category C. *Lactation:* Undetermined. *Children:* Safety and efficacy not established. *Hypocalcemia:* Has occurred. *Renal effects:* Pamidronate has not been tested in patients who have Class Dc renal impairment (creatinine > 5 mg/dl); use with caution. *GI disorders:* Use with caution in patients with active upper GI problems such as dysphagia (difficulty swallowing), symptomatic esophageal diseases, gastritis, duodenitis or ulcers.

NURSING CONSIDERATIONS

Administration/Storage

- Reconstitute powder in vial with 10 ml Sterile Water for Injection. Reconstituted pamidronate is stable for up to 24 hr when stored under refrigeration.
- Hypercalcemia of malignancy: Dilute reconstituted sulution in 1000 ml saline solution or D5W. Solution is stable up to 24 hr if refrigerated. Paget's disease or osteolytic bone lesions of multiple myeloma: Dilute recommended dose in 500 ml of 0.45% or 0.9% saline solution or D5W.
- Hydrate patient adequately during treatment but do not overhydrate, especially patients who have cardiac failure.
- Minimum of 7 days between treatments is recommended.

Assessment/Interventions

- Monitor electrolytes, creatinine, CBC and differentials.
- Carefully monitor patients with preexisting anemia, leukopenia or thrombocytopenia in the first 2 weeks after treatment.
- Obtain patient history, including drug history and any known allergies.
- Monitor hemoglobin, potassium, magnesium and phosphate levels before and during treatment.
- Monitor temperature before and during treatment.
- In patients with hypercalcemia, perform periodic evaluations of renal function.
- If infusion site reaction develops (redness, swelling in duration, pain on palpation), discontinue infusion, elevate site and apply ice pack for 15-20 min q 4-6 hr for 72 hr.
- If fluid overload develops, give diuretics as ordered.

OVERDOSAGE: SIGNS & SYMPTOMS

High fever, hypotension, transient taste perversion

Patient/Family Education

- Instruct patient that if nausea and vomiting develop to adjust diet, restrict activity and take antiemetics.
- Explain that fever is common side effect of this medication but is usually self-limiting. Fatigue or drowsiness are also common.
- Instruct patient to report these symptoms to physician: tingling, numbness, stomach pain, fever, irritation or pain at the injection site, fatigue, swelling, nausea, loss of appetite, constipation, diarrhea, upset stomach, vomiting, sleeplessness, inflammation of the mouth, difficulty breathing, muscle pain, drowsiness, difficult urination.

See Patient Guide, p. 470.

Pancrelipase

(pan-KREE-lih-pace)

Cotazym, Cotazym-S, Creon, Dizymes, Donnazyme, Entozyme, Hi-Vegi-Lip, Ilozyme, Ku-Zyme HP, Pancrease, Pancrease MT 4, Pancrease MT 10, Pancrease MT 16, 4X Pancreatin 600 mg, 8X Pancreatin 900 mg, Protilase, Ultrase MT12, Ultrase MT20, Ultrase MT24, Viokase, Zymase

Class: Digestive enzyme

Action Helps to digest and absorb fats, proteins and carbohydrates from food.

Indications Enzyme replacement therapy in patients who do not produce enough pancreatic enzymes because of cystic fibrosis, chronic pancreatitis, postpancreatectomy, ductal obstructions caused by cancer of pancreas or common bile duct, pancreatic insufficiency; treatment of steatorrhea of malabsorption syndrome; postgastrectomy or after GI surgery; pancreatic function testing.

Contraindications Hypersensitivity to pork protein or enzymes; acute pancreatitis; acute exacerbations of chronic pancreatic disease.

Route/Dosage

Moderate Pancreatic Enzyme Deficiency

ADULTS: **PO** 4000-48,000 U lipase/meal or snack. CHILDREN 7-12 YR: **PO** 4000-12,000 U lipase/meal or snack. CHILDREN 1-6 YR: **PO** 4000-8000 U lipase/meal; 4000 U lipase/snack. CHILDREN 6 MO-1 YR: **PO** 2000 U lipase/meal.

Severe Pancreatic Enzyme Deficiency

ADULTS: **PO** 64,000-88,000 U lipase/meal or more frequently if nausea, cramps or diarrhea do not occur.

Interactions

Antacids: Calcium carbonate or magnesium hydroxide may negate beneficial effect of enzymes. *Iron:* Serum iron response to oral iron may be decreased with concomitant pancreatic enzyme administration.

Lab Test Interferences

None well documented.

Adverse Reactions

GI: Nausea; cramps; diarrhea. *DERM:* Perianal irritation. *OTHER:* Hypersensitivity reaction.

Precautions

Pregnancy: Category C. *Lactation:* Undetermined. *Asthma:* Inhalation of airborne pancrelipase powder can precipitate asthma attack. *Skin irritation:* Contact of pancrelipase with skin can cause irritation.

NURSING CONSIDERATIONS

Administration/Storage

- Do not crush or allow patient to chew enteric-coated formulations.
- Give with or before meals.
- If powder spills on hands, wash with soap and water immediately.
- If patient has difficulty swallowing capsule, open capsule and shake onto small quantity of soft, non-hot food (eg, applesauce, gelatin) that does not require chewing. Have patient swallow immediately without chewing to avoid irritating GI mucosa. Follow with glass of juice or water.
- Be careful not to inhale powder, which can irritate mucosal surfaces and cause asthma attack.
- Store at room temperature in tightly closed container. Protect from moisture.

Assessment/Interventions

- Obtain patient history, including drug history and any known allergies.
- Assess bowel status before and during treatment.
- Maintain growth chart on children.
- Assess for steatorrhea.
- If symptoms of sensitivity occur, discontinue drug and initiate symptomatic and supportive therapy.
- If nausea, abdominal cramps or diarrhea develop, notify physician.

OVERDOSAGE: SIGNS & SYMPTOMS

Nausea, vomiting, abdominal cramps, diarrhea, hyperuricosuria, hyperuricemia

Patient/Family Education

- Tell patient not to change

brands without notifying physician. Products are not bioequivalent.

- Advise patient not to take pancrelipase with antacid containing calcium carbonate or magnesium hydroxide.
- Stress to patient the importance of taking drug before or with meals to enhance effectiveness of drug.
- Instruct patient to avoid inhaling powder to reduce chance of irritating mucous membranes or precipitating asthma attack.
- Advise patient to follow any special dietary recommendations from physician or dietician.

See Patient Guide, p. 471.

Pancuronium Bromide

(PAN-cue-ROW-nee-uhm BROE-mide)

Pavulon

Class: Nondepolarizing neuromuscular blocker

Action Binds competitively to cholinergic receptors on motor end-plate to antagonize action of acetylcholine, resulting in block of neuromuscular transmission.

Indications Adjunct to general anesthesia for induction of skeletal muscle relaxation; facilitation of management of patients undergoing mechanical ventilation; facilitation of tracheal intubation.

Contraindications Hypersensitivity to bromides.

Route/Dosage

Surgical Procedures

ADULTS & CHILDREN > 1 MO: **IV** 0.04-0.1 mg/kg initially. Maintenance: Use incremental doses q 25-60 min beginning with 0.01 mg/kg. NEONATES (< 1 MO): Test dose: **IV** 0.02 mg/kg.

Endotracheal Intubation

ADULTS & CHILDREN: **IV** 0.06-0.1 mg/kg. NEONATES: Test dose: **IV** 0.02 mg/kg.

Interactions *Aminoglycosides, bacitracin, clindamycin, colymycin, polymyxin B, inhalational anesthetics, ketamine, lincomycin, magnesium salts, quinidine, quinine, succinylcholine, vancomycin:* May augment action of pancuronium. *Azathioprine, mercaptopurine:* May cause reversal of neuromuscular blocking effects of pancuronium. *Carbamazepine, hydantoins:* May decrease duration and effect of pancuronium. *Theophyllines:* May cause possible resistance to, or reversal of, effects of pancuronium; cardiac arrhythmias may occur. *Trimethaphan:* May cause prolonged apnea.

Lab Test Interferences None well documented.

Adverse Reactions

CV: Tachycardia; elevated BP. *RESP:* Respiratory insufficiency; apnea. *GI:* Salivation. *DERM:* Transient rash. *OTHER:* Skeletal muscle weakness to complete relaxation; hypersensitivity reactions (bronchospasm, flushing, redness, hypotension, tachycardia).

Precautions

Pregnancy: Category C; do not use in early pregnancy. *Labor:* Reduce dosage in cesarean section if patient is receiving magnesium sulfate. *Children:* Prolonged use in neonates undergoing mechanical ventilation has been associated with severe skeletal muscle weakness and methemoglobinemia. *Altered circulation time (elderly patients, patients with CV disease or edema):* Delay in onset of action. *Electrolyte imbalance:* Neuromuscular blockade may be altered depending on nature of imbalance. *Hepatic or biliary tract disease:* Results in slower onset and prolonged duration. *Myasthenia gravis:* Small doses may have profound effects. *Obesity/neuromuscular disease:* Require special attention to airway maintenance and ventilatory support. *Pain/anxiety:* Pancuronium does not have analgesic or antianxiety effects. Paralyzed patient will still need analgesic or sedative agents if indicated. *Renal disease:* Renally excreted; may require lower doses or less frequent maintenance doses.

NURSING CONSIDERATIONS

Administration/Storage

- May be diluted in 0.9% sodium chloride, D5W, 5% dextrose and sodium chloride and lactated Ringer's solution.
- Have entratracheal equipment, oxygen, suction equipment and mechanical ventilator available for respiratory support.
- Diluted solution is stable for 48 hr at room temperature.
- Store undiluted product in refrigerator (potency maintained for 2 yr) or at room temperature (potency maintained for 6 mo).

Assessment/Interventions

- Obtain patient history, including drug history and any known allergies.
- If patient has myasthenia gravis, small test dose must be administered and patient's response to administration of muscle relaxant must be monitored.
- Provide total care for immobilized patient.
- Turn patient and perform chest physiotherapy q 2 hr.
- Assess I&O.
- Check mechanical ventilator settings often.
- Monitor respiratory status closely and notify physician if changes occur. Ausculate breath sounds to detect wheezes or crackles.
- Monitor vital signs frequently during therapy to detect cardiovascular reactions.
- If respiratory status changes, notify physician.
- If respiratory secretions develop, perform suction.
- If electrolytes and blood gases deteriorate, notify physician immediately.

OVERDOSAGE: SIGNS & SYMPTOMS

Skeletal muscle relaxation, decreased respiratory reserve, low tidal volume, apnea, prolonged neuromuscular blockade

Patient/Family Education

- Reassure patient and family that breathing will return to normal after pancuronium is discontinued.
- Maintain calm environment, provide reassurance regularly and explain all procedures to patient and family.

No patient monograph available.

Papaverine HCl

(pap-PAV-uhr-een HIGH-droe-KLOR-ide)

Pavabid, Pavagen, Pavased, Pavatine, Pavatym

Class: Peripheral vasodilator

Action Directly relaxes tone of all smooth muscle, especially when spasmodically contracted. Causes vasodilatation of blood vessels of the coronary, cerebral, pulmonary and peripheral arteries; relaxes musculature of bronchi, GI tract, ureters and biliary system.

Indications

Oral form: Relief of cerebral and peripheral ischemia associated with arterial spasm and myocardial ischemia complicated by arrhythmias. *Parenteral form:* Vascular spasm associated with acute MI (coronary occlusion), angina pectoris, peripheral and pulmonary embolism, peripheral vascular disease in which there is a vasospastic element, certain cerebral angiospastic states, visceral spasm (eg, ureteral, biliary and GI colic). **Unlabeled use:** Intracavernous injection for impotence.

Contraindications

Complete atrioventricular (AV) heart block; intracorporeal injection for impotence.

Route/Dosage

Ischemia

ADULTS: **PO** 100-300 mg 3-5 times daily (immediate-release tablets) or 150 mg q 8-12 hr or 300 mg q 12 hr (sustained-release capsules).

Vascular Occlusion

ADULTS: **IV/IM** Initial dose: 30 mg. Repeat doses: 30-120 mg q 3 hr prn.

Impotence

ADULTS: **IV** 2.5-60 mg as intracavernous injection (usually combined with phentolamine mesylate).

Interactions

CNS depressants: Effects may be additive. *Levodopa:* May reduce effectiveness of levodopa. INCOMPATIBILITIES: Lactated Ringer's solution incompatible with parenteral formulation; do not mix.

Lab Test Interferences

None well documented.

Adverse Reactions

CV: Increase in heart rate; slight increase in BP. *RESP:* Increased depth of respiration. *CNS:* Depression; dizziness; vertigo; headache; drowsiness; sedation; lassitude; malaise; lethargy. *GI:* Constipation; nausea; diarrhea; abdominal distress; dry mouth; anorexia. *HEPA:* Jaundice; hepatitis. *HEMA:* Eosinophilia. *DERM:* Flushing of face; sweating; pruritus.

Precautions

Pregnancy: Category C. *Lactation:* Unknown. *Children:* Safety and efficacy not established. *Glaucoma:* Use drug with caution. *Hepatic hypersensitivity:* Has been reported.

NURSING CONSIDERATIONS

Administration/Storage

- Give at evenly spaced intervals throughout day.
- Do not crush or allow patient to chew sustained-release capsules.
- Do not administer in lactated Ringer's solution because precipitate will develop.
- Administer parenteral form slowly over 1-2 min to minimize adverse effects.
- Store at room temperature.

Assessment/Interventions

- Obtain patient history, including drug history and any known allergies.
- Assess mental status before and during therapy (lassitude, sedation, malaise, headache, depression).
- Assess bowel status and bowel sounds before administering drug and periodically during treatment.
- Monitor patient's BP, both lying and standing.
- Monitor liver function tests.
- Monitor ECG. If cardiac changes occur on ECG, notify physician immediately.
- If AV block, flushing, headache, jaundice, abdominal distress, constipation or diarrhea develop, notify physician.

OVERDOSAGE: SIGNS & SYMPTOMS

Drowsiness, weakness, diplopia, lassitude, depression, nystagmus, incoordination, coma, cyanosis, respiratory depression, anxiety, ataxia, headache, pruritic skin rashes, nausea, CNS depression, blurred vision, GI upset, vomiting, diaphoresis, sinus tachycardia, metabolic acidosis, hyperventilation, hyperglycemia, hypokalemia

Patient/Family Education

- Instruct patient to take medication at evenly spaced intervals throughout day.
- Advise patient with glaucoma to undergo regular eye examinations.
- Instruct patient to report these symp-

toms to physician: flushing, sweating, headache, tiredness, jaundice, skin rash, nausea, anorexia, abdominal distress, constipation or diarrhea.
- Advise patient to avoid smoking and intake of alcoholic beverages or other CNS depressants.
- Caution patient to avoid sudden position changes to prevent orthostatic hypotension.
- Advise patient that drug may cause dizziness, vertigo and drowsiness and to use caution while driving or performing other tasks requiring mental alertness.

See Patient Guide, p. 472.

Paromomycin Sulfate

(par-oh-moe-MY-sin SULL-fate)

Humatin

Class: Anti-infective/amebicide/aminoglycoside

Action Inhibits production of protein in bacteria, causing bacterial cell death.

Indications Treatment of acute and chronic intestinal amebiasis. Adjunctive therapy in management of hepatic coma. **Unlabeled use:** Treatment of other parasitic infections.

Contraindications Intestinal obstruction; extraintestinal amebiasis; hypersensitivity to aminoglycosides.

Route/Dosage

Intestinal Amebiasis

ADULTS & CHILDREN: PO 25-35 mg/kg/day in 3 divided doses with meals for 5-10 days.

Hepatic Coma

ADULTS: PO 4 g/day in divided doses at regular intervals for 5-6 days.

Interactions

Digoxin: May reduce rate and extent of digoxin absorption; this may be offset by decreased digoxin metabolism. *Methotrexate:* Decreased absorption of methotrexate. *Neuromuscular blockers:* Increased action of both depolarizing and nondepolarizing neuromuscular blocking agents, may prolong need for respiratory support. *Neurotoxic, nephrotoxic or ototoxic medications (eg, polypeptide antibiotics):* Additive adverse effects may occur with concurrent or sequential administration of medications with similar toxic profiles.

Lab Test Interferences

None well documented.

Adverse Reactions

GI: Nausea; vomiting; abdominal cramps; anorexia; epigastric burning; pruritus ani; diarrhea. *OTHER:* Malabsorption syndrome.

Precautions

Pregnancy: Category D. *Lactation:* Excreted in breast milk. *Muscular disorders:* Patients with muscular disorders such as myasthenia gravis or parkinsonism may have worsening of their disease because of potential effect of aminoglycosides on neuromuscular junction. *Ototoxicity and renal damage:* Inadvertent absorption through ulcerative bowel lesions may be associated with significant hearing and kidney damage. *Superinfection:* Prolonged or repeated therapy may result in bacterial or fungal overgrowth of nonsusceptible organisms and secondary infections.

NURSING CONSIDERATIONS

Administration/Storage

- Administer medication with meals.
- Store at room temperature in a tight container.

Assessment/Interventions

- Obtain patient history, including drug history and any known allergies.
- Assess patient for adverse reactions to

paromomycin (eg, altered auditory sensory perception, GI dysfunction, nephrotoxicity, neuromuscular blockage).

- Observe for signs of superinfection.
- If nausea, vomiting or diarrhea occur, give antiemetic or antidiarrheal medication as prescribed.
- If hearing loss occurs or if audiometric testing becomes abnormal or if casts or protein appear in urinalysis, notify physician.

OVERDOSAGE: SIGNS & SYMPTOMS

Neurotoxicity, nephrotoxicity, ototoxicity

Patient/Family Education

- Stress to patient the importance of taking full course of therapy.
- Emphasize to patient the importance of personal hygiene, especially handwashing.
- Explain to patient the symptoms of superinfection and ask patient to watch for symptoms if on prolonged therapy.
- Instruct patient to report these symptoms to physician: ringing in ears, hearing impairment or dizziness.

See Patient Guide, p. 473.

Paroxetine HCl

(puh-ROKS-uh-teen HIGH-droe-KLOR-ide)

Paxil

Class: Antidepressant

Action Blocks reuptake of serotonin, enhancing serotonergic function.

Indications Treatment of depression.

Contraindications Concomitant use in patients taking MAO inhibitors.

Route/Dosage

ADULTS: PO 20 mg/day initially; may increase by 10 mg/day at intervals of ≥ 7 days (maximum 50 mg/day). Administer as single daily dose, usually in morning. ELDERLY OR DEBILITATED PATIENTS OR PATIENTS WITH SEVERE RENAL OR HEPATIC IMPAIRMENT: PO 10 mg/day initially; increase if indicated (maximum 40 mg/day).

Interactions

Alcohol: Causes additive CNS effects; concurrent use is not recommended. *Cimetidine:* May increase paroxetine concentrations. *Digoxin:* May decrease digoxin levels. *MAO inhibitors:* Can cause serious, sometimes fatal reactions. Do not use concomitantly or within 14 days of each other. *Phenobarbital, phenytoin:* May decrease paroxetine concentration; may reduce phenytoin concentration. *Procyclidine:* Reduction of procyclidine dose may be necessary if anticholinergic effects (ie, dry mouth, blurred vision, urinary retention) occur. *Tryptophan:* May cause headache, nausea, sweating and dizziness. *Warfarin:* Increased risk of bleeding.

Lab Test Interferences

None well documented.

Adverse Reactions

CV: Palpitation; orthostatic hypotension; hypertension; syncope; tachycardia; chest pain. *RESP:* Pharyngitis; cough. *CNS:* Drowsiness; dizziness; insomnia; tremor; nervousness; anxiety; paresthesia; agitation; drugged feeling; confusion; amnesia; vertigo; headache; emotional liability; impaired concentration. *EENT:* Blurred vision; tinnitus; rhinitis; taste perversion. *GI:* Nausea; dry mouth; constipation; diarrhea; anorexia; flatulence; vomiting; abdominal pain; dyspepsia; increased appetite. *GU:* Ejaculatory disturbance; genital disorders; decreased libido; urinary frequency; breast atrophy. *HEMA:* Leukopenia; anemia; lymphocytosis; leukocytosis; lymphadenopathy; purpura. *DERM:* Sweating; rash; pruritus.

META: Edema; weight gain or loss; thyroid problems. *OTHER:* Myopathy; myalgia; back pain; asthenia; chills; malaise; fever.

Precautions
Pregnancy: Category B. *Lactation:* Secreted in breast milk. Use with caution. *Children:* Safety and efficacy not established. *Special risk patients:* Use with caution in patients with history of seizure, mania or hypomania, suicidal tendencies, drug abuse or dependence. *Hepatic/renal impairment:* May increase plasma concentrations of paroxetine; adjust dosage. *Hyponatremia:* Has occurred. Use drug with caution in elderly patients, patients taking diuretics and volume-depleted patients.

NURSING CONSIDERATIONS

Administration/Storage
- Do not give within 14 days of MAO inhibitor administration.
- Administer once daily, usually in morning.
- Store at room temperature in well closed container.

Assessment/Interventions
- Obtain patient history, including drug history and any known allergies.
- Review for history of liver or kidney disease or seizure disorder.
- Monitor weight weekly.
- Continue suicide monitoring of high-risk patients.
- If headache, nervousness, nausea, somnolence, insomnia, asthenia, dizziness or sweating occur, report to physician.
- Observe for signs of mood change and report to physician.

OVERDOSAGE: SIGNS & SYMPTOMS
Nausea, vomiting, drowsiness, sinus tachycardia, dilated pupils

Patient/Family Education
- Inform patient that improvement with therapy may not be evident for several weeks.
- Emphasize importance of following drug regimen as prescribed.
- Instruct patient to report these symptoms to physician: headache, nervousness, nausea, somnolence, insomnia, asthenia, dizziness or sweating.
- Advise patient to take sips of water frequently, suck on ice chips or sugarless hard candy or chew sugarless gum if dry mouth occurs.
- Instruct patient to avoid intake of alcoholic beverages.
- Advise patient that drug may cause drowsiness, dizziness and vertigo and to use caution while driving or performing other tasks requiring mental alertness.
- Instruct patient not to take prescription or otc drugs without consulting physician.

See Patient Guide, p. 474.

Pemoline

(PEM-oh-leen)

Cylert

Class: Psychotherapeutic

Action Acts as a CNS stimulant, but with minimal sympathomimetic effects; exact mechanism of action unknown.

Indications Treatment of attention-deficit hyperactivity disorder. **Unlabeled uses:** Treatment of narcolepsy and excessive daytime sedation.

Contraindications Hepatic insufficiency.

Route/Dosage
ADULTS & CHILDREN ≥ 6 YR: PO 37.5 mg/day as a single dose in the morning initially; increase by increments of 18.75 mg weekly until desired

response is obtained (maximum daily dose 112.5 mg/day).

Interactions None well documented.

Lab Test Interferences
None well documented.

Adverse Reactions
CNS: Insomnia; Tourette's syndrome; hallucinations; dyskinetic movements of tongue, lips, face and extremities; abnormal oculomotor function (eg, nystagmus, oculogyric crisis); depression; dizziness; irritability; headache; drowsiness; seizures. *GI:* Anorexia; transient weight loss; stomach ache; nausea. *HEPA:* Elevated liver enzymes; hepatitis; jaundice. *DERM:* Skin rash. *OTHER:* Growth suppression.

Precautions
Pregnancy: Category B. *Lactation:* Undetermined. *Children:* Not recommended for children < 6 yr. *Drug abuse and dependence:* Can occur; use with caution in emotionally unstable patients who may increase the dosage on their own initiative. *Renal impairment:* Use with caution in patients with significantly impaired renal function.

NURSING CONSIDERATIONS

Administration/Storage

- Do not administer if liver function tests are abnormal.
- Administer as a single dose each morning and ensure that chewable tablets are completely chewed and swallowed.
- Administer with caution to emotionally unstable patients. Administration may intensify symptoms of behavior disturbance and thought disorder.
- Administer with caution to patients with impaired renal function.
- Store at room temperature in a tight, dry container.

Assessment/Interventions

- Obtain patient history.
- Clinically assess for tics and Tourette's syndrome in children and their families before use of this drug.
- Monitor growth of children during treatment as long-term administration is associated with growth inhibition.
- Ensure liver function tests are performed prior to and periodically during therapy.
- Assess therapeutic effects of medication. Medication is often interrupted at intervals to determine therapeutic effects to ascertain if there are sufficient behavioral symptoms present to require continued therapy.
- Ensure that dosage is decreased gradually following long-term therapy to prevent withdrawal symptoms.

OVERDOSAGE: SIGNS & SYMPTOMS

Vomiting, agitation, tremors, hyperreflexia, muscle twitching, convulsions (followed by coma), euphoria, confusion, hallucinations, delirium, sweating, flushing, headache, high fever, tachycardia, hypertension, dilated pupils

Patient/Family Education

- Advise patient that clinical improvement is gradual and benefits may not occur until week 3 or 4 of administration.
- Instruct patient to take pemoline as prescribed and not to make up missed doses.
- Caution patient to avoid taking large doses of caffeine or use other stimulants which could adversely potentiate the effects of pemoline.
- Instruct patient to take medication in the morning to avoid sleep disturbance. Notify healthcare provider if problems with sleeping occur.
- Instruct patient to notify healthcare provider of adverse reactions; the dosage may need to be reduced or the drug discontinued.
- Advise patient that medication can cause dizziness or drowsiness and to

avoid driving and other tasks requiring mental alertness.

- Instruct patient not to increase the dose amount or take the medication more frequently because of a high dependence and abuse potential. In addition, psychotic symptoms could occur following long-term misuse of excessive oral doses.
- Instruct patient or family to be aware of the symptoms of overdose and take immediate and appropriate action, such as notifying poison control center.

See Patient Guide, p. 475.

Penbutolol Sulfate

(pen-BYOO-toe-lole SULL-fate)

Levatol

Class: Beta-adrenergic blocker

Action Nonselectively blocks beta-adrenergic receptors, primarily affecting the cardiovascular system (decreased heart rate, decreased cardiac contractility, decreased BP) and lungs (promotes bronchospasm).

Indications Management of mild to moderate hypertension.

Contraindications Greater than first-degree heart block; CHF unless secondary to tachyarrhythmia or untreated hypertension treatable with beta-blockers; overt cardiac failure; sinus bradycardia; cardiogenic shock; hypersensitivity to beta-blockers; untreated bronchial asthma or bronchospasm, including severe COPD.

Route/Dosage

ADULTS: **PO** 20 mg once daily.

Interactions

Clonidine: May attenuate or reverse antihypertensive effect; potentially life-threatening increases in BP, especially on withdrawal. *Epinephrine:* Initial hypertensive episodes followed by bradycardia may occur. *Ergot alkaloids:* Peripheral ischemia, manifested by cold extremities and possible gangrene. *Insulin:* Prolonged hypoglycemia with masking of symptoms. *Lidocaine:* Increased lidocaine levels, leading to toxicity. *Nonsteroidal anti-inflammatory agents:* Some agents may impair antihypertensive effects. *Theophylline:* Elimination of theophylline may be reduced; effects of both drugs may be reduced by pharmacologic antagonism. *Verapamil:* Effects of both drugs may be increased.

Lab Test Interferences

None well documented.

Adverse Reactions

CV: Bradycardia; hypotension; congestive heart failure; edema; worsening angina, atrioventricular (AV) block. *RESP:* Cough; dyspnea; bronchospasm. *CNS:* Dizziness; tiredness; fatigue; headache; insomnia; depression; short-term memory loss; emotional lability. *EENT:* Dry eyes; visual disturbances. *GI:* Diarrhea; nausea; dyspepsia. *GU:* Impotence. *HEMA:* Agranulocytosis; nonthrombocytopenic and thrombocytopenic purpura. *DERM:* Sweating. *META:* May increase or decrease blood sugar.

Precautions

Pregnancy: Category C. *Lactation:* Undetermined. *Children:* Safety and efficacy not established. *CHF:* Administer cautiously in CHF patients controlled by digitalis and diuretics. *Diabetics:* May mask signs and symptoms of hypoglycemia (eg, tachycardia, BP changes). May potentiate insulin-induced hypoglycemia. *Nonallergic bronchospasm:* Give drug with caution to patients with bronchospastic disease. *Thyrotoxicosis:* May mask clinical signs of developing or continuing hyperthyroidism (eg, tachycardia). Abrupt withdrawal may exacerbate symptoms of hyperthyroidism, including thyroid storm. *Abrupt withdrawal:* A beta-blocker withdrawal syndrome (hypertension, tachycardia, anxiety, angina, MI) may occur 1-2 weeks after sudden discontinuation of systemic beta-blockers. If possible, gradually withdraw therapy over 1-2 weeks. *Anaphylaxis:* May be unresponsive to usual doses of epinephrine; aggressive therapy may be required. *Peripheral vascular disease:* May precipitate or aggravate symptoms of arterial insufficiency.

NURSING CONSIDERATIONS

Administration/Storage

- May be taken with or without food.
- Store tablets at room temperature in a tightly closed, light-resistant container.

Assessment/Interventions

- Obtain patient history.
- Evaluate current ECG for signs of bradycardia or heart block.
- Monitor for bradycardia, hypotension, respiratory difficulty and heart block that may indicate need for reduced dosage.
- Avoid use in patients with asthma, chronic bronchitis and other chronic respiratory diseases.
- Monitor I&O and daily weight during therapy for signs of fluid retention. If sudden, severe dyspnea or edema of hands and feet develop, withhold medication and notify physician.
- Notify physician at first sign or symptom of CHF or unexplained respiratory symptoms in any patient.

OVERDOSAGE: SIGNS & SYMPTOMS

Bradycardia, hypotension, CHF, AV block, intraventricular conduction defects, asystole, coma

Patient/Family Education

- Warn patient to never stop taking this medication suddenly. Rebound effects can produce angina, and even MI. Explain that medication will be tapered slowly before discontinuation.
- Instruct patient to take medication at the same time every day.
- Advise patient not to take any over-the-counter medications such as nasal decongestants, diet aids, cold preparations or antihistamines without consulting their healthcare provider first.
- Teach patient and family how to take pulse. Instruct them to check it before taking the medication. If the pulse is irregular or has a rate less than 60 BPM, notify healthcare provider before taking the medication.
- Instruct patient and family on how to take BP. If BP is markedly lower than normal, they should notify healthcare provider.
- Warn patient that sudden position changes may cause dizziness due to postural hypotension.
- Instruct patient to notify healthcare provider if any of the following occurs: confusion, depression, memory loss, rash, shortness of breath, slowed pulse rate, or unusual bruising or bleeding.

No patient monograph available.

Penicillin G

(pen-ih-SILL-in G)

Penicillin G Potassium
Pentids 400, Pentids 800, Pentids 400 for Syrup, Pfizerpen

Penicillin G Sodium
Available as generic only

Penicillin G Procaine
Crysticillin 300 A.S., Crysticillin 600 A.S., Pfizerpen-A.S., Wycillin

Penicillin G Benzathine
Bicillin L-A, Permapen

Class: Antibiotic/penicillin

Action Inhibits mucopeptide synthesis of bacterial cell wall.

Indications Treatment of meningococcal meningitis, actinomycosis, clostridial infections, fusospirochetal infections, rat-bite fever, listeria infections, pasteurella infections, erysipeloid, gram-negative bacillary bacteremia, diphtheria, anthrax, pneumococcal infections, syphilis, gonococcal infections and staphylococcal infections caused by susceptible microorganisms; prophylaxis of bacterial endocarditis and recurrent rheumatic fever. **Unlabeled use:** Treatment of Lyme disease *(Borrelia burgdorferi)*.

Contraindications Hypersensitivity to penicillins. Do not treat severe pneumonia, empyema, bacteremia, pericarditis, meningitis and purulent or septic arthritis with oral penicillin G during acute stage.

Route/Dosage

Penicillin G (Aqueous Potassium or Sodium)

ADULTS: **IV/IM** 1-24 million U/day in divided doses q 4-6 hr. LYME DISEASE: **IV** 200,000-300,000 U/kg/day for 10-20 days. CHILDREN: **IV/IM** 100,000-250,000 U/kg/day in divided doses q 4 hr. INFANTS (OVER 7 DAYS AND > 2000 GM): **IM/IV** 100,000 U/kg/day in divided doses every 6 hr (meningitis: 200,000 U/kg/day in divided doses every 6 hr). INFANTS (UNDER 7 DAYS AND > 2000 GM): **IM/IV** 50,000 U/kg/day in divided doses every 8 hr (meningitis: 150,000 U/kg/day in divided doses every 8 hr). INFANTS (UNDER 7 DAYS AND < 2000 GM): **IM/IV** 50,000 U/kg/day in divided doses every 12 hr (meningitis: 100,000 U/kg/day in divided doses every 12 hr).

Penicillin G Potassium

ADULTS & CHILDREN > 12 YR: **PO** 200,000-500,000 U q 6-8 hr. INFANTS & CHILDREN < 12 YR: **PO** 25,000-90,000 U/kg/day in 3-6 divided doses.

Penicillin G Procaine (Aqueous)

ADULTS & CHILDREN: **IM** 600,000-1.2 million U/day in 1-2 doses. NEWBORNS: **IM** 50,000 U/kg once daily.

Penicillin G Benzathine

ADULTS: **IM** 1.2 million U in one dose. CHILDREN > 27 KG: **IM** 900,000-1.2 million U in one dose. CHILDREN & INFANTS < 27 KG: **IM** 300,000-1.2 million U in one dose. NEONATES: **IM** 50,000 U/kg in one dose.

Penicillin G Benzathine and Procaine Combined

ADULTS & CHILDREN > 27 KG: **IM** 2.4 million U in one dose. CHILDREN 14-27 KG: **IM** 900,000-1.2 million U in one dose. INFANTS & CHILDREN < 14 KG: **IM** 600,000 U in one dose.

Interactions

Anticoagulants, (oral, and heparin): May increase bleeding risks of anticoagulant by prolonging bleeding time. *Beta-blockers:* May potentiate anaphylactic reactions of penicillin. *Chloramphenicol:* May cause synergism or antagonism to develop. *Contraceptives, oral:* May reduce efficacy of oral contraceptives. *Erythromycin:* May cause synergism or antagonism to develop. *Probenecid:* Increases penicillin serum concentration. *Tetracyclines:* May impair bactericidal effects of penicillin G. INCOMPATIBILITIES: *Aminoglycosides, parenteral:* Penicillin may inactivate aminoglycosides in vitro; do not mix in same IV solution. May be used in combination for synergy if administered separately. *Carbohydrate solutions at alkaline pH:* Penicillin solutions is rapidly inactivated.

Lab Test Interferences

Antiglobulin (Coombs') test: Drug may cause false-positive results. *Urine glucose test:* Drug may cause false-positive results with copper sulfate tests (Benedict's test, Fehling's test, or Clinitest tablets); enzyme-based tests (eg, Clinistix, Tes-tape) are not affected. *Urine protein determinations:* Drug may cause false-positive reactions with sulfosalicylic acid and boiling test, acetic acid test, biuret reaction and nitric acid test; bromphenol blue test (Multi-Stix) is not affected.

Adverse Reactions

CNS: Dizziness; fatigue; insomnia; reversible hyperactivity; neurotoxicity (lethargy, neuromuscular irritability, hallucinations, convulsions, seizures). *EENT:* Itchy eyes; stomatitis; gastritis; sore mouth or tongue; furry tongue; black "hairy" tongue; abnormal taste perception. *GI:* Glossitis; dry mouth; nausea; anorexia; vomiting; abdominal pain or cramp; epigastric distress; diarrhea or bloody diarrhea; rectal bleeding; flatulence; enterocolitis; pseudomembranous colitis. *GU:* Interstitial nephritis (eg, oliguria, proteinuria, hematuria, hyaline casts, pyuria); nephropathy; increased BUN and creatinine. *HEMA:* Decreased hemoglobin, hematocrit, RBC, WBC, neutrophils, lymphocytes, platelets; increased lymphocytes, monocytes, basophils, eosinophils and platelets; abnormal coagulation tests. *META:* Elevated serum alkaline phosphatase, hypernatremia; hypokalemia; hyperkalemia. *OTHER:* Hypersensitivity reactions (urticaria, angioneurotic edema, laryngospasm, laryngeal edema, bronchospasm, hypotension, vascular collapse, death, maculopapular to exfoliative dermatitis, vesicular eruptions, erythema multiforme, serum sickness, skin rashes); vaginitis; hyperthermia.

Precautions

Pregnancy: Category B. *Lactation:* Small amount excreted in breast milk. May cause diarrhea, candidiasis or allergic response in nursing infant. *Electrolyte content:* Penicillin G aqueous sodium contains 2 mEq sodium/1 million U. Penicillin G aqueous potassium contains 1.7 mEq potassium and 0.3 mEq sodium/1 million U. Beware of iatrogenic electrolyte abnormalities and fluid overload. *Hypersensitivity:* Reactions range from mild to life threatening. Administer drug with caution to cephalosporin-sensitive patients because of possible cross-reactivity. *Procaine sensitivity:* If sensitivity to procaine in penicillin G procaine is suspected, inject 0.1 ml of 1%-2% procaine solution intradermally. If erythema, wheal, flare or eruption develops, do not use procaine penicillin preparations. *Pseudomembranous colitis:* May occur because of overgrowth of clostridia. *Renal impairment:* Use drug with caution; may require dosage adjustment. *Superinfection:* May result in bacterial or fungal overgrowth of nonsusceptible organisms. *Tartrazine sensitivity:* Some products contain tartrazine, which may cause allergic-type reactions in susceptible individuals.

NURSING CONSIDERATIONS

Administration/Storage

- Depending on route of administration, prepare solution using Sterile Water for Injection, Isotonic Sodium Chloride Injection or Dextrose Injection.
- Administer at regular intervals around clock.
- Give oral form on empty stomach with full glass of water at least 1 hr before or 2 hr after meals.
- Do not administer with acidic juices or carbonated beverages, which may decrease absorption of penicillin G.
- For IM administration, inject deeply into upper outer quadrant of buttock in adults. In infants and small children, inject in midlateral aspect of thigh. With repeated doses, rotate injection sites.
- For IV administration; administer continuously or intermittently. For intermittent infusion, infuse each dose over 1-2 hr (adults) or 15-30 min (neonates and children).
- Solutions prepared for intravenous infusion are stable at room temperature for at least 24 hr.
- Dry powder is stable and does not require refrigeration.
- Sterile solutions may be kept in refrigerator for 1 wk.

Assessment/Interventions

- Obtain patient history, including drug history and any known allergies.
- Assess patient for infection at beginning and throughout therapy (fever, WBC, appearance of wound).
- Obtain specimens for culture and sensitivity before beginning therapy.
- Have emergency medication (eg, epinephrine, antihistamine) and equipment readily available in case of anaphylaxis.
- Observe for anaphylaxis. Persons with no history of hypersensitivity may have allergic response.
- Assess for signs of superinfection (bacterial or fungal overgrowth of nonsusceptible organisms).
- Monitor newborns closely for signs of toxicity or adverse effects.
- Monitor renal function, especially in patients with renal impairment. Monitor I&O strictly. If urinary output is decreased, notify physician.
- If patient develops rash, pruritus, laryngeal edema, evidence of hemolysis, wheezing or other signs of allergic reaction, discontinue drug and notify physician.
- If sudden elevation in temperature develops, notify physician. It may be drug fever.
- Discontinue penicillin G if signs of hemolytic anemia develop (positive Coomb's test).

OVERDOSAGE: SIGNS & SYMPTOMS

Neuromuscular hyperexcitability, convulsions, agitation, confusion, asterixis, hallucinations, stupor, coma, multifocal myoclonus, seizures, encephalopathy, hyperkalemia

Patient/Family Education

- Instruct patient to finish course of therapy even if feeling better.
- Advise patient to take oral penicillin at intervals around clock on empty stomach 1 hr before or 2 hr after meal with full glass of water, not fruit juice or carbonated beverage.
- Instruct penicillin allergic patient to carry Medi-Alert necklace or bracelet.
- Advise patient to use nonhormonal form of contraceptive while taking penicillin.
- Inform patient of signs of hypersensitivity (skin rash, itching, hives, shortness of breath, wheezing) and other side effects, such as black tongue, sore throat, nausea, vomiting, severe diarrhea, fever, swollen joints, and instruct patient to notify physician should they occur.
- Instruct patient to notify physician if there is no improvement in symptoms of infection.
- Advise patient to notify physician of signs of superinfection (eg, vaginitis, black "hairy" tongue).

See Patient Guide, p. 477.

Penicillin V (Phenoxymethyl Penicillin, Penicillin V Potassium)

(pen-ih-SILL-in V)

Beepen-VK, Betapen-VK, Ledercillin VK, Pen-V, Pen-Vee K, Pen VK, Penicillin VK, Robicillin VK, V-Cillin K, Veetids, ♣ *APO-Pen VK, Nadopen-V, Nadopen-V 200, Nadopen-V 400, Novo-Pen-VK, Nu-Pen-VK, Pen-Vee, PVF, PVF K*

Class: Antibiotic/penicillin

Action Inhibits mucopeptide synthesis of bacterial cell wall.

Indications Treatment of upper respiratory tract infections; prevention of bacterial endocarditis; prophylaxis of recurrent rheumatic fever; treatment of pneumococcal, streptococci, and staphylococcal infections and fusospirochetosis (Vincent's infection) of oropharynx caused by susceptible microorganisms. **Unlabeled uses:** Prophylactic treatment of sickle cell anemia in children; treatment of anaerobic infections; treatment of Lyme disease *(Borrelia burgdorferi)*.

Contraindications Hypersensitivity to penicillins. Do not treat severe pneumonia, empyema, bacteremia, pericarditis, meningitis and purulent or septic arthritis with oral penicillin V during acute stage.

Route/Dosage

ADULTS: **PO** 125-500 mg qid. CHILDREN: **PO** 25-50 mg/kg/day in divided doses q 6-8 hr.

Interactions

Beta-blockers: May potentiate anaphylactic reactions of penicillin. *Contraceptives, oral:* May reduce efficacy of oral contraceptives. *Erythromycin:* May cause synergism or antagonism to develop. *Tetracyclines:* May impair bactericidal effects of penicillin V.

Lab Test Interferences

Antiglobulin (Coombs') test: Drug may cause false-positive results. *Urine glucose test:* Drug may cause false-positive results with copper sulfate tests (Benedict's test, Fehling's test or Clinitest tablets); enzyme-based tests (eg, Clinistix, Tes-tape) are not affected. *Urine protein determinations:* Drug may cause false-positive reactions with sulfosalicylic acid and boiling test, acetic acid test, biuret reaction and nitric acid test; bromphenol blue test (Multi-Stix) is not affected.

Adverse Reactions

CNS: Dizziness; fatigue; insomnia; reversible hyperactivity; neurotoxicity (lethargy, neuromuscular irritability, hallucinations, convulsions, seizures). *EENT:* Itchy eyes; furry tongue; black "hairy" tongue; stomatitis; sore mouth or tongue. *GI:* Glossitis; gastritis; dry mouth; nausea; vomiting; abdominal pain or cramp; epigastric distress; diarrhea or bloody diarrhea; rectal bleeding; flatulence; enterocolitis; pseudomembranous colitis. *GU:* Interstitial nephritis (eg, oliguria, proteinuria, hematuria, hyaline casts, pyuria); nephropathy; increased BUN and creatinine. *HEMA:* Decreased hemoglobin, hematocrit, RBC, WBC, neutrophils, lymphocytes, platelets; increased lymphocytes, monocytes, basophils, eosinophils and platelets. *META:* Elevated serum alkaline phosphatase; hypernatremia; hypokalemia; albumin, total proteins and uric acid. *OTHER:* Hypersensitivity reactions (urticaria, angioneurotic edema, laryngospasm, laryngeal edema, bronchospasm, hypotension, vascular collapse, death, maculopapular to exfoliative dermatitis, vesicular eruptions, erythema multiforme, serum sickness, skin rashes, prostration); vaginitis; hyperthermia.

Precautions

Pregnancy: Category B. *Lactation:* Small amount excreted in breast milk. May cause diarrhea, candidiasis or allergic response in nursing infant. *Hypersensitivity:* Reactions range from mild to life threatening. Administer drug with caution to cephalosporin-sensitive patients because of possible cross-reactivity. *Pseudomembranous colitis:* May occur because of overgrowth of clostridia. *Renal impairment:* Use drug with caution; dosage adjustment may be necessary. *Streptococcal infections:* Therapy must be minimum of 10 days. *Superinfection:* May result in bacterial or fungal overgrowth of nonsusceptible organisms.

NURSING CONSIDERATIONS

Administration/Storage

- Administer without regard to food.
- Administer at regular intervals around the clock.
- Reconstituted oral suspension is sta-

ble for 14 days when refrigerated. Shake well before using.

Assessment/Interventions

- Obtain patient history, including drug history and any known allergies.
- Assess patient for infection at beginning and throughout therapy (fever, WBC, appearance of wound).
- Obtain specimens for culture and sensitivity before beginning therapy.
- Observe for anaphylaxis. Persons with no history of hypersensitivity may develop allergic response.
- Assess for signs of superinfection (bacterial or fungal overgrowth of nonsusceptible organisms).
- Monitor renal function, especially in patients with renal impairment.
- If patient develops rash, pruritus, laryngeal edema, wheezing or evidence of hemolytic anemia (positive Coomb's test) or other signs of an allergic reaction, discontinue drug and notify physician.
- If sudden elevation in temperature develops, notify physician. It may be drug fever.
- Discontinue use of penicillin V if signs of hemolytic anemia develop (positive Coomb's test).

OVERDOSAGE: SIGNS & SYMPTOMS

Neuromuscular hyperexcitability, agitation, confusion, asterixis, hallucinations, stupor, coma, multifocal myoclonus, encephalopathy, hyperkalemia

Patient/Family Education

- Instruct patient to complete entire course of therapy even if feeling better.
- Advise patient to use calibrated measuring device for liquid preparation.
- Instruct penicillin allergic patient to carry Medi-Alert necklace or bracelet.
- Advise patient to use nonhormonal form of contraceptive during penicillin V therapy.
- Inform patient of the signs of hypersensitivity (skin rash, itching, hives, shortness of breath, wheezing) and other side effects, such as black tongue, sore throat, nausea, vomiting, severe diarrhea, fever, swollen joints and instruct patient to notify physician should they occur.
- Instruct patient to notify physician if there is no improvement in symptoms of infection.
- Instruct patient to notify physician of signs of superinfection (eg, vaginitis, black "hairy" tongue).

See Patient Guide, p. 478.

Pentamidine Isethionate

(pen-TAM-ih-deen ice-uh-THIGH-uh-nate)

NebuPent, Pentam 300, ♣ *Pentacarinet*

Class: Anti-infective; antiprotozoal

Action Mechanism of action not fully understood. Interferes with synthesis of DNA, RNA, phospholipids and proteins.

Indications

Parenteral form: Treatment of *Pneumocystis carinii* pneumonia (PCP). *Inhalation:* Prevention of PCP in high-risk HIV-infected patients. **Unlabeled uses:** Treatment of trypanosomiasis and visceral leishmaniasis.

Contraindications

Parenteral form: Once diagnosis of PCP is made, there are no absolute contraindications. *Inhalation:* History of anaphylactic reaction to pentamidine.

Route/Dosage

ADULTS & CHILDREN: **IM/IV** 4 mg/kg qd for 14 days. ADULTS: **Inhalation** 300 mg once q 4 wk administered via Respirgard II nebulizer.

Interactions INCOMPATIBILITIES: Do not reconstitute with saline solutions. Do not mix with other drugs.

Lab Test Interferences

None well documented.

Adverse Reactions

CV: Hypotension; ventricular tachycardia; cardiac arrhythmias; chest pain; edema; phlebitis. *RESP:* Shortness of breath; cough; pharyngitis; chest congestion; bronchospasm; pneumothorax (generally associated with inhalation). *CNS:* Confusion; hallucinations; dizziness; fatigue; headache. *EENT:* Bad or metallic taste. *GI:* Nausea; anorexia; vomiting; diarrhea; abdominal pain. *GU:* Acute renal failure; elevated serum creatinine. *HEMA:* Leukopenia; thrombocytopenia; anemia; pancytopenia. *HEPA:* Elevated liver function test results. *DERM:* Stevens-Johnson syndrome; sterile abscess, pain or induration at IM injection site; rash. *META:* Hypoglycemia; hypocalcemia; hyperkalemia. *OTHER:* Neuralgia; myalgia; night sweats, chills.

Precautions

Pregnancy: Category C. *Lactation:* Undetermined. *Children:* Safety and efficacy of inhalation solution not established. *Special risk patients:* Use drug with caution in patients with hypertension, hypotension, hypoglycemia, hyperglycemia, hypocalcemia, leukopenia, thrombocytopenia, anemia, hepatic or renal dysfunction, ventricular tachycardia, pancreatitis, Stevens-Johnson syndrome. *Development of acute PCP:* Acute PCP may develop despite pentamidine prophylaxis. *Fatalities:* Fatalities from severe hypotension (even after one dose), hypoglycemia and cardiac arrhythmias have been reported with IM and IV routes. *Renal failure:* Reduction of dosage, longer infusion time or extension of dosing interval may be required.

NURSING CONSIDERATIONS

Administration/Storage

- For parenteral use, dissolve contents of vial in Sterile Water for Injection or D5W as directed.
- For IV infusion, solution may be diluted further in D5W.
- Infuse pentamidine IV over 1 hr with patient supine to minimize severe hypotension and arrhythmias.
- Monitor BP continuously throughout infusion, every 30 min for 2 hr thereafter and then every 4 hr until BP stabilizes.
- For IM administration, inject deeply and rotate sites.
- Reconstitute medication for inhalation in Sterile Water for Injection, USP. Do not mix with any other drugs.
- Deliver aerosol dose until nebulizer chamber is empty (approximately 30-45 min).
- Reconstituted aerosol preparation is stable up to 48 hr at room temperature, if protected from light source. Discard unused portion.
- IV solutions prepared with D5W are stable at room temperature for up to 48 hr. Discard unused portion.
- Store unopened vial at room temperature. Protect from light.

Assessment/Interventions

- Obtain patient history, including drug history and any known allergies.
- Assess for adverse reactions throughout course of therapy (hypotension, chest pain, neuralgia, phlebitis, edema, headache, nausea, night sweats, chills).
- If patient is coughing, provide physical support to patient's chest. Institute measures to reduce nonproductive coughing to decrease expenditure and chest pain.
- Protect immunocompromised patient from additional infections and stress.
- Consult with nutritionist to maintain optimal diet for patient.
- Inspect injection sites periodically for signs of induration or sterile abscess.

- Obtain prescription for antiemetic agent if needed.
- Keep emergency resuscitation equipment available.
- Monitor lab studies for leukopenia, thrombocytopenia, elevated serum creatinine, elevated liver function studies, hypoglycemia, hypocalcemia or hyperkalemia.
- Monitor vital signs at least every 4 hr during therapy.
- Monitor BP before, during and after pentamidine administration.
- Monitor I&O throughout therapy. If urinary output is decreased, notify physician immediately.
- If patient experiences anorexia, nausea and vomiting, increased hydration will be necessary.
- If vertigo, emotional changes or seizures occur, take safety precautions.
- Notify physician if GI reactions persist or worsen.

Patient/Family Education

- Inform the patient that there may be pain at the injection site with IM administration.
- Caution patient to avoid crowds and persons with known infections.
- Instruct patient to report these symptoms to physician: nausea, vomiting, anorexia, diarrhea, oliguria, dizziness, chest pain or edema.
- Advise patient that drug may cause dizziness and to use caution while driving or performing other tasks requiring mental alertness.

See Patient Guide, pp. 479-480.

Pentazocine

(pen-TAZ-oh-seen)

Talacen, Talwin, Talwin Compound, Talwin NX

Class: Narcotic agonist-antagonist analgesic

Action Produces analgesia by an agonistic effect at the kappa opioid receptor. Weakly antagonizes effects of opiates at mu opioid receptor; does not appear to increase biliary tract pressure.

Indications *Oral and parenteral forms:* Management of moderate to severe pain. *Parenteral form:* Preoperative or preanesthetic medication; supplement to surgical anesthesia.

Contraindications Hypersensitivity to naloxone (in Talwin NX) or sulfites.

Route/Dosage

Moderate to Severe Pain

PENTAZOCINE: ADULTS: **PO** 50 mg q 3-4 hr; increase to 100 mg if necessary (maximum 600 mg/day). **IM/SC/IV** 30 mg q 3-4 hr prn (maximum 360 mg/day). Doses > 30 mg IV or 60 mg SC/IM are not recommended. PENTAZOCINE 12.5 MG WITH ASPIRIN 325 MG (TALWIN COMPOUND): ADULTS: **PO** 2 tablets tid-qid. PENTAZOCINE 25 MG WITH ACETAMINOPHEN 650 MG (TALACEN): ADULTS: **PO** 1 tablet q 4 hr (maximum 6 tablets/day).

Labor

ADULTS: **IM** 30 mg as single dose; alternatively, when contractions are regular, **IV** 20 mg for 2-3 doses given q 2-3 hr.

Interactions *Alcohol:* Causes additive CNS depression. *Barbiturate anesthetics and any other CNS depressants (benzodiazapines, antidepressants, etc.):* Causes increased CNS and respiratory depression. INCOMPATIBILITIES: *Barbiturates:* Do not mix in the same syringe with pentazocine; precipitation will occur.

Lab Test Interferences None well documented.

Adverse Reactions *CV:* Hypotension; hypertension; tachycardia; circulatory depression; shock. *RESP:* Respiratory depression; transient apnea in newborns whose mothers received parenteral pentazocine during labor. *CNS:* Lightheadedness; dizziness; euphoria; hallucinations; disorientation; confusion; seizures. *EENT:* Visual disturbances. *GI:* Nausea. *GU:* Urinary retention. *HEMA:* Granulocytopenia. *DERM:* Nodules, soft tissue induration, depressions, sclerosis and ulceration at injection sites. *OTHER:* Anaphylaxis; tolerance; psychological and physical dependence in long-term use.

Precautions

Pregnancy: Category C. Neonatal abstinence syndrome may develop. *Labor:* Pentazocine rapidly crosses placenta with cord blood levels 40%-70% of maternal serum levels. Use drug with caution in women delivered of premature infants. *Children:* Not recommended for children < 12 yr old. *Special risk patients:* Use with caution in patients with MI, decreased respiratory reserve, asthma, respiratory depression, head injury or increased intracranial pressure. *Abuse/dependence/withdrawal:* Abuse potential exists. Abrupt discontinuation after long-term use may cause withdrawal symptoms. Do not substitute other opiates in pentazocine withdrawal syndrome. Pentazocine may induce withdrawal symptoms in narcotic-dependent patients. *Acute CNS manifestations:* Hallucinations, disorientation, confusion and seizures. *Renal or hepatic impairment:* Duration of action may be prolonged; dosage reduction may be required. *Sulfite sensitivity:* Drug may cause allergic-type reactions (eg, hives, itching, wheezing, anaphylaxis) in susceptible persons. *"Ts and Blues":* Refers to drug abuse by IV injection of oral pentazocine and tripelennamine (antihistamine) as substitute for heroin. Complications of injecting oral pentazocine include pulmonary emboli, vascular occlusion, ulceration, seizures, strokes and CNS infections. Addition of naloxone to pentazocine tablets *(Talwin NX)* prevents this drug abuse; it may cause withdrawal in narcotic-dependent individuals. *Tissue damage:* Severe sclerosis of skin, subcutaneous tissues and underlying muscle have occurred at injection sites.

NURSING CONSIDERATIONS

Administration/Storage

- Pentazocine is schedule IV drug; keep it locked according to hospital policy.
- When anti-inflammatory or antipyretic effects are desired in addition to analgesia, aspirin or acetaminophen can be administered concomitantly with oral form of pentazocine.
- Do not mix barbiturate in same syringe with pentazocine; precipitation will occur.
- If frequent injections are needed, rotate sites.
- For IM administration; inject deep into well-developed tissue.
- For IV administration; inject undiluted by slow bolus. Do not exceed a 30 mg dose.
- Administer SC only when necessary; severe tissue damage is possible at injection sites.
- Store in tightly closed, light-resistant containers.

Assessment/Interventions

- Obtain patient history, including drug history and any known allergies.
- Assess for signs of physical and psychological dependence throughout course of therapy.
- Assess respiratory rate and quality, BP and pulse before administering drug and periodically during therapy.
- Assess for adverse reactions (hypotension, shock, dizziness, hallucinations, seizures, urinary retention, tissue changes from injections).
- Assess newborns whose mothers received parenteral pentazocine for apnea.
- Rate patient's pain before and after each dose. Determine and record on-

set, durations, location, intensity and quality of pain.

- Notify physician if medication does not relieve patient's pain.
- If anaphylaxis occurs, prepare to institute emergency oxygen, mechanical ventilation, intravenous fluids and vasopressors.
- If constipation occurs, give stool softeners or laxative, teach high-fiber diet and increase fluid consumption to 2-3 L/day if tolerated.

OVERDOSAGE: SIGNS & SYMPTOMS

Respiratory depression, hypertension, tachycardia

Patient/Family Education

- For maximum effectiveness, instruct patient to take medication before intolerable pain develops.
- Tell patient to take medication exactly as prescribed, to minimize dependence.
- Teach patient to consume 2-3 L of fluids each day, if tolerated, to prevent constipation.
- Inform patient that aspirin or acetaminophen may be taken concurrenty for additive analgesia as well as its antiinflammatory and antipyretic effects.
- Explain therapeutic value of pentazocine prior to administration to enhance the analgesic effect.
- Caution patient not to stop taking drug abruptly without consulting physician.
- Advise patient to avoid sudden position changes to prevent orthostatic hypotension.
- Instruct patient to avoid intake of alcoholic beverages or other CNS depressants.
- Advise patient that drug may cause dizziness and to use caution while driving or performing other tasks requiring mental alertness.

See Patient Guide, pp. 481.

Pentobarbital Sodium

(pen-toe-BAR-bih-tahl SO-dee-uhm)

Nembutal Sodium, ♣ *Nova Rectal*

Class: Sedative and hypnotic/barbiturate/short-acting; anticonvulsant

Action Depresses sensory cortex, decreases motor activity, alters cerebellar function and produces drowsiness, sedation and hypnosis.

Indications Sedation; short-term treatment of insomnia; preanesthesia; emergency control of convulsions (parenteral form).

Contraindications Hypersensitivity to barbiturates; manifest or latent porphyria.

Route/Dosage

Insomnia

ADULTS: **PO/IV** 100 mg (maximum IV rate 50 mg/min). **IM/PR** 120-200 mg (maximum IM dose 500 mg or 5 ml volume regardless of concentration).

Sedation

ADULTS: **PO/PR** 20-30 mg bid-qid. CHILDREN: **PO/IM** 2-6 mg/kg (maximum 100 mg). **IV** 50 mg.

Convulsions

ADULTS: **IV** Use minimum dose to avoid compounding depression. Administer slowly to allow time for drug to penetrate the blood-brain barrier. Do not exceed 50 mg/min.

Pediatric Patients Unable to Take Orally or by Injection

CHILDREN 12-14 YR (36.4-50 KG): **PR** 60 or 120 mg. CHILDREN 5-12 YR (18.2-36.4 KG); **PR** 60 mg. CHILDREN 1-4 YR (9-18.2 KG): **PR** 30 or 60 mg. CHILDREN 2 MO-1 YR (4.5-9 KG): **PR** 30 mg.

Interactions

Alcohol, CNS depressants: May produce additive depressant effects. *Anticoagulants, beta-blockers, calcium-channel blockers (nifedipine, verapamil), theophylline:* Activity of these drugs may be reduced. *Anticonvulsants:* Serum concentrations of carbamazepine, valproic acid and succinimides may be reduced. Valproic acid may increase barbiturate serum levels. *Corticosteroids:* Effectiveness may be reduced. *Estrogen, estrogen-containing oral contraceptives:* May cause decreased contraceptive and estrogen effect. *Griseofulvin:* Decreased griseofulvin levels.

Lab Test Interferences

Decreased serum bilirubin concentrations, false-positive phentolamine test, decreased response to metyrapone and impaired absorption of radioactive cyanocobalamin.

Adverse Reactions

CV: Bradycardia; hypotension; syncope. *RESP:* Hypoventilation; apnea; laryngospasm; bronchospasm. *CNS:* Drowsiness; agitation; confusion; headache; hyperkinesia; ataxia; CNS depression; paradoxical excitement; nightmares; psychiatric disturbances; hallucinations; insomnia; dizziness. *GI:* Nausea; vomiting; constipation. *HEPA:* Liver damage. *HEMA:* Blood dyscrasias (eg, agranulocytosis, thrombocytopenia). *OTHER:* Hypersensitivity reactions (eg, angioedema, rashes, exfoliative dermatitis); fever; injection site reactions (eg, local pain, thrombophlebitis).

Precautions

Pregnancy: Category D. *Lactation:* Excreted in breast milk. *Children:* May respond with excitement rather than depression. *Elderly patients:* More sensitive to drug effects; dosage reduction is required. *Dependence:* Tolerance or psychological and physical dependence may occur with continued use. *IV administration:* Do not exceed maximum IV rate; respiratory depression, apnea and hypotension may result. Parenteral solutions are highly alkaline; extravasation may cause tissue damage and necrosis. Inadvertent intra-arterial injection may lead to arterial spasm, thrombosis and gangrene. *Renal or hepatic impairment:* Use drug with caution; dosage reduction may be required. *Seizure disorders:* Status epilepticus may result from abrupt discontinuation.

NURSING CONSIDERATIONS

Administration/Storage

- Give IM injections deeply into large muscle. Do not exceed maximum IM dose of 500 mg or 5 ml of volume (regardless of concentration).
- For IV administration, inject into large vein; do not exceed maximum IV rate of 50 mg/min, do not administer into artery and do not allow perivascular extravasation.
- Administer with caution to patients with history of substance abuse.
- Do not use as sleep aid for > 2 wk.
- Store parenteral form at room temperature. Do not use if discolored or if precipitate forms.
- Store suppositories in refrigerator. Do not divide.

Assessment/Interventions

- Obtain patient history, including drug history and any known allergies. Note presence of liver disease, respiratory disease and porphyria.
- Observe for common side effects such as sedation or dizziness and report to physician.
- With prolonged therapy monitor lab test results for liver, renal and hematopoietic functions.
- Monitor patient carefully during IV use for potential respiratory depression.
- Assess infants of lactating mothers and report drowsiness to physician.
- In children, monitor for possible paradoxical response of increased agitation and report to physician.
- Notify physician of signs of barbiturate intoxication: unsteady gait, slurred speech, confusion or irritability.
- Watch for behavior indicative of drug dependency such as inordinate re-

quests for more medication or need to refill prescription early.

OVERDOSAGE: SIGNS & SYMPTOMS

CNS and respiratory depression, Cheyne-Stokes respiration, areflexia, constriction of pupils, oliguria, tachycardia, hypotension, lowered body temperature, coma, apnea, circulatory collapse, respiratory arrest, death

Patient/Family Education

- Warn patient that medication may be habit forming and for this reason it is important to take medicine as directed. Taking too little or too much can have serious complications.
- Instruct patient to report these symptoms to physician: nausea, vomiting, drowsiness, dizziness, fever, sore throat, mouth sores, easy bleeding, bruising, skin irritation or exaggerated sunburn.
- Caution patient to avoid intake of alcoholic beverages or other CNS depressants.
- Advise patient that drug may cause drowsiness and to use caution while driving or performing other tasks requiring mental alertness.

See Patient Guide, p. 482.

Pentostatin (2′-Deoxycoformycin; DCF)

(PEN-toe-STAT-in)

Nipent

Class: Antineoplastic

Action Causes cytotoxicity by inhibiting enzyme adenosine deaminase, which suppresses DNA and RNA synthesis.

Indications Treatment of adults with interferon alfa–refractory hairy-cell leukemia.

Contraindications Standard considerations.

Route/Dosage

ADULTS: IV 2-4 mg/m^2 every other week. Doses should not exceed 4 mg/m^2.

Interactions

Fludarabine: Increases risk of fatal pulmonary toxicity.

Lab Test Interferences

None well documented.

Adverse Reactions

CV: Arrhythmia. *RESP:* Cough; dyspnea; sinusitis; lung disorders; bronchitis; epistaxis; pneumonia. *CNS:* Headache; fever; chills; anxiety; confusion; dizziness; paresthesia; depression; insomnia; nervousness. *EENT:* Abnormal vision; conjunctivitis; ear, eye pain; stomatitis. *GI:* Nausea; vomiting; anorexia; diarrhea; flatulence. *GU:* Increased serum creatinine; hematuria; dysuria. *HEPA:* Elevated liver test results; BUN. *HEMA:* Bleeding; myelosuppression; ecchymosis; petechiae; anemia; thrombocytopenia. *DERM:* Rash; pruritus; skin discoloration; sweating. *META:* Weight loss. *OTHER:* Infection; lymphadenopathy; myalgia; arthralgia; hypersensitivity reactions; increased uric acid.

Precautions

Pregnancy: Category D. *Lactation:* Undetermined. *Children:* Safety and efficacy not established. *Myelosuppression:* Myelosuppression can occur; may increase risk of infection. *Renal toxicity:* Elevations in serum creatinine may occur; patients with renal function impairment may be treated with lower doses. *Rashes:* Can be severe; may worsen with continued treatment.

NURSING CONSIDERATIONS

Administration/Storage

- Wear protective clothing, including polyethylene gloves, during preparation, administration and disposal.
- Administer antiemetics 30-60 min before giving drug. Give prophylactic antibodies as ordered.
- Administer by IV only. May be given by IV bolus or diluted in a larger volume and given over 20-30 min.
- Hydrate with D5W in 0.5 normal saline before administration. Follow with additional 500 ml of fluid.
- Store reconstituted medication at room temperature and ambient light no longer than 8 hours.
- Follow procedures for proper handling and disposal of anticancer drugs.

Assessment/Interventions

- Obtain patient history, including drug history and any known allergies.
- Assess serum creatinine level and creatinine clearance before therapy starts.
- Assess CBC and serum creatinine before each dose of pentostatin and at appropriate periods during therapy.
- Monitor lab results for anemia, leukopenia or thrombocytopenia before and during therapy.
- Assess for extravasation at infusion site.
- Assess patient for rash, fatigue, pain, nausea and vomiting and infection during therapy.
- Withhold drug if severe rash or symptoms of CNS toxicity develop, or if acute infection develops. Temporarily withhold therapy if absolute neutrophil count falls below 200 cells/mm^3 in patient with initial count > 500 cells/mm^3 and resume therapy when cell count returns to pre-dose levels.

OVERDOSAGE: SIGNS & SYMPTOMS

Renal, hepatic, pulmonary and CNS toxicity

Patient/Family Education

- Inform patient that there is no optimal duration of treatment. In absence of toxicity, treatment will continue until response to leukemia is complete–up to 6 months.
- Explain that hair loss may occur.
- Advise patient to avoid crowds and other sources of potential infection.
- Tell patient to report all side effects and potential adverse reactions to physician.

See Patient Guide, p. 483.

Pentoxifylline

(pen-TOX-IH-fill-in)

Trental

Class: Hemorheologic

Action Improves blood flow by decreasing blood viscosity.

Indications Intermittent claudication on basis of chronic occlusive arterial disease of limbs. **Unlabeled uses:** Treatment of psychopathological symptoms in patients with cerebrovascular insufficiency; treatment of diabetic angiopathies; reduction of incidence of stroke in patients with recurrent TIAs.

Contraindications Intolerance to methylxanthines (ie, caffeine, theophylline); recent cerebral or retinal hemorrhage.

Route/Dosage

ADULTS: PO 400 mg controlled-release tablet tid with meals for at least 8 weeks.

Interactions

Cimetidine: Effects of pentoxifylline may be increased.

Lab Test Interferences

None well documented.

Adverse Reactions

CV: Angina; edema; hypotension; dyspnea; arrhythmia; tachycardia. *RESP:* Flu-like symptoms; laryngitis. *CNS:* Dizziness; insomnia; headache; tremor; anxiety; confusion. *EENT:* Blurred vision; conjunctivitis; nosebleed; bad taste; excessive salivation; sore throat. *GI:* Dyspepsia; nausea; vomiting; belching; flatus; bloating; dry mouth. *HEPA:* Hepatitis; jaundice. *HEMA:* Leukopenia; pancytopenia; purpura; thrombocytopenia; decreased serum fibrinogen. *DERM:* Brittle fingernails; pruritus; rash; flushing; urticaria.

Precautions

Pregnancy: Category C. *Lactation:* Excreted in breast milk. *Children:* Safety and efficacy for children < 18 yr not established. *Renal impairment:* Drug may accumulate, producing toxicity; lower dose may be necessary.

NURSING CONSIDERATIONS

Administration/Storage

- Give medication with meals.
- Reduced dosage may be needed if adverse GI or CNS effects develop.
- Store at room temperature in a tightly closed, light-resistant container.

Assessment/Interventions

- Obtain patient history, including drug history and any known allergies.
- Carefully assess for risk of hemorrhage (ie, recent surgery or peptic ulcer), and monitor PT/PTT and Hgb/Hct for indications of bleeding.
- Assess baseline BUN and creatinine, and monitor throughout therapy.
- Monitor patients taking pentoxifylline and anticoagulants for bleeding or changes in PT.

OVERDOSAGE: SIGNS & SYMPTOMS

Symptoms appear to be dose related. They usually occur 4-5 hours after ingestion and last about 12 hours. Symptoms include flushing, hypotension, nervousness, agitation, tremors, convulsions, somnolence, loss of consciousness, fever and agitation. Transient (< 24 hr) bradycardia with first- or second-degree atrioventricular block may be seen

Patient/Family Education

- Explain that improvement in symptoms may take 2-4 wk to notice and up to 8 wk for maximum relief.
- Explain importance of follow-up lab work for patients with high risk of bleeding or taking anticoagulant.
- In patients with occlusive peripheral vasospastic disorders, emphasize use of self-help measures to augment drug therapy (eg, exercise, weight control, no smoking, etc.).
- Review specifics of good foot care, including bathing of feet daily in lukewarm water and drying thoroughly, applying lanolin to feet after bathing, use of lambs wool between toes and feet, avoidance of extremes in temperature, wearing of clean cotton socks daily.
- Instruct patient to report these symptoms to physician: dizziness, chest pain, fainting, excessive bruising or abnormal bleeding.
- Advise patient that drug may cause dizziness and to use caution while driving or performing other tasks requiring mental alertness.

See Patient Guide, p. 484.

Pergolide Mesylate

(PURR-go-lide MEH-sih-LATE)

Permax

Class: Antiparkinson

Action Directly stimulates postsynaptic dopamine receptors in nigrostriatal system.

Indications Adjunctive treatment to levodopa-carbidopa in management of Parkinson's disease.

Contraindications Hypersensitivity to ergot derivatives.

Route/Dosage
Administer in divided doses tid. ADULTS: PO 0.05 mg/day first 2 days. Gradually increase dose by 0.1-0.15 mg/day q 3 days over next 12 days. Dose may then be increased by 0.25 mg/day q 3 days until optimum therapeutic dosage is achieved (mean therapeutic dose is 3 mg/day; maximum 5 mg/day). During titration cautiously decrease levodopa-carbidopa (average daily concurrent dose is 650 mg/day of levodopa).

Interactions *Dopamine antagonists (eg, butyrophenones, metoclopramide, neuroleptics, phenothiazines, thioxanthines)*: May diminish effectiveness of pergolide.

Lab Test Interferences
None well documented.

Adverse Reactions
CV: Orthostatic hypotension; vasodilation; palpitations; hypotension; syncope; hypertension; arrhythmia; MI. *RESP*: Rhinitis; shortness of breath; epistaxis; hiccoughs. *CNS*: Dyskinesia; dizziness; hallucinations; dystonia; confusion; somnolence; insomnia; anxiety; personality disorder; psychosis; extrapyramidal syndrome; incoordination; akinesia; hypertonia; neuralgia. *EENT*: Abnormal vision; diplopia; glaucoma; eye hemorrhage; photophobia; visual field defect; taste perversion. *GI*: Nausea; constipation; diarrhea; dyspepsia; anorexia; dry mouth; vomiting. *GU*: Hematuria. *DERM*: Rash; sweating. *OTHER*: Pains; accidental injury; flu syndrome; chills; peripheral edema; facial edema; edema; weight gain; anemia; bursitis; myalgia; twitching.

Precautions
Pregnancy: Category B. *Lactation*: Unknown. *Children*: Safety and efficacy not established. *Carcinogenesis*: Uterine neoplasia has been observed with high doses of pergolide in animal models and was probably a result of prolactin inhibition. *Cardiac arrhythmias*: Exercise caution in patients with arrhythmias because of possible atrial premature contractions and sinus tachycardia. *Hallucinosis*: Hallucinations may occur in some patients. *Symptomatic hypotension*: Either symptomatic or orthostatic hypotension may occur, especially during initial treatment. With gradual titration, tolerance to hypotension usually develops.

NURSING CONSIDERATIONS

Administration/Storage
- Administer in divided doses 3 times per day.
- Store at room temperature.

Assessment/Interventions
- Obtain patient history, including drug history and any known allergies. Note reports of syncope, irregular heart beats or palpitations.
- If symptomatic orthostatic or sustained hypotension occur, take safety precautions. As dosage is gradually titrated, tolerance to hypotension usually develops.
- Provide regular ophthalmic exams.

OVERDOSAGE: SIGNS & SYMPTOMS
Vomiting, hypotension, agitation, hallucinations, involuntary movements and tingling of extremities, palpitations, ventricular extrasystoles

Patient/Family Education
- Inform patient of risk of hypotension and teach safety measures to prevent falls from orthostatic hypotension (eg, dangling legs before getting out of bed, gradually rising from chairs).
- Instruct patient to report these symptoms to physician: symptomatic or-

thostatic or sustained hypotension, hallucinations, dyskinesia, somnolence, insomnia, nausea, constipation, diarrhea, dyspepsia and rhinitis.

- Tell patient to take sips of water frequently or suck on ice chips or sugarless hard candy or chew sugarless gum if dry mouth occurs.
- Advise patient that drug may cause drowsiness and to use caution while driving or performing other tasks requiring mental alertness.

See Patient Guide, p. 485.

Perphenazine

(per-FEN-uh-zeen)

Trilafon, Trilafon Concentrate

Class: Antipsychotic/phenothiazine; antiemetic

Action Effects apparently caused by postsynaptic dopamine receptor blockade in CNS.

Indications Management of psychotic disorders; control of severe nausea/vomiting; intractable hiccoughs in adults. **Unlabeled uses:** Treatment of Tourette's syndrome; control of acute agitation in elderly; useful in controlling some symptoms of dementia such as agitation, hyperactivity, hallucinations, suspiciousness, hostility and uncooperative behaviors; treatment of hemiballismus (violent writhing/movement of one side of body).

Contraindications Comatose or severely depressed states; allergy to any phenothiazine; presence of large amounts of other CNS depressants; bone marrow depression or blood dyscrasias; liver damage; subcortical brain damage.

Route/Dosage

Psychiatric

ADULT: **PO** 4-64 mg/day, usually in divided doses.

Nausea/Vomiting/Hiccoughs

ADULTS: **PO** 8-16 mg/day in divided doses. (Elderly and debilitated patients should be given lower doses. Administer ⅓ to ½ adult dose.) CHILDREN > 12 YR. May be given lowest limit of adult dosage.

IM

Doses range from 5-10 mg/injection, usually given q 6 hr. Do not exceed 30 mg/day. Administer by deep injection to seated or recumbent patient. IM administration usually reserved for instances in which patient is unwilling or unable to take oral medication.

Oral Liquid Concentrate and IV Form

See Administration/Storage.

Interactions

Alcohol: May result in increased CNS depression and may precipitate extrapyramidal reaction. *Anticholinergics:* May reduce therapeutic effects of perphenazine and worsen anticholinergic effects. Concomitant administration may worsen schizophrenic symptoms and lead to tardive dyskinesia (see Precautions). *Barbiturate anesthetics:* Frequency and severity of neuromuscular excitation and hypotension may increase. *Guanethidine:* Hypotensive action of guanethidine may be inhibited. *Metrizamide:* Possibility of seizure may be increased when subarachnoid metrizamide injection is used.

Lab Test Interferences

May discolor urine pink to red-brown. False-positive pregnancy tests may occur but are less likely to occur with serum test. Increases in protein-bound iodine have been reported.

Adverse Reactions

CV: Orthostatic hypotension; hypertension; tachycardia; bradycardia; syncope; cardiac arrest; circulatory collapse; lightheadedness; faintness; dizziness; ECG changes. *RESP:* Laryngospasm; bronchospasm; dyspnea. *CNS:*

Pseudoparkinsonism dystonia; dyskinesia, motor restlessness; oculogyric crisis; dystonias; hyperreflexia; tardive dyskinesia; drowsiness; headache; fatigue; abnormalities of the cerebrospinal fluid proteins; paradoxical excitement or exacerbation of psychotic symptoms; catatonic-like states; weakness; tremor; paranoid reactions; lethargy; seizures; hyperactivity; nocturnal confusion; bizarre dreams; vertigo; insomnia. *EENT:* Pigmentary retinopathy; glaucoma; photophobia; blurred vision; mydriasis; increased intraocular pressure; dry mouth or throat; nasal congestion. *GI:* Dyspepsia; adynamic ileus (may result in death); nausea; vomiting; constipation. *GU:* Urinary hesitancy or retention; impotence; sexual dysfunction; menstrual irregularities. *HEPA:* Jaundice. *HEMA:* Agranulocytosis; eosinophilia; leukopenia; hemolytic anemia; thrombocytopenic purpura. *DERM:* Photosensitvity; skin pigmentation; dry skin; exfoliative dermatitis; urticarial rash; maculopapular hypersensitivity reaction; seborrhea; eczema. *META:* Hyperglycemia; hypoglycemia; decreased cholesterol. *OTHER:* Increases in appetite and weight; polydipsia; breast enlargement; galactorrhea; increased prolactin levels.

Precautions

Pregnancy: Pregnancy category undetermined. *Lactation:* Undetermined. *Children:* Not recommended in children < 12 yr. *Elderly:* More susceptible to effects; consider lower dose. *Special risk patients:* Use caution in patients with cardiovascular disease or mitral insufficiency, history of glaucoma, EEG abnormalities or seizure disorders, prior brain damage, hepatic or renal impairment. *Antiemetic effects:* Because of suppression of cough reflex, aspiration of vomitus possible. *CNS effects:* May impair mental or physical abilities, especially during first few days of therapy. *Hepatic effects:* Jaundice usually occurs between second and fourth weeks of treatment; considered hypersensitivity reaction. Usually reversible. *Neuroleptic malignant syndrome:* Has occurred with agents of this class; is potentially fatal. Signs and symptoms are hyperpyrexia, muscle rigidity, altered mental status, irregular pulse, irregular blood pressure, tachycardia and diaphoresis. *Pulmonary:* Cases of bronchopneumonia, some fatal, have occurred. *Sudden death:* Has been reported; predisposing factors may be seizures or previous brain damage. Flare-ups of psychotic behavior may precede death. *Tardive dyskinesia:* Syndrome of potentially irreversible involuntary body and facial movements may develop. Prevalence highest in elderly, especially women. Use smallest effective doses for shortest possible time period.

NURSING CONSIDERATIONS

Administration/Storage

- Administer tablets with meals or with full glass of milk or water.

Oral Liquid Concentrate

- Dilute just prior to administration in 60 ml of one of following diluents: water, saline, homogenized milk, carbonated orange beverage, and pineapple, apricot, prune, orange, V-8, tomato or grapefruit juices.
- Do not mix with caffeinated beverages or with drinks containing tannins (tea) or pectinates (apple juice), because physical incompatibilities may occur.
- Shake concentrate before use.
- Dilute each 5 ml of concentrate with at least 60 ml of fluid.
- Protect from light; store at room temperature.

IV

- Give as diluted solution by fractional injection of slow-drip infusion. Slow infusion method is preferred for surgical patients.
- Dilute solution to 0.5 mg/ml (1 ml mixed with 9 ml of saline solution)

and give ≤ 1 mg per injection at not less than 1-2 min intervals. Do not exceed 5 mg.
- Administer injectable form by deep IM to sitting or recumbent patients.
- Protect from light.

Assessment/Interventions
- Obtain patient history, including drug history and any known allergies.
- Monitor for potential signs of pseudoparkinsonism, dystonia, dyskinesia or akathisia and report to physician.
- Monitor for evidence of tardive dyskinesia (involuntary dyskinetic movements of tongue, lip, mouth, face or jaw), and report to physician.
- Be alert for evidence of orthostatic hypotension; take orthostatic blood pressures, and report to physician.
- Report any significant unexplained temperature increase to physician.
- When coadministering anticholinergic drugs, be alert for possible decreased therapeutic effects of perphenazine and increased anticholinergic effects.

OVERDOSAGE: SIGNS & SYMPTOMS

CNS depression, hypotension, extrapyramidal symptoms, agitation, convulsions, fever, hypothermia, ECG changes, cardiac arrhythmias

Patient/Family Education
- Instruct patient to report these symptoms to physician: dizziness, drooling, restlessness, tremors, stiffness, muscle spasms or involuntary face, tongue, mouth or lip movements.
- Caution patient to avoid sudden position changes to prevent orthostatic hypotension.
- Instruct patient to avoid intake of alcoholic beverages or other CNS depressants.
- Advise patient to use caution driving or performing other tasks requiring mental alertness.
- Caution patient to avoid exposure to sunlight and to use sunscreen or wear protective clothing to avoid photosensitivity reaction.

See Patient Guide, p. 486.

Perphenazine/ Amitriptyline

(per-FEN-uh-zeen/am-ee-TRIP-tih-leen)

Triavil, Etrafon, ♣ *PMS-Levazine*

Class: Psychotherapeutic combination

Action Amitriptyline blocks reuptake of serotonin and norepinephrine in CNS. Perphenazine appears to block postsynaptic dopamine receptors.

Indications Treatment of moderate to severe anxiety or agitation and depressed mood; moderate to severe depression and anxiety associated with chronic physical disease; treatment of patients in whom depression and anxiety cannot be clearly differentiated; treatment of schizophrenia with associated depression.

Contraindications Hypersensitivity to phenothiazines; depression of CNS due to drugs (eg, barbiturates, alcohol, narcotics, analgesics, antihistamines); bone marrow depression; hypersensitivity to tricyclic antidepressant. Should not be given concomitantly with MAO inhibitors, suspected or established subcortical brain damage. Not recommended for use during acute recovery phases of myocardial infarction.

Route/Dosage

ADULTS: PO Initially, usual dose is 2-4 mg perphenazine with 10-50 mg amitriptyline tid-qid.

Interactions

Alcohol: May result in increased CNS depression and may precipitate extrapyramidal reaction. *Amphetamines:* May antagonize antipsychotic effects of perphenazine. *Anticholinergics:* May reduce therapeutic effects of perphenazine and worsen anticholinergic effects. Concomitant administration may worsen schizophrenic symptoms and lead to tardive dyskinesia. *Barbiturate anesthetics:* Frequency and severity of neuromuscular excitation and hypotension may increase. *Barbiturates, carbamazepine, charcoal:* May cause decreased amitriptyline blood levels. *Cimetidine, fluoxetine, haloperidol, oral contraceptives:* May cause increased amitriptyline blood levels. *Clonidine:* May result in hypertensive crisis. *CNS depressants:* Depressant effects may be addictive. *Guanethidine:* Hypotensive action may be inhibited. *Lithium:* Possible neurotoxicity with perphenazine and may increase effects of amitriptyline. *MAO inhibitors:* Do NOT use this product with MAO inhibitors as hyperpyretic crisis, severe convulsions and death may result. When switching from MAO inhibitors, wait 14 days and initiate with low doses, increasing dosage gradually until desired response is achieved. *Metrizamide:* Seizure risk may be increased. *Sympathomimetics:* Increased pressor effects.

Lab Test Interferences

May discolor urine pink to red-brown. False positive pregnancy test results may occur, but are less likely to occur with serum test. Increases in protein bound iodine have been reported.

Adverse Reactions

CV: Orthostatic hypotension; hypertension; tachycardia; bradycardia; syncope; cardiac arrest; circulatory collapse; arrhythmias; lightheadedness; faintness; dizziness; EKG changes; palpitations. *RESP:* Laryngospasm; bronchospasm; dyspnea; cough. *CNS:* Sedation; neurologic impairments; extrapyramidal symptoms (eg, pseudoparkinsonism); dystonia; dyskinesia, motor restlessness; oculogyric crisis; opisthotonos; hyperreflexia; tardive dyskinesia; drowsiness; headache; weakness; anxiety; agitation; mania; exacerberation of psychosis; dizziness; tremor; fatigue; slurring of speech; insomnia; vertigo, seizures; abnormalities of CSF proteins; paradoxical excitement or exacerbation of psychotic symptoms; catatonic-like states; paranoid reactions; lethargy; hyperactivity; nocturnal confusion; bizarre dreams. *EENT:* Pigmentary retinopathy; glaucoma; photophobia; rhinitis; pharyngitis; tinnitus; blurred vision; nasal congestion; mydriasis; increased IOP. *GI:* Dyspepsia; adynamic ileus (may cause death); constipation; nausea; vomiting; anorexia; diarrhea; peculiar taste; dry mouth or throat. *GU:* Urinary hesitancy or retention; impotence; sexual dysfunction; menstrual irregularities; nocturia. *HEMA:* Agranulocytosis; eosinophilia; leukopenia; hemolytic anemia; thrombocytopenic purpura. *HEPA:* Jaundice. *DERM:* Photosensitvity reaction; skin pigmentation; dry skin; exfoliative dermatitis; urticarial rash; maculopapular hypersensitivity reaction; seborrhea; eczema; acne; pruritus. *META:* Hyperglycemia; hypoglycemia. *OTHER:* Increases in appetite and weight; polydipsia; breast enlargement; galactorrhea; increased prolactin levels.

Precautions

Pregnancy: Safety not established. *Lactation:* Safety not established. *Elderly:* More susceptible to adverse effects. *Special risk patients:* Use caution in patients with cardiovascular disease or mitral insufficiency, history of glaucoma, EEG abnormalities or seizure disorders, prior brain damage, hepatic or renal impairment. *CNS effects:* May impair mental or physical abilities, especially during first few days of therapy. *Neuroleptic malignant syndrome (NMS):* Has occurred with agents of this class; is potentially fatal. Signs and symptoms are hyperpyrexia, muscle rigidity, altered mental status, irregular pulse, irregular blood pressure, tachycardia and diaphoresis. *Sudden death:* Has been reported; predisposing factors may be seizures or previous brain damage. Flare-up of psychotic behavior may precede death. *Tardive dyskinesia:* Syndrome of potentially irreversible involuntary body and facial movements may develop. Prevalence highest in elderly, especially women. Use smallest effective doses for shortest time possible.

NURSING CONSIDERATIONS

Administration/Storage

- Administer oral medication with meals or with full glass of milk or water.
- Oral concentrate should be used in hospital setting only and diluted with water, milk, fruit juice, soup, saline or lemon-lime carbonated soft drink.
- Store tablets in tightly covered, light-resistant container.

Assessment/Interventions

- Obtain patient history, including drug history and any known allergies.
- Monitor blood cell counts with differential, hepatic, and renal function studies, ECG and ophthalmic status throughout therapy.
- Monitor for jaundice. If present, notify physician immediately.
- Monitor for potential signs of pseudoparkinsonism, dystonia, dyskinesia or akathisia and report to physician.
- Monitor for evidence of tardive dyskinesia, (involuntary dyskinetic movements of tongue, lips, mouth, face or jaw) and report to physician.
- Assess for signs of orthostatic hypotension; take orthostatic blood pressures and report to physician.
- Report any significant unexplained temperature increase to physician.

OVERDOSAGE: SIGNS & SYMPTOMS

Confusion, tachycardia, visual hallucinations, sedation, hypothermia, arrhythmias, congestive heart failure, dilated pupils, seizures, hypotension, coma, hyperpyrexia, muscle rigidity, hyperactive reflexes, death

Patient/Family Education

- Instruct patient to avoid intake of alcoholic beverages or other CNS depressants.
- Tell patient to use caution in driving or operating machinery.
- Advise patient that the medication may take days to weeks before having a full effect.
- Instruct patient to avoid becoming overheated.
- Caution patient to avoid exposure to sunlight and to use sunscreen or wear protective clothing to minimize photosensitivity reaction.
- Teach patient to change position slowly if dizziness occurs.
- Instruct patient to take sips of water frequently, suck on ice chips or sugarless hard candy or chew sugarless gum if dry mouth occurs.
- Instruct patient to report these symptoms to physician: dizziness, drooling, restlessness, tremors, stiffness or muscle spasms.
- Instruct patient to report involuntary face, tongue, mouth or lip movements to physician.
- Explain that urine may turn reddish brown.

See Patient Guide, p. 487.

Phenazopyridine HCl

(fen-AZZ-oh-PIH-rih-deen HIGH-droe-KLOR-ide)

Azo-Standard, Baridium, Eridium, Geridium, Phenazodine, Pyridiate, Pyridium, Urodine, Urogesic, ♣ *Phenazo*

Class: Urinary tract product/analgesic

Action Exerts topical analgesic effect on urinary tract mucosa.

Indications Symptomatic relief of pain, burning, urgency, frequency and other discomforts arising from irritation of lower urinary tract mucosa.

Contraindications Renal insufficiency.

Route/Dosage
ADULTS: **PO** 200 mg tid. CHILDREN (6-12 YR): **PO** 12 mg/kg/24 hr divided into three doses for 2 days.

Interactions None well documented.

Lab Test Interferences
Possible interference with colorimetric lab test procedures and urinalysis based on spectrometry or color reactions.

Adverse Reactions
CNS: Headache. *GI:* Occasional GI disturbances. *GU:* Renal toxicity. *HEMA:* Methemoglobinemia; hemolytic anemia. *HEPA:* Hepatotoxicity. *DERM:* Rash; pruritus. *OTHER:* Anaphylactoid reaction.

Precautions
Pregnancy: Category B. *Lactation:* Unknown. *Renal impairment:* May lead to accumulation, indicated by yellow tinge to skin and sclera.

NURSING CONSIDERATIONS

Administration/Storage

- Administer after meals to avoid GI irritation.
- If patient has renal impairment, dosage reduction may be required.
- If being taken concomitantly with antibiotics for urinary tract infection, this medicine should be taken for only 2 days (6 doses).
- Do not crush tablets or make into a suspension.
- Store at room temperature in a tightly closed container.

Assessment/Interventions

- Obtain patient history, including drug history and any known allergies.
- Obtain BUN and creatinine to assess for renal dysfunction.

OVERDOSAGE: SIGNS & SYMPTOMS

Methemoglobinemia, hemolytic anemia, hemolysis, renal and hepatic impairment and failure

Patient/Family Education

- Inform patient that this drug should not be taken long term for undiagnosed urinary tract pain.
- Advise patient to take drug after meals to avoid GI upset.
- Inform patient that urine may temporarily become reddish-orange in color and may stain fabric.
- Advise patient to wear glasses instead of contact lens while taking this drug; contact lens may become discolored.
- Inform patients with diabetes of possible interference with urine glucose test results.
- Instruct patient not to crush or chew tablets. Permanent teeth discoloration may occur.
- Instruct patient that if skin or sclera become yellowish in color, to discontinue drug and notify physician.
- Instruct patient to notify physician if headache, rash, pruritus, upset stomach, dizziness or difficulty breathing occurs.

See Patient Guide, p. 488.

Phenelzine Sulfate

(FEN-uhl-zeen SULL-fate)

Nardil

Class: Antidepressant/MAO inhibitor

Action Phenelzine blocks activity of enzyme MAO, thereby increasing monoamine (eg, epinephrine, norepinephrine, serotonin) concentrations in CNS.

Indications Treatment of "atypical" ("nonendogenous" or "neurotic") depression; management of depression in patients unresponsive to other antidepressant drugs. **Unlabeled uses:** Treatment of bulimia; treatment of cocaine addiction; control of panic disorder with agoraphobia.

Contraindications Hypersensitivity to MAO inhibitors; pheochromocytoma; CHF; abnormal liver function; history of liver disease; severe renal impairment; cerebrovascular defect; concurrent use of dextromethorphan or CNS depressants (eg, alcohol); sympathomimetic drugs (eg, amphetamine, dopamine, norepinephrine) or related drugs (eg, methyldopa); cardiovascular disease.

Route/Dosage

ADULTS: **PO** 15 mg tid initially; may titrate up to 90 mg/day. Elderly should receive no more than 60 mg daily. After maximum benefit is achieved, dose can be slowly decreased over several weeks to maintenance dose. Doses as low as 15 mg q od may be used for maintenance.

Interactions

Amine-containing foods: May cause severe hypertension or hemorrhagic strokes. *Anorexiants:* May cause exaggerated pharmacologic effects (eg, severe headaches, hypertension, hyperpyrexia) of anorexiants (amphetamines and related compounds). *CNS depressants:* May enhance CNS effects. *Dextromethorphan:* Concurrent use has been associated with severe reactions (hyperpyrexia, hypotension, death). *Fluoxetine, paroxetine, sertraline trazodone:* Although data are limited, interactions comparable to those of the tricyclic antidepressants and phenelzine may occur. *Guanethidine:* MAO inhibitors may antagonize the antihypertensive effect. *Insulin, sulfonylureas:* May enhance hypoglycemic action. *Levodopa:* May cause hypertensive reactions. *Meperidine:* May lead to severe reactions, including hypotension, convulsions, respiratory depression and vascular collapse. *Sympathomimetics:* May cause severe headache, hypertensive crisis and hyperpyrexia. *Tricyclic antidepressants, buspirone, cyclobenzaprine, carbamazepine, maprotiline, guanethidine, CNS stimulants, tyramine.* May lead to potentially fatal reactions, including seizures and hypertensive crisis; mental status changes, hyperthermia.

Lab Test Interferences

None well documented.

Adverse Reactions

CV: Orthostatic hypotension; edema; hypertensive crisis. *CNS:* Dizziness; headache; sleep disturbances; tremors; hyperflexemia; manic symptoms; convulsions; toxic delirium; coma. *EENT:* Blurred vision; glaucoma. *GI:* Constipation; nausea; GI disturbances; anorexia. *GU:* Sexual dysfunction; urinary retention; incontinence. *HEMA:* Anemia; leukopenia; agranulocytosis; thrombocytopenia. *HEPA:* Fatal progressive necrotizing hepatocellular damage; elevated serum transaminases; hepatitis. *DERM:* Rash; sweating; photosensitivity. *META:* Weight gain; hypermetabolic syndrome (eg, fever, tachycardia, rapid breathing, rigidity, metabolism, acidosis, coma); hypernatremia. *OTHER:* Transient respiratory and circulatory depression following electroconvulsive therapy.

Precautions

Pregnancy: Category C. *Lactation:* Undetermined. *Children:* Not recommended in patients < 16 yr. *Elderly patients:* Drug should be used cautiously in patients > 60 yr because of possibility of existing cerebral sclerosis with damaged vessels. If hypertension develops, the risk of stroke may be increased. *Depression associated with drug abuse/alcoholism:* Use with caution; increased risk of serious drug interactions. *Epilepsy:* May lower seizure threshold. *Diabetes:* May alter glucose control. *Hypotension:* Orthostatic hypotension is significant side effect and may lead to falling and changes in heart rate. *Pyridoxine:* Phenelzine may cause pyridoxine deficiency, with symptoms of numbness, paresthesias and edema. Supplements may be required. *Suicidal patients:* Strict supervision may be necessary in patients at risk.

NURSING CONSIDERATIONS

Administration/Storage

- Tablets may be crushed if patient is unable to swallow them whole.
- Give no more than 60 mg/day to elderly.
- Do not administer several days before surgery. If possible, discontinue 7-14 days before elective surgery.
- Wait 14 days after discontinuing tricyclic antidepressants, other MAO inhibitors, carbamazepine, maprotiline, guanethidine, paroxetine, sertraline cyclobenzaprine or CNS stimulants to administer this medication. Wait 5 wk after discontinuing fluoxetine before starting phenelzine.
- Do not administer unless patient has been on tyramine-free diet for at least 2-3 days. Continue on this diet for 2 wk after discontinuation of MAOI.
- Store in tightly closed container and protect from heat and light.

Assessment/Interventions

- Obtain patient history, including drug history and any known allergies. Note CHF, cardiovascular disease, cerebrovascular disease, hypertension, abnormal liver or renal function, pheochromocytoma or severe headaches.
- Monitor patient's lying and standing BP before initiating therapy.
- Monitor liver function if jaundice or other signs of liver dysfunction occur, discontinue drug and notify physician.
- Obtain baseline CBC and liver function tests.
- During initial therapy, monitor BP and pulse.
- Monitor I&O carefully until dosage is stabilized.
- Observe for onset of therapeutic effect (ie, improved mood, improved sleep patterns, socialization) in depressed patients in 7-14 days and full response in up to 6 wk.
- Continue to monitor potentially suicidal patients until they demonstrate definite significant, lasting improvement.
- Be alert for evidence of orthostatic hypotension, monitor orthostatic BP and report to physician.
- Monitor for signs of hypertensive crisis (high BP, severe headache, palpitations, severe chest pain, sweating, nausea and vomiting, dilated pupils, photophobia). If signs occur, discontinue drug and notify physician. Have readily available alpha-adrenergic blocking agent (eg, phentolamine) to lower BP and external cooling mechanisms for hyperpyrexia.
- Monitor blood sugars of patients receiving insulin or other antidiabetic agents; coadministration may enhance hypoglycemic effect.

OVERDOSAGE: SIGNS & SYMPTOMS

Excitement, hypotension, dizziness, movement disorders, irritability, insomnia, weakness, severe headache, anxiety, restlessness, drowsiness, coma, convulsions, flushing, hypertension, sweating, tachypnea, acidosis, hyperpyrexia, tachycardia, cardiorespiratory arrest, incoherence, agitation, mental confusion, shock

Patient/Family Education

- Inform patient that it may be 4 wk before improvement in mood is noticed.
- Instruct patient that antidepressant medications will not make him or her high or elevate mood; antidepressants restore depressed people to normal state.
- Instruct patient to avoid sudden position changes to prevent orthostatic hypotension.
- Instruct patient that it is important to consult physician before taking any medication and that it is especially important that he/she avoids otc cold, hay fever or weight reduction preparations.
- Instruct patient to avoid tyramine- or tryptophan-containing foods while taking drug and for 2 wk after discontinuing medication. These are protein foods that are aged or fermented and include cheeses, pickled herring, liver, hard sausage (eg, Genoa salami or pepperoni), pods of broad beans, beer, red wine, yeast extract, yogurt, ginseng, soy sauce, bananas, raisins and avocados. Advise patient to consult dietitian.
- Instruct patient to ingest caffeine and chocolate in moderation.
- Advise patient to weigh self 2-3 times weekly and report unusual gains.
- Instruct patient to stop taking phenelzine and to notify physician immediately if severe headache, severe chest pain, change in heart rate, photophobia, increased sweating, nausea and vomiting or stiff or sore neck occurs.
- Advise patient not to use alcohol or any abuse drug.
- Advise patient that drug may cause drowsiness and to use caution while driving or performing other tasks requiring mental alertness.

See Patient Guide, p. 489.

Phenobarbital

(fee-no-BAR-bih-tahl)

Phenobarbital

Solfoton

Phenobarbital Sodium

Luminal Sodium

Class: Sedative and hypnotic/barbiturate/anticonvulsant

Action Depresses sensory cortex, decreases motor activity, alters cerebellar function and produces drowsiness, sedation and hypnosis.

Indications Short-term treatment of insomnia; long-term treatment of generalized tonic-clonic and cortical focal seizures; emergency control of acute convulsions; preanesthetic sedation. **Unlabeled uses:** Treatment of febrile seizures in children; treatment and prevention of hyperbilirubinemia in neonates; management of chronic cholestasis.

Contraindications Hypersensitivity to barbiturates; history of addiction to sedative/hypnotic drugs; history of porphyria; severe liver impairment; respiratory disease with dyspnea; nephritic patients.

Route/Dosage

Insomnia

ADULTS: **PO/IM/IV** 100-320 mg.

Sedation

ADULTS: **PO** 30-120 mg/day in 2-3 divided doses.

Epilepsy

ADULTS: **PO** 60-250 mg/day.

Convulsions
ADULTS: **IV** 100-320 mg. Repeat if needed (maximum 600 mg/24 hr).

Status Epilepticus
ADULTS: **IV** 10-20 mg/kg. Repeat if needed. CHILDREN: **IV** 15-20 mg/kg over 10-15 min.

Preoperative Sedation
CHILDREN: **PO/IM/IV** 1-3 mg/kg.

Anticonvulsant
CHILDREN: **IM/IV** 4-6 mg/kg/day. For 10 days, then adjust to blood level. Alternatively, use IM/IV 10-15 mg/kg/day to reach therapeutic level more quickly. Maximum IV rate 60 mg/min. Maximum adult IM dose 500 mg or 5 ml volume regardless of concentration.

Interactions

Alcohol, CNS depressants: May enhance CNS depressant effects. *Anticoagulants (eg, warfarin), beta-blockers (eg, metoprolol, propranolol), doxycycline, metronidazole, quinidine, theophyllines, verapamil:* Activity of these drugs may be reduced. *Anticonvulsants:* Serum concentrations of carbamazepine, valproic acid and succinimides may be reduced. Valproic acid may increase barbiturate serum levels. *Corticosteroids:* May reduce effectiveness of corticosteroids. *Estrogens, estrogen-containing oral contraceptives:* May reduce contraceptive effectiveness. *Phenytoin:* May increase phenobarbital levels while phenytoin levels may increase or decrease.

Lab Test Interferences

May cause decreased serum bilirubin concentrations; false-positive phentolamine test results; decreased response to metyrapone; impaired absorption of radioactive cyanocobalamin.

Adverse Reactions

CV: Bradycardia; hypotension; syncope. *RESP:* Hypoventilation; apnea; laryngospasm; bronchospasm. *CNS:* Drowsiness; agitation; confusion; anxiety; headache; hyperkinesia; ataxia; CNS depression; paradoxical excitement; nightmares; psychiatric disturbances; hallucinations; insomnia; dizziness. *GI:* Nausea; vomiting; constipation. *HEMA:* Blood dyscrasias (eg, agranulocytosis, thrombocytopenia). *HEPA:* Liver damage. *OTHER:* Hypersensitivity reactions (eg, angioedema, rashes, exfoliative dermatitis); fever; injection site reactions (eg, local pain, thrombophlebitis).

Precautions

Pregnancy: Category D. *Lactation:* Excreted in breast milk. *Children:* May respond with excitement rather than depression. *Elderly patients:* More sensitive to drug effects; dosage reduction is required. *Debilitated patients:* Use drug with extreme caution. *Abuse:* Administer drug with caution to patients with history of drug abuse. *Dependence:* Tolerance or psychologic and physical dependence may occur with continued use. *Renal or hepatic impairment:* Use drug with caution; dosage reduction may be required. *Seizure disorders:* Status epilepticus may result from abrupt discontinuation.

NURSING CONSIDERATIONS

Administration/Storage

- For oral administration, tablets may be crushed and mixed with fluid or food.
- For IM administration, inject deeply into large muscle. Do not exceed maximum IM dose of 500 mg or 5 ml of volume (regardless of concentration).
- For IV administration, inject into large vein. Do not exceed maximum IV rate of 60 mg/min; respiratory depression, apnea and hypotension may result.
- Do not base IV administration on response as there may be more than 15-min delay in peak concentrations in brain.
- Avoid inadvertent intra-arterial injection; arterial spasm, thrombosis and gangrene may result.

- Do not use as sleeping aid for more than 2 wk.
- Store at room temperature. Protect from light.

Assessment/Interventions

- Obtain patient history, including drug history and any known allergies. Evaluate for history of substance abuse, liver disease, respiratory disease and porphyria.
- Monitor vital signs of patient undergoing IV administration at least every hour if indicated. Keep resuscitation equipment and drugs readily available.
- After IM administration (1 g dose), observe patient closely for at least 30 min to ensure that necrosis is not excessive.
- Observe for common side effects such as sedation and dizziness and, if excessive, report to physician. Institute safety precautions for elderly patients to prevent accidental falls.
- In children monitor for possible paradoxical response of increased agitation and notify physician.
- Be alert for evidence of barbiturate intoxication (unsteady gait, slurred speech, confusion or irritability) and report to physician.
- Watch for behavior indicative of drug dependence such as inordinate requests for more medication or need to refill prescription early.
- With prolonged therapy monitor lab tests for liver, renal and hematopoietic functions.

OVERDOSAGE: SIGNS & SYMPTOMS

CNS and respiratory depression, Cheyne-Stokes respiration, areflexia, constriction of pupils, oliguria, tachycardia, hypotension, lowered body temperature, coma, shock syndrome, pneumonia, pulmonary edema, cardiac arrhythmias, CHF, renal failure

Patient/Family Education

- Advise patient to increase intake of vitamin D–fortified foods (eg, milk products) while taking this medication.
- Explain importance of maintaining adequate intake of folic acid: fresh vegetables, fruits, whole grains, liver.
- Instruct patient to report these symptoms to physician: nausea, vomiting, drowsiness, dizziness, fever, sore throat, mouth sores or easy bleeding or bruising.
- Caution patient to avoid intake of alcoholic beverages or other CNS depressants.
- Warn patient that medication may be habit forming and for that reason it is important to take medicine as directed.
- Advise patient that drug may cause drowsiness and to use caution while driving or performing other tasks requiring mental alertness.
- Instruct patient not to stop taking medication abruptly without consulting physician.

See Patient Guide, p. 490.

Phenolphthalein

(fee-nahl-THAY-leen)

Alophen Pills No. 973, Espotabs, Evac-U-Gen, Evac-U-Lax, Ex-Lax, Feen-A-Mint, Lax Pills, Medilax, Modane, Phenolax, Prulet, Laxative Pills

Class: Laxative

Action Directly acts on intestinal mucosa by altering water and electrolyte secretion, inducing defecation.

Indications Short-term treatment of constipation.

Contraindications Nausea, vomiting or other symptoms of appendicitis; acute surgical abdomen; fecal impaction; intestinal obstruction; undiagnosed abdominal pain.

Route/Dosage

ADULTS & CHILDREN > 12 YR:

PO 60-194 mg preferably at bedtime. CHILDREN (6-11 YR): PO 30-60 mg. Note: Yellow phenolphthalein is 2-3 times more potent than white phenolphthalein.

Interactions None well documented.

Lab Test Interferences None well documented.

Adverse Reactions CV: Palpitations. *CNS:* Dizziness; fainting. *GI:* Excessive bowel activity (gripping, diarrhea, nausea, vomiting); perianal irritation; bloating; flatulence; abdominal cramping. *DERM:* Pruritis; rash. *OTHER:* Sweating; weakness.

Precautions *Pregnancy:* Pregnancy category undetermined. *Lactation:* Unknown. *Abuse/dependency:* Chronic use may lead to laxative dependency, which may result in fluid and electrolyte imbalances, steatorrhea, osteomalacia and vitamin and mineral deficiencies. Cathartic colon, a poorly functioning colon, results from chronic abuse of stimulant cathartics. Pathologic presentation may resemble ulcerative colitis. *Discoloration of alkaline urine:* May occur, causing pink-red, red-violet or red-brown urine. *Fluid and electrolyte imbalance:* Excessive laxative use may lead to significant fluid and electrolyte imbalance. *Rectal bleeding or failure to respond:* May indicate serious condition that may require further medical attention. *Skin hypersensitivity:* Drug may cause fixed drug eruption, requiring drug discontinuation. *Tartrazine sensitivity:* Some products may contain tartrazine, which may cause allergic-type reactions (including bronchial asthma) in susceptible individuals.

NURSING CONSIDERATIONS

Administration/Storage

- Administer at bedtime with full glass of water or juice.
- Store at room temperature.

Assessment/Interventions

- Obtain patient history, including drug history and any known allergies.
- Assess patient's living habits that affect bowel function such as diet and exercise.
- Assess color, consistency and amount of stool produced.
- Monitor pattern of bowel function.

OVERDOSAGE: SIGNS & SYMPTOMS

Nausea, vomiting, diarrhea, abdominal cramping

Patient/Family Education

- Instruct patient that laxatives are for short-term treatment of constipation (≤ 1 wk).
- Caution patient not to use laxatives in presence of abdominal pain, nausea or vomiting.
- Teach importance of modifying living habits to avoid constipation. Explain need for adequate fluid intake (4-6 full glasses of water every day), proper dietary habits including sufficient fiber or roughage, daily exercise and importance of responding to urge to defecate.
- Instruct patient that if regular bowel function has not resumed in 1 wk, to discontinue laxative use and notify physician.
- Advise patient to avoid exposure to sunlight and to use sunscreen or wear protective clothing to avoid photosensitivity reaction.
- Instruct patient to report these symptoms to physician: unrelieved constipation, rectal bleeding or symptoms of electrolyte imbalance (eg, muscle cramps or pain, weakness, dizziness).
- Advise patient that while taking laxatives urine may change color to pink-red, red-violet or red-brown color.

See Patient Guide, p. 491.

Phenoxybenzamine HCl

(fen-ox-ee-BEN-zuh-meen HIGH-droe-KLOR-ide)

Dibenzyline

Class: Antihypertensive/agent for pheochromocytoma

Action Irreversibly blocks alpha-adrenergic receptors.

Indications Control of episodes of hypertension and sweating in patients with pheochromocytoma. **Unlabeled uses:** Treatment of micturition disorders resulting from neurogenic bladder; treatment of functional outlet obstruction and partial prostatic obstruction.

Contraindications Conditions in which fall in BP may be undesirable.

Route/Dosage

ADULTS: PO 10 mg bid initially. Usual dosage range is 20-40 mg bid-tid. CHILDREN: PO 1-2 mg/kg/day in 3-4 divided doses.

Interactions

Epinephrine: Exaggerated hypotensive response and tachycardia may occur when epinephrine, or other agents that stimulate both alpha- and beta-receptors, are given concomitantly with phenoxybenzamine.

Lab Test Interferences

None well documented.

Adverse Reactions

CV: Orthostatic hypotension; tachycardia. *RESP:* Nasal congestion. *CNS:* Drowsiness; fatigue. *EENT:* Miosis. *GI:* Gastrointestinal irritation. *GU:* Inhibition of ejaculation.

Precautions

Pregnancy: Safety not established. *Lactation:* Undetermined. *Special risk patients:* Administer drug with caution to patients with marked cerebral or coronary arteriosclerosis or renal damage. Adrenergic blocking effects may aggravate respiratory infections.

NURSING CONSIDERATIONS

Administration/Storage

- Give drug with milk or in divided doses to reduce GI irritation.
- Store in airtight container and protect from light.

Assessment/Interventions

- Obtain patient history, including drug history and any known allergies.
- Instruct patient to change position slowly, especially from lying to sitting up or standing, and to dangle and move legs before standing.
- Assess for adverse reactions: orthostatic hypotension, tachycardia, nasal congestion.
- Assess for effectiveness (lowering of BP) periodically.
- Take safety precautions if patient develops lightheadedness.
- If shocklike state develops, place patient in Trendelenburg position. Notify physician and begin emergency interventions.
- During dosage adjustments, monitor BP and pulse (quality, rate, rhythm) with patient in lying and standing position for 4 days.
- In patients with peripheral vasospastic problems, observe for improvement in skin color, temperature and quality of peripheral pulses.

OVERDOSAGE: SIGNS & SYMPTOMS

Orthostatic hypotension, dizziness, fainting, tachycardia, vomiting, lethargy, shock

Patient/Family Education

- Advise patient to avoid alcoholic beverages.
- Stress to patient importance of weight reduction, sodium and alcohol restriction, discontinuation of smok-

ing, regular exercise and behavior modification.

- Instruct patient to avoid otc cough, cold or allergy medications containing sympathomimetics without consulting physician.
- Instruct patient to avoid sudden position changes to prevent orthostatic hypotension. Warn patient that taking a hot bath or shower may aggravate dizziness.
- Inform patient that drug may cause nasal congestion and constricted pupils.
- Advise patient that inhibition of ejaculation may occur, but reassure patient that this condition generally decreases with continued therapy.
- Advise patient that drug may cause drowsiness and to use caution while driving or performing other tasks requiring mental alertness.

See Patient Guide, p. 492.

Phentolamine

(fen-TOLE-uh-meen)

Regitine, *Rogitine*

Class: Antihypertensive/agent for pheochromocytoma

Action Decreases total peripheral resistance and venous return to heart by competitive blockade of presynaptic and postsynaptic alpha-adrenergic receptors.

Indications Prevention or control of hypertensive episodes in patients with pheochromocytoma; pharmacologic test for pheochromocytoma (not method of choice); prevention and treatment of dermal necrosis and sloughing following IV administration or extravasation of norepinephrine or dopamine. **Unlabeled uses:** Control of hypertensive crises secondary to MAO inhibitor–sympathomimetic amine interactions or withdrawal of clonidine, propranolol or other antihypertensives; in conjunction with papaverine as intracavernous injection for impotence.

Contraindications Hypersensitivity to phentolamine or related compounds; MI, coronary insufficiency, angina or other evidence suggestive of coronary artery disease.

Route/Dosage

Hypertensive Episodes in Pheochromocytoma

ADULTS: **IM/IV** 5 mg 1-2 hr before surgery. Repeat if necessary. During surgery, **IV** 5 mg as indicated. CHILDREN: **IM/IV** 1 mg 1-2 hr before surgery. During surgery, **IV** 1 mg as indicated.

Prevention of Dermal Necrosis and Sloughing

ADULTS: **IV** add 10 mg/1 L of solution containing norepinephrine.

Treatment of Dermal Necrosis or Sloughing After Norepinephrine Extravasation

ADULTS: 5-10 mg in 10 ml saline solution in area of extravasation within 12 hr. CHILDREN: **Infiltrate area** 0.1-0.2 mg/kg (maximum 10 mg).

Diagnosis of Pheochromocytoma

ADULTS: **IV/IM** 2.5-5 mg. CHILDREN: **IV** 1 mg *or* **IM** 3 mg.

Interactions

Epinephrine, ephedrine: Vasoconstricting and hypertensive effects of epinephrine and ephedrine are antagonized by phentolamine.

Lab Test Interferences

None well documented.

Adverse Reactions

CV: Acute and prolonged hypotensive episodes; tachycardia; cardiac arrhythmias; orthostatic hypotension. *CNS:* Weakness; dizziness. *EENT:* Nasal stuffiness. *GI:* Nausea; vomiting; diarrhea. *OTHER:* Flushing.

Precautions

Pregnancy: Category C. *Lactation:* Undetermined. *Cardiovascular effects:* Marked hypotensive episodes and shocklike states may follow use of phentolamine and lead to MI, cerebrovascular spasm or cerebrovascular occlusion. *Screening tests:* Urinary assays of catecholamines or other biochemical assays have largely supplanted phentolamine and other pharmacologic tests for pheochromocytoma. Phentolamine is usually used as confirmation. Follow specific guidelines for use of phentolamine.

NURSING CONSIDERATIONS

Administration/Storage

- Have patient remain supine during IV therapy.
- Dilute 5 mg in 1 ml Sterile Water for Injection. May dilute further with 5-10 ml Sterile Water for Injection.
- Use reconstituted solution immediately; do not store.
- Store unopened vial in light resistant container at room temperature.
- When using phentolamine for managing hypertensive crisis or as a diagnostic test, inject drug by rapid IV bolus.

Assessment/Interventions

- Obtain patient history, including drug history and any known allergies.
- Obtain baseline lying and standing BP and pulse before starting therapy.
- Assess IV site for infiltration.
- Monitor BP every 2 min when beginning IV therapy until BP is stable.
- Notify physician immediately if symptoms of severe hypotension or shock develop.
- If chest pain develops during infusion, notify physician.
- If patient develops dizziness, take safety precautions (bed in low position, supervise ambulation).

OVERDOSAGE: SIGNS & SYMPTOMS

Severe hypotension, shock, tachycardia, flushing

Patient/Family Education

- Instruct patient to avoid sudden position changes to prevent orthostatic hypotension.
- Instruct patient to notify physician if chest pain develops during infusion.
- Tell patient to report these symptoms to physician: dizziness, fainting spells or weakness.

No patient monograph available.

Phenylephrine HCl

(fen-ill-EFF-rin HIGH-droe-KLOR-ide)

AK-Dilate, AK-Nefrin, Alconefrin, Children's Nostril, Isopto Frin, Mydfrin, Neo-Synephrine, Nostril, Phenoptic, Prefrin, Relief, Rhinall, Sinex, ♣ *Diophenyl-T, Novahistine Decongestant*

Class: Vasopressor; decongestant

Action Stimulates postsynaptic alpha-receptors, resulting in rise in intense arterial peripheral vasoconstriction. Causes marked increase in systolic, diastolic and pulmonary pressures as well as reflex bradycardia. Slightly decreases cardiac output and increases coronary blood flow.

Indications Treatment of vascular failure in shock, shocklike states, drug-induced hypotension or hypersensitivity; correction of paroxysmal supraventricular tachycardia; prolongation of spinal anesthesia; vasoconstriction in regional analgesia; maintenance of adequate level of BP during spinal and inhalation anesthesia; temporary relief of nasal congestion and of minor eye irritations; pupil dilation in uveitis; treatment of open-angle glaucoma; use in diagnostic procedures (funduscopy) and before surgery.

Contraindications Severe hypertension; ventricular tachycardia; pheochromocytoma; 10% ophthalmic solution contraindicated in infants and patients with aneurysms.

Route/Dosage

Mild or Moderate Hypotension
ADULTS: **SC/IM** 1-10 mg (usually 2-5 mg); do not exceed initial dose of 5 mg. **IV** 0.1-0.5 mg (usually 0.2 mg); do not exceed initial dose of 0.5 mg. Avoid repeat injections more often than q 10-15 min.

Severe Hypotension and Shock
ADULTS: Initial dose: **IV continuous infusion** 100-180 mcg/min of 1:25,000 or 1:50,000 solution (10 mg/250-500 ml D5W or Sodium Chloride); once BP has stabilized to low normal level, decrease to maintenance rate of 40-60 mcg/min. If prompt initial vasopressor response is not obtained, increase dosage in increments ≥ 10 mg and add to infusion; adjust rate until desired BP is obtained.

Hypotension of Spinal Anesthesia
ADULTS: **SC/IM** 2-3 mg 3-4 min before injection of anesthetic. For hypotensive emergencies during spinal anesthesia, inject 0.2 mg, increasing by no more than 0.1-0.2 mg/dose (maximum 0.5 mg/dose). CHILDREN: **SC/IM** 0.5-1 mg/25 lb (55 kg).

Prolongation of Spinal Anesthesia
ADULTS: 2-5 mg added to anesthetic solution increases duration of motor block by up to 50%.

Vasoconstriction for Regional Analgesia
ADULTS: ≥ 2 mg added to local anesthetic solution in concentration of 1:20,000 (1 mg/20 ml).

Paroxysmal Supraventricular Tachycardia
ADULTS: Initial dose: **IV** ≤ 0.5 mg via rapid IV push (within 20-30 sec); subsequent doses should not exceed preceding dose by more than 0.1-0.2 mg (maximum 1 mg/dose).

Nasal Congestion
ADULTS & CHILDREN ≥ 12 YR.: **Intranasal** 1-2 sprays or 3 gtt of 0.25%, 0.5% or 1% solution q 4 hr. CHILDREN 6-12 YR: **Intranasal** 2-3 sprays of 0.25% solution in each nostril q 3-4 hr. CHILDREN 6 MO-6 YR: **Intranasal** 1-2 gtt of 0.16% solution in each nostril q 3 hr.

Vasoconstriction/Pupil Dilation
ADULTS: **Ophthalmic** Instill 1 gtt 2.5% or 10% on upper limbus. If necessary, repeat after 1 hr.

Uveitis/Prevention of Synechiae
ADULTS: **Ophthalmic** Instill 2.5% or 10% phenylephrine plus atropine.

To Free Recently Formed Posterior Synechiae
ADULTS: **Ophthalmic** Instill 1 gtt of 2.5% or 10% to upper surface of cornea.

Wide-Angle Glaucoma
ADULTS: **Ophthalmic** Instill 1 gtt of 10% on upper surface of cornea prn.

Open-Angle Glaucoma
ADULTS: **Ophthalmic** Instill 2.5% or 10% solution in conjunction with miotics.

Surgery
ADULTS: **Ophthalmic** Instill 2.5% or 10% solution 30-60 min before operation as short-acting mydriatic.

Refraction
ADULTS: **Ophthalmic** Instill 1 gtt 2.5% solution. CHILDREN: **Ophthalmic** Instill 1 gtt 2.5% solution.

Ophthalmascopic Examination
ADULTS: **Ophthalmic** Instill 1 gtt 2.5% solution in each eye.

Diagnostic Procedures/Provocative Test for Angleblock in Glaucoma
ADULTS: **Ophthalmic** Instill 2.5%.

Retinoscopy
ADULTS: **Ophthalmic** Instill 2.5% solution.

Blanching Test
ADULTS: **Ophthalmic** Instill 1-2 gtt of 2.5% solution.

Minor Eye Irritations
ADULTS: **Ophthalmic** Instill 1-2 gtt of 0.12% solution up to 4 times daily.

Interactions

Beta-blockers: Decrease phenylephrine's effect. *General anesthetics:* Arrhythmias. *Guanethidine:* May increase pressor response of phenylephrine; resulting in severe hypertension. *Halogenated hydrocarbon anesthetics:* May sensitize myocardium to effects of catecholamines. Use extreme caution to avoid arrhythmias. *MAO inhibitors, furazolidone:* May significantly increase pressor response resulting in hypertensive crisis and intracranial hemorrhage. *Oxytoxic drugs:* May cause severe persistent hypertension. *Tricyclic antidepressants:* May decrease or increase response; use with caution.

Lab Test Interferences

None well documented.

Adverse Reactions

CV: Reflex bradycardia; hypertension; angina; arrhythmias. *CNS:* Headache; excitability; restlessness; tremor. *EENT:* With ophthalmic and intranasal forms: Transitory stinging on initial instillation; blurring of vision; rebound congestion.

Precautions

Pregnancy: Category C. *Lactation:* Undetermined. *Children:* Ophthalmic use of phenylephrine 10% is contraindicated in infants. *Special risk patients:* Administer drug with caution to patients with hyperthyroidism, bradycardia, partial heart block, myocardial disease, prostatic hypertrophy, diabetes mellitus, increased IOP or severe arteriosclerosis. *Hypovolemia:* Avoid use in uncorrected hypovolemic states unless used as temporary emergency measure to maintain coronary and cerebral flow and in patients with tachyarrhythmias or ventricular fibrillation. *Sulfite sensitvity:* Use drug with caution in sulfite-sensitive individuals; some commercial preparations contain sodium bisulfite. *Narrow-angle glaucoma:* Ordinarily any mydriatic is contraindicated in patients with glaucoma. However, when temporary dilation of pupil may free adhesions or when vasoconstriction of intrinsic vessels may lower intraocular tension, these advantages may temporarily outweigh danger from coincident dilation of pupil. *Corneal effects:* If corneal epithelium has been denuded or damaged, corneal clouding may occur if phenylephrine 10% is instilled. *Rebound congestion:* May occur with extended use of intranasal or ophthalmic forms.

NURSING CONSIDERATIONS

Administration/Storage

- For vasopressor use, administer medication via continuous pump infusion. Administer intravenously through large vein, preferably central vein. Titrate carefully to avoid hypotension.
- With intranasal administration, do not share container. Instill spray into nose with head upright. Have patient sniff hard for a few minutes after administration. To instill drops, have patient recline on bed, hang head over edge and instill drops. Have patient remain in this position for several minutes after using and turn head from side to side. Do not allow tip of container to touch nasal passage. Discard after medication is no longer needed.
- To instill ophthalmic solution tilt patient's head back, hold dropper over eye, drop medication inside lower lid, apply pressure to inside corner of eye for 1 min. Take care not to touch dropper to eye.
- Prolonged exposure of ophthalmic solution to air or strong light may cause oxidation and discoloration. Do not use if solution is discolored or cloudy or contains precipitate.
- Store parenteral and nasal solution at room temperature and protect from light.

Assessment/Interventions

- Obtain patient history, including drug history and any known allergies. Note history of cardiovascular disease such as hypertension and assess for MAO inhibitor use.

- For ocular or ophthalmic use, assess for intraocular lens implants due to possibility of dislodging lens. Also assess for history of damaged corneal epithelium.
- Check BP and pulse frequently.
- Monitor hemodynamic function.
- Observe IV site for extravasation and infiltration.

OVERDOSAGE: SIGNS & SYMPTOMS

Severe hypertension, vomiting, ventricular extrasystoles, short paroxysms of ventricular tachycardia, sensation of fullness in head, tingling of extremities, somnolence, sedation, coma, profuse sweating, hypotension, shock

Patient/Family Education

Intranasal

- Advise patient that intranasal form is for short-term use only and should not be used for more than 3-5 days.
- Inform patient that stinging, burning or drying of the nose or an increase in nasal discharge may occur with intranasal form.
- Instruct patient to gradually stop taking intranasal form of this medicine rather than abruptly discontinuing it because rebound congestion can occur with sudden withdrawal. First stop using drug in one nostril and then in both nostrils.

Ophthalmic

- Caution patient that ophthalmic form of drug can cause discoloration of contact lenses and advise patient to wear glasses during therapy.
- Instruct patient not to use ophthalmic form for more than 72 hr without consulting physician.
- Advise patient to discontinue drug and notify physician if severe eye pain, headache, vision changes, floating spots, acute eye redness, pain with light exposure, insomnia, dizziness, weakness, tremor or irregular heartbeat occur.
- Advise patient that drug may cause temporary blurred or unstable vision and to use caution while driving or performing other tasks requiring mental alertness.

See Patient Guide, pp. 493-494.

Phenylpropanolamine HCl

(fen-ill-pro-pan-OLE-uh-meen HIGH-droe-KLOR-ide)

Acutrim II Maximum Strength, Acutrim Late Day, Control, Dex-A-Diet Maximum Strength, Dexatrim Pre-Meal, Phenyldrine, Prolamine, Propagest, Rhindecon, Unitrol

Class: CNS stimulant/anorexiant; nasal decongestant

Action Causes appetite suppression; stimulates adrenergic receptors and smooth muscle (reducing nasal congestion).

Indications Short-term (8-12 wk) adjunct to diet plan to reduce weight; relief of nasal congestion. **Unlabeled use:** Treatment of stress incontinence in women.

Contraindications Hypersensitivity to sympathomimetic amines; cardiovascular disease; hypertension; hyperthyroidism; kidney disease; diabetes; glaucoma; depression; during or within 14 days following MAO inhibitor use.

Route/Dosage

Appetite Suppressant

ADULTS: **PO** 25 mg tid ½ hr before meals (immediate release tablets) *or* 75 mg in morning (sustained release capsules).

Nasal Decongestant

ADULTS: **PO** 25 mg q 4 hr (maximum 150 mg/day) *or* **PO** 75 mg (sustained release capsules) q 12 hr. CHILDREN 6-12 YR: **PO** 12.5 mg q 4 hr (maximum 75 mg/day). CHILDREN 2-6 YR: **PO** 6.25 mg q 4 hr.

Interactions

Guanethidine: May decrease hypotensive effect. *Indomethacin:* May cause severe hypertensive episode. MAO *inhibitors, furazolidone:* May cause hypertensive crisis and intracranial hemorrhage. *Methyldopa:* May cause hypertension.

Lab Test Interferences

None well documented.

Adverse Reactions

CV: Palpitations; tachycardia; arrhythmias; hypertensive crisis and possible renal failure that may include rhabdomyolysis. CNS: Restlessness; dizziness; insomnia; tremor; headache; bizarre behavior. *EENT:* Nasal dryness. *GI:* Dry mouth; nausea. *GI:* Dysuria.

Precautions

Pregnancy: Category C. *Lactation:* Undetermined. *Children:* Safety and efficacy as anorexiant not established. *Special risk patients:* Patients with hypertension or other cardiovascular diseases, hyperthyroidism, diabetes mellitus, prostatic hypertrophy or increased intraocular pressure should use these products only with medical advice. *Cardiovascular effects:* Acute BP elevation may occur. *Tartrazine sensitivity:* Some products contain tartrazine, which may cause allergic-type reactions in susceptible individuals.

NURSING CONSIDERATIONS

Administration/Storage

- Do not crush or allow patient to chew sustained release or precision release capsules.
- Administer immediate release tablets for appetite suppression ½ hr before meals.
- Administer sustained release capsules once a day in the morning. Administer precision release capsules once a day after breakfast.
- Store in tightly closed, light-resistant container.

Assessment/Interventions

- Obtain patient history, including drug history and any known allergies.
- If drug is administered as diet aid, monitor patient's weight and nutritional intake.
- If drug is administered as nasal decongestant, assess nasal congestion periodically.

> **OVERDOSAGE: SIGNS & SYMPTOMS**
>
> Restlessness, tremor, hyperreflexia, tachypnea, confusion, assaultive behavior, convulsions, hallucinations, arrhythmias, hypertension, nausea, vomiting

Patient/Family Education

- Caution patient not to take medication immediately before bedtime to avoid insomnia.
- Warn patient not to exceed recommended dosage.
- When drug is prescribed as diet aid, remind patient that drug must be used in conjunction with restricted-calorie diet to be effective.
- Advise patient to avoid excessive intake of caffeine-containing foods and beverages.
- Instruct patient to discontinue drug and notify physician if rapid pulse, dizziness, nervousness, insomnia, weakness, tremor or palpitations occur.
- Advise patient to notify physician if no improvement in symptoms or if high fever occurs.
- Instruct patient not to take otc medications without consulting physician.

See Patient Guide, p. 495.

Phenylpropanolamine HCl/Guaifenesin

(fen-ill-pro-pan-OLE-uh-meen HIGH-droe-KLOR-ide/GWH-fen-ah-sin)

Ami-Tex LA, Dura-Vent, Entex LA, Exgest, Guaipax, Partuss LA, Phenylfenesin LA, Rymed-TR, SINUvent Stamoist LA, ULR-LA, Vanex-LA

Class: Nasal decongestant and expectorant

Action Phenylpropanolamine, a sympathomimetic amine, causes constriction and shrinkage of mucous membranes, resulting in less nasal stuffiness and improved drainage and ventilation. Guaifenesin enhances output of respiratory tract fluid by reducing adhesiveness and surface tension of viscous mucus.

Indications Symptomatic relief of respiratory conditions characterized by nasal congestion and dry, nonproductive cough in presence of mucus in respiratory tract.

Contraindications Hypersensitivity or idiosyncrasy to sympathomimetic amines manifested by insomnia, dizziness, weakness, tremor or arrhythmias; hypersensitivity to guaifenesin; MAO inhibitor therapy during or within 14 days of administration; severe hypertension and coronary artery disease.

Route/Dosage

ADULTS: **PO** 25 mg phenylpropanolamine/100-400 mg guaifenesin q 4 hr (immediate release tablets) *or* 75 mg phenylpropanolamine/100-600 mg guaifenesin q 12 hr (sustained release tablets). CHILDREN: **PO** 6.25-12.5 mg phenylpropanolamine/50-200 mg guaifenesin q 4 hr.

Interactions

Guanethidine: May inhibit effect of decongestant and reverse hypotension action of guanethidine. MAO *inhibitors, furazolidone:* May result in severe headache, hypertension and hyperpyrexia, possibly resulting in hypertensive crisis. *Methyldopa:* May cause hypertension.

Lab Test Interferences

May cause color interference with certain laboratory determinations of 5-hydroxyindoleacetic acid (5-HIAA) and vanillylmandelic acid (VMA).

Adverse Reactions

CV: Arrhythmias and cardiovascular collapse with hypotension; palpitations; tachycardia; transient hypertension; bradycardia. *RESP:* Respiratory difficulty. *CNS:* Fear; anxiety; tenseness; restlessness; headache; lightheadedness; dizziness; drowsiness; tremor; insomnia; hallucinations; psychological disturbances; prolonged psychosis (paranoia, terror, delusions); convulsions; CNS depression; anorexia; weakness. *EENT:* Blepharospasm (ocular irritation, tearing, photophobia); nasal dryness. *GI:* Nausea; vomiting; dry mouth. *GU:* Dysuria. *DERM:* Pallor; sweating; rash; urticaria. *OTHER:* Orofacial dystonia.

Precautions

Pregnancy: Category C. *Lactation:* Undetermined. *Elderly patients:* May be more likely to experience adverse reactions. *Special risk patients:* Administer drug with caution to patients with hyperthyroidism, diabetes mellitus, cardiovascular disease, coronary artery disease, ischemic heart disease, increased IOP or prostatic hypertrophy. *Hypertension:* Avoid administering drug to patients with hypertension. *Persistent cough:* Not indicated for cough associated with smoking, asthma or emphysema. If cough persists for > 1 wk, is recurring, or is accompanied by high fever, rash or persistent headache, notify physician. *Sulfite sensitivity:* Some of these products contain sulfites, which can cause allergic-like reactions.

NURSING CONSIDERATIONS

Administration/Storage

- Patient should be withdrawn from MAO inhibitor therapy 2 wk before taking this drug.
- Do not crush or allow patient to chew sustained release preparations.
- Give each dose of expectorant with glass of water or fluid.
- Store at room temperature.

Assessment/Interventions

- Obtain patient history, including drug history and any known allergies.
- Encourage patient to increase fluid intake. Provide room humidification to liquefy secretions.
- Evaluate patient's cough: type, frequency, character (including sputum).

OVERDOSAGE: SIGNS & SYMPTOMS

Restlessness, tremor, hyperreflexia, tachypnea, confusion, assaultive behavior, convulsions, hallucinations, arrhythmias, hypertension, hypotension, nausea, vomiting, drowsiness, lethargy

Patient/Family Education

- Teach patient the importance of adequate fluid intake to help to liquefy mucus. Recommend use of humidifier.
- Advise patient that this product is not for persistent or chronic cough such as occurs with smoking, asthma, chronic bronchitis or emphysema unless prescribed by physician.
- Instruct patient to notify physician if symptoms persist for more than 1 wk, tend to recur, or are accompanied by fever, rash or persistent headache.
- Advise patient that drug may cause drowsiness and to use caution while driving or performing other tasks requiring mental alertness.
- Caution patient to avoid smoking, smoke–filled rooms, perfume, dust, environmental pollutants and cleansers.

See Patient Guide, p. 496.

Phenytoin

(FEN-ih-toe-in)

Phenytoin

Dilantin Infatab, Dilantin Injection, Dilantin-125, Dilantin-30 Pediatric, Dilantin Injection

Phenytoin Sodium

Dilantin Kapseals, Diphenylan Sodium

Class: Anticonvulsant/hydantoin

Action Appears to act at motor cortex in inhibiting spread of seizure activity. Possibly works by promoting sodium efflux from neurons, thereby stabilizing threshold against hyperexcitability. Also decreases post-tetanic potentiation at synapse.

Indications Control of grand mal and psychomotor seizures; prevention and treatment of seizures occurring during or after neurosurgery; control of grand mal type of status epilepticus (parenteral administration). **Unlabeled uses:** Control of arrhythmias, (particularly cardiac glycoside-induced arrhythmias); control of convulsions in severe preeclampsia; treatment of trigeminal neuralgia (tic douloureux), recessive dystrophic epidermolysis bullosa and junctional epidermolysis bullosa.

Contraindications Hypersensitivity to phenytoin or other hydantoins; sinoatrial block; sinus bradycardia; second- and third-degree atrioventricular block; Adams-Stokes syndrome.

Route/Dosage

Individualize dose within clinically effective therapeutic serum level of 10-20 mcg/ml.

Seizures
ADULTS: **PO** 100 mg (or 125 mg of suspension) tid initially. Maintenance: 300-400 mg/day (maximum 600 mg/day). Sometimes initial 1 g loading dose is divided into 3 doses (400 mg, 300 mg and 300 mg) and is given at 2 hr interval). Once seizure control is established, extended release form (300 mg) may be administered for once-a-day dosing. CHILDREN: **PO** 5 mg/kg/day in 2-3 divided doses initially. Maintenance: 4-8 mg/kg/day (maximum 300 mg/day).

Status Epilepticus
ADULTS: **IV** Loading dose of 10-15 mg/kg via slow IV. Then **PO/IV** 100 mg q 6-8 hr. CHILDREN: **IV** Loading dose of 15-20 mg/kg at rate not exceeding 1-3 mg/kg/min.

Neurosurgery Prophylaxis
ADULTS: **IM** 100-200 mg at 4-hr intervals during surgery and postoperatively.

Interactions
Acetaminophen: May increase hepatotoxicity potential with chronic phenytoin use. *Amiodarone, chloramphenicol, disulfiram, estrogens, felbamate, fluconazole, isoniazid, cimetidine, trimethoprim, phenylbutazone, oxyphenbutazone, phenacemide, sulfonamides:* May increase phenytoin serum levels. *Carbamazepine, sucralfate, antineoplastic agents, rifampin, rifabutin:* May decrease phenytoin serum levels. *Corticosteroids, coumarin anticoagulants, doxycycline, estrogens, levodopa, felodipine, methadone, loop diuretics, oral contraceptives, quinidine, rifampin, rifabutin:* May impair effects of these agents. *Cyclosporine:* May reduce cyclosporine levels. *Disopyramide:* May cause decreased disopyramide levels and bioavailability and may enhance anticholinergic actions. *Enteral nutritional therapy:* May reduce phenytoin concentrations. *Folic acid:* May cause folic acid deficiency. *Metyrapine:* Phenytoin may cause subnormal response to metyrapone. *Mexiletine:* May decrease mexiletine levels and effects. *Nondepolarizing muscle relaxants:* May cause these agents to have shorter duration or decreased effects. *Phenobarbital, sodium valproate, valproic acid:* May increase or decrease phenytoin levels. Phenytoin may increase pheobarbital and decrease valproic acid levels. *Primidone:* May increase concentrations of primidone and metabolites. *Sympathomimetics (eg, dopamine):* May cause profound hypotension and possibly cardiac arrest. *Theophyllines:* Effects of either agent may be decreased.

Lab Test Interferences
Phenytoin may interfere with metapyrone and dexamethasone tests, causing inaccurate results because of increased metabolism of these agents. Drug may cause decreases in serum levels of protein-bound iodine. It may cause increased levels of glucose, alkaline phosphatase and gamma glutamyl transpeptidase. INCOMPATIBILITIES: Do not mix with other drugs in syringe.

Adverse Reactions
CV With IV use: CV collapse; hypotension; atrial and ventricular conduction depression; ventricular fibrillation. *CNS:* Nystagmus; ataxia; dysarthria; slurred speech; mental confusion; dizziness; insomnia; transient nervousness; motor twitching; diplopia; fatigue; irritability; drowsiness; depression; numbness; tremor; headache; choreoathetosis (with IV use). *EENT:* Conjunctivitis. *GI:* Nausea; vomiting; diarrhea; constipation. *HEMA:* Thrombocytopenia; leukopenia; granulocytopenia; agranulocytosis; pancytopenia; macrocytosis; megaloblastic anemia; eosinophilia; monocytosis; leukocytosis; simple anemia; hemolytic anemia; aplastic anemia. *HEPA:* Toxic hepatitis and liver damage; hepatocellular degeneration and necrosis; hepatitis; jaundice; nephrosis. *DERM:* Rashes, sometimes accompanied by fever; bullous, exfoliative or purpuric dermatitis; lupus erythematosus; Stevens-Johnson syndrome; toxic epidermal necrolysis; hirsutism; alopecia. *OTHER:* Gingival hyperplasia;

coarsening of facial features; lip enlargement; Peyronie's disease; polyarthropathy; hyperglycemia; weight gain; chest pain; IgA depression; fever; photophobia; gynecomastia; periarteritis nodosa; pulmonary fibrosis; tissue injury at injection site; lymph node hyperplasia; hypothyroidism.

Precautions

Pregnancy: Pregnancy category undetermined. Consult physician. Possible risk of birth defects must be considered along with risk of seizures to fetus in untreated epileptic mothers. *Lactation:* Excreted in breast milk. *Special risk patients:* Use drug with caution with hepatic impairment, acute intermittent poryphria, alcohol abuse, hypotension and severe myocardial insufficiency. *Bioavailability:* Because products vary in bioavailability, brand interchange is not recommended. *Hypersensitivity reactions:* Rapid substitution of alternate therapy may be necessary. *Seizures:* Drug should not be given to treat seizures due to hypoglycemia or other metabolic causes or petit mal (absence) epilepsy. *Withdrawal:* Abrupt withdrawal may precipitate status epilepticus. Dosage must be reduced or other anticonvulsant medicine substituted gradually.

NURSING CONSIDERATIONS

Administration/Storage

- Shake oral suspension well.
- Do not administer discolored capsules.
- Administer oral forms with food.
- Only extended release capsules are recommended for once-a-day dosage.
- Do not crush or allow patient to chew extended release capsules.
- Do not substitute one brand for another; bioequivalence problems exist.
- For parenteral administration, direct IV administration is recommended.
- Administer via IV into large vein via large-gauge needle or cannula. Do not exceed rate of 50 mg/min for adults or 1-3 mg/kg/min in neonates. Immediately flush with normal saline solution. Avoid continuous infusion.
- Monitor BP for possible hypotension during IV infusion. Rate of infusion may need to be decreased.
- Avoid IM route when possible. If IM administration is needed for more than 1 wk, consider alternatives such as gastric intubation.
- When patient is stabilized with oral phenytoin and switched from oral to IM route, dose must be increased by 50%. When patient returns to oral form after IM administration, ½ original oral dose should be given for 1 wk.
- Do not abruptly discontinue medication; withdrawal must be slowly tapered.
- Do not use parenteral solution if precipitates form that will not dissolve at room temperature.
- Do not use parenteral solution if it is hazy; faint, clear yellow color is acceptable for use.

Assessment/Interventions

- Obtain patient history, including drug history and any known allergies. Note hepatic impairment, cardiac disease and porphyria.
- Perform blood counts and urinalyses on initiation of therapy and at monthly intervals for several months.
- Observe for rash, which may signify hypersensitivity reaction that can lead to serious dermatological reactions. If rash occurs, withhold drug and notify physician.
- Monitor ECG and BP continuously.
- Monitor for elevated blood glucose values in diabetic patients and report to physician.
- Observe for side effects including nystagmus, ataxia, drowsiness, severe nausea or vomiting, gingival hyperplasia or jaundice and report to physician.

OVERDOSAGE: SIGNS & SYMPTOMS

Nystagmus, ataxia, dysarthria, hypotension, diminished mental capacity, coma, unresponsive pupils, respiratory and cardiovascular depression

Patient/Family Education

- Advise patient to take medication with food.
- Teach patient to shake oral suspension well.
- Instruct patient taking capsules not to use discolored ones.
- Tell patient to notify physician if skin rash develops.
- Instruct patient to report these symptoms to physician: nystagmus, ataxia, drowsiness, severe nausea or vomiting, gingival hyperplasia or jaundice.
- Caution patient to consult with physician before using alcohol or taking any other drug including otc medications.
- Warn patient that stopping medication too quickly may precipitate seizures. Stress that dose should be changed only under physician's direction.
- Inform patient that it is important to maintain good oral hygiene and to inform dentist of phenytoin therapy.
- Instruct diabetic patient that changes may occur in blood sugars and to monitor and report any abnormal results to physician.
- Inform patient that urine may turn pink.
- Advise patient to carry identification such as Medi-Alert that identifies illness and medication.
- Warn patient to inform surgeon, physician or dentist about this medication before any surgical, emergency or dental procedure.
- Advise patient that drug may cause drowsiness and to use caution while driving or performing other tasks requiring mental alertness.

See Patient Guide, p. 497.

Phytonadione (K$_1$; Phylloquinone; Methylphytyl Naphthoquinone)

(fye-toe-nuh-DIE-ohn)

AquaMEPHYTON, Konakion, Mephyton

Class: Blood modifier/Vitamin K

Action Promotes hepatic synthesis of active prothrombin (factor II), proconvertin (factor VII), plasma thromboplastin component (factor IX) and Stuart factor (factor X).

Indications Management of coagulation disorders due to faulty formation of factors II, VII, IX and X when due to vitamin K deficiency or interference with vitamin K activity. *Oral/parenteral:* Treatment of anticoagulant-induced prothrombin deficiency; treatment of hypoprothrombinemia secondary to salicylates or antibacterial therapy or secondary to obstructive jaundice and biliary fistulas, provided bile salts are also given. *Parenteral:* Treatment of hypoprothrombinemia secondary to conditions limiting absorption or synthesis of vitamin K prophylaxis and therapy of hemorrhagic disease of the newborn.

Contraindications Standard considerations.

Route/Dosage

ADULTS & CHILDREN: **PO/SC/IM** 2.5-10 mg (in adults, up to 25 mg for serious bleeding; rarely, 50 mg), may repeat oral dose based on response in 6-8 hr or 12-48 hr; avoid oral route when disorder would prevent adequate absorption. NEONATES (HEMORRHAGIC DISEASE): Prophylaxis: Single dose **IM** 0.5-1 mg within 1 hr of birth. Treatment: **SC/IM,** 1 mg accompanied by laboratory evaluation. INFANTS: **PO/SC/IM** 2 mg.

Interactions

Oral anticoagulants: Effects are

antagonized by vitamin K, particularly in patients with advanced liver disease.

Lab Test Interferences

Paradoxical prolongation of prothrombin time (PT) after maximum doses of vitamin K.

Adverse Reactions

CV: Hypotension; cyanosis. *CNS:* Headache; dizziness. *DERM:* Pruritic erythematous plaques at IM injection site; rash; urticaria. *HEPA:* Hyperbilirubinemia, including kernicterus, in newborns. *OTHER:* Anaphylactoid reactions; pain, swelling and tenderness at injection site; death after IV injection.

Precautions

Pregnancy: Category C. *Lactation:* Vitamin K excreted in breast milk. *Anticoagulation:* Patient may be refractory to oral anticoagulants, particularly large doses. *Bleeding:* Giving vitamin K has no immediate coagulant effect. Management of bleeding involves standard measures (eg, transfusions). *Hypersensitivity:* Rash and urticaria; anaphylactoid reactions. *Impaired hepatic function:* Giving vitamin K to correct hypoprothrombinemia associated with severe hepatitis or cirrhosis may further depress prothrombin concentration. *IV administrtion:* Deaths have occurred; this route should be restricted to situations in which other routes of administration are not feasible.

NURSING CONSIDERATIONS

Administration/Storage

- After initial dose, determine subsequent doses by PT response or clinical condition. If in 6-8 hr after parenteral administration or 12-48 hr after oral administration, PT has not been shortened satisfactorily, repeat dose.
- Give SC or IM when possible. For adults and older children, inject IM in upper outer quadrant of buttocks. In infants and young children, anterolateral aspect of thigh or deltoid region is preferred.
- Protect from light at all times.
- Avoid IV route unless risk outweighs benefit. If IV administration is unavoidable, inject very slowly, not exceeding 1 mg/min.

Assessment/Interventions

- Obtain patient history, including drug history and any known allergies.
- When given for oral anticoagulant–induced hypoprothrombinemia, remember that phytonadione promotes synthesis of prothrombin by liver, but does not directly counteract effects of oral anticoagulants. Do not expect immediate coagulant effect; it takes minimum of 1-2 hr for measurable improvement in PT.
- Check PT prior to and after treatment with phytonadione.
- For prophylaxis or treatment of hemorrhagic disease of newborn, phytonadione (vitamin K_1) is safer than menadiol sodium diphosphate (vitamin K_4). A prompt response (shortening of the PT in 2-4 hr) is usually diagnostic of hemorrhagic disease of newborn; failure to respond indicates another diagnosis or coagulation disorder.

OVERDOSAGE: SIGNS & SYMPTOMS

Parenteral administration: Hypotension, asystole, chest pain, dyspnea, nausea, rash, pruritus

Patient/Family Education

- Explain that patient may experience temporary "flushing sensations" and "peculiar" sensations of taste. Rarely dizziness, rapid weak pulse, profuse sweating, or difficulty breathing may occur. Another rare occurrence is pain, swelling or tenderness at injection site.
- Remind patients on anticoagulant and phytonadione therapy of importance of regular lab work to check PT.

Anticoagulant effects are antagonized by vitamin K so temporary resistance to oral anticoagulants may result, especially when larger doses are used.

- Instruct patient to report any symptoms of bleeding.

See Patient Guide, pp. 498-499.

Pilocarpine

(pie-low-CAR-peen)

Pilocarpine HCl

Adsorbocarpine, Akarpine, Isopto-Carpine, Pilocar, Piloptic, Pilopine HS, Pilostat

Pilocarpine Nitrate

Pilagan

Pilocarpine Ocular Therapeutic System

Ocusert Pilo-20, Ocusert Pilo-40, ✦ *Diocarpine, Miocarpine, R.O.-Carpine, Spersacarpine*

Class: Ophthalmic/antiglaucoma; mouth and throat product

Action Decreases IOP by constricting pupil and stimulating ciliary muscles to open trabecular meshwork spaces and facilitate outflow of aqueous humor. *Oral use:* Stimulates exocrine glands including mucous cells of respiratory tract and salivary glands in oral cavity.

Indications *Ophthalmic use:* Treatment of chronic simple glaucoma, chronic angle-closure glaucoma, acute angle-closure glaucoma; pre- and postoperative management of intraocular tension; treatment of mydriasis. *Oral use:* Treatment of xerostomia in patients with malfunctioning salivary glands due to radiotherapy for cancer of head and neck.

Contraindications Hypersensitivity; conditions in which cholinergic effects such as constriction are undesirable. Oral use also contraindicated in uncontrolled asthma, acute iritis, narrow-angle glaucoma, acute inflammatory disease of anterior segment of eye.

Route/Dosage

Solution

ADULTS: Instill 1-2 drops of 1% or 2% solution in affected eye(s) up to 6 times daily. More concentrated solutions are sometimes used.

Gel

ADULTS: Apply 0.5 inch ribbon in lower conjunctival sac of affected eye(s) once daily at bedtime.

Ocular Therapeutic System

ADULTS: Place system into conjunctival cul-de-sac of affected eye(s) at bedtime. Replace each unit q 7 days. **PO** 5 mg tid; may titrate up to 10 mg tid.

Interactions *Anticholinergics:* May antagonize action of pilocarpine (oral and ophthalmic). *Beta-blockers:* Potential for conduction disturbances with oral pilocarpine.

Lab Test Interferences None well documented.

Adverse Reactions *EENT: Ophthalmic use:* Transient stinging and burning; tearing; ciliary spasm; conjunctival vascular congestion; temporal, peri- or supraorbital headache; superficial keratitis-induced myopia; blurred vision; poor dark adaptation; conjunctival hyperemia; reduced visual acuity in poor illumination; lens opacity; subtle corneal granularity; conjunctival irritation, ciliary spasm; precipitation of angle closure; irritation; corneal abrasion; visual impairment. *Oral use:* Rhinitis. *CV:* Hypertension; tachycardia; dizziness; headache; asthenia; chills; flushing. *RESP:* Bronchiolar spasm; pulmonary edema. *GI:* Excessive salivation; nausea; vomiting; diarrhea. *GU: Oral use:* Urinary frequency. *DERM:* Sweating.

Precautions

Pregnancy: Category C. *Lactation:* Undetermined. *Children:* Safety and efficacy not established. *Special risk patients:* Use oral with caution in acute cardiac failure, bronchial asthma, peptic ulcer, hypertension, hyperthyroidism, retinal disease, GI or biliary tract spasm or obstruction, urinary tract obstruction or Parkinson's disease.

NURSING CONSIDERATIONS

Administration/Storage

Oral

- Give medication with food if GI distress occurs.

Optic

- To avoid contamination, do not touch tip of container to any surface. Replace cap after administration. Gently apply pressure over nasolacrimal drainage system (bridge of nose) for 1-2 min.
- Keep bottle tightly closed when not in use.
- Wash hands before and after using.
- Keep out of reach of children.
- Solution: Store at room temperature and protect from light.
- Gel: Refrigerate until time of dispensation. Do not freeze.

Ocular Therapeutic System (A Small Device That Releases Pilocarpine Through a Membrane When Placed in the Cul-De-Sac of the Eye.)

- Wash hands with soap and water before touching or manipulating system.
- Read and follow directions on package insert.
- Check for presence of system at end and beginning of each shift.
- If displaced system contacts unclean surfaces, rinse with cool tap water before replacing. Discard contaminated systems and replace with fresh unit.
- Refrigerate. Do not freeze.
- Place system into eye at bedtime. If keeping unit in eye is problem, move unit from lower to upper lid by gentle lid massage. If unit slips out during night, its effects continue for period of time similar to that following instillation of eyedrops.

Assessment/Interventions

- Obtain patient history, including drug history and any known allergies.
- During early treatment of adult glaucoma, perform hourly tonometric tests to monitor for transitory increase in IOP.
- Use physician- or manufacturer-recommended technique for application for patient with contact lenses.
- Monitor for changes in vision, which could indicate potential retinal detachment.

OVERDOSAGE: SIGNS & SYMPTOMS

Oral: Salivation, lacrimation, nausea, vomiting, diarrhea, cramping, sweating, frequent urination, bradycardia, asystole, death

Patient/Family Education

- For treatment of glaucoma, emphasize need to adhere to medical regimen to prevent blindness.
- Explain that long-term therapy may be required.
- Instruct patient to wash hands thoroughly before and after using ophthalmic preparation.
- Review proper procedure for administration of ophthalmic preparations.
- Explain that ophthalmic preparations may sting upon instillation, especially with first few doses.
- Tell patient to discard solution after expiration date.
- Explain that medication may cause headache or browache and that because of blurring, altered distance vision and night vision; patient should use caution while night driving or performing hazardous tasks.
- Explain that during acute phases miotic (agent that causes pupil to

constrict) also must be instilled into unaffected eye to prevent occurrence of angle-closure glaucoma.

- Tell patients using oral form to report these symptoms to physician: sweating, nausea, nasal congestion, chills, flushing, frequent urination, dizziness, weakness, headache, indigestion, tearing, diarrhea, fluid retention.
- Tell patients using Therapeutic Ocular System that signs of irritation, including mild redness with or without slight increase in mucus secretion may be noticed with first use but that these symptoms tend to lessen or disappear after first week of therapy.
- Instruct patient to check for placement of system before retiring and on arising.

See Patient Guide, pp. 500-501.

Pindolol

(PIN-doe-lahl)

Visken, ♣ *APO-Pindol, Gen-Pindolol, Novo-Pindol, Nu-Pindol, Syn-Pindolol*

Class: Beta-adrenergic blocker

Action Nonselectively blocks beta receptors, which primarily affect heart (slows rate), vascular musculature (decreases blood pressure) and lungs (reduces function).

Indications Management of mild to moderate hypertension.

Contraindications Greater than first-degree heart block; congestive heart failure unless secondary to tachyarrhythmia treatable with beta-blockers; overt cardiac failure; sinus bradycardia; cardiogenic shock; hypersensitivity to beta-blockers; bronchial asthma or bronchospasm, including severe COPD.

Route/Dosage

Hypertension

ADULTS: **PO** 5 mg bid. May be increased by 10 mg q 3-4 wk until desired response; maximum dose is 60 mg/day.

Interactions

Clonidine: May enhance or reverse antihypertensive effect; potentially life-threatening situations may occur, especially on withdrawal. *Epinephrine:* Initial hypertensive episode followed by bradycardia may occur. *Ergot alkaloids:* Peripheral ischemia, manifested by cold extremities and possible gangrene, may occur. *Impaired liver function:* Dosage may need to be reduced. *Insulin:* Prolonged hypoglycemia with masking of symptoms may occur. *Lidocaine:* Lidocaine levels may increase, leading to toxicity. *Nonsteroidal anti-inflammatory agents:* Some agents may impair antihypertensive effect. *Prazosin:* Orthostatic hypotension may be increased. *Theophyllines:* Elimination of theophylline may be reduced. Also, effects of both drugs may be reduced by pharmacologic antagonism. *Verapamil:* Effects of both drugs may be increased.

Lab Test Interferences

None well documented.

Adverse Reactions

CV: Bradycardia; hypotension; congestive heart failure; edema; worsening angina. *RESP:* Wheezing; bronchospasm; difficulty breathing (at higher doses). *CNS:* Depression; visual disturbances; short-term memory loss; dizziness. *EENT:* Dry eyes; visual disturbances. *GI:* Nausea; vomiting; diarrhea. *GI:* Impotence; urinary retention; difficulty with urination. *HEMA:* Agranulocytosis. *HEPA:* May increase AST or ALT; rarely increases LDH or alkaline phosphatase. *DERM:* Skin rash; increased sensitivity to cold. *META:* May increase or decrease blood glucose, uric acid.

Precautions

Pregnancy: Category B. *Lactation:* Excreted in breast milk. *Children:* Safety and efficacy not established. *Anaphylaxis:* Deaths have occurred; aggressive therapy may be required.

Diabetics: May mask signs and symptoms of hypoglycemia (eg, tachycardia, BP changes). May potentiate insulin-induced hypoglycemia. *Peripheral vascular disease:* May precipitate or aggravate symptoms of arterial insufficiency. *Thyrotoxicosis:* May mask clinical signs of developing or continuing hyperthyroidism (eg, tachycardia). Abrupt withdrawal may exacerbate symptoms of hyperthyroidism, including thyroid storm. *Congestive heart failure:* Administer cautiously in CHF patients controlled by digitalis and diuretics. Notify physician at first sign or symptom of CHF or unexplained respiratory symptoms in any patient. *Renal/hepatic function impairment:* Reducing daily dose advised.

NURSING CONSIDERATIONS

Administration/Storage

- Give orally.
- Give medication at same time each day.
- May be taken without regard to meals.
- Store at room temperature and protect from moisture, light and air.

Assessment/Interventions

- Obtain patient history, including drug history and any known allergies.
- Assess pulse and BP prior to initiation of therapy.
- Monitor BP, apical and radial pulses, intake and output, daily weight, respiration and circulation in extremities.
- Review baseline serum glucose level, results of liver and renal function studies and monitor lab data throughout therapy.
- Monitor blood glucose closely for diabetic patients.
- Notify physician if symptoms of CHF occur (difficulty breathing, cough or swelling in extremities).
- Report bothersome side effects to physician, especially new-onset depression.
- Reduce dose gradually upon discontinuation of therapy. Abrupt withdrawal is associated with adverse effects, including precipitation or worsening of angina.

OVERDOSAGE: SIGNS & SYMPTOMS

Bradycardia, hypotension, seizures, respiratory depression

Patient/Family Education

- Teach patient and family technique for measuring BP and pulse rates and to keep written record.
- Instruct patient to notify physician if pulse rate is < 50 bpm or systolic BP is < 90 mm Hg.
- Warn patient not to engage in activities that require mental alertness until drug effects are apparent because it may cause blurred vision, drowsiness and dizziness.
- Explain that decreased blood supply to extremities may cause patient to be more sensitive to cold temperatures.
- Encourage patients with diabetes to monitor blood glucose carefully.
- Advise patient to report these symptoms to physician: any asthma-like symptoms, cough or nasal stuffiness, skin rash, fever, sore throat, unusual bleeding or bruising.
- Instruct patient not to take any otc medications without consulting physician.
- Instruct patient to sit or lie down immediately if dizziness or faintness occurs.

See Patient Guide, p. 502.

Piperacillin Sodium

(PIH-per-uh-SILL-in SO-dee-uhm)
Pipracil
Class: Antibiotic/penicillin

Action Inhibits bacterial cell wall mucopeptide synthesis.

Indications Treatment of intra-abdominal, urinary tract, gynecologic, lower respiratory tract infections, septicemia, skin and skin structure infections, bone and joint infections and gonococcal urethritis; surgical prophylaxis; treatment of infection due to susceptible microorganisms including infections caused by *Streptococcus* and *Pseudomonas* species.

Contraindications Hypersensitivity to penicillins or cephalosporins.

Route/Dosage
ADULTS: **IM/IV** 3-4 g q 4-6 hr (maximum 24 g/day). CHILDREN: **IM/IV** 200-500 mg/kg/day divided q 4-6 hr. NEONATES: **IM/IV** 100 mg/kg/dose q 12 hr.

Interactions
Aminoglycosides, parenteral: May inactivate aminoglycosides in vitro; do not mix in same IV solution. May be used in combination for synergy. *Anticoagulants:* May increase bleeding risks by prolonging bleeding time. *Chloramphenicol:* Synergism or antagonism may develop. *Contraceptives, oral:* May reduce efficacy of oral contraceptives. Use additional form of contraception during piperacillin therapy. *Erythromycin:* Synergism or antagonism may develop. *Heparin:* May increase bleeding risks of heparin by prolonging bleeding time. *Tetracyclines:* May impair bactericidal effects of piperacillin.

Lab Test Interferences
May cause false-positive urine glucose test results with Benedict's solution, Fehling's solution, or Clinitest tablets but not with enzyme-based tests (eg, Clinistix, Tes-tape); false-positive direct Coombs' test result in certain patient groups; positive direct antiglobulin tests (DAT); false-positive protein reactions with sulfosalicylic acid and boiling test, acetic acid test, biuret reaction and nitric acid test but not with the bromphenol blue test (Multi-Stix).

Adverse Reactions
CNS: Neurotoxicity (lethargy, neuromuscular irritability, hallucinations, convulsions and seizures) especially with large dose or patient with renal failure; dizziness; fatigue; insomnia; reversible hyperactivity; prolonged muscle relaxation. *EENT:* Itchy eyes. *GI:* Nausea; vomiting; abdominal pain or cramping; epigastric distress; diarrhea or bloody diarrhea; rectal bleeding; flatulence; enterocolitis; pseudomembranous colitis; anorexia. *GU:* Interstitial nephritis (oliguria, proteinuria, hematuria, hyaline casts, pyuria); nephropathy; elevated creatinine or BUN; vaginitis; moniliasis. *HEMA:* Anemia; hemolytic anemia; thrombocytopenia; thrombocytopenic purpura; eosinophilia; leukopenia; granulocytopenia; neutropenia; bone marrow depression; agranulocytosis; reduced Hgb or Hct; prolongation of bleeding and prothrombin time; decrease in WBC and lymphocyte counts; increase in lymphocytes, monocytes, basophils and platelets. *HEPA:* Elevated SGPT or SGOT and bilirubin; transient hepatitis; cholestatic jaundice. *DERM:* Ecchymosis. *META:* Elevated serum alkaline phosphatase; hypernatremia; hypokalemia, reduced albumin, total proteins and uric acid. *OTHER:* Hypersensitivity reactions (urticaria, angioneurotic edema, laryngospasm, bronchospasm, hypotension, vascular collapse, death, maculopapular to exfoliative dermatitis, vesicular eruptions, erythema multiforme, serum sickness, laryngeal edema, skin rashes, prostration); vaginitis; hyperthermia; pain at site of injection; deep vein thrombosis; hematomas; vein irritation; phlebitis; hyperthermia; sciatic neuritis.

Precautions
Pregnancy: Category B. *Lactation:* Excreted in breast milk. *Bleeding abnormalities:* Hemorrhagic manifestations associated with abnormalities of coagulation tests (bleeding time, prothrombin time, platelet aggregation) may occur. Abnormalities should revert to normal once drug is discontinued. *Cystic fibrosis patients:* May experience higher incidence of side effects when treated with piperacillin. *Hypersensitiv-*

ity: Reactions range from mild to life-threatening. Administer cautiously to cephalosporin-sensitive patients due to possible cross-reactivity. *Pseudomembranous colitis:* May occur due to overgrowth of clostridia. *Renal failure:* Dosage adjustment required. *Superinfection:* May result in bacterial or fungal overgrowth of nonsusceptible organisms.

NURSING CONSIDERATIONS

Administration/Storage

- Obtain culture and sensitivity before administering first dose.
- IM or IV route.
- For IM use, dilute to 1 g/2.5 ml. Lidocaine (0.5-1%) may be used to dilute (for IM use only).
- Give no more than 2 g IM at any one site.
- For IV injection, reconstitute each gram with at least 5 ml compatible dilutent.
- IV infusion is diluted further with 50-100 ml of D5W or normal saline and infused over 20-30 min.
- Time doses for even distribution throughout 24 hours.

Assessment/Interventions

- Obtain patient history, including drug history and any known allergies.
- Assess for drug reactions especially in patients with asthma, hay fever, urticaria or allergy to cephalosporins.
- Assess baseline CBC and liver and renal function study results prior to initiating therapy and monitor throughout therapy.
- Monitor results of diagnostic cultures and sensitivity tests.
- Monitor patient for at least 20 min after administering penicillin to observe for signs or symptoms of anaphylaxis. Notify physician if skin rash, hives, wheezing, nausea or vomiting occur.

OVERDOSAGE: SIGNS & SYMPTOMS

Agitation, confusion, asterixis, hallucinations, stupor, coma, seizures, hyperexcitability

Patient/Family Education

- Instruct patient to notify physician if symptoms of potential superinfection (nausea/vomiting, diarrhea, black tongue, swollen joints, unusual bleeding or bruising).
- Explain signs and symptoms of allergic reaction (hives, wheezing, skin rash or itching) and importance of seeking medical supervision as soon as possible.
- Emphasize need for good hygiene to avoid superinfections.
- If patient develops allergy to piperacillin, advise patient to notify future caregivers of penicillin allergy and patient should wear Medi-Alert identification.

See Patient Guide, p. 503.

Pirbuterol Acetate

(pihr-BYOO-tuh-role ASS-uh-TATE)

Maxair

Class: Bronchodilator/ sympathomimetic

Action Produces bronchodilation by relaxing bronchial smooth muscle through beta-2 receptor stimulation.

Indications Prevention and treatment of reversible bronchospasm associated with asthma or other obstructive pulmonary diseases.

Contraindications Hypersensitivity to drug components; cardiac arrhythmias associated with tachycardia.

Route/Dosage

ADULTS & CHILDREN ≥ 12 YR:

Inhalation 1-2 inhalations q 4-6 hr; not to exceed 12 inhalations/day.

Interactions

MAO inhibitors, tricyclic antidepressants: May increase the effects of pirbuterol.

Lab Test Interferences

None well documented.

Adverse Reactions

CV: Palpitations; tachycardia; BP changes. *RESP:* Cough; throat irritation. *CNS:* Tremor; anxiety; confusion; fatigue; dizziness; nervousness; headache. *EENT:* Dry nose; throat irritation. *GI:* GI distress; dry mouth.

Precautions

Pregnancy: Category C. *Lactation:* Undetermined. *Elderly:* Lower doses may be required. *Cardiovascular effects:* Toxic symptoms in patients with cardiovascular disorders may occur. *CNS effects:* CNS stimulation may occur; use cautiously in patients with history of seizure or hyperthyroidism. *Diabetes:* Dosage adjustment of insulin or oral hypoglycemic agent may be required. *Excessive use:* Paradoxical bronchospasm and cardiac arrest have been associated with excessive inhalant use. *Hypokalemia:* Decreases in potassium levels have occurred. *Labor and delivery:* May inhibit uterine contractions and delay preterm labor. *Tolerance:* If previously effective dose fails to provide relief therapy may need to be reassessed.

NURSING CONSIDERATIONS

Administration/Storage

- Give pressurized inhalation during second half of breath intake.
- If more than one inhalation is needed, wait 1-2 minutes before administering second dose.
- Discard any discolored solutions of drug.
- Store at room temperature in light-resistant container.

Assessment/Interventions

- Obtain patient history, including drug history and any known allergies.
- Obtain baseline ABGs prior to initiation of therapy.
- Assess BP and pulse before and after each dose.
- Assess for CNS response and adjust dose and frequency accordingly.
- To prevent respiratory depression, administer oxygen based on ABGs and symptoms.
- Assess vital capacity and forced expiratory volume.
- If 3-5 aerosol treatments have been given within 6-12 hours with minimal relief, notify physician and do not give further treatment.

OVERDOSAGE: SIGNS & SYMPTOMS

Tremor, palpitations, tachycardia, elevated blood pressure, anginal pain, hypokalemia, seizures

Patient/Family Education

- Advise patient to take drug early in day to prevent insomnia.
- Explain that implementing therapy in morning and after meals may reduce fatigue and improve lung ventilation.
- Encourage patient to increase fluid intake to help liquefy secretions.
- Tell patient to report these symptoms to physician: dizziness, chest pain, palpitations, muscle spasms, headache, difficult urination, dyspnea or nervous tremor.
- Explain that if no relief is obtained from normal daily dose, patient should call physician instead of increasing dose. Also if more than three aerosol treatments are needed in 24 hours, patient should notify physician.
- Tell patient to wait at least 1-2 min before administering second inhalation.
- Instruct patient that regular, consistent use of medication is required for maximum benefits.

- Explain benefits of and demonstrate technique for postural drainage and chest vibration.
- Instruct patient not to take any otc medications without consulting physician.
- Emphasize that it is important to avoid getting aerosol medication in eyes.
- Tell patient to avoid smoking, smoke-filled rooms and persons with respiratory infections.
- Explain how to use and care for inhalers and any other respiratory equipment.

See Patient Guide, p. 504.

Piroxicam

(pihr-OX-ih-kam)

Feldene, ♣ *Novo-Pirocam, Nu-Pirox*

Class: Analgesic/NSAID

Action Decreased inflammation, pain and fever, probably through inhibition of cyclooxygenase activity and prostaglandin synthesis.

Indications Treatment of acute and chronic rheumatoid arthritis and osteoarthritis. **Unlabeled uses:** Symptomatic relief of primary dysmenorrhea, pain, sunburn.

Contraindications Known allergy or hypersensitivity to aspirin, iodides or any NSAID, including piroxicam.

Route/Dosage

Rheumatoid Arthritis, Osteoarthritis

ADULTS: PO Initiate and maintain at 20 mg/day in 1-2 divided doses.

Interactions

Alcohol: May augment risk of GI bleeding. *Anticoagulants:* May increase effect of anticoagulants due to decreased plasma protein binding and inhibition of platelet aggregation. May increase risk of gastric erosion and bleeding. *Beta-blockers:* Antihypertensive effect may be decreased. *Cholestyramine:* Effects of piroxicam may be decreased. *Lithium:* May decrease lithium clearance. *Methotrexate:* May increase methotrexate levels and methotrexate toxicity.

Lab Test Interferences

May prolong bleeding time. May reversibly increase BUN and serum creatinine.

Adverse Reactions

CV: Edema; weight gain; CHF; alterations in BP; vasodilation; palpitations; tachycardia. *RESP:* Bronchospasm; laryngeal edema; dyspnea; hemoptysis; shortness of breath. *CNS:* Headache; malaise; dizziness; somnolence; vertigo; depression; insomnia; nervousness. *EENT:* Tinnitus; swollen eyes; blurred vision; eye irritation; rhinitis; pharyngitis. *GI:* Epigastric distress; nausea; vomiting; anorexia; constipation; stomatitis; abdominal discomfort; diarrhea; flatulence; abdominal pain; indigestion; toxicity (bleeding, ulceration, perforation). *HEMA:* Increased bleeding time; decreased Hgb and Hct; anemia; leukopenia; eosinophilia, thrombocytopenia. *HEPA:* Increased liver function tests. *GU:* Hematuria; proteinuria; increased BUN and serum creatinine; acute renal insufficiency and failure; papillary necrosis; interstitial nephritis; nephrotic syndrome; hyperkalemia; hyponatremia. *DERM:* Pruritus; rash; sweating; erythema; bruising; desquamation; erythema multiforme; toxic epidermal necrolysis.

Precautions

Pregnancy: Pregnancy category undetermined. *Lactation:* Undetermined. *Children:* Safety and efficacy not established. *Elderly patients:* Increased risk of adverse reactions. May require decreased dosage. *Asthma:* In certain patients (aspirin-allergic, nasal polyps) may precipitate asthma attacks. *Cardiovascular disease:* May worsen CHF and hypertension. *Coagulation disorders:* Increases risk of bleeding. *GI effects:* Serious GI toxicity can occur at any time, with or without warning symptoms. *Renal disease:* Drug may accumulate, increasing the risk of toxicity.

NURSING CONSIDERATIONS

Administration/Storage

- Give after meals to reduce GI effects.
- Store at room temperature.

Assessment/Interventions

- Obtain patient history, including drug history and any known allergies.
- Obtain baseline vital signs, weight and lab results and monitor throughout therapy.
- Notify physician of any changes in creatinine and electrolyte values and of any signs of renal or liver dysfunction, bleeding, GI discomfort or vision changes.

OVERDOSAGE: SIGNS & SYMPTOMS

Drowsiness, dizziness, mental confusion, disorientation, lethargy, paresthesia, numbness, vomiting, GI irritation, headache, tinnitus, seizure, increased BUN

Patient/Family Education

- Explain that increased response may be seen after weeks of therapy.
- Caution patient to avoid exposure to sunlight and to use sunscreen or wear protective clothing to avoid photosensitivity reaction.
- Identify signs and symptoms patient should report to physician, including changes in how food tastes, nausea, vomiting, constipation, diarrhea, cramping, black or red stool, discolored urine, changes in urination, fever, rash, unusual bruising or bleeding.
- Explain that taking medication with food will minimize GI distress.
- Inform patient to avoid aspirin and alcohol during therapy.
- Instruct patient not to take any otc medications without consulting physician.
- Advise patient that drug may cause drowsiness and to use caution while driving or performing other tasks requiring mental alertness until the effects of the drug are known.
- Encourage patient to maintain adequate fluid intake.

See Patient Guide, p. 505.

Plicamycin (Mithramycin)

(PLY-kae-MY-sin)

Mithracin

Class: Antineoplastic/antibiotic

Action Suppresses cellular division by complexing with DNA, causing inhibition of DNA-dependent RNA synthesis; decreases serum calcium concentrations.

Indications Treatment of malignant testicular tumors when surgery or radiation is impossible; management of hypercalcemia and hypercalciuria associated with advanced neoplasms.

Contraindications Thrombocytopenia; thrombocytopathy, coagulation disorders or increased bleeding susceptibility; impaired bone marrow function; pregnancy.

Route/Dosage Use ideal body weight to calculate dose if abnormal fluid retention present.

Testicular Tumors

ADULTS: **IV** 25-30 mcg/kg/day for 8-10 days unless significant side effects occur. Do not use > 10 daily doses. Do not exceed 30 mcg/kg/day. Treatment may be repeated at monthly intervals.

Hypercalcemia of Malignancy

ADULTS: **IV** 25 mcg/kg/dose/day over

4-6 hr for 3-4 days or 1-3 doses/wk. May repeat treatment at weekly intervals.

Interactions None well documented.

Lab Test Interferences
None well documented.

Adverse Reactions
CNS: Fever; drowsiness; weakness; headache. *GI:* Stomatitis; anorexia; nausea; vomiting; diarrhea. *GU:* Increased serum creatinine and BUN; proteinuria. *HEMA:* Bleeding syndrome; thrombocytopenia; leukopenia; anemia; increased prothrombin times. *HEPA:* Increased liver function test results. *OTHER:* Hypocalcemia; hypokalemia; hypophosphatemia; rash; facial flushing.

Precautions
Pregnancy: Category X. *Lactation:* Undetermined. *Electrolyte imbalance:* Hypocalcemia, hypokalemia, and hypophosphatemia can occur. *Hemorrhagic syndrome:* Clotting factor abnormalities may occur; severe thrombocytopenia and bleeding episodes resulting in death have occurred. Risk of bleeding may be increased by use of aspirin or oral anticoagulants. *Renal and hepatic toxicity:* May cause renal and hepatic function impairment; patients with pre-existing disease have greatest risk.

NURSING CONSIDERATIONS

Administration/Storage

- Wear disposable nonpermeable surgical gown (with closed front) and latex gloves during preparation.
- Prepare solution under laminar flow hood, and cover work area with disposable plastic liner.
- Add sterile water to vial and shake to dissolve drug.
- Administer slowly, over 4-6 hr.
- Store unreconstituted vials in refrigerator.

Assessment/Interventions

- Obtain patient history, including drug history and any known allergies.
- Assess patient for evidence of hemorrhage (epistaxis, hemoptysis, hematemesis, purpura, marked facial flushing or ecchymosis).
- Assess patient regularly for stomatitis, oral mucositis.
- Evaluate IV site regularly for signs or symptoms of infiltration.
- Stop IV if infiltration occurs and apply heat to site to reduce pain and tissue damage.
- Obtain baseline blood work, and monitor hematologic parameters, blood count, chemistry values and prothrombin times.
- Continually assess for changes in patient morale. Provide psychosocial supports as necessary.
- Assess baseline nutritional status and monitor I&O. Report any nausea, vomiting, anorexia, dehydration or electrolyte imbalance.
- Assess for alterations in skin integrity.
- Administer prescribed antiemetics as needed for nausea and vomiting.
- Monitor body temperature and administer antipyretic as prescribed.
- Provide oral care every 4-6 hours to prevent mouth deterioration.
- When injections are necessary, apply pressure for 3-5 minutes to prevent leakage or hematoma.
- Dispose of urine, feces and vomitus using double-glove technique.

OVERDOSAGE: SIGNS & SYMPTOMS

Severe bleeding, renal or liver toxicity

Patient/Family Education

- Caution patient that this medication must not be taken during pregnancy or when pregnancy is possible. Advise patient to use reliable form of birth control while taking this drug.
- Stress importance of compliance with all aspects of regimen.
- Provide family with literature appro-

priate to type of cancer or patient illness.

- Describe side effects (alopecia, nausea, vomiting, oral ulceration, skin alterations) and tell patient to report them to physician.
- Advise patient to notify physician if fever, chills, sore throat, signs of infection or bleeding gums occur.
- Caution patient to avoid taking aspirin or aspirin-containing products.
- Instruct family on proper disposal of urine, feces and vomitus if patient is receiving drug at home.
- Provide literature about local cancer support groups.

See Patient Guide, p. 506.

Pneumococcal Vaccine, Polyvalent

(new-moe-KAH-kuhl vaccine)

Pneumovax 23, Pnu-Imune 23

Class: Vaccine, inactivated bacteria

Action Induces antibodies against 23 capsular types of *Streptococcus pneumoniae*. Type-specific antibody facilitates bacterial destruction by complement-mediated lysis.

Indications Protection against pneumococcal pneumonia, pneumococcal bacteremia and other pneumococcal infections.

Contraindications Patients with Hodgkin's disease who have received extensive chemotherapy or nodal irradiation; patients with Hodgkin's disease cannot have immunization < 10 days before or during chemotherapy; children < 2 yr. Some packages contain thimerosal as preservative; use cautiously in mercury-sensitive patients or choose different brand.

Route/Dosage

ADULTS & CHILDREN: **SC/IM** 0.5 ml. *Booster dose:* Revaccinate recipients of 14-valent pneumococcal vaccine (distributed from 1977 to 1983) who are also at highest risk of fatal penumococcal infection (eg, asplenic patients), using 23-valent vaccine. Revaccinate adults who received 23-valent vaccine 6 or more yr earlier if they are also at highest risk or are likely to have rapid decline in antibody levels (eg, patients with asplenia, patients with nephrotic syndrome, renal failure or transplant recipients). Consider revaccination of children with nephrotic syndrome, asplenia or sickle-cell anemia after 3 to 5 yr, if these children would be < 10 yr of age at time of revaccination.

Interactions In patients anticipating immunosuppression, response to pneumoccal vaccine is best if administered 10-14 days prior to immunosuppressive chemotherapy or radiation. Pneumococcal and influenza vaccines and HIB, meningococcal and pneumococcal vaccines may safely and effectively be administered simultaneously at separate injection sites. As with other drugs administered by IM injection, give pneumococcal vaccine with caution to persons receiving anticoagulant therapy.

Lab Test Interferences

None well documented.

Adverse Reactions

Local: Erythema and soreness at injection site, usually < 48 hr in duration. Local induration occurs less commonly. *Systemic:* Rash, arthralgia, adenitis, fever > 39° C (102° F), malaise, myalgia and asthenia occur rarely. Low-grade fever (< 38.3° C or 100.9° F) occurs occasionally and usually subsides within 24 hr. Patients with otherwise stabilized immune thrombocytopenic purpura may rarely experience relapse in thrombocytopenia, 2-14 days after vaccination, lasting up to 2 wk. Anaphylactoid reactions have been rarely reported.

Precautions

Pregnancy: Category C. Vaccinate if risk of disease outweighs risk to patients. *Lactation:* Undetermined.

NURSING CONSIDERATIONS

Administration/Storage

- Administer via SC or IM route only.
- Keep medication under refrigeration.

Assessment/Interventions

- Obtain patient history, including drug history and any known allergies. Note if patient is receiving immunosuppressive therapy or scheduled for surgery. Vaccine should be administered at least 2 weeks prior to these procedures when possible.
- If needed, give one dose of acetaminophen to reduce pain at injection site and to prevent fever.

Patient/Family Education

- Instruct parents on risks and benefits of vaccination.
- Explain that tepid bath may reduce pain at injection site.
- Advise parents to complete all immunizations.
- Explain that low-grade fever is transient and should subside in 24 hr.
- Tell patient or parents to notify physician immediately if any serious adverse reactions occur (shortness of breath, hives, wheezing).
- This vaccine is usually only needed once.

No patient monograph available.

Poliovirus Vaccine, Inactivated (IPV)

(POE-lee-oh-VYE-russ vaccine)

IPOL, Poliovax

Class: Vaccine, inactivated virus

Action Induces protective antipoliovirus antibodies, reducing pharyngeal excretion of poliovirus types 1, 2 and 3.

Indications Routine use in infants and children is not recommended; OPV is generally preferred. Prophylaxis for individuals traveling to regions where poliomyelitis is endemic or epidemic (eg, developing countries), who routinely are exposed to patients who may be excreting polioviruses or to laboratory specimens that may contain polioviruses, and for members of communities with disease caused by wild polioviruses. Offer IPV to individuals who decline OPV or in whom OPV is contraindicated. In household with immunocompromised member or close contacts, or in household with unimmunized adult, use only IPV for all those requiring poliovirus immunization. Previous clinical poliomyelitis (usually due to single poliovirus type) or incomplete immunization with OPV are not contraindications to completing primary series of immunization with IPV.

Contraindications History of hypersensitivity to any component of vaccine, including neomycin, streptomycin and polymyxin B. Patients with acute febrile illness should not receive IPV until after recovery.

Route/Dosage

CHILDREN: **SC** 0.5 ml in deltoid region. In infants and small children, preferred site is anterolateral thigh muscle. CHILDREN: Primary series consists of 3 doses of 0.5 ml. Separate first 2 doses by at least 4 wk, but preferably 8 wk; commonly given at 2 and 4 mo of age. Give third dose at least 6 mo, but preferably 12 mo, after second dose, commonly given at 15-18 mo of age. Give all children who received primary series of IPV or combination of IPV and OPV booster dose of OPV or IPV before entering school, unless third dose of primary series was administered on or after fourth birthday. ADULTS: For unvaccinated adults at increased risk of exposure to poliovirus, give primary series of IPV: 2 doses at 1-2-mo interval, with third dose 6-12 mo later. If < 3 mo, but > 2 mo remain before protection is needed (eg, planned international travel), give 3 doses of IPV at least 1 mo apart.

Likewise, if only 1 or 2 mo remain, give 2 doses of IPV 1 mo apart. If < 4 wk remain, give single dose of either OPV or IPV. Give adults at increased risk of exposure who have had at least 1 dose of OPV, < 3 doses of conventional IPV (available before 1988) or combination of conventional IPV and OPV totaling < 3 doses, at least 1 dose of OPV or IPV. Give any additional doses needed to complete primary series if time permits. Give adults who have completed primary series with any poliovirus vaccine and who are at increased risk of exposure to poliovirus single dose of either OPV or IPV.

Interactions Several routine pediatric vaccines may safely and effectively be administered simultaneously at separate injection sites (eg, DTP, MMR, OPV, Hib, hepatitis B, influenza). National authorities recommend simultaneous immunization at separate sites as indicated by age or health risk.

Lab Test Interferences
None well documented.

Adverse Reactions
Local: IPV administration may result in erythema, induration and pain at injection site. *Systemic:* Temperatures 39° C (102° F) or higher reported in 38% of IPV vaccinees.

Precautions
Pregnancy: Category C. Vaccinate if risk of disease outweighs risk to patients. *Lactation:* Undetermined.

NURSING CONSIDERATIONS

Administration/Storage

- Give 0.5 ml subcutaneously in deltoid for adults; preferred site for infants is vastus lateralis.
- If blood appears in syringe after aspiration, do not inject. Withdraw needle and discard syringe. Use new dose injected at different site.
- Document manufacturer and lot number of vaccine, date of administration and name, address and title of person administering vaccine in permanent record according to federal regulations.
- Store under refrigeration.

Assessment/Interventions

- Obtain patient history, including drug history and any known allergies.
- Advise adult patients to be vaccinated before traveling to developing country.
- Note if patient is immunocompromised or in household with unimmunized adult.
- If patient has acute febrile illness, notify physician and do not administer until after recovery.
- Assess patient for any adverse reactions and document properly in patient record. Report as required by Vaccine Adverse Event Reporting System (VAERS) (800-822-7967).

Patient/Family Education

- Advise patient to observe for fever, erythema, induration or pain at injection site and to report to physician immediately.
- Explain risks and benefits of vaccination.
- Advise patient and family about vaccine schedule. Explain that the series must be completed to offer full protection.

No patient monograph available.

Poliovirus Vaccine, Live, Oral, Trivalent (OPV)

(POE-lee-oh-VYE-russ vaccine)
Orimune
Class: Vaccine, live virus

Action Induces protective antibodies, reducing intestinal and pharyngeal excretion of poliovirus. OPV administration simulates natural infection, inducing active mucosal and systemic immunity against poliovirus types 1, 2 and 3.

Indications Prevention of poliomyelitis. Infants as young as 6-12 wk and all unimmunized children and adolsecents up to 18 yr are usual candidates for routine OPV prophylaxis. OPV is also recommended for control of epidemic poliomyelitis. *Adults:* Primary immunization with inactivated polio vaccine is recommended whenever feasible for unimmunized adults subject to increased risk of exposure, such as by travel to or contact with epidemic or endemic areas (eg, developing countries) and for those employed in medical and sanitation facilities. If < 4 wk remain before protection is needed, single dose of OPV is recommended, with remaining vaccine doses given later if person remains at increased risk. Immunization with IPV may be indicated for unimmunized parents and those in other special situations in which protection may be needed. In household with immunocompromised member or other close contacts or in household with unimmunized adult, use only IPV for all those requiring poliovirus immunization.

Contraindications Do not administer OPV to any person with immunosuppression or to any household member of immunodeficient person. This includes combined immunodeficiency, hypogammaglobulinemia, agammaglobulinemia, thymic abnormalities, leukemia, lymphoma, generalized malignancy, lowered resistance to infection from therapy with corticosteroids, alkylating drugs, antimetabolites or radiation. Advise vaccine recipients to avoid contact with such persons for at least 6-8 wk. Do not give OPV to member of household in which there is family history of immunodeficiency until immune status of intended recipient and other children in family is determined to be normal. IPV is preferred for immunizing all persons in these circumstances.

Route/Dosage
OLDER CHILDREN, ADOLESCENTS & ADULTS: **PO** 0.5 ml. Give 2 doses no less than 6 wk apart (or no more than 8 wk apart) followed by third dose 6-12 mo later. INFANTS: **PO** 0.5 ml. Administer at 2, 4 and 15-18 mo. A fourth dose is given when child begins school if third dose of primary series was administered before child's fourth birthday. OPV may be administered with any of following: Distilled water, chlorinated tap water, simple syrup, milk, bread, sugar cube or cake.

Interactions Immune globulin (IG) does not interfere with immunity following OPV. However, do not administer OPV < 7 days after IG administration unless unavoidable, such as unexpected travel to or contact with epidemic or endemic areas or persons. If OPV is given within 1 wk after IG, the OPV dose should probably be repeated 3 mo later, if immunity is still needed. Like all live viral vaccines, administration to patients or contacts of patients receiving immunosuppressant drugs, including steroids or radiation may predispose patients to disseminated infections or insufficient response to immunization. They may remain susceptible despite immunization. Several routine pediatric vaccines may safely and effectively be administered simultaneously at separate injection sites (eg, DTP, MMR, IPV, Hib, hepatitis B, influenza). National authorities recommend simultaneous immunization at separate sites as indicated by age or health risk. Live virus vaccines may cause delayed-hypersensitivity skin test results (eg, tuberculin, histoplasmin) to appear falsely negative. Effect may persist for several weeks after vaccination. Give tuberculin tests either prior to live-virus vaccination, simultaneously with it, or 6 or more wk after vaccination.

Lab Test Interferences None well documented.

Adverse Reactions Vaccine-associated paralysis occurs with frequency of 1 case per 2.6 million OPV vaccine doses distributed.

Precautions Do not use OPV in immunodeficient persons, including persons with congenital or acquired immune deficiencies, whether due to genetics, disease or drug or radiation therapy. Contains live viruses. Avoid use in HIV-positive persons, regardless of whether symptomatic or asymptomatic. Poliovirus is shed for 6-8 wk in vaccinees' stool and by pharyngeal route. *Pregnancy:* Category C. Use OPV in pregnancy if exposure is imminent and immediate protection is needed. *Lactation:* Breast-feeding does not generally interfere with successful immunization of infants, despite IgA antibody secretion in breast milk.

NURSING CONSIDERATIONS

Administration/Storage

- Give medication orally.
- Administer directly or mix with distilled water, plain tap water, syrup, milk or sugar cube. Changes in color of product are of no significance as long as product remains clear.
- Store in freezer. Drug may remain in liquid state to 14° C (7° F) because of sorbital content.
- If frozen, vaccine must be thawed completely before use.
- Follow recommended schedule for immunization (2, 4, 15 or 18 mo and at 4-6 yr).
- Discard poliovirus pipettes in manner that will inactivate live virus (eg, autoclave, incinerator).
- Maximum of 10 freeze-thaw cycles are permitted provided (1) temperature dose not exceed 8° C (46° F) and (2) vaccine remains thawed for no more than 24 hr total.

Assessment/Interventions

- Obtain patient history, including drug history and any known allergies.
- Note if patient has had hypersensitivity test within 48 hr. Live virus could cause false-negative result.
- Document manufacturer, lot number, date of administration, name, address and title of person administering on patient's chart.
- Adhere to guidelines of Vaccine Adverse Event Reporting System (VAERS) for reporting adverse effects (800/822-7967).

Patient/Family Education

- Advise women to abstain from breastfeeding 2-3 hr before and after vaccination of infants to permit establishment of viruses in gut.
- Explain risks and benefits of vaccination. Point out to parents or patient that vaccine produces protective antibodies against poliomyelitis.
- Tell parents that child should receive dose at 2, 4, and 15 or 18 mo and at 4-6 yr to be fully immunized.
- Explain that attenuated live virus vaccine may be shed for a few weeks following vaccination. This virus is not harmful to normal individuals but may cause disease in immumocompromised patients. Therefore vaccine recipient must stay away from immunocompromised individuals.

No patient monograph available.

Polyethylene Glycol-Electrolyte Solution (PEG-ES)

(poli-eth-uh-leen gli-cawl)

Colovage, CoLyte, GoLYTELY, OCL

Class: Laxative

Action Induces diarrhea, which rapidly cleanses bowel, usually within 4 hr.

Indications Bowel cleansing prior to GI examination. **Unlabeled use:** Management of acute iron overdose in children.

Contraindications GI obstruction; gastric retention; bowel perforation; toxic colitis; toxic megacolon or ileus.

Route/Dosage

ADULTS: **PO/Nasogastric** 4 L prior to GI examination. Give orally as 240 ml q 10 min or via NG tube as 1.2-1.8 L/hr until 4 L are consumed or until rectal effluent is clear. Via nasogastric (NG) tube, use rate of 1.2-1.8 L/hr.

Interactions

Oral medication given within 1 hr of starting therapy: Medication may be flushed from GI tract and not absorbed.

Lab Test Interferences

None well documented.

Adverse Reactions

EENT: Rhinorrhea. *GI:* Nausea; abdominal fullness; bloating; abdominal cramps; vomiting; anal irritation. *DERM:* Urticaria; dermatitis.

Precautions

Pregnancy: Category C. *Children:* Safety and efficacy not established. *Regurgitation/aspiration:* Use with caution in patients with impaired gag reflex. *Severe ulcerative colitis:* Use with caution. If GI obstruction or perforation is suspected, rule out these contraindications before administration.

NURSING CONSIDERATIONS

Administration/Storage

- May be given via NG tube for patients unable or unwilling to drink solution.
- Reconstitute solution with tap water and shake container until powder is dissolved.
- Do not add flavorings or additional ingredients to solution before use. Chilling solution before administration improves palatability.
- Refrigerate reconstituted solution. Use within 48 hr.
- Minimum of 3 L of solution should be administered to achieve satisfactory bowel evacuation.

Assessment/Interventions

- Obtain patient history, including drug history and any allergies. Note history of ulcerative colitis.
- Do not administer if patient has, or is suspected to have, GI obstruction, gastric retention, bowel perforation, toxic colitis, toxic megacolon or ileus.
- Observe patients with impaired gag reflex or patient who is otherwise prone to regurgitation or aspiration during administration, especially if solution is given via NG tube.
- Notify physician if patient is unable to tolerate solution or if rectal bleeding occurs.
- If patient complains of bloating, abdominal pain or distention, slow solution or discontinue until symptoms abate.

OVERDOSAGE: SIGNS & SYMPTOMS

Diarrhea, bloating, abdominal pain

Patient/Family Education

- Explain that solution is given to cleanse bowel as preparation for GI examination.
- Explain that if discomfort becomes intolerable patient should stop drinking solution temporarily or allow

longer intervals between drink portions.

- Instruct patient not to eat or drink anything for 3-4 hr before ingestion and explain that only clear liquids are allowed after ingestion of solution.
- Tell patient to continue drinking solution until watery stool is clear and free of solid material.
- Instruct patient to report the following symptoms to physician: severe bloating, distention or abdominal pain.

See Patient Guide, p. 507.

Potassium Chloride

(poe-TASS-ee-uhm KLOR-ide)

Cena-K, Gen-K, K + Care, K-Dur, K-Lor, K-Lyte/Cl, K-Norm, K-Tab, Kaochlor, Kaon-Cl, Kato, Kay Ciel, Klor-Con, Klorvess, Klotrix, K-Lease, Micro-K, Potassium Chloride (for injection), Rum-K, Slow-K, Ten-K, K + 10, Potasalan, ♣ *APO-K, Kalium, K-Lor, K-Med 900, Roychlor*

Class: Electrolyte

Action Major intracellular cation, essential in maintaining acid-base balance and isotonicity within cells. Functions in muscle contraction, nerve impulse transmission, gastric secretion, renal function and metabolism.

Indications Treatment of hypokalemia; prevention of potassium depletion in certain conditions. Parenterally, as prophylaxis and/or treatment of moderate to severe potassium loss when oral therapy is not adequate or feasible. **Unlabeled use:** Treatment of thallium poisoning; with anticholinesterase agents in myasthenia gravis.

Contraindications Severe renal impairment with concomitant azotemia or oliguria; hyperkalemia; diseases in which high potassium levels may be present include: renal failure and conditions in which potassium retention is present; anuria; trauma with muscle destruction; severe hemolytic reactions; adrenocortical insufficiency; heat cramps; acute dehydration; adynamica episodica hereditaria; early postoperative oliguria (except during GI drainage); use of potassium-sparing diuretics.

Route/Dosage

ADULTS: **PO** 20-100 mEq in divided doses. **IV** 10-40 mEq/hr. INFANTS: **PO** 2-3 mEq/kg in divided doses.

Interactions

Digitalis: Cardiac arrhythmias may occur with potassium imbalance. *Potassium-sparing diuretics:* Severe hyperkalemia may occur.

Lab Test Interferences

None well documented.

Adverse Reactions

GI: Abdominal discomfort or distention; GI obstruction; bleeding; ulceration or perforation; nausea; vomiting; flatulence. *GU:* Oliguria; anuria. *DERM:* Rashes. *OTHER:* Hyperkalemia (symptoms may include paresthesia of extremities; listlessness; confusion; weak or heavy limbs; flaccid paralysis; hypotension; arrhythmias; heart block; cardiac arrest; prolonged QT interval; wide QRS complex; peaked T waves; ST depression.

Precautions

Pregnancy: Category C. *Lactation:* Undetermined. *Children:* Safety and efficacy not established. *Special risk patients:* Administer with caution to elderly patients or patients with decreased renal function. Use with caution in patients with cardiac disease. *GI lesions:* May cause stenotic or ulcerative lesions of the small bowel and death. Discontinue immediately if bowel obstruction or perforation is suspected. *Hyperkalemia:* May produce hyperkalemia or cardiac arrest in patients with impaired potassium excretion.

NURSING CONSIDERATIONS

Administration/Storage

- Do not give tablets to patients who have physical conditions that may slow or stop tablet in GI track; use properly diluted concentrate form.
- Use whole tablets; do not crush or split tablets. Do not allow patient to chew or suck tablets.
- Administer tablets after meals or with food and full glass of water.
- Mix or dissolve completely oral liquids, soluble powders, or effervescent tablets in 3-8 oz of cold water, juice or other beverage and have patient drink slowly to minimize GI irritation.
- Do not give via IM route.
- Generally, do not begin IV administration until renal flow is established.
- Do not exceed IV administration rate of 20 mEq/hr and concentration of 40 mEq/L without performing cardiac monitoring. Rapid infusion may cause local pain; reduce rate to relieve irritation.
- Dilute parenteral concentrates before use. Direct injection may be instantly fatal.
- Maximum 24 hr dose should not exceed 200 mEq if serum potassium is > 2.5 mEq/L; 400 mEq, if serum potassium is < 2 mEq/L.

Assessment/Interventions

- Obtain patient history, including drug history and any known allergies. Note renal cardiac disease, untreated Addison's disease, dehydration or other conditions that may place patient at risk.
- Ensure that potassium level has been obtained before beginning therapy. Monitor potassium levels regularly during treatment. Cardiac monitoring is recommended when giving parenteral potassium at rates > 20 mEq/hr.
- Monitor serum potassium levels closely in patients with renal impairment.
- Watch for ECG changes such as peaking of T waves, loss of P wave, depression of ST segment, prolongation of QT interval, lengthened P-R interval or widened QRS complex during cardiac monitoring.
- Observe for overt signs of hyperkalemia: decreased BP, parasthesia, muscle weakness and flaccid paralysis of extremities, listlessness, mental confusion, shock, cardiac arrhythmias or heart block. Notify physician immediately if these symptoms occur.
- Observe for phlebitis (IV) and for possible GI distress including abdominal discomfort, nausea, vomiting and diarrhea. Notify physician if these symptoms occur.
- Do not abruptly discontinue drug in patients who are also receiving digitalis; digitalis toxicity may occur.

OVERDOSAGE: SIGNS & SYMPTOMS

ECG changes, ventricular fibrillation, death, muscle weakness that may progress to paralysis of diaphragm

Patient/Family Education

- Instruct patient to take oral medication after meals or with food and full glass of water.
- Advise patient to swallow tablets whole, without chewing, sucking or crushing.
- Warn patient not to use salt substitutes and to avoid "salt-free" food unless approved by physician.
- Advise patients taking time-released drug that wax matrix may appear in stool. Emphasize that this is normal.
- Explain importance of avoiding ingestion of large amounts of potassium through excessive intake of foods such as avocados, bananas, broccoli, dried fruits, grapefruit, oranges, beans, nuts, spinach, tomatoes and sunflower seeds.
- Instruct patient to promptly report these symptoms to physician: severe nausea or vomiting, abdominal pain,

black stools, tingling of hands and feet, unusual fatigue or weakness or feeling of heaviness in legs.

See Patient Guide, p. 508.

Pravastatin Sodium

(PRUH-vuh-stuh-tin SO-dee-uhm)

Pravachol

Class: Antihyperlipidemic/HMG-CoA reductase inhibitor

Action Increases rate at which body removes cholesterol from blood and reduces production of cholesterol in body by inhibiting enzyme that catalyzes early rate-limiting step in cholesterol synthesis.

Indications Reduction of elevated cholesterol and low-density lipoprotein (LDL) cholesterol levels in patients with primary hypercholesterolemia (types IIa and IIb). **Unlabeled uses:** Lowers elevated cholesterol levels in patients with heterozygous familial hypercholesterolemia, familial combined hyperlipidemia, diabetic dyslipidemia in non-insulin-dependent diabetics, hypercholesterolemia secondary to nephrotic syndrome and homozygous familial hypercholesterolemia in patients who are not completely devoid of LDL receptors but have reduced level of LDL receptor activity.

Contraindications Active liver disease or unexplained persistent elevations of liver function tests; pregnancy; lactation.

Route/Dosage

ADULTS: **PO** 10-40 mg at bedtime.

Interactions

Bile acid sequestrants: Large decrease in pravastatin bioavailability. *Gemfibrozil:* Severe myopathy or rhabdomyolysis; decreased urinary excretion and protein binding of pravastatin.

Lab Test Interferences

None well documented.

Adverse Reactions

CV: Chest pain. *RESP:* Common cold; rhinitis; cough; influenza. *CNS:* Headache; dizziness. *EENT:* Dysfunction of certain cranial nerves (including alteration of taste, impairment of extraocular movement, facial paresis); lens opacities. *GI:* Nausea; vomiting; diarrhea; abdominal pain; constipation; flatulence; heartburn; dyspepsia; pancreatitis. *HEPA:* Hepatitis; jaundice; fatty changes in liver; cirrhosis; fulminant hepatic necrosis; hepatoma; increased serum transaminases. *GU:* Urinary abnormality. *DERM:* Rash; pruritus. *OTHER:* Localized pain; myalgia; myopathy; rhabdomyolysis; fatigue; paresthesia; peripheral neuropathy. An apparent hypersensitivity syndrome has been reported rarely that has included one or more of these features: anaphylaxis; angioedema; lupus erythematous–like syndrome; polymyalgia rheumatica; vasculitis; purpura; thrombocytopenia; leukopenia; hemolyticanemia; positive anti-nuclear antibodies; increase in erythrocyte sedimentation rate; arthritis; arthralgia; urticaria; asthenia; photosensitivity; fever; chills; flushing; malaise; dyspnea; toxic epidermal necrolysis; erythema multiforme, including Stevens-Johnson syndrome.

Precautions

Pregnancy: Category X. *Lactation:* Excreted in breast milk. *Children:* Use in children not recommended. *Liver dysfunction:* Use with caution in patients who consume substantial quantities of alcohol or those with history of liver disease. Marked, persistent increases in serum transaminases have occurred. *Renal impairment:* Monitor patients closely. *Skeletal muscle effects:* Rhabdomyolysis with renal dysfunction secondary to myoglobinuria has occurred.

NURSING CONSIDERATIONS

Administration/Storage

- Administer at bedtime for best results. Hepatic cholesterol production is highest during night.
- Store at room temperature in tightly closed container.

Assessment/Interventions

- Obtain patient history, including drug history and any known allergies. Assess dietary history.
- Ensure that total cholesterol and LDL levels have been obtained before beginning therapy and reassess periodically during therapy.
- Assess for side effects (nausea and vomiting, diarrhea, abdominal pain, headache).

Patient/Family Education

- Caution patient that this medication must not be taken during pregnancy or when pregnancy is possible. Advise patient to use reliable form of birth control while taking this drug.
- Explain that full effectiveness of drug may not occur for up to 4 wk after initiation of therapy.
- Teach dietary habits that reduce cholesterol and saturated fats.
- Instruct patient to report these symptoms to physician: any unexplained muscle pain, tenderness or weakness, especially if accompanied by fever or malaise; yellowing of skin or eyes.
- Emphasize importance of follow-up visits to monitor drug effectiveness.

See Patient Guide, p. 509.

Praziquantel

(pray-zih-KWAHN-tuhl)
Biltricide
Class: Anti-infective/antihelmintic

Action Increases cell membrane permeability in susceptible worms, resulting in loss of intracellular calcium, massive contractions and paralysis of their musculature. Phagocytes are thus able to attach to worm, causing its death.

Indications Infections caused by *Schistosoma mekongi*, *S japnicum*, *S mansoni*, *S hematobium*, liver flukes, *Clonorchis sinensis* and *Opisthorchis viverrini*. **Unlabeled uses:** Treatment of neurocysticercosis, tissue flukes (opisthorchis, felineus, *Paragonimus westermani*, *Fasciola hepatica*), intestinal flukes (*Heterophyes heterophyes*, *Fasciolopsis buski*) and intestinal cestodes (*Diphyllobothrium latum*, *Taenia saginata*, *T solium*, *Dipylidium canium*, *Hymenolepsis nana*), and schistomiasis (in concurrent use with oxamniquine).

Contraindications Ocular cysticercosis.

Route/Dosage

Schisosomiasis

ADULTS & CHILDREN > 4 YR: **PO** 60 mg/kg in 3 equally divided doses q 4-6 hr for 1 day.

Clonorchiasis and Opisthorchiasis

ADULTS: **PO** 75 mg/kg in 3 equally divided doses q 4-6 hr for 1-2 days.

Larval Cysticercosis

ADULTS & CHILDREN: 10-25 mg/kg in single dose; 50 mg/kg in 3 divided doses for 14 days.

Interactions None well documented.

Lab Test Interferences None well documented.

Adverse Reactions
CNS: Malaise; headache; fever; drowsiness; dizziness. *GI:* Abdominal discomfort, with or without nausea. *HEPA:* Increased liver enzymes. *DERM:* Urticaria.

Precautions
Pregnancy: Category B. *Lactation:* Excreted in breast milk. Lactating women should avoid breastfeeding on day of treatment and for subsequent 72

hr. *Children:* Safety and efficacy not established in children < 4 yr.

NURSING CONSIDERATIONS

Administration/Storage

- Administer tablets during meals with liquids.
- Instruct patient not to chew tablets.
- Store at room temperature.

Assessment/Interventions

- Obtain patient history, including drug history and any known allergies. Note history of seizures.
- Monitor for side effects, especially malaise, headache, dizziness, abdominal pain, nausea or fever.

Patient/Family Education

- Explain that treatment lasts only 1 day for most parasitic infections.
- Instruct patient to take drug with liquids during meals and not to chew tablets.
- Advise patient to have all family members examined for infestation.
- Emphasize need for follow-up examinations.
- Instruct patient to report these symptoms to physician: malaise, headache, dizziness, abdominal pain, nausea, urticaria or fever.
- Advise patient that drug may cause drowsiness and to use caution while driving or performing other tasks requiring mental alertness.

See Patient Guide, p. 510.

Prazosin

(PRAY-zoe-sin)

Minipress, ♣ *APO-Prazo, Novo-Prazin, Nu-Prazo*

Class: Antihypertensive/antiadrenergic, peripherally acting

Action Selectively blocks postsynaptic alpha-1-adrenergic receptors, resulting in dilation of arterioles and veins.

Indications Treatment of hypertension. **Unlabeled uses:** Refractory CHF; Raynaud's vasospasm; prostatic outflow obstruction; ergotamine-induced peripheral ischemia.

Contraindications Hypersensitivity to doxazosin or terazosin.

Route/Dosage

ADULTS: **PO** 1 mg bid-tid initially. Maintenance: 6-20 mg/day in divided doses (maximum 40 mg/day). CHILDREN: **PO** 0.5-7 mg tid has been suggested.

Interactions

Beta-blockers: Enhanced acute orthostatic hypotensive reaction after first dose of prazosin. *Verapamil:* Increased serum prazosin levels and increased sensitivity to orthostatic hypotension.

Lab Test Interferences

May cause false elevation in vanillylmandelic acid.

Adverse Reactions

CV: Palpitations; orthostatic hypotension; hypotension; tachycardia. *RESP:* Dyspnea. *CNS:* Depression; dizziness; nervousness; paresthesia; asthenia; drowsiness; headache. *EENT:* Blurred vision; conjunctivitis; tinnitus; nasal congestion; epistaxis. *GI:* Nausea; vomiting; dry mouth; diarrhea; constipation; abdominal discomfort or pain. *GU:* Impotence; urinary frequency; incontinence; priapism. *DERM:* Pruritus; rash; sweating; alopecia; lichen planus. *OTHER:* Arthralgia; edema; fever.

Precautions

Pregnancy: Category C. *Lactation:* Excreted in breast milk. *Children:* Safety and efficacy not established. *Concomitant therapy:* When adding a diuretic or other antihypertensive agent, reduce dosage to 1-2 mg tid and then retitrate. *First-dose effect:* May cause marked hypotension (especially orthostatic) and syncope at 30 min after first few doses, after reintroduction, with rapid increase (≥ 2 mg) in dosing or after addition of another antihypertensive. To avoid, initiate dosing with low dose (1 mg or ≤ 2 mg) and gradually increase after 2 wk. *Lipids:* May decrease total cholesterol levels and LDLs and increase HDLs.

NURSING CONSIDERATIONS

Administration/Storage

- Give initial dose at bedtime to avoid syncope.
- Dosage is increased slowly, usually q 2 wk, with increase given in hs dose.
- Give maintenance therapy in divided doses.
- Note that efficacy does not increase when dosage exceeds 20 mg/day.
- Store at room temperature in tightly closed, light-resistant container.

Assessment/Interventions

- Obtain patient history, including drug history and any known allergies. Note current use of antihypertensives.
- Obtain baseline BP and pulse.
- Observe for possible retention of water and sodium.
- Monitor closely for first-dose effect. If syncope occurs, place patient in recumbent position and notify physician.
- If patient complains of dizziness, palpitations, drowsiness, fatigue, tiredness, nausea or headache, notify physician.

OVERDOSAGE: SIGNS & SYMPTOMS

Drowsiness, depressed reflexes, hypotension

Patient/Family Education

- Advise patient to take medication at same time each day.
- Warn patient about possibility of syncope or orthostasis.
- Instruct patient to report these symptoms to physician: dizziness, palpitations, drowsiness, fatigue, nausea, or headache.
- Caution patient to avoid sudden position changes to prevent orthostatic hypotension.
- Advise patient to avoid driving or performing other tasks requiring mental alertness for 12-24 hr after first dose, after dosage increase, and after resuming treatment after interruption. After the 12-24 hr period, advise patient to use caution.
- Instruct patient not to take otc medications (eg, nonprescription weight loss products or cough, cold or allergy medications) without consulting physician.

See Patient Guide, p. 511.

Prednisolone

(pred-NISS-oh-lone)

Prednisolone

Delta-Cortef, Prelone, ♣ *Minims Prednisolone, Novo-Prednisolone*

Prednisolone Acetate

Articulose-50, Econopred, Econopred Plus, Key-Pred 25, Key-Pred 50, Predcor-25, Predcor-50, Predaject-50, Predalone 50, Pred Forte, Pred Mild, ♣ *Diopred, Ophtho-Tate*

Prednisolone Sodium Phosphate

AK-Pred, Hydeltrasol, Inflamase Forte, Inflamase Mild, Key-Pred-SP, Pediapred, ♣ *R.O.-Predphate*

Prednisolone Tebutate

Hydeltra-T.B.A., Predalone T.B.A., Prednisol TBA

Class: Corticosteroid

Action Intermediate-acting glucocorticoid that depresses formation, release and activity of endogenous mediators of inflammation including prostaglandins, kinins, histamine, liposomal enzymes and complement system. Also modifies body's immune response.

Indications

Oral/parenteral administration: Endocrine disorders; rheumatic disorders; collagen diseases; dermatologic diseases; allergic and inflammatory ophthalmic processes; respiratory diseases; hematologic disorders; neoplastic diseases; edematous states caused by nephrotic syndrome; GI diseases; multiple sclerosis; tuberculous meningitis; trichinosis with neurologic or myocardial involvement. *Intra-articular or soft tissue administration:* Short-term adjunctive therapy of synovitis of osteoarthritis, rheumatoid arthritis, bursitis, acute gouty arthritis, epicondylitis, acute nonspecific tenosynovitis, posttraumatic osteoarthritis. *Intralesional administration:* Treatment of following lesions: keloids; localized hypertrophic, infiltrated, inflammatory lesions of lichen planus, psoriatic plaques, granuloma annulare, lichen simplex chronicus; discoid lupus erythematosus; necrobiosis lipoidica diabeticorum; alopecia areata; cystic tumors of aponeurosis or tendon. *Ophthalmic administration:* Treatment of steroid-responsive inflammatory conditions of palpebral and bulbar conjunctiva, lid, cornea and anterior segment of globe. **Unlabeled use:** Adjunctive therapy for tuberculous pleurisy.

Contraindications

Oral/parenteral: Systemic fungal infections; administration of live virus vaccines. *IM:* Idiopathic thrombocytopenic purpura; sulfite sensitivity. *Ophthalmic:* Acute superficial herpes simplex keratitis; fungal diseases of ocular structures, vaccinia, varicella and most other viral diseases of cornea and conjunctiva; ocular tuberculosis.

Route/Dosage

ADULTS: **PO** 5-60 mg/day (prednisolone, prednisolone sodium phosphate). **IM** 4-60 mg/day (prednisolone acetate). **IV/IM** 4-60 mg/day (prednisolone sodium phosphate). **Ophthalmic** 1-2 gtt into conjunctival sac q hr during day and q 2 hr during night (prednisolone acetate, prednisolone sodium phosphate).

Intra-Articular, Intralesional or Soft Tissue Administration

ADULTS: 4-100 mg (prednisolone acetate); 4-30 mg or lesions (prednisolone tebutate), or 2-30 mg prednisolone sodium phosphate.

Multiple Sclerosis

ADULTS: **PO** 200 mg/day for 1 wk then 80 mg qod for 1 mo (prednisolone, prednisolone sodium phosphate). **IM** 200 mg/day for 1 wk then 80 mg qod for 1 mo (prednisolone acetate).

Tuberculous Pleurisy

ADULTS: **PO** 0.75 mg/kg/day then taper as tolerated until patient is drug-free (prednisolone).

Interactions

Anticholinesterases: May antagonize anticholinesterase effects in myasthenia gravis. *Barbiturates:* May decrease pharmacologic effect of prednisolone. *Contraceptives (oral), estrogens, ketoconazole:* May decrease clearance of prednisolone. *Hydantoins, rifampin:* May increase clearance and decrease efficacy of prednisolone. *Salicylates:* May reduce serum levels and efficacy of salicylates. *Troleandomycin:* May increase prednisolone effects.

Lab Test Interferences

May cause increased serum cholesterol; decreased serum levels of potassium, T_3 and T_4; decreased uptake of thyroid I^{131}; false-negative results of nitroblue-tetrazolium test for systemic bacterial infection; suppression of skin test reactions.

Adverse Reactions

CV: Thromboembolism or fat embolism; thrombophlebitis; necrotizing angiitis; cardiac arrhythmias or ECG changes; syncopal episodes; hypertension; myocardial rupture; CHF. *CNS:* Convulsions; pseudotumor cerebri (increased intracranial pressure with papilledema); vertigo; headache; neuritis; paresthesias; psychosis. *EENT:* Posterior subcapsular cataracts; increased intraocular pressure; glaucoma; exophthalmos. With ophthalmic use: glaucoma with optic nerve damage; visual acuity and field defects; posterior subcapsular cataract formation; secondary ocular infections; transient stinging or burning; perforation of globe. *GI:* Pancreatitis; abdominal distention; ulcerative esophagitis; nausea; vomiting; increased appetite and weight gain; peptic ulcer with perforation and hemorrhage; small and large bowel perforation. *GU:* Increased or decreased motility and number of spermatozoa. *HEMA:* Leukocytosis. *DERM:* Impaired wound healing; thin, fragile skin; petechiae and ecchymoses; erythema; lupus erythematosus–like lesions; subcutaneous fat atrophy; striae; hirsutism; acneiform eruptions; allergic dermatitis; urticaria; angioneurotic edema; perineal irritation; hyperpigmentation or hypopigmentation. *META:* Sodium and fluid retention; hypokalemia; hypokalemic alkalosis; metabolic alkalosis; hypocalcemia; negative nitrogen balance. *OTHER:* Musculoskeletal effects (eg, weakness, myopathy, muscle mass loss, tendon rupture, osteoporosis, aseptic necrosis of femoral and humoral heads, spontaneous fractures); endocrine abnormalities (eg, menstrual irregularities, cushingoid state, growth suppression in children, sweating, decreased carbohydrate tolerance, hyperglycemia, glycosuria, increased insulin or sulfonylurea requirements in diabetic patients, hirsutism); anaphylactoid or hypersensitivity reactions; aggravation or masking of infections; fatigue; insomnia. With intra-articular administration: osteonecrosis; tendon rupture; infection, skin atrophy; postinjection flare; hypersensitivity; facial flushing.

Precautions

Pregnancy: Category C (prednisolone sodium phosphate). Safety not established. *Lactation:* Excreted in breast milk. *Children:* Observe growth and development of infants and children on prolonged therapy. *Elderly patients:* May require lower doses. *Adrenal suppression:* Prolonged therapy may lead to hypothalamic-pituitary-adrenal suppression. *Cardiovascular effects:* Use drug with great caution in patient who has suffered recent MI. *Hepatitis:* Drug may be harmful in patients with chronic active hepatitis positive for hepatitis B surface antigen. *Hypersensitivity:* Reactions may occur, including anaphylaxis. *Immunosuppression:* Do not administer live virus vaccines during treatment. *Infections:* Drug may mask signs of infection. May decrease host-defense mechanisms to prevent dissemination of infection. *Ocular effects:* Use systemic drug with caution in ocular herpes simplex because of possible corneal perforation. *Ophthalmic use:* Prolonged use may result in cataracts, glaucoma or other complications. *Peptic ulcer:* May contribute to peptic ulceration, especially in large doses. *Renal impairment:* Use drug with caution. *Repository injections:* Do not inject SC. Avoid injection into deltoid muscle and repeated IM injection into same site. *Stress:* Increased dosage of rapidly acting corticosteroid may be needed before, during and after stressful situations. *Withdrawal:* Abrupt discontinuation may result in adrenal insufficiency.

NURSING CONSIDERATIONS

Administration/Storage

- Check drug name carefully to avoid confusion with prednisone.
- Administer oral medication with food.
- For long-term use, alternate-day regimen may be used.
- Do not inject SC or IM doses into deltoid muscle. IM injection should be given in gluteal muscle. Rotate injection sites.

- Do not administer if patient has had live vaccine within last month.
- Discontinuation of drug must be done gradually.
- If giving ophthalmic solution, do not touch eye with dropper, place drops in lower lid and wait 5 min between drops. Apply pressure on lacrimal sac to prevent systemic effects. Wash hands before and after administering.
- Store dosage forms at room temperature and protect from light.

Assessment/Interventions

- Obtain patient history, including drug history and any known allergies. Note MI, diabetes, renal impairment, hepatitis, peptic ulcer disease, ocular herpes simplex or current infections.
- If patient is at increased risk for herpes, chickenpox or other viruses, notify physician.
- Ensure that baseline lab tests have been obtained before beginning therapy. Monitor for possible hyperglycemia, hypoglycemia and hypocalcemia during treatment.
- Be aware that drug may mask signs of infection and that resistance to infection may be diminished.
- In patients with diabetes, monitor blood glucose carefully.
- Monitor renal function, especially in patients with renal impairment.
- Observe for possible delayed wound healing.
- If menstrual irregularities, muscle wasting or weakness, moon face, fluid retention, GI bleeding or mental status changes occur, notify physician.
- Assess for signs of adrenal insufficiency (fever, myalgia, arthralgia, malaise, anorexia, nausea, orthostatic hypotension, dizziness, fainting) and notify physician immediately if suspected.

OVERDOSAGE: SIGNS & SYMPTOMS

Cushingoid changes, moonface, striae, central obesity, hirsutism, acne, ecchymoses, hypertension, osteoporosis, myopathy, sexual dysfunction, diabetes mellitus, hyperlipidemia, peptic ulcer, GI bleeding, increased susceptibility to infection, electrolyte and fluid imbalance, psychosis

Patient/Family Education

- Advise patient to take single daily or alternate-day doses in morning before 9 AM and to take multiple doses at evenly spaced intervals throughout day.
- Instruct patient to take medication with meals or snacks to avoid GI irritation.
- Caution patient not to take drug with aspirin or other otc medications containing salicylates unless directed by physician.
- Instruct patient to check weight at home daily at same time of day.
- Advise patient on chronic steroid therapy to wear Medi-Alert identification indicating condition and drug regimen.
- Remind patient to wash hands before and after instillation.
- Teach patient correct method for instilling eye drops.
- Instruct patient not to rub eyes or touch dropper into eye.
- Inform patient of increased appetite and counsel patient on appropriate diet management (diet high in protein, calcium and potassium but low in sodium and carbohydrates).
- Advise family that medication may slow growth in children.
- Inform patient of the possible side effects of moonface, mood swings and increased emotions.
- Teach patient to monitor for infection, eye burning or increased bruising.
- Instruct patient not to drive soon after using eye drops because vision may be blurred initially.

- Inform patient that ophthalmic preparation may cause sensitivity to bright light and recommend use of sunglasses to minimize this effect.
- Instruct patient to report these symptoms to physician: unusual weight gain, swelling of lower extremities, muscle weakness, black tarry stools, vomiting of blood, puffing of face, menstrual irregularities, prolonged sore throat, fever, cold or infection.
- Tell patient to notify physician if these symptoms occur after dosage reduction or withdrawal of therapy: fatigue, anorexia, nausea, vomiting, diarrhea, weight loss, weakness, dizziness or low blood sugar.

See Patient Guide, pp. 512-513.

Prednisone

(PRED-nih-sone)

Deltasone, Liquid Pred, Meticorten, Orasone, Panasol-S, Prednicen-M, Sterapred, Sterapred DS, ♣ *Winpred*

Class: Corticosteroid

Action Intermediate-acting glucocorticoid that depresses formation, release and activity of endogenous mediators of inflammation, including prostaglandins, kinins, histamine, liposomal enzymes and complement system. Also modifies body's immune response.

Indications Endocrine disorders; rheumatic disorders; collagen diseases; dermatologic diseases; allergic states; allergic and inflammatory ophthalmic processes; respiratory diseases; hematologic disorders; neoplastic diseases; edematous states (because of nephrotic syndrome); GI diseases; multiple sclerosis; tuberculous meningitis; trichinosis with neurologic or myocardial involvement. **Unlabeled uses:** COPD; Duchenne's muscular dystrophy; Graves ophthalmopathy.

Contraindications Systemic fungal infections; administration of live virus vaccines.

Route/Dosage
ADULTS: PO 5-60 mg/day.

COPD
ADULTS: PO 30-60 mg/day for 1-2 wk, then taper.

Duchenne's Muscular Dystrophy
ADULTS: PO 0.75-1.5 mg/kg/day.

Graves Ophthalmopathy
ADULTS: PO 60 mg/day; taper to 20 mg/day.

Interactions *Anticholinesterases:* Antagonizes anticholinesterase effects in myasthenia gravis. *Anticoagulants, oral:* Alters anticoagulant dose requirements. *Barbiturates, hydantoins (eg, phenytoin), rifampin:* Decreased pharmacologic effect of prednisone. *Cyclosporine:* Enhanced cyclosporine toxicity. *Estrogens, ketoconazole, oral contraceptives:* Decreased clearance of prednisone. *Nondepolarizing muscle relaxants:* May potentiate, counteract or have no effect on neuromuscular blocking action. *Salicylates:* Reduced serum levels and efficacy of salicylates. *Somatrem:* Inhibition of growth-promoting effects of somatrem. *Theophylline:* Alterations in pharmacologic activity of either agent.

Lab Test Interferences May increase serum cholesterol; decrease serum levels of T_3 and T_4; decrease uptake of thyroid I^{131}; and cause false-negative result on nitroblue-tetrazolium test for systemic bacterial infection and suppression of skin test reactions.

Adverse Reactions CV: Thromboembolism or fat embolism; thrombophlebitis; necrotizing angiitis; cardiac arrhythmias or ECG changes; syncopal episodes; hypertension; myocardial rupture; CHF. *CNS:* Convulsions; pseudotumor cerebri (increased intracranial pressure with papilledema); vertigo; headache; neuritis/paresthesias; psychosis. *EENT:* Posterior subcapsular cataracts; increased intra-ocular pressure; glaucoma; exophthalmos. *GI:* Pancreatitis; abdominal distention; ulcerative esophagitis; nausea; vomiting; increased appetite and weight gain; peptic ulcer with perforation and hemorrhage; small and large bowel perforation. *GU:* Increased or decreased motility and number of spermatozoa. *HEMA:* Leukocytosis. *DERM:* Impaired wound healing; thin fragile skin; petechiae and ecchymoses; erythema; lupus erythematosus–like lesions; subcutaneous fat atrophy; purpura; striae; hirsutism; acneiform eruptions; allergic dermatitis; urticaria; angioneurotic edema; perineal irritation. *META:* Sodium and fluid retention; hypokalemia; hypokalemic alkalosis; metabolic alkalosis; hypocalcemia. *OTHER:* Musculoskeletal effects (muscle weakness, steroid myopathy, muscle mass loss, tendon rupture, osteoporosis, aseptic necrosis of femoral and humeral heads, spontaneous fractures, including vertebral compression fractures and pathologic fracture of long bones); endocrine abnormalities (menstrual irregularities, cushingoid state, growth suppression in children secondary to adrenocortical and pituitary unresponsiveness, increased sweating, decreased carbohydrate tolerance, hyperglycemia, glycosuria, increased insulin or sulfonylurea requirements in diabetics, negative nitrogen balance because of protein catabolism, hirsutism); anaphylactoid/hypersensitivity reactions; aggravation or masking of infections; malaise; fatigue; insomnia.

Precautions

Pregnancy: Category C. *Lactation:* Excreted in breast milk. *Children:* Observe growth and development of infants and children on prolonged therapy. *Elderly:* May require lower doses. *Adrenal suppression:* Prolonged therapy may lead to hypothalamic-pituitary-adrenal suppression. *Cardiovascular effects:* Use drug with great caution in patients who have suffered recent MI. *Hepatitis:* Drug may be harmful in patients with chronic active hepatitis positive for hepatitis B surface antigen. *Hypersensitivity:* May occur, including anaphylaxis. *Immunosuppression:* Do not administer live virus vaccines during treatment. *Infections:* May mask signs of infection. May decrease host-defense mechanisms to prevent dissemination of infection. *Ocular effects:* Use systemic drug cautiously in ocular herpes simplex because of possible corneal perforation. *Ophthalmic use:* Prolonged use may result in glaucoma, cataracts or other complications. *Peptic ulcer:* May contribute to peptic ulceration, especially with large doses. *Renal impairment:* Use with caution; monitor renal function. *Stress:* Increased dosage of rapidly acting corticosteroid may be needed before, during and after stressful situations. *Withdrawal:* Abrupt discontinuation may result in adrenal insufficiency.

NURSING CONSIDERATIONS

Administration/Storage

- Administer with meal or snack.
- Give single daily dose before 9 AM; space multiple doses evenly throughout day.
- Do not administer to patients who have received live virus vaccine within last month.

Assessment/Interventions

- Obtain patient history, including drug history and any known allergies. Note MI, diabetes, renal impairment, hepatitis, tuberculosis, peptic ulcer disease, ocular herpes simplex or current infections.
- Ensure that baseline laboratory tests have been obtained before beginning therapy, and monitor for possible hyperglycemia, hypokalemia and hypocalcemia during treatment.
- Be aware that drug may mask signs of infection and that resistance to infection may be diminished.

- Observe for possible delayed wound healing.
- Monitor blood glucose of diabetic patient carefully.
- If menstrual irregularities, muscle wasting or weakness, rounded moon facies, fluid retention, GI bleeding or mental status changes occur, notify physician.
- Assess for signs of adrenal insufficiency (fever, myalgia, arthralgia, malaise, anorexia, nausea, orthostatic hypotension, dizziness, fainting). Notify physician immediately if this condition is suspected.

OVERDOSAGE: SIGNS & SYMPTOMS

Cushingoid changes, moonface, striae, central obesity, hirsutism, acne, ecchymoses, hypertension, osteoporosis, myopathy, sexual dysfunction, diabetes mellitus, hyperlipidemia, peptic ulcer, GI bleeding, increased susceptibility to infection, electrolyte and fluid imbalance, psychosis

Patient/Family Education

- Advise patient to take single daily doses or alternate day doses in morning (before 9 AM) and to take multiple doses at evenly spaced intervals throughout day.
- Instruct patient to take medication with meals or snack to avoid GI irritation.
- Caution patient not to discontinue drug suddenly, to avoid withdrawal syndrome. Explain that dosage will be tapered slowly (until ≤ 5 mg/day) before stopping.
- Warn patient to avoid persons with known viral infections, particularly chickenpox or measles, and to inform physician if exposure occurs.
- Explain that patient should not receive live virus vaccinations.
- Instruct diabetic patients to monitor blood glucose closely.
- Advise patient to notify health care providers of drug regimen before any surgical procedure, emergency treatment, immunization or skin test.
- Tell patient to carry medical identification card at all times describing medication being taken.
- Tell patient about symptoms of adrenal insufficiency (fever, myalgia, malaise, anorexia, nausea, orthostatic hypotension, dizziness, fainting) and need to report these symptoms to physician immediately.
- Instruct patient to report these symptoms to physician: black tarry stools, vomiting of blood, menstrual irregularities, unusual weight gain, swelling of lower extremities, puffy face, muscle weakness, prolonged sore throat, fever or cold.

See Patient Guide, p. 514.

Primaquine Phosphate

(PRIM-uh-kween FOSS-fate)

Available as generic only

Class: Anti-infective/antimalarial

Action Disrupts metabolic processes of parasitic organism, eliminating tissue (exoerythrocytic) infection and preventing development of blood (erythrocytic) forms of parasite responsible for relapses of vivax malaria.

Indications Radical cure or prevention of relapse in vivax malaria; after termination of chloroquine phosphate suppressive therapy in areas where vivax malaria is endemic. **Unlabeled use:** With clindamycin, treatment of *Pneumocystis carinii* pneumonia associated with AIDS.

Contraindications Concomitant administration of quinacrine and primaquine; acutely ill patient with systemic disease manifested by granulocytopenia (eg, rheumatoid arthritis, lupus erythematosus); concurrent administration of other potentially hemolytic or bone marrow depressant medications.

Route/Dosage

Begin therapy during last 2 wk of or after course of suppression with chloroquine or comparable drug. ADULTS: PO 26.3 mg (15 mg base) for 14 days. CHILDREN: PO 0.5 mg/kg/day (0.3 mg/kg/day of base) for 14 days (maximum 15 mg/day of base).

Interactions

Quinacrine: May potentiate toxicity of antimalarial compounds that are structurally related to primaquine.

Lab Test Interferences

None well documented.

Adverse Reactions

GI: Nausea; vomiting; epigastric distress; abdominal cramps. *HEMA:* Leukopenia; hemolytic anemia in G-6-PD deficiency; methemoglobinemia in NADH methemoglobin reductase deficiency.

Precautions

Pregnancy: Pregnancy category undetermined. *Lactation:* Undetermined. To aoid adverse effects in the infant, do not give to lactating women. *Hemolytic anemia:* May occur in patients with following conditions: G-6-PD deficiency, NADH methemoglobin reductase deficiency; idiosyncratic reactions (leukopenia, methemoglobinemia; hemolytic anemia). Discontinue drug if marked darkening of urine or sudden decrease in hemoglobin or leukocyte count occurs. *Maximum dose:* Hemolytic reactions may occur with doses of drug exceeding recommended dose.

NURSING CONSIDERATIONS

Administration/Storage

- Do not begin administration unless patient has completed or is within 2 wk of completing course of suppression with chloroquine or comparable drug.
- Do not administer to patient who is taking or has recently received quinacrine within past 3 mo.
- Administer with food if medicine causes GI upset.
- Store at room temperature in tightly closed, light-resistant container.

Assessment/Interventions

- Obtain patient history, including drug history and any known allergies. Note recent use of quinacrine and other antimalarial agents.
- Ensure that CBC with differentials have been obtained before beginning therapy and are performed routinely during therapy.
- Monitor for hemolytic reactions (marked darkening of urine or sudden decrease in hemoglobin concentration or leukocyte or erythrocyte count); notify physician if these reactions occur.

OVERDOSAGE: SIGNS & SYMPTOMS

Anemia, methemoglobinemia, leukopenia, acute abdominal cramps, vomiting, epigastric distress, CNS and cardiovascular disturbances, granulocytopenia, hemolytic anemia

Patient/Family Education

- Tell patient that medicine may be taken with food if stomach upset (nausea, vomiting, abdominal cramps) occurs, and advise to contact physician if upset persists.
- Emphasize importance of compliance with drug regimen.
- Advise patient to report marked darkening of urine to physician.

See Patient Guide, p. 515.

Primidone

(PRIM-ih-dohn)

Mysoline

Class: Anticonvulsant

Action

Drug and its metabolites (phenobarbital and phenylethylmalonamide) have anticonvulsant activity, raising seizure threshold and altering seizure patterns.

Indications Control of grand mal, psychomotor or focal epileptic seizures; may control grand mal seizures refractory to other anticonvulsants. **Unlabeled use:** Treatment of benign familial tremor (essential tremor).

Contraindications Hypersensitivity to barbiturates; porphyria.

Route/Dosage

ADULTS & CHILDREN > 8 YR: If no previous treatment, initiate as follows: **PO** Days 1-3: 100-125 mg at bedtime; days 4-6: 100-125 mg bid; days 7-9: 100-125 mg tid; day 10 through maintenance: 250 mg tid or qid. May increase to 250 mg 5-6 times/day, but do not exceed 500 mg qid (2 g/day). CHILDREN < 8 YR: **PO** Days 1-3: 50 mg at bedtime; days 4-6: 50 mg bid; days 7-9: 100 mg bid; day 10 through maintenance: 125-250 mg tid or 10-25 mg/kg/day in divided doses.

Patients Already Taking Anticonvulsants

Initiate at 100-125 mg at bedtime, gradually increasing dose to maintenance level as other drug is gradually decreased. Complete switch to primidone should occur over > 2 wk.

Interactions

Anticoagulants: Decreased anticoagulant effects. *Beta-blockers:* Decreased bioavailability of beta-blockers. *Carbamazepine:* Decreased primidone levels; increased concentrations of carbamazepine. *Corticosteroids:* Decreased effect of corticosteroids. *Doxycycline:* Decreased doxycycline serum levels. *Estrogens, oral contraceptives:* Contraceptive failure. *Ethanol:* Additive CNS suppression. *Felodipine:* Decreased effect of felodipine. *Griseofulvin:* Decreased serum griseofulvin levels. *Hydantoins, valproic acid:* Increased primidone serum levels. *Methoxyflurane:* Enhanced renal toxicity. *Metronidazole:* Therapeutic failure of metronidazole. *Nifedipine:* Decreased nifedipine levels. *Phenylbutazone, oxyphenbutazone:* Shortened elimination rate of these agents. *Quinidine:* Decreased quinidine serum levels. *Succinimides:* Decreased primidone levels. *Theophyllines:* Decreased theophylline levels.

Lab Test Interferences

None well documented.

Adverse Reactions

CNS: Ataxia; vertigo; fatigue; hyperirritability; emotional disturbances; drowsiness; personality deterioration; mood changes; paranoia. *EENT:* Diplopia; nystagmus. *GI:* Nausea; anorexia; vomiting. *GU:* Impotence; crystalluria. *HEMA:* Megaloblastic anemia; thrombocytopenia. *DERM:* Morbiliform or maculopapular skin eruptions.

Precautions

Pregnancy: Pregnancy category undetermined. Consult physician regarding anticonvulsant use during pregnancy. *Lactation:* Excreted in breast milk. *Status epilepticus:* May be precipitated by abrupt withdrawal.

NURSING CONSIDERATIONS

Administration/Storage

- Administer in divided doses.
- For patients with swallowing difficulties, crush tablets or use suspension.
- Do not reach maximum dose in < 10 days (maximum adult dose: 2 g day; maximum pediatric dose: 25 mg/kg/day).
- Do not substitute one brand of drug for another; bioequivalence problems exist.
- Shake suspension well, do not freeze.
- Store at room temperature in tightly closed, light-resistant container.

Assessment/Interventions

- Obtain patient history, including drug history and any known allergies. Note liver disease, renal disease or porphyria.
- Ensure that complete blood cell count and sequential multiple analyzer 12 tests have been obtained

before beginning therapy; repeat q 6 mo throughout treatment.
- Monitor drug blood level (5-12 mcg/ml) periodically during therapy.
- Observe for common side effects such as ataxia, vertigo or somnolence; notify physician if these symptoms occur.

OVERDOSAGE: SIGNS & SYMPTOMS
CNS depression (drowsiness to coma), respiratory depression, shock, crystalluria

Patient/Family Education
- Instruct patient to take with food if GI distress occurs.
- Explain that full effectiveness of drug may not occur for several weeks after initiation of drug therapy.
- Warn the patient that discontinuing medication too quickly may precipitate status epilepticus; explain that dosage will be tapered slowly before stopping.
- Advise patient to notify physician or dentist of medication regimen before treatment or surgery.
- Instruct patient to report these symptoms to physician: ataxia, vertigo, drowsiness, nausea, vomiting or loss of appetite. Advise patient that ataxia or vertigo are common side effects, but usually resolve with continued therapy.
- Caution patient to avoid intake of alcoholic beverages, other CNS depressants or otc medications unless authorized by physician.
- Advise patient that drug may cause drowsiness and to use caution while driving or performing other tasks requiring mental alertness.

See Patient Guide, p. 516.

Probenecid

(pro-BEN-uh-sid)
Benemid, Probalan
Class: Analgesic/gout/uricosuric

Action Inhibits tubular reabsorption of urate, thus increasing urinary excretion of uric acid. Inhibits tubular secretion of most penicillin and cephalosporin antibiotics.

Indications Treatment of hyperurecemia associated with gout and gouty arthritis; adjunctive therapy with penicillins or cephalosporins to elevate and prolong serum levels.

Contraindications Children < 2 yr; blood dyscrasias or uric acid kidney stones. Do not start therapy until acute gout attack subsides.

Route/Dosage
Gout
ADULTS & CHILDREN > 110 LB: **PO** 250 mg bid initially (for 1 wk), followed by 500 mg bid. Maintenance: May reduce by 500 mg q 6 mo until serum uric acid increases. IN CONJUNCTION WITH ANTIBIOTIC THERAPY: **PO** 2 g/day in divided doses. CHILDREN 2-14 YR (< 110 LB): **PO** 25 mg/kg or 0.7 g/m^2 initially. Maintenance: 40 mg/kg/day or 1.2 g/m^2, divided into 4 doses.

Interactions Interacts with many other drugs by altering their clearance and elimination. *Barbiturate anesthetics, dyphylline, methotrexate, oral hypoglycemic agents, zidovudine:* Increased serum levels and effects of these drugs. *Salicylates:* Inhibition of uricosuric effect of either drug.

Lab Test Interferences
May produce false-positive results for glycosuria in some urine glucose tests and falsely high assays for theophylline with Schack and Waxler technique. May inhibit renal excretion of phenosulfophthalein, 17-ketosteroids and sulfobromophthalein.

Adverse Reactions
CNS: Headaches; dizziness. *GI:* Anorexia; nausea; GI distress; vomiting; sore gums. *HEPA:* Hepatic necrosis. *GU:* Urinary frequency; hematuria; re-

nal colic; nephrotic syndrome. *DERM:* Dermatitis; pruritus. *HEMA:* Anemia; hemolytic anemia (possibly related to G-6-PD deficiency); aplastic anemia. *OTHER:* Hypersensitivity reactions; anaphylaxis; fever; flushing; exacerbation of gout; uric acid stones; costovertebral pain.

Precautions

Pregnancy: Pregnancy category undetermined. Probenecid crosses placenta and appears in cord blood. *Children:* Not recommended for children < 2 yr. *Alkalinization of urine:* May be needed to prevent hematuria, renal colic, costovertebral pain, formation of uric acid stones. *Exacerbation of gout:* May occur; appropriate drug therapy (eg, colchicine or other appropriate therapy) is advisable. *History of peptic ulcer:* Use with caution. *Hypersensitivity:* Severe allergic reactions and anaphylaxis, although rare, have occurred. These have usually been associated with prior probenecid use. *Renal impairment:* May require increased doses for gout (not to exceed 2 g/day). Probenecid may be ineffective in chronic renal insufficiency (ie, glomular filtration rate of < 30 ml/min). Drug is not recommended for use with penicillin in cases of known renal impairment.

NURSING CONSIDERATIONS

Administration/Storage

- Do not start therapy during acute gout attack; wait until attack subsides.
- Give with food or antacid to reduce GI upset.
- Colchicine is sometimes prescribed concurrently for first 3-6 mo of therapy since probenecid alone may aggravate gout.

Assessment/Interventions

- Obtain patient history, including drug history and any known allergies. Note renal impairment, blood dyscrasias, peptic ulcers or uric acid kidney stones.
- Encourage liberal fluid intake and give sodium bicarbonate or potassium citrate to prevent urate crystallization in kidney.
- Monitor BUN and renal function test results.
- Monitor for GI tolerance. If nausea, vomiting or diarrhea becomes problem, notify physician.
- Observe for possible exacerbation of gout. If symptoms of exacerbation occur, notify physician; adjunctive therapy may be needed.
- Observe for possible allergic reaction. If reaction occurs, withhold drug and notify physician.

OVERDOSAGE: SIGNS & SYMPTOMS

Nausea, vomiting, diarrhea, seizure

Patient/Family Education

- Instruct patient to take drug with food or antacids if GI upset occurs.
- Advise patient that drinking 6-8 full glasses of water daily may help prevent formation of kidney stones.
- If physician has recommended restriction of intake of foods high in purine, review foods to be avoided (eg, organ meats, meat gravy, anchovies and sardines). Explain that moderate amounts of purine are found in other meats, fish and other seafood, asparagus, spinach, peas, dried legumes and wild game.
- Inform patient to notify physician if GI upset, anorexia or headaches become bothersome.
- Instruct patient to report these symptoms to physician: painful urination, bloody urine, severe lower back pain, difficulty breathing or rash.

- Advise patient to avoid intake of alcoholic beverages.
- Instruct patient not to take otc medications (including aspirin) without consulting physician.
- Caution patient not to discontinue drug without consulting physician.

See Patient Guide, p. 517.

Procainamide HCl

(pro-CANE-uh-mide HIGH-droe-KLOR-ide)

Procan SR, Pronestyl, Pronestyl-SR
Class: Antiarrhythmic

Action Increases effective refractory period of atria and bundle of His–Purkinje system; reduces impulse conduction velocity and myocardial excitability in atria, Purkinje fibers and ventricles.

Indications Treatment of documented ventricular arrhythmias that are life threatening.

Contraindications Complete heart block; idiosyncratic hypersensitivity; lupus erythematosus; torsade de pointes.

Route/Dosage
ADULTS: **PO** 50 mg/kg/day in divided doses (q 3 hr for regular release; q 6 hr for sustained release). **IV** 20 mg/min for 25-30 min as loading dose, then 2-6 mg/min for maintenance. **IM** 50 mg/kg/day in divided doses q 3-6 hr until oral therapy is possible. CHILDREN: Safety not established. Following doses have been used: **PO** 15-50 mg/kg/day in divided doses q 3-6 hr maximum of 4 g/day; **IM** 20-30 mg/kg/day in divided doses q 4-6 hr, maximum 4 g/day; **IV** 3-6 mg/kg/dose over 5 min for loading dose, then 20-80 mcg/kg/min continuous infusion (maximum 100 mg/dose or 2 g/day).

Interactions
Amiodarone, cimetidine, trimethoprim: May increase procainamide and NAPA concentrations.

Lab Test Interferences
None well documented.

Adverse Reactions
CV: Proarrhythmic effects; hypotension. *CNS:* Dizziness; weakness; depression; psychosis with hallucinations. *EENT:* Bitter taste. *GI:* Nausea; vomiting; anorexia; abdominal pain. *DERM:* Angioneurotic edema; urticaria; pruritus; flushing; rash. *HEMA:* Neutropenia; thrombocytopenia; hemolytic anemia; agranulocytosis. *OTHER:* Lupus erythematosus–like syndrome.

Precautions
Pregnancy: Category C. *Lactation:* Excreted in breast milk. *Children:* Safety and efficacy not established. *Special risk patients:* Elderly patients and patients with renal, hepatic or cardiac insufficiency will require smaller or less frequent doses. Individual dosage adjustment will be necessary. *Asymptomatic PVCs:* Avoid use of product in treatment of patients with this condition. *Blood dyscrasias:* Agranulocytosis, bone marrow depression, neutropenia, hypoplastic anemia and thrombocytopenia have been reported; monitor carefully. *Cardiovascular effects:* Procainamide has proarrhythmic effects. May cause or aggravate CHF or produce severe hypotension especially in patients with CHF, acute ischemic heart disease or cardiomyopathy. *Complete heart block:* Do not administer to patients with complete heart block because of effects in suppressing nodal or ventricular pacemakers and hazard of asystole. *Concurrent antiarrhythmic agents:* May see enhanced prolongation of conduction or depression of contractility and hypotension. *Digitalis intoxication:* Use with caution treating arrhythmias associated with digitalis intoxication. *First-degree heart block:* Use with caution if first degree heart block develops during procainamide therapy. *Myasthenia gravis:* Pa-

tients may experience increase of muscle weakness. Observe closely. *Renal impairment:* Individual dose adjustment may be necessary. *Predigitalization for atrial flutter or fibrillation:* Cardiovert or digitalize patient prior to procainamide therapy to avoid enhancement of atrioventricular conduction. *Sulfite sensitivity:* Parenteral forms contain sulfites. *Tartrazine sensitivity:* Some tablet forms contain tartrazine. *Antinuclear antibodies (ANA):* Approximately 50% of patients will develop ANA within 2-18 mo of starting therapy. Some of these patients may develop lupus-like syndrome.

NURSING CONSIDERATIONS

Administration/Storage

- Give sustained-release forms whole. Do not crush or allow patient to bite or chew them.
- Digitalize or cardiovert patients with atrial flutter or fibrillation as prescribed prior to administration.
- Prepare IV infusion solution using D5W. Use controlled infusion device.
- IV solutions may turn slightly yellow or light amber on standing but potency is not affected.
- For direct IV injection, do not exceed maximal IV rate of 50 mg/min and do not give more than 100 mg in any 5-min period.
- Wait 3-4 hr after last IV dose before first oral dose.
- IV solutions may be stored at room temperature for 24 hr or for 7 days if refrigerated. Discard IV infusion solutions that are darker than light amber.
- Store oral dosage forms at room temperature in tightly closed container.

Assessment/Interventions

- Obtain patient history, including drug history and any known allergies.
- Repeat ECG as ordered.
- Be aware that patients with decreased renal function and elderly patients will metabolize drug more slowly.
- Monitor ECG and blood pressure regularly during parenteral administration.
- Monitor muscle weakness in patients with myasthenia gravis.
- Monitor results of complete blood cell counts (including white blood cell differential and platelet count) weekly during first 3 months of therapy and periodically thereafter as well as at any time patient develops signs of infection, bruising or bleeding.
- Monitor procainamide and NAPA levels as ordered.
- Report diarrhea, vomiting, anorexia, abdominal pain, dizziness or altered mental status to physician.
- In prolonged therapy observe for lupus erythematosus–like syndrome with arthralgia, pleural or abdominal pain, and possible fever, chills, myalgia, pericarditis, pleural effusion, arthritis or skin lesions and report to physician.

OVERDOSAGE: SIGNS & SYMPTOMS

Hypotension, widening of QRS complex, prolonged QT and PR intervals, ventricular tachyarrhythmias

Patient/Family Education

- Tell patient to take medication with full glass of water.
- Caution patient not to crush or chew sustained release capsules.
- Explain that this medication should be taken throughout 24 hr period.
- Explain importance of informing other physicians or dentist about therapy before surgical or dental procedures.
- Emphasize importance of drug compliance. Caution patient not to make up for missed doses.
- Instruct patient to report these symptoms to physician immediately: difficulty breathing, pounding or irregular heartbeat, joint pain, fever, chills, skin rash or continued dizziness.
- Explain that diarrhea, nausea, dizzi-

ness or loss of appetite may occur and to contact physician if symptoms are bothersome.

- Advise patient that drug may cause dizziness and to use caution when driving or performing other tasks requiring mental alertness.

See Patient Guide, p. 519.

Procarbazine HCl (N-Methylhydrazine; MIH)

(pro-CAR-buh-ZEEN HIGH-droe-KLOR-ide)

Matulane, ✤ *Natulan*

Class: Antineoplastic

Action May inhibit protein, RNA and DNA synthesis, which prevents cancer cell growth.

Indications In combination with other antineoplastic agents for treatment of stage III and IV Hodgkin's disease; used as part of MOPP (nitrogen mustard, vincristine, procarbazine, prednisone) regimen.

Contraindications Inadequate marrow reserve demonstrated by bone marrow aspiration. Possibility of this state should be considered in patients with leukopenia, thrombocytopenia or anemia.

Route/Dosage

As Single Agent

ADULTS: **PO** 2-4 mg/kg/day for first week. Maintain 4-6 mg/kg/day until leukopenia or thrombocytopenia develops or maximum response obtained. Treatment is restarted at 1-2 mg/kg/daily when bone marrow recovery is adequate. Maintenance: 1-2 mg/kg/day after maximum response is obtained. CHILDREN: **PO** 50 mg/m^2 daily for first week. Maintain 100 mg/m^2/day until leukopenia or thrombocytopenia develops or maximum response is obtained. Treatment is restarted at 50 mg/m^2/daily when bone marrow recovery is satisfactory.

Interactions

Alcohol: Facial flushing (disulfiram-like reactions) may occur. *Digitalis glycosides:* Combination chemotherapy may result in decrease in digoxin plasma levels, even several days after stopping chemotherapy. Procarbazine possesses weak MAO inhibitor activity and may interact with following agents: *Levodopa:* Coadministration may result in flushing and significant rise in blood pressure within 1 hour of levodopa administration. *Narcotics:* Concomitant use may result in depressant effects on CNS. *Sympathomimetics and ingestion of foods high in tyramine (red wine, yogurt, ripe cheese, bananas):* May cause abrupt increase in blood pressure. *Tricyclic antidepressants:* Excitability, fluctuations in blood pressure.

Lab Test Interferences

None well documented.

Adverse Reactions

CV: Hypotension; tachycardia; syncope. *RESP:* Pleural effusion; pneumonitis. *CNS:* Paresthesias; neuropathies; headache; dizziness; depression; apprehension; nervousness; insomnia; nightmares; hallucinations; falling; weakness; fatigue; lethargy; slurred speech; drowsiness; unsteadiness; ataxia; foot drop; decreased reflexes; tremors; coma; confusion; convulsions. *EENT:* Retinal hemorrhage; nystagmus; photophobia; diplopia; inability to focus; papilledema; stomatitis; hearing loss; hoarseness. *GI:* Nausea; vomiting; anorexia; dry mouth; dysphagia; abdominal pain; diarrhea; constipation. *HEPA:* Jaundice; hepatic dysfunction. *GU:* Hematuria; urinary frequency; nocturia. *HEMA:* Leukopenia; anemia; thrombocytopenia; pancytopenia; eosinophilia; hemolytic anemia; bleeding tendencies. *DERM:* Dematitis; pruritus; rash; urticaria; herpes; hyperpigmentation; photosensitivity; flushing; alopecia. *OTHER:* Arthralgias; myalgias; pyrexia; diaphoresis;

chills; intercurrent infection secondary to leukopenia; edema; fainting; generalized allergic reactions; secondary nonlymphoid malignancy; gynecomastia.

Precautions

Pregnancy: Category D. *Lactation:* Undetermined. *Dosing in patients with fluid retention:* Use estimated lean body weight (dry weight) if patient is obese or has edema, ascites or other form of abnormal fluid retention. *Radiation/bone marrow suppressive chemotherapy:* Procarbazine therapy may be delayed for 1 month or longer to allow bone marrow recovery. *Renal and hepatic function impairment:* Increased toxicity may occur.

NURSING CONSIDERATIONS

Administration/Storage

- Cautiously handle drug, following National Institutes of Health Division of Safety guidelines.
- Give only under supervision of physician experienced in using potent antineoplastic agents.
- Administer as single daily dose. Dose may be divided if nausea or vomiting occurs.
- Store at room temperature.

Assessment/Interventions

- Obtain patient history, including drug history and any known allergies.
- Assess baseline renal and hepatic function and hemoglobin, hematocrit, CBC with differential, reticulocyte and platelet counts prior to therapy; monitor every 3-4 days during therapy and for 2 weeks after recovery period.
- Check results of urinalysis and serum levels of transaminase, alkaline phosphatase and BUN weekly during therapy and for 2 weeks after recovery period.
- Notify physician if patient develops paresthesias, neuropathies, confusion, stomatitis, diarrhea, bleeding tendencies, hypersensitivity reaction or has white blood count < 4000 or platelet count < 100,000.
- Report depression, loss of appetite, sweating, headache, nausea, vomiting, constipation, drowsiness, dizziness, fever, chills, shortness of breath, increased bronchial secretions or hypotension to physician.
- Watch for possible decreased digoxin plasma levels when drug is used in combination chemotherapy; this action may continue for several days after stopping drug.

OVERDOSAGE: SIGNS & SYMPTOMS

Nausea, vomiting, diarrhea, hypotension, tremors, seizures, hematologic toxicity, coma

Patient/Family Education

- Instruct patient to avoid tyramine-containing foods; these include protein foods that are aged or fermented and include cheeses, pickled herring, liver, hard sausage (such as Genoa salami or pepperoni), pods of broad beans, beer, wine, yeast extract and yogurt.
- Advise patient to maintain adequate fluid intake (2-3 L/day).
- Explain importance of added precautions against infection, because drug may decrease resistance.
- Instruct patient to report these symptoms to physician immediately: shortness of breath, fever, chills, unusual bleeding or bruising, vomiting of blood or black tarry stools.
- Tell patient to report these symptoms to physician: nausea, vomiting, sweating, tiredness, headache, loss of hair, loss of appetite, constipation or depression.
- Advise patient to avoid intake of alcoholic beverages.
- Advise patient that drug may cause drowsiness and dizziness and to use caution while driving or performing other tasks requiring mental alertness.

- Caution patient to avoid exposure to sunlight or to use sunscreen or wear protective clothing to prevent photosensitvity reaction.
- Instruct patient not to take any otc medications (especially nosedrops, cough medicines or weight-control medication) without consulting physician.

See Patient Guide, p. 520.

Prochlorperazine

(pro-klor-PURR-uh-zeen)

Compazine, Compazine Spansules, Prochlorperazine Edisylate, Prochlorperazine Maleate, ✤ *PMS-Prochlorperazine, Stemetil*

Class: Antipsychotic/phenothiazine; antiemetic

Action Effects apparently related to dopamine receptor blocking in CNS. Antiemetic activity may be caused by direct inhibition on medullary chemoreceptor trigger zone.

Indications Management of psychotic disorders; short-term treatment of generalized nonpsychotic anxiety; control of severe nausea and vomiting. **Unlabeled uses:** Treatment of severe vascular or tension headaches (IV), Tourette's syndrome, acute agitation in elderly patients and some symptoms of dementia.

Contraindications Coma or severely depressed states; allergy to any phenothiazine; presence of large amounts of other CNS depressants; bone marrow depression or blood dyscrasias; liver damage; cerebral arteriosclerosis; coronary artery disease; severe hypotension or hypertension; subcortical brain damage; surgery in pediatric patients.

Route/Dosage Individualize dosage. SC administration is not advised because of local irritation.

Psychiatric

ADULTS: **PO** 20-150 mg/day, usually in divided doses. **IM** 10-20 mg. May repeat every 2-4 hr.

Nonpsychotic Anxiety

ADULTS: **PO** 5 mg tid-qid; 15 mg (sustained-release formulation) in morning or 10 mg (sustained-release formation) q 12 hr. Do not exceed 20 mg/day or give for longer than 12 wk. CHILDREN 2-12 YR: **PO/PR** 2.5 mg bid-tid. CHILDREN 2-5 YR: Do not exceed 20 mg/day. CHILDREN 6-12 YR: Do not exceed 25 mg/day. CHILDREN < 12 YR: **IM** 0.03 mg/kg by deep injection.

Nausea and Vomiting

ADULTS: **PO** 5 or 10 mg tablet tid-qid; 15 mg (sustained-release formulation) on arising or 10 mg q 12 hr. **PR** 25 mg bid, **IM** 5-10 mg. May repeat q 3-4 hr. Do not exceed 40 mg/day. CHILDREN: Adjust according to patient response and severity of symptoms. CHILDREN 40-85 LB: 2.5 mg tid or 5 mg bid; do not exceed 15 mg/day. **IM** 0.03 mg/kg given by deep IM injection. CHILDREN 30-39 LB: **PO/PR** 2.5 mg given bid-tid; do not exceed 10 mg/day. CHILDREN 20-29 LB: **PO/PR** 2.5 mg given once or twice daily; do not exceed 7.5 mg/day.

Nausea and Vomiting (Surgery)

ADULTS: **IM** 5-10 mg 1-2 hr prior to induction of anesthesia (may repeat once in 30 min) or to control acute symptoms during and after surgery (may repeat once). **IV** 2.5-10 mg by slow IV injection or infusion, at rate not to exceed 5 mg/min. Single dose should not exceed 10 mg. Daily dose IV should not exceed 40 mg. **IV injection** 5-10 mg 15-30 min before induction of anesthesia or to control acute symptoms during or after surgery. Repeat once if necessary. **IV infusion** 20 mg/L of isotonic solution. Add to IV infusion 15-30 min before induction of anesthesia.

Interactions
Alcohol: May result in increased

CNS depression and may precipitate dystonic reactions. *Anticholinergics:* May reduce therapeutic effects of prochlorperazine and worsen anticholinergic effects. *Barbiturate anesthetics:* Frequency and severity of neuromuscular excitation and hypotension may be increased. *Guanethidine:* Hypotensive action of guanethidine may be inhibited. *Metrizamide:* Possibility of seizure may be increased when subarachnoid metrizamide injection is used. INCOMPATIBILITIES: Do not mix prochlorperazine injection with other agents in syringe. Do not dilute with any diluent containing parabens as preservative.

Lab Test Interferences

May discolor urine pink to red-brown. False-positive pregnancy tests may occur but are less likely to occur with serum test. Increases in protein-bound iodine have been reported.

Adverse Reactions

CV: Orthostatic hypotension; hypertension; tachycardia; bradycardia, syncope; cardiac arrest; circulatory collapse; lightheadedness; faintness; dizziness; ECG changes. *RESP:* Laryngospasm; bronchospasm; dyspnea. *CNS:* Pseudoparkinsonism; dystonia; dyskinesia; motor restlessness; oculogyric crises; opisthotonos; hyperreflexia; tardive dyskinesia; drowsiness; headache; weakness; tremor; fatigue; slurring of speech; insomnia; vertigo; abnormalities of CSF proteins; paradoxical excitement or exacerbation of psychotic symptoms; catatonic-like states; paranoid reactions; lethargy; seizures; hyperactivity; nocturnal confusion; bizarre dreams. *EENT:* Pigmentary retinopathy; glaucoma; photophobia; blurred vision; mydriasis; glaucoma; dry mouth or throat; nasal congestion. *GI:* Nausea; vomiting; dyspepsia, adynamic ileus (which may result in death); constipation. *GU:* Urinary hesitancy or retention; impotence, sexual dysfunction; menstrual irregularities. *HEPA:* Jaundice. *HEMA:* Agranulocytosis; eosinophilia; leukopenia; hemolytic anemia; thrombocytopenic purpura. *DERM:* Photosensitivity; skin pigmentation; dry skin; pruritus; exfoliative dermatitis; urticarial rash; maculopapular hypersensitivity reaction; seborrhea; eczema. *META:* Hyperglycemia; hypoglycemia; increased cholesterol levels. *OTHER:* Increases in appetite and weight; polydipsia; breast enlargement; galactorrhea; increased prolactin levels; heat stroke.

Precautions

Pregnancy: Safety not established. *Lactation:* Safety not established. *Children:* Do not give to children < 20 lb or < 2 yr. Do not use in pediatric surgery. Extrapyramidal side effects may develop even at moderate doses. Use lowest effective dose. Some children respond with restlessness and excitement; do not give additional doses. Use with caution in children with acute illnesses or dehydration. *Elderly:* More susceptible to effects; consider lower dose. *Special risk patients:* Use caution in patients with cardiovascular disease or mitral insufficiency, history of glaucoma, EEG abnormalities or seizure disorders, prior brain damage, hepatic or renal impairment. *Aspiration:* As result of suppression of cough reflex, aspiration of vomitus possible. *CNS effects:* May impair mental or physical abilities, especially during first few days of therapy. *Hepatic effects:* Jaundice usually occurs between weeks 2 and 4 of treatment; considered hypersensitivity reaction. Usually reversible. *Neuroleptic malignant syndrome:* Has occurred with agents in this class; is potentially fatal. Signs and symptoms are hyperpyrexia, muscle rigidity, altered mental status, irregular pulse, fluctuating blood pressure, tachycardia and diaphoresis. *Pulmonary:* Cases of bronchopneumonia, some fatal, have occurred. *Sudden death:* Has been reported; predisposing factors may be seizures or previous brain damage. Flare ups of psychotic behavior may precede death. *Sulfite sensitivity:* Some parenteral products contain sulfites. *Tardive dyskinesia:* Syndrome of potentially irreversible involuntary body and facial movements may develop. Prevalence highest in elderly, especially women. Use smallest effective doses for shortest possible time.

NURSING CONSIDERATIONS

Administration/Storage

- Give sustained-release forms whole; do not crush, and do not allow patient to bite or chew.
- Double-check pediatric dosage for suppositories (2.5 mg) to avoid confusion with adult dose (25 mg).
- Give IM deeply in upper outer quadrant of buttock; do not administer SC.
- Do not mix injectable form with other drugs in syringe and do not dilute with any diluent containing parabens.
- Give IV injection at rate not to exceed 5 mg/min. May be administered undiluted or diluted in isotonic solution. May be given undiluted at 5 mg/min or diluted at rate of 5 mg/ml/min. Do not give as bolus and do not give more than 10 mg/dose.
- Prepare IV infusion by adding 20 mg to no less than 1 L of isotonic solution.
- Total daily parenteral dose should not exceed 40 mg.
- Store oral and injectable dosage forms at room temperature and protect from light.
- Store suppositories at room temperature.
- Avoid freezing solution or injectable products.

Assessment/Interventions

- Obtain patient history, including drug history and any known allergies.
- Carefully position patient to prevent aspiration of vomitus after surgery.
- Report possible side effects to physician: extrapyramidal reactions (pseudoparkinsonism, dystonia, dyskinesia), urinary retention or hesitancy, jaundice, orthostatic hypotension, dizziness, drowsiness, dry mouth or throat, drooling, blurry vision, increases in weight or appetite or breast enlargement.
- Immediately report to physician symptoms of possible neuroleptic malignant syndrome, including hyperpyrexia, muscle rigidity, altered mental status, irregular pulse or blood pressure, tachycardia and diaphoresis.
- In patients chronically treated with this drug, observe for signs of tardive dyskinesia (rhythmical involuntary movements of tongue, face, mouth or jaw) and report to physician.
- Notify physician of possible allergic reaction.

OVERDOSAGE: SIGNS & SYMPTOMS

CNS depression (somnolence to coma); hypotension, extrapyramidal effects, circulatory collapse, seizures, arrhythamias

Patient/Family Education

- Explain potential problems during long-term treatment with this drug, and identify signs of tardive dyskinesia.
- Explain that urine may turn reddish-brown color.
- Advise patient to use caution in hot weather because of increased possibility of heat stroke.
- Instruct patient to report these symptoms to physician: pseudoparkinsonism (dystonia, dyskinesia, akathisia), urinary retention or hesitancy, jaundice, orthostatic hypotension, dizziness, drowsiness, dry mouth or throat, drooling, blurry vision, increases in weight or appetite, fever, skin rash, breast enlargement.
- Caution patient to sudden position changes to minimize problems with dizziness or light headedness.
- Instruct patient to avoid intake of alcoholic beverages or other CNS depressants.
- Advise patient that drug may cause

drowsiness or dizziness and to use caution while driving or performing other tasks requiring mental alertness.

- Caution aptient to avoid exposure to sunlight or to use sunscreen or wear protective clothing.

See Patient Guide, p. 521.

Procyclidine

(pro-SIGH-klih-deen)

Kemadrin, *Procyclid*

Class: Antiparkinson/anticholinergic

Action Has atropine-like action and exerts antispasmodic effect on smooth muscle. Is potent mydriatic and inhibits salivation and normally has no sympathetic ganglion-blocking activity.

Indications Treatment of parkinsonism, including postencephalitic, arteriosclerotic and idiopathic types. Usually more efficacious in relief of rigidity than of tremor and can be used alone in mild to moderate cases. Also can be given to treat drug-induced extrapyramidal symptoms of phenothiazine or rauwolfia therapy and to control sialorrhea associated with neuroleptic medication.

Contraindications Angle-closure glaucoma; pyloric and duodenal obstruction; stenosing peptic ulcers; prostatic hypertrophy; bladder neck obstruction; achalasia; myasthenia gravis; megacolon.

Route/Dosage

Parkinsonism (No Prior Therapy)

ADULTS: **PO** 2.5 mg tid after meals initially. If well tolerated, dose may be gradually increased to 5 mg tid. Bedtime dose can be added if necessary.

Transferring from Prior Therapy

Substitute 2.5 mg tid for all or part of original agent. Increase prn while other drug is lowered or omitted. Individualize (maximum dose 60 mg/day).

Drug-Induced Extrapyramidal Symptoms

ADULTS: Begin with 2.5 mg tid; increase by 2.5 mg increments until symptoms are relieved. Usually 10-20 mg daily is adequate.

Interactions

Haloperidol: Schizophrenic symptoms may worsen, haloperidol levels may decrease and tardive dyskinesia may develop. *Phenothiazines:* Actions of phenothiazines may be decreased. Anticholinergic side effects may increase.

Lab Test Interferences

None well documented.

Adverse Reactions

CV: Tachycardia; palpitations; orthostatic hypotension. *CNS:* Disorientation; confusion; memory loss; hallucinations; agitation; nervousness; depression; drowsiness; giddiness; lightheadedness. *EENT:* Mydriasis; blurred vision. *GI:* Dry mouth; nausea; vomiting; epigastric distress; constipation; paralytic ileus. *GU:* Urinary retention; urinary hesitancy. *DERM:* Rash; urticaria; decreased sweating. *OTHER:* Muscle weakness; acute suppurative parotitis; hyperthermia; heat stroke.

Precautions

Pregnancy: Category C. *Lactation:* Undetermined. *Children:* Safety and efficacy not established. *Elderly:* More susceptible to adverse effects. Occasionally may exhibit confusion, disorientation, agitation, hallucinations and psychotic-like symptoms. *Special risk patients:* Use caution in concurrent illness in which anticholinergic effects may be undesirable (ie, tachycardia, urinary retention, marked prostatic hypertrophy). Closely observe hypotensive patients. *Anticholinergic effects:* Administration of other drugs with anticholinergic effects will increase incidence and severity of these effects. *CNS:* Psychotic episode may be precipitated in treating drug-induced extrapyramidal side effects of phenothiazines or rauwolfia derivatives. *Heat illness:* Give with caution during hot weather. *Ophthalmic:* Incipient narrow-angle glaucoma may be precipitated.

NURSING CONSIDERATIONS

Administration/Storage

- Give with food if GI upset is experienced.
- Give before meals if excessive drying of mouth occurs.
- Offer water or ice chips to aid patient comfort.
- Give with caution during hot weather (anhidrosis and hyperthermia may occur).
- Store at room temperature in tightly closed containers.

Assessment/Interventions

- Obtain patient history, including drug history and any known allergies.
- Observe hypotensive patients closely.
- Inform physician of dizziness, orthostatic hypotension, tachycardia or mild bradycardia, dry mouth, constipation, blurred vision, disorientation, confusion, urinary retention or hesitancy or other side effects.
- Observe elderly patients for signs of mental confusion and disorientation.

OVERDOSAGE: SIGNS & SYMPTOMS

Circulatory collapse, respiratory depression or arrest, CNS depression preceded or followed by stimulation, psychosis, stupor, coma, seizures, fever, hot/dry/flushed skin, dry mucous membranes, paralytic ileus

Patient/Family Education

- Advise patient to use caution in hot weather as drug increases susceptibility to heat stroke.
- Instruct patient to report these symptoms to physician immediately: pounding heartbeat, eye pain, confusion or skin rash. Also tell patient to report bothersome side effects including blurred vision, urinary retention or hesitancy, nausea, vomiting, constipation, dizziness, drowsiness or dry mouth, nose or throat.
- Tell patient to take sips of water frequently, suck on ice chips or sugarless hard candy or chew sugarless gum if dry mouth occurs.
- Instruct patient to avoid intake of alcoholic beverages or other CNS depressants.
- Advise patient that drug may cause drowsiness or dizziness and to use caution while driving or performing tasks requiring mental alertness.
- Instruct patient not to take any otc medications without consulting physician.

See Patient Guide, p. 522.

Progesterone

(pro-JESS-ter-ohn)

Gesterol, Progestaject, Progestasert
Class: Progestin

Action Inhibits secretion of pituitary gonadotropins, thereby preventing follicular maturation and ovulation (contraceptive effect); inhibits spontaneous uterine contraction; transforms proliferative endometrium into secretory endometrium.

Indications Treatment of amenorrhea and functional uterine bleeding; intrauterine contraception in women who have had at least one child. **Unlabeled uses:** Treatment of PMS (suppository), premature labor in late stages of pregnancy and menorrhagia (intrauterine).

Contraindications

IM, suppository, intrauterine: Hypersensitivity to progestins; thrombophlebitis, thromboembolic disorders, cerebral hemorrhage (or history of these disorders); impaired liver function; breast cancer; undiagnosed vaginal bleeding; missed abortion; diagnostic test for pregnancy; pregnancy or suspected pregnancy. *Intrauterine:* Previous ectopic pregnancy; presence or history of PID; IV drug abuse.

Route/Dosage

Amenorrhea

IM 5-10 mg daily for 6-8 days.

Functional Uterine Bleeding

IM 5-10 mg daily for 6 days.

Contraceptive

Intrauterine 1 intrauterine system inserted into uterine cavity once yearly.

PMS

Intravaginal/PR Insert suppository 200-400 mg bid.

Interactions

Anticoagulants: Use intrauterine system with caution in patients receiving anticoagulant therapy.

Lab Test Interferences

Altered metyrapone test.

Adverse Reactions

CNS: Depression; headache; migraine; fatigue; nervousness; dizziness; insomnia. *GI:* Abdominal pain or discomfort; nausea. *GU:* Breakthrough bleeding; spotting; change in menstrual flow; amenorrhea; vaginal candidiasis; pruritus vulvae; changes in cervical erosion and secretions. *Intrauterine:* Endometritis; spontaneous abortion; pelvic infection. *HEPA:* Cholestatic jaundice. *DERM:* Rash; acne; melasma; chloasma; photosensitivity. *OTHER:* Pain at injection site; breast tenderness; masculinization of female fetus; edema; weight changes; decreased libido.

Precautions

Pregnancy: Category X. *Lactation:* Excreted in breast milk. *Depression:* Carefully observe patients with history of depression. *Embedment:* Partial penetration or lodging of intrauterine system in endometrium can result in difficult removal. *Fluid retention:* Use cautiously when conditions that might be affected by this factor are present (eg, asthma, cardiac or renal dysfunction, epilepsy). *Intrauterine system:* Postpone insertion in patients who have cervicitis or vaginitis. Do not insert postpartum or postabortion until involution of uterus is complete. Use with caution in patients who have anemia or history of menorrhagia. Bleeding and cramps may occur during first few weeks after insertion. Prophylactic antibiotics may be considered prior to insertion to decrease risk of PID. *Ophthalmic effects:* Discontinue medication if there are any sudden changes in vision or other serious ophthalmic effects. *Pelvic infection:* Increased risk of PID with intrauterine devices has been reported. *Perforation:* Partial or total perforation of uterine wall or cervix may occur. *Thrombotic disorders:* Discontinue if these conditions occur or are suspected.

NURSING CONSIDERATIONS

Administration/Storage

- When progesterone is used with estrogen, begin progesterone 2 wk after estrogen therapy.
- When progesterone is used for functional uterine bleeding, discontinue therapy when menstrual flow begins.
- Parenteral form is for IM use only. Inject into large muscle.
- Rotate injection sites.
- Store parenteral preparation at room temperature. Avoid freezing.

Assessment/Interventions

- Obtain patient history, including drug history and any known allergies.
- Perform thorough physical assessment prior to therapy. Include breasts and pelvic organs and Pap smear at

6-12 mo intervals while patient is undergoing therapy.
- Before insertion of IUD be certain that gonorrhea and chlamydia cultures and other tests for sexually transmitted diseases are completed and that sounding of uterus is done.
- Assess for breakthrough bleeding, spotting, changes in menstrual flow, amenorrhea, breast changes, cholestatic jaundice or rash and report to physician.
- Monitor I&O and patient's weight.
- Observe for signs of fluid retention (especially in patients with epilepsy, migraine, asthma, cardiac or renal dysfunction) and report to physician.
- Notify physician of signs of suspected thrombophlebitis, cerebrovascular disorders, retinal thrombosis or pulmonary embolism.
- Notify physician in cases of sudden, painful or complete loss of vision or if there is sudden onset of diplopia, proptosis or migraine.
- Assess for signs of depression (especially in patients with prior history of depression) and report to physician.
- Assess diabetic patients for possible reduction in glucose tolerance.

Patient/Family Education

- Caution patient that this medication must not be taken during pregnancy or when pregnancy is possible. Advise patient to use reliable form of birth control while taking this drug.
- Tell patient to take oral forms with food if GI distress occurs.
- Advise diabetic patients that glucose tolerance may decrease and to monitor blood or urine sugars closely, reporting abnormalities to physician.
- Instruct patient not to smoke. Offer information on smoking cessation programs.
- Teach patients with IUD to recognize symptoms of pelvic inflammatory disease and ectopic pregnancy and to report these symptoms to physician.
- Advise patients with IUD that displacement can occur.
- Teach patients with IUD to check after each menstrual period for string protruding from uterus and to contact physician if it cannot be located.
- Instruct patient to report these symptoms to physician immediately: pain in calves with swelling, warmth and redness or sudden severe headache, visual disturbance or numbness in arm or leg.
- Tell patient to report these symptoms to physician: depression, steady weight gain, edema, decreased libido, breakthrough bleeding, spotting, changes in menstrual flow, amenorrhea, breast changes, jaundice or rash.
- Caution patient to avoid exposure to sunlight and to use sunscreen or wear protective clothing to avoid photosensitivity reaction.

See Patient Guide, pp. 523-524.

Promethazine HCl

(pro-METH-uh-zeen HIGH-droe-KLOR-ide)

Anergan 50, K-Phen 50, Pentazine, Phenameth, Phenazine 25, Phenazine 50, Phencen-50, Phenergan, Phenergan Fortis, Phenergan Plain, Phenoject-50, Pro-50, Prometh-50, Prorex-25, Prorex-50, Prothazine, Prothazine Plain, V-Gan 25, V-Gan 50, ✤ Histantil

Class: Antihistamine; antiemetic and antivertigo

Action Competitively antagonizes histamine at H_1 receptor sites. Produces sedative and antiemetic effects.

Indications

Oral/rectal: Temporary relief of runny nose and sneezing caused by common cold; symptomatic relief of perennial and seasonal allergic rhinitis, vasomotor rhinitis, allergic conjunctivitis, allergic and non-allergic pruritic symptoms, mild, uncomplicated skin manifestations of urticaria and angioedema; amelioration of allergic reactions to blood or plasma; treatment of dermographism; adjunctive therapy in anaphylactic reactions; preoperative, postoperative or obstetric sedation; prevention and control of nausea and vomiting associated with certain types of anesthesia and surgery; adjunctive therapy to analgesics for postoperative pain; sedation and relief of apprehension; induction of light sleep; active and prophylactic treatment of motion sickness; antiemetic therapy in postoperative patients. *Parenteral:* Treatment of motion sickness; prevention and control of nausea and vomiting associated with anesthesia and surgery; allergic reactions. *Intravenous:* Adjunct to anesthesia and analgesia with reduced amounts of meperidine or other narcotic analgesics in special surgical situations (eg, repeated bronchoscopy, ophthalmic surgery, poor-risk patients).

Contraindications Hypersensitivity to antihistamines; narrow-angle glaucoma; stenosing peptic ulcer; symptomatic prostatic hypertrophy; asthmatic attack; bladder neck obstruction; pyloroduodenal obstruction; comatose patients; CNS depression from barbiturates, general anesthetics, tranquilizers, alcohol, narcotics or narcotic analgesics; previous phenothiazine idiosyncrasy, jaundice or bone marrow depression; acutely ill or dehydrated children; intra-arterial injection.

Route/Dosage

Allergy

ADULTS: **PO/PR** 25 mg at bedtime. **IM/IV** 25 mg; repeat within 2 hr if needed. CHILDREN > 2 YR: **PO/PR** 25 mg at bedtime *or* 6.25-12.5 mg tid.

Motion Sickness

ADULTS: **PO** 25 mg bid with initial dose taken ½-1 hr before travel and repeated in 8-12 hr if needed. Thereafter 25 mg on rising and before evening meal. CHILDREN > 2 YR: **PO/PR** 12.5-25 mg bid.

Nausea and Vomiting

ADULTS: **PO/PR** 25 mg. Repeat doses of 12.5-25 mg prn q 4-6 hr. **IM/IV** 12.5-25 mg not more than q 4 hr. CHILDREN > 2 YR: **PO/PR** 1 mg/kg q 4-6 hr prn.

Prophylaxis of Nausea and Vomiting

ADULTS: **PO/PR** 25 mg q 4-6 hr prn. CHILDREN > 2 YR: **PO/PR** 1 mg/kg q 4-6 hr prn.

Nighttime Sedation

ADULTS: **PO/PR/IM/IV** 25-50 mg. CHILDREN > 2 YR: **PO/PR/IM/IV** 12.5-25 mg.

Preoperative Sedation

ADULTS: **PO/PR** 50 mg night before surgery. **IM/IV** 25-50 mg night before surgery. CHILDREN > 2 YR: **PO/PR/IM/IV** 12.5-25 mg night before surgery.

Postoperative Sedation and Adjunctive Use with Analgesics

ADULTS: **PO/PR/IM/IV** 25-50 mg. CHILDREN > 2 YR: **PO/PR/IM/IV** 12.5-25 mg.

Sedation During Labor

ADULTS: **IM/IV** 50 mg in early stages of labor. When labor is established, 25-75 mg with reduced dose of narcotic (maximum total dose 100 mg/24 hr).

Interactions

Anticholinergics: May decrease action of promethazine. *Barbiturate anesthetics:* Risk of neuromuscular excitation and hypotension may increase. *CNS depressants (eg, alcohol, narcotics):* May have additive CNS depressant effects. *MAO inhibitors:* May prolong and intensify anticholinergic effects; may cause hypotension and extrapyramidal effects. *Metrizamide:* May increase risk of seizure.

Lab Test Interferences

Diagnostic pregnancy tests based on immunologic reactions between hcg and anti-hcg may result in false-negative or false-positive interpretations. Following interferences have also occurred: increased serum cholesterol, blood glucose, spinal fluid protein, and urinary urobilinogen concentrations; decreased protein-bound iodine; false positive urine bilirubin tests; interference with urinary ketone and steroid determinations; false-positive phenylketonuria test results.

Adverse Reactions

CV: Orthostatic hypotension; palpitations; bradycardia; tachycardia; reflex tachycardia; extrasystoles. *RESP:* Thickening of bronchial secretions; chest tightness; wheezing; respiratory depression. *CNS:* Drowsiness; sedation; dizziness; faintness; disturbed coordination; extrapyramidal effects (usually dose related and include three forms: pseudoparkinsonism, akathisia, dystonias); tardive dyskinesia; adverse behavioral effects. *EENT:* Blurred vision; nasal stuffiness; dry nose; dry or sore throat. *GI:* Epigastric distress; dry mouth; nausea; vomiting; diarrhea; constipation. *GU:* Urinary retention/frequency. *HEMA:* Hemolytic anemia; thrombocytopenia; agranulocytosis. *META:* Increased appetite, weight gain. *OTHER:* Hypersensitivity reactions; photosensitivity; elevated prolactin levels; neuroleptic malignant syndrome.

Precautions

Pregnancy: Category C. Do not use during third trimester. *Lactation:* Undetermined. Contraindicated in nursing mothers. *Children:* Contraindicated in children who are acutely ill or dehydrated. Tablets and suppositories are not recommended in children < 2 yr. Antihistamines may diminish mental alertness and may produce paradoxical excitation. Administer IV form with caution. Not recommended for treatment of uncomplicated vomiting in children; use only when vomiting is prolonged and of unknown cause. Extrapyramidal symptoms that can occur secondary to IV use may be confused with CNS signs of undiagnosed primary disease (eg, encephalopathy, Reye's syndrome). Avoid use in children with history of sleep apnea, family history of SIDS or hepatic diseases and in children with Reye's syndrome. *Elderly patients:* Greater likelihood of dizziness, excessive sedation, syncope, toxic confusional states and hypotension in patients > 60 yr. Dosage reduction may be required. *Special risk patients:* Use drug with caution in patients with predisposition to urinary retention, history of bronchial asthma, increased intraocular pressure, hyperthyroidism, sleep apnea, cardiovascular disease or hypertension, bone marrow depression, liver dysfunction, ulcer disease or respiratory impairment. *Hypersensitivity:* May occur. Have 1:1000 epinephrine immediately available. *Lower seizure threshold:* Drug may lower seizure threshold; use drug with caution in persons with known seizure disorders or when giving in combination with narcotics or local anesthetics that may alter seizure control. *Respiratory disease:* Drug is generally not recommended to treat lower respiratory tract symptoms including asthma. *Skin test procedures:* May prevent or diminish positive reactions to dermal reactivity indicators. If possible, discontinue 4 days prior to skin test.

NURSING CONSIDERATIONS

Administration/Storage

- Give oral form with food if GI upset occurs.
- When administering drug parenterally, preferred route is IM injection.
- If drug must be administered IV, use caution; do not inject directly into vein and inject through appropriate site in IV tubing. Promethazine may be mixed with meperidine in same syringe.
- Do not exceed IV concentration of 25 mg/ml and do not exceed IV rate of 25 mg/min.
- Do not administer SC or intra-arterially.
- Dose of barbiturates must be reduced

by ½ and of narcotics by ¼-½ when using this drug concomitantly.
- Avoid use of this drug in cases of vomiting of unknown origin.
- Discontinue drug 4 days before skin testing procedures.
- Store suppositories in refrigerator and use while cold and firm.
- Store oral dosage form at room temperature in tightly closed, light-resistant container.
- Store parenteral form at room temperature, protected from light. Do not freeze.

Assessment/Interventions

- Obtain patient history, including drug history and any known allergies. Note presence of glaucoma, ulcer disease, urinary retention, hypertension, seizure disorder, bone marrow depression, history of bronchial asthma, hyperthyroidism, cardiovascular disease or liver dysfunction.
- Monitor for possible increased blood glucose.
- In children check for history of sleep apnea, Reye's syndrome, hepatic disease or family history of SIDS.
- Observe for sedation, fatigue, insomnia, dry mouth, sore throat, thickening of mucus, unusual bleeding or nervousness and report to physician.

OVERDOSAGE: SIGNS & SYMPTOMS

CNS depression (sedation to coma), apnea, diminished mental alertness, cardiovascular collapse, insomnia, hallucinations, tremors, convulsions, profound hypotension, respiratory depression, dizziness, ataxia, tinnitus, blurred vision, fixed dilated pupils, flushing, dry mouth, fever, oral and facial dystonic reactions

Patient/Family Education

- Instruct patient using drug for motion sickness to take drug 30 min-1 hr before travel.
- Teach patient to store suppositories in refrigerator and to use while cold and firm.
- Advise patient to notify all health professionals of this drug therapy.
- Inform patient that drug may cause dryness of mouth, nose or throat and to notify physician if this dryness continues for more than 2 wk.
- Instruct patient to report these symptoms to physician: sore throat, thickening of mucus, fever, unusual bleeding, drowsiness or unusual weakness.
- Advise patient to take sips of water frequently or to suck on ice chips or sugarless candy or chew sugarless gum if dry mouth occurs.
- Caution patient to avoid sudden position changes to prevent orthostatic hypotension.
- Instruct patient to avoid intake of alcoholic beverages and other CNS depressants.
- Advise patient that drug may cause drowsiness and to use caution while driving or performing other tasks requiring mental alertness.
- Caution patient to avoid exposure to sunlight and to use sunscreen or wear protective clothing to avoid photosensitvity reaction.

See Patient Guide, p. 525.

Propantheline Bromide

(pro-PAN-thuh-leen BROE-mide)

Pro-Banthine

Class: Anticholinergic; antispasmodic

Action Exerts anticholinergic effects, resulting in GI smooth muscle relaxation and diminished volume and acidity of GI secretions.

Indications Adjunctive therapy in treatment of peptic ulcer.

Unlabeled use: Treatment of secretory and spastic disorders of GI tract, biliary tract, urinary tract and bladder.

Contraindications Hypersensitivity to anticholinergic drugs; narrow-angle glaucoma; adhesions between iris and lens; obstructive uropathy; obstructive disease of GI tract; paralytic ileus; intestinal atony of elderly or debilitated patient; severe ulcerative colitis; toxic megacolon complicating ulcerative colitis; hepatic or renal disease; tachycardia; myocardial ischemia; unstable cardiovascular status in acute hemorrhage; myasthenia gravis.

Route/Dosage

Peptic Ulcer

ADULTS: PO 15 mg 30 min before meals and 30 mg at bedtime. PATIENTS WITH MILD MANIFESTATIONS, ELDERLY PATIENTS OR THOSE OF SMALL STATURE: PO 7.5 mg tid.

Secretory Disorders

ADULTS: PO 1.5 mg/kg/day in 3-4 divided doses.

Spastic Disorders

ADULTS: PO 2-3 mg/kg/day in divided doses q 4-6 hr and at bedtime.

Interactions

Antacids: Decrease absorption of propantheline if given together. *Drugs with anticholinergic effects (eg, antihistamines, antiparkinson drugs, tricyclic antidepressants):* Additive peripheral anticholinergic side effects. *Haloperidol:* May cause decreased serum haloperidol levels, worsened schizophrenic symptoms and tardive dyskinesia. *Phenothiazines:* May decrease antipsychotic effectiveness of phenothiazines; may produce additive anticholinergic effects.

Lab Test Interferences

None well documented.

Adverse Reactions

CV: Palpitations; tachycardia. *CNS:* Headache; flushing; nervousness; drowsiness; weakness; dizziness; confusion; insomnia; fever; mental confusion or excitement; restlessness; tremor. *EENT:* Blurred vision; mydriasis; photophobia; cycloplegia; increased intraocular pressure; dilated pupils; nasal congestion; altered taste perception. *GI:* Dry mouth; nausea; vomiting; dysphagia; heartburn; constipation; bloated feeling; paralytic ileus. *GU:* Urinary hesitancy and retention; impotence. *DERM:* Severe allergic reactions including anaphylaxis, urticaria and dermal manifestations. *OTHER:* Suppression of lactation; decreased sweating.

Precautions

Pregnancy: Category C. *Lactation:* Undetermined. *Children:* Safety and efficacy not established. *Elderly or debilitated patients:* Drug may cause excitement, agitation, drowsiness and other untoward manifestations, even in small doses. *Special risk patients:* Use drug with caution in patients with glaucoma, autonomic neuropathy, hepatic or renal disease, ulcerative colitis, hyperthyroidism, coronary artery disease, CHF, cardiac tachyarrhythmias, tachycardia, hypertension, prostatic hypertrophy and hiatal hernia associated with reflux esophagitis. *Diarrhea:* May be symptom of incomplete intestinal obstruction, especially in patients with ileostomy or colostomy. Treatment of diarrhea with drug is inappropriate and possibly harmful. *Gastric ulcer:* May delay gastric emptying rate and complicate therapy. *Heat prostration:* Can occur in presence of high environmental temperature.

NURSING CONSIDERATIONS

Administration/Storage

- Do not crush or allow patient to chew tablets.
- Administer antacids 1 hr before or after propantheline.
- Administer 30 min before meals and

at bedtime (at least 2 hr after last meal) unless otherwise directed.
- Store at room temperature in tight container.

Assessment/Interventions
- Obtain patient history, including drug history and any known allergies.
- Check patient's vital signs.
- Monitor I&O.
- Observe for drowsiness, dizziness, urinary hesitancy or retention, blurred vision, diarrhea or constipation and other anticholinergic side effects and report to physician.

OVERDOSAGE: SIGNS & SYMPTOMS

Dry mouth, thirst, vomiting, nausea, abdominal distention, paralytic ileus, difficulty swallowing, muscular weakness, paralysis, CNS stimulation (restlessness, anxiety), delirium (disorientation, hallucinations), drowsiness, stupor, fever, dizziness, headache, seizures, ataxia, coma, circulatory failure, rapid pulse and respiration, vasodilation, tachycardia with weak pulse, hypertension, hypotension, respiratory depression, palpitations, urinary urgency with difficulty in micturition, blurred vision, photophobia, dilated pupils, leukocytosis, flushed hot dry skin, rash

Patient/Family Education
- Advise patient to take drug 30 min before meals and at bedtime unless directed otherwise by physician.
- Instruct patient not to chew or crush tablets.
- Warn patient that drug increases risk of heat prostration and caution patient to avoid becoming overheated by exercise or high environmental temperatures.
- Instruct patient to report these symptoms to physician: drowsiness, dizziness, urinary hesitancy and retention, blurred vision, diarrhea or constipation, skin rash, flushing or eye pain.
- Tell patient to take sips of water frequently, suck on ice chips or sugarless hard candy or chew sugarless gum if dry mouth occurs.
- Advise patient that drug may cause drowsiness and to use caution while driving or performing other tasks requiring mental alertness.

See Patient Guide, p. 526.

Propofol

(PRO-puh-FOLE)

Diprivan

Class: General anesthetic

Action Produces sedation/hypnosis rapidly (within 40 sec) and smoothly with minimal excitation; decreases intraocular pressure and systemic vascular resistance; rarely is associated with malignant hyperthermia and histamine release; suppresses cardiac output and respiratory drive.

Indications Induction and maintenance of anesthesia in adults and children ≥ 3 yr; initiation and maintenance of monitored anesthesia care sedation in adults; sedation in intubated or respiratory-controlled adult ICU patients.

Contraindications Situations in which general anesthesia or sedation are contraindicated.

Route/Dosage

Anesthesia

ADULTS < 55 YR: **IV** Induction: 40 mg q 10 sec until onset. (Usual dose: 2-2.5 mg/kg total). Maintenance infusion: Titrate to 100-200 mcg/kg/min (6-12 mg/kg/hr). Maintenance intermittent bolus: 25-50 mg increments, as needed. ELDERLY, DEBILITATED OR ASA

III/IV*: **IV** 20 mg q 10 sec until onset. (Usual dose: 1-1.5 mg/kg). Maintenance infusion: Titrate to 50-100 mcg/kg/min (3-6 mg/kg/hr). NEUROSURGICAL PATIENTS: **IV** Induction: 20 mg q 10 sec until onset. (Usual dose: 1-2 mg/kg). Maintenance infusion: 100-200 mcg/kg/min (6-12 mg/kg/hr). CHILDREN (≥ 3 YR): **IV** Induction: 2.5-3.5 mg/kg over 20-30 sec. Maintenance infusion: Titrate to 125-300 mcg/kg/min (7.5-18 mg/kg/hr).

Sedation

ADULTS (< 55 YR): **IV** Initiation: 100-150 mcg/kg/min (6-9 mg/kg/hr) for 3-5 min (preferred method) or slow injection of 0.5 mg/kg over 3-5 min; follow by maintenance infusion. Maintenance: 25-75 mcg/kg/min (1.5-4.5 mg/kg/hr) (preferred method) or incremental bolus doses of 10-20 mg. ELDERLY, DEBILITATED, OR ASA III/IV: **IV** Initiation: Same as adults; not as rapid bolus. Maintenance: 20% reduction of adult dose; avoid rapid bolus doses.

ICU Sedation

ADULTS: **IV** Initiation: 5 mcg/kg/min (0.3 mg/kg/hr) for ≥ 5 min; increments of 5-10 mcg/kg/min (0.2-0.6 mg/kg/hr) over 5-10 min may be used until desired level of sedation is achieved. Maintenance: 5-50 mcg/kg/min (0.3-3 mg/kg/hr) or higher may be required; use minimum dose required for sedation.

Interactions

CNS depressants (eg, barbiturates, benzodiazepines, narcotics): Increased CNS depression. IV INCOMPATIBILITIES: Do not mix with other therapeutic agents prior to administration. Avoid mixing blood or plasma in same IV catheter.

Lab Test Interferences

None well documented.

Adverse Reactions

CV: Myocardial ischemia; hypotension; bradycardia; decreased cardiac output; hypertension (especially in children). *RESP*: Apnea; cough; respiratory acidosis during weaning. *CNS*: Amorous behavior; movement hypotonia; hallucinations; neuropathy; opisthotonos. *EENT*: Conjunctival hyperemia; nystagmus. *DERM*: Rash. *META*: Hyperlipidemia. *OTHER*: Asthenia; burning, stinging or pain at injection site; fever.

Precautions

Pregnancy: Category B. *Lactation*: Excreted in breast milk. *Labor/delivery*: Not recommended for obstetrical anesthesia (neonatal depression). *Children*: Not recommended for children < 3 yr. *Special risk patients*: Use lower induction and maintenance doses in elderly, debilitated and ASA III/IV patients and monitor continuously for sign of hypotension or bradycardia. Use with caution in patients with lipid metabolism disorders, because propofol is an emulsion. Epileptics may be at risk of convulsions during recovery phase. Avoid significant decreases in mean arterial pressure (and cerebral perfusion) in patients with increased intracranial pressure or impaired cerebral circulation. *Anaphylaxis*: Has occurred rarely; relationship to drug has not been established.

*(American Society of Anesthesiologists classification of heart disease, cardiac function, angina and physical status used to assign risk for anesthesia.)

NURSING CONSIDERATIONS

Administration/Storage

- Should be administered only by personnel who are trained in administration of general anesthesia and familiar with drug.
- Administer only in settings in which resuscitation equipment is immediately available.
- Shake well before use. Do not use if

there is evidence of separation of phases of emulsion.

- Maintain strict aseptic technique in handling; rapid growth of organisms may occur if contaminated.
- Dilute with 5% Dextrose Injection, but do not dilute to concentration < 2 mg/ml. Drug is compatible with 5% Dextrose, USP; Lactated Ringers Injection, USP; Lactated Ringers and 5% Dextrose Injection; 5% Dextrose and 0.45% Sodium Chloride Injection, USP; 5% Dextrose and 0.2% Sodium Chloride Injection, USP.
- Minimize pain associated with administration by infusing into larger veins.
- Discard any unused portions of drug or solution at end of anesthetic procedure; do not keep for > 6 hr.
- In ICU sedation discard after 12 hr if administered directly from vial or after 6 hr if transferred to syringe or other container.
- Store at room temperature. Do not refrigerate. Protect from light.

Assessment/Interventions

- Obtain patient history, including drug history and any known allergies. Note epilepsy, cardiac and respiratory status and lipid disorders.
- Monitor patient carefully; be especially alert for apnea, hypotension or cardiovascular depression (bradycardia). Notify physician if these symptoms occur.
- Be prepared for possible alterations in mental status including confusion, combativeness and hallucinations and for possible neurological changes, including increases in movement, hypertonia, clonic/myoclonic movement and bucking, jerking or thrashing.
- Monitor for increases in serum triglycerides or serum turbidity in patients at risk of hyperlipidemia and notify physician.
- Observe for possible respiratory acidosis during weaning after prolonged administration.

OVERDOSAGE: SIGNS & SYMPTOMS

Cardiorespiratory and cardiovascular depression

Patient/Family Education

- Advise patient that mental alertness, coordination and physical dexterity may be impaired for some time after administration of this drug.

No patient monograph available.

Propoxyphene

(pro-POX-ee-feen)

Propoxyphene Hydrochloride

Darvon Pulvules, Dolene

Propoxyphene Napsylate

Darvon-N

Class: Narcotic analgesic

Action Relieves pain by stimulating opiate receptors in CNS; also causes respiratory depression, peripheral vasodilation, inhibition of intestinal peristalsis, sphincter of Oddi spasm, stimulation of chemoreceptors that cause vomiting and increased bladder tone.

Indications Relief of mild to moderate pain.

Contraindications Upper airway obstruction; acute asthma; diarrhea caused by poisoning or toxins.

Route/Dosage

Propoxyphene Hydrochloride

ADULTS: PO 65 mg q 4 hr prn; not to exceed 390 mg/day.

Propoxyphene Napsylate

ADULTS: PO 100 mg q 4 hr prn; not to exceed 600 mg/day.

Interactions

Carbamazepine: Increased carbamazepine serum concentrations. *Cigarette smoking:* Decreased propoxyphene effect caused by liver enzyme induction. *CNS depressants (eg, Alcohol, barbiturate anesthetics, sedatives, tranquilizers):* Additive CNS depression. *Warfa-*

rin: Potentiation of hypoprothrombinemic effect.

Lab Test Interferences

Increased amylase and lipase for up to 24 hr after administration.

Adverse Reactions

CV: Hypotension. *RESP:* Depression of cough reflex. *CNS:* Lightheadedness; dizziness; sedation; disorientation; incoordination; paradoxical excitement; hallucinations; euphoria; dysphoria; insomnia. *GI:* Nausea; vomiting; constipation; abdominal pain. *GU:* Urinary retention or hesitancy. *HEPA:* Jaundice; abnormal liver function tests. *DERM:* Sweating; pruritus; urticaria. *OTHER:* Tolerance; psychological and physical dependence with chronic use; weakness.

Precautions

Pregnancy: Category C. Category D–if used for long periods. *Lactation:* Excreted in breast milk. *Children:* Not recommended for children. *Special risk patients:* Use with caution in patients with myxedema, acute alcoholism, acute abdominal conditions, ulcerative colitis, decreased respiratory reserve, head injury or increased intracranial pressure, hypoxia, supraventricular tachycardia, depleted blood volume or circulatory shock. *Drug dependence:* Has abuse potential. *Fatalities:* Excessive doses of propoxyphene alone or with other CNS depressants (including alcohol) are major cause of drug-induced death. Do not use in patients who are suicidal or addiction prone. *Hepatic or renal impairment:* Duration of action may be prolonged; may need to reduce dose.

NURSING CONSIDERATIONS

Administration/Storage

- Administer with food if GI upset occurs.
- Be aware that 65 mg of HCl form is equivalent to 100 mg of napsylate form in delivering same amount of propoxyphene.
- Store in light-resistant container at room temperature.

Assessment/Interventions

- Obtain patient history, including drug history and any known allergies. Note potential for suicide or drug dependence.
- Assess pain prior to and 30-60 min after administration.
- Provide safety measures (accessible call bell, side rails, night light) and assist with ambulation.
- Monitor for prolonged duration of action in cases of hepatic or renal impairment and report to physician; dose may need to be reduced.
- Observe for respiratory depression, dizziness, sedation, nausea, vomiting, or constipation; notify physician if these symptoms occur.

OVERDOSAGE: SIGNS & SYMPTOMS

CNS depression (stupor to coma), respiratory depression, hypotension, seizures, pulmonary edema, cardiac arrhythmias, respiratory-metabolic acidosis

Patient/Family Education

- Advise patient to take drug with food if GI upset occurs.
- Explain that increasing fluid and fiber intake may help decrease constipation. Use of stool softeners and laxatives may also be suggested.
- Advise patient not to wait until pain level is high to self-medicate because drug will not be as effective.
- For long-term therapy, explain that dosage will be tapered gradually to prevent withdrawal symptoms.
- Tell patient to notify physician if drug does not provide pain relief.
- Instruct patient to report these symptoms to physician: shortness of breath or difficulty breathing, nausea, vomiting, constipation or other effects of drug.

- Caution patient to avoid sudden position changes to prevent orthostatic hypotension.
- Instruct patient to avoid intake of alcoholic beverages or other CNS depressants.
- Advise patient that drug may cause drowsiness or dizziness and to use caution while driving or performing other tasks requiring mental alertness.

See Patient Guide, p. 527.

Propoxyphene/Acetaminophen

(pro-POX-ee-feen/ass-cet-ah-MEE-noe-fen)

Propoxyphene HCl/Acetaminophen
E-Lor, Genagesic, Wygesic

Propoxyphene Napsylate/Acetaminophen
Darvocet-N 50, Darvocet-N 100, Propacet 100

Class: Narcotic analgesic combination

Action Propoxyphene relieves pain by stimulating opiate receptors in CNS; also causes respiratory depression; peripheral vasodilation, inhibition of intestinal peristalsis, sphincter of Oddi spasm, stimulation of receptors that cause vomiting, increased bladder tone. Acetaminophen inhibits synthesis of prostaglandins; does not have significant anti-inflammatory effects or antiplatelet effects; produces antipyresis by direct action on the hypothalamic heat-regulating center.

Indications Relief of mild to moderate pain; as analgesic-antipyretic in presence of aspirin allergy, hemostatic disturbances, bleeding diatheses, upper GI disease and gouty arthritis.

Contraindications Standard considerations.

Route/Dosage

Propoxyphene Napsylate

ADULTS: PO 100 mg (with 650 mg acetaminophen) q 4 hr prn; not to exceed 600 mg/day.

Propoxyphene Hydrochloride

ADULTS: PO 65 mg (with 650 mg acetaminophen) q 4 hr; not to exceed 390 mg/day.

Interactions

Carbamazepine: Increased carbamazepine serum levels; increased risk of acetaminophen hepatotoxicity. *Charcoal:* Decreased propoxyphene absorption. *Cigarette smoking:* Decreased propoxyphene effect because of liver enzyme induction. *CNS depressants (alcohol, antidepressants, barbiturates, muscle relaxants, sedatives, tranquilizers):* Increased CNS and respiratory depression. *Hydantoins:* Increased risk of acetaminophen hepatotoxicity. *Sulfinpyrazone:* Increased risk of acetaminophen hepatotoxicity. *Warfarin:* Potentiation of hypoprothrombinemic effect.

Lab Test Interferences

Increased amylase and lipase for up to 24 hr after administration.

Adverse Reactions

CV: Hypotension. *RESP:* Dyspnea; depression of cough reflex. *CNS:* Lightheadedness; weakness; fatigue; sedation; dizziness; disorientation; uncoordination; paradoxical excitement; euphoria; dysphoria; insomnia. *GI:* Nausea; vomiting; constipation; anorexia; stomach pain; biliary spasm. *GU:* Urinary retention or hesitancy. *OTHER:* Tolerance; psychological and physical dependence with long-term use; histamine release; pain at injection site.

Precautions

Pregnancy: Category C (D if used for prolonged periods). *Lactation:* Excreted in breast milk. *Children:* Safety and efficacy not established. *Special risk patients:* Use with caution in patients with myxedema, acute alcoholism, acute abdominal conditions, ulcerative colitis, decreased respiratory reserve, head injury or increased cranial pressure, hypoxia, supraventricular tachycardia, depleted blood volume or circulatory shock. *Drug dependence:* Has abuse potential. *Fatalities:* Excessive doses, either alone or in combination with other CNS depressants (including alcohol), are major cause of drug-induced death. Do not use in patients who are suicidal or addiction prone. *Hepatic and renal impairment:* Use drug with caution; reduce total daily dosage; advise chronic alcoholics to limit acetaminophen intake to < 2 g/day.

NURSING CONSIDERATIONS

Administration/Storage

- Give with food or milk if GI upset occurs.
- Be aware that 65 mg of HCl form is equivalent to 100 mg of napsylate form in delivering same amount of propoxyphene.
- Store in light-resistant container at room temperature.

Assessment/Interventions

- Obtain patient history, including drug history and any known allergies. Note potential for suicide or drug dependence.
- Assess pain prior to and 30-60 min after administration.
- Observe for respiratory depression, dizziness, sedation, nausea, vomiting or constipation; notify physician if these symptoms occur.
- Provide safety measures (accessible call bell, side rails, night light) and assist with ambulation.
- Monitor for prolonged duration of action in cases of hepatic or renal impairment and report to physician, since dose may need to be reduced.

OVERDOSAGE: SIGNS & SYMPTOMS

CNS depression (stupor to coma), respiratory depression, hypotension, seizures, pulmonary edema, cardiac arrhythmias, respiratory-metabolic acidosis, hepatitis

Patient/Family Education

- Advise patient to take drug with food if GI upset occurs.
- For long term therapy, explain that dosage will be tapered slowly before stopping to prevent withdrawal symptoms.
- Advise patient not to take any other medications (prescription or otc) containing acetaminophen except on advice of physician.
- Tell patient not to wait until pain level is high to self-medicate because drug will not be as effective.
- Advise patient to notify physician if drug does not provide pain relief.
- Explain that increasing fluid and fiber intake may help decrease constipation; stool softeners and laxatives may also be suggested.
- Instruct patient to report these symptoms to physician: shortness of breath, difficulty breathing, nausea, vomiting, constipation or other side effects.
- Caution patient to avoid sudden position changes to prevent orthostatic hypotension.
- Instruct patient to avoid intake of alcoholic beverages or other CNS depressants.
- Advise patient that drug may cause drowsiness and to use caution while driving or performing other tasks requiring mental alertness.

See Patient Guide, p. 528.

Propranolol HCl

(pro-PRAN-oh-lahl HIGH-droe-KLOR-ide)

Betachron E-R, Inderal, Inderal LA, Propranolol HCl Intensol, ♣ APO-Propranolol, PMS-Propranolol

Class: Beta-adrenergic blocker

Action Blocks beta receptors, primarily affecting the cardiovascular system (decreased heartrate, decreased cardiac contractility and decreased BP) and lungs (promotes bronchospasm).

Indications Treatment of hypertension; angina pectoris; hypertrophic subaortic stenosis; MI; pheochromocytoma; migraine prophylaxis; essential tremor; some ventricular and supraventricular arrhythmias. **Unlabeled uses:** Treatment of alcohol withdrawal syndrome; esophageal varices rebleeding; anxiety; thyrotoxicosis symptoms.

Contraindications Hypersensitivity to beta-blockers; greater than first-degree heart block; CHF unless secondary to tachyarrhythmia or untreated hypertension treatable with beta-blockers; overt cardiac failure; sinus bradycardia; cardiogenic shock; untreated bronchial asthma or bronchospasm, including severe COPD.

Route/Dosage

Hypertension

ADULTS: **PO** Initial dose: 40 mg bid initially or 80 mg sustained-release medication/day; titrate to response. Maintenance: 120-240 mg/day in 2-3 divided doses or 120-160 mg/day sustained-release medication. Do not exceed 640 mg/day. CHILDREN: **PO** 0.5 mg/kg bid; titrate q 3-5 days to maximum dose of 1 mg/kg bid.

Angina

ADULTS: **PO** 80-320 mg/day in 2-4 divided doses or 160 mg/day of sustained-release medication.

Arrhythmias

ADULTS: **PO** 10-30 mg 3-4 times/day before meals and at bedtime.

Hypertrophic Aortic Stenosis

ADULTS: **PO** 20-40 mg 3-4 times/day before meals and at bedtime or 80-160 mg sustained-release medication one time/day.

MI

ADULTS: **PO** 180-240 mg/day in 3-4 divided doses up to 240 mg/day.

Pheochromocytoma

ADULTS: **PO** 60 mg/day for 3 days prior to surgery, given with alpha-blocker.

Migraine

ADULTS: **PO** 80 mg in divided doses daily or once daily (sustained release); titrate to response (maximum dose: 240 mg/day); discontinue after 6 wk if no response.

Arrhythmias (Life Threatening)

ADULTS: **IV** 1-3 mg at rate of 1 mg/min; may repeat after 2 min; give subsequent doses q 4 hr.

Essential Tremor

ADULTS: **PO** 40 mg bid initially; titrate to response. Maintenance: 120-320 mg/day in 2-3 divided doses.

Interactions *Barbiturates:* Decreased bioavailability of propranolol. *Cimetidine:* Increased propranolol levels. *Clonidine:* Attenuation or reversal of antihypertensive effect; potentially life-threatening increases in BP, especially on withdrawal. *Epinephrine:* Initial hypertensive episode followed by bradycardia. *Ergot alkaloids:* Peripheral ischemia, manifested by cold extremities and possible gangrene. *Hydralazine:* Increased serum levels of both drugs. *Insulin:* Prolonged hypoglycemia with masking of symptoms. *Lidocaine:* Increased lidocaine levels, leading to toxicity. *NSAIDs:* Some agents may impair antihypertensive effect. *Phenothiazines:* Increased effects of either drug. *Prazosin:* Increased orthostatic hypotension. *Propafenone,* *quinidine, thioamines:* Increased effects of propranolol. *Rifampin:* Decreased effects of propranolol. *Theophylline:* Reduces elimination of theophylline; pharmacologic antagonism. *Verapamil:* Increased effects of both drugs.

Lab Test Interferences

May interfere with glaucoma screening tests; may increase BUN, serum transaminases, alkaline phosphatase or LDH.

Adverse Reactions

CV: Bradycardia; hypotension; CHF; atrioventricular (AV) block; worsening angina; torsades de pointes; edema; peripheral ischemia. *RESP:* Wheezing; dyspnea; bronchospasm; difficulty breathing. *CNS:* Depression; tiredness; fatigue; lethargy; sleep disturbances;. bizarre dreams; short-term memory loss; dizziness. *EENT:* Dry eyes; visual disturbances. *GI:* Dyspepsia; nausea; vomiting; diarrhea; dry mouth. *GU:* Impotence; urinary retention; difficulty with urination. *HEMA:* Agranulocytosis. *HEPA:* Elevated liver enzymes. *DERM:* Rash; pruritus. *META:* Hyperglycemia; hypoglycemia. *OTHER:* Increased sensitivity to cold (Raynaud's phenomenon); psoriasis-like eruptions; skin necrosis; systemic lupus erythematosus; decreased exercise tolerance.

Precautions

Pregnancy: Category C. *Lactation:* Excreted in breast milk. *Children:* Safety and efficacy not established. IV use is not recommended, but oral propranolol has been used. *Abrupt withdrawal:* A beta blocker withdrawal syndrome (hypertension, tachycardia, anxiety, angina, MI) may occur 1-2 weeks after sudden discontinuation of systemic beta blockers. If possible, gradually withdraw therapy over 1-2 weeks. *Anaphylaxis:* Deaths have occurred; aggressive therapy may be required. *CHF:* Should be administered cautiously in patients whose CHF is controlled by digitalis and diuretics. *Diabetes mellitus:* May mask symptoms of hypoglycemia (eg, tachycardia, BP changes). May potentiate insulin-induced hypoglycemia. *Nonallergic bronchospastic diseases:* Give drug with caution in patients with bronchospastic diseases. *Peripheral vascular disease:* May precipitate or aggravate symptoms of arterial insufficiency. *Renal/hepatic impairment:* Dose should be reduced. *Thyrotoxicosis:* May mask clinical signs (eg, tachycardia) of developing or continuing hyperthyroidism. Abrupt withdrawal may exacerbate symptoms of hyperthyroidism, including thyroid storm. *Wolff-Parkinson-White syndrome:* In several cases, tachycardia was replaced by severe bradycardia requiring a demand pacemaker.

NURSING CONSIDERATIONS

Administration/Storage

- Administer consistently either with or without food.
- Patients who are taking sustained-released capsules should swallow them whole; instruct patient not to bite, open or chew capsules.
- Administer via IV route only in cases of life-threatening arrhythmias or those occurring under anesthesia and only under careful monitoring (eg, central venous pressure, ECG).
- Store tablets/capsules/oral solution at room temperature in tight, light-resistant containers.
- Protect injectable solution from light.
- Administer IV form undiluted or diluted with 10 ml D5W for Injection. Give 1 mg or less/min; may be diluted in 50 ml sodium chloride and 1 mg given over 10-15 min.

Assessment/Interventions

- Obtain patient history, including drug history and any known allergies. Note diabetes; respiratory, liver or cardiac disease or sensitivity to other beta blockers.
- Review baseline ECG.
- Assess pulse and BP before and during

administration. If pulse rate is below 60 bpm or if patient hypotensive, withhold medication and notify physician.

- If renal damage is present, obtain creatinine clearance.
- Obtain hepatic enzyme levels before and during administration.
- Monitor I&O and daily weight during therapy for signs of fluid retention.
- Monitor for headache, light-headedness and decreased BP, which may indicate need for reduced dosage.
- If sudden severe dyspnea or edema of hands and feet develops, withhold medication and notify physician.
- If chest pain occurs, assess for location, intensity, duration and radiation, and notify physician.

OVERDOSAGE: SIGNS & SYMPTOMS

Bradycardia, hypotension, CHF, AV block, intraventricular conduction defects, asystole, coma

Patient/Family Education

- Explain that dosage will be tapered slowly before stopping. Warn that sudden discontinuation can cause chest pain or heart attack.
- Instruct patient to take medication at same time each day.
- Teach patient how to take pulse and instruct to check before taking drug. Warn patient not to take drug if pulse is < usual rate (or < 60 bpm) and to call physician.
- Educate patient or family to take BP and advise to take on regular basis.
- Inform diabetic patient to monitor blood glucose level carefully.
- Instruct patient to report these symptoms to physician: difficulty breathing, night cough, slowed pulse rate, dizziness, rash, fever, sore throat, confusion, depression, drowsiness, unusual bruising or bleeding.
- Caution patient to avoid sudden position changes to prevent orthostatic hypotension.
- Advise patient that drug may cause drowsiness and to use caution while driving or performing other tasks requiring mental alertness.
- Instruct patient not to take otc medications (including nasal decongestants, diet aids, or cold preparations) without consulting physician.

See Patient Guide, p. 529.

Propylthiouracil (PTU)

(pro-puhl-thigh-oh-YOU-rah-sill)

Available as generic only, ♣ *Propyl-Thyracil*

Class: Antithyroid

Action Inhibits synthesis of thyroid hormones.

Indications Long-term therapy of hyperthyroidism; amelioration of hyperthyroidism in preparation for subtotal thyroidectomy or radioactive iodine therapy; when thyroidectomy is contraindicated or not advisable. **Unlabeled use:** Management of alcoholic liver disease.

Contraindications Hypersensitivity to antithyroid drugs; lactating women.

Route/Dosage

ADULTS: **PO** Initial dose: 300 mg/day in 3 equal doses q 8 hr. In patients with severe hyperthyroidism or very large goiters, initial dose is usually 400 mg/day, occasionally up to 600-900 mg/day. Maintenance: 100-150 mg/day in divided doses q 8 hr. CHILDREN > 10 YR: **PO** Initial dose: 150-300 mg/day in divided doses q 8 hr. Maintenance: Determined by response. CHILDREN 6-10 YR: **PO** Initial dose: 50-150 mg/day in divided doses q 8 hr. ALTERNATE DOSING FOR CHILDREN: **PO** Initial dose: 5-7 mg/kg/day in divided doses q 8 hr. Maintenance: $\frac{1}{3}$-$\frac{2}{3}$ initial dose, beginning when patient is euthyroid.

Interactions

Anticoagulants: Altered anticoagulant action. *Beta blockers:* Increased effects of beta blockers. *Digitalis glycosides:* Increased digitalis levels, resulting in toxicity. *Theophylline:* Altered theophylline clearance in hyperthyroid or hypothyroid patients.

Lab Test Interferences

None well documented.

Adverse Reactions

CNS: Paresthesias; neuritis; headache; vertigo; drowsiness; neuropathies; CNS stimulation; depression. *EENT:* Loss of taste; sialadenopathy. *GI:* Nausea; vomiting; epigastric distress. *HEPA:* Jaundice; hepatitis. *GU:* Nephritis. *HEMA:* Inhibition of myelopoiesis (eg, agranulocytosis, leukopenia, granulocytopenia, thrombocytopenia); aplastic anemia; hypoprothrombinemia; periarteritis. *DERM:* Rash; urticaria; pruritus; erythema nodosum; skin pigmentation; exfoliative dermatitis; lupus-like syndrome (splenomegaly, hepatitis, periarteritis; hypoprothrombinemia; bleeding). *OTHER:* Abnormal hair loss; arthralgia; myalgia; edema; lymphadenopathy; drug fever; interstitial pneumonitis; insulin autoimmune syndrome (hypoglycemia).

Precautions

Pregnancy: Category D. *Lactation:* Avoid nursing. However, if antithyroid drug is essential, PTU is preferred antithyroid agent while nursing. *Children:* Hepatotoxicity has occurred in pediatric patients. Discontinue drug immediately if signs and symptoms of hepatic dysfunction develop. *Agranulocytosis:* Potentially most serious side effect. Discontinue drug if agranulocytosis, aplastic anemia, hepatitis, fever or exfoliative dermatitis occur. *Hemorrhagic effects:* May cause hypoprothrombinemia and bleeding.

NURSING CONSIDERATIONS

Administration/Storage

- Give with meals to minimize GI irritation.
- Administer q 8 hr to maintain serum drug levels.
- Encourage fluid intake of 3-4 L/day, unless contraindicated.
- Store in tight, light-resistant container at room temperature.

Assessment/Interventions

- Obtain patient history, including drug history and any known allergies.
- Obtain baseline weight, BP, body temperature and pulse rate and monitor periodically during therapy.
- Ensure that baseline thyroid function has been evaluated prior to therapy and reassess q 2-3 mo during therapy.
- Determine baseline WBC count and differential before administration and monitor for agranulocytosis during first 3 mo of therapy.
- Monitor I&O and check for edema.
- Before discharge, obtain dietary consult for patient regarding iodine intake; shellfish and iodine-containing foods may be restricted.
- Assess for signs of hypoprothrombinemia; monitor prothrombin time during therapy, especially during surgical procedures.
- Assess patient for development and tolerance of symptoms of hyperthyroidism or hypothyroidism.
- If symptoms of hypersensitivity occur (swollen lymph nodes, skin eruption or itching), notify physician. Drug may be discontinued.

OVERDOSAGE: SIGNS & SYMPTOMS

Nausea, vomiting, epigastric distress, headache, fever, arthralgia, pruritis, edema, pancytopenia; most serious effect: agranulocytosis

Patient/Family Education

- Instruct patient to take resting pulse daily and encourage patient to keep recorded chart.
- Advise patient to monitor weight at least 2-3 times/wk or per physician instruction, obtaining weight at same

time, using same scale. Encourage patient to keep recorded chart.
- Emphasize importance of following dietary restrictions regarding shellfish, iodized salt and other foods high in iodine.
- Explain that desired response may take several months if the thyroid is greatly enlarged.
- Advise patient to carry Medi-Alert identification at all times describing medications.
- Instruct patient to notify dentist or physician of drug regimen before surgical or dental procedures.
- Emphasize importance of follow-up visits to monitor effectiveness of drug therapy.
- Caution patient not to stop taking medication abruptly to avoid thyroid crisis.
- Instruct patient to report these symptoms to physician: sore throat, fever, rash, mouth sores; cold intolerance, mental depression; tachycardia, irritability; persistent nausea, steatorrhea or vomiting, drowsiness, yellowing of skin or whites of eyes; unusual bleeding or bruising.
- Advise patient that drug may cause drowsiness and to use caution while driving or performing other activities requiring mental alertness.
- Instruct patient not to take otc medications without consulting physician.

See Patient Guide, p. 530.

Protamine Sulfate

(PRO-tuh-meen SULL-fate)

Available as generic only

Class: Heparin antagonist

Action Neutralizes heparin by forming heparin-protamine complex.

Indications Treatment of heparin overdose.

Contraindications Standard considerations.

Route/Dosage
ADULTS: **IV** 1 mg for each 90 USP units of heparin derived from lung tissue or 115 USP units of heparin derived from intestinal mucosa. Because heparin disappears rapidly from circulation, the dose of protamine required decreases rapidly with time following IV injection of heparin. For example, if protamine is administered 30 min after heparin, ½ the usual dose may be sufficient. The dose of protamine should be determined by blood coagulation studies.

Interactions None well documented. INCOMPATIBILITIES: Protamine should not be mixed with other drugs without knowledge of their compatibility.

Lab Test Interferences
None well documented.

Adverse Reactions
CV: Hypotension; bradycardia; circulatory collapse. *RESP:* Shortness of breath; pulmonary edema; acute pulmonary hypertension. *CNS:* Lassitude. *GI:* Nausea; vomiting. *OTHER:* Anaphylaxis (severe respiratory distress, circulatory collapse, capillary leak, noncardiogenic pulmonary edema); transient flushing and feeling of warmth; back pain.

Precautions
Pregnancy: Category C. *Lactation:* Undetermined. *Children:* Safety and efficacy not established. *Circulatory collapse:* Can occur along with myocardial failure and reduced cardiac output. *Heparin rebound:* When used to neutralize large doses of heparin, protamine can be inactivated by blood; treatment consists of giving additional protamine. *Hypersensitivity:* Fatal anaphylaxis may occur. *Pulmonary edema:* High-protein noncardiogenic pulmonary edema has occurred with use of protamine in patients on cardiopulmonary bypass undergoing cardiovascular surgery. *Too-*

rapid administration: Can result in severe hypotension and anaphylactoid reactions.

NURSING CONSIDERATIONS

Administration/Storage

- Discontinue IV heparin infusion and maintain IV route access.
- Flush IV line completely to clear previously administered medications.
- When given via direct IV injection, use 10 mg/ml concentration and administer slowly over 1-3 min. No more than 50 mg should be given in any 10 min period.
- Protamine sulfate injection is not intended to be further diluted. If further dilution is desired, dilute with D5W or normal saline.
- Store protamine sulfate injection in refrigerator. Do not freeze.

Assessment/Interventions

- Obtain patient history, including drug history and any known allergies, particularly hypersensitivity to drug, fish (salmon) or previous reaction to or use of isophane or protamine insulins. Note if male patient has had vasectomy or history of infertility (either can increase risk of hypersensitivity reaction).
- Assess for hypovolemia before initiating therapy, because peripheral vasodilation of protamine sulfate can result in cardiovascular collapse if hypovolemia is uncorrected.
- Have resuscitation equipment available.
- Monitor patient for urticaria, edema, rash, wheezing and coughing (hypersensitivity symptoms).
- Monitor activated clotting time, activated partial thromboplastin time, and thrombin time 5-15 min after therapy is begun and prn.
- Monitor vital signs frequently.
- Assess for bleeding during and after therapy (heparin rebound can precipitate hemorrhage 8-9 hr after therapy; after cardiopulmonary bypass, rebound can occur as late as 18 hr after therapy). Monitor for severe headache, gingival erythema or bleeding, complaint of abdominal or back pain, petechiae or bruises and excessive bleeding from cuts or venipuncture sites. Check urine and stool for visible and occult blood. Ask female patient about increased amount of menstrual discharge.
- To prevent bleeding, avoid injections and rectal temperatures and provide gentle mouth care.

OVERDOSAGE: SIGNS & SYMPTOMS
Bleeding

Patient/Family Education

- Instruct patient to notify physician immediately if any bleeding occurs.
- Tell patient to report these symptoms to physician: shortness of breath, dizziness or swelling.
- Advise patient to avoid activities that could damage blood vessels or precipitate bleeding (shaving, vigorous brushing of teeth, ambulation) until risk of hemorrhage has passed.

No patient monograph available.

Protriptyline HCl

(pro-TRIP-tih-leen HIGH-droe-KLOR-ide)

Vivactil, ♣ *Triptil*

Class: Tricyclic antidepressant

Action Inhibits reuptake of norepinephrine and serotonin in CNS.

Indications Relief of symptoms of depression. **Unlabeled uses:** Treatment of obstructive sleep apnea and panic disorder.

Contraindications Hypersensitivity to tricyclic antidepressants. Generally not to be given in combination with or within 14 days of treatment with MAO inhibitor, nor during acute recovery phases of MI.

Route/Dosage
ADULTS: PO 15-60 mg/day in divided doses. Maintenance dose may be given as a single daily dose. ELDERLY & ADOLESCENTS: PO Initial dose: 5 mg tid. Increase slowly if needed.

Interactions
Cimetidine, fluoxetine: Increased protriptyline blood levels and effects. *CNS depressants:* Additive depressant effects. *Clonidine:* Hypertensive crisis. *Dicumarol:* Increased anticoagulant actions. *Guanethidine:* Inhibition of hypotensive action by guanethidine. *MAO inhibitors:* Hyperexcitability, hyperthermia, convulsions, and death may occur. *Sympathomimetics (direct-acting, eg, norepinephrine, phenylephrine):* Increased pressor response. *Sympathomimetics (indirect-acting, eg, dopamine, ephedrine):* Decreased pressor response.

Lab Test Interferences
None well documented.

Adverse Reactions
CV: Orthostatic hypotension; hypertension; tachycardia; palpitations; arrhythmias; ECG changes; heart block; CHF. *RESP:* Pharyngitis, rhinitis; sinusitis; laryngitis; cough. *CNS:* Confusion; hallucinations; disorientation; delusions; nervousness; restlessness; anxiety; agitation; panic; insomnia; nightmares; mania; exacerbaton of psychosis; drowsiness; dizziness; weakness; fatigue; emotional lability; seizures; tremors. *EENT:* Mydriasis; blurred vision; increased intraocular pressure; tinnitus; peculiar taste. *GI:* Nausea; vomiting; anorexia; GI distress; diarrhea; flatulence; dry mouth; constipation. *GU:* Impotence; sexual dysfunction; nocturia; dysmenorrhea; amenorrhea; urinary retention and hesitancy. *HEMA:* Bone marrow depression, including agranulocytosis; eosinophilia; purpura; thrombocytopenia; leukopenia. *DERM:* Rash; pruritus; photosensitivity reaction; dry skin; acne; itching. *META:* Elevation or depression of blood glucose. *OTHER:* Numbness; breast enlargement; extrapyramidal symptoms (eg, pseudoparkinsonism, movement disorders, akathesia).

Precautions
Pregnancy: Pregnancy category undetermined. *Lactation:* Excreted in breast milk. *Children:* Safety and efficacy not established. *Special risk patients:* Use drug with caution in patients with history of seizures, urinary retention, urethral or ureteral spasm, angle-closure glaucoma or increased intraocular pressure, cardiovascular disorders, hyperthyroid patients or those receiving thyroid medication, hepatic or renal impairment, schizophrenic or paranoid patients. *Anticholinergic effects:* Additive with other medications with anticholinergic effects.

NURSING CONSIDERATIONS

Administration/Storage

- Give with food or milk to minimize GI irritation.
- Maintenance doses may be given as a single daily dose, in the morning and not at night, because of the mild stimulant effect of the drug.
- Store at room temperature in tightly closed, light-resistant container.

Assessment/Interventions

- Obtain patient history, including drug history and any known allergies. Note recent MI, seizure disorder or prostatic hypertrophy.
- Ensure that baseline CBC with differential, ECG and hepatic studies have been obtained before beginning therapy and monitor regularly.
- Obtain baseline weight, BP (standing and lying), and pulse.
- Supervise patient closely during initiation of therapy. Assess appearance,

behavior, speech pattern, level of interest, and mood.

- Monitor for weight gain (appetite may increase), dysrhythmias, and drop in BP. Withhold drug and notify physician if systolic pressure drops 20 mm Hg.
- Closely monitor cardiovascular response of elderly patients receiving > 20 mg/day.
- Assist with ambulation at start of therapy and provide safety measures (eg, siderails up), especially for elderly patients.
- Monitor for headache, nausea, vertigo, malaise, and nightmares (symptoms of withdrawal when drug is abruptly discontinued or dose reduced).
- Monitor pattern of daily bowel activity, stool consistency, and urinary output. Modify fluid and bulk in diet to offset constipation.

OVERDOSAGE: SIGNS & SYMPTOMS

CNS stimulation (agitation, irritability, delirium) followed by depression (drowsiness to coma), hypertension followed by hypotension, hyperpyrexia followed by hypothermia, cardiac arrhythmias, seizures

Patient/Family Education

- Explain that therapeutic effect of drug may be seen within 2-5 days, but full effectiveness of drug may not occur for 2-3 wk.
- Tell patient that dosage will be tapered slowly before stopping to prevent withdrawal symptoms.
- Warn patient to monitor food intake: weight gain can occur because of increased appetite.
- Emphasize importance of follow-up visits to monitor effectiveness of therapy.
- Instruct patient to report these symptoms to physician: visual disturbances, mental status changes (especially increase in depression or panic), urinary retention and extrapyramidal symptoms (frequently noted in elderly) such as rigidity or fine hand tremors.
- Advise patient to take sips of water frequently or to suck on ice chips, sugarless hard candy or chew sugarless gum to relieve dry mouth.
- Caution patient to avoid sudden position changes to avoid dizziness.
- Instruct patient to avoid intake of alcoholic beverages or other CNS depressants.
- Advise patient that drug may cause drowsiness and to use caution while driving or performing other activities requiring mental alertness while dose is being stabilized.
- Caution patient to avoid exposure to sunlight and use sunscreen or wear protective clothing to avoid photosensitivity reaction.
- Instruct patient to avoid taking otc medications without consulting physician.

See Patient Guide, p. 531.

Pseudoephedrine (d-Isoephedrine)

(SUE-doe-eh-FED-rin)

Afrin, Allermed, Cenafed, Children's Congestion Relief, Congestion Relief, Decofed, Defed-60, Dorcol Children's Decongestant, Drixoral Non-Drowsy, Genaphed, Halofed, Novafed, Pedia Care Infant's Decongestant, Propagest, Pseudo, Pseudo-Gest, Rhindecon, Seudotabs, Sinustop Pro, Sudafed, Sudafed Pediatric Nasal Decongestant Oral Drops, ♣ *Balminil Decongestant Syrup, Benylin Decongestant, Durafedrin, Eltor 120 Caplets, Maxenal Caplets, Robidrine*

Class: Nasal decongestant

Action Causes vasoconstriction and subsequent shrinkage of nasal mucous membranes by alpha-adrenergic stimulation, promoting nasal drainage.

Indications Relief of nasal or eustachian tube congestion.

Contraindications Hypersensitivity to sympathomimetic amines; severe hypertension; coronary artery disease; MAO inhibitor therapy; breastfeeding mothers.

Route/Dosage

Pseudoephedrine Sulfate

ADULTS & CHILDREN > 12 YR: **PO** 120 mg sustained-release q 12 hr.

Pseudoephedrine HCl

ADULTS: **PO** 60 mg q 4-6 hr or 120 mg sustained-release q 12 hr. Not to exceed 240 mg/day. CHILDREN 6-12 YR: **PO** 30 mg q 4-6 hr. Not to exceed 120 mg/day. CHILDREN 2-5 YR: **PO** 15 mg q 4-6 hr. Not to exceed 60 mg/day. CHILDREN 1-2 YR: **PO** 7 drops (0.2 ml)/kg q 4-6 hr. Not to exceed 4 doses/day. CHILDREN 3-12 MO: **PO** 3 drops/kg q 4-6 hr. Not to exceed 4 doses/day.

Interactions

Furazolidone, guanethidine, methyldopa: Increased BP. MAO *inhibitors:* Severe headache, hypertension and hyperpyrexia; can cause hypertensive crisis. *Urinary acidifiers (eg, ammonium chloride):* Increased elimination of pseudoephedrine. *Urinary alkalinizers (eg, sodium bicarbonate):* Decreased elimination of pseudoephedrine.

Lab Test Interferences

None well documented.

Adverse Reactions

CV: Arrhythmias; cardiovascular collapse with hypotension; tachycardia; bradycardia; transient hypertension. *CNS:* Nervousness; excitability; dizziness; tremor; insomnia; restlessness; depression. *GI:* Anorexia; nausea; vomiting; dry mouth. *GU:* Difficulty urinating. *DERM:* Pallor.

Precautions

Pregnancy: Category C. *Lactation:* Do not give to breastfeeding mothers. *Children:* Use drug only under physician's advice in children < 3 mo. *Elderly:* Ensure that short-acting product is tolerated before giving sustained-release product. *Special risk patients:* Use drug with caution in patients with hyperthyroidism, diabetes, cardiovascular disease, increased intraocular pressure or prostatic hypertrophy. Patients with hypertension should use only under medical advice. *Excessive use:* Systemic effects (nervousness, dizziness, sleeplessness) are more common in elderly and infants.

NURSING CONSIDERATIONS

Administration/Storage

- Tell patient to swallow sustained-release preparations whole, and not to break, crush or chew.
- Contents of capsule may be mixed with food (eg, jelly, applesauce) if patient has difficulty swallowing.
- Administer at least 2 hr before bedtime to diminish insomnia.
- Store at room temperature.

Assessment/Interventions

- Obtain patient history, including drug history, special risk factors (eg, hypertension) and any known allergies. Note hypersensitivity to pseudoephedrine or other sympathomimetic amines.
- Assess congestion (nasal, sinus, eustachian tubes), vital signs, lung sounds and characteristics of respiratory secretions prior to and during therapy.
- Provide sufficient fluid intake to liquify secretions and maintain hydration.

OVERDOSAGE: SIGNS & SYMPTOMS

Somnolence; sedation, which may be accompanied by profuse sweating, hypotension or shock; coma. Symptoms in elderly include hallucinations, seizures, CNS depression, and death

Patient/Family Education

- Advise patient not to exceed recommended dose.

- Instruct patient not to chew or crush sustained release form.
- Teach patient to use calibrated measuring device to administer liquid and calibrated dropper to administer drops.
- Instruct patient to report these symptoms to physician: breathing difficulties, hallucinations, seizures (symptoms of overdose); lack of improvement within 7 days; high fever.
- Instruct patient to take sips of water frequently or suck on ice chips, sugarless hard candy or chew sugarless gum if dry mouth occurs.
- Advise patient to avoid taking other otc medications containing sympathomimetic amines.

See Patient Guide, pp. 532-533.

Pyrazinamide

(peer-uh-ZIN-uh-mide)

Available as generic only, *Tebrazid*

Class: Anti-infective/antitubercular

Action Pyrazine analog of nicotinamide may be bacteriostatic or bactericidal against *Mycobacterium tuberculosis*.

Indications Initial treatment of active tuberculosis in adults and selected children when combined with other antituberculosis agents.

Contraindications Severe hepatic damage; acute gout.

Route/Dosage
ADULTS: **PO** 15-30 mg/kg one time/day (maximum 2 gm/day) or 50-70 mg/kg 2 times/week (maximum 4 gm/dose). CHILDREN: **PO** 15-30 mg/kg once daily (maximum 2 gm/day).

Interactions None well documented.

Lab Test Interferences
May interfere with Acetest and Ketostix urine tests, producing pink-brown color.

Adverse Reactions
GI: Nausea; vomiting; anorexia. *HEPA:* Hepatotoxicity. *DERM:* Rash; acne; photosensitivity. *META:* Gout; porphyria. *OTHER:* Arthralgia and myalgia; hypersensitivity reactions (urticaria, pruritus); fever.

Precautions
Pregnancy: Category C. *Lactation:* Excreted in breast milk. *Children:* Safety and efficacy not established. Use only if therapy is essential. *Diabetes mellitus:* Management of diabetes mellitus may be more difficult. *Hepatic function impairment:* Closely follow patients with pre-existing liver disease or patients at increased risk (eg, alcohol abusers). It may be necessary to discontinue drug; do not resume therapy if signs of hepatocellular damage appear. *Hyperuricemia:* May inhibit renal excretion of urates, resulting in hyperuricemia.

NURSING CONSIDERATIONS

Administration/Storage

- Drug should always be part of multi-drug therapy to decrease chance of resistant organisms. Question doses > 35 mg/kg/day.
- Administer with food to decrease GI irritation.
- Store at room temperature in tightly closed, light-resistant container.

Assessment/Interventions

- Obtain patient history, including drug history and any known allergies.
- Assess for signs of anemia (hematocrit, hemoglobin and evidence of fatigue).
- Ensure that serum AST, ALT and uric acid concentration have been determined before beginning therapy and repeated q 2-4 wk.

- Obtain culture and sensitivity monthly to detect resistance and ensure sensitivity to medication.
- Monitor patient for signs of liver disease or gout.

OVERDOSAGE: SIGNS & SYMPTOMS
Abnormal liver function tests

Patient/Family Education
- Emphasize need to be compliant with regimen and to not miss any doses.
- Explain that long-term therapy (6 mo-2 yr) will be necessary.
- Inform diabetic patients that drug may interfere with urine ketone values.
- Emphasize importance of follow-up examinations to monitor effectiveness of therapy and identify side effects.
- Instruct patient to report these symptoms to physician: fever; loss of appetite; malaise; nausea and vomiting; darkened urine, yellowish skin or eye discoloration; pain or swelling joints.
- Advise patient to avoid intake of alcoholic beverages and alcohol-containing products.

See Patient Guide, p. 534.

Pyridoxine HCl (B6)

(peer-ih-DOX-een HIGH-droe-KLOR-ide)

Beesix, Nestrex, ♣ *Hexa-Betalin*
Class: Vitamin

Action Vitamin B6 functions as coenzyme in amino acid, carbohydrate and lipid metabolism.

Indications Pyridoxine deficiency, including inadequate diet, drug-induced causes (eg, isoniazid, oral contraceptives) or inborn errors of metabolism. Parenteral use is indicated when oral therapy is not feasible. **Unlabeled uses:** Treatment of hydrazine poisoning, PMS, hyperoxaluria type I, nausea and vomiting in pregnancy, sideroblastic anemia associated with high serum iron.

Contraindications Standard considerations.

Route/Dosage
Dietary Deficiency
ADULTS: **PO/IM/IV** 10-20 mg/day for 3 wk.

Drug-Induced Deficiency Anemia or Neuritis
ADULTS: **PO/IM/IV** 100-200 mg/day for 3 wk; follow with 25-100 mg/day.

Neuropathy
ADULTS: **PO/IM/IV** 50-200 mg/day.

Vitamin B6 Dependency Syndrome
ADULTS: **PO/IM/IV** 600 mg, followed by 30 mg/day for life. PYRIDOXINE-DEPENDENT INFANTS: **IM/IV** 10-100 mg, followed by 2-100 mg/day.

Metabolic Disorders
ADULTS: **PO/IM/IV** 100-500 mg/day.

Isoniazid (INH) Poisoning
ADULTS & CHILDREN: **IV** 4 gm IV followed by 1 gm IM q 30 min until pyridoxine dose equal to INH dose has been given.

Interactions
Cycloserine, INH, hydralazine, oral contraceptives, penicillamine: Increased need for pyridoxine. *Levodopa:* Decreased effect of levodopa. (Interaction does not occur with levodopa/carbidopa in combination with pyridoxine.) PARENTERAL INCOMPATIBILITIES: Incompatible with alkaline solutions, iron salts and oxidizing agents.

Lab Test Interferences
May result in false-positive urobilinogen in the spot test using Ehrlich's reagent.

Adverse Reactions
CNS: Neuropathy; unstable gait; drowsiness; somnolence. *EENT:* Perioral numbness. *OTHER:* Numbness of feet; decreased sensation to touch, tem-

perature or vibration; paresthesia; low serum folic acid levels; burning/stinging at IM injection site.

Precautions
Pregnancy: Category A. *Lactation:* Excreted in breast milk; may inhibit lactation. *Children:* Safety and efficacy not established in doses exceeding nutritional requirements.

NURSING CONSIDERATIONS

Administration/Storage
- Instruct patient to swallow sustained-release preparation whole and not to break, crush or chew.
- When giving via IM route, rotate sites.
- IV preparation may be given undiluted or added to standard compatible IV solutions.
- Store all forms of drug at room temperature in tightly closed, light-resistant containers. Avoid freezing injection.

Assessment/Interventions
- Obtain patient history, including drug history and any known allergies.
- Assess for signs of vitamin B6 deficiency (irritability, seizures, anemia, dermatitis, nausea and vomiting) prior to and during therapy.
- Institute seizure precautions in pyridoxine-dependent infants.
- Obtain dietary consultation to review importance of well-balanced meals and sources of B6 prior to discharge home.

OVERDOSAGE: SIGNS & SYMPTOMS
Ataxia, sensory neuropathy

Patient/Family Education
- Emphasize importance of complying with prescribed dietary recommendations.
- Teach patient about foods high in B6 (whole grain cereals, meat [eg, liver], potatoes, green vegetables, legumes [eg, lima beans], yeast and bananas).
- If patient is self-medicating with vitamin supplements, caution that megadosing may cause side effects such as unsteady gait, impaired hand coordination and numbness of feet.

See Patient Guide, p. 535.

Quazepam

(KWAY-zuh-pam)
Doral
Class: Sedative and hypnotic/ benzodiazepine

Action Potentiates action of GABA, an inhibitory neurotransmitter, resulting in increased neuronal inhibition and CNS depression, especially in limbic system and reticular formation.

Indications Short-term management of insomnia.

Contraindications Hypersensitivity to benzodiazepines; pregnancy; sleep apnea.

Route/Dosage
ADULTS: PO 15 mg at bedtime initially; may reduce to 7.5 mg once individual response is determined. ELDERLY OR DEBILITATED PATIENT: Attempt dosage reduction after 1-2 nights.

Interactions
Alcohol, CNS depressants: May cause additive CNS depressant effects. *Cimetidine, disulfiram, omeprazole:* May increase quazepam effects. *Digoxin:* May increase serum digoxin concentrations. *Theophylline:* May antagonize sedative effects.

Lab Test Interferences
None well documented.

Adverse Reactions
CV: Palpitations, tachycardia.

CNS: Daytime drowsiness; dizziness; lethargy; confusion; memory impairment; euphoria; relaxed feeling; falling, ataxia; hallucinations; paradoxical reactions (eg, anger, hostility, mania); headache. *EENT:* Blurred vision; difficulty focusing. *GI:* Anorexia; diarrhea; abdominal cramping; constipation; nausea and vomiting. *DERM:* Rash. *HEPA:* Hepatic dysfunction. *HEMA:* Leukopenia; agranulocytopenia. *OTHER:* Tolerance; physical and psychological dependence; weakness; slurred speech.

Precautions

Pregnancy: Category X. *Lactation:* Excreted in breast milk. *Children:* Contraindicated in children < 18 yr. *Special risk patients:* Use drug with caution in patients with renal or hepatic impairment, depression or suicidal tendencies, drug abuse and dependence, chronic pulmonary insufficiency, seizure disorders. *Dependence/withdrawal:* Prolonged use can lead to psychologic or physical dependence. Withdrawal syndrome may occur; dose must be tapered gradually.

NURSING CONSIDERATIONS

Administration/Storage

- Administer ½-1 hr before bedtime with full glass of water. If GI upset occurs, administer with snack.
- Check to see that medication is swallowed.
- After long-term use, drug must be discontinued gradually. When drug is discontinued, expect nighttime sleep to be disturbed briefly (a few days).
- Store in tight container in cool area.

Assessment/Interventions

- Obtain patient history, including drug history and any known allergies. Note potential for suicide or drug dependence.
- Assess type of sleep difficulty: falling asleep, remaining asleep.
- Assess sleep pattern prior to and during therapy.
- Assess mental status: sensorium, affect, mood and long-term and short-term memory.
- Provide safety measures (removal of cigarettes, side rails up, night light, easily accessible call bell) and assistance with ambulation.

OVERDOSAGE: SIGNS & SYMPTOMS

Somnolence, confusion with reduced or absent reflexes, respiratory depression, apnea, hypotension, impaired coordination, slurred speech, seizures, coma

Patient/Family Education

- Caution patient that this medication must not be taken during pregnancy or when pregnancy is possible. Advise patient to use reliable form of birth control while taking this drug.
- Discuss with patient ways to facilitate sleep (quiet, darkened room; avoidance of caffeine and nicotine; warm bath; warm milk; deep breathing; relaxation, self-hypnosis).
- Instruct patient *not* to increase dose.
- Emphasize importance of follow-up evaluation with physician to monitor progress of therapy. Instruct patient to inform physician if drug does not seem to be working.
- Instruct patient not to discontinue medication abruptly after prolonged therapy (eg, > 2 wk).
- Advise patient that disturbed nocturnal sleep may be experienced for 1-2 nights after discontinuing drug.
- Instruct patient to report these symptoms to physician: sudden onset of vision changes, irregular heart beat, fever, sore throat, bruising, rash, jaundice, unusual bleeding (eg, epistaxis) or if pregnancy is detected.
- Advise patient to avoid intake of alcoholic beverages or other CNS depressants.
- Advise patient that drug may cause drowsiness and to use caution while

driving or performing other tasks requiring mental alertness.

See Patient Guide, p. 536.

Quinacrine HCl

(KWIN-uh-kreen HIGH-droe-KLOR-ide)

Atabrine Hydrochloride

Class: Anti-infective/antimalarial and anthelmintic

Action Interferes with DNA so that it is unable to replicate or serve for transcription of RNA. Protein synthesis is impaired in susceptible parasites.

Indications Treatment of giardiasis and cestodiasis; treatment and suppression of malaria. **Unlabeled use:** Intrapleurally as sclerosing agent in prevention of pneumothorax recurrence.

Contraindications Concomitant primaquine therapy.

Route/Dosage

Dwarf Tapeworm

ADULTS: **PO** 1 tbsp sodium sulfate dissolved in water on night prior to treatment. On day 1, 900 mg on empty stomach in 3 portions 20 min apart with sodium sulfate purge 1½ hr later. On following 3 days, 100 mg tid. CHILDREN 11-14 YR: **PO** ½ tbsp sodium sulfate night before treatment. On day 1, 400 mg; next 3 days, 100 mg tid. CHILDREN 8-10 YR: **PO** ½ tbsp sodium sulfate night before treatment. On day 1, 300 mg; next 3 days 100 mg tid. CHILDREN 4-8 YR: **PO** ½ tbsp sodium sulfate night before treatment. On day 1, 200 mg; next 3 days 100 mg after breakfast.

Beef, Pork or Fish Tapeworm

ADULTS: **PO** 4 doses of 200 mg 10 min apart (800 mg total) with sodium bicarbonate 600 mg each dose. CHILDREN 11-14 YR: **PO** 600 mg in 3-4 divided doses 10 min apart with 300 mg sodium bicarbonate with each dose. CHILDREN 5-10 YR: **PO** 400 mg in 3-4 divided doses 10 min apart with 300 mg sodium bicarbonate with each dose.

Giardiasis

ADULTS: **PO** 100 mg tid for 5-7 days. CHILDREN: **PO** 7 mg/kg/day in 3 divided doses (maximum 300 mg/day) after meals for 5 days. May repeat 2 wk later if indicated.

Malaria Treatment

ADULTS & CHILDREN > 8 YR: **PO** 200 mg with 1 g sodium bicarbonate q 6 hr for 5 doses; then 100 mg tid for 6 days (total dose, 2.8 gm in 7 days). CHILDREN 4-8 YR: **PO** 200 mg tid first day; then 100 mg q 12 hr for 6 days. CHILDREN 1-4 YR: **PO** 100 mg tid first day; then 100 mg/day in single dose for 6 days.

Malaria Suppression

ADULTS: **PO** 100 mg/day for 1-3 mo. CHILDREN: **PO** 50 mg/day for 1-3 mo.

Interactions

Primaquine: Increases primaquine toxicity.

Lab Test Interferences

None well documented.

Adverse Reactions

CNS: Headache; dizziness; neuropsychiatric disturbances (nervousness, vertigo, irritability, emotional change, nightmares, transient psychosis); seizures. *EENT:* Reversible corneal edema or deposits (visual halos, focusing difficulty, blurred vision); retinopathy. *GI:* Diarrhea; anorexia; nausea; abdominal cramps; vomiting. *HEPA:* Hepatitis. *HEMA:* Aplastic anemia. *DERM:* Pleomorphic skin eruptions; exfoliative dermatitis; contact dermatitis; lichen planus-like eruptions; temporary yellowing of skin (not jaundice). *OTHER:* Intense yellow color to urine.

Precautions

Pregnancy: Pregnancy category undetermined. *Lactation:* Unknown. *El-*

derly or debilitated patients: Transitory psychosis may occur in patients > 60 yr or those with history of psychosis. *Hepatic impairment:* Because quinacrine concentrates in liver, patients with hepatic disease or alcoholism or taking other hepatotoxic drugs may be at risk for adverse effects. *Psoriasis or porphyria:* Severe attack or exacerbation of condition could occur.

NURSING CONSIDERATIONS

Administration/Storage

- For children administer in jam or honey to disguise bitter taste of pulverized tablets.
- For dwarf tapeworm treatment, the night before medication give adult 1 tbsp of sodium sulfate dissolved in water. After medication follow with sodium sulfate purge 1½ hr later. For child, administer ½ tbsp of sodium sulfate on night before medication. For beef, pork or fish tapeworm, provide bland, semisolid, nonfat diet or milk diet on day before medication. Have patient fast after evening meal. Administer saline purge or purge and cleansing enema before treatment if ordered. Administer saline purge 1-2 hr after treatment. The expelled worm is stained yellow, facilitating identification of scolex.
- Administer sodium bicarbonate 600 mg (300 mg for child) with each dose of quinacrine to reduce nausea and vomiting.
- For giardiasis treatment, administer after meals with fluids (water, tea, fruit juice). Examine stools 2 wk after medication and repeat medication regimen if necessary.
- For malaria treatment or suppression, administer after meals with fluids (water, tea, fruit juice). Administration for 1-3 mo is necessary for malaria suppression.
- Store in tightly closed container.

Assessment/Interventions

- Obtain patient history, including drug history and any known allergies. Note presence of hepatic disease and alcoholism and history of psoriasis or porphyria.
- Assess all stools for scolex (yellow tapeworms).
- Assess for infection in other family members.
- Assess mental status (affect, mood, behavioral changes), especially in patient > 60 yr or with history of psychosis.
- Monitor CBC if used for long-term therapy.
- Notify physician of adverse reactions.

OVERDOSAGE: SIGNS & SYMPTOMS

CNS excitation, restlessness, insomnia, psychic stimulation, convulsions, GI disorders, nausea, vomiting, abdominal cramps, diarrhea, vascular collapse, hypotension, shock, cardiac arrhythmias or arrest, yellow pigmentation of skin

Patient/Family Education

- Advise patient that medication may temporarily turn skin and urine yellow.
- Teach patient/family proper hygiene to be performed after bowel movement (ie, handwashing). Tell patient not to put fingers in mouth.
- Explain need for compliance with dosage schedule and duration of treatment.
- Inform patient at risk of possible risk of severe attack or exacerbation of psoriasis and porphyria.
- Instruct patient receiving prolonged therapy to undergo periodic complete ophthalmologic examinations.
- If used to treat tapeworm, advise patient that the worms will be passed in the stool and may be visible as yellow-colored scolex.
- Instruct patient to report any visual disturbances to physician promptly.
- Advise patient that drug may cause dizziness and to use caution while

driving or performing other tasks requiring mental alertness.

See Patient Guide, p. 537.

Quinapril HCl

(KWIN-uh-PRILL HIGH-droe-KLOR-ide)

Accupril

Class: Antihypertensive/angiotensin-converting enzyme (ACE) inhibitor

Action Competitively inhibits angiotensin I–converting enzyme, resulting in prevention of angiotensin I conversion to angiotensin II, a potent vasoconstrictor that also stimulates aldosterone release. Clinical consequences are decrease in BP, reduced sodium resorption and potassium retention.

Indications Treatment of hypertension; adjunctive therapy of CHF.

Contraindications Hypersensitivity to ACE inhibitors.

Route/Dosage

Hypertension

ADULTS: **PO** 10 mg qd initially; may increase after 1-2 wk. Maintenance: 20, 40 or 80 mg/day as single dose or 2 equally divided doses. In presence of renal impairment, recommended initial dose varies based on creatinine clearance: > 60 ml/min = 10 mg; 30-60 ml/min = 5 mg; 10-30 ml/min = 2.5 mg.

CHF

ADULTS: **PO** 5 mg bid initially; may increase dose weekly for clinical control.

Interactions *Allopurinol:* Greater risk of hypersensitivity possible with coadministration. *Antacids:* Quinipril bioavailability may be decreased. Separate administration times by 1 to 2 hr. *Capsaicin:* Cough may be exacerbated. *Digoxin:* May cause increased digoxin levels. *Diuretics:* Increased risk of hypotension. *Food:* Food (especially fat) reduces bioavailability of quinapril. *Indomethacin:* May reduce hypotensive effects, especially in low-renin or volume-dependent hypertensive patients. *Lithium:* May cause increased lithium levels and symptoms of lithium toxicity. *Loop diuretics:* Effects of loop diuretics may be decreased. *Phenothiazines:* Enhanced hypotensive effect. *Potassium supplements and potassium-sparing diuretics:* Hyperkalemia. *Tetracycline:* Decreased tetracycline absorption.

Lab Test Interferences False elevation of liver enzymes, serum bilirubin, uric acid and blood glucose may occur.

Adverse Reactions *CV:* Hypotension; orthostatic hypotension. *RESP:* Cough; asthma; bronchospasm. *CNS:* Headache; dizziness; fatigue; nervousness. *GI:* Nausea; abdominal pain; vomiting; diarrhea. *DERM:* Pruritus. *META:* Hyperkalemia; hyponatremia. *OTHER:* Hypersensitivity; angioedema.

Precautions *Pregnancy:* Category D (second, third trimester); Category C (first trimester). Avoid use in pregnant patients and discontinue drug as soon as pregnancy is detected; closely observe infants with histories of *in utero* exposure. *Lactation:* Undetermined. *Children:* Safety and efficacy not established. *Elderly patients:* May show higher peak blood levels of metabolite. *Angioedema:* May occur and is potentially fatal if laryngeal edema occurs. Use drug with extreme caution in patients with hereditary angioedema. *Cough:* Chronic cough may occur during treatment; more common in women. *Hepatic impairment:* Use drug with caution; dosage reduction may be necessary because of impaired metabolism. *Hypotension/first-dose effect:* Significant decreases in BP may occur after first dose, especially in severely salt- or volume-depleted patients (eg, patients on aggressive diuretic therapy) or in those with heart failure. *Neutropenia and agranulocytosis:* Have occurred rarely; risk appears greater with renal dysfunction, heart failure or immunosuppression. *Proteinuria:* Has occurred with similar agents, especially with high doses or prior renal disease. *Renal impairment:* May further decrease renal function with elevations in BUN and serum creatinine because of decreased renal perfusion. Furthermore, dosage should be reduced to compensate for reduced drug elimination.

NURSING CONSIDERATIONS

Administration/Storage

- Give 1 hr before meals.
- Do not administer antacids within 1-2 hours of this medication.
- Dose is adjusted at 2-wk intervals based on BP response at trough (predose) and peak (2-6 hr after dose) blood levels.
- If possible, diuretic therapy should be discontinued and salt intake increased about 1 wk prior to quinapril initiation to prevent severe hypotension precipitated by first dose. If diuretic cannot be discontinued, initial dose must be decreased to 5 mg.
- Monitor patient closely for 2 hr after first dose and for next 2 wk for hypotension.
- Store in light-resistant container at room temperature.

Assessment/Interventions

- Obtain patient history, including drug history and any known allergies.
- Note liver and renal disease, CHF and concurrent use of diuretics or dialysis.
- Obtain baseline renal function tests (serum BUN, protein, creatinine and urine dipstick for protein) and hepatic function tests prior to therapy.
- Caution patient to change position slowly; assist with ambulation.
- Monitor BP and pulse frequently during initial dose and during therapy.
- Monitor for hyperkalemia in patients with impaired renal function or diabetes mellitus and patients receiving potassium supplementation or potassium-sparing diuretics.
- Monitor BUN, creatinine and electrolytes during therapy. Expect potassium to increase and BUN and creatinine to transiently increase; sodium may decrease.
- Monitor for lightheadedness, dizziness and fainting. Provide for safety during first few days of therapy.
- Monitor renal function. Reduced dose is necessary in patients with renal impairment.
- Monitor WBC counts frequently.
- If severe hypotension occurs after first dose, if not medically contraindicated, administer IV infusion of normal saline (0.9% Sodium Chloride) as ordered as volume expander.
- If sudden severe dyspnea, swelling of lips or eyes or edema of hands and feet develops, withhold medication and notify physician.

OVERDOSAGE: SIGNS & SYMPTOMS

Hypotension

Patient/Family Education

- Remind patient that quinapril controls, not cures, high BP.
- Emphasize importance of other BP-controlling activities (weight loss, regular exercise, smoking cessation, moderate alcohol intake, stress management).
- Teach patient/family proper BP measurement technique. If possible, have patient/family demonstrate use of monitor they will be using at home. Stress that BP should be checked weekly (at least) and that patient should report significant changes to physician immediately.
- Advise patient that persistent dry, nonproductive cough should be reported. Remind patient not to self-medicate cough with otc medications

unless instructed to do so by physician.

- Emphasize need for ongoing medical follow up, even in absence of side effects or problems related to this medication therapy.
- Advise CHF patient to avoid rapid increases in physical activity. Emphasize importance of adequate fluid intake.
- Warn patient that excessive perspiration, dehydration, vomiting and diarrhea may lead to fall in BP.
- Caution patient not to use salt substitute containing potassium without consulting physician.
- Instruct patient to report these symptoms to physician immediately: rash, mouth sores, taste impairment, fever, sore throat, swelling of face or mouth, swelling, numbness or tingling of hands or feet, chest pain, breathing difficulty or jaundice.
- Caution patient to avoid sudden position changes to prevent orthostatic hypotension.

See Patient Guide, p. 538.

Quinidine

(KWIN-ih-deen)

Quinidine Sulfate
Quinidex Extentabs, Quinora,
✤ *Biquin Durules*

Quinidine Gluconate
Quinaglute Dura-Tabs, Quinalan,
✤ *Quinate*

Quinidine Polygalacturonate
Cardioquin

Class: Antiarrhythmic

Action Depresses myocardial excitability, conduction velocity and contractility; prolongs effective refractory period and increases conduction time; indirect anticholinergic effects; may decrease vagal tone at low doses paradoxically increasing conduction through the AV node.

Indications Treatment of premature atrial, atrioventricular junctional and ventricular contractions; treatment of paroxysmal supraventricular tachycardia, paroxysmal atrioventricular junctional rhythm, atrial flutter, paroxysmal and chronic atrial fibrillation and paroxysmal ventricular tachycardia not associated with complete heart block; maintenance therapy after electrical conversion of atrial fibrillation or flutter. *Quinidine gluconate (IV administration)*: Treatment of life-threatening *Plasmodium falciparum* malaria.

STOP **Contraindications** Myasthenia gravis; history of thrombocytopenic purpura associated with quinidine administration; digitalis intoxication; complete heart block; left bundle branch block; complete atrioventricular (AV) block with AV nodal or idioventricular pacemaker; aberrant ectopic impulses and abnormal rhythms because of escape mechanisms; history of drug-induced torsade de pointes; history of long QT syndrome.

Route/Dosage
The following oral doses are expressed as quinidine sulfate salt:

Premature Atrial and Ventricular Contractions
ADULTS: **PO** 200-300 mg tid/qid. CHILDREN: **PO** 30 mg/kg/day *or* 900 mg/m^2/day in 5 divided doses.

Paroxysmal Supraventricular Tachycardia
ADULTS: **PO** 400-600 mg q 2-3 hr until event is abated.

Atrial Flutter
Administer after digitalization and individualize dose.

Conversion of Atrial Fibrillation
ADULTS: **PO** 200 mg q 2-3 hr for 5-8 doses, then maintain with 200-300 mg tid-qid (immediate release tablets) *or* 300-600 mg bid-tid (sustained-release tablets); do not exceed 3-4 gm/day.

Quinidine Gluconate
ADULTS: **PO** 324-648 mg (1-2 tablets) q 8-12 hr.

Quinidine Polygalacturonate
ADULTS: **PO** Maintenance dose 275 mg q 8-12 hr.

Parenteral Quinidine Gluconate
ACUTE TACHYCARDIA: ADULTS: **IM** 600 mg initially, then 400 mg prn up to q 2 hr. CHILDREN: **IV** 2-10 mg/kg/dose q 3-6 hr prn. P. FALCIPARUM MALARIA: ADULTS: **IV** 15 mg/kg infused over 4 hr initially, then 7.5 mg/kg over 4 hr q 8 hr for 7 days or until oral therapy can be instituted *or* 10 mg/kg over 1-2 hr initially, then 0.02 mg/kg/min for up to 72 hr or until oral therapy can be instituted.

Interactions

Amiodarone, antacids, cimetidine, verapamil: May increase quinidine levels. *Anticoagulants*: May increase effect of anticoagulant; may cause hemorrhage. *Barbiturates, nifedipine, primidone, sucralfate*: May decrease quinidine levels. *Beta-blockers*: May increase effect of beta-blocker. *Dextromethorphan*: May increase plasma dextromethorphan concentrations. *Digitoxin, digoxin*: May increase digoxin plasma levels. *Hydantoins*: May reduce therapeutic effect of quinidine. *Nondepolarizing neuromuscular blocking agents, succinylcholine*: May increase neuromuscular blockade effect. *Propofenone*: Increased propofenone levels. *Rifampin*: May increase quinidine metabolism.

Lab Test Interferences

Triamterene will interfere with the fluorescent measurement of quinidine levels.

Adverse Reactions

CV: Widening of QRS complex; cardiac asystole; ventricular ectopy; hypotension; paradoxical tachycardia. *CNS*: Headache; fever; vertigo; excitement; confusion; delerium; syncope. *EENT*: Mydriasis; blurred vision; photophobia, diplopia, night blindness; tinnitus. *GI*: Nausea; vomiting; anorexia; abdominal pain; diarrhea. *GU*: Lupus nephritis. *HEPA*: Hepatitis. *HEMA*: Acute hemolytic anemia; agranulocytosis; thrombocytopenic purpura. *DERM*: Rash; urticaria; pruritus; flushing; photosensitivity. *OTHER*: Lupus erythematosus–like syndrome; cinchonism (headache, tinnitus, nausea, disturbed vision, deafness, dizziness, vertigo, lightheadedness); hypersensitivity reactions; arthralgia; myalgia.

Precautions

Pregnancy: Category C. *Lactation*: Excreted in breast milk. *Children*: Safety and efficacy not established. *Atrial flutter or fibrillation*: Pretreat these patient with digitalis preparation. *Bioequivalency*: Different salts have different amounts of quinidine base. Do not interchange without taking this into consideration. *Cardiotoxicity*: May occur; immediately discontinue drug. *Hepatotoxicity (including granulomatous hepatitis)*: Has occurred. Consider possibility if unexplained fever or elevated hepatic enzymes develop. *Hypersensitivity reactions*: May occur; administer single 200 mg tablet of quinidine sulfate or 200 mg IM injection of quinidine gluconate before starting therapy to determine if patient has idiosyncrasy to quinidine. *Malaria*: Dose schedules may result in hypotension, ECG changes and cinchonism. *Parenteral therapy*: Use only when oral therapy is not possible or when rapid therapeutic effect is required. *Potassium balance*: Effect of quinidine is enhanced by potassium and reduced if hypokalemia is present. *Renal, hepatic or cardiac impairment*: Use drug with caution because of potential for toxicity. *Syncope*: Occasionally occurs in patients on long-term therapy; may be fatal. Often caused by torsades de pointes. *Vagolytic effects*: May antagonize vagal maneuvers or administration of cholinergic drugs used to terminate paroxysmal supraventricular tachycardia.

NURSING CONSIDERATIONS

Administration/Storage

- Use IV route only when rapid response is needed or oral route is not feasible.
- Give test dose of 200 mg as ordered to evaluate intolerance/sensitivity.
- Position patient supine during IV administration to minimize hypotension.
- For direct IV push, administer slowly at 1 ml/min.
- For intermittent IV infusion, dilute 800 mg/50 ml or more with D5W; give at a rate of 16 mg/min or less. Use infusion device for accuracy/safety.
- Administer IM injection in deltoid muscle.
- Give oral preparation with full glass of water on empty stomach (1 hr before or 2 hr after other medication) to enhance absorption; if GI distress develops, administer with or just after meal.
- Do not break or crush or allow patient to chew sustained-release preparations. Instruct patient to swallow whole.
- Store vial at room temperature. Parenteral solution must be clear and colorless. Solution is stable for 24 hr.
- Store tablets in tight, light-resistant container.

Assessment/Interventions

- Obtain patient history, including drug history and any known allergies.
- Determine if patient has myasthenia gravis.
- When drug is used as antiarrhythmic agent, assess ECG prior to and continuously throughout therapy. Therapy is discontinued if severe heart block occurs (50% widening of QRS complex, PR or QT interval are prolonged) or tachycardia or frequent ventricular ectopic beats develops.
- Obtain baseline BP and pulse and assess continuously during therapy.
- Monitor CBC and hepatic and renal function tests during long-term therapy.
- When drug is used as antimalarial agent, monitor BP, ECG and plasma quinidine levels closely during therapy, especially if drug is being administered parenterally.
- If patient had been receiving digoxin, measure digoxin concentration to ensure it does not increase to toxic levels.
- Observe for hypotension, tachycardia and arrhythmias.

OVERDOSAGE: SIGNS & SYMPTOMS

Cardiorespiratory depression, lethargy, confusion, coma, seizures, headache, paresthesia, vertigo, vomiting, abdominal pain, diarrhea, nausea, tachyarrhythmias, depressed automaticity and conduction, hypotension, syncope, heart failure, cinchonism, hypokalemia, visual/auditory disturbances, tinnitus, acidosis

Patient/Family Education

- Instruct patient/family to administer medication around clock as directed and to continue taking medication even if feeling better.
- Advise patient to take with food if GI upset occurs.
- Tell patient that sustained-release tablet should not be crushed or chewed.
- Instruct patient/family how to take pulse. Advise them to check pulse prior to each dose and to contact physician if rate or rhythm changes.
- Advise patient to carry identification (eg, Medi-Alert) indicating disease and drug therapy at all times.
- Advise patient to notify other physicians/dentist prior to other therapy/surgery.
- Emphasize importance of regular medical follow-up, even in absence of side effects or problems related to this drug therapy.
- Caution patient to wear dark glasses as needed to decrease light sensitivity

and inform patient that dark glasses may be needed both indoors and outside.

- Instruct patient to report these symptoms to physician immediately: visual disturbances (eg, blurring), tinnitis, bleeding, bruising, fever, headache, dizziness, severe diarrhea or skin rash/eruption.
- Advise patient that drug causes dizziness and blurred vision and to use caution while driving or performing other tasks requiring mental alertness.
- Caution patient to avoid exposure to sunlight and to use sunscreen or wear protective clothing to avoid photosensitivity reaction.
- Instruct patient not to take otc medications without consulting physician.

See Patient Guide, p. 539.

Quinine Sulfate

(KWIE-nine SULL-fate)

Formula-Q, Legatrin, M-KYA, Q-vel, Quinam, Quiphile

Class: Anti-infective/antimalarial

Action Causes pH elevation in intracellular organelles of parasites; also has skeletal muscle relaxant effects and cardiovascular effects similar to those of quinidine.

Indications Treatment of chloroquine-resistant falciparum malaria; alternative treatment for chloroquine-sensitive strains of *P. falciparum*, *P. malariae*, *P. ovale* and *P. uivae*; prevention and treatment of nocturnal recumbency leg cramps.

Contraindications G-6-PD deficiency; optic neuritis; tinnitus; history of blackwater fever and thrombocytopenic purpura associated with previous quinine ingestion; pregnancy.

Route/Dosage

Chloroquine-Resistant P. Falciparum Malaria

ADULTS: **PO** 650 mg q 8 hr for 5-7 days. CHILDREN: **PO** 25 mg/kg/day in divided doses q 8 hr for 5-7 days.

Chloroquine-Sensitive Malaria

ADULTS: **PO** 600 mg q 8 hr for 5-7 days. CHILDREN: **PO** 10 mg/kg q 8 hr for 5-7 days.

Nocturnal Leg Cramps

ADULTS: **PO** 260-300 mg at bedtime.

Interactions

Aluminum-containing antacids: Causes delayed or decreased quinine absorption. *Anticoagulants, oral:* May cause depression of hepatic enzyme system that synthesizes vitamin K–dependent clotting factors and may enhance action of oral anticoagulants. *Cimetidine:* May reduce quinine's clearance and prolong its half-life in body. *Digoxin:* May cause increased digoxin serum concentration. *Mefloquine:* May cause ECG abnormalities or cardiac arrest and may increase risk of convulsions. Do not use concurrently. Delay administration 12 hr after last dose of quinine. *Neuromuscular blocking agents:* May potentiate neuromuscular blockade and may result in respiratory difficulties. *Urinary alkalinizers:* May increase quinine serum concentrations and potentiate toxicity.

Lab Test Interferences

Urinary 17-ketogenic steroids may have elevated values with Zimmerman method.

Adverse Reactions

CV: Anginal symptoms. *CNS:* Vertigo; dizziness; headache; fever; apprehension; restlessness; confusion; syncope; excitement; delirium; hypothermia; seizures. *EENT:* Visual disturbances (photophobia; blurred vision with scotomata; night blindness; amblyopia; diplopia; diminished visual fields; mydriasis; optic atrophy) tinnitus; deafness. *GI:* Nausea; vomiting; diarrhea; epigastric pain. *GU:* Renal tubular damage; anuria. *HEPA*: Hepatitis. *HEMA*: Acute hemolysis; hemolytic anemia; thrombocytopenic purpura; agranulocytosis; hypoprothrombinemia. *OTHER*: Cinchonism (headache, tinnitus, nausea, diarrhea, disturbed vision, skin, CV and CNS symptoms at very high doses); hypersensitivity (rash, pruritus, flushing, sweating, facial edema, asthmatic symptoms).

Precautions

Pregnancy: Category X. *Lactation*: Excreted in breast milk. *Cardiac disease*: Patients with cardiac arrhythmias may have exacerbation of symptoms with quinine, which acts similarly to quinidine. May cause cardiotoxicity. In patients with atrial fibrillation, quinine requires same precautions as for quinidine. *Hemolysis*: Has been associated with G-6-PD deficiency. Discontinue immediately if hemolysis appears.

NURSING CONSIDERATIONS

Administration/Storage

- Give with food or after meals to minimize GI irritation; give bedtime dose with milk or snack.
- Administer around clock (every 8 hr) to maintain serum drug levels if being used to treat malaria.
- Administer at bedtime if being used to treat or prevent nocturnal leg cramps.
- Do not crush tablets; have patient swallow tablets whole.
- Store in tight, light-resistant container.

Assessment/Interventions

- Obtain patient history, including drug history and any known allergies.
- Determine whether patient has any contraindications to quinine (eg, G-6-PD deficiency, pregnancy).
- Obtain baseline ECG, hepatic studies and CBC prior to therapy.
- Assess pulse and ECG during therapy to detect arrhythmias.
- Assess for evidence of hematological abnormalities (sore throat, fever, bleeding/bruising, fatigue or weakness).
- Assess for signs of cinchonism: blurred vision, headache, tinnitus, vertigo, lightheadedness, nausea. Report these adverse effects immediately to physician.

OVERDOSAGE: SIGNS & SYMPTOMS

Tinnitus, dizziness, skin rash, GI disturbance, diarrhea, arrhythmias, convulsions, blurred vision, headache, nausea/vomiting, fever, confusion

Patient/Family Education

- Caution patient that this medication must not be taken during pregnancy or when pregnancy is possible. Advise patient to use reliable form of birth control while taking this drug.
- If medication is being used to treat malaria, advise patient to take medication around clock and to take full course of treatment even if feeling better.
- Emphasize importance of medical follow-up when this course of therapy has been completed to ensure that therapy has been successful.
- If medication is being used to treat nocturnal leg cramps, advise patient to take drug before bedtime.
- Instruct patient to consult physician before combining any new medications with this drug.
- Advise patient to take medication with or after meals or snack to minimize GI distress.
- Instruct patient to report these symptoms to physician: flushing, itching, rash, fever, difficulty breathing, vision problems, ringing in ears, diarrhea, nausea/vomiting or vertigo.

- Advise patient that drug may cause dizziness and vision problems and to use caution while driving or performing other tasks requiring mental alertness.
- Instruct patient not to take otc medications (especially cold preparations) without consulting physician.

See Patient Guide, p. 540.

Rabies Immune Globulin (RIG), Human

(RAY-beez ih-MYOON GLAB-byoo-lin)

Hyperab, Imogam

Class: Immune serum

Action Directly neutralizes rabies virus.

Indications Passive, transient postexposure prevention of rabies infection in susceptible individuals.

Contraindications Repeated doses once vaccine treatment has been initiated. RIG may theoretically be contraindicated in persons who have had life-threatening reactions in human IgG antibody products or any of its components. Previous complete immunization with rabies vaccine and presence of adequate antibody titer.

Route/Dosage

ADULTS & CHILDREN: **IM** 20 IU/kg (0.133 ml/kg) as soon as possible after exposure, preferably with first dose of vaccine.

Interactions

Measles, mumps, polio or rubella live vaccines: Other antibodies in RIG preparation may interfere with response to these live vaccines.

Lab Test Interferences

None well documented.

Adverse Reactions

GU: Nephrotic syndrome. *DERM:* Urticaria; skin rash. *OTHER:* Local tenderness, soreness or stiffness at injection site; low-grade fever; angioedema; sensitization to repeated injections; anaphylactic shock.

Precautions

Pregnancy: Category C. Use only if clearly needed. *Lactation:* Unknown. *Hypersensitivity to thimerosal or human immunoglobulins:* Give drug with caution. *Live vaccines:* To avoid inactivating live vaccines, do not give live vaccines within 4 mo after RIG.

NURSING CONSIDERATIONS

Administration/Storage

- Use up to ½ dose to infiltrate wound site if nature and location of wound site permits. Administer balance of dose IM at different site and in different extremity from rabies vaccine, preferably in gluteal muscle (upper outer quadrant only) or deltoid muscle.
- Administer as soon as possible after exposure up to 8 days after first vaccine dose.
- RIG is used in conjunction with rabies vaccine. Administer human diploid cell culture (HDCV) rabies vaccine as soon as possible after rabies exposure.
- Do not give more than 5 ml in one injection site.
- Store under refrigeration; do not freeze.

Assessment/Interventions

- Obtain complete history, including drug history and any known allergies. Verify that prior vaccine treatment has not been initiated and that hypersensitivity to human immune globulins and thimerosal (chemical found in contact lens solutions) does not exist.
- Assess for signs of immediate (within 15 min) and delayed allergic reaction: shortness of breath, rash, pruritus and

fever. Report symptoms to physician immediately.
- Note date of last tetanus immunization. Vaccinate if needed.

Patient/Family Education
- Advise patient that pain, itching and swelling may temporarily occur at injection site.
- Advise patient to take acetaminophen to alleviate headache, fever and pain.
- Teach patient wound care and signs of infection (fever, wound drainage, increased pain at wound) if applicable prior to discharge.
- Encourage patient to return for medical follow-up within 7-10 days after discharge.

No patient monograph available.

Rabies Vaccine, Human Diploid Cell Cultures (HDCV)

(RAY-beez vaccine)

Imovax Rabies Vaccine, Imovax Rabies I.D. Vaccine

Class: Vaccine, inactivated virus

Action Induces neutralizing antibodies and cellular immunity.

Indications Induction of active immunity against rabies virus either before or after viral exposure.

Contraindications May theoretically be contraindicated in persons who have had life-threatening allergic reactions to rabies vaccine or any of its components. Pre-exposure treatment: developing febrile illness.

Route/Dosage

Preexposure Prophylaxis

ADULTS & CHILDREN: **IM** 1 ml *or* **Intradermal** 0.1 ml (*Imovax ID* only) on days 0, 7, and 21 or 28.

Postexposure Prophylaxis

ADULTS & CHILDREN: Following RIG administration, **IM** 1 ml on days 0, 3, 7, 14 and 28. Patients who previously received preexposure prophylaxis: **IM** 1 ml on only days 0 and 3. Do not give RIG.

Interactions

Chloroquine: Long-term therapy with chloroquine may suppress immune response to intradermal rabies vaccine. Complete pre-exposure rabies vaccination 1-2 mo before starting chloroquine administration. *Immunosuppressant drugs (including high-dose corticosteroids):* May result in insufficient response to immunization. If possible, do not give immunosuppressive agents during post-exposure therapy.

Lab Test Interferences

None well documented.

Adverse Reactions

CNS: Headache; dizziness. *GI:* Nausea; abdominal pain. *Local:* Swelling, erythema, pruritis, local pain and discomfort. *OTHER:* Muscle aches; slight fever; fatigue; serum-sickness–like reactions with intradermal booster doses.

Precautions

Pregnancy: Category C. Vaccinate if risk of disease outweighs risk to patients. *Lactation:* Unknown. *Hypersensitivity reactions:* In persons who experience immune-complex–like (or serum-sickness–like) hypersensitivity reactions during pre-exposure prophylaxis, do not give further doses of rabies vaccine unless they are exposed to rabies or they are likely to be unapparently or unavoidably exposed to rabies virus and have unsatisfactory antibody titers. *Intradermal route:* Indicated only for pre-exposure immunization. *Pre-exposure immunization:* Those at high risk of exposure to the rabies virus require pre-exposure immunization: veterinarians, certain laboratory workers, animal handlers, forest rangers, spelunkers and persons staying > 1 mo in other countries where rabies is constant threat (eg, India). *Postexposure prophylaxis:* If bite from animal is unprovoked, animal is not apprehended and rabies is present in that species in area, administer RIG and rabies vaccine. Consider vaccine recipients adequately immunized if they previously completed preexposure or postexposure prophylaxis with either current rabies vaccine (but not Wyvac brand from Wyeth) or have documented adequate antibody response. *Radiation therapy:* Persons undergoing radiation therapy may experience insufficient response to immunization and remain susceptible. *Travelers:* Travelers to endemic areas may receive vaccine by intradermal route if 3-dose series can be completed ≥ 30 days before departure; otherwise give vaccine IM.

NURSING CONSIDERATIONS

Administration/Storage

- Reconstitute vaccine with 1 ml of diluent using a needle longer than the intradermal needle used for administration. Stir contents until dissolved and withdraw amount needed. Remove reconstitution needle and replace with smaller needle for administration.
- For postexposure vaccination, do not administer intradermally; administer intramuscularly in deltoid area in older child and adult and in vastis lateralis in young child. Never administer rabies vaccine in gluteal area; this may result in inadequate immune response.
- May administer pre-exposure prophylaxis vaccine intradermally. Intradermal injections in lateral aspect of upper arm are less likely to cause adverse reactions than intradermal injections in forearm.
- Follow careful recordkeeping when administering vaccine: note manufacturer, lot number, expiration date of vaccine, date of administration and signature of person administering vaccine.
- Report severe reaction to FDA through local/state health departments; note reaction on patient chart.
- Store under refrigeration; do not freeze.

Assessment/Interventions

- Obtain patient history, including drug history and any known allergies. Note previous life-threatening allergic reaction to rabies vaccine or any of its components.
- Determine if patient is receiving immunosuppressive therapy.
- Assess for allergic reaction (urticaria, breathing difficulty, nausea and vomiting, fever) within 15 min of administration and document patient tolerance of vaccine.
- Have epinephrine and antihistamines (eg, diphenhydramine) readily available.

Pre-exposure Prophylaxis

- Assess temperature; withhold pre-exposure dose if patient has febrile illness.

Postexposure Prophylaxis

- Immediately and thoroughly scrub wounds/scratches with antibacterial soap and water. Dress wound as necessary.
- Give tetanus prophylaxis and control bacterial infection (wound management, antibiotics) as ordered.

Patient/Family Education

- Advise patient at risk for ongoing rabies exposure to receive rabies booster every 2 yr or more often (per serology q 6 mo) if very high risk (eg, veterinarians).
- Advise patient to seek immediate medical attention should future rabies exposure occur. Emphasize danger of wound infection and need to evaluate rabies antibody response.
- Teach patient/family wound care and signs of infection (fever, wound drainage, increased pain at wound) prior to discharge.
- Advise patient that aspirin/

antihistamines can be taken to treat mild local or systemic reactions.

- Encourage medical follow-up within 7-10 days after discharge for wound evaluation.

No patient monograph available.

Ramipril

(ruh-MIH-prill)

Altace

Class: Antihypertensive/angiotensin-converting enzyme (ACE) inhibitor

Action Competitively inhibits angiotensin I-converting enzyme, resulting in prevention of angiotensin I conversion to angiotensin II, a potent vasoconstrictor. Clinical consequences are decrease in BP and indirectly (by inhibiting aldosterone) decrease in sodium and fluid retention and increase in diuresis.

Indications Treatment of hypertension. **Unlabeled use:** Treatment of CHF.

Contraindications Hypersensitivity to ACE inhibitors (particularly history of angioedema).

Route/Dosage

Hypertension

ADULTS: PO 2.5 mg qd initially. Maintenance: 2.5-20 mg/day as single dose or in 2 equally divided doses.

Patients with Renal Impairment

PO 1.25 mg qd in patients with creatinine clearance < 40 ml/min (serum creatinine > 2.5 mg/dl) (maximum 5 mg/day).

CHF

ADULTS: PO 2.5 mg bid. Switch to 1.25 mg bid if hypotension occurs. Titrate to target dose of 5 mg bid.

Interactions *Allopurinol:* Greater risk of hypersensitivity possible with coadministration. *Antacids:* Ramipril bioavailability may be decreased. Separate administration times by 1 to 2 hr. *Capsaicin:* May exacerbate cough. *Digoxin:* Increased digoxin levels. *Indomethacin:* May reduce hypotensive effects, especially in low-renin or volume-dependent hypertensive patients. *Lithium:* May cause increased lithium levels and symptoms of lithium toxicity. *Loop diuretics.* Effects of loop diuretics may be decreased. *Phenothiazines:* Enhanced hypotensive effects. *Potassium supplements, potassium-sparing diuretics:* May cause increased potassium serum levels.

Lab Test Interferences False elevation of liver enzymes, serum bilirubin, uric acid and blood glucose may occur.

Adverse Reactions CV: Hypotension. *RESP:* Angioneurotic edema with dyspnea; asthma; bronchospasm; upper respiratory infection; cough. *CNS:* Headache; dizziness; fatigue. *GI:* Nausea; vomiting. *HEMA:* Decreases in Hgb or Hct; leukopenia; eosinophilia; proteinuria. *DERM:* Rash; pruritis. *META:* Hyperkalemia. *OTHER:* Asthenia, fever, hypersensitivity, flu-like syndrome, anaphylactoid reaction.

Precautions *Pregnancy:* Category D (second, third trimester); Category C (first trimester). Discontinue use in pregnant patients, fetal/neonatal injury and death have occurred; closely observe infants with histories of in utero exposure. *Lactation:* Undetermined. *Children:* Safety and efficacy not established. *Elderly patients:* May show higher blood levels of active metabolite. *Angioedema:* May occur. Use drug with extreme caution in patients with hereditary angioedema. *Cough:* Chronic cough may occur during treatment; it is more common in women. *Hepatic impairment:* Use drug with caution. Dosage reduction may be required due to impaired metabolism. *Hypotension/first-dose effect:* Significant decreases in BP may occur following first dose, especially in severely salt- or volume-depleted patients (such as those receiving diuretics) or those with heart failure. *Neutropenia and agranulocytosis:* Have occurred with similar agents; risk appears greater in presence of renal dysfunction, heart failure or immunosuppression. *Proteinuria:* Has occurred with agents in this class, especially with high doses or prior renal disease. *Renal impairment:* Dosage reduction is required. May further decrease renal function with elevations in BUN and serum creatinine due to decreased renal perfusion.

NURSING CONSIDERATIONS

Administration/Storage

- Alternative route of administration: Ramipril capsules are usually swallowed whole. However, the capsules may be opened and the contents sprinkled on a small amount of approximately 4 oz applesauce or mixed in apple juice or water. Entire mixture should be consumed. Pre-prepared mixtures can be stored for up to 24 hours at room temperature for for up to 48 hours under refrigeration.
- Diuretics should be discontinued 2-3 days prior to ramipril therapy, if possible. If diuretic cannot be discontinued, dose reduction of ramipril is required.
- Store at room temperature in tightly closed container.

Assessment/Interventions

- Obtain patient history, including drug history and any known allergies.
- Obtain baseline CBC, potassium level and WBC counts and monitor at regular intervals.
- Obtain baseline orthostatic BP prior to first dose. Monitor frequent intervals during first 2 wk of therapy.
- Obtain baseline renal and liver function tests. Monitor renal function test results at regular intervals during drug therapy, especially in patients with renal impairment.
- Note that patients with severe CHF may experience renal failure during ACE inhibitor therapy.
- Assess for proteinuria at monthly intervals.
- Notify physician if patient develops hypotension, nausea, vomiting, headache, dizziness, fatigue, angioedema, fever, infection or mouth sores.

OVERDOSAGE: SIGNS & SYMPTOMS

Hypotension

Patient/Family Education

- Advise patient that chronic dry cough may develop and to notify physician if cough becomes bothersome.
- Instruct patient to maintain adequate fluid status and to avoid excess dehydration or perspiration or overhydration.
- Advise patient to consult physician prior to using salt substitutes containing potassium.
- Instruct patient to notify physician of persistent rash, angioedema, abdominal pain, jaundice, excessive fatigue, irregular heart rate or chest pain.
- Teach family member or friend how to take BP and instruct patient to keep written record.
- Encourage patient to follow nonmedical interventions to control hypertension: weight control, sodium and alcohol restriction, smoking cessation and regular exercise.
- Instruct patient not to take otc medications without first consulting with physician.
- Advise patient to avoid sudden position changes to prevent orthostatic hypotension. Advise patient that hot bath or shower may aggravate dizziness.
- Tell patient to avoid abrupt discontinuation of therapy unless instructed by physician.
- Inform patient that drug may cause drowsiness and to use caution while

driving or performing other tasks requiring mental alertness.

See Patient Guide, p. 541.

Ranitidine

(ran-EYE-tih-DEEN)

Zantac, ✦ *Nu-Ranit, Zantac-C, Novo-Ranidine*

Class: Histamine H_2 antagonist

Action Reversibly and competitively blocks histamine at H_2 receptors, particularly those in gastric parietal cells, leading to inhibition of gastric acid secretion.

Indications Treatment and maintenance of duodenal ulcer; management of gastroesophageal reflux disease (GERD; including erosive or ulcerative disease); short-term treatment of benign gastric ulcer; treatment of pathologic hypersecretory conditions (Zollinger-Ellison). **Unlabeled uses:** Prevention of upper GI bleeding; treatment of aspiration pneumonia; stress ulcer; and gastric NSAID damage. Used as a part of a mulit-drug regimen to eradicate *Helicobacter pylori* in the treatment of peptic ulcer; protection against aspiration of acid during anesthesia; prevention of gastro duodenal mucosal damage that may be associated with long-term NSAIDS; to control acute upper GI bleeding; prevention of stress ulcers.

Contraindications Hypersensitivity to ranitidine or other H_2 antagonists.

Route/Dosage

Duodenal Ulcer (Active)

ADULTS: **PO** 150 mg bid or 300 mg at bedtime. Maintenance: 150 mg at bedtime. **IM/IV/Intermittent IV** 50 mg q 6-8 hr.

Acute Benign Gastric Ulcer and GERD

ADULTS: **PO** 150 mg bid. **IM/IV/Intermittent IV** 50 mg q 6-8 hr.

Pathologic Hypersecretory Conditions

ADULTS: **PO** 150 mg bid. Individualize.

Erosive Esophagitis

ADULTS: **PO** 150 mg qid. **IM/IV/Intermittent IV** 50 mg q 6-8 hr. **Continuous IV** 6.25 mg/hr. For patients with Zollinger-Ellison, start infusion at rate of 1 mg/kg/hr and adjust upward in 0.5 mg/kg/hr increments according to gastric acid output (maximum 2.5 mg/kg/hr; infusion rate 220 mg/hr).

Renal Insufficiency (Creatinine Clearance < 50 ml/min)

ADULTS: **PO** 150 mg q 24 hr. **IM/IV** 50 mg q 18-24 hr.

Interactions

Diazepam: Pharmacolgic effects may be decreased due to decreased GI absorption by ranitidine. Staggering administration times may avoid this reaction. *Ethanol:* May increase plasma ethanol levels. *Glipizide:* Possible increased hypoglycemia effect. *Ketoconazole:* May decrease effects of ketoconazole. *Lidocaine:* May cause increased lidocaine levels. *Warfarin:* Ranitidine may interfere with warfarin clearance. Hypoprothombinemic effects may increase; may need adjustment.

Lab Test Interferences

False-positive test results for urine protein with Multistix may occur during ranitidine therapy; testing with sulfosalicyclic acid is recommended.

Adverse Reactions

CV: Cardiac arrhythmias; bradycardia. *CNS:* Headache; somnolence; fatigue; dizziness; hallucinations; depression; insomnia. *GI:* Nausea; vomiting; abdominal discomfort; diarrhea; constipation; pancreatitis. *HEMA:* Agranulocytosis; autoimmune hemolytic or aplastic anemia; thrombocytopenia, granulocytopenia. *HEPA:* Cholestatic or hepatocellular effects. *DERM:* Alopecia; rash; erythema multiforme. *OTHER:* Hypersensitivity reactions.

Precautions

Pregnancy: Category B. *Lactation:* Excreted in breast milk. *Children:* Safety and efficacy not established. *Elderly patients:* May have reduced renal function, therefore decreased drug clearance may be more common. *Hepatic impairment:* Use drug with caution; decreased clearance may occur. *Hepatocellular injury:* May occur, manifested as reversible hepatitis, hepatocellular or hepatocanalicular or mixed, with or without jaundice. *Hypersensitivity:* Rare cases of anaphylaxis have occurred as well as rare episodes of hypersensitivity. *Rapid IV administration:* May rarely result in bradycardia, tachycardia or premature ventricular beats, usually in patients predisposed to cardiac rhythm disturbances. *Renal impairment:* Decreased clearance may occur; dosage reduction may be needed. Hemodialysis reduces level of ranitidine–dosage timing must be adjusted so that scheduled dose coincides with end of hemodialysis.

NURSING CONSIDERATIONS

Administration/Storage

Intravenous

- For IV use, medication is stable in 5% or 10% Dextrose Injection, 0.9% Sodium Chloride or Lactated Ringer's Solution.
- Administer without regard to meals.
- When administering via IV push, dilute to volume of 20 ml with Saline for Injection and inject over at least 5 min.
- For intermittent infusion, dilute 50 mg in 50-100 ml D5W and infuse over 15-20 min.
- Do not mix with other IV medications.
- Administer continuous infusion at rate of 6.25 mg/hr except for patients with Zollinger-Ellison syndrome.
- Store diluted IV solutions at room temperature. Discard after 48 hr.

Oral

- Do not give oral drug at same time as other antacids. Separate administration by at least 1 hr.
- Store syrup form in refrigerator.
- Dissolve EFFERdose tablets in 6-8 oz of water.

Assessment/Interventions

- Obtain patient history, including drug history and any known allergies.
- Obtain baseline CBC, renal and liver function test results and monitor at regular intervals.
- Assess mental status before starting drug and monitor for changes.
- Notify physician if patient develops right upper quadrant abdominal pain, nausea, vomiting, change in color or consistency of stools, and jaundice.
- Slow rate of IV administration if bradycardia, tachycardia or premature ventricular contractions develop. If these conditions persist, stop infusion and notify physician.
- Notify physician if patient has arrhythmias, headache, fatigue, dizziness, hallucinations, depression, insomnia, alopecia, rash or erythema multiforme, or severe or persistent diarrhea.

OVERDOSAGE: SIGNS & SYMPTOMS

Rapid respiration, respiratory failure, tachycardia, muscle tremors, vomiting, restlessness, pallor of mucous membranes, redness of mouth and ears, hypotension, collapse, lacrimation, salivation, diarrhea, miosis

Patient/Family Education

- Instruct patient not to take antacids at same time as drug. Separate administration by at least 1 hr.
- Advise patient to report these symptoms to physician: abdominal pain, nausea, vomiting, change in color or consistency of stools, black stools or coffeeground emesis; jaundice, headache, excessive fatigue, dizziness, un-

usual bruising or bleeding, petechiae, rash or shortness of breath.
- Discuss necessary dietary changes or restrictions appropriate for patient. Refer patient to dietitian if indicated.
- Advise patient with ulcers to avoid alcohol and smoking.
- Discuss stress reduction with patient if indicated.
- Instruct patient to dissolve effervescent formulation in 6-8 oz of water before drinking.
- Advise patient that drug may cause dizziness and to use caution while driving or performing other tasks requiring mental alertness.

See Patient Guide, p. 542.

Rh_0(D) Immune Globulin (RhIG); Rh_0(D) Immune Globulin Intravenous (RhIGIV)

([RH_0D] ih-MYOON GLAB-byoo-lin)

Gamulin Rh, HypRho-D, HypRho-D Mini-Dose, MICRhoGAM, Mini-Gamulin Rh, Rhesonativ, RhoGAM, WinRho SD

Class: Immune serum

Action By binding Rh_0(D) antigen on red blood cells (RBCs), RhIG prevents production of anti-Rh_0(D) antibodies in Rh_0(D) antigen–negative persons. Prevention of Rh sensitization, in turn, prevents hemolytic disease of fetus and newborn in subsequent Rh_0(D) antigen–positive children.

Indications Passive, transient protection against development of endogenous anti-Rh antibodies (isoimmunization) in nonsensitized Rh antigen–negative persons who receive Rh antigen–positive blood. Such exposure may result from fetomaternal hemorrhage occurring during delivery, spontaneous or induced abortion, abdominal trauma, ectopic pregnancy, chorionic villus sampling (CVS), percutaneous umbilical cord blood sampling (PUBS), amniocentesis, fetal surgery or manipulation or as result of transfusion accident. RhIG/RhIGV prevents hemolytic disease of fetus and newborn (including erythroblastosis fetalis and hydrops fetalis) in subsequent Rh antigen–positive children. If Rh typing of fetus is not possible, assume fetus is Rh antigen–positive and give mother RhIG/RhIGV. Do not perform Rh cross-match prior to administration. *Term delivery:* To warrant RhIG/RhIGV. administration, (1) mother must be Rh antigen–negative, (2) mother should not have been previously sensitized to Rh factor [and thus produce her own anti-Rh antibodies], and (3) infant must be Rh antigen–positive and direct antiglobulin negative. (4) If father can be determined to be Rh antigen–negative, RhIG/RhIGV need not be given. *Other obstetric conditions:* Administer RhIG/RhIGV to all nonsensitized Rh antigen–negative women after spontaneous or induced abortions, after ruptured ectopic pregnancies, amniocentesis, other abdominal trauma, CVS, PUBS, fetal surgery or manipulation or any transplacental hemorrhage, unless blood type of fetus has been determined to be Rh antigen–negative. Sensitization occurs more frequently in women undergoing induced abortions than in those aborting spontaneously. *Transfusion accidents:* RhIG/RhIGV can be used to prevent Rh sensitization in Rh antigen–negative patients who accidentally receive transfusions with RBCs or blood components containing RBCs, platelets or granulocytes prepared from Rh antigen–positive blood. Administer within 72 hours following Rh-incompatible transfusion. *Intravenous preparation (WinRho SD) only:* Immune thrombocytopenia purpura.

STOP **Contraindications** Hypersensitivity to thimerosal, any immune globulin, or any of the product's components.

Route/Dosage

For IM administration only except for *WinRho SD*, which may be used IM or IV. Contents of total dose may be injected as divided dose at different injection sites at same time, or total dosage may be divided and injected at intervals, provided total dosage to be given is injected within 72 hr.

Postpartum Prophylaxis, Miscarriage, Abortion or Ectopic Pregnancy

1 full-dose vial or syringe of RhIG prevents maternal sensitization if RBC volume that entered mother's circulation is < 15 ml. When fetomaternal hemorrhage exceeds 15 ml of RBCs, administer > 1 container of RhIG. One minidose container of RhIG will prevent formation of anti-Rh antibodies resulting from spontaneous or induced abortion up to 12 wk gestation. After 12 wk gestation, give full-dose container.

Antepartum Prophylaxis

1 full-dose container of RhIG at 28 weeks gestation and again within 72 hr after Rh-incompatible delivery is highly effective in preventing Rh isoimmunization during pregnancy.

Threatened Abortion

Following threatened abortion at any stage of gestation with continuation of pregnancy, give 1 full-dose container of RhIG, unless larger dose is needed.

Amniocentesis or Abdominal Trauma

Following amniocentesis at either 15-18 wk gestation or during third trimester, or following abdominal trauma in second or third trimester, give 1 full-dose container of RhIG, unless larger dose is needed.

Transfusion Accidents

Dose of RhIG is dependent on volume of red cells or whole blood transfused. To determine amount of RhIG needed, multiply volume (measured in ml) of Rh antigen–positive whole blood administered by Hct of donor unit. This value equals volume of RBCs transfused. Divide volume of RBCs by 15 to obtain dose of RhIG needed. If dose calculation results in fraction, administer next higher whole number of full-dose vials or syringes of RhIG. Rh antigen–negative patients who receive Rh antigen–positive blood have received as many as 15-33 vials of RhIG without adverse reaction. If any event requires administration of RhIG at 13-18 wk gestation, give another full dose at 26-28 wk gestation. Give additional full dose of RhIG within 72 hr after delivery if infant is Rh antigen–positive. If delivery occurs within 3 wk after last dose, postpartum dose may be withheld, unless there is fetomaternal hemorrhage of > 15 ml RBCs.

Rh_O(D) Immune Globulin Intravenous

Pregnancy

Administer IM or IV 1,500 IU (300 mcg) at 28 weeks gestation. If administered early in pregnancy, give at 12 week intervals. Administer 600 IU (120 mcg) as soon as possible after delivery of a confirmed Rh_O(D) antigen positive baby and within 72 hours after delivery. If Rh status of baby is not known at 72 hours, administer Rh_O(D) immune globulin to mother at 72 hours after delivery. If >72 hours have elapsed, administer as soon as possible, up to 28 days after delivery.

Other Obstetric Conditions

Administer IM or IV 600 IU (120 mcg) immediately after abortion, amniocentesis (after 34 weeks gestation) or any other manipulation late in pregnancy (after 34 weeks gestation) associated with increased risk of Rh isoimmunization. Administraton should take place within 72 hours after the event. Administer IM or IV 1,500 IU (300 mcg) dose immediately after amniocentesis before 34 weeks gestation or after chorionic vilus sampling. Repeat this dose every 12 weeks during pregnancy. In case of threatened abortion, give as soon as possible.

Transfusion
Administer within 72 hours after exposure for treatment of incompatible blood transfusion or massive fetal hemorrhage. IV 3,000 IU (600 mcg) every 8 hours until the total dose is administered (Rh + blood/ml = 45 IU [9 mcg] or Rh + red cells/ml cells = 90 IU [18 mcg]). IM 6,000 IU (1,200 mcg) every 12 hours until the total dose is administered (administered Rh + blood/ml blood = 60 IU [12 mcg] or Rh + red cells/ml cells = 120 IU [24 mcg]).

Immune thrombocytopenia Purpura (ITP)
ADULTS and CHILDREN: IV only [Rh_0(D) IGIV (WinRho SD) must be used IV for the treatment of ITP]. Initial dose 250 IU (50 mcg) per kg, given as a single dose or in two divided doses on separate days. If patient has a hemoglobin level <10 g/dl, give reduced dose of 125 to 200 IU (25 to 40 mcg) per kg. If subsequent therapy is needed to elevate platelet counts, an IV dose of 125 to 300 IU (25 to 60 mcg) per kg is recommended. Frequency and dose of maintenance therapy is determined by patient's clinical response.

Interactions Antibodies in RhIG/RhIGV may interfere with response to live vaccines. Do not give live vaccines within 14-30 days before or 3 mo after RhIG/RhIGV administration. Nonetheless, RhIG/RhIGV does not usually impair response to rubella vaccine. Rubella-susceptible postpartum women who received blood products or RhIG/RhIGV may receive rubella vaccine prior to discharge, provided that rubella antibody titer is drawn 6-8 wk after vaccination to assure seroconversion.

Lab Test Interferences
Infants born of women given RhIG/RhIGV antepartum may have weakly positive antiglobulin (Coombs') test result at birth. Anti-Rh antibodies may be detected in maternal serum within several weeks of administration of RhIG/RhIGV. Such finding does not preclude further RhIG/RhIGV doses. Presence of RhIG/RhIGV antibodies in maternal blood sample can affect interpretation of tests to identify patient as candidate for RhIG/RhIGV. In case of doubt as to patient's Rh group or immune status, give RhIG/RhIGV. Significant fetomaternal hemorrhage late in pregnancy or following delivery may cause weak, mixed field positive D^u test result. If there is any doubt about mother's Rh type, give RhIG/RhIGV. Screening test for fetal RBCs may help in such cases.

Adverse Reactions As with most IgG products, adverse reactions are infrequent, usually mild in nature and generally confined to site of injection. Occasional patient may react more strongly with localized tenderness, erythema or low-grade fever. Fever, splenomegaly, myalgia, lethargy and elevated bilirubin levels occurred in some individuals receiving multiple doses of RhIG/RhIGV following mismatched transfusions. This latter reaction may be due to relatively rapid rate of foreign red cell destruction, not to RhIG/RhIGV. Hypersensitivity and systemic reactions and induced sensitization with repeated injections occur rarely. *ITP:* Adverse effects related to the destruction of Rh_0(D) antigen-positive red cells, such as decreased hemoglobin. Additional adverse reactions associated with use of RhIGIV include: headache; chills; fever.

Precautions
Pregnancy: Category C. *Lactation:* Undetermined. *Children:* For suppression of Rh isoimmunization in the mother. Do not administer to infants. *IM administration:* As with other drugs administered by IM injection, give RhIG/RhIGV with caution to persons on anticoagulant therapy.

NURSING CONSIDERATIONS

Administration/Storage

- Administer IM only.
- If desirable, divide total dose and give at different injection sites or inject at intervals.
- Give total dosage within 72 hours.
- Store in refrigerator.
- Confirm mother is $Rh_0(D)$ negative prior to administration.
- Obtain blood type and direct antiglobulin test on infant immediately post partum prior to administration.

Assessment/Interventions

- Obtain patient history, including drug history and any known allergies.
- Observe injection site for tenderness or erythema.
- Administer with caution if patient receiving anticoagulants.
- Notify physician if fever, splenomegaly, myalgia or lethargy develops.
- Assess bilirubin levels prior to and following treatment.

Patient/Family Education

- Tell patient to report fever, myalgia, lethargy, abdominal pain or jaundice to physician.
- Instruct patient not to receive any live vaccines within 30 days before or 3 mo after administration of drug.
- Explain how future Rh_0-positive infants will be protected.

No patient monograph available.

Ribavirin

(rye-buh-VIE-rin)

Virazole

Class: Anti-infective/antiviral

Action Has antiviral inhibitory activity against respiratory syncytial virus (RSV), influenza virus and herpes simplex virus. Exact mechanism is unknown.

Indications Treatment of carefully selected hospitalized infants and young children with severe lower respiratory tract infections due to RSV. **Unlabeled uses:** Treatment of influenza A and B infection and of other viral diseases including acute and chronic hepatitis, herpes genitalis, measles and Lassa fever.

Contraindications Infants requiring assisted ventilation because drug may precipitate in the equipment, interfering with safe and effective ventilation; females who are or may become pregnant.

Route/Dosage

RSV

INFANTS & CHILDREN: **Inhalation** 6 gm reconstituted with 300 ml Sterile Water aerosolized and administered over 12-18 hr/day for 3-7 days.

Interactions None well documented.

Lab Test Interferences None well documented.

Adverse Reactions

CV: Cardiac arrest; hypotension; digitalis toxicity. *RESP:* Worsening of respiratory status; bacterial pneumonia; pneumothorax; apnea; ventilator dependence. *EENT:* Conjunctivitis. *HEMA:* Anemia (IV or orally); reticulocytosis. *DERM:* Rash.

Precautions

Pregnancy: Category X. *Lactation:* Unknown.

NURSING CONSIDERATIONS

Administration/Storage

- Administer by aerosol using only Small Particle Aerosol Generator (SPAG-2) aerosol generator. Refer to manufacturer instructions for use of device.

- Reconstitute with 100 ml of preservative-free Sterile Water for Injection, then transfer solution to reservoir.
- Dilute to final volume of 300 ml with Sterile Water for Injection. Concentration should be 20 mg/ml.
- Do not administer with other aerosol medications.
- Discard solutions placed in SPAG-2 unit at least every 24 hr and when liquid level is low before adding newly reconstituted solution.
- Store reconstituted solution at room temperature and discard after 24 hr.
- Store powder form of drug at room temperature.
- Minimize environmental exposure to ribavirin by use of an aerosol delivery hood or other shielding techniques. Do not allow pregnant women near the patient when the aerosol is being delivered.

Assessment/Interventions

- Obtain patient history, including drug history and any known allergies.
- Obtain baseline reticulocyte count and monitor daily.
- Monitor I&O.
- Obtain baseline vital signs and monitor at regular intervals during administration.
- Assess respiratory status prior to starting drug and monitor closely during treatment.
- If respiratory status deteriorates rapidly, discontinue treatment and notify physician.
- Obtain baseline digoxin levels on patients who are concomitantly receiving digoxin and monitor for digoxin toxicity.
- Assess skin prior to starting drug and observe for changes.

Patient/Family Education

- Caution patient that this medication must not be taken during pregnancy or when pregnancy is possible.
- Tell family to notify physician if change in respiratory status or rash occurs.

No patient monograph available.

Riboflavin (Vitamin B_2)

(RYE-boh-FLAY-vin)

Available as generic only

Class: Vitamin

Action Is converted in body to coenzyme necessary in oxidation-reduction. Also necessary in maintaining integrity of RBCs.

Indications Prevention and treatment of riboflavin deficiency.

Contraindications Standard considerations.

Route/Dosage

Supplement

ADULTS: **PO** 1.4-1.8 mg (men), 1.2-1.3 mg (women), 1.6-1.8 mg (pregnant or lactating women). CHILDREN: **PO** 0.8-1.2 mg/day.

Treatment of Deficiency

ADULTS: **PO** 5-100 mg/day. CHILDREN: **PO** 2-10 mg/day.

Interactions None well documented.

Lab Test Interferences

Large doses produce bright-yellow urine, which may contain fluorescent substances and interfere with urinalysis based on spectrometry or color reactions.

Adverse Reactions

GU: Yellow-orange discoloration of urine.

Precautions

Deficiency: Riboflavin deficiency rarely occurs alone; often associated with deficiency of other B vitamins and protein.

NURSING CONSIDERATIONS

Administration/Storage

- May be given IM or IV as component of multivitamin.
- Administer with food for optimal absorption.
- Store in cool place in light-resistant container.

Assessment/Interventions

- Obtain patient history, including drug history and any known allergies.
- Assess for deficiency of other B vitamins and protein.
- Evaluate diet history.
- Perform nutritional assessment if indicated.

Patient/Family Education

- Instruct patient to take medication with meals to increase drug absorption.
- Inform patient that urine may turn yellow-orange color.
- Advise patient to take only recommended dose.
- Teach patient about nutritious diet and refer to dietitian if necessary.
- Review diet of foods high in riboflavin (B_2): eggs, organ meats, whole-grain cereals and breads, green vegetables, mushrooms, avocadoes, kidney beans, cashews, chestnuts, cheeses.

See Patient Guide, p. 543.

Rifabutin

(RIFF-uh-BYOO-tin)

Mycobutin

Class: Anti-infective/antitubercular

Action Inhibits DNA-dependent RNA polymerase in susceptible strains of bacteria.

Indications Prevention of disseminated *Mycobacterium avium* complex (MAC) disease in patients with advanced HIV infection.

Contraindications Hypersensitivity to rifabutin or other rifamycins; active tuberculosis.

Route/Dosage

ADULTS: PO 300 mg once daily. INFANTS & CHILDREN: PO Up to 5 mg/kg/day.

Interactions

Oral anticoagulants, benzodiazepines, beta-blockers, chloramphenicol, oral contraceptives, corticosteroids, cyclosporine, digitoxin, disopyramide, estrogens, hydantoins, methadone, mexiletine, quinidine, sulfonylureas, theophyllines, tocainide, verapamil: Therapeutic efficacy may be decreased due to live enzyme-inducing properties of rifabutin. *Zidovudine:* May decrease plasma levels of zidovudine.

Lab Test Interferences

None well documented.

Adverse Reactions

CV: Chest pain. *CNS:* Asthenia; headache; insomnia. *EENT:* Taste perversion. *GI:* Anorexia; diarrhea; dyspepsia; abdominal pain; eructation; flatulence; nausea; vomiting. *GU:* Discolored urine. *HEMA:* Anemia; eosinophilia, leukopenia, neutropenia, thrombocytopenia. *DERM:* Rash. *META:* Increased alkaline phosphatase, AST and ALT. *OTHER:* Myalgia; fever; discolored saliva, sputum, tears, skin.

Precautions

Pregnancy: Category B. *Lactation:* Unknown. Discontinue nursing or discontinue drug. *Children:* Safety and efficacy not established. Based on the limited data available, there is no evidence that doses greater than 5 mg/kg daily are useful.

NURSING CONSIDERATIONS

Administration/Storage

- Administer on empty stomach. If nausea and vomiting develop, may give in divided doses mixed with food such as applesauce.
- Store at room temperature, in tightly closed container.

Assessment/Interventions

- Obtain patient history, including drug history and any known allergies.
- Obtain baseline CBC and monitor at regular intervals during drug therapy. Report decreased neutrophil count.
- Inform physician if signs or symptoms of MAC or tuberculosis develops.
- Obtain baseline liver function test results and monitor during treatment.

Patient/Family Education

- Inform patient that body fluids (urine, feces, saliva, sputum, perspiration, tears) may be brown-orange in color and that soft contact lenses may be permanently stained. Suggest use of glasses during drug therapy.
- Instruct patient to use nonhormonal methods of birth control while taking drug.
- Instruct patient to notify physician of rash, nausea, vomiting, anorexia, diarrhea, abdominal pain, change in color or consistency of stools, jaundice, arthralgias, myositis, chest pressure or pain with shortness of breath, seizure activity, parathesia, aphasia, confusion, insomnia, excessive fatigue, fever or infection.
- Instruct patient to report photophobia, excessive tearing, or eye pain immediately.

See Patient Guide, p. 544.

Rifampin

(RIFF-am-pin)

Rifadin, Rimactane, ♣ *Rofact*

Class: Anti-infective/antitubercular

Action Inhibits DNA-dependent RNA polymerase in susceptible strains of bacteria.

Indications Adjunctive treatment of tuberculosis; short-term management to eliminate meningococci from nasopharynx in *Neisseria meningitidis* carriers. **Unlabeled uses:** Treatment of infections caused by *Staphylococcus aureus* and *Staphylococcus epidermidis;* treatment of gram-negative bacteremia in infancy; treatment of Legionella; management of leprosy; prophylaxis of *Haemophilus influenzae* meningitis.

Contraindications Hypersensitivity to any rifamycin.

Route/Dosage

Tuberculosis

ADULTS: **PO/IV** 600 mg once daily. CHILDREN: **PO/IV** 10-20 mg/kg/day (maximum 600 mg/day).

Meningococcal Carriers

ADULTS: **PO/IV** 600 mg once daily for 4 consecutive days. CHILDREN ≥ 1 MO OF AGE: **PO/IV** 10 mg/kg q 12 hr for 2 consecutive days. CHILDREN < 1 MO OF AGE: 5 mg/kg q 12 hr for 2 consecutive days.

Interactions

Oral anticoagulants, benzodiazepines, beta-blockers, chloramphenicol, oral contraceptives, corticosteroids, cyclosporine, digitoxin, disopyramide, estrogens, hydantoins, methadone, mexiletine, quinidine, sulfonylureas, theophyllines, tocainide, verapamil: Therapeutic efficacy may be decreased due to live enzyme–inducing properties of rifampin. *Digoxin:* May decrease digoxin serum concentrations. *Enalapril:* May significantly increase BP. *Halothane:* Hepatotoxicity and hepatic encephalopathy have been reported with concomitant administration. *Isoniazid:* May result in higher rate of hepatotoxicity. *Ketoconazole:* May cause treatment failure of either ketoconazole or rifampin. *Probenicid.* Elevates rifampin levels.

Lab Test Interferences

May inhibit standard microbiological assays for serum folate and vitamin B_{12}. Thus, use alternate assay methods. Transient abnormalities in liver function tests (elevation in serum bilirubin, abnormal bromsulfophthalein excretion, alkaline phosphatase and serum transaminases) and reduced biliary excretion of contrast media used for visualization of gallbladder may occur. Therefore, perform these tests before the morning dose of rifampin.

Adverse Reactions

CV: Hypotension; shock. *RESP:* Shortness of breath; wheezing. *CNS:* Headache; drowsiness; fatigue; dizziness; inability to concentrate; mental confusion; generalized numbness; behavioral changes; myopathy. *EENT:* Visual disturbances; exudative conjunctivitis. *GI:* Heartburn; epigastric distress; anorexia; nausea; vomiting; gas; cramps; diarrhea; sore mouth and tongue; pseudomembranous colitis; pancreatitis. *GU:* Hemoglobinuria; hematuria; renal insufficiency; acute renal failure. *HEMA:* Eosinophilia; transient leukopenia; hemolytic anemia; decreased hemoglobin; hemolysis; thrombocytopenia. *HEPA:* Asymptomatic elevations of liver enzymes and hepatitis. *DERM:* Rash; pruritus; urticaria; pemphigoid reaction; flushing. *OTHER:* Ataxia; muscular weakness; pain in extremities; osteomalacia; myopathy; menstrual disturbances; fever; elevations in BUN; elevated serum uric acid; possible immunosuppression; abnormal growth of lung tumors; reduced 25-hydroxycholecalciferol levels; edema of face and extremities; discoloration of body fluids.

Precautions

Pregnancy: Category C. *Lactation:* Excreted in breast milk. Discontinue nursing or discontinue drug. *Body fluids:* Medication may cause harmless red-orange discoloration of urine, feces, saliva, sputum, sweat and tears. Soft contact lenses may be permanently stained. *Hepatic impairment:* Dosage adjustment is necessary.

NURSING CONSIDERATIONS

Administration/Storage

- Administer oral form 1 hr before or 2 hr after meals.
- Observe IV site closely for extravasation.
- For IV infusion, reconstitute powder in 10 ml of Sterile Water for Injection and swirl gently. Reconstituted solution is stable at room temperature for 24 hr. Withdraw appropriate dose of drug, mix with 500 ml of D5W and infuse over 3 hr. If ordered, drug may be added to 100 ml and infused over 30 min. A less concentrated solution infused over a longer period is preferred.
- If D5W is contraindicated, use sterile saline. Do not mix with other solutions.
- Initial dilutions of drug in vial are stable for 24 hr at room temperature.
- Final dilution (500 or 100 ml volumes) should be used within 24 hr because precipitation may occur after this time period.
- Administer solution for injection by IV route only. Do not administer IM or SC.

Assessment/Interventions

- Obtain patient history, including drug history, history of medication noncompliance, and any known allergies.
- Obtain baseline CBC and liver and renal function test results and monitor at regular intervals.
- Assess skin prior to starting drug and during treatment for rash, pruritus, flushing, urticaria and jaundice.
- Assess baseline neurologic status and observe for changes.

- Monitor I&O and assess for development of edema.

OVERDOSAGE: SIGNS & SYMPTOMS

Nausea, vomiting, increasing lethargy, unconsciousness, liver enlargement, jaundice, increased direct and total bilirubin levels, altered hepatic enzyme levels

Patient/Family Education

- Instruct patient to take drug on empty stomach, 1 hr before or 2 hr after meals.
- Inform patient that body fluids may turn red-orange in color and that soft contact lenses may become permanently stained. Advise patient to wear glasses during course of therapy.
- Instruct patient to notify physician of persistent anorexia, nausea, vomiting, diarrhea, jaundice, fever, change in color or consistency of stools, malaise or right upper quadrant abdominal pain, unusual bleeding or bruising, petechiae, hematuria, bleeding gums or pallor.
- Tell patient to notify physician of drowsiness, fatigue, dizziness, inability to concentrate, confusion or visual or behavioral changes.
- Advise patient who uses oral contraceptives to use nonhormonal form of contraception during therapy.
- Advise patient that drug may cause drowsiness and to use caution while driving or performing other tasks requiring mental alertness.
- Advise patient of importance of medication compliance in treatment of TB. Medication non-compliance reduces efficacy and promotes resistance.
- Caution patient to avoid alcohol.

See Patient Guide, p. 545.

Riluzole

(RILL-you-zole)

Rilutek

Class: Neuroprotective

Action Unknown; however, the following properties may be related to effects: Inhibits glutamate release; inactivates voltage-dependent sodium channels; interferes with intracellular events following transmitter binding at excitatory amino acid receptors. These effects may protect neural tissues against degenerative changes.

Indications Treatment of patients with amyotrophic lateral sclerosis (ALS; Lou Gehrig's disease).

Contraindications Standard considerations.

Route/Dosage

ADULTS: PO 50 mg q 12 hr.

Interactions

Caffeine, theophylline, amitriptyline, quinolones: May reduce riluzole elimination. *Cigarette smoke, rifampin, omeprazole:* May enhance riluzole elimination.

Lab Test Interferences

None well documented.

Adverse Reactions

CV: Hypertension; tachycardia; palpitations; peripheral edema. *RESP:* Decreased lung function; cough. *CNS:* Headache; hypertonia; depression; dizziness; insomnia; somnolence; vertigo; circumoral paresthesia; aggravation reaction; agitation; tremor. *EENT:* Rhinitis; sinusitis. *GI:* Nausea; vomiting; dyspepsia; anorexia; diarrhea; constipation; flatulence; abdominal pain; stomatitis; dry mouth; oral moniliasis. *GU:* Urinary tract infection; dysuria. *DERM:* Pruritus; eczema; alopecia; exfoliative dermatitis. *META:* Weight loss. *HEPA:* Abnormal liver function tests. *OTHER:* Asthenia; arthralgia; back pain; malaise.

Precautions

Pregnancy: Category C. *Lactation:* Undetermined. *Children:* Safety and efficacy not established. *Elderly:* Age-related compromised renal and hepatic function may cause a decrease in clearance of riluzole. *Renal impairment:* Use with caution in patients with renal impairment. *Hepatic function impairment:* Use with caution in patients with current evidence or history of abnormal liver function indicated by significant elevations of liver enzymes. Baseline elevations of several LFTs (especially elevated bilirubin) should preclude use of riluzole. *Monitoring:* Measure serum aminotransferases before and during therapy. Evaluate serum SGPT levels every month during the first 3 months of treatment, every 3 months during the remainder of the first year and periodically thereafter. *Special populations:* Females and Japanese patients may possess a lower metabolic capacity to eliminate riluzole as compared to males and Caucasian subjects respectively.

NURSING CONSIDERATIONS

Administration/Storage

- Medication is most effective on an empty stomach. Take at least 1 hour before or 2 hours after a meal for best effect.
- Store at room temperature; protect from bright light.

Assessment/Interventions

- Obtain patient history.
- Obtain baseline laboratory tests, including BUN, SGPT, Hgb and Hct. Perform and evaluate these tests periodically during treatment, (eg, SGPT levels monthly for 3 months, every 3 months during the remainder of the year and periodically thereafter).
- Monitor for effectiveness and reduction in symptom progression of the disease.
- Assess patient for development of asthenia, nausea, dizziness, diarrhea, decreased level of consciousness and respiratory distress.

OVERDOSAGE: SIGNS & SYMPTOMS

None reported

Patient/Family Education

- Instruct patient to take medication 30 minutes before or 2 hours after a meal.
- Take with a full glass of water.
- Instruct patient to take medicine at same time each day. If a dose is missed, take the next dose as originally planned.
- Instruct patient not to change dose or discontinue medication without consulting healthcare provider. Larger than prescribed doses do not increase effectiveness, but do increase the side effects.
- Instruct patient to check with healthcare provider before taking any over-the-counter or prescription medications, and vaccinations.
- Have patient report any serious side effects to healthcare provider, including: asthenia, nausea, dizziness, diarrhea, decreased level of consciousness and respiratory distress.
- Inform patient of need for frequent laboratory tests while taking medication. Be sure to keep appointments.
- Instruct patient to report any fevers to healthcare provider.
- Instruct patient to avoid drinking alcohol in excess while taking this medication.
- Advise patient that drug may cause dizziness, vertigo or somnolence and not to drive or operate machinery until patient has gained enough experience to gauge whether or not it affects their mental or motor performance adversely.

See Patient Guide, p. 546.

Rimantadine HCl

(rih-MAN-tuh-deen HIGH-droe-KLOR-ide)

Flumadine

Class: Anti-infective/antiviral

Action Inhibits viral replication cycle in various strains of influenza A virus.

Indications
Adults: Prophylaxis and treatment of infection caused by various strains of influenza A virus. *Children:* Prophylaxis against influenza A virus.

Contraindications Hypersensitivity to drugs of adamantine class including rimantadine and amantadine.

Route/Dosage
Prophylaxis and Treatment
ADULTS: PO 100 mg bid. ELDERLY NURSING HOME PATIENTS, HEPATIC AND RENAL IMPAIRMENT (CREATININE CLEARANCE < 10 ML/MIN): Reduce to 100 mg daily.

Prophylaxis
CHILDREN ≥ 10 YR: PO 100 mg bid. CHILDREN 1-10 YR: PO 5 mg/kg daily (maximum 150 mg/dose).

Interactions
Acetaminophen, aspirin: Decreased peak serum concentration of rimantadine. *Cimetidine:* Increased serum concentration due to decreased clearance.

Lab Test Interferences
None well documented.

Adverse Reactions
CNS: Insomnia; dizziness; headache; nervousness; asthenia; impaired concentration. *EENT:* Eye pain. *GI:* Nausea; vomiting; anorexia; dry mouth; abdominal pain.

Precautions
Pregnancy: Category C. *Lactation:* Undetermined. Should not be administered to nursing mothers. *Elderly patients:* CNS symptoms may occur more frequently. *Seizures:* Increased incidence of seizures in patients with seizure history and who receive amantadine.

NURSING CONSIDERATIONS

Administration/Storage
- Administer orally only.
- Store at room temperature.

Assessment/Interventions
- Obtain patient history, including drug history and any known allergies.
- Assess baseline renal and liver function test results.
- Notify physician if patient has seizure activity, severe or persistent diarrhea, dizziness, impaired concentration, asthenia or dyspnea.

> **OVERDOSAGE: SIGNS & SYMPTOMS**
> Agitation, cardiac arrhythmias

Patient/Family Education
- Tell patient with history of seizures to discontinue drug and notify physician if seizure activity develops.
- Tell patient to report insomnia, dizziness, headache, nervousness, asthenia, impaired concentration, nausea, vomiting, anorexia, persistent diarrhea, dry mouth, abdominal pain, dyspnea, cough, palpitations or syncope.
- Caution patient to avoid driving or operating hazardous equipment if dizziness or confusion develops.
- Advise patient to take drug several hours before going to bed if insomnia develops.

See Patient Guide, p. 547.

Risperidone

(RISS-PURR-ih-dohn)
Risperdal
Class: Antipsychotic/benzisoxazole

Action Has antipsychotic effect, apparently due to dopamine and serotonin receptor blocking in CNS.

Indications Management of psychotic disorders.

Contraindications Standard considerations.

Route/Dosage
ADULTS: **PO** 1 mg bid on first day, 2 mg bid on second day and 3 mg bid on third day. Dosage adjustment thereafter should occur at intervals of at least 1 wk in increments of 1 mg bid. Range is 4-16 mg/day.

Renal or Hepatic Impairment
ELDERLY PATIENTS: **PO** 0.5 mg bid initially; increase in 0.5 mg increments bid thereafter.

Interactions
Alcohol, CNS depressants: May cause additive CNS depressant effects. *Antihypertensives:* Risperidone may enhance hypotensive effects of some antihypertensives. *Carbamazepine:* May increase clearance of risperidone. *Clozapine:* May decrease clearance of risperidone. *Levodopa:* The effects of levodopa may be antagonized.

Lab Test Interferences
None well documented.

Adverse Reactions
CV: Orthostatic hypotension; tachycardia; palpitations; hypertension; cardiac arrhythmias; syncope; angina pectoris; lightheadedness; ECG changes. *RESP:* Coughing; upper respiratory infection; shortness of breath. *CNS:* Tardive dyskinesia; extrapyramidal symptoms such as pseudoparkinsonism, akathesia, and dystonias; drowsiness; increased sleep duration; headache; insomnia; agitation; anxiety; aggressive reaction; dizziness; seizure. *EENT:* Abnormal vision; abnormal accommodation; tinnitus; rhinitis; sinusitis; pharyngitis. *GI:* Constipation; nausea; dyspepsia; vomiting; abdominal pain; increased salivation; toothache; anorexia; reduced salivation. *GU:* Menorrhagia; orgasmic dysfunction; dry vagina; erectile dysfunction. *HEMA:* Epistaxis; purpura; anemia. *HEPA:* Hepatic failure; hepatitis. *DERM:* Rash; dry skin; seborrhea; photosensitivity. *META:* Increased AST and ALT. *OTHER:* Arthralgia; back pain; chest pain; fever; polyuria or polydipsia; increased weight; elevated prolactin levels.

Precautions
Pregnancy: Category C. *Lactation:* Undetermined. Therefore, should not breastfeed. *Children:* Safety and efficacy not established. *Elderly and debilitated patients:* May have reduced ability to eliminate risperidone. At increased risk of tardive dyskinesia, especially elderly women. *Cardiac effects:* Appears to have proarrhythmic effects. Orthostatic hypotension may also occur. *Change in drug therapy:* When patient is switched from another antipsychotic to risperidone, it is recommended that the other antipsychotic be discontinued before starting risperidone therapy or to minimize period of overlap. *Hepatic/renal impairment:* Patients with hepatic/renal impairment may experience enhanced effect of risperidone because of reduced ability to eliminate risperidone. Dose adjustment may be required. *Long-term use (> 8 wk):* Long-term use not well evaluated. Periodically reevaluate usefulness. *Neuroleptic malignant syndrome (NMS):* Has occurred with antipsychotics; is potentially fatal. Signs and symptoms are hyperpyrexia, muscle rigidity, altered mental status, irregular pulse, irregular BP, tachycardia and diaphoresis. *Tardive dyskinesia:* A potentially irreversible syndrome of involuntary body and facial movements may occur. *Renal*

or hepatic impairment: May need dose adjustment.

NURSING CONSIDERATIONS

Administration/Storage

- May be given without regard to meals.
- Administer with full glass of water.
- Dosage will be adjusted daily for first 3 days and then at weekly intervals as indicated.
- Store at room temperature, protected from light and moisture.

Assessment/Interventions

- Obtain patient history, including drug history and any known allergies.
- Obtain baseline renal and liver function test results.
- Obtain baseline BP and monitor postural BP at regular intervals, especially after dosages changes.
- Inform physician immediately if hyperpyrexia, muscle rigidity, altered mental status, irregular pulse and BP, tachycardia and diaphoresis develop.
- Assess baseline neurologic status and observe during treatment for involuntary body and facial movements, drowsiness, headache, insomnia, agitation, anxiety, aggressive reaction, dizziness or seizure activity.
- Monitor cardiac patients during initiation of drug for prolongation of QT interval; notify physician if this occurs.
- Notify physician if any of the following develops: tachycardia, chest pain, arrhythmias, hypertension, nausea, vomiting, abdominal pain, upper respiratory infection, cough, shortness of breath, epistaxis, purpura, rash, visual disturbances, arthralgias or fever.
- Monitor patient for suicidal tendencies often associated with schizophrenia. Assess medication compliance.

OVERDOSAGE: SIGNS & SYMPTOMS

Drowsiness, tachycardia, hypotension, extrapyramidal symptoms, hyponatremia, hypokalemia, prolonged QT and widened QRS intervals, seizures

Patient/Family Education

- Tell patient to immediately report hyperpyrexia, muscle rigidity, altered mental status, irregular pulse, tachycardia and diaphoresis to physician.
- Instruct patient to drink adequate liquids while taking drug.
- Advise patient that drug may cause photosensitivity and to use sunscreen or wear protective clothing until tolerance to the sun/UV light is determined.
- Instruct patient to avoid alcoholic beverages.
- Instruct patient to get up slowly from lying or sitting position and to avoid sudden position changes to prevent postural hypotension. Advise patient to report dizziness with position changes to physician. Caution patient to avoid hot tubs and hot showers and baths.
- Advise patient taking antihypertensives to monitor BP at regular intervals.
- Instruct patient to notify physician of drowsiness, insomnia, increased agitation or anxiety, seizures, excessive fatigue, involuntary body and facial movements, constipation, nausea, vomiting, polyuria, excessive thirst, cough, shortness of breath, upper respiratory infection, angina, palpitations, fever, rash, visual disturbances, sexual problems, vaginal dryness, menorrhagia, epistaxis, purpura, abdominal pain, change in color or consistency of stools or arthralgias.
- Instruct patient to take sips of water

frequently or to suck on ice chips, sugarless hard candy or chewing gum if dry mouth occurs.

- Advise patient that drug may cause drowsiness and to use caution while driving or performing other tasks requiring mental alertness.
- Advise patient about potential weight gain.

See Patient Guide, p. 548.

Ritodrine HCl

(RIH-toe-dreen HIGH-droe-KLOR-ide)

Yutopar, ✱ *Yutopar S.R.*

Class: Uterine relaxant

Action Inhibits contractility of uterine smooth muscle through beta-adrenergic receptor stimulation.

Indications Management of preterm labor in suitable patients.

Contraindications Before 20th week of pregnancy and when continuation of pregnancy is hazardous to mother or fetus; hypersensitivity; pre-existing maternal conditions that would be seriously affected by pharmacologic properties of betamimetic agent.

Route/Dosage

ADULTS: **IV** 0.05 mg/min initially, increasing by 0.05 mg/min q 10 min until desired result is obtained. The usual effective dose is between 0.15-0.35 mg/min, continued for at least 12 hr after uterine contractions cease.

Interactions

Atropine: Systemic hypertension may be exaggerated. *Beta-adrenergic blockers:* Effects are antagonistic; avoid coadministration. *Corticosteroids:* Concomitant use may lead to pulmonary edema. *Magnesium sulfate; diazoxide; meperidine; general anesthetics:* Cardiovascular effects of ritodrine may be potentiated. *Sympathomimetics:* Effects may be additive or potentiated.

Lab Test Interferences

None well documented.

Adverse Reactions

CV: Palpitations; chest pain or tightness; heart murmur; angina pectoris; myocardial ischemia; alterations in BP; pulmonary edema; sinus bradycardia upon drug withdrawal; arrhythmias; drowsiness; weakness; mild tachycardia. *CNS:* Tremor, headache (including migraines); nervousness; jitteriness; restlessness; emotional upset; anxiety; malaise; hyperventilation. *GI:* Nausea; constipation; diarrhea; vomiting; epigastric distress; ileus; bloating. *DERM:* Erythema; rash *HEPA:* Hemolytic icterus; impaired liver function. *META:* Lactic acidosis; glycosuria. *RESP:* Dsypnea. *HEMA:* Leukopenia; agranalocytosis. *OTHER:* Sweating; chills; hypokalemia; hyperglycemia.

Precautions

Pregnancy: Contraindicated before 20th week of pregnancy; otherwise, Category B. *Lactation:* Undetermined. *Cardiovascular responses:* Are common and more pronounced with IV administration. *Maternal pulmonary edema:* Has been reported. Closely monitor and avoid fluid overload. *Mild to moderate preeclampsia, hypertension or diabetes:* Do not use in these patients unless benefits clearly outweigh risks. *Advanced labor:* Safety and efficacy in advanced labor (cervical dilation > 4 cm or effacement > 80%) are not established. *Sulfite sensitivity:* May cause allergic-type reaction in susceptible patients.

NURSING CONSIDERATIONS

Administration/Storage

- 150 mg in 500 ml fluid yields a final concentration of 0.3 mg/ml. When fluid restriction is desirable, may prepare a more concentrated solution. Dilute with 5% Dextrose. Because of increased probability of pulmonary edema, reserve saline diluents for cases where D5W is undesirable.

- Do not use if solution is discolored or contains any precipitate.
- Administer IV infusion with patient in left lateral position to minimize risk of hypotension.
- Use controlled infusion device to deliver medication.
- Use diluted drug within 48 hr. Store at room temperature and avoid excessive heat.
- Store at room temperature, protected from excessive heat.

Assessment/Interventions

- Obtain patient history, including drug history and any known allergies.
- Monitor maternal HR, BP, lung sounds and fetal HR frequently during IV administration.
- Evaluate strength and frequency of contractions at regular intervals.
- Notify physician if patient develops persistent tachycardia or tachypnea or increased systolic BP with widening pulse pressure.
- Discontinue drug, notify physician and obtain ECG if chest pain or tightness develops.
- Assess baseline serum glucose (in patients with diabetes) and electrolytes and monitor at regular intervals with IV administration.
- Assess baseline ECG prior to starting drug.
- Notify physician if palpitations, tremor, nausea, vomiting, headache, erythema, nervousness, restlessness, anxiety or malaise develops.
- Monitor I&O for possible fluid overload.
- Assess neonate for ileus and hypotension.
- Monitor glucose and electrolytes of neonate.

OVERDOSAGE: SIGNS & SYMPTOMS

Symptoms relate to excessive beta-adrenergic stimulation and include tachycardia, palpitations, cardiac arrhythmias, hypotension, dyspnea, nervousness, tremor, nausea, vomiting

Patient/Family Education

- Tell patient to report palpitations, chest pain or tightness, tremor, headache, nervousness, emotional upset, anxiety, malaise, hyperventilation, nausea, vomiting, epigastric distress, bloating, chills or sweating.

See Patient Guide, p. 549.

Ritonavir

(rih-TON-a-veer)

Norvir

Class: Antiviral

Action Inhibits human immunodeficiency virus (HIV) protease, the enzyme required to form functional proteins in HIV-infected cells.

Indications Treatment of HIV infection. May be given in combination with nucleoside analogues (eg, zidovudine) or as monotherapy.

Contraindications Concomitant therapy with amiodarone, astemizole, bepridil, bupropion, cisapride, clozapine, encainide, flecainide, meperidine, piroxicam, propafenone, propoxyphene, quinidine, rifabutin and terfenadine. Concurrent administration of alprazolam, clorazepate, diazepam, estazolam, flurazepam, midazolam, triazolam and zolpidem.

Route/Dosage ADULTS & CHILDREN ≥ 12 YR: **PO** 600 mg bid. If nausea occurs, relief may be provided by dose titration: 300 mg bid for 1 day, 400 mg bid for 2 days, 500 mg bid for 1 day, then 600 mg bid.

Interactions *Amiodarone, astemizole, bepridil, bupropion, cisapride, clozapine, encainide, flecainide, meperidine, piroxicam, propafenone, propoxyphene, quinidine, rifabutin,* *terfenadine*: Ritonavir may elevate blood levels of these drugs, which may increase the risk of arrhythmias, hematologic abnormalities, seizures or other potential serious adverse effects. *Alprazolam, clorazepate, diazepam, estazolam, flurazepam, midazolam, triazolam, zolpidem*: Ritonavir may increase blood levels of these drugs, which may produce extreme sedation and respiratory depression. Do not co-administer. *Carbamazepine, dexamethasone, phenobarbital, phenytoin, rifabutin, rifampin*: May decrease plasma concentrations of ritonavir. *Desipramine*: Desipramine levels may be increased. *Disulfiram, metronidazole*: Ritonavir contains alcohol and may produce a disulfiram-like reaction with these drugs. *Oral contraceptives*: Concentrations of ethinyl estradiol, a component of oral contraceptives, may be reduced. *Saquinavir*: Ritonavir may inhibit saquinavir metabolism and increase saquinavir levels. *Theophylline*: Theophylline levels may be decreased. *Warfarin*: The risk of bleeding may be increased.

Lab Test Interferences

None well documented.

Adverse Reactions

CV: Vasodilation; hemorrhage; hypotension; palpitations, postural hypotension; tachycardia. *CNS*: Headache; malaise; circumoral paresthesia; paresthesia; dizziness; insomnia; somnolence; abnormal thinking. *EENT*: Pharyngitis; sore throat; abnormal taste. *GI*: Anorexia; constipation; diarrhea; dyspepsia; flatulence; nausea; vomiting; abdominal pain. *GU*: Impotence; dysuria; kidney failure. *HEPA*: Hepatitis; hepatomegaly; abnormal liver function tests. *DERM*: Rash; swelling. *META*: Increased creatinine phosphokinase; hyperlipidemia; diabetes mellitus. *OTHER*: Asthenia; fever; myalgia.

Precautions

Pregnancy: Category B. *Lactation*: Undetermined. HIV-infected mothers should not breastfeed their infants. *Children*: Not recommended for children < 12 yr. *Hepatic function impairment*: Use caution; decreased ritonavir clearance may occur.

NURSING CONSIDERATIONS

Administration/Storage

- The medication should be taken with food.
- The oral solution may be mixed with chocolate milk, Ensure or Advera within 1 hour of dosing to improve the taste.
- Store capsules in the refrigerator in a light-resistant container.
- Oral solution should be stored in refrigerator until opened. It may be stored at room temperature after opening, if used within 30 days. Keep in original container with cap tightly closed.
- Do not switch between oral solution and capsules as the absorption rates are different.

Assessment/Interventions

- Obtain patient history.
- Assess for history of impaired hepatic function. This medication is metabolized in, and toxic to, the liver.
- Obtain baseline triglycerides, SGOT, SGPT, GGT, CPK and uric acid. Monitor periodically during treatment.
- Monitor WBC and differential. Note any significant changes.
- Monitor Hct and Hgb frequently (severe anemia may require blood transfusions).

OVERDOSAGE: SIGNS & SYMPTOMS

Paresthesia

Patient/Family Education

- Advise patient to take medication exactly as prescribed.
- Warn patient not to alter the dose or discontinue the medication without consulting the healthcare provider.
- If patient misses a dose, the next dose

should be taken as soon as possible. If a dose is skipped, the patient should NOT double the next dose.

- Instruct patient not to take any other medications, including over-the-counter medications, without checking with their healthcare provider first. This medication interacts with a wide range of all types of medications.
- Explain that the patient will be required to have frequent follow-up blood and urine tests during the course of the treatment and to keep appointments.
- Inform patient that this medication is NOT a cure for HIV infection and they may continue to acquire secondary illnesses associated with the disease.
- Emphasize to patient, family and significant others that this medication does NOT reduce the risk of transmitting HIV to others through sexual contact or blood contamination.
- Inform patient to report symptoms associated with paresthesia (sensations of burning, prickling, formication, etc) to the healthcare provider for a possible reduction in dosage.
- Inform patient to report any other serious side effects to the healthcare provider.
- Explain that the long-term effects of this medication are not known at this time.

See Patient Guide, p. 550.

Salicylate Combination (Choline magnesium trisalicylate)

(suh-LIS-ih-late)

Trisilate

Class: Analgesic/salicylate combination

Action Relieves pain by inhibiting prostaglandin synthesis and release; reduces fever by vasodilation of peripheral vessels. Unlike aspirin, does not inhibit platelet aggregation.

Indications Relief of mild to moderate pain; treatment of rheumatic fever and rheumatoid arthritis including juvenile arthritis and osteoarthritis; management of fever.

Contraindications Hypersensitivity to nonacetylated salicylates, NSAIDs or aspirin; advanced chronic renal insufficiency; bleeding disorders; GI bleeding.

Route/Dosage

Inflammatory Conditions

ADULTS: **PO** 1500 mg bid *or* 3000 mg qd. ELDERLY PATIENTS: **PO** 750 mg tid.

Fever, Mild to Moderate Pain

ADULTS: **PO** 1000-1500 mg bid. CHILDREN < 37 KG: **PO** 50 mg/kg/day in 2 divided doses. CHILDREN > 37 KG: **PO** 2250 mg/day in 2 divided doses. Doses are adjusted based on patient's response, tolerance and serum salicylate concentration.

Interactions

Carbonic anhydrase inhibitors (eg, acetazolamide): Accumulation of carbonic anhydrase inhibitor and toxicity. *Corticosteroids*: Decreased plasma salicylate concentration. *Methotrexate*: Could cause methotrexate toxicity. *Oral hypoglycemics or insulin*: Could cause hypoglycemia. *Urinary acidifiers*: Increased salicylate serum concentration. *Urinary alkalinizers (eg, chronic antacids)*: Decreased salicylate serum concentration. *Warfarin*: Enhanced anticoagulant activity of oral anticoagulants. Creates potential for increased prothrombin time due to protein-binding displacement.

Lab Test Interferences

Phenolsulfonphthalein: Salicylates decrease renal excretion. *Thyroid function tests*: Drug causes increased free T_4 and decreased total T_4; thyroid function is not affected. *Urine glucose*: Drug causes false-negative results by glucose oxidase method and false-positive results by copper reduction method with moderate to high doses of salicylates. *Urine 5-HIAA:* Salicylates interfere with fluorescent method. *Urine ketones:* Drug causes interference with ferric chloride (Gerhardt) method by turning urine a reddish color. *Urine vanillylmandelic acid:* Salicylates can interfere with determination.

Adverse Reactions

RESP: Bronchospasm. *EENT:* Tinnitus. *GI:* Nausea; dyspepsia; gastric ulceration. *HEMA:* Prolonged bleeding time. *HEPA:* Hepatotoxicity. *DERM:* Hives; rash; angioedema. *META:* Uric acid levels elevated by salicylate concentrations < 10 mg/dl and decreased by levels > 10 mg/dl. *OTHER:* Anaphylaxis; salicylism may occur with large doses or chronic therapy (symptoms include dizziness, tinnitus, vomiting, diarrhea, confusion, CNS depression, headache, sweating, hyperventilation and lassitude); fever.

Precautions

Pregnancy: Category C. Do not use during third trimester; could prematurely close ductus arteriosus in the fetus. *Lactation:* Excreted in breast milk. *Children:* May increase risk of Reye's syndrome; do not use in individuals < 18 yr if chickenpox or flu symptoms are suspected. *Special risk patients:* Use drug with caution in patients with renal or hepatic dysfunction, peptic ulcer disease or gastritis. *Aspirin or NSAID hypersensitivity:* Nonacetylated salicylates have been tolerated in aspirin-sensitive asthmatic patients; however, cases of cross-sensitivity including bronchospasm have been reported.

NURSING CONSIDERATIONS

Administration/Storage

- May cause GI upset; take with food or after meals. Take with a full glass of water.
- Store in tight, light-resistant container.

Assessment/Interventions

- Obtain patient history, including drug history and any known allergies.
- Assess quality of pain (location, onset, type and duration) or temperature prior to therapy.
- Monitor pain relief and temperature after medication administration.
- Inspect affect joints. Assess mobility, swelling/deformities and skin condition.
- Monitor improvement during therapy (fever reduction, relief from joint tenderness and pain; increased movement).
- Assess areas of bruising prior to and during therapy. Report increased bruising immediately to physician.
- If tinnitus, flushing, tachycardia, hyperventilation, sweating or thirst occurs, withhold medication and immediately notify physician.
- Obtain baseline hepatic and renal studies and CBC, PT and PTT. Monitor periodically if patient is undergoing long-term therapy.
- Monitor salicylate serum levels as ordered by physician.

OVERDOSAGE: SIGNS & SYMPTOMS

Respiratory alkalosis, hyperpnea, tachypnea, nausea, vomiting, hypokalemia, tinnitus, neurologic abnormalities (disorientation, irritability, lethargy, stupor), dehydration, hyperthermia, seizures, coma

Patient/Family Education

- Advise patient to take medication with food or after meals with full glass of water.
- Emphasize need to avoid alcohol ingestion and use of NSAIDs during therapy (which increase risk of GI irritation/GI bleeding), especially if patient is undergoing long-term therapy.
- Instruct patients with diabetes to

monitor blood levels closely during treatment.

- Instruct patient to call physician immediately if ringing in ears or persistent GI pain occurs while taking this medication.

See Patient Guide, p. 551.

Salmeterol Xinafoate

(sal-MEET-ah-rahl zin-AF-oh-ate)

Serevent

Class: Bronchodilator/sympathomimetic

Action Produces bronchodilation by relaxing bronchial smooth muscle through beta-2 receptor stimulation.

Indications Maintenance treatment of asthma and prevention of bronchospasm in patients with reversible obstructive airway disease; prevention of exercise-induced bronchospasm.

Contraindications Cardiac tachyarrhythmias.

Route/Dosage

Asthma/Bronchospasm

ADULTS & CHILDREN ≥ 12 YR: **Inhalation** 2 inhalations twice daily, approximately 12 hours apart.

Exercise-induced bronchospasm

ADULTS & CHILDREN ≥ 12 YR: **Inhalation** 2 inhalations at least 30 to 60 minutes before exercise; additional doses should not be used for up to 12 hours.

Interactions

MAO inhibitors, tricyclic antidepressants: May increase cardiovascular effects of salmeterol.

Lab Test Interferences

None well documented.

Adverse Reactions

CV: Tachycardia; palpitations. *RESP:* Cough; paradoxical bronchospasm. *CNS:* Tremor; anxiety; malaise; fatigue; dizziness; vertigo; nervousness; headache. *EENT:* Rhinitis; throat dryness/irritation. *GI:* GI distress; nausea; vomiting; diarrhea. *META:* Hyponatremia.

Precautions

Pregnancy: Category C. *Children:* Not recommended for children < 12 yr. *Acute asthma seizures:* Do not use to treat acute symptoms. *Cardiovascular disease:* Use with caution in patients with cardiovascular disease, toxic symptoms may occur. *Excessive use:* Paradoxical bronchospasm and cardiac arrest have been associated with excessive inhalant use. *Hypokalemia:* Decreases in potassium levels may occur.

NURSING CONSIDERATIONS

Administration/Storage

- This medication is available only in a pressurized, metered-dose inhalation aerosol unit.
- Use only with supplied aerosol actuator. Do not use the actuator with other medications.
- Store at room temperature. The therapeutic effects are reduced when cold; the container may explode if exposed to temperatures above 120° F. Protect from freezing and direct sunlight.
- Store canister with nozzle end down.
- Do not puncture or incinerate canister.
- Shake well before using.

Assessment/Interventions

- Obtain patient history.
- Closely monitor patients with a history of arrhythmias, seizures or peptic ulcers.
- Obtain baseline pulmonary function tests.
- Note frequency and severity of asthma attacks.

OVERDOSAGE: SIGNS & SYMPTOMS

Tremor, palpitations, tachycardia, headache, hypokalemia, hyperglycemia, cardiac arrest

Patient/Family Education

- Instruct patient on the proper storage and use of the aerosol inhaler, referring patient to the instruction sheet included with the medication.
- Advise patient not to exceed the recommended dosage and frequency of the medication.
- Warn patient not to alter the dose or discontinue the medication without consulting the healthcare provider.
- Instruct patient to check with his/her physician first before taking any over-the-counter or prescription medications.
- Emphasize to patient that this medication is NOT to be used for the treatment of acute or deteriorating asthma.
- Inform patient that this medication is NOT a substitute for other medications he/she may be on, including oral or inhaled corticosteroids.
- Instruct patient to call the healthcare provider if the medication seems to be less effective.
- Alert patient that this medication may be used 30 to 60 minutes BEFORE exercise to reduce or prevent exercise-induced bronchospasm.
- Have patient report any serious side effects to the healthcare provider, including: tachycardia, palpitations, tremors, change in personality, insomnia, shortness of breath and stomach cramps.

See Patient Guide, p. 552.

Saquinavir Mesylate

(sack-KWIN-uh-vihr MEH-sih-LATE)

Invirase

Class: Antiviral

Action Inhibits human immunodeficiency virus (HIV) protease, the enzyme required to form functional proteins in HIV-infected cells.

Indications Treatment of advanced HIV infection. Saquinavir is given in combination with nucleoside analogs (eg, zidovudine).

Contraindications Standard considerations.

Route/Dosage

ADULTS & CHILDREN ≥ 16 YR: **PO** Three 200 mg capsules (600 mg) tid within 2 hours after a full meal.

Interactions

Food: Enhance bioavailability of saquinavir. *Rifabutin, rifampin:* May increase metabolism of saquinavir and decrease serum levels. *Terfenadine, astemizole:* Possible elevation of terfenedine/astemizole serum levels with toxicity. Avoid concurrent use.

Lab Test Interferences

None well documented.

Adverse Reactions

CNS: Paresthesia; numbness; confusion; seizures; headache; ataxia. *GI:* Diarrhea; abdominal discomfort; nausea. *DERM:* Rash; photosensitivity. *OTHER:* Ataxia; weakness.

Precautions

Pregnancy: Category B. *Lactation:* Undetermined. HIV infected mothers should not breastfeed their infants. *Children:* Not recommended for children < 16 yr. *Clinical chemistry:* Clinical chemistry tests should be performed prior to and at appropriate intervals during therapy. *Dosage adjustment:* Do not reduce dose; lower doses do not exhibit antiviral activity. *Hepatic function impairment:* Exercise caution when administering to patients with hepatic insufficiency (liver function tests > 5 times upper limit of normal). *Nucleoside analog therapy:* Saquinavir must be used in combination with nucleoside analog (eg, AZT, ddC) therapy. *Photosensitivity:* May occur; take protective measures against exposure to ultraviolet or sunlight until tolerance is determined.

NURSING CONSIDERATIONS

Administration/Storage

- The medication should be taken within 2 hours after a full meal.
- Doses less than 600 mg tid are not effective.
- Capsules should be stored at room temperature in a tightly closed bottle.

Assessment/Interventions

- Obtain patient history.
- Assess for history of impaired hepatic function.
- Obtain baseline triglycerides, SGOT, SGPT, GGT, CPK and uric acid. Monitor periodically during treatment.
- Monitor WBC and differential. Note any significant changes.
- Monitor Hct and Hgb frequently (severe anemia may require blood transfusions).

OVERDOSAGE: SIGNS & SYMPTOMS

No acute toxicities or sequelae have been reported

Patient/Family Education

- Advise patient to take the medication exactly as prescribed.
- Advise patient regarding importance of taking after a meal.
- Warn patient not to alter the dose or discontinue the medication without consulting the healthcare provider.
- Instruct patient not to take any other medications, including over the counter medications, without checking with their healthcare provider first.
- Explain that the patient will be required to have frequent followup blood and urine tests during the course of the treatment and to keep appointments.
- Inform patient that this medication is NOT a cure for HIV infection and they may continue to acquire secondary illnesses associated with the disease.
- Emphasize to patient, family and significant others that this medication does NOT reduce the risk of transmitting HIV to others through sexual contact or blood contamination.
- Inform patient to report any serious side effects to the healthcare provider.
- Explain that the long-term effects of this medication are not known at this time, and the initial results have not demonstrated a reduction in symptoms or prolongation of life.
- Caution patient regarding possibility of photosensitivity and to use protective measures until tolerance is determined.

See Patient Guide, p. 553.

Sargramostim

(sar-GRUH-moe-STIM)

Leukine, Prokine

Class: Colony-stimulating factor

Action Supports survival, proliferation and differentiation of hematopoietic progenitor cells; induces partially committed progenitor cells to divide and differentiate in granulocyte-macrophage pathways; activates mature granulocytes and macrophages; promotes proliferation of megakaryocytic and erythroid progenitors.

Indications Myeloid reconstitution after autologous bone marrow transplantation and after bone marrow transplantation failure or graft failure; promotion of early engraftment or engraftment delay; treatment of neutropenia associated bone marrow transplant. **Unlabeled uses:** Increase WBC counts in patients with myelodysplastic syndromes and in AIDS patients receiving zidovudine; decrease nadir of leukopenia secondary to myelosuppressive chemotherapy; decrease myelosuppression in preleukemic patients; correct neutropenia in aplastic anemia patients; decrease transplantation-associated organ system damage.

Contraindications Excessive leukemic myeloid blasts in bone marrow or peripheral blood; hypersensitivity to granulocyte-macrophage colony-stimulating factor, yeast-derived products or any component of product.

Route/Dosage

Bone Marrow Transplant Failure or Engraftment Delay

ADULTS: IV 250 mcg/m^2/day for 14 days.

Myeloid Reconstitution After Bone Marrow Transplantation

ADULTS: IV 250 mcg/m^2/day for 21 days (first dose given 2-4 hr after transplant).

Interactions

Antineoplastics: Do not use concomitantly. *Corticosteroids or lithium:* May potentiate myeloproliferative effects of sargramostim.

Lab Test Interferences

None well documented.

Adverse Reactions

CV: Transient supraventricular arrhythmia. *GI:* Diarrhea. *GU:* Urinary tract disorder. *DERM:* Rash. *OTHER:* Peripheral edema.

Precautions

Pregnancy: Category C. *Lactation:* Undetermined. *Children:* Safety and efficacy not established. However, available data indicate that sargramostim does not exhibit any greater toxicity in children than in adults. *Concomitant chemotherapy and radiotherapy:* Since rapidly dividing cells are particularly sensitive to cytotoxic chemotherapy and radiotherapy, sargramostim should not be given within 24 hr of chemotherapy or within 12 hr of radiotherapy. *Growth factor potential:* Administer with caution in patients with myeloid malignancies. *Hypersensitivity:* Reactions are infrequent and have ranged from serious allergic or anaphylactic reactions to transient rashes and local injection site reactions. *Renal hepatic and cardiac patients:* Monitor patients closely and use with caution. *Respiratory symptoms:* It may be necessary to decrease rate of infusion by 50% if dyspnea occurs during administration.

NURSING CONSIDERATIONS

Administration/Storage

- Reconstitute with 1 ml Sterile Water for Injection (without preservative); do not re-enter vial. Discard any unused portion.
- During reconstitution, direct sterile water at side of vial and gently swirl contents to prevent foaming during dissolution. Avoid excessive or vigorous agitation; do not shake.
- Dilute in 0.9% Sodium Chloride Injection to prepare IV infusion. If final concentration is < 10 mcg/ml, add human albumin to make final concentration of 0.1% to saline before adding sargramostim to prevent absorption to drug delivery system. For final concentration of 0.1% albumin, add 1 mg human albumin/1 ml 0.9% saline injection. Give within 6 hr after reconstitution. Discard any unused portion after 6 hr.
- Administer each dose over 2 hr as IV infusion.
- Do not use in-line membrane filter for IV infusion.
- Do not add other medications to IV solution.
- Administer 2-4 hr after autologous bone marrow infusion, not less than 24 hr after last dose of antineoplastics, and 12 hr after last dose of radiotherapy, bone marrow transplantation failure or engraftment delay.

- Refrigerate sterile powder, reconstituted solution and diluted solution for injection. Do not freeze or shake.

Assessment/Interventions

- Obtain patient history, including drug history and any known allergies.
- Monitor CBC and differential biweekly during therapy. If ANC > 20,000/mm^3 or platelet count > 500,000 cells/mm^3, discontinue or reduce dose by one half. Leukocytosis may occur.
- Monitor renal and hepatic studies before treatment, including BUN, creatinine, urinalysis, AST, ALT, alkaline phosphatase, and monitor biweekly during therapy if renal or hepatic disease is present.
- Observe for hypersensitivity reactions, including rashes and local injection site reactions, which are usually transient.
- Monitor I&O, hydration status and weight. Observe for fluid retention or edema; pleural and pericardial effusions have occurred.
- Monitor vital signs during therapy; supraventricular arrhythmias have occurred in patients with cardiac disease. Hypotension with flushing and syncope has rarely occurred with first dose.
- Monitor for respiratory symptoms during and immediately following infusion, especially in patients with history of pulmonary disease. If dyspnea occurs during infusion, reduce rate by one half. If symptoms worsen, notify physician and discontinue infusion.

OVERDOSAGE: SIGNS & SYMPTOMS

Dyspnea, malaise, nausea, fever, rash, sinus tachycardia, headache and chills

Patient/Family Education

- Reassure patient that hypotension with flushing and syncope has rarely occurred with first dose.
- Stress importance of follow-up for laboratory tests.
- Instruct patient to inform nurse or physician of dyspnea, malaise, nausea, fever, rash, rapid heart rate, headache or chills.

See Patient Guide, p. 554.

Scopolamine HBr (Hyoscine HBr)

(skoe-PAHL-uh-meen HIGH-droe-BRO-mide)

Isopto

Class: Antiemetic and antivertigo/anticholinergic

Action Competitively inhibits action of acetylcholine at muscarinic receptors. Principal effects are on iris and ciliary body (pupil dilations and blurred vision), secretory glands (dry mouth), drowsiness, euphoria, fatigue, decreased nausea and vomiting.

Indications Accomplishment of cycloplegia and mydriasis for diagnostic procedures and for preoperative and postoperative states in treatment of iridocyclitis (ophthalmic use); prevention of nausea and vomiting associated with motion sickness (transdermal); preanesthetic sedation and obstetric amnesia in conjunction with analgesics and to calm delirium (parenteral).

Contraindications Hypersensitivity to any product component, glaucoma; adhesions between iris and lens; children with previous severe reaction to atropine.

Route/Dosage

Ophthalmic

ADULTS: 1-2 gtt of 1% solution into eye 1 hr prior to refraction; or 1-2 gtt up to qid for uveitis. CHILDREN: 1-2 gtt of 0.5% solution into eye 1 hr prior to refraction; or 1-2 gtt of 0.5% solution up to tid for uveitis.

Parenteral
ADULTS: **IM/SO/IV** 0.32-0.65 mg. CHILDREN: 0.006 mg/kg (maximum 0.3 mg).

Transdermal
ADULTS: One transdermal patch placed behind ear at least 4 hr prior to event. Wear only 1 patch at a time. 0.5 mg will be delivered over 3 days.

Interactions
Haloperidol: Worsened schizophrenia, decreased haloperidol levels and tardive dyskinesia may occur. *IV incompatibilities:* Solutions are incompatible with alkalies. *Phenothiazines:* Actions of phenothiazines may be decreased.

Lab Test Interferences
None well documented.

Adverse Reactions
CV: Increased heart rate. *RESP:* Decreased respiratory rate. *CNS:* Drowsiness; disorientation; delirium. *EENT:* Blurred vision; stinging; increased IOP; photophobia; conjunctivitis. *GI:* Dry mouth. *DERM:* Contact dermatitis; erythema.

Precautions
Pregnancy: Category C. *Lactation:* Undetermined. *Children:* Safety and efficacy not established for transdermal use. Use with caution in children, infants, geriatric patients, those with diabetes, thyroid abnormalities or glaucoma. *Hypersensitivity:* Contact dermatitis for transdermal system has been reported. Potentially alarming idiosyncratic reactions may occur with therapeutic doses. *Other:* Dizziness, nausea, vomiting, headache and disturbances with equilibrium have been reported upon discontinuation after several days of use.

NURSING CONSIDERATIONS

Administration/Storage

- *Direct IV:* Dilute with Sterile Water for Injection and give slowly; position patient recumbent and keep in bed for 1 hr after administration to prevent orthostatic hypotension.
- *Transdermal route:* Apply patch 4 hr prior to expected motion. Apply to clean, hairless, dry area behind ear. Do not touch exposed adhesive area of patch; wash hands thoroughly before and after application. Rotate application sites; place only one patch at a time; change patch every 72 hr.
- *Ophthalmic route:* Wash hands before and after instillation. Position patient supine or with head tilted back in "star-gazing" position (looking at ceiling) to administer drops. Pull down lower lid to form pocket and instill solution as ordered. Avoid contact between dispenser and eye. Close eye gently and apply pressure to inner canthus for 1-2 min to prevent systemic absorption and drainage into nose/throat. Blot excessive solution from around eye with tissue. Wait 5 min before instilling additional ophthalmic solutions.
- Store transdermal patches in packages until ready for use; note expiration date; store ophthalmic and parenteral solutions at room temperature and protect from light.

Assessment/Interventions

- Obtain patient history, including drug history and any known allergies.
- Assess vital signs (heart rate, BP), presence of pain and intake/output ratio (watch for urinary retention) prior to and during therapy.
- Provide pain medication concomitantly as needed; remember medication alone can precipitate behavior changes such as excitation and delirium.
- Assess mouth for dryness; provide mouth care, hard candy or frequent sips of water as needed.
- Assess for blurred vision, drowsiness and dizziness; implement safety pre-

cautions (call bell, side rails) and assist with ambulation.

OVERDOSAGE: SIGNS & SYMPTOMS

Somnolence, dry mouth, dilated pupils, delirium, disorientation, memory disturbances, dizziness, restlessness, hallucinations

Patient/Family Education

Oral/Parenteral/Transdermal

- Tell patient if dose is missed to take as soon as remembered, but caution against doubling doses.
- Advise patient to avoid use of alcohol or other CNS depressants (sedatives, antihistamines) while taking this medication.
- Advise patient that drug may cause drowsiness or dizziness and to use caution while driving or performing other tasks requiring mental alertness.
- Explain that rinsing mouth, good oral hygiene and sugarless gum or candy will help to counteract mouth dryness.
- Encourage medical follow-up to monitor effects of therapy.
- Instruct patient and family in correct technique for application of patches; explain that patch is waterproof and not affected by showering or bathing.
- Remind patient to wash hands before and after applying patch.
- Explain that if patch is dislodged it should be replaced with a new unit at a different site.

Ophthalmic Preparation

- Instruct patient to wash hands before and after instillation.
- Instruct patient and family in correct technique for instillation of drops for ophthalmic use.
- Explain that blurring of vision will decrease with repeated use of drug and to avoid hazardous activities until vision clears.
- Explain that eyes may become sensitivie to light and advise use of dark glasses indoors and outdoors.
- Emphasize need to contact physician immediately if patient notices change in vision, eye pain, loss of sight, inability to breath or flushing.
- Tell patient to notify physician if light sensitivity persists longer than 1 wk after medication has been discontinued.

See Patient Guide, pp. 555-557.

Secobarbital Sodium

(see-koe-BAR-bih-tahl SO-dee-uhm)

Available as generic only

Class: Sedative and hypnotic/ barbiturate

Action Depresses sensory cortex, decreases motor activity, alters cerebellar function and produces drowsiness, sedation and hypnosis.

Indications Short-term (up to 2 wk) treatment of insomnia; induction of basal hypnosis before anesthesia (parenteral form); sedation (parenteral form). **Unlabeled use:** Control of status epilepticus or acute seizure episodes.

Contraindications Hypersensitivity to barbiturates; history of addiction to sedative/hypnotic drugs; history of porphyria; severe liver impairment; respiratory disease with dyspnea; nephritic patients.

Route/Dosage

Insomnia

ADULTS: **PO** At bedtime 100 mg.

Hypnotic

ADULTS: **IM** 100-200 mg; **IV** 50-250 mg.

Sedation

ADULTS: **PO** 30-50 mg tid or qid. CHILDREN: **PO/PR** 2-6 mg/kg. For rectal administration, dilute to 1%-1.5% solution.

Preoperative Sedation
ADULTS: **PO** 200-300 mg 1-2 hr before surgery. CHILDREN: **PO** 2-6 mg/kg (maximum 100 mg) 1-2 hr before surgery.

Sedation/Preanesthesia
ADULTS: **IM** (light sedation) 1 mg/kg 15 min before procedure. CHILDREN: **IM** 4-5 mg/kg.

Convulsions
ADULTS: **IM/IV** 1.1-2.2 mg/kg. Maximum IV rate 50 mg/15 sec. Maximum adult IM dose 500 mg or 5 ml volume regardless of concentration.

Interactions

Alcohol, CNS depressants: May produce additive CNS depressant effects. *Anticoagulants (eg, warfarin), beta-blockers (eg, metoprolol, propranolol), verapamil, quinidine, theophyllines:* May reduce activity of these drugs. *Anticonvulsants:* May reduce serum concentrations of carbamazepine, valproic acid and succinimides. Valproic acid may increase barbiturate serum levels. *Corticosteroids:* May reduce effectiveness of corticosteroids. *Estrogens, estrogen-containing oral contraceptives:* May reduce contraceptive effect and estrogen effect.

Lab Test Interferences

May increase bromsulphalein retention; may cause decreased serum bilirubin concentrations; false-positive phentolamine test results; decreased response to metyrapone; impaired absorption of radioactive cyanocobalamin.

Adverse Reactions

CV: Bradycardia; hypotension; syncope. *RESP:* Hypoventilation; apnea; laryngospasm; bronchospasm. *CNS:* Drowsiness; agitation; confusion; headache; hyperkinesia; ataxia; CNS depression; paradoxical excitement; nightmares; psychiatric disturbances; hallucinations; insomnia; dizziness. *GI:* Nausea; vomiting; constipation. *HEMA:* Blood dyscrasias (eg, agranulocytosis, thrombocytopenia). *OTHER:* Hypersensitivity reactions (eg, angioedema, rashes, exfoliative dermatitis); fever; liver damage; injection site reactions (eg, local pain, thrombophlebitis).

Precautions

Pregnancy: Category D. *Lactation:* Excreted in breast milk. *Children:* May respond with excitement rather than depression. *Elderly or debilitated patients:* More sensitive to drug effects; dosage reduction is required. *Dependence:* Tolerance or psychological and physical dependence may occur with continued use. *IV administration:* Do not exceed maximum IV rate 50 mg/15 sec; respiratory depression, apnea and hypotension may result. Parenteral solutions are highly alkaline; extravasation may cause tissue damage and necrosis. Inadvertent intra-arterial injection may lead to arterial spasm, thrombosis and gangrene. *Renal or hepatic impairment:* Use drug with caution; dosage reduction may be required. *Seizure disorders:* Status epilepticus may result from abrupt discontinuation.

NURSING CONSIDERATIONS

Administration/Storage

- Administer on empty stomach with full glass of water to enhance absorption. Tablet may be crushed and mixed with food or swallowed whole.
- For insomnia, give ½-1 hr before bedtime.
- Check to see that medication is swallowed.
- For IM administration: inject deep into large muscle using Z-track technique to diminish tissue irritation and potential sloughing. Do not inject subcutaneously. Do not exceed 5 ml at any 1 site. Rotate injection sites.
- For direct IV administration, may give undiluted or diluted with Sterile Water for Injection, normal saline (0.9% Sodium Chloride) or Ringer's solution. Do not use lactated Ringer's solution.

- Administer intravenously no faster than 50 mg/15 sec; too rapid administration can cause respiratory depression and hypotension. Have resuscitative equipment readily available.
- Use diluted solution within 30 min of mixing. Rotate, do not shake vial.
- For rectal administration in children preoperatively, after cleansing enema, give diluted parenteral solution (1%-1.5%) as ordered.
- Store oral preparation at room temperature. Refrigerate parenteral form. Use only clear solution; discard if precipitate forms or solution becomes cloudy.

Assessment/Interventions

- Obtain patient history, including drug history and any known allergies. Note history of respiratory disease with dyspnea or hypersensitivity to barbiturates or sedative/hypnotic drug addiction.
- Assess type of sleep difficulty: falling asleep, remaining asleep.
- Assess sleep pattern prior to and during therapy.
- Assess vital signs q 15-30 min after parenteral administration for 2 hr and then prn.
- Assess mental status: sensorium, affect, mood and long-term and short-term memory.
- Obtain baseline Hct, Hgb, RBC and liver function test results (transaminase levels and bilirubin). Periodically evaluate those results if patient is on long-term therapy.
- Provide safety measures (removal of cigarettes, side rails up, night light, easily accessible call-bell) and assistance with ambulation.

OVERDOSAGE: SIGNS & SYMPTOMS

CNS and respiratory depression, Cheyne-Stokes respiration, areflexia, oliguria, tachycardia, hypotension, lowered body temperature, coma, pulmonary edema, death

Patient/Family Education

- Explain that this medication may cause psychological and physical dependence. Emphasize that it is important not to increase dose without consulting physician.
- Discuss ways to facilitate sleep (quiet, darkened room; avoidance of caffeine and nicotine; warm bath, warm milk; deep breathing; relaxation; self-hypnosis).
- Inform patient that it may take a few doses to achieve noticeable sleep benefit.
- Instruct patient to notify physician immediately of sudden onset of fever, sore throat, bruising, rash, jaundice, or unusual bleeding (eg, epistaxis).
- Instruct patient to avoid intake of alcoholic beverages or other CNS depressants (eg, pain relievers, antihistamines, sedatives) to prevent serious CNS depression.
- Emphasize importance of follow-up evaluation with physician to monitor progress of therapy.
- Inform patient that after discontinuation of drug, nighttime sleeping might be disturbed for a few days and increased dreaming may occur.
- Advise patient that drug may cause daytime drowsiness and to use caution while driving or performing other tasks requiring mental alertness.
- Instruct patient not to discontinue medication abruptly without consulting physician.

See Patient Guide, p. 558.

Selegiline HCl (L-Deprenyl)

(seh-LEH-jih-leen HIGH-droe-KLOR-ide)

Eldepryl

Class: Antiparkinson

Action Selective type B monamine oxidase (MAO) inhibitor thought to increase dopaminergic activity. MAO enzyme breaks down catecholamines and serotonin. Selegiline may also interfere with dopamine reuptake at synapse.

Indications Adjunct to levodopa/carbidopa in idiopathic Parkinson's disease, postencephalic parkinsonism/symptomatic parkinsonism.

Contraindications Standard considerations.

Route/Dosage
ADULTS: **PO** 10 mg/day as divided dose of 5 mg each taken at breakfast and lunch. Do not exceed 10 mg/day. After 2-3 days of treatment, try reducing levodopa/carbidopa dose by 10-30%. Further reductions may be possible during continued selegiline therapy.

Interactions
Fluoxetine: May produce a "serotinin" syndrome (CNS irritability, increased muscle tone, altered consciousness). *Meperidine:* Could result in agitation, seizures, diaphoresis and fever, which may progress to coma, apnea and death. Reactions may occur several weeks following withdrawal of selegiline.

Lab Test Interferences
None well documented.

Adverse Reactions
CV: Palpitations; orthostatic hypotension; arrhythmia; hypertension; new or increased angina; syncope. *CNS:* Dizziness; lightheadedness; fainting; confusion; hallucinations; vivid dreams; headache; anxiety; tension; insomnia; lethargy; depression; loss of balance; delusions; dyskinesias; increased akinetic involuntary movements; bradykinesia; chorea. *EENT:* Diplopia; blurred vision. *GI:* Nausea; abdominal pain; dry mouth; diarrhea. *GU:* Sexual dysfunction; urinary retention, frequency, hesitancy. *DERM:* Sweating; rash; photosensitivity. *OTHER:* Generalized ache; leg pain; low back pain; weight loss.

Precautions
Pregnancy: Category C. *Lactation:* Undetermined. *Children:* Effects have not been evaluated. *Maximum:* Do not exceed recommended daily dose of 10 mg/day because of risks associated with nonselective inhibition of MAO (potentially serious food or drug interactions may occur at higher doses). *Hypertensive crisis risk:* Selegiline can be given with active amine-containing medications and tyramine foods as long as recommended dose is not exceeded. However, report any possible symptoms suggestive of hypertensive crisis.

NURSING CONSIDERATIONS

Administration/Storage

- Administer 5 mg with breakfast and with lunch.
- Do not exceed 10 mg daily.

Assessment/Interventions

- Obtain patient history, including drug history and any known allergies.
- Monitor vital signs, especially BP and respirations.
- Assess patient for decrease in akathisia and mood.
- Assess patient's mental status: affect, mood, behavioral changes, depression.
- Dosage of levodopa/carbidopa may be reduced after 2-3 days of treatment.
- Assess for side effects, particularly nausea, dizziness, lightheadedness, abdominal pain, confusion, hallucination.

- Assist patient with ambulation at beginning of therapy.
- Assess diet for tyramine-containing foods.
- Implement safety measures to prevent falls, especially during initial treatment.

> **OVERDOSAGE: SIGNS & SYMPTOMS**
> Hypotension, psychomotor agitation

Patient/Family Education

- Encourage patient to change position slowly to prevent orthostatic hypotension.
- Instruct patient to avoid driving or other potentially hazardous activities until effect of medication is determined.
- Explain that dosage of levodopa/carbidopa may be reduced after initiation of adjunctive therapy.
- Identify tyramine-containing foods; explain rationale for exclusion from diet.
- Instruct patient to report these side effects: twitching, eye spasms.
- Caution patient to use drug exactly as prescribed. Explain that if drug is discontinued, parkinsonian crisis may occur.
- Advise patient not to exceed 10 mg/day dose.
- Inform patient and family of symptoms of hypertensive crisis and when to call physician. Instruct them to report severe headache or other unusual symptoms.

See Patient Guide, p. 559.

Senna

(SEN-ah)

Black-Draught, Dr. Caldwell Senna Laxative, Fletcher Castoria, Gentlax, Senexon, Senna-Gen, Senokot, Senokotxtra, Senolax, X-prep, ♣ *Glysennid, Mucinum Herbal*

Class: Laxative

Action Directly acts on intestinal mucosa by altering water and electrolyte secretion, inducing peristalsis and defecation.

Indications Short-term treatment of constipation; preoperative and preradiographic bowel evacuation for procedures involving GI tract.

Contraindications Nausea, vomiting or other symptoms of appendicitis; acute surgical abdomen; fecal impaction; intestinal obstruction; undiagnosed abdominal pain.

Route/Dosage

ADULTS: **PO** 2 tablets, 1 tsp of granules or 10-15 ml of syrup, usually at bedtime. **PR** 1 suppository at bedtime; may repeat in 2 hr. CHILDREN: Generally, for children 6-12 yr or > 60 lb, give (at bedtime) 1 tablet or ½ tsp granules **PO** or ½ suppository **PR.** Liquid dose ranges from 1.25-15 ml depending on age and product formulation.

Interactions None well documented.

Lab Test Interferences

None well documented.

Adverse Reactions

CV: Palpitations. *CNS:* Dizziness; fainting. *GI:* Excessive bowel activity (eg, griping, diarrhea, nausea, vomiting); perianal irritation; bloating; flatulence; abdominal cramping. *OTHER:* Sweating; weakness.

Precautions

Pregnancy: Category C. *Lactation:* Undetermined. *Abuse/dependency:* Long-term use may lead to laxative dependency, which may result in fluid and electrolyte imbalances, steatorrhea, osteomalacia and vitamin and mineral deficiencies. Cathartic colon, a poorly functioning colon, results from long-term abuse. Pathologic presentation may resemble ulcerative colitis. *Discoloration of acidic urine:* May result in yellow-brown urine. *Discoloration of alkaline urine:* May result in pink to red urine. *Fluid and electrolyte imbalance:* Excessive laxative use may lead to significant fluid and electrolyte imbalance. *Melanosis coli:* Darkened pigmentation of colonic mucosa may occur after long-term use, usually resolving within 5-11 months of discontinuation. *Rectal bleeding or failure to respond:* May indicate serious condition requiring further attention.

NURSING CONSIDERATIONS

Administration/Storage

- Administer at bedtime on empty stomach.
- Shake liquid solution before administering.
- Dissolve granules before administering.
- For preoperative or prediagnostic bowel preparation, give between 2-4 PM on day before procedure.
- Limit patient's diet to clear liquids until after procedure.
- Give oral dosages with full glass of water or juice.
- Administer suppository with patient lying on left side.

Assessment/Interventions

- Obtain patient history, including drug history and any known allergies.
- Assess bowel function, including normal frequency, type, last bowel movement, bowel sounds, abdominal distention.
- Assess for presence of abdominal pain, nausea, vomiting.
- Assess for fluid and electrolyte imbalance associated with long-term laxative use.
- Identify factors potentially contributing to constipation, ie, opoid analgesics, inactivity.
- Monitor effectiveness of therapy.
- Implement measures to prevent constipation, ie, fluids, activity, dietary bulk.

OVERDOSAGE: SIGNS & SYMPTOMS

Gripping pain, diarrhea

Patient/Family Education

- Explain potential hazards (eg, dependence) associated with long-term laxative use.
- Advise that senna may result in discolored yellow-brown or reddish urine.
- Explain that bowel patterns are very individual.
- Identify measures to improve bowel function, ie, fluids, activity, dietary bulk.
- Caution against taking laxatives in presence of acute abdominal pain or in presence of nausea or vomiting.

See Patient Guide, p. 560.

Sertraline HCl

(SIR-truh-leen HIGH-droe-KLOR-ide)

Zoloft

Class: Antidepressant

Action Selectively blocks reuptake of serotonin, enhancing serotonergic function .

Indications Treatment of depression. **Unlabeled use:** Control of obsessive-compulsive disorder.

Contraindications Standard considerations.

Route/Dosage

ADULTS: **PO** 50-200 mg once daily.

Interactions

Alcohol, CNS depressants: May enhance CNS depressant effects. MAO *inhibitors:* May cause serious, even fatal reactions. Discontinue MAO inhibitors at least 14 days before starting sertraline.

Lab Test Interferences

None well documented.

Adverse Reactions

CV: Palpitations. *CNS:* Agitation; anxiety; nervousness; headache; insomnia; dizziness; tremor; fatigue; tingling; diminished sensation; twitching; hypertonia; decreased concentration; confusion. *EENT:* Abnormal vision; ringing in the ears; rhinitis; pharyngitis; change in taste perception. *GI:* Nausea; diarrhea; dry mouth; anorexia; vomiting; flatulence; constipation; abdominal pain; increased appetite. *GU:* Sexual dysfunction; urinary frequency; urinary disorder; menstrual disorder; pain. *HEMA:* Lymphadenopathy; purpura. *DERM:* Sweating, rash. *META:* Dehydration; hypoglycemia. *OTHER:* Muscle pain; weight loss or gain.

Precautions

Pregnancy: Category B. *Lactation:* Undetermined. *Children:* Safety and efficacy not established. *Elderly or debilitated patients:* Dosage reduction may be required. *Renal and hepatic impairment:* Use drug with caution. Lower or less frequent dosing schedule may be required. *Seizures:* Use drug with caution in patients with history of seizures. *Suicide:* Depressed patients at risk should be supervised during initial therapy.

NURSING CONSIDERATIONS

Administration/Storage

- Administer once daily in either morning or afternoon.
- Dosage changes should not be changed at intervals of < 1 wk.
- Do not administer to patients who have used MAO inhibitor in past 14 days.
- Store at room temperature.

Assessment/Interventions

- Obtain patient history, including drug history and any known allergies. Determine whether any MAO inhibitors have been used in past 14 days. Note history of seizure disorders and renal and hepatic impairment.
- Observe for common side effects (agitation, insomnia, somnolence, dizziness, headache, tremor, anorexia, diarrhea/loose stools, nausea and fatigue) and notify physician.
- Take appropriate safety measures because possibility of suicide may persist until significant remission occurs.

OVERDOSAGE: SIGNS & SYMPTOMS

Somnolence, nausea, vomiting, tachycardia, ECG changes, anxiety, dilated pupils

Patient/Family Education

- Discuss with family members precautionary measures to be taken to prevent suicide attempt.
- Inform patient that improvement may not be evident for 2-4 weeks after treatment has started.
- Advise female patient to notify physician if she becomes pregnant, intends to become pregnant or is breastfeeding an infant.
- Inform male patient of possible sexual dysfunction (primarily ejaculatory delay) and advise patient to notify physician if it occurs.
- Explain that anorexia, nausea, diarrhea and weight loss may occur. Advise patient to notify physician if these symptoms persist.
- Instruct patient to report these symptoms to physician: agitation, insomnia, somnolence, dizziness, headache, tremor, anorexia, diarrhea/loose stools, nausea, fatigue or other physical complaints.
- Tell patient to avoid intake of alcoholic beverages or other CNS depressants.
- Advise patient that drug may cause drowsiness and dizziness and to use caution while driving or performing other tasks requiring mental alertness.

See Patient Guide, p. 561.

Simethicone

(sih-METH-ih-kone)

Flatulex, Gas Relief, Gas-X, Gas-X (Extra Strength), Major-Con, Maximum Strength Phazyme 125, Mylanta Gas, Mylanta Gas (Maximum Strength), Mylicon, Phazyme, Phazyme 95, ♣ *Ovol-40, Ovol-80, Ovol Drops, Phazyme-55*

Class: Antiflatulent

Action Relieves flatulence by dispersing and preventing formation of mucus-surrounded gas pockets in GI tract.

Indications Relief of painful symptoms and pressure of excess gas in digestive tract. Adjunct in treatment of many conditions in which gas retention may be problem, such as postoperative gaseous distention and pain, endoscopic examination, air swallowing, functional dyspepsia, peptic ulcer, spastic or irritable colon, diverticulosis. **Unlabeled use:** Treatment of infant colic.

Contraindications Standard considerations.

Route/Dosage

Capsules

ADULTS: **PO** 125 mg qid after meals and at bedtime.

Tablets

ADULTS: **PO** 40-125 mg qid after meals and at bedtime.

Liquid (Drops)

ADULTS: **PO** 40-80 mg qid (up to 500 mg/day). CHILDREN 2-12 YR: **PO** 40 mg qid. CHILDREN < 2 YR: **PO** 20 mg qid (up to 240 mg/day).

Interactions None well documented.

Lab Test Interferences None well documented.

Adverse Reactions None well documented.

Precautions None well documented.

NURSING CONSIDERATIONS

Administration/Storage

- Tablets: Be certain patient chews tablet thoroughly or allows tablet to dissolve in mouth.
- Liquid: Shake well before using.
- Store tablets/capsules at room temperature in well closed container.
- Store suspension at room temperature in tight, light-resistant container. Do not freeze.

Assessment/Interventions

- Obtain patient history, including drug history and any known allergies.
- Assess baseline bowel sounds and gastrointestinal status prior to therapy, and continue to monitor bowel sounds throughout therapy.
- Assess for belching and flatus as evidence of drug action.
- Monitor effectiveness of therapy, documenting decreased abdominal distention and discomfort.

Patient/Family Education

- Advise patient to report any worsening of GI symptoms to physician.

See Patient Guide, p. 562.

Simvastatin

(SIM-vuh-STAT-in)
Zocor
Class: Antihyperlipidemic/HMG-CoA reductase inhibitor

Action Increases rate at which body removes cholesterol from blood and reduces production of cholesterol by inhibiting enzyme that catalyzes early rate-limiting step in cholesterol synthesis.

Indications Adjunct to diet for reducing elevated total cholesterol and LDL cholesterol levels in patients with primary hypercholesterolemia (types IIa and IIb) when response to diet and other nonpharmacologic measures alone are inadequate. **Unlabeled uses:** Lower elevated cholesterol levels in patients with heterozygous familial hypercholesterolemia, familial combined hyperlipidemia, diabetic dyslipidemia in non-insulin-dependent diabetics, hyperlipidemia secondary to nephrotic syndrome and homozygous familial hypercholesterolemia in patients who have defective, rather than absent, LDL receptors.

Contraindications Active liver disease or unexplained persistent elevations of liver function values; pregnancy; lactation.

Route/Dosage
ADULTS: PO 5-40 mg/day in evening.

Interactions
Cyclosporine, erythromycin, gemfibrozil, niacin: Severe myopathy or rhabdomyolysis may occur.

Lab Test Interferences
None well documented.

Adverse Reactions
RESP: Upper respiratory infection. *CNS:* Headache; asthenia; paresthesia; peripheral neuropathy. *EENT:* Dysfunction of certain cranial nerves (including alteration of taste, impairment of extra-ocular movement, facial paresis); progression of cataracts. *GI:* Nausea; vomiting; diarrhea; abdominal pain; constipation; flatulence; dyspepsia; pancreatitis. *HEPA:* Hepatitis; jaundice; fatty change in liver; cirrhosis; fulminant hepatic necrosis; hepatoma; increased serum transaminases. *OTHER:* Myopathy; rhabdomyolysis; fatigue. Apparent hypersensitivity syndrome has been reported rarely which has included one or more of following features: anaphylaxis; angioedema; lupus erythematous–like syndrome; polymyalgia rheumatica; vasculitis; purpura; thrombocytopenia; leukopenia; hemolytic anemia; positive ANA; ESR increase; arthritis; arthralgia; urticaria; asthenia; photosensitivity; fever; chills; flushing; malaise; dyspnea; toxic epidermal necrolysis; erythema multiforme, including Stevens-Johnson syndrome.

Precautions
Pregnancy: Category X. A reliable form of birth control should be used. *Lactation:* Undetermined. *Children:* Use in children not recommended. *Liver dysfunction:* Use drug with caution in patients who consume substantial quantities of alcohol or who have history of liver disease. Marked, persistent increases in serum transaminases have occurred. *Renal impairment:* High doses may result in severe renal insufficiency. *Skeletal muscle effects:* Rhabdomyolysis with renal dysfunction secondary to myoglobinuria has occurred in this class of drugs. Consider myopathy in any patient with diffuse myalgias, muscle tenderness or weakness, or marked elevation of CPK.

NURSING CONSIDERATIONS

Administration/Storage

- Adjust dosage as indicated, usually at 4 wk intervals.
- Administer at bedtime for best results. Hepatic cholesterol production highest during night.
- Store at room temperature.

Assessment/Interventions

- Obtain patient history, including drug history and any known allergies.
- Maintain patient on standard cholesterol diet for at least 3-6 mo.
- Determine baseline serum cholesterol and triglyceride levels and monitor at 4-6 wk intervals and again at 3 mo.
- Determine baseline liver function test values and monitor q 6 wk for first 3 mo, q 8 wk for remainder of first year, then q 6 mo thereafter.
- In patients with renal impairment, monitor for possible severe renal insufficiency.
- Periodic CPK determinations may be necessary.
- Notify physician if cholesterol levels are unchanged or if there is significant rise in trigylceride levels.

Patient/Family Education

- Caution patient that this medication must not be taken during pregnancy or when pregnancy is possible. Advise patient to use reliable form of birth control while taking this drug.
- Advise patient to control weight and to adhere to prescribed dietary regimen.
- Tell patient to notify physician or pharmacist if taking, will be taking or stop taking any prescription or nonprescription medication.
- Advise patient that exercise and diet that reduces intake of cholesterol and saturated fats are helpful.
- Instruct patient to report these symptoms to physician: any unexplained muscle pain, tenderness or weakness, especially if accompanied by fever or malaise; yellowing of skin or eyes.
- Tell patient to avoid intake of alcoholic beverages.

See Patient Guide, p. 563.

Sodium Bicarbonate

(SO-dee-uhm by-CAR-boe-nate)

Bell/ans, Neut

Class: Urinary tract product/alkalinizer; electrolyte; antacid

Action Increases plasma bicarbonate; buffers excess hydrogen ion concentrations; raises blood pH; reverses metabolic acidosis.

Indications Treatment of metabolic acidosis; promotion of gastric, systemic and urinary alkalinization; replacement therapy in severe diarrhea; used to reduce incidence of chemical phlebitis (used as neutralizing additive solution).

Contraindications Loss of chloride from vomiting or continuous GI suction when patient is receiving diuretics known to produce hypochloremic alkalosis; metabolic and respiratory alkalosis; hypocalcemia in which alkalosis may produce tetany, hypertension, convulsions or CHF; when administration of sodium could be clinically detrimental.

Route/Dosage

ADULTS & CHILDREN > 2 YR: **IV** Administration performed in concentrations ranging from 1.5% (isotonic)-8.4% depending on clinical condition and requirements of patient. **SC** After dilution to isotonicity (1.5%). The dose depends on the clinical condition and requirements of the patient (including age and weight). **PO** 325 mg-2 g 1-4 times daily (patients < 60 yr, maximum dose 16 g/day; patients > 60 yr maximum dose 8 g/day). INFANTS ≤ 2

YR: **IV** 4.2% solution at rate ≤ 8 mEq/kg/day.

Interactions

Amphetamine, dextroamphetamine, ephedrine, flecainide, mecamylamine, methamphetamine, pseudoephedrine, quinidine: Sodium bicarbonate can decrease elimination of these drugs, thus increasing their therapeutic effects. *Chlorpropamide, lithium, methotrexate, salicylates, tetracyclines:* Sodium bicarbonate can increase elimination of these drugs, thus decreasing their therapeutic effect. *Ketoconazole:* PO sodium bicarbonate may decrease the dissolution of ketoconazole in the GI tract, reducing the effectiveness. INCOMPATIBILITIES: Do not mix with IV solutions containing catecholamines, such as dobutamine, dopamine and norepinephrine.

Lab Test Interferences

None well documented.

Adverse Reactions

CV: Exacerbation of CHF. *GI:* Rebound hyperacidity; milk-alkali syndrome. *META:* Hypernatremia; alkalosis. *OTHER:* Extravasation with cellulitis, tissue necrosis, ulceration and sloughing; local pain; venous irritation; tetany; edema.

Precautions

Pregnancy: Category C. *Lactation:* Undetermined. *Neonates and children < 2 yr:* Administration of ≥ 10 ml/min of hypertonic sodium bicarbonate may produce hypernatremia, decreased CSF pressure and possible intracranial hemorrhage. *Special risk patients:* Use drug with caution in edematous sodium-retaining states, CHF, liver cirrhosis, toxemia of pregnancy or renal impairment. *Sodium content:* May be significant, especially in patients with hypertension or CHF or in patients on low-sodium diets.

NURSING CONSIDERATIONS

Administration/Storage

- For IV solution preparation, use Sterile Water for Injection, Sodium Chloride Injection, 5% Dextrose or other standard electrolyte solutions as diluent.
- With chewable tablets instruct patient to chew thoroughly before swallowing and then to drink a glass of water.
- Do not administer other oral drugs within 1-2 hr of oral sodium bicarbonate (antacid) administration.

Assessment/Interventions

- Obtain patient history, including drug history and any known allergies.
- Evaluate pH and electrolytes with preadministration values. If there is evidence of alkalosis, notify physician.
- Assess baseline BP and respiratory rate and rhythm.
- Assess serum pH, PaO_2, $PaCO_2$ and serum electrolytes frequently during therapy. Inform physician of results.
- Test urine to determine pH.
- If patient has edematous tendency, notify physician.
- If patient exhibits shortness of breath and hyperpnea, notify physician.
- If patient is vomiting, withhold medication and notify physician.
- Notify physician if relief is not obtained or if patient demonstrates any symptoms that suggest bleeding, such as black tarry stools or coffee ground emesis.

OVERDOSAGE: SIGNS & SYMPTOMS

Alkalosis, hyperirritability, tetany, nausea, vomiting

Patient/Family Education

- Instruct patient not to take medication with milk because renali calculi can develop.
- Explain need to avoid otc medications containing sodium bicarbonate, such as Alka-Seltzer. Excessive use of sodium bicarbonate can result in

increase acid secretion or systemic alkalosis.

- Instruct patient not to use maximum dose of antacids for more than 2 wk except under supervision of physician.
- Advise patient not to take sodium bicarbonate on routine or long-term basis. Tell patient to notify physician if symptoms of gastric distress continue.
- Caution patient to report these symptoms to physician immediately: nausea, vomiting and anorexia.

See Patient Guide, p. 564.

Sodium Phosphate/ Sodium Biphosphate

(SO-dee-uhm FOSS-fate/SO-dee-uhm by-FOSS-fate)

Fleet (enema), Fleet Phospho-soda, Sodium Phosphates

Class: Laxative

Action Attracts and retains water in intestinal lumen, thereby increasing intraluminal pressure and inducing urge to defecate.

Indications Short-term treatment of constipation; evacuation of colon for rectal and bowel evaluations.

Contraindications Nausea, vomiting or other symptoms of appendicitis; acute surgical abdomen; fecal impaction; intestinal obstruction; undiagnosed abdominal pain; megacolon; imperforate anus; congestive heart failure; patients on sodium-restricted diet; edema; hypertension.

Route/Dosage

Sodium Phosphate Oral Solution (Fleet Phospho-soda)

Give orally only. ADULTS & CHILDREN > 12 YR: **PO** 20 ml (4 teaspoonfuls) mixed with ½ glass cool water. CHILDREN 10- < 12 YR: **PO** 10 ml (2 teaspoonfuls). CHILDREN 5- < 10 YR: **PO** 5 ml (1 teaspoonful).

Disposable Enema

Give rectally. ADULTS & CHILDREN > 12 YR: **PR** 118 ml (contents of 1 disposable adult enema). CHILDREN ≥ 2 YR: **PR** ½ adult dose (contents of 1 disposable pediatric enema).

Interactions None well documented.

Lab Test Interferences None well documented.

Adverse Reactions

CV: Palpitations. *CNS:* Dizziness; fainting. *GI:* Excessive bowel activity (griping, diarrhea, nausea, vomiting); perianal irritation; bloating; flatulence; abdominal cramping. *META:* Fluid and electrolyte imbalances. *OTHER:* Sweating; weakness.

Precautions

Pregnancy: Consult physician. Improper use of saline cathartics can lead to dangerous electrolyte imbalances. *Lactation:* Consult physician before use. *Children:* Do not administer enemas to children < 2 yr. *Abuse/dependency:* Chronic use of laxatives may lead to laxative dependency, which may result in fluid and electrolyte imbalances, steatorrhea, osteomalacia and vitamin and mineral deficiencies. *Fluid and electrolyte imbalance:* Excessive laxative use may lead to significant fluid and electrolyte imbalance. *Rectal bleeding or failure to respond:* May indicate serious condition that may require further medical attention. *Renal impairment:* Use drug with caution; hyperphosphatemia, hypernatremia, acidosis and hypocalcemia may occur.

NURSING CONSIDERATIONS

Administration/Storage

- Use oral or rectal form according to patient needs.
- Administer alone for better absorption. Do not give within 1 hr of other drugs.
- Store at room temperature.

Assessment/Interventions

- Obtain patient history, including drug history and any known allergies.
- Use with caution in patients with large hemorrhoids or anal excoriations.
- Determine if patient has adequate fluid intake prior to initiating therapy.
- Monitor I&O.
- Assess bowel sounds daily.
- Evaluate effectiveness of therapy daily. Enemas usually elicit response within 10-15 minutes.
- Assess for abdominal pain, distention, nausea and vomiting.

OVERDOSAGE: SIGNS & SYMPTOMS

Excessive bowel activity, dehydration (hypotension, tachycardia), electrolyte abnormalities (hypernatremia, hypocalcemia, hyperphosphatemia), metabolic acidosis

Patient/Family Education

- Explain importance of adequate daily fluid intake.
- Tell patient to increase dietary sources of bulk, including cereals, fresh fruit and vegetables.
- Caution against prolonged or excessive use, which could result in laxative dependence.
- Encourage daily exercise.
- Instruct patient not to take medication if abdominal pain or nausea and vomiting are present.
- Tell patient to report these symptoms to physician: abdominal pain, rectal bleeding, unrelieved constipation, symptoms of electrolyte imbalances (muscle cramps, pain, weakness, dizziness, excessive thirst).

See Patient Guide, p. 565.

Sodium Polystyrene Sulfonate

(SO-dee-uhm pah-lee-STYE-reen SULL-fuh-nate)

Kayexalate, SPS

Class: Potassium-removing resin

Action Resin that exchanges sodium ions for potassium in large intestine.

Indications Treatment of hyperkalemia.

Contraindications Hypokalemia.

Route/Dosage

ADULTS: **PO or via NG tube** 15 g 1-4 times/day. **PR** 30-50 g q 6 hr has been given as daily enema. CHILDREN: **PO** Calculate children's dose by exchange ratio of 1 mEq potassium per gram of resin. (1 g/kg q 6 hr has been recommended.)

Interactions

Digitalis: If hypokalemia occurs, likelihood of toxic effects of digoxin may be increased. *Nonabsorbable cation donating antacids and laxatives (eg, aluminum carbonate, magnesium hydroxide):* Systemic alkalosis has occurred. Potassium exchange capability of sodium polystyrene sulfonate may be reduced. Intestinal obstruction due to concretions of aluminum hydroxide when used in combination has occurred.

Lab Test Interferences

None well documented.

Adverse Reactions

GI: Gastric irritation; anorexia;

nausea; vomiting; constipation; fecal impaction. *META:* Hypokalemia; hypocalcemia; sodium retention.

Precautions

Pregnancy: Category C. *Lactation:* Undetermined. *Electrolyte abnormalities:* Serious potassium deficiency can occur. Sodium polystyrene sulfonate is not totally selective for potassium and small amounts of magnesium and calcium can be lost. Use with caution in patients who cannot tolerate even small increase in sodium load (ie, severe congestive heart failure, severe hypertension, marked edema). *Severe hyperkalemia:* Treatment with this drug alone may be insufficient to rapidly correct severe hyperkalemia associated with states of rapid tissue breakdown (eg, burns, renal failure) or hyperkalemia so marked as to constitute medical emergency.

NURSING CONSIDERATIONS

Administration/Storage

- Oral powder: Shake bottle well before administration. Give each dose as suspension in water or, for greater palatability, in syrup. Use sorbitol to combat constipation. Oral suspensions contain sorbitol and sodium. Resin may be introduced into stomach through plastic tube; if desired, mixed with appropriate diet. Never mix with orange juice because of high potassium content.
- Retention enema: After initial cleansing enema, insert soft, large (28 F) rubber tube into the rectum about 20 cm, with tip well into sigmoid colon, and tape in place. Elevate hips to prevent leakage. After administration, flush suspension with 50-100 ml of fluid, clamp tube and leave in place. Keep suspension in sigmoid colon for several hours. Then irrigate colon with approximately 2 L of non-sodium-containing solution. Drain return through Y-tube connection.
- Store at room temperature. Store repackaged product in refrigerator and use within 14 days. Do not store freshly prepared suspensions longer than 24 hr. Do not heat, because this may alter exchange of properties of resin.

Assessment/Interventions

- Obtain patient history, including drug history and any known allergies.
- Assess GI function. Use caution in elderly because of predisposition to fecal impaction.
- Assess electrolyte levels including sodium, potassium, calcium and magnesium.
- Use caution with patients who have tendencies toward hypernatremia or hypertension or who are receiving digitalis preparations.
- Assess vital signs each shift.
- Monitor serum potassium and sodium daily and observe for signs and symptoms of hypokalemia, including irritability, confusion, cardiac arrhythmias, ECG changes and muscle weakness.
- Observe for signs of sodium overload, such as edema.
- Closely monitor patients on sodium restriction.
- Monitor serum calcium levels. If deficient, patient may require supplements.
- Observe for changes in bowel function. Report to physician if patient becomes constipated.

OVERDOSAGE: SIGNS & SYMPTOMS

Nausea, vomiting, constipation (fecal impaction), hypokalemia, hypocalcemia, sodium retention

Patient/Family Education

- Tell patient not to mix medication with fruit juice.
- Instruct patient to shake bottle well before taking medication.
- Advise patient to report any water retention or edema.

- Instruct patient to report these symptoms to physician: anorexia, nausea, vomiting and any changes in bowel function.
- Tell patient not to take otc medications without consulting physician.

See Patient Guide, p. 566.

Somatrem

(so-muh-TREM)

Protropin

Class: Growth hormone

Action Mimics actions of naturally occurring growth hormone to stimulate linear and skeletal growth; increases number and size of muscle cells; increases RBC mass and internal organ size; increases cellular protein synthesis; reduces body fat stores and lipid mobilization; increases plasma fatty acids.

Indications Long-term treatment of children with growth failure caused by lack of adequate endogenous growth hormone secretion.

Contraindications Benzyl alcohol sensitivity; closed epiphyses; evidence of tumor activity; intracranial lesions must be inactive and antitumor therapy complete prior to instituting therapy.

Route/Dosage
CHILDREN: **SC/IM** Up to 0.1 mg/kg 3 times weekly.

Interactions
Glucocorticoids: May inhibit growth-promoting effects of somatrem.

Lab Test Interferences
None well documented.

Adverse Reactions
OTHER: Persistent antibodies to growth hormone.

Precautions
Pregnancy: Category C. *Lactation:* Undetermined. *Hypothyroidism:* May develop during therapy. *Insulin resistance:* May be induced with therapy. *Intracranial hypertension:* Intracranial hypertension with papilledema, visual changes, headache, nausea or vomiting has been reported in a few patients. *Intracranial lesion:* Frequently examine patient with history of intracranial lesion for progression or recurrence of lesion. *Slipped capital epiphysis:* May occur more frequently in patients treated with growth hormone.

NURSING CONSIDERATIONS

Administration/Storage

- Reconstitute with Bacteriostatic Water for Injection, USP (Benzyl Alcohol Preserved) only. Roll or swirl gently; do not shake.
- Use syringe small enough to permit accurate measurement of drug. Needle should be 1 inch or longer to ensure ability to reach muscle layer.
- Reconstitute with Water for Injection when administering to newborns. Use only one dose per vial. Discard unused portion.
- Rotate injection sites.
- Do not use if solution is cloudy.
- Store before and after reconstitution in the refrigerator. Store reconstituted drug in refrigerator for up to 14 days. Avoid freezing.

Assessment/Interventions

- Obtain patient history, including drug history and any known allergies. Determine if epiphyses are closed and if intracranial lesions and tumor activity are present.
- Examine patients with intracranial lesions frequently to make sure that the lesions are not active.
- Check thyroid function periodically to detect possible hypothyroidism.
- Monitor for signs of acromegaly and report to physician.

- Monitor for glucose intolerance; insulin resistance may develop.
- Monitor patient's growth.
- Observe for common side effects of headache, weakness, localized muscle pain or mild transient edema and report to physician.
- Notify physician of any limp or complaints of hip or knee pain in children; these symptoms indicate slipped capital femoral epiphyses.

OVERDOSAGE: SIGNS & SYMPTOMS
Hypoglycemia, hyperglycemia, acromegaly

Patient/Family Education

- Instruct diabetic patient to monitor blood sugars closely and to report variations to physician.
- Teach children and parents to report any limp or complaints of hip or knee pain to physician as soon as possible.
- Instruct patient to report these symptoms to physician: headache, weakness, localized muscle pain or mild transient edema.

See Patient Guide, p. 567.

Somatropin

(SO-muh-TROE-pin)
Humatrope, Nutropin
Class: Growth hormone

Action Mimics actions of naturally occurring growth hormone to stimulate linear and skeletal growth; increases number and size of skeletal muscle cells; increases RBC mass and internal organ size; increases cellular protein synthesis; reduces body fat stores and lipid mobilization and increases plasma fatty acids.

Indications Long-term treatment of children with growth failure caused by lack of adequate endogenous growth hormone secretion. Nutropin is used for treatment of children with growth failure associated with chronic renal insufficiency up to time of renal transplantation.

Contraindications Closed epiphyses; evidence of tumor activity, or active neoplasm; intracranial lesion must be inactive and antitumor therapy complete prior to instituting therapy; sensitivity to benzyl alcohol (Nutropin diluent) glycerin or M-cresol (Humatrope diluent).

Route/Dosage

Growth Hormone Inadequacy

CHILDREN: *(Humatrope)* **IM/SC** 0.06 mg/kg 3 times/wk. *(Nutropin)* **SC** 0.03 mg/kg daily.

Chronic Insufficiency

CHILDREN: *(Nutropin)* **SC** 0.035 mg/kg daily.

Interactions

Glucocorticoids: May inhibit growth promoting effects of somatropin.

Lab Test Interferences

None well documented.

Adverse Reactions

CNS: Headache; weakness; recurrent growth of intracranial tumor. *GU:* Glucosuria; hypercalciuria. *DERM:* Rash; urticaria; pain; inflammation at injection site. *META:* Hypothyroidism; hyperglycemia. *OTHER:* Localized muscle pain; mild, transient edema; antibodies to growth hormone.

Precautions

Pregnancy: Category C. *Lactation:* Undetermined. *Concomitant glucocorticoid therapy:* May inhibit growth-promoting effects. *Hypothyroidism:* May develop during therapy; monitor thyroid function. *Insulin resistance:* May be induced with therapy; monitor for glucose intolerance. *Intracranial hypertension:* Intracranial hypertension, with papilledema, visual changes, headache, nausea or vomiting has been reported in few patients. *Intracranial lesion:* Frequently examine patients with history of lesion. *Slipped capital epiphysis:* May be seen in children with advanced renal osteodystrophy; may be affected by growth hormone. Be alert to development of limp or complaints of hip or knee pain.

NURSING CONSIDERATIONS

Administration/Storage

- Reconstitute each 5 mg vial with 1 to 5 ml or each 10 mg vial with 1 to 10 ml of Bacteriostatic Water for Injection, USP (benzyl alcohol preserved) only.
- Store before and after administration in refrigerator. Use reconstituted drug within 14 days; refrigerate until used; avoid freezing.
- In patients with sensitivity to m-cresol, glycerin or benzyl alcohol reconstitute with Sterile Water for Injection; use reconstituted dose within 24 hours; refrigerate until used; do not freeze; use only 1 dose per vial; discard unused portion.

Assessment/Interventions

- Obtain patient history, including drug history and any known allergies.
- Be aware that use of product with glucocorticoid therapy may inhibit growth-promoting effects.
- Examine patients with history of intracranial lesion frequently for evidence of recurrence or progression of lesion.
- Monitor thyroid function test results.
- Be aware that insulin resistance may develop and monitor for signs of glucose intolerance.
- Be alert for signs of acromegaly and report to physician.
- Assess for common side effects of headache, weakness, localized muscle pain or transient edema and report to physician.
- Report any limp or complaints of hip or knee pain in children to physician; this may indicate slipped epiphyses.

OVERDOSAGE: SIGNS & SYMPTOMS

Overdosage: Hypoglycemia followed by hyperglycemia. Chronic overdosage: Acromegaly

Patient/Family Education

- Instruct diabetic patients to monitor blood sugar closely and to report variations to physician.
- Tell children and parents to report limp or complaints of hip or knee pain to physician as soon as possible.
- Instruct patient to report these symptoms to physician: headache, weakness, localized muscle pain or mild, transient edema.

See Patient Guide, p. 568.

Sotalol HCl

(SOTT-uh-lahl HIGH-droe-KLOR-ide)

Betapace

Class: Beta-adrenergic blocker

Action Blocks beta receptors, which primarily affects heart (slows rate), vascular musculature (decreases blood pressure) and lungs (reduces function).

Indications Management or prevention of life-threatening ventricular arrhythmias.

Contraindications Hypersensitivity to beta-blockers; greater than first-degree heart block; CHF unless secondary to tachyarrhythmia treatable with beta-blockers; overt cardiac failure; sinus bradycardia; cardiogenic shock; bronchial asthma or bronchospasm, including severe COPD; congenital or acquired long QT syndromes.

Route/Dosage

Ventricular Arrhythmias

ADULTS: PO 80 mg bid; may increase up to 320 mg/day given in 2 or 3 divided doses.

Interactions

Amiodarone, disopyramide, procainamide, quinidine: May prolong cardiac refractoriness. *Calcium channel blockers:* Increase risk of hypotension; possible increased effect on atrioventricular conduction or ventricular function. *Clonidine:* May enhance or reverse antihypertensive effects; may enhance clonidine rebound hypertension. *Guanethidine, reserpine:* Increase hypotension or bradycardia. *Insulin, oral sulfonylurea hypoglycemic agents:* Hyperglycemia; symptoms of hypoglycemia may be masked. *NSAIDS:* Some agents may impair antihypertensive effect.

Lab Test Interferences

May interfere with glucose or insulin tolerance tests.

Adverse Reactions

CV: Arrhythmias; torsade de pointes; sustained ventricular tachycardia or fibrillation. *RESP:* Wheezing; bronchospasm; difficulty breathing. *CNS:* Depression; dizziness; lethargy; vivid dreams; depression; paresthesias; headache. *GI:* Nausea; vomiting; diarrhea; flatulence; dry mouth; constipation; anorexia; dyspepsia. *GU:* Impotence; decreased libido; dysuria; urinary tract infection; nocturia; urinary retention or frequency. *HEPA:* Elevated liver enzymes. *DERM:* Rash. *META:* May increase or decrease blood glucose.

Precautions

Pregnancy: Category B. *Lactation:* Excreted in breast milk. *Children:* Safety and efficacy not established. *Abrupt withdrawal:* Has been associated with adverse effects; gradually decrease dose over 1-2 wk. *Anaphylaxis:* Deaths have occurred; aggressive therapy may be required. *CHF:* Administer cautiously in patients CHF controlled by digitalis and diuretics. *Diabetic patients:* Drug may mask signs and symptoms of hypoglycemia (eg, tachycardia, BP changes). Drug may potentiate insulin-induced hypoglycemia. *Nonallergic bronchospasm:* Give drug with caution in patients with bronchospastic disease. *Peripheral vascular disease:* May precipitate or aggravate symptoms of atrial insufficiency. *Proarrhythmia:* May provoke new or worsened arrhythmias. Correct hypokalemia or hypomagnesemia before administering sotalol. Anticipate proarrhythmic events with initial dose and with every dose adjustment. *Renal/hepatic function impairment:* Alteration of dosage interval and reduced daily dose are advised. *Thyrotoxicosis:* May mask clinical signs, eg, tachycardia, of developing or continuing hyperthyroidism. Abrupt withdrawal may exacerbate symptoms of hyperthyroidism, including thyroid storm.

NURSING CONSIDERATIONS

Administration/Storage

- Adjust dosage gradually to attain steady-state plasma concentrations.
- Before initiating therapy, carefully monitor response to withdrawal of previous antiarrhythmic therapy.
- Give on empty stomach.
- Store at room temperature.

Assessment/Interventions

- Obtain patient history, including drug history and any known allergies.
- Obtain complete cardiac assessment prior to initiation of therapy.
- Closely monitor patient during initiation of therapy and with each dosage change.
- Monitor pulse and BP, ECG and heart rate and rhythm routinely.
- Monitor potassium, magnesium and glucose levels routinely.
- Assess apical pulse and blood pressure prior to each dose.
- If you detect extremes in pulse rates, withhold medication and call physician immediately.
- Notify physician immediately of any signs of CHF or of any unexplained respiratory symptoms.

OVERDOSAGE: SIGNS & SYMPTOMS

Bradycardia, CHF, hypotension, bronchospasm, prolongation of QT interval, torsade de pointes, ventricular tachycardia, premature ventricular complexes, hypoglycemia

Patient/Family Education

- Explain importance of not discontinuing drug suddenly, and advise that dosage will be decreased over 1-2 weeks.
- Explain that drug may mask signs and symptoms of hypoglycemia.
- Teach patient to take pulse daily and to notify physician if pulse drops below 60.
- Tell patient to call physician if adverse reaction occurs.
- Instruct patient not to take otc medications without consulting physician.

See Patient Guide, p. 569.

Spironolactone

(SPEER-oh-no-LAK-tone)

Aldactone, ♣ *Novo-Spiroton, Novo-Spirozine*

Class: Potassium-sparing diuretic

Action Competitively inhibits aldosterone in distal tubules, resulting in increased excretion of sodium and water and decreased excretion of potassium.

Indications Short-term preoperative treatment of primary hyperaldosteronism; long-term maintenance therapy for idiopathic hyperaldosteronism; management of edematous conditions in CHF, cirrhosis of liver and nephrotic syndrome; management of essential hypertension; treatment of hypokalemia. **Unlabeled uses:** Treatment of hirsutism; relief of PMS symptoms; short-term treatment of familial male precocious puberty; and short-term treatment of acne vulgaris.

Contraindications Anuria; acute renal insufficiency; impaired renal excretory function; hyperkalemia.

Route/Dosage

Diagnosis of Primary Hyperaldosteronism

ADULTS: **PO** 400 mg/day for 4 days (short test) or 3-4 wk (long test).

Maintenance Therapy for Hyperaldosteronism

ADULTS: **PO** 100-400 mg daily in single or divided doses.

Edema

ADULTS: **PO** 25-200 mg/day in single or divided doses. CHILDREN: **PO** 3.3 mg/kg/day in single or divided doses.

Essential Hypertension

ADULTS: **PO** 50-100 mg/day in single or divided doses. CHILDREN: **PO** 1-2 mg/kg bid.

Diuretic-Induced Hypokalemia

ADULTS: **PO** 25-100 mg/day when oral potassium or other potassium-sparing regimens are inappropriate.

Interactions

ACE inhibitors: May result in severely elevated serum potassium levels. *Digitalis glycosides:* May decrease digoxin clearance, resulting in increased serum digoxin levels and toxicity; may attenuate inotropic action of digoxin. *Mitotane:* May decrease therapeutic response to mitotane. *Potassium preparations:* May severely increase serum potassium levels, possibly resulting in cardiac arrhythmias or cardiac arrest. Do not take with potassium preparations. *Salicylates:* May result in decreased diuretic effect.

Lab Test Interferences

Drug may cause falsely elevated serum digoxin values with radioimmunoassay (assay specific) for measuring digoxin.

Adverse Reactions

CNS: Drowsiness; lethargy; headache; mental confusion; ataxia. *GI:* Cramping; diarrhea; gastric bleeding; gastric ulceration; gastritis; vomiting. *GU:* Inability to achieve or maintain erection. *HEMA:* Agranulocytosis. *DERM:* Maculopapular or erythematous cutaneous eruptions; urticaria. *META:* Hyperchloremic metabolic acidosis in decompensated hepatic cirrhosis. *OTHER:* Gynecomastia; irregular menses or amenorrhea; postmenopausal bleeding; hirsutism; deepening of voice; drug fever; carcinoma of breast.

Precautions

Pregnancy: Category D. *Lactation:* Excreted in breast milk. *Electrolyte imbalances and BUN increase:* Hyperkalemia (serum potassium > 5.5 mEq/L), hyponatremia, hypochloremia and increases in BUN may occur.

NURSING CONSIDERATIONS

Administration/Storage

- If single dose is prescribed, administer in morning.
- Take medication with food.
- May crush tablets and administer as suspension.
- Suspension is stable for 30 days under refrigeration. Protect from light.
- Store tablets at room temperature.

Assessment/Interventions

- Obtain patient history, including drug history and any known allergies.
- Assess fluid and electrolyte status prior to therapy.
- Monitor potassium levels. If level is > 5.5 mEq/L, withhold medication and notify physician.
- Monitor serum electrolytes, I&O, weight and BP daily.
- Monitor ABGs, liver and renal function studies.
- If deep rapid respirations or headaches develop, notify physician.
- Assess urinary status. If patient develops frequency, dysuria, edema or reduced urinary output, notify physician.
- Assess for any changes in hepatic status. If patient appears jaundiced and mentally confused, notify physician.
- If nausea, vomiting, distention, diarrhea or anorexia occur, notify physician.
- Note any changes in neurologic status. If drowsiness, ataxia, lethargy, confusion or headache occurs, notify physician.

OVERDOSAGE: SIGNS & SYMPTOMS

Electrolyte imbalance

Patient/Family Education

- Explain that medication's full diuretic effect may not be achieved for 1-2 wk.
- Instruct patient to avoid large quantities of potassium-rich foods or potassium salt substitutes.
- For patient being treated for hypertension, explain that patient may feel tired for several weeks because body needs to adjust to lowered BP.
- Instruct patient to take drug with food to minimize GI irritation.
- Tell patient to weigh self twice weekly and to notify physician of any increase.
- Instruct patient to notify physician if new symptoms develop.
- Tell patient to report these symptoms to physician: GI cramping, diarrhea, lethargy, thirst, headache, skin rash, menstrual abnormalities, deepening of voice and breast enlargement in men.
- Advise patient that drug may cause drowsiness and to use caution while driving or performing other tasks requiring mental alertness.
- Instruct patient not to take prescription or otc medications without consulting physician.

See Patient Guide, p. 570.

Streptokinase

(strep-toe-KYE-nase)
Kabikinase
Class: Thrombolytic enzyme

Action Acts with plasminogen to convert plasminogen to proteolytic enzyme plasmin, which degrades fibrin clots, fibrinogen and other plasma proteins.

Indications Treatment of acute evolving transmural MI; treatment of deep vein thrombosis, arterial thrombosis and embolism; clearance of occluded arteriovenous cannulae.

Contraindications Active internal bleeding; recent cerebrovascular accident; intracranial or intraspinal surgery; intracranial neoplasm; severe uncontrolled hypertension.

Route/Dosage
ADULTS: **IV** 20,000-1,500,000 IU.

Interactions
Anticoagulants, antiplatelet agents: Increase risk of bleeding complications.

INCOMPATIBILITIES: Do not add other medications to streptokinase.

Lab Test Interferences
May decrease plasminogen and fibrinogen; increases TT, APTT and PT.

Adverse Reactions
HEMA: Minor and major bleeding. *OTHER:* Allergy (eg, minor breathing difficulty, bronchospasm, periorbital swelling, angioneurotic edema, urticaria, itching, flushing, nausea, headache, musculoskeletal pain); delayed hypersensitivity (eg, vasculitis, interstitial nephritis); fever; Guillain-Barré syndrome.

Precautions
Pregnancy: Category C. *Lactation:* Undetermined. *Children:* Safety and efficacy not established. *Arrhythmias:* Rapid lysis of coronary thrombi may cause atrial or ventricular arrhythmias. *Hypersensitivity:* Anaphylactic and anaphylactoid reactions may occur. *Noncardiogenic pulmonary edema:* Increased risk in patients experiencing large MIs and undergoing intracoronary thrombolytic therapy. *Severe hypotension:* May occur.

NURSING CONSIDERATIONS

Administration/Storage
Acute Myocardial Infarction

- IV infusion: Administer as soon as possible after symptom onset. Use 1,500,000 IU vial diluted to volume of 45 ml. Administer total dose within 60 min.
- Note that IM injection is contraindicated.
- Intracoronary infusion: Use 250,000 IU vial diluted to total volume of 125 ml. Administer 20,000 IU (10 ml) by bolus followed by 2000 IU/min for 60 min (60 ml/hr) for total dose of 140,000 IU.
- Store at room temperature.

Pulmonary Embolism, Deep Vein Thrombosis, Arterial Thrombosis or Embolism

- IV infusion: Use 1,500,000 vial diluted to total volume of 90 ml. Institute treatment as soon as possible after onset of thrombotic event. Follow with 100,000 IU/hr (6 ml/hr) for 24-72 hr for arterial thrombosis or embolism, 72 hr for deep vein thrombosis and 24 hr for pulmonary embolism. If TT after 4 hr of therapy is not significantly different from control, discontinue infusion.
- Intracoronary infusion: Use 1,500,000 infusion bottle diluted to volume of 45 ml and infuse at 15 ml/hr for 30 min, followed by 3 ml/hr.
- Continuous IV infusion of heparin has been recommended after termination of streptokinase infusion for

treatment of pulmonary embolism or deep vein thrombosis.

Arteriovenous Cannulae Occlusion

- Instill 250,000 IU in 2 ml solution into each occluded limb of cannula slowly and clamp cannula limb(s) for 2 hr. Then aspirate contents of infused cannula limb(s), flush with saline solution, reconnect cannula.

Reconstitution/Dilution

- Slowly add 5 ml Sodium Chloride or Dextrose 5% Injection into vial or bottle, directing diluent at side of bottle or vial. Roll and tilt gently. Do not shake. Store unopened vials at controlled room temperature.
- Reconstitute immediately before use. Solution may be used within 8 hr of reconstitution if refrigerated. Discard unused reconstituted drug. Do not add other medication to streptokinase. Use electronic infusion device to administer streptokinase.
- If patient has had recent streptococcal infection or recent treatment with streptokinase, a higher loading dose may be necessary.
- Have emergency drugs, including packed RBCs and plasma expanders, and equipment available. Also have corticosteroids and aminocaproic acid available in case excessive bleeding occurs.

Assessment/Interventions

- Obtain patient history, including drug history and any known allergies. Evaluate history of bleeding tendencies.
- Complete baseline bleeding studies, type and crossmatch prior to initiation of therapy.
- Maintain involved extremity in straight alignment to prevent bleeding from infusion site.
- Avoid unnecessary venipunctures; use pressure dressing on puncture sites for at least 15 min.
- Avoid unnecessary handling of patient to prevent bruising.
- Monitor for arrhythmias during and immediately after intracoronary administration.
- Monitor patient for excessive bleeding q 15 min for 1 hr, q 30 min for 2-8 hr, then once every shift.
- Monitor TT q 4-12 hr.
- Assess pulses, color and sensation of extremities q hr.
- Monitor vital signs frequently.
- If bleeding occurs, withhold therapy and notify physician.
- Observe for hypersensitivity. If hypersensitivity occurs, notify physician immediately.

OVERDOSAGE: SIGNS & SYMPTOMS

Bleeding

Patient/Family Education

- Advise patient and family to avoid excessive handling of patient to prevent bruising.
- Instruct patient to report these symptoms to physician: bleeding, bruising, dyspnea and hypersensitivity reactions.

No patient monograph available.

Streptozocin

(STREP-toe-ZOE-sin)

Zanosar

Class: Antineoplastic/alkylator

Action Inhibits DNA synthesis. Cell cycle nonspecific.

Indications Treatment of symptomatic or progressive metastatic islet cell carcinoma of pancreas.

Contraindications Concomitant administration of other potential nephrotoxins.

Route/Dosage

ADULTS: **IV** May be given daily at dose of 500 mg/m^2 of body surface area (BSA) for 5 consecutive days q 6 weeks or at initial dose of 1000 mg/m^2 BSA q wk for first 2 wk. Monitor for favorable response or signs of toxicity.

When given weekly, subsequent courses of therapy may be increased but not to exceed single dose of 1500 mg/m^2 BSA.

Interactions

Nephrotoxic drugs (eg, gentamicin): Increased risk of nephrotoxicity.

Lab Test Interferences

None well documented.

Adverse Reactions

CNS: Confusion; lethargy; depression. *GI:* Nausea; vomiting; diarrhea. *HEPA:* Hepatotoxicity; hypoalbuminemia. *GU:* Dose-related, cumulative renal toxicity with azotemia; anuria; hypophosphatemia; glycosuria; renal tubular acidosis; nephrogenic diabetes insipidus. *HEMA:* Decreased hematocrit; reduced leukocyte and platelet counts. *META:* Abnormal glucose tolerance; insulin shock with hypoglycemia. *OTHER:* Tissue damage caused by extravasation; burning after IV injection.

Precautions

Pregnancy: Category C. *Lactation:* Undetermined. *Monitoring:* Perform CBCs and liver function tests at least weekly. Obtain serial urinalysis, BUN, plasma creatinine, serum electrolytes and creatinine clearance prior to treatment and then at least weekly during and for 4 weeks after drug administration to determine potential renal toxicity. *Renal toxcity:* Common in patients receiving streptozocin; dose-related and cumulative and may be severe or fatal. Reduce dose or discontinue drug in presence of significant renal toxicity. Determine risk-benefit in patients with pre-existing renal disease. Do not use with other known nephrotoxins. *Topical exposure:* Dermal exposure may pose carcinogenic hazard. Use caution in handling (ie, gloves); immediately wash affected areas after exposure.

NURSING CONSIDERATIONS

Administration/Storage

- Give antiemetic 30-60 min before administering drug.
- Reconstitute with 9.5 ml of Dextrose Injection or 0.9% Sodium Chloride Injection. Solution will appear pale gold in color. May be further diluted in 50-250 ml. May be given directly over 5-15 min.
- Do not mix with any other drug.
- Exercise caution and wear gloves when preparing solution. If powder or solution contacts skin or mucosa, immediately wash affected area with soap and water.
- Limit handling and preparation of product to individuals who have been trained in preparation of chemotherapeutic agents.
- Store reconstituted Streptozocin no longer than 12 hr because of lack of preservative; however, drug will remain stable for at least 48 hr at room temperature or 96 hr if refrigerated.
- Refrigerate unopened vials and protect from light.

Assessment/Interventions

- Obtain patient history, including drug history and any known allergies.
- Assess injection site for signs of irritation and extravasation.
- Assess urinalysis, BUN, creatinine, serum electrolytes and creatinine clearance before therapy begins and monitor weekly during therapy and for 4 weeks after each course of therapy.
- Monitor intake and output each shift. Encourage several liters of fluids per day. If output decreases, suspect renal toxicity and notify physician.
- Test urine for protein each shift. If mild proteinuria exists, suspect renal toxicity. Notify physician immediately. If proteinuria is determined, start 24-hr quantitative urine collection.
- Use serial monitoring of fasting insu-

lin levels to determine biochemical response to therapy.
- If nausea and vomiting occur, ensure patient is being treated with antiemetic.
- Perform finger sticks or test urine for glucose daily and observe for symptoms of hypoglycemia.
- Institute neutropenic precautions if WBC levels are low.

OVERDOSAGE: SIGNS & SYMPTOMS
Nausea, vomiting, renal toxicity

Patient/Family Education
- Explain reason for avoiding otc products containing aspirin.
- Explain that nausea and vomiting occur in almost all patients. Advise patient to follow dietary regimen, reduce activity and take antiemetic as prescribed.
- Instruct patient to report these symptoms to physician: anemia or bleeding (bruising, bleeding gums, melena) and infection (fatigue, fever).

See Patient Guide, p. 572.

Sucralfate

(sue-KRAL-fate)

Carafate, *Sulcrate*

Class: Gastrointestinal

Action Adheres to ulcer in acidic gastric juice, forming protective layer that serves as barrier against acid, bile salts and enzymes present in stomach and duodenum.

Indications Short-term treatment of duodenal ulcer; maintenance therapy of duodenal ulcer. **Unlabeled uses:** Treatment of gastric ulcers; reflux and peptic esophagitis; treatment of NSAID- or aspirin-induced GI symptoms and mucosal damage; prevention of stress ulcers and GI bleeding in critically ill patients; treatment of oral and esophageal ulcers caused by radiation, chemotherapy and sclerotherapy; treatment of oral ulcerations and dysphagia in patients with epidermolysis bullosa.

Contraindications Standard considerations.

Route/Dosage
Active Duodenal Ulcer
ADULTS: **PO** 1 g qid on empty stomach (1 hr before meals and at bedtime) for 4-8 wk. Maintenance: 1 g bid.

Interactions
Aluminum containing antacids: May increase total body burden of aluminum. *Cimetidine, ciprofloxacin (and other quinolone antibiotics), digoxin, hydantoins (eg, phenytoin), ketoconazole, pencillamine, ranitidine, tetracycline, theophylline:* Oral absorption and pharmacologic action of these agents may be reduced if given with sucralfate. Administer 2 hr apart from sucralfate.

Lab Test Interferences
None well documented.

Adverse Reactions
CNS: Dizziness; insomnia; vertigo; headache. *GI:* Constipation; diarrhea; nausea; vomiting; dry mouth; indigestion; flatulence. *DERM:* Rash; pruritus. *OTHER:* Back pain.

Precautions
Pregnancy: Category B. *Lactation:* Undetermined. *Children:* Safety and efficacy not established. *Chronic renal failure/dialysis:* Small amounts of aluminum may be absorbed from sucralfate, and concomitant use of other aluminum containing products may increase total body burden of aluminum. Aluminum is not removed by dialysis and excretion through kidneys is impaired in patients with chronic renal failure. Aluminum accumulation and toxicity (eg, aluminum osteodystrophy, osteomalacia, encephalopathy) have occurred.

NURSING CONSIDERATIONS

Administration/Storage

- Administer with glass of water, on empty stomach, at least 1 hr before meals and at bedtime (maintenance therapy may be twice daily).
- Administer other medications 2 hr before or after giving sucralfate to minimize effect on absorption.
- Do not administer antacids within ½ hr of giving this drug.
- Use with caution in patients with chronic renal failure; avoid concomitant use of other products containing aluminum (eg, some antacids).
- Store at room temperature.

Assessment/Interventions

- Obtain patient history, including drug history and any known allergies.
- Report constipation, diarrhea, nausea, rash, pruritus or other side effects to physician.
- Observe for signs of GI bleeding or GI distress and report to physician.
- Be alert to possibility of aluminum accumulation and toxicity in patients with chronic renal failure (evidenced by drowsiness and seizures); excretion of aluminum through kidneys will be impaired and aluminum is not removed by dialysis.

Patient/Family Education

- Caution patient not to crush or chew tablets.
- Tell patient to take with glass of water, on empty stomach at least 1 hr before meals.
- If patient is taking other medications, instruct patient to take these drugs 2 hr before or after taking sucralfate, if possible.
- Instruct patient to use antacids only with physician permission and not to use within ½ hr of taking this drug.
- Advise patient to consult physician or pharmacist before taking any other medication (including over the counter).
- Explain that increase in fluid and fiber intake, and exercise may prevent drug-induced constipation.
- Instruct patient to report these symptoms to physician: drowsiness, constipation, diarrhea, nausea, rash, pruritus or other side effects (including signs of GI bleeding).

See Patient Guide, p. 573.

Sufentanil Citrate

(sue-FEN-tuh-nill SIH-trate)

Sufenta

Class: Narcotic analgesic

Action Relieves pain by stimulating opiate receptors in CNS; causes respiratory depression, peripheral vasodilation, inhibition of intestinal peristalsis, sphincter of Oddi spasm, stimulation of chemoreceptors that cause vomiting and increased bladder tone.

Indications Adjunct for surgical analgesia; induction of primary anesthesia for major surgical procedures requiring favorable myocardial or cerebral oxygen balance or when extended postoperative ventilation is anticipated; epidural analgesia with bupivacaine during labor and vaginal delivery.

Contraindications Upper airway obstruction; acute asthma; diarrhea caused by poisoning or toxins.

Route/Dosage

General Surgery (with Nitrous Oxide/Oxygen)

ADULTS: IV 1-2 mcg/kg initially; 10-25 mcg prn for maintenance.

Major Surgical Procedures (with Nitrous Oxide/Oxygen)

ADULTS: IV 2-8 mcg/kg initially; 10-50 mcg prn for maintenance.

Major Cardiovascular Surgery/Neurosurgery (with 100% Oxygen)
ADULTS: **IV** 8-30 mcg/kg initially; 25-50 mcg prn for maintenance. CHILDREN < 12 YR: **IV** 10-25 mcg/kg initially; 25-50 mcg prn for maintenance.

Labor and Delivery
ADULTS: **Epidural** 10-15 mcg sufentanil mixed with 10 ml bupivacaine 0.125% with or without epinephrine. Can give total of 3 doses ≥ 1 hr intervals until delivery.

Interactions

Barbiturate anesthetics: May cause increased CNS and respiratory depression.

Lab Test Interferences

Increased amylase and lipase for up to 24 hr after dose may occur.

Adverse Reactions

CV: Hypotension; orthostatic hypotension; hypertension; bradycardia; tachycardia; arrhythmias. *RESP:* Bronchospasm; depression of cough reflex; respiratory depression; postoperative respiratory depression; chest wall rigidity. *CNS:* Sedation. *GI:* Nausea; vomiting. *DERM:* Pruritus. *OTHER:* Chills; intraoperative muscle movement; tolerance.

Precautions

Pregnancy: Category C. *Lactation:* Undetermined. *Children:* Safety and efficacy have been demonstrated in limited number of children < 2 yr undergoing cardiovascular surgery. *Elderly or debilitated patients:* May require dosage reduction. *Special risk patients:* Use drug with caution in patients with decreased respiratory reserve, head injury or increased intracranial pressure or hypoxia. *Drug dependence:* Has abuse potential. *Hypoventilation:* Naloxone and intubation equipment must be available in case hypoventilation occurs. *Obese patients:* If patient is > 20% above ideal weight, dose must be adjusted based on ideal body weight. *Renal or hepatic impairment:* Duration of action may be prolonged; dosage reduction may be required.

NURSING CONSIDERATIONS

Administration/Storage

- For direct IV administration, administer slowly over 1-2 min.
- Store at room temperature. Protect from light.

Assessment/Interventions

- Obtain patient history, including drug history and any known allergies.
- Assess patient for head injury, pulmonary disease or decreased respiratory reserve.
- Maintain narcotic antagonist and resuscitative equipment at bedside.
- Monitor respiratory rate and BP closely during administration.
- Observe for evidence of effective induction of anesthesia.
- Monitor vital signs at frequent intervals postoperatively.

OVERDOSAGE: SIGNS & SYMPTOMS

Miosis, respiratory and CNS depression, circulatory collapse, seizures, cardiopulmonary arrest, death

Patient/Family Education

- Inform patient that nausea, vomiting or constipation may occur and advise patient to notify physician should these symptoms become prominent.
- Advise patient to ask for assistance with ambulation.
- Instruct patient to report these symptoms to physician: shortness of breath or difficulty breathing.
- Caution patient to avoid sudden position changes to prevent orthostatic hypotension.

No patient monograph available.

Sulfasalazine

(SULL-fuh-SAL-uh-zeen)

Azulfidine, Azulfidine EN-tabs, ♣ *S.A.A.-500, Salazopyrin, Salazopyrin Desensitizing Kit, Salazopyrin EN-Tabs, S.A.S. Enteric-500*

Class: Anti-infective/sulfonamide

Action Competitively antagonizes PABA, an essential component in folic acid synthesis.

Indications Treatment of ulcerative colitis. **Unlabeled uses:** Treatment of ankylosing spondylitis, collagenous colitis, Crohn's disease, rheumatoid arthritis.

Contraindications Hypersensitivity to sulfonamides or chemically related drugs (eg, sulfonylureas, thiazide and loop diuretics, carbonic anhydrase inhibitors, sunscreens containing PABA, local anesthetics); pregnancy at term; lactation; infants < 2 mo; porphyria; hypersensitivity to salicylates; intestinal or urinary obstruction.

Route/Dosage

ADULTS: **PO** 3-4 g/day in evenly divided doses. More than 4 g/day is associated with higher incidence of side effects. May begin with 1-2 g/day to lessen GI effects. Maintenance: **PO** 2 g/day in four divided doses. CHILDREN > 2 YEARS: **PO** 40-60 mg/kg/24 hr initially in 4-6 divided doses. Maintenance: **PO** 20-30 mg/kg/day in 4 divided doses. Maximum 2 g/day.

Interactions

Folic acid: Signs of folate deficiency have occurred, but specific symptoms related to deficiency have not been reported. *Methotrexate:* Risk of methotrexate-induced bone marrow suppression may be enhanced. *Sulfonylureas:* Increased sulfonylurea half-lives and hypoglycemia have occurred.

Lab Test Interferences

May produce false-positive urinary glucose tests when performed by Benedict's method.

Adverse Reactions

RESP: Pulmonary infiltrates. *CNS:* Headache; insomnia; peripheral neuropathy; depression; convulsions. *GI:* Nausea; vomiting; abdominal pain; diarrhea; anorexia; pancreatitis; impaired folic acid absorption; pseudomembranous enterocolitis. *GU:* Orange-yellow urine; crystalluria; hematuria; proteinuria; elevated creatinine; nephrotic syndrome; toxic nephrosis with oliguria and anuria. *HEMA:* Agranulocytosis; aplastic anemia; thrombocytopenia; leukopenia; hemolytic anemia; purpura; hypoprothrombinemia; methemoglobinemia; megaloblastic (macrocytic) anemia; Heinz body anemia. *HEPA:* Hepatitis; hepatocellular necrosis. *DERM:* Orange-yellow discoloration of skin. *OTHER:* Drug fever; chills; pyrexia; arthralgia; myalgia; periarteritis nodosum; lupus erythematosus phenomenon. *Hypersensitivity reactions:* May present as erythema multiforme of Stevens-Johnson type; generalized skin eruptions; allergic myocarditis; epidermal necrolysis, with or without corneal damage; urticaria; serum sickness; pruritus; exfoliative dermatitis; anaphylactoid reactions; periorbital edema; photosensitization; arthralgia; transient pulmonary changes with eosinophilia and decreased pulmonary function.

Precautions

Pregnancy: Category B. *Lactation:* Excreted in breast milk. *Children:* Do not use in infants < 2 mo. *Allergy or asthma:* Use drug with caution in patients with severe allergy or bronchial asthma. Hemolytic anemia may occur in G-6-PD deficient individuals. *Contact lenses:* May permanently stain soft contact lenses yellow. *Porphyria:* May precipitate acute attack of porphyria. *Renal or hepatic impairment:* Use drug with caution in renal or hepatic function impairment. *Severe reactions:* Reactions, including deaths, have been associated with hypersensitivity reactions, agranulocytosis, aplastic anemia, other blood dyscrasias and renal and hepatic damage. Irreversible neuromuscular and CNS changes and fibrosing alveolitis may occur. *Sulfonamides:* Bear chemical similarities to some goitrogens, diuretics (acetazolamide and thiazides) and oral hypoglycemic agents. Goiter production, diuresis, and hypoglycemic have occurred rarely in patients receiving sulfonamides. Cross-sensitivity may exist.

NURSING CONSIDERATIONS

Administration/Storage

- Have resuscitative equipment readily available during administration.
- Give after meals or with food (to minimize GI irritation and prolong intestinal passage). Administer around clock (q 6-8 hr) in evenly spaced doses.
- Give each dose with full glass of water; encourage fluids between meals up to 2000 ml/day (to maintain hydration and decrease crystallization in kidneys).
- Do not allow patient to chew or crush enteric-coated tablet.
- Shake oral suspension well prior to administration; measure dose accurately with calibrated device.
- Store tables in tight, light-resistant container at room temperature; refrigerate suspension after opening and discard unused portion after 14 days.

Assessment/Interventions

- Obtain patient history, including drug history and any known allergies.
- Assess results of CBC, hepatic function and renal function studies (BUN, creatinine, urinalysis) prior to and during therapy if on long-term regimen.
- Assess stool pattern (frequency, consistency [dose increased if diarrhea recurs/continues] and quantity) and document abdominal pain prior to and during therapy; sigmoidoscopy and proctoscopy may be used to verify response or adjust dosage.
- Monitor I&O; note urine color, pH and character (high urine acidity may require alkalinization).
- Assess skin for rash, bleeding, bruising, jaundice; note fever, sore throat, mouth sores or joint pain. Report any of these symptoms to physician (may require medication discontinued).

OVERDOSAGE: SIGNS & SYMPTOMS

Anuria, nausea, vomiting, gastric distress, drowsiness, seizures

Patient/Family Education

- Advise patient to take with or after meals if GI intolerance occurs.
- Instruct patient and family to adhere to around the clock schedule as directed. Explain that if dose is missed, patient should take it as soon as remembered. Emphasize that patient should not double up doses.
- Tell patient to notify other physicians/dentist of therapy prior to other treatments/surgery.
- Explain that medication may cause urine and skin to have yellow-orange discoloration (expected effect) and that may permanently stain soft contact lenses yellow.
- Encourage medical followup to ensure success of therapy and to evaluate continuing symptoms.
- Advise patient to take each oral dose with full glass of water to prevent crystalluria.
- Instruct patient to report these symptoms to physician immediately: difficulty breathing, skin rash, fever, chills, mouth sores, sore throat, ringing in ears or unusual bleeding/bruising.
- Advise patient that drug may cause dizziness and to use caution while driving or performing other activities requiring mental alertness.
- Caution patient to avoid exposure to sunlight and to wear protective clothing or use sunscreen to avoid photosensitivity reaction.

- Instruct patient not to take otc medications (even vitamins) without consulting physician.

See Patient Guide, p. 574.

Sulfinpyrazone

(sull-fin-PEER-uh-zone)

Anturane, ✤ *Novo-Pyrazone*

Class: Uricosuric/gout

Action Potent uricosuric agent that inhibits renal tubular reabsorption of uric acid and reduces renal tubular secretion of other organic anions; possesses antithrombotic and platelet-inhibiting effects.

Indications Treatment of chronic and intermittent gouty arthritis. Not intended for relief of acute attack of gout. **Unlabeled uses:** Post MI treatment (within 1-6 mo of acute MI) to decrease incidence of sudden cardiac death. May also be used to reduce frequency of systemic embolism in rheumatic mitral stenosis.

Contraindications Active peptic ulcer or symptoms of GI inflammation or ulceration; hypersensitivity to phenylbutazone or other pyrazoles; blood dyscrasias.

Route/Dosage

ADULTS: **PO** Initial: 200-400 mg daily in 2 divided doses with meals or milk, gradually increasing to full maintenance dosage in 1 wk. Maintenance: 200-800 mg daily, given in 2 divided doses; may increase or decrease after serum urate level is controlled. In case of acute exacerbations, administer concomitant treatment with indomethacin (or another NSAID) or colchicine.

Interactions

Acetaminophen: Increased hepatotoxicity and reduced efficacy of acetaminophen may occur. *Anticoagulants, sulfonylureas (eg, tolbutamide):* Blood levels and toxicity of these agents may increase. *Salicylates:* Uricosuric action of sulfinpyrazone may be reduced. *Verapamil:* Reduced efficacy of verapamil may occur.

Lab Test Interferences

None well documented.

Adverse Reactions

RESP: Bronchoconstriction (in aspirin-sensitive patients). *GI:* Nausea; vomiting; epigastric distress. *HEMA:* Blood dyscrasias, including anemia; leukopenia; agranulocytosis; thrombocytopenia; aplastic anemia. *DERM:* Rash.

Precautions

Pregnancy: Use only when clearly needed. *Lactation:* Undetermined. *Children:* Safety and efficacy not established. *Alkalinization of urine:* Sulfinpyrazone use may precipitate acute gouty arthritis, urolithiasis and renal colic. Adequate fluid intake (10-12 8 oz glasses of fluid) and alkalinization of urine are recommended to reduce potential for renal complications. *Healed peptic ulcer:* Administer with care to these patients. *Renal function impairment:* Periodically assess renal function.

NURSING CONSIDERATIONS

Administration/Storage

- Administer with food or milk; add antacid if needed.

Assessment/Interventions

- Obtain patient history, including drug history and any known allergies.
- Maintain adequate fluid intake and alkalinization of urine. Monitor I&O.
- Monitor blood uric acid levels to evaluate efficacy of treatment.
- Monitor complete blood cell counts for evidence of blood dyscrasias.
- In patients with impaired renal func-

tion, monitor renal function test values.
- Observe for upper GI disturbances, rash, or bronchoconstriction and report to physician.

OVERDOSAGE: SIGNS & SYMPTOMS

Nausea, vomiting, diarrhea, epigastric pain, ataxia, labored respiration, convulsions, coma

Patient/Family Education

- Tell patient that medication is taken on daily basis to provide long-term protection from attacks of gout.
- Point out that gout attacks may worsen during initial treatment but continue the drug.
- Explain that other medications may be needed to control attacks of gout.
- Explain that drug may cause GI distress and to take with food or milk and antacid if needed.
- Instruct patient to report these symptoms to physician: rash, difficulty breathing, unusual bleeding or bruising, sore throat, fatigue or fever.
- Explain importance of adequate hydration and instruct patient to drink 10-12 full glasses of fluid each day.
- Advise patient to consult physician before using aspirin or other salicylates, acetaminophen or drinking alcohol.
- Tell patient to notify physician if GI distress continues.

See Patient Guide, p. 575.

Sulfisoxazole

(sull-fih-SOX-uh-zole)

Gantrisin, Gantrisin Ophthalmic Solution, Gantrisin Pediatric

Class: Anti-infective/sulfonamide

Action Exerts bacteriostatic action by competing with PABA, an essential component in folic acid synthesis, thus preventing synthesis of folic acid, needed by bacteria for growth.

Indications *Oral:* Treatment of UTI, chancroid, inclusion conjunctivitis, malaria, meningitis caused by *Haemophilus influenze* or meningococci, nocardiosis, acute otitis media, toxoplasmosis and trachoma. *Ophthalmic:* Treatment of conjunctivitis, corneal ulcer and superficial ocular infections, adjunct to systemic sulfonamide therapy of trachoma. **Unlabeled use:** *Oral:* Treatment of recurrent otitis media.

Contraindications Hypersensitivity to sulfonamides or chemically related drugs (eg, sulfonylureas, thiazide and loop diuretics, carbonic anhydrase inhibitors, sunscreens containing PABA, local anesthetics); hypersensitivity to salicylates; porphyria; children < 2 mo; pregnancy at term.

Route/Dosage ADULTS: **PO** 2-4 g initially, then 4-8 g/day in 4-6 divided doses. **Ophthalmic** Instill 1-2 gtt into lower conjunctival sac q 1-3 hr daily. CHILDREN & INFANTS > 2 MO: **PO** 75 mg/kg initially, then 120-150 mg/kg/day in 4-6 divided doses (maximum 6 g/day).

Interactions *Anticoagulants, oral:* May enhance anticoagulant action. *Cyclosporine:* Reduced concentration of cyclosporine and increased risk of toxicity. *Hydantoins:* May increase hydantoin serum levels. *Methotrexate:* May enhance risk of methotrexate-induced bone marrow suppression. *Sulfonylureas:* May increase sulfonylurea half-life and produce hypoglycemia.

Lab Test Interferences May produce false-positive urinary glucose test results when performed by Benedict's method; may interfere with Urobilistix test; may produce false-positive results with sulfosalicylic acid tests for urinary protein.

Adverse Reactions

RESP: Pulmonary infiltrates. *CNS:* Headache; peripheral neuropathy; depression; convulsions; dizziness; ataxia. *GI:* Nausea; vomiting; abdominal pain; diarrhea; anorexia; pancreatitis; impaired folic acid absorption; pseudomembranous enterocolitis. *GU:* Crystalluria; hematuria; proteinuria; elevated creatinine; nephrotic syndrome; toxic nephrosis with oliguria and anuria. *HEPA:* Hepatitis; hepatocellular necrosis. *HEMA:* Agranulocytosis; aplastic anemia; thrombocytopenia; leukopenia; hemolytic anemia; purpura; hypoprothrombinemia; anemia; methemoglobinemia; megaloblastic (macrocytic) anemia. *OTHER:* Drug fever; chills; pyrexia; arthralgia; myalgia; periarteritis nodosum; lupus erythematosus phenomenon. Hypersensitivity reactions may present as erythema multiforme of Stevens-Johnson type, generalized skin eruptions, allergic myocarditis, epidermal necrolysis with or without corneal damage, urticaria, serum sickness; pruritus, exfoliative dermatitis, anaphylactoid reactions, periorbital edema, photosensitization, arthralgia and transient pulmonary changes with eosinophilia and decreased pulmonary function. *Ophthalmic:* Browache; local irritation; transient epithelial keratitis; reactive hyperemia; conjunctival edema; burning; stinging; sensitivity to bright light.

Precautions

Pregnancy: Category C. Sulfonamides cross placenta and can produce jaundice, hemolytic anemia and kernicterus in newborn; therefore they are contraindicated at term. *Lactation:* Excreted in breast milk in low concentrations. Do not nurse premature infants or those with hyperbilirubinemia or G-6-PD deficiency. *Children:* Contraindicated in infants < 2 mo. *Allergy or asthma:* Use drug with caution in patients with severe allergy or bronchial asthma. *Dry eye (ophthalmic):* Use with caution in patients with severe dry eye. *Group A beta-hemolytic streptococcal infections:* Do not use drug for these infections. *Hemolytic anemia:* May occur in G-6-PD–deficient individuals. *Photosensitivity:* Photosensitization may occur. *Porphyria:* Drug may precipitate acute attack of porphyria. *Renal or hepatic impairment:* Use drug with caution. *Severe reactions:* Reactions, including deaths, have been associated with hypersensitivity reactions, agranulocytosis, aplastic anemia, other blood dyscrasias and renal and hepatic damage. Irreversible neuromuscular and CNS changes and fibrosing alveolitis may occur. *Sulfonamides:* Have chemical similarities to some goitrogens, diuretics (acetazolamide and the thiazides) and oral hypoglycemic agents. Goiter production, diuresis and hypoglycemia have occurred rarely in patients receiving sulfonamides. Cross-sensitivity may exist.

NURSING CONSIDERATIONS

Administration/Storage

Oral Administration

- Give on empty stomach with full glass of water 1 hr before meal or 2 hr after meal for best absorption.
- Administer around clock at equal intervals.
- May crush tablet and mix with liquid for ease of swallowing. May allow patient to chew tablet.
- Shake oral suspension well prior to administration. Measure dose accurately with calibrated device.
- Store oral suspension in refrigerator.

Ophthalmic Solution

- Do not use solution if it is discolored or contains precipitate.
- Wash hands thoroughly before and after instillation.
- Position patient supine or have patient tilt head back in "star-gazing" position (looking at ceiling). Pull

down lower lid to form pocket and instill drops as ordered. Avoid contact between dispensing container and eye. Close eye gently and apply pressure to inner canthus for 1-2 minutes to prevent systemic absorption and draining into nose/throat.

- Store at room temperature and protect from light.

Assessment/Interventions

- Obtain patient history, including drug history and any known allergies. Note hypersensitivity to salicylates, sulfonamides or chemically related drugs (eg, thiazides, acetazolamide, probenecid); severe hepatic/renal dysfunction; G-6-PD deficiency; porphyria.
- Assess patient for infection (vital signs; appearance of wound, sputum, urine and stool).
- Obtain CBC and culture and sensitivity. First dose may be given before results are available.
- Culture and sensitivity may be repeated when full course of therapy is completed.
- Encourage fluids between meals (up to 2000 ml/day) to maintain hydration and decrease crystallization in kidneys.
- Assess diabetic patients taking oral hypoglycemic agents frequently for hypoglycemia prior to and during therapy.
- Monitor I&O. Note urine color, pH and character.
- Assess skin for rash, bleeding, bruising and jaundice. Note fever, chills, sore throat, mouth sores or joint pain. Report any of these symptoms immediately to physician.

OVERDOSAGE: SIGNS & SYMPTOMS

Anorexia, nausea, vomiting, abdominal cramping, dizziness, headache, drowsiness, coma

Patient/Family Education

Oral

- Advise patient to administer medication around clock.
- Advise patient to notify other physicians and dentist of this drug therapy prior to other treatments or surgery.
- Instruct patient to report these symptoms to physician immediately: difficulty breathing, skin rash, fever, chills, mouth sores, sore throat, ringing in ears or unusual bleeding/bruising.
- Caution patient to avoid exposure to sunlight and to use sunscreen or wear protective clothing to avoid photosensitivity reaction. Inform patient that photosensitivity may persist for several months after therapy is completed.
- Advise patient not to take otc medications without consulting physician.

Ophthalmic

- Instruct patient/family in correct instillation of drops. Inform patient that stinging, burning and blurred vision may occur after instillation of ophthalmic preparations. Advise patient to avoid hazardous activities until vision clears. Emphasize need for patient to contact physician immediately if patient notices a change in vision, eye pain, increased redness, itching, swelling, loss of sight, inability to breath or flushing after ophthalmic application of this medication.
- Advise patient to note color change or precipitate in container and to discard if these are present.
- Tell patient to notify physician if improvement is not noted within 7 days.

See Patient Guide, p. 576.

Sulindac

(sull-IN-dak)

Clinoril, ♣ *APO-Sulin, Novo-Sundac*

Class: Analgesic/NSAID

Action Decreases inflammation, pain and fever, probably through inhibition of cyclooxygenase activity and prostaglandin synthesis.

Indications Treatment of acute and chronic rheumatoid and osteoarthritis, ankylosing spondylitis, acute gouty arthritis, acute painful shoulder, tendinitis, bursitis. **Unlabeled uses:** Treatment of juvenile rheumatoid arthritis and sunburn.

Contraindications Hypersensitivity to aspirin, iodides or any NSAID.

Route/Dosage

Osteoarthritis, Rheumatoid Arthritis, Ankylosing Spondylitis

ADULTS: **PO** 150 mg bid.

Acute Painful Shoulder, Acute Gouty Arthritis

ADULTS: **PO** 200 mg bid for 7-14 days. Maximum dose 400 mg/day.

Interactions

Anticoagulants: May increase effect of anticoagulants because of decreased plasma protein binding. May increase risk of gastric erosion and bleeding. *Lithium:* May decrease lithium clearance. *Loop diuretics:* Decreased diuresis may result. *Methotrexate:* May increase methotrexate levels.

Lab Test Interferences

May prolong bleeding time.

Adverse Reactions

CV: Edema; weight gain; congestive heart failure; alterations in blood pressure; vasodilation; palpitations; tachycardia; arrhythmia. *RESP:* Bronchospasm; laryngeal edema; rhinitis, dyspnea, pharyngitis; hemoptysis; shortness of breath. *CNS:* Dizziness; headaches; nervousness; anxiety; vertigo; lightheadedness; drowsiness; somnolence; tiredness; insomnia; depression; psychic disturbances; seizures; syncope; aseptic meningitis. *EENT:* Tinnitus; blurred vision; visual disturbances; decreased hearing. *GI:* Peptic ulceration; GI bleeding; GI pain; dyspepsia; nausea; vomiting; diarrhea; constipation; pancreatitis; flatulence; anorexia; GI cramps. *HEPA:* Increase liver function tests; hepatitis; hepatic failure; cholestasis; jaundice. *GU:* Discoloration of urine; dysuria; proteinuria; hematuria; interstitial nephritis; nephrotic syndrome; acute renal insufficiency; hyperkalemia; hyponatremia; renal papillary necrosis. *HEMA:* Increased bleeding time; thrombocytopenia; purpura; leukopenia; agranulocytosis; neutropenia; bone marrow depression. *DERM:* Rash; pruritus; ecchymosis; sweating; photosensitivity; alopecia; erythema multiforme; toxic epidermal necrolysis; exfoliative dermatitis. *OTHER:* Dry mucous membranes.

Precautions

Pregnancy: Pregnancy category undetermined. *Lactation:* Undetermined. *Children:* Safety and efficacy not established. *Elderly:* Increased risk of adverse reactions. *GI effects:* Serious GI toxicity (eg, bleeding, ulceration, perforation) can occur at any time, with or without warning symptoms. Do not give to patients with active GI lesions or history of recurrent lesions, except in special circumstances and with close monitoring. *Hepatic impairment:* Use with caution. *Hypersensitivity:* May occur; use caution in aspirin-sensitive individuals because of possible cross-sensitivity. Potentially fatal reaction. *Renal function impairment:* Assess function before and during therapy, because NSAID metabolites are eliminated renally.

NURSING CONSIDERATIONS

Administration/Storage

- Give with food, milk or antacids if needed to minimize GI irritation.
- Crush tablet and mix with food for patient with swallowing difficulty.
- Store in tight, light-resistant container at room temperature.

Assessment/Interventions

- Obtain patient history, including drug history and any known allergies, noting chronic alcohol use, fluid retention, nasal polyps, bronchospastic disease or hypersensitivity to aspirin or NSAIDs.
- Assess hearing and vision (audiometry, ophthalmic exam) prior to and during therapy if long-term.
- Assess areas of bruising prior to and during therapy; report increased bruising immediately to physician.
- Assist with ambulation if drowsiness or dizziness is present; provide for safety at all times (call bell, side rails).
- Assess quality of pain (location, onset, type and duration) and body temperature prior to therapy; monitor pain relief and body temperature after medication administration.
- Assess affected joints (mobility, swelling/deformities, skin condition); monitor improvement during therapy (relief from joint tenderness and pain; increased movement and improved strength of upper extremities).
- Monitor for fever, chills and joint pain (symptoms of acute hypersensitivity reaction); withhold medication and report symptoms immediately to physician.
- Monitor CBC, renal and liver function test results periodically if on long-term therapy.

OVERDOSAGE: SIGNS & SYMPTOMS

Drowsiness, dizziness, confusion, disorientation, lethargy, vomiting, abdominal pain, headache, tinnitus, sweating, seizures, stupor, coma

Patient/Family Education

- Advise patient/family to take medication with food or after meals.
- Tell patient to take medication with full glass of water to prevent medication from lodging in esophagus.
- Emphasize importance of regular medical followup, even in absence of side effects or problems related to drug therapy.
- Instruct patient to report these symptoms of toxicity to physician immediately: ringing in ears, blurred vision or change in urine (pattern, blood in urine).
- Tell patient to avoid intake of alcoholic beverages or other NSAIDs/ASA during therapy (increases risk of GI irritation/GI bleeding), especially during long-term therapy.
- Advise patient that drowsiness or dizziness may occur and to use caution while driving or performing other activities requiring mental alertness.
- Caution patient to avoid exposure to sunlight and to use sunscreen or wear protective clothing to prevent photosensitivity reaction.

See Patient Guide, p. 577.

Sumatriptan Succinate

(SUE-muh-TRIP-tan SOOS-in-ate)

Imitrex

Class: Analgesic/migraine

Action Selective agonist for vascular serotonin (5-HT) receptor subtype, causing vasoconstriction of cranial arteries.

Indications Short-term treatment of migraine attacks with/without aura. **Unlabeled use:** Treatment of cluster headaches.

Contraindications IV use (causes coronary vasospasm); SC use in patients with ischemic heart disease or in patients with Prinzmetal's angina; symptoms consistent with possible ischemic heart disease; uncontrolled hypertension; concurrent use of ergotamine-containing preparations; management of hemiplegic or basilar migraine.

Route/Dosage

ADULTS: **PO:** Recommended dose is 25 mg taken with fluids; maximum recommended single dose is 100 mg. If a satisfactory response has not been obtained at 2 hours, a second dose of up to 100 mg may be given. If headache returns, additional doses may be taken at intervals of at least 2 hours up to a daily maximum of 300 mg. If headache returns following an initial dose with the injection, additional doses of single tablets (up to 200 mg/day) may be given with an interval of at least 2 hours between tablet doses. **SC** Administer as soon as symptoms appear. Maximum single adult dose is 6 mg. Maximum dose per 24 hr is two 6 mg injections separated by at least 1 hr. Available in autoinjection prefilled syringe devices that deliver 6 mg for easy use; however, lower doses should be used in patients who have untoward side effects at usual dose.

Interactions

Ergot-containing drugs: May cause additive prolonged vasospastic reactions. Avoid use within 24 hr of each other.

Lab Test Interferences

None well documented.

Adverse Reactions

CV: Hypertension; hypotension; bradycardia; tachycardia; palpitations; pulsating sensations; various transient ECG changes; syncope; arrhythmia; angina; coronary vasospasm in patients with history of CAD. *CNS:* Dizziness; vertigo; drowsiness; sedation; headache; anxiety; malaise; fatigue. *EENT:* Eye irritation; vision alterations; photophobia; lacrimation; throat or mouth discomfort; nasal cavity or sinus discomfort. *GI:* Abdominal discomfort; dysphagia. *OTHER:* Tingling; warm or hot sensation; burning sensation; feeling of heaviness; numbness; feeling strange; tight feeling in head; cold sensation; weakness; neck pain or stiffness; myalgia; muscle cramp; tightness or pressure in chest; injection site reaction; flushing; sweating; abnormalities in liver function tests.

Precautions

Pregnancy: Category C. *Lactation:* Undetermined. *Children:* Safety and efficacy not established. *Elderly:* Safety and efficacy in patients > 65 yr not thoroughly evaluated. *Cardiac events/vasoconstriction:* Serious coronary events, though extremely rare, can occur after sumatriptan use. Administer first dose in physician's office to patients at possible risk of unrecognized coronary disease. If symptoms consistent with angina occur, conduct ECG evaluation for ischemic changes. May cause coronary vasospasm in patients with history of CAD. Rare reports of major arrhythmias and angina symptoms. *Hepatic or renal function impairment:* Use caution.

NURSING CONSIDERATIONS

Administration/Storage

Injection

- Administer via SC route. Do not give IV (can cause coronary vasospasm).
- Store at room temperature and protect from light.
- Discard any unused portion.

Oral

- Should be taken with plenty of fluids.

Assessment/Interventions

- Obtain patient history, including drug history and any known allergies.
- Assess pain location, intensity and duration and associated symptoms of migraine attack.
- Administer initial dose in physician's office to patients with potential for

coronary artery disease (CAD) including postmenopausal women, men > 40 yr, patients with risk factors for CAD (hypertension, hypercholesterolemia, obesity, diabetes, smokers, family history). Monitor BP prior to and for 1 hr after initial injection; transient increases in BP may occur during first hr. If angina occurs, monitor ECG for ischemic changes.

- Provide quiet, calm environment. Decrease stimuli, noise, light.
- Monitor for side effects and local injection site reactions.

> **OVERDOSAGE: SIGNS & SYMPTOMS**
>
> Convulsions, tremor, inactivity, erythema of extremities, reduced respiratory rate, cyanosis, ataxia, mydriasis, injection site reactions (desquamation, hair loss, scab formation), paralysis

Patient/Family Education

- Instruct patient and family on proper technique for loading, administering medication and disposing of autoinjector.
- Provide patient information pamphlet.
- Explain that drug is to be used during migraine attack and does not prevent or reduce number of attacks. Emphasize only to treat actual migraine attack.
- Teach patient to inject dose SC as soon as symptoms of migraine occur, but explain that may be given at any time during attack. If symptoms return, explain that second injection may be given. Tell patient to allow at least 1 hr between injections and not to use more than 2 doses in 24 hr.
- Advise patient if pain or tightness in chest or throat occurs when using sumatriptan, to notify physician prior to using drug again. If chest pain is severe or does not go away, tell patient to notify physician immediately.
- Advise patient that pain or redness at injection site usually lasts less than 1 hr.
- Tell patient to notify physician immediately if wheezing, heart throbbing, swelling of eyelids, face or lips, skin rash, skin lumps or hives occurs.
- Instruct patient to report these symptoms to physician: tingling, heat, flushing, heaviness, pressure, drowsiness, dizziness, tiredness or sickness.
- Advise patient that drug may cause drowsiness or dizziness and to use caution while driving or performing other activities requiring mental alertness.
- Advise patients that oral sumatriptan should be taken as soon as symptoms of migraine appear; a second dose may be taken if symptoms return, but no sooner than 2 hours following the first dose. For a given attack, if there has been no response to the first tablet, do not take a second tablet without first consulting your healthcare provider. Do not take more than 300 mg in any 24-hour period.

See Patient Guide, p. 578.

Tacrine HCl
(Tetrahydroaminoacridine; THA)

(TAK-reen HIGH-droe-KLOR-ide)

Cognex

Class: Psychotherapeutic

Action Believed to inhibit (reversibly) cholinesterase in CNS, leading to increased concentrations of acetylcholine.

Indications Treatment of mild to moderate dementia of Alzheimer's type.

Contraindications Hypersensitivity to acridine derivatives; previous treatment with tacrine that resulted in jaundice (confirmed by elevated total bilirubin > 3 mg/dl).

Route/Dosage

ADULTS: PO 10 mg qid for 6 wk,

then 20 mg qid. May increase in 6-wk intervals up to 40 mg qid.

Interactions

Cimetidine: Increased tacrine concentrations. *Levodopa:* The antiparkinsonism effects of levodopa may be inhibited. *Theophylline:* Increased theophylline concentrations.

Lab Test Interferences

None well documented.

Adverse Reactions

CV: Hypotension; hypertension; chest pain; edema; heart failure; MI; cerebrovascular accident; pulmonary embolism. *RESP:* Cough; bronchitis; pneumonia; shortness of breath. *CNS:* Headache; dizziness; agitation; confusion; ataxia; insomnia; depression; anxiety; drowsiness; tremor; convulsions; fainting; hyperkinesia; tingling; coma. *EENT:* Conjunctivitis; sinusitis; pharyngitis. *GI:* Nausea; vomiting; diarrhea; upset stomach; anorexia; abdominal pain; flatulence; constipation; GI hemorrhage. *GU:* Urinary frequency; UTI; urinary incontinence; urinary retention. *HEMA:* Purpura; anemia; lymphadenopathy; leukopenia; thrombocytopenia; hemolysis; pancytopenia. *HEPA:* Elevated transaminases. *DERM:* Rash; facial and skin flushing; sweating. *OTHER:* Fatigue; weight decrease; back or muscle pain; cholinergic crisis.

Precautions

Pregnancy: Category C. *Lactation:* Undetermined. *Children:* Safety and efficacy not established in any dementing illness. *Anesthesia:* Use of muscle relaxants such as succinylcholine during anesthesia while receiving tacrine may lead to exaggerated effects. *Carcinogenesis:* May be carcinogenic. *Concomitant medical conditions:* Increases cholinergic activity and therefore can affect other organ systems, possibly leading to bradycardia, bladder outflow obstruction, increased gastric acid secretion or bronchoconstriction. Use drug with caution in patients susceptible to these effects. *Hepatic effects:* Use drug with caution in patients with history of abnormal liver function. *Neurologic conditions:* Drug may contribute to seizures. Cognitive function may worsen after discontinuation or large dose reductions.

NURSING CONSIDERATIONS

Administration/Storage

- Give between meals when possible. May be taken with meals to minimize GI irritation; however, food reduces absorption.
- Check to see that medication is swallowed.
- Store in tight, light-resistant container.

Assessment/Interventions

- Obtain patient history, including drug history and any known allergies.
- Determine whether jaundice developed when patient was previously treated with tacrine or whether patient has history of hepatic dysfunction.
- Assess baseline mental status: sensorium, appearance, behavior, mood and short-term and long-term memory.
- Obtain baseline weight, heart rate and BP.
- Monitor for weight gain and fluctuations in vital signs. Report abnormal findings immediately to physician.
- Monitor mental status frequently.
- Determine baseline hepatic function (especially transaminase levels, bilirubin). Monitor serum tacrine level and hepatic function weekly for first 18 wk and then every 3 mo. Observe for evidence of hepatic damage. Return to weekly testing for 6 wk after every dose increase or as results warrant. Total bilirubin > 3 mg/dl indicates tacrine intolerance; withhold drug and notify physician. Notify physician if transaminase levels are

noted to be ≥ 3 times upper limit of normal.

- Monitor daily bowel activity and stool quality (consistency, color and presence of blood). Expect loose stool; explain this to patient/family. Report abnormal findings immediately to physician.
- Inspect oropharynx (lips, mouth, tongue, gums, throat) for irritation/ulceration. Provide frequent mouth care.

> **OVERDOSAGE: SIGNS & SYMPTOMS**
> Cholinergic crisis, severe nausea, vomiting, salivation, sweating, bradycardia, hypotension, collapse, convulsions

Patient/Family Education

- Instruct patient/family to administer medication at regular intervals and between meals if possible. Drug may be taken with meals if GI upset occurs. Encourage consistency in dosage schedule (eg, every dose with meals or every dose between meals) because drug level can be decreased when taken with food. Instruct family to ensure that medication is swallowed.
- Caution patient/family that drug dosage changes will be required during therapy and not to discontinue this medication abruptly or change dose without direct physician order.
- Emphasize need for continuing monitoring of physical and mental status of patient. Home care or supervised living arrangements must be made prior to discharge.
- Instruct family to modify fluid and bulk in patient's diet to offset diarrhea/constipation.
- Advise patient to carry identification (Medi-Alert bracelet or written drug regimen in wallet) indicating drug regimen and condition.
- Instruct patient to notify other physicians and dentist prior to other therapy or surgery.
- Explain to patient/family that this drug is not cure but that it may slow progressive memory loss of Alzheimer's type.
- Emphasize importance of regular medical follow-up to monitor lab values and evaluate effectiveness of drug.
- Instruct family or persons responsible for patient to report these symptoms to physician: changes in cognitive function (decreased alertness, deterioration of previous intact memory, behavior change, mood swings), rash, flushing of skin/face, wheezing and yellowing of skin and whites of eyes (jaundice).
- Tell patient to take sips of water frequently, suck on ice chips or sugarless hard candy or chew sugarless gum if dry mouth occurs.
- Advise patient/family that drug may cause dizziness and drowsiness and to use caution while driving or performing other tasks requiring mental alertness.

See Patient Guide, p. 620.

Tacrolimus (FK506)

(tack-CROW-lih-muss)

Prograf

Class: Immunosuppressive

Action Suppresses cell-mediated immune reactions and some humoral immunity, but exact mechanism is not known.

Indications Prophylaxis of organ rejection in patients receiving allogenic liver transplants. Is used in conjunction with adrenal corticosteroids. **Unlabeled uses:** Prophylaxis of rejection for patients receiving kidney, bone marrow, cardiac, pancreas, pancreatic island cell and small bowel transplantation.

Contraindications Hypersensitivity to polyoxyl 60 hydrogenated castor oil, which is present in the injection.

Route/Dosage

ADULTS: **PO** 0.15-0.3 mg/kg/day in 2 divided daily doses every 12 hr. **IV** 0.05-0.1 mg/kg/day as continuous infusion. CHILDREN: **PO** 0.3 mg/kg/day in 2 divided daily doses every 12 hr. **IV** 0.1 mg/kg/day as continuous infusion.

Interactions

Macrolide antibiotics, clotrimazole, fluconazole: May elevate tacrolimus concentrations, increasing toxicity. *Cyclosporine:* Additive nephrotoxicity. Do not use concurrently. *Food:* Decreased absorption of tacrolimus.

Lab Test Interferences

None well documented.

Adverse Reactions

CV: Hypertension; edema. *RESP:* Pleural effusion; atelectasis; dyspnea. *CNS:* Tremor; headache; insomnia; paresthesia; weakness; abnormal dreams; agitation; anxiety; confusion. *EENT:* Abnormal vision; tinnitus. *GI:* Diarrhea; nausea; constipation; anorexia; vomiting; abdominal pain. *GU:* Renal dysfunction; urinary tract infection; oliguria. *HEMA:* Anemia; leukocytosis; thrombocytopenia. *HEPA:* Abnormal liver function tests. *DERM:* Pruritus; rash. *META:* Hyperkalemia; hypomagnesemia; hyperuricemia; hyperglycemia. *OTHER:* Fever; ascites; pain; back pain.

Precautions

Pregnancy: Category C. *Lactation:* Excreted in breast milk. Avoid nursing. *Children:* Generally require higher doses to maintain trough tacrolimus levels similar to adults. *Anaphylactic reactions:* May occur with IV injection. *Hepatic disease:* May require reduced doses. *Renal impairment:* May require reduced doses; monitor closely. *Hyperglycemia:* Frequently occurs with tacrolimus; may require treatment.

NURSING CONSIDERATIONS

Administration/Storage

- Dilute IV form of the medication prior to use with 0.9% normal saline or 5% dextrose injection to a concentration between 0.004 mg/ml and 0.02 mg/ml.
- Diluted solution must be stored in glass or polyethylene containers for no more than 24 hours after mixing. Storage in PVC containers reduces stability.
- Solutions that contain particulate matter or are discolored should not be used.
- The initial IV or oral dose of this medication should be no sooner than 6 hours after transplantation.
- Patients should be switched to the oral form of the medication as soon as possible.
- When converting from IV to oral dosage form, the first oral dose should be no sooner than 8 to 12 hours after discontinuation of IV administration.
- Oral medication is most effective on an empty stomach.
- This medication should not be used simultaneously with cyclosporine. Discontinue cyclosporine at least 24 hours before administering this drug.
- Diluted IV solution may be stored at controlled room temperature.
- Store capsules at room temperature.

Assessment/Interventions

- Obtain patient history. Note hypersensitivity to other antirejection drugs such as cyclosporine and polyoxyethylated castor oil.
- Obtain baseline laboratory tests, including BUN, creatinine, lipid levels, potassium, WBC with diff and CBC. Perform and evaluate these tests periodically during treatment.
- Assess for pre-existing hypertension, particularly in children.
- Assess for any signs of infection, bleeding or bruising.
- Remain with patient for the first 30 minutes of the initial IV administration of this medication and assess for symptoms of anaphylactic reac-

tion. Assess frequently during all IV administrations.
- Maintain medical asepsis and eliminate any potential sources of environmental contamination.
- Monitor patient and lab tests for evidence of organ rejection.

OVERDOSAGE: SIGNS & SYMPTOMS
No acute toxicities have been reported

Patient/Family Education
- Warn patient not to alter the dose or discontinue the medication without consulting the healthcare provider.
- Instruct patient to check with his/her healthcare provider before taking any over-the-counter or prescription medications, or receiving any vaccinations.
- Inform patient to report any serious side effects to the healthcare provider.
- Inform patient of the need for frequent laboratory tests to assess the effectiveness of the treatment regimen and the need to keep appointments.
- Direct patient to avoid contact with others who may have any type of infection.
- Direct patient to take the medication 30 minutes before or 2 hours after meals. If the medication causes GI upset, take with a full glass of water. May be taken with food, but is less effective.

See Patient Guide, p. 580.

Tamoxifen Citrate

(ta-MOX-ih-fen SIH-trate)
Nolvadex, ♣ *APO-Tamox, Nolvadex-D, Tamofen, Tamone, Tamoplex*
Class: Antineoplastic/antiestrogen

Action Nonsteroidal agent with potent antiestrogenic properties related to ability to compete with estrogen for binding sites in target tissues such as breast.

Indications Treatment of advanced metastatic breast cancer in women and men particularly if tumor is estrogen-receptor positive. Effective as adjuvant therapy in delaying recurrence after total mastectomy and axillary dissection or segmental mastectomy, axillary dissection and breast irradiation in women with axillary node–negative breast cancer and after total mastectomy and axillary dissection in postmenopausal women with breast cancer. **Unlabeled uses:** Treatment of mastalgia; decrease degree and pain of gynecomastia; treatment of pancreatic carcinoma.

Contraindications Standard considerations.

Route/Dosage
ADULTS: **PO** 10 or 20 mg bid (morning & evening) as ordered by physician.

Interactions
Anticoagulants (eg, warfarin): Increased anticoagulant effect. *Bromocriptine:* May increase tamoxifen levels.

Lab Test Interferences
May produce transient increase in serum calcium. T^4 elevations also were observed to occur in few postmenopausal patients but were not accompanied by clinical hyperthyroidism. Variations in karyopyknotic index on vaginal smears and various degrees of estrogen effect on Pap smears have been seen infrequently in postmenopausal patients.

Adverse Reactions
CV: Hot flushes (most frequent); thromboembolic events (infrequent). *CNS:* Headache; lighheadedness; depression. *EENT:* Decreased visual acuity; retinopathy. *GI:* Nausea; vomiting; anorexia. *GU:* Vaginal bleeding; vaginal discharge; menstrual irregularities; pruritus vulvae; ovarian cysts. *HEMA:* Thrombocytopenia; leukopenia.

DERM: Rash; partial alopecia. *META*: Hypercalcemia. *OTHER*: Peripheral edema; food distaste.

Precautions

Pregnancy: Category D. *Lactation*: Undetermined. *Blood disorders*: Use cautiously in leukeopenia or thrombocytopenia. Transient decreases in platelet counts have occurred but usually returned to normal with continued treatment. Perform periodic platelet and complete blood cell counts. *Hypercalcemia*: Has occurred within few weeks of starting tamoxifen therapy in some breast cancer patients with bone metastases. If occurs, institute appropriate measures, and if severe, discontinue drug. *Hyperlipidemia*: Has occurred infrequently. Periodic monitoring of plasma triglycerides and cholesterol may be indicated in patients with pre-existing hyperlipidemias. *Ophthalmologic effects*: A few patients treated with extended high doses had retinopathy, corneal changes and decreased visual acuity. A few cases of ocular changes have also occurred at recommended doses. *Tumor response*: Increased bone and tumor pain and local disease flare are sometimes associated with good tumor response shortly after starting tamoxifen, and generally subside rapidly. Increased lesion size, development of new lesions or localized erythema may also occur.

NURSING CONSIDERATIONS

Administration/Storage

- Administer medication in morning and after evening meal, before bedtime.
- Give antiemetic 30-60 min before giving drug to prevent vomiting if patient becomes nauseated.
- Store at room temperature in light-resistant container.

Assessment/Interventions

- Obtain patient history, including drug history and any known allergies.
- Assess results of periodic monitoring of plasma triglycerides and cholesterol in patients with pre-existing hyperlipidemias.
- Review periodic complete blood counts, including platelet counts, especially in patients with leukopenia/thrombocytopenia. Notify physician of results.
- Monitor I&O. Increase fluid intake to prevent dehydration.
- Report to physician any nausea, vomiting, hot flashes, vaginal bleeding, vaginal discharge, menstrual irregularities, rash, decreased visual acuity, peripheral edema, weight gain and other side effects.
- Be alert for signs of thromboembolic event and notify physician; however, such events are infrequent with this drug.
- Watch for possible hypercalcemia, especially in patients with breast cancer with bone metastases; discontinuation of the drug may be necessary (a transient increase in serum calcium may occur in other patients).
- In postmenopausal women, watch for possible infrequent variations in karyopyknotic index on vaginal smears and various degrees of estrogen effect on Pap smears.
- Be aware of possibility of ovarian cysts developing in pre-menopausal women with advanced breast cancer who have been treated with this drug.

OVERDOSAGE: SIGNS & SYMPTOMS

Nausea, vomiting, cardiac arrhythmias, tremor, hyperreflexia, dizziness, seizure

Patient/Family Education

- Explain that tumor flare may occur (increase in tumor size, increased bone pain) but will subside rapidly. Tell patient that analgesics may be taken for pain.
- Advise patient to follow liquid diet if severe nausea and vomiting occur.

- Warn patient to immediately contact physician regarding signs of thromboembolic event (pain or swelling in legs, shortness of breath or difficulty breathing).
- Instruct patient to report these symptoms to physician: nausea, vomiting, hot flushes, vaginal bleeding, vaginal discharge, menstrual irregularities, rash, decreased visual acuity, peripheral edema, weight gain, confusion, drowsiness, symptoms of infection and other side effects.

See Patient Guide, p. 579.

Temazepam

(tem-AZE-uh-pam)

Restoril

Class: Sedative and hypnotic/benzodiazepine

Action Potentiates action of GABA (gamma-aminobutyric acid), an inhibitory neurotransmitter, resulting in increased neuronal inhibition and CNS depression, especially in limbic system and reticular formation.

Indications Short-term management of insomnia.

Contraindications Hypersensitivity to benzodiazepines; pregnancy.

Route/Dosage
ADULTS: **PO** 15-30 mg at bedtime; individualize. ELDERLY OR DEBILITATED PATIENTS: **PO** 15 mg until individual response is determined.

Interactions
Alcohol, other CNS depressants: Additive CNS depressant effects. *Digoxin:* Serum digoxin concentrations may increase. *Theophylline:* May antagonize sedative effects.

Lab Test Interferences
None well documented.

Adverse Reactions
CV: Palpitations; tachycardia. *CNS:* Drowsiness; dizziness; lethargy; confusion; euphoria; weakness; falling; ataxia; hallucinations; paradoxical reactions (eg, excitement, agitation); headache; memory impairment. *EENT:* Blurred vision; difficulty focusing. *GI:* Anorexia; diarrhea; abdominal cramping; constipation; nausea; vomiting. *HEMA:* Leukopenia; agranulocytopenia. *OTHER:* Tolerance; physical and psychological dependence; slurred speech; elevated AST, ALT, bilirubin.

Precautions
Pregnancy: Category X. *Lactation:* Similar drugs excreted in breast milk. *Children:* Not for use in children < 18 yr. *Elderly/debilitated:* Increased side effects; start with lowest dose. *Anterograde amnesia:* Has occurred with similar drugs. Alcohol may increase risk. *Dependence/withdrawal:* Prolonged use can lead to psychological or physical dependence. Withdrawal syndrome may occur; dose must be tapered gradually. *Renal or hepatic impairment:* Observe caution. Abnormal liver function test results and blood dyscrasias have occurred.

NURSING CONSIDERATIONS

Administration/Storage
- Administer ½ hr before bedtime with full glass of water.
- If GI upset occurs, administer with food.
- Store in tightly closed container at cool temperature.

Assessment/Interventions
- Obtain patient history, including drug history and any known allergies. Note drug dependence and potential for suicide.
- Assess type of sleep difficulty (eg, falling asleep, remaining asleep, etc.).
- Provide safety measures (siderails up,

nightlight, call bell accessible) and assist with ambulation.

- Carefully document response to initial dose; dose may be increased to 30 mg.
- Assess results of baseline liver and kidney function test and complete blood count with differential. Periodically reevaluate these values throughout long-term therapy.
- Assess and document mental and psychological parameters such as hallucinations, dreaming and nightmares, depression, euphoria, apprehension affect, mood and memory. Report potential problems to physician.
- Notify physician if any of these symptoms occur: palpitations, increased heart rate, visual disturbances along with nausea and vomiting or headache, excitation, dermatitis, sweating, flushing, pruritus, body or joint pain, tinnitus and nasal congestion.

OVERDOSAGE: SIGNS & SYMPTOMS

Symptoms of decreased CNS function: somnolence, confusion, respiratory depression; decreased blood pressure; seizures, coma, impaired coordination, slurred speech

Patient/Family Education

- Caution patient that this medication must not be taken during pregnancy or when pregnancy is possible. Advise patient to use reliable form of birth control while taking this drug.
- Discuss with patient ways to facilitate sleep: quiet, avoidance of caffeine and nicotine, warm baths, deep breathing, relaxation techniques.
- Explain that disturbed nocturnal sleep may occur for first or second night after discontinuing use.
- Tell patient not to discontinue medication abruptly after prolonged therapy (> 2 wk).
- Explain safety precautions with regard to falls, especially for elderly and debilitated patients.
- Instruct patient to report these symptoms to physician: visual disturbances, abdominal pain or palpitations, fever, sore throat, bruising, rash, jaundice, unusual bleeding.
- Advise patient to avoid intake of alcoholic beverages or other CNS depressants.
- Caution patient that drug may cause drowsiness and to use caution while driving or performing other tasks requiring mental alertness.

See Patient Guide, p. 582.

Teniposide (VM-26)

(TEN-ih-POE-side)

Vumon

Class: Antineoplastic/mitotic inhibitor

Action Prevents cells from entering mitosis by inhibiting topoisomerase type II activity and causing breaks in DNA cross-links.

Indications Combination induction therapy for refractory childhood acute lymphoblastic leukemia (ALL). **Unlabeled use:** Refractory childhood acute lymphocytic leukemia.

Contraindications Hypersensitivity to etoposide or Cremophor EL (polyoxyethylated castor oil).

Route/Dosage

Individualize dosage. CHILDREN: **IV** over 30-60 min or longer. Sample regimens: 165 mg/m^2 twice weekly or 250 mg/m^2 once weekly. DOWN SYNDROME PATIENTS: For first course, give 50% of usual dose.

Interactions

Sodium salicylate, sulfamethazole, tolbutamide: Increased free drug concentration of teniposide; possible increased toxicity. INCOMPATIBILITIES: *Heparin:*

Precipitate will form. Do not mix teniposide with other drugs unless specific compatibility data are available.

Lab Test Interferences
None well documented.

Adverse Reactions
CV: Hypotension; phlebitis. *CNS:* Fever. *GI:* Mucositis; nausea; vomiting; diarrhea. *HEMA:* Myelosuppression. *HEPA:* Hepatic dysfunction. *DERM:* Alopecia; rash. *OTHER:* Anaphylactic reactions; infection.

Precautions
Pregnancy: Category D. *Lactation:* Undetermined. *Anaphylaxis:* May occur with first or subsequent doses; patients with brain tumors and neuroblastoma have greatest risk. Generally manifested by chills, fever, tachycardia, bronchospasm, shortness of breath, facial flushing, hypertension or hypotension. *Benzyl alcohol:* Associated with fatal "gasping" syndrome in premature infants. *CNS depression:* Alcohol content may increase risk for CNS depression, especially with high doses. *Hepatic impairment:* May cause increased teniposide levels and toxicity. *Hypotension:* May occur with rapid IV injection. *Myelosuppression:* Bone marrow suppression is most significant toxicity. May result in infection or bleeding; if severe, dosage reduction may be indicated. Downs syndrome patient may be more sensitive.

NURSING CONSIDERATIONS

Administration/Storage

- Wear gloves while handling and preparing solution. If solution contacts skin, wash thoroughly with soap and water.
- For IV preparation, dilute with D5W or 0.9% Sodium Chloride Injection to final concentration of 0.1, 0.2, 0.4 or 1 mg/ml. Prepare and administer solution in non-DEHP–containing large volume parenteral containers such as glass or polyolefin plastic bags or containers. Use of PVC containers is not recommended.
- Administer IV infusion over 30-60 min or longer. Do not give as rapid IV infusion (hypotension may occur).
- In Down syndrome, 50% of usual dose is given for first course of therapy.
- Avoid contact of undiluted teniposide with plastic equipment, which can cause softening and cracking of plastic and possible drug leakage.
- Store unopened vial in refrigerator in original package.
- Diluted solutions (concentrations of 0.1-0.4 mg/ml) are stable for 24 hr at room temperature but should be used within 4 hr. Do not use if precipitate is present.

Assessment/Interventions

- Obtain patient history, including drug history and any allergies.
- Assess for symptoms of anaphylaxis. Patients with brain tumors and neuroblastoma are at the greatest risk. Symptoms include chills, fever, increased heart rate, bronchospasm, shortness of breath, facial flushing or increased or decreased BP. Have epinephrine 1:1000 readily available.
- Obtain baseline blood chemistry, hematologic, renal and liver function test results and monitor levels throughout therapy.
- Monitor patient for evidence of GI toxicity (eg, mucositis, nausea, vomiting) and report these signs to physician. Consider use of antiemetics prior to administration.

OVERDOSAGE: SIGNS & SYMPTOMS
Severe bone marrow depression

Patient/Family Education

- Advise patient to avoid alcohol ingestion.
- Caution patient to avoid crowds and persons with known infections.
- Advise patient to use electric razor and soft toothbrush.
- Explain that patient should not re-

ceive any vaccines during this therapy.

- Inform patient of possibility of hair loss.
- If nausea and vomiting are a problem, advise patient to discuss need for antiemetic with physician.
- Tell patient to notify physician immediately if fever or anaphylaxis occurs.
- Instruct patient to report these symptoms to physician: nausea, vomiting, diarrhea or symptoms of hepatic dysfunction (dark urine, pruritus, or jaundice), rapid heartbeat or difficulty in breathing.
- Caution patient to avoid sudden position changes to avoid orthostatic hypotension.

See Patient Guide, p. 583.

Terazosin

(ter-AZE-oh-sin)

Hytrin

Class: Antihypertensive/antiadrenergic, peripherally acting

Action Selectively blocks postsynaptic alpha$_1$-adrenergic receptors, resulting in dilation of arterioles and veins.

Indications Management of hypertension and symptomatic benign prostatic hyperplasia.

Contraindications Hypersensitivity to doxazosin or prazosin.

Route/Dosage

Hypertension

ADULTS: **PO** Initial: 1 mg at bedtime. (*Do not* exceed this as initial dose to avoid severe hypotensive effects; reinstitute at this dose if drug is discontinued for several days). Maintenance: 1-5 mg q day; may consider bid dosing (maximum 20 mg/day).

Benign Prostatic Hyperplasia

ADULTS: **PO** Initial: 1 mg at bedtime. (*Do not* exceed this as initial dose); increase dose in stepwise fashion. Usual maintenance: 10 mg q day for minimum of 4-6 wk (maximum 20 mg/day).

Interactions None well documented.

Lab Test Interferences
None well documented.

Adverse Reactions
CV: Palpitations; orthostatic hypotension; hypotension; tachycardia; arrhythmias; vasodilation. *RESP:* Dyspnea; bronchitis; bronchospasm; flu symptoms; increased cough. *CNS:* Dizziness; nervousness; paresthesia; somnolence; anxiety; headache; insomnia; weakness; drowsiness. *EENT:* Blurred or abnormal vision; conjunctivitis; tinnitus; nasal congestion; sinusitis; epistaxis; pharyngitis. *GI:* Nausea; vomiting; dry mouth; diarrhea; constipation; abdominal discomfort or pain; flatulence. *GU:* Impotence; urinary frequency; urinary tract infection. *DERM:* Pruritus; rash; sweating. *OTHER:* Shoulder; neck; back or extremity pain; arthralgia; edema; fever; weight gain.

Precautions
Pregnancy: Category C. *Lactation:* Undetermined. *Children:* Safety and efficacy not established. *BPH complications:* Long-term effects on incidence of surgery, acute urinary obstruction or other complications of BPH have not been determined. *First-dose effect:* May cause marked hypotension (especially orthostatic) and syncope at 15-90 min after first few doses, after reintroduction, with rapid increase in dosing, or after addition of another antihypertensive; to avoid, initiate dosing with low dose and gradually increase after 2 weeks; monitor patients carefully. *Hemodilution:* Small decreases in hematocrit, hemoglobin, WBCs, total protein and albumin may occur, possibly because of hemodilution.

NURSING CONSIDERATIONS

Administration/Storage

- Give orally. Maximum dosage should not exceed 20 mg.
- For benign prostatic hypertrophy, increase dose in stepwise fashion, as prescribed.
- Store in tight container in cool location.

Assessment/Interventions

- Obtain patient history, including drug history and any known allergies.
- Assess BP response and pulse after administration to aid dosage adjustment.
- Check weight daily.
- Monitor I&O.
- Implement safety precautions for patients who experience dizziness. Fainting occasionally occurs after the first dose.
- Observe for symptoms of decreased blood pressure, such as dizziness.
- Assess for potential respiratory side effects, including dyspnea, bronchospasm or cough.

> **OVERDOSAGE: SIGNS & SYMPTOMS**
> Severe hypotension

Patient/Family Education

- Explain to patient that first few doses may cause hypotension and syncope. Therefore, initially, terazosin should be taken at bedtime and patient should be warned to stay prone after taking dose. After first few doses, orthostatic hypotension with syncope is rare.
- Advise patient to avoid otc cough, cold, and allergy medicines containing sympathomimetics, and identify common examples.
- Instruct patient to avoid driving or other activities that require alertness for first 24 hours after initial dose.
- Advise patient to follow up with physician to monitor BP.
- Caution patient to rise slowly from lying or sitting position to minimize dizziness.
- Instruct patient to report these symptoms to physician: dizziness, visual changes or palpitations.
- Alert male patients that impotence may be side effect.
- Explain potential adverse reactions: arthralgia, weight gain, tinnitus, pruritus, epistaxis, and blurred vision. Be certain patient understands that physician should be made aware of any significant adverse reactions.
- Caution patient to avoid sudden position changes to prevent orthostatic hypotension.

See Patient Guide, p. 584.

Terbutaline Sulfate

(ter-BYOO-tuh-leen SULL-fate)

Brethaire, Brethine, Bricanyl, ♣ *Bricanyl Turbuhaler*

Class: Bronchodilator/ sympathomimetic

Action Produces bronchodilation by relaxing bronchial smooth muscle through beta$_2$-receptor stimulation.

Indications Treatment of reversible bronchospasm associated with asthma, bronchitis and emphysema. **Unlabeled use:** Inhibits premature labor.

Contraindications Cardiac arrhythmias associated with tachycardia.

Route/Dosage

ADULTS & CHILDREN ≥ 12 YR: **Inhalation** 2 inhalations (separated by 60 sec interval) q 4-6 hr. Do not repeat more than q 4 hr. ADULTS & CHILDREN ≥ 15 YR: **PO** 2.5-5 mg at 6 hr intervals, 3 times per day during waking hours. Do not exceed 15 mg in 24 hr. CHILDREN 12-15 YR: **PO** 2.5 mg tid. Do not exceed 7.5 mg in 24 hr. **SC** 0.25 mg given in lateral deltoid area. May repeat in 15-30 min. Do not exceed 0.5 mg in 4 hr.

Premature Labor Inhibition
ADULTS: **IV** 10-80 mcg/min for 4 hr has shown some success. Maintenance: **PO** 2.5 mg q 4-6 hr.

Interactions
Beta-blockers: Block bronchodilator effect of terbutaline. MAO *inhibitors:* Hypertension may occur. *Tricyclic antidepressants:* Cardiovascular effects of terbutaline may be enhanced.

Lab Test Interferences
None well documented.

Adverse Reactions
CV: Palpitations; tachycardia; chest discomfort or pain; arrhythmias. *RESP:* Dyspnea. *CNS:* Stimulation; tremor; dizziness; nervousness; drowsiness; headache. *GI:* Nausea; vomiting; GI distress. *HEPA.* Elevated liver enzymes. *META:* Hypokalemia (with high doses). *OTHER:* Flushing; sweating; muscle cramps; hypersensitivity vasculitis.

Precautions
Pregnancy: Category B. *Lactation:* Excreted in breast milk. *Labor and delivery:* May inhibit uterine contractions and delay preterm labor. *Children:* Safety and efficacy in children < 12 years not established. *Elderly:* Lower doses may be required. *Cardiovascular effects:* Toxic symptoms in patients with cardiovascular disorders may occur. *CNS effects:* CNS stimulation may occur; use cautiously in patients with history of seizures or hyperthyroidism. *Diabetes:* Dosage adjustment of insulin or oral hypoglycemic agent may be required. *Excessive use:* Paradoxical bronchospasm and cardiac arrest have been associated with excessive inhalant use. *Hypokalemia:* Decreases in potassium levels have occurred. *Tolerance:* If previously effective dose fails to provide relief, therapy may need to be reassessed.

NURSING CONSIDERATIONS

Administration/Storage

- For IV administration, obtain baseline potassium level prior to administration and place patient on cardiac monitor to assess for tachycardia or arrhythmias. Toxic symptoms have been documented in patients with cardiovascular disorders.
- Do not allow patient to use inhaler form of medication more than 6 times/day.
- Limit subcutaneous doses to no more than 0.5 mg in 4 hours.
- For patients who are also using steroid inhaler, make sure that terbutaline is used first and 5 min elapse before steroid inhaler is used.
- Do not use medication if discolored.
- Store at room temperature. Protect from light.

Assessment/Interventions

- Obtain patient history, including drug history and any known allergies.
- Be alert for drug tolerance, which may occur with long-term use.

OVERDOSAGE: SIGNS & SYMPTOMS
Tremor, palpitations, increased heart rate, decreased blood pressure, seizures, hypokalemia, muscle cramps, headache, hyperglycemia

Patient/Family Education

- Instruct patient on proper technique for use of inhalers and evaluate return demonstration.
- Demonstrate use of spacer or peak flow meter if prescribed.
- Caution patient not to use inhaler form of medication more than 6 times/day.
- Advise patient to take tablets with food to avoid gastrointestinal upset.
- Inform patient that the drug can stop working over time. If this is noted or if the inhalation makes breathing worse, the physician should be notified at once.

- Instruct patient to report these symptoms to physician: chest pain, dizziness or headache or persisting symptoms of asthma.

See Patient Guide, p. 585.

Terconazole

(ter-CONE-uh-zole)

Terazole 7, Terazole 3

Class: Topical/antifungal

Action May alter permeability of fungus cell membrane, allowing leakage of essential intracellular components.

Indications Local treatment of vulvovaginal candidiasis.

Contraindications Standard considerations.

Route/Dosage

ADULTS: **Intravaginal** 1 suppository at bedtime for 3 days *or* 1 applicatorful of 0.4% cream at bedtime for 7 days *or* 1 applicatorful of 0.8% cream for 3 days.

Interactions None well documented.

Lab Test Interferences

None well documented.

Adverse Reactions

CNS: Headache. *GI:* Abdominal pain. *GU:* Dysmenorrhea; genitalia pain; vulvovaginal burning; itching; irritation; burning. *OTHER:* Body pain; fever; chills.

Precautions

Pregnancy: Category C; avoid during first trimester due to absorption possibility. *Lactation:* Undetermined. *Children:* Safety and efficacy not established. *Recurrent infections:* May indicate underlying medical cause, including diabetes or HIV infection.

NURSING CONSIDERATIONS

Administration/Storage

- Insert applicator high in vagina.
- Store at room temperature.

Assessment/Interventions

- Obtain patient history, including drug history and any known allergies.
- Ask patient about local reactions. If reactions are severe or symptoms of infection persist or worsen, notify physician.

Patient/Family Education

- Instruct patient to complete full course of therapy. This medication must be used continuously even through menses.
- Alert patient to potential side effects of vulvovaginal itching or burning, head or body aches. Advise patient to discontinue medication and notify physician if irritation occurs.
- Instruct patient to insert applicator high into vagina.
- Wash hands before and after application. Also, maintain external clean genitalia but avoid use of douches or other vaginal otc products while using the medication.
- Advise patient to wash applicator with mild soap and rinse thoroughly.
- Caution patient to refrain from sexual intercourse during course of therapy in order to help to prevent reinfection.
- Advise patient that sanitary napkin or minipad may be used to prevent stains on clothing.
- Instruct patient to consult with physician if infection recurs. Diabetes, AIDS and chronic antibiotic or steroid therapy place patient at increased risk for recurrent infection.
- Explain that ingredients in product may interact with latex and weaken latex condoms and diaphragms. Ad-

vise patient to avoid use of these forms of birth control for 72 hr after application of medication.

See Patient Guide, p. 586.

Terfenadine

(ter-FEN-uh-deen)

Seldane

Class: Antihistamine

Action Competitively antagonizes histamine at H_1 receptor sites.

Indications Symptomatic relief of seasonal allergic rhinitis. **Unlabeled uses:** Symptomatic relief of chronic idiopathic urticaria, dermatographism; relief of histamine-induced bronchoconstriction in asthmatics, exercise and hyperventilation-induced bronchospasm.

Contraindications Significant hepatic dysfunction; concomitant erythromycin, clarithromycin, troleandomycin, ketoconazole or itraconazole therapy; hypersensitivity to antihistamines.

Route/Dosage

ADULTS & CHILDREN > 12 YR: **PO** 60 mg bid. The following pediatric doses have been suggested: CHILDREN 6-12 YR: **PO** 30-60 mg bid. CHILDREN 3-6 YR: **PO** 15 mg bid.

Interactions

Fluconazole, itraconazole, ketaconazole, miconazole, macrolide antibiotics (eg, erythromycin): May increase terfenadine plasma levels leading to serious cardiovascular effects. Other drugs that prolong QT interval may also increase risk for these cardiovascular effects (see precautions).

Lab Test Interferences

Skin testing procedures. Antihistamines may prevent or diminish an otherwise positive reaction to dermal reactivity indicators.

Adverse Reactions

CV: Rare cases of serious cardiovascular adverse events, including death, cardiac arrest, torsades de pointes and other ventricular arrhythmias have been observed in overdose and in patients with significant hepatic dysfunction or concomitant administration of azole antifungals or macrolide antibiotics (see contraindications). *RESP:* Bronchospasm; cough. *CNS:* Depression; dizziness; terfenadine appears to have little to no sedative effects. *EENT:* Visual disturbances. *GI:* Dry mouth. *HEPA:* Mild or moderate serum transaminase elevations; jaundice; cholestatic hepatitis, hepatitis (rare). *DERM:* Angioedema; skin eruption and itching. *OTHER:* Alopecia; galactorrhea; menstrual disorders (eg, dysmenorrhea); musculoskeletal pain; nightmares. Terfenadine appears to have little or no anticholinergic effects.

Precautions

Pregnancy: Category C. *Lactation:* Unknown. *Children:* Safety not established in children < 12 yr. *Cardiovascular toxicity:* Rare cases of serious cardiovascular adverse events, including death, cardiac arrest, torsades de pointes and other ventricular arrhythmias have been observed in overdose and in patients with significant hepatic dysfunction or concomitant administration of azole antifungals or macrolide antibiotics (see contraindications). In some cases arrhythmias have been preceded by episodes of syncope. Syncope should lead to discontinuation of treatment and full evaluation of potential arrhythmias, including ECG testing. Terfenadine should be avoided in patients receiving drugs or who have conditions that prolong QT interval. These include patients taking certain antiarrhythmics, bepridil, certain psychotropics, probucol, or astemizole; patients with electrolyte abnormalities such as hypokalemia or hypomagnesemia, or patients taking diuretics with potential for inducing electrolyte abnormalities; and patients with congenital QT syndrome. *Hepatic impairment:* Use drug caution in patients with cirrhosis or other liver diseases; contraindicated in patients with significant hepatic dysfunction.

NURSING CONSIDERATIONS

Administration/Storage

- Give orally.
- Store in tight, light-resistant container.

Assessment/Interventions

- Obtain patient history, including drug history and any known allergies.
- Assess baseline hematologic and LFT results.
- Monitor for any adverse effects, including syncope, torsades de pointes, other ventricular arrhythmias, cardiac arrest, sudden death; bronchospasm, angioedema, visual disturbances, alopecia and musculoskeletal pain.
- Monitor elderly patients closely, as they tend to be more susceptible to adverse reactions.

OVERDOSAGE: SIGNS & SYMPTOMS

Mild CNS depression, headache, nausea, confusion, ventricular arrhythmias, cardiovascular collapse, seizures

Patient/Family Education

- Have patient or family notify physician of any symptoms of liver impairment (jaundice, pruritus or dark urine).
- Caution patient to avoid exposure to sunlight and to use sunscreen or wear protective clothing to avoid photosensitvity reaction.
- Tell patient to alert physician immediately of any symptoms of anaphylaxis, dizziness, palpitations, confusion, sedation or hypotension.
- Alert male patients of possibility of impotence.
- Tell patient that urinary frequency, dysuria or urinary retention may be experienced.
- Advise patient not to increase dose or use more frequently than prescribed.
- Inform patient of potential for drug interactions and to report use of terfenadine whenever a new medication is prescribed.

See Patient Guide, p. 587.

Testolactone

(TESS-toe-lak-TONE)

Teslac

Class: Antineoplastic/androgen

Action Principal action appears to be inhibition of steroid aromatase activity and consequent reduction in estrone synthesis from adrenal androstenedione, the major source of estrogen in postmenopausal women. Inhibition may be noncompetitive and irreversible. This action inhibits growth of estrogen-dependent tumors such as breast carcinoma.

Indications Adjuvant therapy in palliative treatment of advanced or disseminated breast carcinoma in postmenopausal women when hormonal therapy is indicated and in premenopausal women with disseminated breast carcinoma in whom ovarian function has been terminated.

Contraindications Carcinoma of male breast.

Route/Dosage

ADULTS: PO 250 mg qid for minimum of 3 mo, unless there is active disease progression.

Interactions
Anticoagulants: May increase effects of oral anticoagulants.

Lab Test Interferences
May result in decreased estradiol concentrations with radioimmunoassays for estradiol, increased plasma calcium concentrations and increased 24-hr excretion of creatine and 17-ketosteroids.

Adverse Reactions
CV: Increases in BP. *CNS:* Paresthesias. *GI:* Glossitis; anorexia; nausea; vomiting. *DERM:* Maculopapular erythema; alopecia; nail growth disturbances. *OTHER:* Aches and edema of extremities.

Precautions
Pregnancy: Category C. *Lactation:* Undetermined. *Children:* Safety and efficacy not established. *Androgenic effects:* Consider precautions associated with other androgenic agents. *Monitoring:* Routinely monitor plasma calcium levels, particularly during active remission of bone metastases. Manage hypercalcemia accordingly.

NURSING CONSIDERATIONS

Administration/Storage
- Administer without regard to food.
- Store at room temperature.

Assessment/Interventions
- Obtain patient history, including drug history and any known allergies.
- Assess need for concomitant antiemetic therapy for anorexia, nausea or vomiting. Glossitis may also occur.
- Monitor for complaints or signs of paresthesias, maculopapular erythema, arthralgia and edema of extremities, alopecia, disturbances in nail growth and increase in BP.
- Monitor fluids and electrolytes.
- Assess baseline prothrombin time/partial thromboplastin time as oral anticoagulant effects may increase.
- Assess baseline hepatic and renal function test results.
- Alert physician to signs of virilization.

Patient/Family Education
- Explain that therapeutic response is not immediate and may not be noted for 2-3 mo.
- Tell patient to notify physician if numbness or tingling of face, toes or fingers occurs.
- Tell patient to notify physician if gastrointestinal symptoms are pronounced.

See Patient Guide, p. 588.

Testosterone

(teh-STAHS-tuh-RONE)

Testosterone
Histerone 100, Tesamone, Testandro, Testoderm

Testosterone Cypionate
depAndro 100, depAndro 200, Depo-Testosterone, Depotest 100, Depotest 200, Duratest-100, Duratest-200

Testosterone Enanthate
Andro L.A. 200, Andropository-200, Delatestryl, Durathate-200, Everone 200

Testosterone Propionate
Available as generic only
Class: Androgen

Action Promotes growth and development of male reproductive organs, maintains secondary sex characteristics, increases protein anabolism and decreases protein catabolism.

Indications
Men: Replacement therapy in primary hypogonadism and hypogonadotropic hypogonadism; stimulation of puberty in delayed puberty; treatment of impotence and male cli-

macteric symptoms. *Women:* Ablation of ovaries in metastatic breast cancer; management of postpartum breast pain or engorgement. **Unlabeled use:** Reversible contraception in men.

Contraindications Serious cardiac, hepatic or renal disease; men with carcinoma of breast or prostate; women who are or may become pregnant.

Route/Dosage

Androgen Replacement Therapy

ADULTS: **IM** 25-50 mg 2-3 times/wk (testosterone, testosterone propionate). **IM** 50-400 mg q 2-4 wk (testosterone enanthate, testosterone cypionate). **Transdermal** 6 mg/day system applied daily *or* 4 mg/day system applied daily if scrotal area is small.

Delayed Puberty

ADOLESCENTS: **IM** 40-50 mg/m^2/dose for 6 mo (testosterone, testosterone propionate) *or* **IM** 50-200 mg q 2-4 wk for limited duration (testosterone enanthate, testosterone cypionate) *or* **IM** 40-50 mg/m^2/dose monthly until growth rate falls to prepubertal levels (testosterone, testosterone propionate).

Breast Cancer

ADULTS: **IM** 50-100 mg 3 times weekly (testosterone, testosterone propionate) *or* **IM** 200-400 mg q 2-4 wk (testosterone enanthate, testosterone cypionate).

Postpartum Breast Engorgement

ADULTS: **IM** 25-50 mg per day for 3-4 days (testosterone, testosterone propionate).

Interactions

Anticoagulants: May potentiate anticoagulant effects. *Insulin, oral hypoglycemics:* May decrease glucose levels and antidiabetic drug requirements.

Lab Test Interferences

Thyroid function tests: Testosterone may cause decreased levels of thyroid hormones. *Clotting factors II, V, VII, X:* Testosterone may suppress expression.

Adverse Reactions

CV: Edema. *CNS:* Depression; headache; increased or decreased libido; anxiety. *GI:* Nausea. *GU:* Men: Gynecomastia; penile erections; decreased ejaculatory volume. Women: Amenorrhea; virilization (deepening of voice and clitoral enlargement). *HEPA:* Cholestatic jaundice (elevated LFT results). *DERM:* Acne; hirsutism; male pattern baldness; seborrhea; rash. *META:* Increased cholesterol; decreased serum glucose. *OTHER:* Inflammation at injection site; fluid and electrolyte retention.

Precautions

Pregnancy: Category X. *Lactation:* Undetermined. *Children:* Use drug with great caution; may affect bone maturation. *Elderly patients:* Elderly men may be at increased risk of developing prostatic hypertrophy or carcinoma. *Acute intermittent porphyria:* Has been reported. Use drug with caution in patients known to have this condition. *Athletic performance:* Abuse of these agents to enhance athletic performance has potential risk of serious side effects. *Breast cancer and immobilized patients:* May cause hypercalcemia. *Edema:* Use drug with caution in patients with conditions that might be affected by fluid retention (eg, asthma, cardiac or renal dysfunction, epilepsy). *Gynecomastia:* Frequently occurs and may persist. Use drug with caution in patients with preexisting gynecomastia. *Hepatic effects:* Prolonged use of high doses of androgens may result in potentially life-threatening hepatitis, hepatic neoplasms or hepatocellular carcinoma. *Oligospermia and reduced ejaculatory volume:* May occur after prolonged use. *Product interchange:* Do not interchange products because of their differences in duration of action, especially testosterone cypionate and testosterone propionate. *Serum cholesterol:* Levels may increase with androgen use; use drug with caution in patients with history of MI or coronary artery disease.

NURSING CONSIDERATIONS

Administration/Storage

- Administer IM injections deep in gluteal muscle. Rotate sites.
- Shake vial well before withdrawing solution. Warming and shaking vial dissolves crystals that may have formed.
- Using wet needle or syringe may cause solution to become cloudy; however, this does not affect potency of drug.
- Ascertain whether physician desires aqueous suspension or oil-based testosterone. Do not interchange products. Different salt forms have different duration of action.
- Wear gloves while handling transdermal patches. Apply transdermal patches to clean, dry and shaved scrotal skin. Patch should be worn 22-24 hr/day. Fold used patches with adhesive edges together. Discard patches so that they cannot be handled.
- Store IM preparation at room temperature.

Assessment/Interventions

- Obtain patient history, including drug history and any known allergies.
- Determine if patient has serious cardiac, hepatic or renal disease, carcinoma of breast or prostate, clotting problems, epilepsy or migraine headaches.
- Monitor and record I&O. Notify physician of fluid retention.
- Report jaundice or inflamed injection site to physician.
- Monitor serum cholesterol and report to physician if total cholesterol has increased and is > 200 mg/dl.
- In male adolescents being treated for delayed puberty, monitor bone maturation by assessing bone age of the wrist and hand every 6 mo by x-ray evaluation.
- Perform periodic LFTS.
- Observe for hypercalcemia, especially in breast cancer patients and immobilized patients.
- Monitor for signs of virilization in women.

OVERDOSAGE: SIGNS & SYMPTOMS

Chronic overdose: virilization, MI, thrombosis, movement disorders, hepatitis, nausea, vomiting, acne, seborrheic dermatitis

Patient/Family Education

- Caution patient that this medication must not be taken during pregnancy or when pregnancy is possible. Advise patient to use reliable form of birth control while taking this drug.
- Advise patient to consult with physician before taking otc or prescription drugs.
- Instruct patient to remain as active as possible. Hypercalcemia may result if patient is inactive and therapy will have to be discontinued.
- Advise patient to report these symptoms to physician: depression, headache, nausea, yellow skin or yellowing of whites of eyes, swelling of ankles, painful or difficult urination, severe acne or painful or prolonged penile erections.
- Inform patient of potential side effects: increased facial or body hair and loss of scalp hair (in both men and women), breast enlargement and decreased ejaculatory volume (in men) and deep voice, enlarged clitoris and cessation of menses (in women).
- Warn patients being treated for hypogonadism that gynecomastia caused by testosterone therapy may persist.
- Caution patient to neither take this drug without prescription nor increase prescribed dosage in effort to increase athletic performance. Side effects can be very serious.
- Instruct patient not to accept brands, types or forms of drug different from one originally prescribed.
- Advise patient using transdermal patches to wear briefs instead of boxer

shorts underwear to keep the patch from falling off.

- Instruct patient using the transdermal scrotal patch to shave scrotum with dry disposable razor about once a week. Apply patch to dry scrotum. Patch should be temporarily removed while bathing or swimming. Patch is adhesive-free and clings to skin by an electrostatic effect.

See Patient Guide, p. 589.

Tetanus and Diphtheria Toxoids (adult strength, Td)

(TET-ah-nus and diff-THEER-ee-uh toxoids)

Available as generic only

Class: Vaccine, inactivated bacteria

Action Induces antibodies against toxins made by *Corynebacterium diphtheriae* and *Clostridium tetani*.

Indications Achievement of active immunity against diphtheria and tetanus. Tetanus and diphtheria toxoids for adult use (Td) is preferred agent for immunizing most adults and children after age 7.

Contraindications Immediate hypersensitivity to product, to thimerosal or to any components; during immunosuppression, acute respiratory infection (except for emergency booster recall doses).

Route/Dosage

Primary Immunizing Series

ADULTS & CHILDREN ≥ 7 YR: **IM** A total of 3 doses (0.5 ml each): 1 dose now followed by 1 dose 4-8 wk later and then 1 dose 6-12 mo after first dose.

Booster Doses

ADULTS: **IM** 0.5 ml at 10-yr intervals throughout life to maintain immunity.

Interactions None well documented.

Lab Test Interferences
None well documented.

Adverse Reactions

Local: Small amount of erythema, induration, pain, tenderness, heat and edema surrounding injection site, persisting for few days, is not unusual. Nodule may be palpable at injection site for few weeks. Allow such nodules to recede spontaneously. Sterile abscess and SC atrophy occur rarely. Adverse reactions often associated with multiple prior booster doses may be manifested 2 to > 12 hr after administration by erythema, boggy edema, pruritus, lymphadenopathy and induration surrounding point of injection. Pain and tenderness, if present, are usually not primary complaints. *Systemic:* Transient low-grade fever (temperatures > 38° C [100° F]) following Td administration are unusual, chills, malaise, generalized aches and pains, headaches, flushing, generalized urticaria or pruritus, tachycardia, anaphylaxis, hypotension, neurologic complications. Persons developing significant adverse reactions should not be given Td, even emergency doses, more frequently than every 10 years.

Precautions

Pregnancy: Category C. *Lactation:* Undetermined. *Anticoagulant therapy:* As with all IM injections, give drug with caution to persons receiving anticoagulant therapy. *Susceptibility:* Like all inactivated vaccines, administration of Td to persons receiving immunosuppressant drugs, including high-dose corticosteroids or radiation therapy may result in insufficient response to immunization. They may remain susceptible despite immunization.

NURSING CONSIDERATIONS

Administration/Storage

- Shake vial before withdrawing dose.
- Give IM only, do not administer IV or SC.
- Inject into deltoid muscle. Take care to avoid major peripheral nerve trunks.
- Several routine vaccines may safely and effectively be administered simultaneously at separate injection sites (eg, measles-mumps-rubella, oral polio vaccine, inactivated poliomyelitis vaccine, *Haemophilus influenzae* type b, hepatitis B, influenza). Authorities recommend simultaneous immunization at separate sites as indicated by age or health risk.
- Document in patient's medical record manufacturer name and lot number, date of administration, and name, address and title of person administering vaccine.
- Report adverse events to Vaccine Adverse Event Reporting System (VAERS), 1-800-822-7967.
- Store under refrigeration.

Assessment/Interventions

- Obtain patient history, including drug history and any known allergies.
- Use caution when administering to patient on anticoagulant therapy.
- Observe patient after injection for symptoms of anaphylaxis. Have 1:1000 epinephrine on hand.
- Monitor for significant side effects, including tachycardia, hypotension, neurologic complications, fever, chills, generalized arthralgias, headache and flushing.

Patient/Family Education

- Explain that pain, edema or pruritus may be experienced at site of injection.
- Stress to family that patient must receive all 3 doses for immunization to be effective.
- Explain need for booster at 10-yr intervals.

No patient monograph available.

Tetanus Immune Globulin (TIG)

(TET-ah-nus ih-MYOON GLAH-byoo-lin)

Hyper-Tet

Class: Immune serum

Action Directly neutralizes toxin excreted by *Clostridium tetani*, cause of tetanus.

Indications Passive, transient protection against tetanus in any person with wound that may be contaminated with tetanus spores when: (1) patient's personal history of immunization with tetanus toxoid is unknown or uncertain, (2) person received < 2 prior doses of tetanus toxoid or (3) person received 2 prior doses of tetanus toxoid, but delay of > 24 hours occurred between time of injury and initiation of tetanus prophylaxis. **Unlabeled use:** Treatment of clinical tetanus.

Contraindications Hypersensitivity to human antibody product, thimerosal or other components; circulating anti-IgA antibodies.

Route/Dosage

ADULTS: Prophylactic dose: **IM** 250 units. Give 500 units if wounds are severe or treatment is delayed. Dosage may be increased to 1000-2000 units. For therapy of tetanus, give 500-3000 or 6000 units. Give deep IM, preferably in upper outer quadrant of gluteal muscle. CHILDREN: **IM** dose is calculated on basis of body weight (4 units/kg); however, it may be advisable to administer 250 units regardless of the size of the child. The same amount of toxin is produced by the bacteria in adults and children.

Interactions There is no significant interaction between TIG and tetanus toxoid if given at different injection sites. To avoid inactivating vaccines containing live viruses or bacteria, give live vaccines 2-4 wk before or 12 wk after TIG.

Lab Test Interferences None well documented.

Adverse Reactions Local and systemic reactions following TIG are infrequent and usually mild. Expect some pain, tenderness and muscle stiffness at injection site, persisting for several hours. Hives, angioedema, nephrotic syndrome and local inflammation occur occasionally. Anaphylactic reactions are very infrequent.

Precautions *Pregnancy:* Category C. *Lactation:* Undetermined. Use TIG as soon as possible after tetanus-prone injuries. Do not inject IV.

NURSING CONSIDERATIONS

Administration/Storage

- Administer by IM injection only; do not give IV.
- Refer to appropriate immunization schedule or CDC wound management guideline for correct dosing.
- Use different syringe and injection site for the tetanus toxoid.
- Remember that prior history of tetanus "shots" is not reliable unless it can be confirmed that these shots were tetanus toxoid. However, U.S. Armed Forces personnel since 1940 have received at least 1 dose and probably complete immunizing series. If tetanus toxoid is needed, give in a separate site.
- Store in the refrigerator.

Assessment/Interventions

- Obtain patient history, including drug history and any known allergies.
- Observe patient for possible anaphylactic reaction after administration.

Patient/Family Education

- Alert patient that pain, soreness, inflammation or stiffness at site of injection may be experienced.
- Advise patient who is also receiving tetanus toxoid series to complete pending immunizations since TIG protection is only temporary.

No patient monograph available.

Tetracycline HCl

(teh-truh-SIGH-kleen HIGH-droe-KLOR-ide)

Achromycin, Achromycin V, Ala-Tet, Panmycin, Nor-Tet, Robitet, Sumycin, Sumycin 250, Sumycin 500, Teline, Teline 500, Tetracap, Tetralan, Topicycline, ♣ *APO-Tetra, Novo-Tetra, Tetracyn*

Class: Antibiotic/tetracycline

Action Inhibits bacterial protein synthesis.

Indications Treatment of infections due to susceptible strains of gram-positive and gram-negative bacteria; treatment of Rickettsiae, *Mycoplasma* pneumonia; chlamydial infections including treatment of trachoma; treatment of susceptible infections when penicillins are contraindicated; treatment of acute intestinal amebiasis. *Ophthalmic:* Prophylaxis of ophthalmia neonatorum; treatment of superficial ocular infections due to susceptible organisms. *Topical:* Treatment of acne vulgaris; infection prophylaxis in minor cuts, wounds, burns, and abrasions. **Unlabeled use:** Treatment of acne.

Contraindications Hypersensitivity to tetracyclines or any component; Ophthalmic use is contraindicated in epithelial herpes simplex keratitis, fungal disease of ocular structure and after removal of corneal compound.

Route/Dosage

ADULTS: **PO** 1-2 g daily in 2-4 equal doses. CHILDREN > 8 YR: **PO** 25-50 mg/kg in 4 equal doses.

Acute Gonococcal Infection

ADULTS: **PO** 1.5 g initially, then 500 mg q 6 hr to total 9 g.

Syphilis

ADULTS: **PO** 30-40 g in equally divided doses over 10-15 days.

Chlamydia

ADULTS: **PO** 500 mg qid for at least 7 days.

Ocular Infections

ADULTS: **Ophthalmic** acute infections: 1-2 gtt q 15-30 min initially or 0.5-inch ointment q 3-4 hr; moderate infections: 1-2 gtt 4-6 times daily or 0.5-inch ointment bid-tid.

Ophthalmia Neonatorium Prevention

NEONATES: **Ophthalmic** 0.5-inch ointment to eyes once.

Acne Vulgaris

ADULTS: **Topical** Apply am and pm 1-4 times daily to affected area. **PO** 125-500 mg once daily.

Interactions

Digoxin: May increase digoxin serum levels. *Food, dairy products, iron salts, antacids (containing aluminum, zinc, calcium, magnesium), bismuth salts, activated charcoal, divalent or trivalent cations:* May decrease oral absorption of tetracycline. *Lithium:* May see altered lithium levels; monitor therapy. *Methoxyflurane:* Increased potential for nephrotoxicity exists; do not use together. *Oral contraceptives:* May reduce effect of oral contraceptives. *Penicillins:* May interfere with bactericidal action of penicillins. *Zinc salts, urinary alkalinizers:* May decrease serum tetracycline levels.

Lab Test Interferences

None well documented.

Adverse Reactions

CV: Pericarditis. *GI:* Diarrhea; nausea; vomiting; abdominal pain or discomfort; anorexia; bulky, loose stools; sore throat; glossitis; anorexia. *GU:* Increased BUN. *HEMA:* Hemolytic anemia; thrombocytopenia; neutropenia. *HEPA:* Increased liver function test results. *DERM:* Rash; urticaria; photosensitivity. *OTHER:* Hypersensitivity, including anaphylaxis; local reactions (eg, stinging or burning sensation with topical application).

Precautions

Pregnancy: Avoid during pregnancy. *Lactation:* Excreted in breast milk. *Children:* Avoid in children < 8 yr because abnormal bone formation and discoloration of teeth may occur. *Outdated product:* Do not use since degradation products are highly nephrotoxic. *Ophthalmic use:* May retard corneal epithelial healing. *Pseudotumor cerebri (benign intracranial hypertension):* Has been reported in adults. Usual manifestations are headache and blurred vision. *Renal impairment:* Excessive accumulation may occur in patients with renal impairment, resulting in possible liver toxicity; dosage reduction may be required. *Superinfection:* Prolonged use may result in bacterial or fungal overgrowth.

NURSING CONSIDERATIONS

Administration/Storage

- Administer oral form with full glass of water 1 hr before or 2 hr after meals to enhance absorption. Give at least 1 hr before bedtime to prevent esophagitis.
- Do not expose drug to light or heat.
- Store suspension form in refrigerator.

Assessment/Interventions

- Obtain patient history, including drug history and any known allergies.
- Assess baseline liver function test results and blood chemistry as tetracycline may cause LFT results and BUN to increase.

- Observe patient for anaphylactic reaction after administration.

> **OVERDOSAGE: SIGNS & SYMPTOMS**
> Nausea, vomiting, headache, increased intracranial pressure, skin pigmentation

Patient/Family Education
- Tell patient to take oral doses with full glass of water 1 hr before or 2 hr after meals to enhance absorption.
- Alert patient to potential side effects, such as photosensitivity and nausea, vomiting and diarrhea.
- Advise patient to avoid dairy products, antacids and iron supplements while taking this drug.
- Caution patient to avoid exposure to sunlight and to use sunscreen or wear protective clothing to avoid photosensitivity reaction.
- Instruct patient to watch for signs of superinfection.
- Notify patient that topical use may result in burning sensation. Explain that if this persists or if infection occurs, physician should be notified and use should be discontinued.
- Explain that topical medication may stain clothing.
- Demonstrate proper administration technique for ophthalmic installation and have patient provide return demonstration.
- Instruct patient to discard old oral tetracycline products as the product becomes toxic when outdated.

See Patient Guide, p. 590.

Theophylline

(thee-AHF-ih-lin)

Accurbron, Aerolate, Aquaphyllin, Asmalix, Bronkodyl, Constant-T, Elixomin, Elixophyllin, Elixophyllin SR, Lanophyllin, Quibron-T Dividose, Quibron-T/SR Dividose, Respbid, Slo-bid, Gyrocaps, Slo-Phyllin, Slo-Phyllin Gyrocaps, Sustaire, T-Phyl, Theo-24, Theo-Dur, Theo-Sav, Theobid Duracaps, Theobid Jr. Duracaps, Theochron, Theoclear L.A., Theoclear-80 Syrup, Theolair, Theolair-SR, Theospan-SR, Theostat 80, Theovent, Uniphyl, ♣ *Pulmophylline, Somophyllin-12, Theo-SR*

Class: Bronchodilator/Xanthine derivative

Action Relaxes bronchial smooth muscle and stimulates central respiratory drive.

Indications Prevention or treatment of reversible bronchospasm associated with asthma or chronic obstructive pulmonary disease. **Unlabeled uses:** Treatment of apnea and bradycardia of prematurity; reduction of essential tremor.

Contraindications Hypersensitivity to xanthines; seizure disorders not adequately controlled with medication.

Route/Dosage Dosage based on lean body weight.

Acute Therapy in Patients Not Currently Receiving Theophylline
Loading dose: ADULTS & CHILDREN: **PO** 5 mg/kg. Maintenance: CHILDREN 9-16 YR & YOUNG ADULT SMOKERS: **PO** 3 mg/kg q 6 hr. CHILDREN 1-9 YR: **PO** 4 mg/kg q 6 hr. ELDERLY & COR PULMONALE PATIENTS: **PO** 2 mg/kg q 8 hr. PATIENTS WITH CHF: **PO** 1-2 mg/kg q 12 hr. NONSMOKING ADULTS: **PO** 3 mg/kg q 8 hr.

Acute Therapy in Patients Receiving Theophylline
Each 0.5 mg/kg theophylline administered as a loading dose will increase serum theophylline concentration by about 1 mcg/ml. If a serum theophylline concentration can be obtained rapidly, defer the loading dose. If this is not possible, clinical judgment must be exercised, using close monitoring. Maintenance doses as per above.

Chronic Therapy
Slow clinical titration preferred. Initial

dose: 16 mg/kg/24 hr or 400 mg/24 hr, whichever is less. Increasing dose: Increase the above dosage by 25% increments at 3 day intervals as long as the drug is tolerated or until the following maximum dose is reached (not to exceed 900 mg, whichever is less). MAXIMUM DOSE (WHERE SERUM CONCENTRATION IS NOT MEASURED): Do not attempt to maintain any dose that is not tolerated. ADULTS & CHILDREN > 16 YR: 13 mg/kg/day. CHILDREN 12-16 YR: 18 mg/kg/day. CHILDREN 9-12 YR: 20 mg/kg/day. CHILDREN 1-9 YR: 24 mg/kg/day.

Adjustments Based on Serum Theophylline Concentrations (Recommended for Final Adjustments in Dosage)

If serum theophylline concentration is within the desired range (10-20 mcg/ml), maintain dosage if tolerated. If too high (20-25 mcg/ml) decrease doses by about 10% and recheck in 3 days; (25-30 mcg/ml) skip the next dose, decrease subsequent doses by about 25% and recheck after 3 days; (over 30 mcg/ml) skip the next 2 doses, decrease subsequent doses by about 50% and recheck in 3 days. If too low (< 10 mcg/ml) increase dosage by 25% at 3 day intervals until either the desired clinical response or serum concentration is achieved.

Infant Guidelines

INFANTS 26-52 WK: Dosing interval is q 6 hr. INFANTS ≤ 26 WK: Dosing interval is q 8 hr. INFANTS 6-52 WK: **PO** 24 hr dose in mg [(0.2 × age in wk) + 5] × weight in kg. PREMATURE INFANTS > 24 DAYS: **PO** 1.5 mg/kg q 12 hr. PREMATURE INFANTS ≤ 24 DAYS: **PO** 1 mg/kg q 12 hr. Final dosage guided by serum concentration after steady state is achieved.

Interactions *Allopurinol, nonselective beta-blockers, calcium channel blockers, cimetidine, oral contraceptives, corticosteroids, disulfiram, ephedrine, influenza virus vaccine, interferon, macrolide antibiotics (eg, erythromycin), mexiletine, quinolone antibiotics (eg, ciprofloxacin), thyroid hormones:* Increase theophylline levels. *Aminoglutethimide, barbiturates, hydantoins, ketoconazole, rifampin, smoking (cigarettes and marijuana), sulfinpyrazone, sympathomimetics:* Decrease theophylline levels. *Benzodiazepines and propofol:* Theophylline may antagonize sedative effects. *Beta-agonists:* Cardiovascular adverse effects may be additive. However, may be used together for additive beneficial effects. *Carbamazepine, isoniazid and loop diuretics:* May increase or decrease theophylline levels. *Halothane:* Coadministration has caused catecholamine-induced arrhythmias. *Ketamine:* Coadministration may result in seizures. *Lithium:* Theophylline may reduce lithium levels. *Nondepolarizing muscle relaxants:* Theophylline may antagonize neuromuscular blockade. INCOMPATIBILITIES: Do not mix following solutions with theophylline in IV fluids: ascorbic acid; chlorpromazine; corticotropin; dimenhydrinate; epinephrine HCl; erythromycin gluceptate; hydralazine; hydroxyzine HCl; insulin; levorphanol tartrate; meperidine; methadone; methicillin sodium; morphine sulfate; norepinephrine bitartrate; oxytetracycline; papaverine; penicillin G potassium; phenobarbital sodium; phenytoin sodium; procaine; prochlorperazine maleate; promazine; promethazine; tetracycline; vancomycin; vitamin B complex with C.

Lab Test Interferences None well documented.

Adverse Reactions *CV:* Palpitations; tachycardia; hypotension; arrhythmias. *RESP:* Tachypnea; respiratory arrest. *CNS:* Irritability; headache; insomnia; muscle twitching; seizures. *GI:* Nausea; vomiting; gastroesophageal reflux; epigastric pain. *GU:* Proteinuria; diuresis. *OTHER:* Fever; flushing; hyperglycemia; inappropriate antidiuretic hormone secretion; sensitivity reactions (exfoliative dermatitis and urticaria).

Precautions

Pregnancy: Category C. *Lactation:* Excreted in breast milk. *Cardiac effects:* Theophylline may cause or worsen pre-existing arrhythmias. *GI effects:* Theophylline may cause or worsen pre-existing ulcers or gastroesophageal reflux. *Toxicity:* Patients with liver impairment, cardiac failure or > 55 yrs of age are at greatest risk; monitor theophylline levels to prevent toxicity.

NURSING CONSIDERATIONS

Administration/Storage

- Some sustained release preparations should be given on empty stomach to avoid rapid drug release.
- Do not crush or allow patient to chew sustained release preparations.
- If GI irritation occurs, give with food or full glass of water.
- When administering parenterally, use a pump or controller to maintain a constant infusion rate.

Assessment/Interventions

- Obtain patient history, including drug history and any known allergies.
- Carefully monitor patients with history of arrhythmias, seizures, peptic ulcer or gastroesophageal reflux.
- Monitor theophylline levels. The usual therapeutic range is 7 to 20 mcg/ml but some toxicity may be noted at the upper end of this range.
- Assess baseline LFT results.
- Implement cardiac monitoring as ordered for patients receiving IV form of theophylline.
- Monitor vital signs and I&O.

OVERDOSAGE: SIGNS & SYMPTOMS

Anorexia, nausea and vomiting, nervousness, insomnia, agitation, irritability, headache, tachycardia, extrasystoles, tachypnea, fasciculations, seizures, ventricular arrhythmias, and hyperamylasemia

Patient/Family Education

- Emphasize importance of follow-up with physician to monitor drug levels.
- Explain to patient that the medication is used to prevent asthma attacks and should be used continuously.
- Explain that some sustained release forms should be taken on empty stomach. Sustained release products should not be crushed or chewed.
- Explain that low-protein, high-carbohydrate diets may increase theophylline levels while high-protein, low-carbohydrate diets and charcoal-broiled foods may decrease theophylline levels.
- Alert patients to common adverse reactions including stomach upset, nausea, insomnia, tremors, palpitations, exfoliative dermatitis and urticaria.
- Tell patient to avoid food products containing caffeine.
- Instruct patient not to take extra doses of theophylline for acute asthma attack.
- Advise patient to consult with physician before taking any otc preparations.

See Patient Guide, p. 591.

Thiabendazole

(THIGH-uh-BEND-uh-zole)

Mintezol

Class: Anti-infective/anthelmintic

Action Inhibits helminth-specific enzyme fumarate reductase; suppresses egg or larval production and may inhibit subsequent development of eggs or larvae that are passed in the stool.

Indications Treatment of strongyloidiasis (threadworm infection), cutaneous larva migrans (creeping eruption) and visceral larva migrans alone or in conjunction with enterobiasis (pinworm). Secondary therapy for uncinariasis (hookworm: *Necator americanus* and *Ancylostoma duodenale*), trichuriasis (whipworm) and ascariasis (large roundworm); alleviation of symptoms of trichinosis during invasive phase.

Contraindications Standard considerations.

Route/Dosage
ADULTS ≥ 150 LB (68 KG): **PO** 1.5 g/dose bid (maximum 3 g/day). ADULTS & CHILDREN 30-150 LB (13.6-68 KG): **PO** 10 mg/lb/dose (22 mg/kg/dose) (maximum 3 g/day).

Strongyloidiasis, Ascariasis, Uncinariasis, Trichuriasis, Cutaneous Larva Migrans
2 doses daily for 2 successive days (may repeat for some indications).

Trichinosis
2 doses daily for 2-4 successive days.

Visceral Larva Migrans
2 doses daily for 7 successive days.

Interactions
Xanthines: Thiabendazole may increase serum concentrations of theophylline to potentially toxic levels.

Lab Test Interferences
None well documented.

Adverse Reactions
CV: Hypotension. *CNS:* Dizziness; fatigue; drowsiness; giddiness; headache; numbness; hyperirritability; seizures; collapse. *EENT:* Tinnitus; abnormal sensation in eyes; xanthopsia; blurring of vision; drying of mucous membranes; appearance of live ascaris in mouth and nose. *GI:* Anorexia; nausea; vomiting; diarrhea; epigastric distress. *GU:* Hematuria; enuresis; malodor of urine; crystalluria. *HEMA:* Transient leukopenia. *HEPA:* Jaundice; cholestasis; parenchymal liver damage, transient rise in cephalin flocculation and AST. *OTHER:* Hypersensitivity reaction (pruritus, fever, facial flush, chills, conjunctival injection (red eye), angioedema, anaphylaxis, skin rashes, erythema multiforme, lymphadenopathy).

Precautions
Pregnancy: Category C. *Lactation:* Unknown. *Children:* Safety and efficacy in children weighing < 13.6 kg (30 lb) not established. *Mixed infections with* Ascaris lumbricoides: Thiabendazole may cause these worms to migrate. Drug should not be used prophylactically. *Supportive therapy:* Anemic, dehydrated or malnourished patients may need concomitant therapy to reverse these conditions.

NURSING CONSIDERATIONS

Administration/Storage
- Shake suspension before administering.
- Administer with food to reduce stomach upset.
- Instruct patient to chew tablets thoroughly before swallowing.
- Store at room temperature.

Assessment/Interventions
- Obtain patient history, including drug history and any known allergies. Monitor patient closely for signs of hypersensitivity reactions: Stevens-Johnson syndrome and erythema multiforme.
- If anemic, dehydrated or malnourished, provide supportive measures.
- If patient is taking theophylline or aminophylline, monitor theophylline serum levels; dosage adjustment may be necessary.
- Assess patient for possible hypotension after administration.
- Obtain baseline LFTs.

OVERDOSAGE: SIGNS & SYMPTOMS
Transient visual disturbances, psychic alterations

Patient/Family Education
- Instruct patient to take medicine with food. No special diets are needed.
- Advise patient that all family members should be treated and that treatment may need to be repeated in 7 days to prevent reinfection.
- Instruct patient to bathe daily and to launder bedlinens, clothes and towels daily. Instruct patient on proper technique for hygiene and hand-washing.
- Advise patient to avoid consuming excessive amounts of caffeine-containing beverages, such as coffee.
- Instruct patient to inform physician immediately of any symptoms of hypersensitivity or overdosage.
- Advise patient that drug can cause drowsiness and dizziness and to use caution while driving or performing other tasks requiring mental alertness.

See Patient Guide, p. 592.

Thiamine HCl (B_1)

(THIGH-uh-min HIGH-droe-KLOR-ide)

Biamine, Thiamilate, ♣ *Betaxin, Bewon*
Class: Vitamin

Action Thiamine, after conversion to thiamine pyrophosphate, functions with adenosine triphosphate (ATP) in carbohydrate metabolism. Deficiencies result in beriberi, characterized by GI manifestations, peripheral neuropathy and cerebral deficits.

Indications Prophylaxis or treatment of thiamine deficiency (beriberi). Parenteral use indicated when oral therapy not feasible or advisable. **Unlabeled uses:** Mosquito repellant; treatment of ulcerative colitis, chronic diarrhea, cerebellar syndrome, polyneuritis; appetite stimulant; prevention of Wernicke-Korsakoff syndrome.

Contraindications Standard considerations.

Route/Dosage
ADULTS: **PO** 0.5 mg/1000 kcal intake. RDA is 1.2-1.5 mg (adult males), 1.1 mg (adult females) 1.2 mg (CHILDREN 6-10 YR), 0.8-1 mg (CHILDREN < 6 YR), and 0.3-0.5 mg (infants).

Wet Beriberi with Myocardial Failure
ADULTS: **IV** 10-30 mg tid. Treat as emergency cardiac condition.

Beriberi
ADULTS: **IM** 10-20 mg tid for 2 wk, then **PO** 5-10 mg (as part of multivitamin) for 1 mo. CHILDREN: **IV** 10 mg initially followed by **IM** 10 mg bid for 3 days, then 10 mg daily for 6 wk.

Thiamine Deficiency Secondary to Alcoholism (Wernicke's Encephalopathy)
ADULTS: **IV** 50-100 mg; then **IM/IV** 50-100 mg/day until consuming normal diet; then **PO** 40 mg/day.

Metabolic Disorders
ADULTS: **PO** 10-20 mg daily; maximum doses of 4 g daily have been used.

Interactions
IV incompatibilities: Unstable in neutral or alkaline solutions. Incompatible with sulfite containing solutions. Incompatible with barbiturates, erythromycin, lactobionate, citrates.

Lab Test Interferences
None well documented.

Adverse Reactions
CV: Cardiovascular collapse; hypotension; death. *RESP:* Pulmonary edema; cyanosis. *CNS:* Weakness; restlessness. *EENT:* Tightness of throat. *GI:* Nausea; hemorrhage into GI tract. *DERM:* Pruritus; urticaria. *OTHER:* Feeling of warmth; sweating; anaphylaxis; angioneurotic edema; local tenderness and induration (after IM use).

Precautions

Pregnancy: Category A. *Lactation:* Undetermined. *Hypersensitivity:* Can occur. Deaths have resulted from IV administration. Intradermal test dose is recommended if sensitivity is suspected. *Deficiency:* Single vitamin B_1 deficiency is rare; suspect multiple vitamin deficiencies. *Wernicke's encephalopathy:* May occur or worsen suddenly in thiamine-deficient patients given glucose. If deficiency is suspected, give thiamine before or with dextrose-containing fluids.

NURSING CONSIDERATIONS

Administration/Storage

- As a nutritional supplement, calculate dosage based on standard dose of 0.5 mg/1000 kcal daily intake.
- For IV infusion, give at rate of ≤ 100 mg/≥ 5 min.
- For IM injection, rotate injection sites if pain and inflammation occur. Administer via Z-track method to minimize pain. Application of cold may decrease pain.
- Store in light-resistant container.

Assessment/Interventions

- Obtain patient history, including drug history and any known allergies.
- Give intradermal test dose first if hypersensitivity is suspected.
- Assess the patient for other nutritional deficiencies, since single vitamin deficiencies are rare.
- Administer thiamine before giving IV solutions containing glucose as glucose administration may cause sudden worsening of Wernicke's encephalopathy.
- Monitor for adverse reactions, and notify physician of signs of weakness, restlessness, cardiovascular collapse, pulmonary edema, throat tightness, nausea, gastrointestinal hemorrhage, pruritus, urticaria, feeling of warmth, diaphoresis, cyanosis, angioneurotic edema.

Patient/Family Education

- Alert patient to potential lab test abnormalities.
- Inform patient of all potential adverse reactions and of importance of reporting problems to physician.
- Teach patient about proper nutritional balance needed in diet. Thiamine-rich foods are yeast, beef, liver, legumes, beans and whole grains.

See Patient Guide, p. 593.

Thioguanine (TG; 6-Thioguanine)

(THIGH-oh-GWAHN-een)

Available as generic only

Class: Antineoplastic/antimetabolite

Action Thioguanine, a nucleic acid analog, interferes with synthesis of guanine nucleotides. Furthermore, thioguanine nucleotides are incorporated into both RNA and DNA by producing cytotoxic effect.

Indications Remission, induction, consolidation and maintenance therapy of acute nonlymphocytic leukemias. Usually given in combination chemotherapy for induction of remission. *Other neoplasms:* Thioguanine is not effective in chronic lymphocytic leukemia, Hodgkin's lymphoma, multiple myeloma or solid tumors. It may have benefit as second line therapy (after busulfan) in treatment of chronic myelogenous leukemia.

Contraindications Prior resistance to drug. Cross resistance with mercaptopurine is common.

Route/Dosage

ADULTS & CHILDREN: Initial dose: **PO** 2 mg/kg/day. If after 4 wk there is no clinical improvement and no leukocyte depression, dosage may be cautiously increased to 3 mg/kg/day. Total dose may be given at one time. *Combi-*

nation therapy: Complete remission has been achieved using multiple-drug protocol including thioguanine, prednisone, cytarabine, cyclophosphamide and vincristine in children with acute nonlymphocytic leukemia and combination of thioguanine and cytarabine in adults.

Interactions Unlike azathioprine and mercaptopurine, thioguanine does not appear to interact with allopurinol. *Busulfan:* Increased risk of liver injury and esophageal varices.

Lab Test Interferences
None well documented.

Adverse Reactions
GI: Stomatitis; nausea; vomiting; anorexia; intestinal necrosis and perforation in multi-drug chemotherapy. *HEMA:* Bone marrow toxicity/myelosuppression; bone marrow hypoplasia; anemia; leukopenia; thrombocytopenia. *HEPA:* Jaundice; veno-occlusive hepatic disease; toxic hepatitis; hepatomegaly; anorexia. *OTHER:* Hyperuricemia.

Precautions
Pregnancy: Category D. *Lactation:* Undetermined. *Hyperuricemia:* Frequently occurs due to rapid cell lysis. Minimize side effects by increasing hydration, urine alkalinization and prophylactic administration of allopurinol. *Hepatic dysfunction:* Thioguanine may be hepatotoxic further compromising liver function.

NURSING CONSIDERATIONS

Administration/Storage

- Implement appropriate precautions for handling antineoplastic product.
- Store at room temperature in a dry place.

Assessment/Interventions

- Obtain patient history, including drug history and any known allergies.
- Evaluate Hgb, Hct, WBC and quantitative platelet count frequently during therapy.
- Assess results of baseline LFTs prior to therapy, and monitor weekly at start of therapy and monthly thereafter.
- Monitor for symptoms of bone marrow suppression such as fever, sore throat, nausea and vomiting, jaundice, symptoms of infection or bleeding. Notify physician if any symptoms are noted.
- Monitor for and report joint pain, headache, dizziness and swelling of feet and legs.
- Monitor serum uric acid levels.

OVERDOSAGE: SIGNS & SYMPTOMS

Immediate: Nausea, vomiting, malaise, hypertension, diaphoresis; *delayed:* myelosuppression and azotemia

Patient/Family Education

- Inform patient of symptoms of liver function abnormality, including jaundice, dark urine or pruritus.
- Inform patient of symptoms of potential toxicity, including nausea and vomiting, malaise and diaphoresis. Have patient alert physician immediately if these symptoms are present.
- Explain that if patient misses dose, next dose should be taken as soon as possible. However, patients should be cautioned against doubling doses in attempt to "catch up" unless advised to do so by physician. If more than one dose is missed, tell patient to inform physician.
- Tell patient to alert physician immediately for any symptoms of infection or bleeding.

See Patient Guide, p. 594.

Thiopental Sodium

(thigh-oh-PEN-tahl SO-dee-uhm)
Pentothal
Class: General anesthetic/barbiturate

Action Depresses CNS to produce hypnosis and anesthesia without analgesia.

Indications Induction of anesthesia; supplementation of other anesthetic agents; IV anesthesia for short surgical procedures with minimal painful stimuli; induction of hypnotic state; control of convulsions and increased intracranial pressure (IV administration); induction of preanesthetic sedation or basal narcosis (rectal administration).

Contraindications Hypersensitivity to barbiturates; variegate or acute intermittent porphyria; absence of suitable veins for IV administration; status asthmaticus. *Rectal administration:* Patients undergoing rectal surgery; lesions of bowel.

Route/Dosage

Test Dose
ADULTS: **IV** 25-75 mg; observe for 60 sec.

Anesthesia
ADULTS: **IV** 50-75 mg slowly q 20-40 sec until anesthesia is established then 25-50 mg prn *or* continuous infusion of 0.2% or 0.4%. CHILDREN: **IV** 5-6 mg/kg then 1 mg/kg prn. INFANTS: **IV** 5-8 mg/kg then 1 mg/kg prn. NEONATES: **IV** 3-4 mg/kg then 1 mg/kg prn.

Convulsive States
ADULTS: **IV** 75-125 mg; may need 125-250 mg over 10 min. CHILDREN: **IV** 2-3 mg/kg/dose; repeat prn.

Increased Intracranial Pressure
ADULTS: **IV** 1.5-3.5 mg/kg. CHILDREN: **IV** 1.5-5 mg/kg/dose; repeat prn.

Psychiatric Disorders
ADULTS: **IV** 100 mg/min slowly with patient counting backwards *or* as infusion of 50 ml/min of 0.2% solution.

Preanesthetic Sedation
ADULTS: **PR** 1 g/34 kg (30 mg/kg).

Basal Narcosis
ADULTS: **PR** 1 g/22.5 kg (44 mg/kg) (maximum 3.4 g for adults weighing > 90 kg). CHILDREN > 3 MO: **PR** 25 mg/kg/dose; if not sedated within 15-20 min, may repeat with single dose of 15 mg/kg/dose (maximum 1.15 g for children > 34 kg). CHILDREN < 3 MO: **PR** 15 mg/kg/dose; if not sedated within 15-20 min, may repeat with single dose of < 7.5 mg/kg/dose.

Interactions
Narcotics: May cause additive barbiturate effects and increase risk of apnea. *Phenothiazines:* May increase frequency and severity of neuromuscular excitation and hypotension. *Probenecid:* May extend barbiturate effects or effects may be achieved at lower doses. *Sulfisoxazole:* May enhance barbiturate effects. INCOMPATIBILITIES: Tubocurarine, succinylcholine or other acid pH solutions.

Lab Test Interferences
LFTs: Drug may falsely elevate results. *Serum potassium:* Drug may falsely elevate results.

Adverse Reactions
CV: Myocardial depression; arrhythmias. *RESP:* Apnea; laryngospasm; bronchospasm; hiccoughs; sneezing; coughing. *CNS:* Delirium, headache; amnesia; seizures. *GI:* Abdominal pain; rectal irritation; diarrhea; cramping; rectal bleeding (rectal suspension). *DERM:* Rash. *OTHER:* Thrombophlebitis; pain at injection site; salivation; shivering.

Precautions
Pregnancy: Category C; readily crosses placental barrier. *Lactation:* Excreted in breast milk. *Elderly or debilitated patients:* At increased risk of prolonged or potentiated hypnotic effects. Dosage reduction is required when administered rectally. *Special risk patients:* Use drug with caution in patients with

severe cardiovascular, respiratory, renal, hepatic or endocrine disease, hypotension or shock, conditions in which hypnotic effects may be prolonged or potentiated, potential rectal surgery (rectal suspension) or presence of inflammatory, ulcerative, bleeding or neoplastic lesions of lower bowel (rectal suspension). *Repeated doses:* May result in prolonged drug effect due to accumulation. *Severe renal impairment:* Dosage reduction is required (75% of normal dose if creatinine clearance < 10 ml/min).

NURSING CONSIDERATIONS

Administration/Storage

- Use Sterile Water for Injection, Sodium Chloride Injection, or 5% Dextrose Injection as diluent.
- Avoid extravascular or intra-arterial injection since ulceration, necrosis and gangrene may result.
- Patients with renal dysfunction require dosage reduction.
- Use freshly prepared solutions promptly. Discard unused portions after 24 hr.
- When preparing rectal suspension, observe caution when filling applicator. Cleansing enema is not required.
- Dosage reduction of thiopental may be required if thiopental is administered concomitantly with narcotic analgesics.
- Store at room temperature, protected from light.

Assessment/Interventions

- Obtain patient history, including drug history and any known allergies.
- Give test dose to assess reaction.
- Monitor vital signs before, during and after administration.
- Monitor ventilation carefully when drug is being administered to neurosurgical patients with increased intracranial pressure who are not receiving mechanical ventilation.
- Maintain airway patency at all times and have oxygen and resuscitation equipment nearby.
- Monitor respiration rate carefully.
- If patient is receiving drug intravenously, monitor cardiac function on cardiac monitor to assess for arrhythmias.
- Observe for thrombophlebitis, which may occur with IV administration.
- Observe for symptoms of anaphylaxis including pruritus, urticaria, and erythema.

OVERDOSAGE: SIGNS & SYMPTOMS

Respiratory depression, hypotension, shock, apnea, occasional laryngospasm, coughing, respiratory difficulties

Patient/Family Education

- Instruct patient to notify physician of any signs of hypersensitivity to barbiturates.
- Inform patient to avoid alcohol or other CNS depressants for 24 hr.
- Advise patient that drug can continue to impair abilities for 24 hr following administration and caution patient to avoid driving or performing other tasks requiring mental alertness.

No patient monograph available.

Thioridazine HCl

(THIGH-oh-RID-uh-zeen HIGH-droe-KLOR-ide)

Mellaril, Mellaril-S, Thioridazine HCl Intensol, ♣ *APO-Thioridazine*

Class: Antipsychotic/phenothiazine; antiemetic

Action Effects apparently due to dopamine receptor blocking in CNS.

Indications Management of psychotic disorders (eg, schizophrenia); short-term treatment of moderate to marked depression with variable degrees of anxiety in adults; treatment of multiple symptoms (eg, agitation, anxiety, depressed mood, tension, sleep disturbances and fears) in geriatric patients; treatment of severe behavioral problems in children marked by combativeness or explosive hyperexcitable behavior; short-term treatment of hyperactive children who show excessive motor activity with accompanying conduct disorders. **Unlabeled uses:** Treatment of Tourette's syndrome, acute agitation in elderly and some symptoms of dementia.

Contraindications Comatose or severely depressed states; allergy to this or any phenothiazine; presence of large amounts of other CNS depressants; bone marrow depression or blood dyscrasias; liver damage; extensive cerebral arteriosclerosis; severe coronary artery disease; severe hypotension or hypertension; subcortical brain damage.

Route/Dosage

ADULTS: **PO** 200-800 mg/day in divided doses. For moderate disorders, start with 10 mg bid-tid. Do not exceed 800 mg/day. CHILDREN 13-18 YR: **PO** 25-800 mg/day. CHILDREN 7-12 YR: **PO** 25-500 mg/day. CHILDREN 3-6 YR: **PO** 10-100 mg/day. CHILDREN 2-12 YR: **PO** Usually 0.5-3 mg/kg/day. HOSPITALIZED, SEVERELY DISTURBED, OR PSYCHOTIC CHILDREN: **PO** 25 mg bid-tid. ELDERLY: **PO** 20-200 mg/day.

Interactions

Alcohol and other CNS depressants: May result in increased CNS depression and may precipitate extrapyramidal reaction. *Anticholinergics:* May reduce therapeutic effects of thioridazine and worsen anticholinergic effects of thioridazine. May lead to tardive dyskinesia. *Barbiturate anesthetics:* Frequency and severity of neuromuscular excitation and hypotension may increase. *Beta-blockers:* May result in increased plasma levels of beta-blocker and thioridazine. *Epinephrine:* May antagonize effects of epinephrine. *Lithium:* May cause disorientation, unconsciousness and extrapyramidal effects.

Lab Test Interferences

May discolor urine pink to red-brown. False-positive pregnancy test results may occur, but are less likely to occur with serum test. Increases in protein bound iodine have been reported.

Adverse Reactions

CV: Orthostatic hypotension; hypertension; tachycardia; bradycardia; syncope; cardiac arrest; circulatory collapse; lightheadedness; faintness; dizziness; EKG changes. *RESP:* Laryngospasm; respiratory depression; bronchospasm; dyspnea. *CNS:* Pseudoparkinsonism; dystonias; motor restlessness; headache; weakness; tremor; fatigue; slurring; insomnia; vertigo; seizures; tardive dyskinesia; drowsiness; paradoxical excitement; headache; confusion. *EENT:* Pigmentary retinopathy; glaucoma; photophobia; blurred vision; mydriasis; increased IOP; dry throat; nasal congestion. *GI:* Dyspepsia; constipation; dry mouth; adynamic ileus. *GU:* Urinary hesitancy or retention; impotence; sexual dysfunction; dysmenorrhea; menstrual irregularities. *HEMA:* Agranulocytosis; eosinophilia; leukopenia; hemolytic anemia; thrombocytopenic purpura. *HEPA:* Jaundice. *DERM:* Photosensitivity; skin pigmentation; dry skin; exfoliative dermatitis; urticarial rash; maculopapular hypersensitivity reaction; seborrhea; eczema. *META:* Decreased cholesterol. *OTHER:* Increases in appetite and weight; polydipsia; breast enlargement; galactorrhea; neuroleptic malignant syndrome.

Precautions

Pregnancy: Safety not established. *Lactation:* Safety not established. *Children:* Not recommended in children < 2 yr. *Elderly patients:* More susceptible to effects; consider lower dose. *Special risk patients:* Use caution in patients with cardiovascular disease or mitral insufficiency, history of glaucoma, EEG abnormalities or seizure disorders, prior brain damage, hepatic or renal impairment. *CNS effects:* May impair mental or physical abilities, especially during first few days of therapy. *Hepatic effects:* Jaundice usually occurs between 2nd and 4th weeks of treatment; considered hypersensitivity reaction. Usually reversible. *Neuroleptic malignant syndrome (NMS):* Has occurred with agents of this class; is potentially fatal. Signs and symptoms are hyperpyrexia, muscle rigidity, altered mental status, irregular pulse, irregular blood pressure, tachycardia and diaphoresis. *Pulmonary:* Cases of bronchopneumonia, some fatal, have occurred. *Sudden death:* Has been reported; predisposing factors may be seizures or previous brain damage. Flare-ups of psychotic behavior may precede death.

NURSING CONSIDERATIONS

Administration/Storage

- If using concentrate, do not mix with beverages containing caffeine, tannins or apple juice. Examples of possible mixing solutions include milk, saline, pineapple, orange-flavored soda, tomato juice, apricot or grapefruit juice.
- Avoid contact with skin.
- Store in tight, light-resistant container.

Assessment/Interventions

- Obtain patient history, including drug history and any known allergies.
- Assess mental status before initial administration.
- Check to ensure patient has swallowed drug.
- Monitor vital signs and check orthostatic BP and pulse before treatment and q 4 hr during therapy.
- Assess for signs of liver dysfunction (jaundice, light-colored stools, palpable liver).
- Monitor bilirubin, CBC and LFTs monthly.
- Assess alcohol consumption.
- Monitor for signs of tardive dyskinesia and other extrapyramidal symptoms and assess need for antiparkinson agent.
- Assess ECG for rhythm disturbances.
- Notify physician of changes in vital signs, ECG, or cardiac status.
- Notify physician if patient demonstrates psychiatric changes.
- Monitor I&O. Palpate bladder if urine output is decreased.
- Supervise ambulation until patient is stable.
- Increase fluid intake to prevent constipation.
- Provide sips of water, sugarless candy or sugarless gum to relieve dry mouth.

OVERDOSAGE: SIGNS & SYMPTOMS

Decreased consciousness, arrhythmias, extrapyramidal effects, confusion, agitation, respiratory depression, anticholinergic effects

Patient/Family Education

- Caution patient not to consume alcohol and to avoid otc medications while taking drug.
- Explain changes in urine color that may occur with this medication.
- Tell patient to report flank pain or changes in urination other than expected color changes.
- Tell patient to report signs of liver dysfunction, such as light-colored stools or jaundice.
- Explain type and potential significance of tardive dyskinesia such as changes in control of facial muscles.
- Instruct patient to avoid sudden position changes to prevent orthostatic hypotension.
- Caution patient to avoid hot tubs and hot showers and baths since hypotension may occur.
- Tell patient/family to report seizures, headaches, faint feeling, dizziness, or changes in mental function.
- Tell patient to use precautions against photosensitivity reactions. Advise use of sunscreen.

- Stress good oral hygiene.
- Caution patient not to drive while on medication, as may cause drowsiness or dizziness.
- Inform patient that in hot weather patient may have increased risk of heat stroke and increased sensitivity to sun.

See Patient Guide, p. 595.

Thiotepa (Triethylenethiophosphoramide; TSPA; TESPA)

(thigh-oh-TEP-uh)

Thioplex

Class: Antineoplastic/alkylator

Action Cell cycle–nonspecific alkylating agent related to nitrogen mustard that works by releasing ethylenimine radicals, which disrupt bonds of DNA.

Indications Treatment of adenocarcinoma of breast or ovary; control of intracavitary effusions secondary to treatment of superficial papillary carcinoma of urinary bladder. Previously used in treatment of lymphomas and Hodgkin's disease; other treatments more common now.

Contraindications Existing hepatic, renal or bone marrow damage.

Route/Dosage Note: Parenteral administration is most reliable route. IV doses may be given directly and rapidly. Drug may also be given directly into tumor mass. Individualize dosage. Do not give more frequently than weekly. Initial dose is usually higher, with maintenance dose adjusted weekly based on blood counts. ADULTS: **IV** 0.3-0.4 mg/kg at 1-4 wk intervals by rapid infusion.

Intratumor Administration

ADULTS: Initial doses of 0.6-0.8 mg/kg injected directly into tumor. Give local anesthetic first using same syringe. Dilute drug in Sterile Water for Injection 10 mg/ml. Maintenance doses, given at 1-4 wk intervals, range from 0.07-0.8 mg/kg.

Intracavitary Administration

ADULTS: Administer 0.6-0.8 mg/kg through same tubing used to remove cavitary fluid.

Intravesical Administration

ADULTS: Dehydrate patient with papillary bladder carcinoma for 8-12 hr pretreatment. Instill 60 mg in 30-60 ml of Sterile Water for Injection into bladder by catheter and retain solution for 2 hr. Usual course is once/wk for 4 wk. May be repeated 2nd and 3rd time; use caution due to possible bone marrow suppression.

Interactions *Pancuronium, succinylcholine:* Prolonged muscle paralysis and respiratory depression.

Lab Test Interferences None well documented.

Adverse Reactions *CNS:* Dizziness; blurred vision; headache. *GI:* Nausea; vomiting; anorexia. *GU:* Amenorrhea; interference with spermatogenesis. *HEMA:* Bone marrow suppression; leukopenia; thrombocytopenia; anemia. *DERM:* Allergic reactions; hives; rash; alopecia; pain at injection site. *OTHER:* Febrile reaction; subcutaneous lesion weeping.

Precautions *Pregnancy:* Not recommended. Pregnancy category D. *Lactation:* Undetermined. *Hematopoietic toxicity:* Rapidly falling WBC or platelet count indicates need to discontinue or reduce dosage. Do not combine with other alkylating agents having same mechanism of action or with irradiation due to increased risk of toxicity. Provide adequate recovery time, indicated by WBC, before instituting similar therapy.

NURSING CONSIDERATIONS

Administration/Storage

- Before bladder instillation, dehydrate patient for 8-10 hr before administration.
- For bladder instillation, change patient position q 15 min.
- Reconstitute to 10 mg/ml with Sterile Water. Reconstituted solution will remain stable for 5 days if refrigerated.
- Refrigerate unreconstituted solution and protect from light.

Assessment/Interventions

- Obtain patient history, including drug history and any known allergies.
- Assess CBC with platelets results at least weekly during therapy and for at least 3 wk after therapy discontinuation. Check with physician before giving if white blood count is $< 3,000/mm^3$ or platelets $< 150,000/mm^3$.
- Monitor vital signs.
- Monitor nutritional status.
- Assess for signs of infection and report significant findings to physician.
- Premedicate patient with antiemetics, as ordered. Monitor effectiveness of antiemetics.
- Report lab results not within normal range to physician.
- Report signs of liver, renal, GI, GU, skin or CNS dysfunction to physician.

OVERDOSAGE: SIGNS & SYMPTOMS

Hematopoietic toxicity

Patient/Family Education

- Caution patient that this medication should not be taken during pregnancy or when pregnancy is possible. Advise patient to use reliable form of birth control while taking this drug.
- Tell patient to report fever, chills, yellow skin, skin rashes, uncontrolled nausea and vomiting, diarrhea, black or bloody stools, changes in or discolored urine, vaginal bleeding or yeast-like discharge, mouth sores, recurrent headaches or dizziness to physician.
- Teach patient and caregiver about basic function of components of CBC and platelets and therapeutic effect of drug.
- Advise patient about precautions against infection.
- If patient has low platelet count, explain appropriate precautions to prevent bleeding.
- Inform patient regarding hair loss and head-covering options.
- Instruct patient to avoid otc products that contain aspirin.

See Patient Guide, p. 596.

Thiothixene

(THIGH-oh-THIX-een)

Navane, Navane Concentrate

Class: Antipsychotic/thioxanthene

Action Produces antipsychotic effects apparently due to dopamine receptor blocking in CNS.

Indications Management of psychotic disorders such as schizophrenia. **Unlabeled uses:** Treatment of Tourette's syndrome; control of acute agitation in elderly; treatment of some symptoms of dementia.

Contraindications Comatose or severely depressed states; presence of large amounts of CNS depressants; circulatory collapse; liver damage; subcortical brain damage; CNS depression from any cause; bone marrow depression or blood dyscrasias.

Route/Dosage

ADULTS: **PO** Up to 60 mg/day. **IM** 4 mg bid-qid (maximum 30 mg/day). ELDERLY OR DEBILITATED PATIENTS: **PO** Up to 30 mg/day. CHILDREN 12-18 YR: **PO** 0.3 mg/kg/day (usual range 5-42 mg/day).

Interactions

Alcohol, other CNS depressants: May cause additive CNS depressant effects. *Anticholinergics:* May reduce therapeutic effects and increase anticholinergic effects of thiothixene; may lead to tardive dyskinesia. *Guanethidine:* May inhibit hypotensive effect of guanethidine.

Lab Test Interferences

False-positive pregnancy test results may occur, but are less likely to occur with serum test. Increases in protein-bound iodine have been reported.

Adverse Reactions

CV: Orthostatic hypotension; tachycardia; syncope; lightheadedness; ECG changes. *RESP:* Laryngospasm; bronchospasm; increased depth of respiration. *CNS:* Tardive dyskinesia; extrapyramidal symptoms (eg, pseudoparkinsonism, akathesia, dystonias); drowsiness; insomnia; restlessness; agitation; seizures; paradoxical exacerbation of psychotic symptoms. *EENT:* Pigmentary retinopathy; lenticular pigmentation; blurred vision; nasal congestion. *GI:* Dry mouth; anorexia; diarrhea; nausea; vomiting; constipation. *GU:* Impotence, sexual dysfunction; amenorrhea. *HEMA:* Leukopenia; leukocytosis. *DERM:* Rash; pruritus; urticaria; photosensitivity. *META:* Elevations of serum transaminase and alkaline phosphatase. *OTHER:* Breast enlargement; lactation; gynecomastia; hypoglycemia; hyperglycemia; glycosuria; polydipsia; increase in appetite and weight; peripheral edema; elevated prolactin levels; increased sweating or salivation.

Precautions

Pregnancy: Pregnancy category undetermined. *Lactation:* Undetermined. *Children:* Not recommended in children < 12 yr. *Elderly patients:* More susceptible to adverse effects. *Special risk patients:* Use drug with caution in patients with cardiovascular disease or mitral insufficiency, history of glaucoma, EEG abnormalities or seizure disorders, prior brain damage or hepatic or renal impairment. *CNS effects:* Drug may impair mental or physical abilities, especially during first few days of therapy. *Hepatic effects:* Jaundice (usually reversible) may occur, usually between second and fourth wk of treatment, and is considered hypersensitivity reaction. *Neuroleptic malignant syndrome:* Has occurred with similar agents and is potentially fatal. Signs and symptoms are hyperpyrexia, muscle rigidity, altered mental status, irregular pulse, irregular BP, tachycardia and diaphoresis. *Pulmonary effects:* Cases of bronchopneumonia, some fatal, have occurred. *Sudden death:* Has been reported; predisposing factors may be seizures or previous brain damage. Flareups of psychotic behavior may precede death. *Tardive dyskinesia:* Potentially irreversible involuntary body and facial movements may occur. Prevalence highest in elderly, especially women.

NURSING CONSIDERATIONS

Administration/Storage

- Administer at bedtime to minimize effects of sedation and orthostatic hypotension if prescribed as a single daily dose.
- If using liquid concentrate, measure each dose and mix with a small amount of water for each administration.
- If patient is reluctant to take medicine, observe that medication is taken and not hoarded.
- Reconstitute powder for IM injection with 2.2 ml Sterile Water for Injection. Reconstituted powder can be stored at room temperature for up to 48 hr before discarding.
- Deep IM injection should be given in gluteal muscle.

Assessment/Interventions

- Obtain patient history, includ-

ing drug history and any known allergies.

- Assess for history of breast enlargement.
- Assess vital signs (including orthostatic BP) and blood glucose.
- Monitor weight.
- Obtain ECG as ordered by physician.
- If signs of changes in baseline psychiatric condition occur, notify physician.
- Monitor LFTs periodically during therapy.
- If hypotension, tachycardia, faint feeling, chest pain, nausea, vomiting, diarrhea, constipation, menstrual changes, sexual dysfunction, vision changes, mouth dryness, nasal blockage or skin changes occur, notify physician.
- Notify physician of increasing breast size, increased appetite, salivation and sweating or changes in lab results.
- Monitor patient for onset of extrapyramidal side effects, and notify physician if these occur.

OVERDOSAGE: SIGNS & SYMPTOMS

Somnolence, coma, hypotension, extrapyramidal symptoms, agitation, restlessness, convulsions, fever, hypothermia, ECG changes, cardiac arrhythmias

Patient/Family Education

- Caution patient to avoid alcohol and other CNS depressants while taking this medication.
- Advise patient not to take otc medications without consulting physician.
- Instruct patient/family to notify physician of mental changes, chest pain, faint feeling, swelling, vision changes, headaches, skin changes, menstrual changes, stool discoloration or yellowing of skin or eyes.
- Instruct patient to take sips of water frequently or to suck on ice chips, sugarless candy or chewing gum if dry mouth occurs.
- Caution patient to avoid exposure to sunlight and to use sunscreen or wear protective clothing to avoid photosensitivity reaction.
- Inform patient that patient may experience increased sweating while taking this medication.
- Instruct family to call emergency number if patient has seizure.
- Instruct patient to avoid sudden position changes to prevent orthostatic hypotension.
- Advise patient that drug causes lightheadedness and drowsiness and to use caution while driving or performing other tasks requiring mental alertness.
- Advise patient that medication increases sensitivity to heat and to avoid exposure to high ambient temperatures.

See Patient Guide, p. 597.

Thyroid, Desiccated
(Thyroid USP)

(THIGH-royd, DESS-ih-KATE-uhd)

Armour Thyroid, S-P-T, Thyrar, Thyroid Strong

Class: Thyroid

Action Increases metabolic rate of body tissues.

Indications Replacement or supplemental therapy in hypothyroidism; TSH suppression (in thyroid cancer, nodules, goiters and enlargement in chronic thyroiditis); diagnostic agent to differentiate suspected hyperthyroidism from euthyroidism.

STOP **Contraindications** Hypersensitivity to any ingredient; acute MI and thyrotoxicosis uncomplicated by hypothyroidism. Also contraindicated when hypothyroidism and hypoadrenalism (Addison's disease) coexist, unless treatment of hypoadrenalism with adrenocortical steroids precedes initiation of thyroid therapy.

Route/Dosage

Optimal dosage determined by clinical response and laboratory findings.

Hypothyroidism

ADULTS: **PO** 30 mg/day initially, increasing by 15 mg increments every 2-3 wk. In patients with long-standing myxedema, 15 mg/day, particularly if cardiovascular impairment is suspected. Reduce dosage if angina occurs. Maintenance: 60-120 mg/day. CHILDREN: **PO** See table for recommended dose in congenital hypothyroidism.

CONGENITAL HYPOTHYROIDISM DOSE

Age	Dose per day (mg)	Daily dose per kg (mg)
>12 yr	>90	1.2-1.8
6 to 12 yr	60-90	2.4-3
1 to 5 yr	45-60	3-3.6
6-12 mo	30-45	3.6-4.8
0-6 mo	15-30	4.8-6

Thyroid Cancer

Larger doses required.

Interactions

Anticoagulants: Anticoagulant effects may be increased. *Cholestyramine:* May decrease thyroid efficacy. *Digitalis glycosides:* Digitalis levels may increase, resulting in toxicity. *Theophyllines:* Theophylline clearance may be altered in hyperthyroid or hypothyroid patients.

Lab Test Interferences

Consider changes in thyroid-binding globulin concentration when interpreting T_4 and T_3 values. Medicinal or dietary iodine interferes with all in vivo tests of radioiodine uptake, producing low uptakes that may not reflect true decrease in hormone synthesis.

Adverse Reactions

Adverse reactions generally indicate hyperthyroidism due to therapeutic overdosage. *CV:* Palpitations; tachycardia; cardiac arrhythmias; angina pectoris; cardiac arrest. *CNS:* Tremors; headache; nervousness; insomnia. *GI:* Diarrhea; vomiting. *GU:* Menstrual irregularities. *OTHER:* Hypersensitivity; weight loss; sweating; heat intolerance; fever.

Precautions

Pregnancy: Category A. *Lactation:* Excreted in breast milk. *Children:* Congenital hypothyroidism: Routine determinations of serum T_4 or TSH are strongly advised in neonates. Initiate treatment immediately on diagnosis and continue for life, unless transient hypothyroidism is suspected. In infants, excessive doses of thyroid hormone preparations may produce craniosynostosis. Children may experience transient partial hair loss in first few months of thyroid therapy. *Cardiovascular disease:* Use caution when integrity of CV system, particularly coronary arteries is suspect (eg, angina, elderly). Development of chest pain or worsening CV disease requires decrease in dosage. Observe patients with coronary artery disease during surgery, since possibility of cardiac arrhythmias may be greater in those treated with thyroid hormones. *Endocrine disorders:* Therapy in patients with concomitant diabetes mellitus or insipidus or adrenal insufficiency (Addison's disease) exacerbates intensity of symptoms. Therapy of myxedema coma requires simultaneous administration of glucocorticoids. In patients whose hypothyroidism is secondary to hypopituitarism, adrenal insufficiency, if present, should be corrected with corticosteroids before administering thyroid hormones. *Hyperthyroid effects:* May rarely precipitate hyperthyroid state or may aggravate existing hyperthyroidism. *Morphologic hypogonadism and nephrosis:* Rule out before therapy. *Myxedema:* Patients are particularly sensitive to thyroid preparations. Begin with small doses. *Obesity:* Should not be used for weight reduction; may produce serious or even life-threatening toxicity in larger doses, particularly when given with anorexiants.

NURSING CONSIDERATIONS

Administration/Storage

- Assess baseline T_4 or TSH as ordered by physician.
- When administered as single dose, give in morning to avoid sleeplessness.
- Adjust dose to administer lowest dose possible to relieve symptoms.
- Do not interchange different thyroid products. Absorption may vary.
- Store at room temperature in tightly closed container.

Assessment/Interventions

- Obtain patient history, including drug history and any known allergies.
- Before each dose, assess BP and pulse.
- Monitor vital signs and weight.
- In children, monitor height and weight to document normal growth rate.
- Notify physician of any changes from baseline status in physical assessment or laboratory testing.

OVERDOSAGE: SIGNS & SYMPTOMS

Tachycardia, arrhythmias, hypertension, angina, fever, tremor, vomiting, diarrhea, insomnia, headache, seizures, coma

Patient/Family Education

- Explain that children may have short-term temporary hair loss at start of therapy.
- Tell patient to report fever, weight loss, menstrual irregularity, palpitations, chest pain, headache, faint feeling, sweatiness, diarrhea, vomiting, inability to sleep, excitability, irritability, anxiety, nervousness or any changes to physician.
- Teach patient to avoid otc preparations and food with iodine: iodinated salt, soy beans, tofu, turnips, some seafood, some types of bread.
- Instruct patient not to switch drug brands unless physician approves.

See Patient Guide, p. 598.

Ticarcillin (Ticarcillin disodium)

(TIE-car-sill-in)

Ticar

Class: Antibiotic/penicillin

Action Inhibits bacterial cell wall mucopeptide synthesis.

Indications Treatment of bacterial septicemia, skin and soft tissue infections, acute and chronic respiratory tract infections and genitourinary tract infections caused by susceptible strains of anaerobic bacteria, *Pseudomonas aeruginosa*, *Proteus* species, and *Escherichia coli*.

Contraindications Hypersensitivity to penicillins.

Route/Dosage

Serious Urinary Tract and Systemic Infections

ADULTS & CHILDREN: **IV** 200-300 mg/kg/day in divided doses q 4-6 hr. In adults, the usual dose is **IV** 3-4 g q 4-6 hr.

Uncomplicated Urinary Tract Infections

ADULTS: **IM/IV** 1 g q 6 hr. CHILDREN < 40 KG: **IM/IV** 50-100 mg/kg/day in divided doses q 6-8 hr. NEONATES: **IM/IV** 75-100 mg/kg q 8-12 hr.

Interactions

Anticoagulants: May increase bleeding risks of anticoagulant by prolonging bleeding time. *Chloramphenicol:* Synergism or antagonism may develop. *Contraceptives, oral:* May reduce efficacy of oral contraceptives. Use additional form of contraception during ticarcillin therapy. *Erythromycin:* Synergism or antagonism may develop. *Heparin:* May increase bleeding risks of heparin by prolonging bleeding time. *Probenecid:* May increase ticarcillin concentration. *Tetracyclines:* May impair bactericidal effects of ticarcillin. INCOMPATIBILITIES: *Aminoglycosides, parenteral:* May inactivate aminoglycosides in vitro; do not mix in same IV solution. May be used in combination for synergy.

Lab Test Interferences

May cause false-positive urine glucose test results with Benedict's Solution, Fehling's Solution or Clinitest tablets but not with enzyme-based tests (e.g., Clinistix, Tes-tape); false-positive direct Coombs' test result in certain patient groups; false-positive protein reactions with sulfosalicylic acid and boiling test, acetic acid test, biuret reaction and nitric acid test but not with bromphenol blue test (Multi-Stix).

Adverse Reactions

CV: Phlebitis; vein irritation; deep vein thrombosis. *CNS:* Neurotoxicity (lethargy, neuromuscular irritability, hallucinations, convulsions and seizures). *EENT:* Itchy eyes. *GI:* Nausea; vomiting; diarrhea or bloody diarrhea; pseudomembranous colitis. *GU:* Elevated creatinine or BUN; vaginitis. *HEMA:* Anemia; hemolytic anemia; thrombocytopenia; thrombocytopenic purpura; eosinophilia; leukopenia; granulocytopenia; neutropenia; bone marrow depression; prolongation of bleeding and prothrombin time; increase in platelets. *HEPA:* Transient hepatitis (elevated AST). *DERM:* Rash; pruritis; urticaria. *META:* Elevated serum alkaline phosphatase; hypernatremia; reduced serum potassium. *OTHER:* Hypersensitivity reactions; hyperthermia; pain at site of injection; hematomas.

Precautions

Pregnancy: Category B. *Lactation:* Excreted in breast milk. *Bleeding abnormalities:* Hemorrhagic manifestations associated with abnormalities of coagulation tests (bleeding time, prothrombin time, platelet aggregation) may occur. Abnormalities should revert to normal once drug is discontinued. *Hypersensitivity:* Reactions range from mild to life-threatening. Administer drug with caution to cephalosporin-sensitive patients due to possible cross-reactivity. *Pseudomembranous colitis:* May occur due to overgrowth of clostridia. *Renal insufficiency:* Dosage and interval adjustments are necessary. *Sodium content:* Contains 4.7-5 mEq sodium per gram. *Superinfection:* May result in bacterial or fungal overgrowth of nonsusceptible organisms.

NURSING CONSIDERATIONS

Administration/Storage

IM

- Reconstitute with sterile water, sodium chloride or 1% lidocaine HCl solution (without epinephrine) to obtain 1 g ticarcillin per 2.6 ml solution.
- Use promptly after reconstitution.
- Inject into relatively large muscle.
- Do *not* exceed 1 g/injection.

IV

- Do *not* mix gentamicin, amikacin or tobramycin in same IV solution.
- Administer slowly over 30 min-2 hr to avoid vein irritation.
- To reconstitute: Add 4 ml of Sodium Chloride Injection, Dextrose Injection 5% or Lactated Ringer's Injection to each gram of ticarcillin powder to obtain 200 mg/ml. When dissolved, dilute further to desired volume.
- Reconstitute 3 g piggyback bottles with minimum of 30 ml of desired IV solution. A dilution of 50 mg/ml or less will reduce incidence of vein irritation.
- After reconstitution, may be stored frozen for up to 30 days.
- Store IV solutions mixed in Sodium Chloride or Dextrose no longer than 72 hr at room temperature or 14 days under refrigeration.
- Store IV solutions mixed in Ringer's Solution no longer than 48 hr at room temperature or 14 days under refrigeration.

Assessment/Interventions

- Obtain patient history, including drug history and any known allergies.
- Obtain urine and culture and sensitivity specimens and send to lab. Therapy may be initiated before results are received, but cultures should be collected prior to drug therapy.
- Request WBC and differential counts prior to initiation of therapy and at least weekly during therapy.
- Request AST & ALT, H&H, BUN and creatinine studies at appropriate intervals during therapy.
- Perform periodic hemoccult tests on stool.
- Monitor and record skin integrity, report ecchymosis, bleeding, rashes.
- Assess neurologic status, and report lethargy and irritability.
- Asses GI status and report changes in appetite or bowel habits.
- Assess GU status and report hematuria, oliguria and proteinuria.
- Monitor lab results and report abnormal H&H, potassium, WBC & differential counts, blood coagulation tests, and LFTs.
- Monitor results of culture and sensitivity to ensure bacteria is sensitive to ticarcillin.
- Monitor IV site and report signs of vein irritation.
- Monitor I&O and report imbalances. Ensure adequate fluid intake, especially if patient has diarrhea episodes.
- Apply ice pack if pain and induration occur at injection site.
- Monitor for signs of superinfection.

OVERDOSAGE: SIGNS & SYMPTOMS

May result in neuromuscular hyperexcitability or seizures

Patient/Family Education

- Advise patient to report rash, hives, fever, itching, severe diarrhea, shortness of breath, wheezing, black tongue, sore throat, nausea, vomiting, swollen joints, unusual bleeding or bruising.
- Tell diabetic patients to use Clinistix or Tes-tape for urine monitoring. Solutions used for urine glucose testing may indicate false positive results if taking penicillin therapy over period of time.

See Patient Guide, p. 599.

Ticarcillin/Clavulanate (Ticarcillin Disodium and Clavulanate Potassium)

(TIE-car-sill-in/CLAV-you-luh-nate)

Timentin

Class: Antibiotic/penicillin

Action Ticarcillin inhibits bacterial cell wall mucopeptide synthesis. Clavulanate lactamase enzymes commonly found in microorganisms resistant to ticarcillin.

Indications Treatment of bacterial septicemia, skin and soft tissue infections, acute and chronic respiratory tract infections, bone and joint infections, and genitourinary and gynecologic infections caused by susceptible strains of bacteria.

Contraindications Hypersensitivity to penicillin.

Route/Dosage

Systemic and Urinary Tract Infections

ADULTS ≥ 60 KG: **IV** 3.1 g q 4-6 hr. ADULTS & CHILDREN ≤ 60 kg: **IV** 200-300 mg/kg/day in divided doses q 4-6 hr.

Gynecologic Infections

ADULTS: **IV** 200-300 mg/kg/day in divided doses q 4-6 hr.

Interactions

Anticoagulants: May increase bleeding risks of anticoagulant by prolonging bleeding time. *Chloramphenicol:* Synergism or antagonism may develop. *Contraceptives, oral:* May reduce efficacy of oral contraceptives. Use additional form of contraception during ticarcillin/clavulanate therapy. *Erythromycin:* Synergism or antagonism may develop. *Heparin:* May increase bleeding risks of heparin by prolonging bleeding time. *Probenecid:* May increase ticarcillin levels. *Sodium bicarbonate:* Ticarcillin/clavulanate is incompatible with sodium bicarbonate; not recommended as diluent. *Tetracyclines:* May impair bactericidal effects of ticarcillin/clavulanate. INCOMPATIBILITIES: *Aminoglycosides, parenteral:* May inactivate aminoglycosides in vitro; do not mix in same IV solution. May be used in combination for synergy.

Lab Test Interferences

May cause false-positive urine glucose test results with Benedict's Solution, Fehling's Solution, or Clinitest tablets but not with enzyme-based tests (e.g., Clinistix, Tes-tape); false-positive direct Coombs' test in certain patient groups; positive direct antiglobulin tests (DAT); false-positive protein reactions with sulfosalicylic acid and boiling test, acetic acid test, biuret reaction and nitric acid test but not with bromphenol blue test (Multi-Stix).

Adverse Reactions

CV: Deep vein thrombosis; vein irritation; phlebitis. *CNS:* Neurotoxicity (lethargy, neuromuscular irritability and seizures). *GI:* Nausea; vomiting; abdominal pain or cramp; diarrhea; pseudomembranous colitis. *GU:* Elevated creatinine or BUN; vaginitis. *HEMA:* Anemia; hemolytic anemia; thrombocytopenia; eosinophilia; leukopenia; granulocytopenia; neutropenia; prolongation of bleeding and prothrombin time. *HEPA:* Transient hepatitis; cholestatic jaundice. *DERM:* Rash; pruritis; urticaria; ecchymosis. *META:* Elevated serum alkaline phosphatase; hypernatremia; reduced serum potassium. *OTHER:* Hypersensitivity reactions; pain at site of injection; hematomas; hyperthermia.

Precautions

Pregnancy: Category B. *Lactation:* Excreted in breast milk. *Bleeding abnormalities:* Hemorrhagic manifestations associated with abnormalities of coagulation tests (bleeding time, prothrombin time, platelet aggregation) may occur. Abnormalities should revert to normal once drug is discontinued. *Hypersensitivity:* Reactions range from mild to life-threatening. Administer cautiously to cephalosporin-sensitive patients due to possible cross-reactivity. *Hypokalemia:* Ticarcillin has rarely decreased potassium levels. *Pseudomembranous colitis:* May occur due to overgrowth of clostridia. *Renal insufficiency:* Dosage and interval adjustments necessary. *Sodium content:* Powder for injection contains 4.75 mEq Na/gram of ticarcillin. *Superinfection:* May result in bacterial or fungal overgrowth of nonsusceptible organisms.

NURSING CONSIDERATIONS

Administration/Storage

- To reconstitute: Add approximately 13.0 ml of Sterile Water for Injection or Sodium Chloride Injection. Then dilute further to concentrations of 10-100 mg/ml with NaCl, 5% Dextrose or Lactated Ringer's.
- Administer IV over 30 min by direct infusion or by piggyback.
- Discontinue other solutions while this drug is being infused via piggyback.
- Do *not* mix sodium bicarbonate, gentamicin, amikacin or tobramycin in same IV solution.
- Store concentrated stock solution (200 mg/ml) no longer than 6 hr at room temperature or 72 hr under refrigeration.
- Store concentrations of 10-100 mg/ml in Sodium Chloride for Injection or Lactated Ringer's no longer than 24 hr at room temperature; 7 days under refrigeration or 30 days frozen. Store solutions made with 5% Dextrose no longer than 24 hr at room

temperature, 3 days under refrigeration or 7 days frozen.

- Thaw premixed, frozen solutions at room temperature or in refrigerator.
- Do *not* immerse in water baths or microwave to thaw.
- After thawing, store refrigerated no longer than 7 days or 24 hr at room temperature.
- Do *not* refreeze.

Assessment/Interventions

- Obtain patient history, including drug history and any known allergies.
- Assess results of AST & ALT, H&H, BUN and creatinine studies at appropriate intervals during therapy.
- Send urine and culture and sensitivity specimens to lab. Therapy may be initiated before results are received, but cultures should be collected prior to drug therapy.
- Request WBC and differential counts prior to initiation of therapy and at least weekly during therapy.
- Perform periodic hemoccult tests on stool.
- Monitor and record skin integrity. Report ecchymosis, bleeding and rashes.
- Assess neurologic status and report lethargy and irritability.
- Assess GI status and report changes in appetite or bowel habits. If patient has diarrhea, consider possibility of pseudomembranous colitis.
- Assess GU status and report hematuria, oliguria and proteinuria.
- Monitor data throughout therapy and report abnormalities to physician.
- Monitor I&O and report imbalances to physician. Ensure adequate fluid intake, especially if client has diarrhea episodes.
- Assess IV site regularly and report signs of vein irritation to physician.
- If pain and induration occur at injection site, apply ice pack.
- Monitor for signs of superinfection.

OVERDOSAGE: SIGNS & SYMPTOMS

Neuromuscular hyperexcitability, seizures

Patient/Family Education

- Advise patient to report rash, hives, fever, itching, severe diarrhea, shortness of breath, wheezing, black tongue, sore throat, nausea, vomiting, fever, swollen joints, unusual bleeding or bruising.
- Explain that intermittent urinalysis may be required several months after treatment.
- Tell diabetic patients to use Clinistix or Tes-tape for urine monitoring. Solutions used for urine glucose testing may indicate false-positive results if taking penicillin therapy over period of time.

No patient monograph available.

Ticlopidine HCl

(tie-KLOE-pih-DEEN HIGH-droe-KLOR-ide)

Ticlid

Class: Antiplatelet

Action Produces time- and dose-dependent inhibition of both platelet aggregation and release of platelet granule constituents as well as prolongation of bleeding time; interferes with platelet membrane function by inhibiting platelet-fibrinogen binding and subsequent platelet-platelet interactions.

Indications Reduction of risk of thrombotic stroke in patients who have experienced stroke precursors and in patients who have had completed thrombotic stroke. Reserved for patients intolerant to aspirin because of greater risk of adverse reactions. **Unlabeled uses:** Improved walking distance in intermittent claudication; vascular improvement in chronic arterial occlusion; reduced incidence of neurologic deficit in subarachnoid hemorrhage; reduced incidence of vascular occlusion in uremic patients with arteriovenous shunts or fistulas; control of platelet count in open heart surgery; decreased graft occlusion in coronary artery bypass grafts; reduced degree of proteinuria and hematuria in primary glomerulonephritis; reduced incidence, duration and severity of infarctive crises in sickle cell disease.

Contraindications Presence of hematopoietic disorders (eg, neutropenia, thrombocytopenia); presence of hemostatic disorder or active pathologic bleeding (eg, bleeding, peptic ulcer, intracranial bleeding, hemophilia, other coagulation defects); severe liver impairment.

Route/Dosage

ADULTS: PO 250 mg bid with food.

Interactions

Antacids: May reduce ticlopidine absorption. *Aspirin:* Increased effect of aspirin on collagen-induced platelet aggregation. *Cimetidine:* Elevated ticlopidine levels with possible increase in therapeutic and toxic effects. *Theophylline:* Elevated serum theophylline concentrations, increasing risk of toxicity.

Lab Test Interferences

None well documented.

Adverse Reactions

CV: Vasculitis. *CNS:* Headache; peripheral neuropathy. *EENT:* Tinnitus. *GI:* Diarrhea; nausea; fullness. *GU:* Nephrotic syndrome. *HEMA:* Prolonged bleeding time; bleeding complications (ecchymosis, epistaxis, hematuria, conjunctival hemorrhage, GI bleeding, perioperative bleeding); neutropenia; pancytopenia; hemolytic anemia; serum sickness; immune thrombocytopenia; thrombocytopenic thrombotic purpura. *HEPA:* Hepatitis; cholestatic jaundice, increased alkaline phosphotase; serum transaminases and bilirubin. *DERM:* Maculopapular or urticarial rash. *META:* Increased cholesterol and triglycerides. *OTHER:* Weakness; pain; allergic pneumonitis; systemic lupus erythematosus; arthropathy; myositis; hyponatremia.

Precautions

Pregnancy: Category B. *Lactation:* Undetermined. *Children:* Safety and efficacy in children < 18 yr not established. *Elderly patients:* Require dosage reduction. *Hematologic effects:* Fatal reactions (eg, pancytopenia) have occurred. *Hypersensitivity:* Reactions range from minor to life-threatening. *Liver disease:* Use not recommended because patient may have pre-existing bleeding diathesis. *Renal impairment:* Dosage reduction or discontinuation of therapy may be required if hemorrhagic or hematopoietic complications occur.

NURSING CONSIDERATIONS

Administration/Storage

- Administer medication with food.
- Anticoagulant or fibrinolytic drugs must be discontinued before initiation of ticlopidine administration.
- Ticlopidine must be discontinued 10-14 days before surgery.
- Store at room temperature.

Assessment/Interventions

- Obtain patient history, including drug history and any known allergies. Note ulcers and bleeding problems.
- Ensure that patient does not have pre-existing bleeding tendency by monitoring PT/PTT. Measure periodically during therapy.
- Check results of CBC with platelets and ANC (absolute neutropil count).
- Take vital signs including orthostatic BP and pulse.
- Assess for signs of infection.
- Obtain CBC with platelets and ANC as baseline and then every 2 wk dur-

ing first 3 mo of therapy. Assess more frequently if ANC decreases constantly or is 30% less than baseline. After 3 mo, if CBC, platelet and ANC are stable, assess these values only if there are signs of infection or bleeding.

- When drug is discontinued, perform CBC with platelet and ANC 1-3 wk after last dose.
- Monitor LFTs periodically during therapy.
- Monitor for nausea, vomiting or diarrhea.
- Monitor for signs of bleeding, including petechiae or unusual bruising.

OVERDOSAGE: SIGNS & SYMPTOMS

Increased bleeding time, increased ALT

Patient/Family Education

- Instruct patient to take with food.
- Inform patient of increased risk of bleeding and caution patient to take precautionary measures (eg, not to use manual razor, to use soft toothbrush, to handle knives carefully, to always wear shoes when walking).
- Instruct patient to report signs of infection (eg, fever, white overgrowth in mouth, vaginal yeast, nonhealing wounds or wounds that appear red with drainage) to physician.
- Advise patient to notify physician of signs of blood or changes in stool or urine, unusual bruising, decreased appetite, dark urine, light-colored stools or yellow skin color.
- Instruct patient to inform physicians and dentist of drug regimen before undergoing any treatments or surgery or receiving new drugs.
- Suggest that patient carry identification (eg, Medi-Alert) indicating drug regimen and condition.
- Advise patient to separate administration of ticlopidine and antacids by at least 2 hr.

See Patient Guide, p. 600.

Timolol Maleate

(TI-moe-lahl MAL-ee-ate)

Blocadren, Timoptic, Timoptic Ocudose, ♣ *Apo-Timol, Apo-Timop*

Class: Beta-adrenergic blocker

Action Blocks beta-receptors, which primarily affects heart (slows rate), vascular musculature (decreases blood pressure) and lungs (reduces function). Reduces both elevated and normal IOP via decreasing production of aqueous humor or increasing flow.

Indications Treatment of hypertension, alone or in combination with other agents; reduction of risk of reinfarction post-MI; migraine prophylaxis; topical management of chronic open angle glaucoma; management of ocular hypertension. **Unlabeled uses:** Treatment of ventricular arrhythmias and tachycardias, essential tremors, anxiety; management of chronic stable angina pectoris.

Contraindications Hypersensitivity to beta-blockers; greater than first-degree heart block; CHF unless secondary to tachyarrhythmia treatable with beta-blockers; overt cardiac failure; sinus bradycardia; cardiogenic shock; bronchial asthma or bronchospasm, including severe COPD.

Route/Dosage

Hypertension

ADULTS: PO 10 mg bid, titrate to response q 7 days (maximum 60 mg/day).

MI Prophylaxis

ADULTS: PO 10 mg bid.

Migraine Prophylaxis

ADULTS: PO 10 mg bid (maximum 30 mg/day); if no response in 6 weeks then discontinue.

Essential Tremor

ADULTS: PO 10 mg/day.

Glaucoma

ADULTS: **Ophthalmic** 1 gtt 0.25-0.5% solution in affected eye(s) bid.

Interactions

Clonidine: May enhance or reverse antihypertensive effect; potentially life-threatening situations may occur, especially on withdrawal. *Epinephrine:* Initial hypertensive episode followed by bradycardia may occur. *Ergot alkaloids:* Peripheral ischemia, manifested by cold extremities and possible gangrene, may occur. *Insulin:* Prolonged hypoglycemia with masking of symptoms may occur. *NSAIDs:* Some agents may impair antihypertensive effect. *Prazosin:* Orthostatic hypotension may be increased. *Theophyllines:* Elimination of theophylline may be reduced. Effects of both drugs may be reduced. *Verapamil:* Effects of both drugs may be increased.

Lab Test Interferences

None well documented.

Adverse Reactions

CV: Hypotension; heart palpitations; bradycardia; heart failure, edema. *RESP:* Wheezing; cough; breathing difficulties, especially in asthmatics or patients with COPD. *CNS:* Dizziness; depression; lethargy; headache; insomnia; anxiety; tremor; paresthesia. *EENT (topical use):* Transient irritation, burning, tearing and conjunctival edema; blurred vision; light sensitivity. *GI:* Abdominal pain; diarrhea; nausea. *GU:* Impotence; sexual dysfunction; decreased libido; dysuria; urinary retention or frequency; nocturia; increased BUN. *HEMA:* Decreased Hgb, Hct. *DERM:* Increased sensitivity to cold; rash; pruritus; alopecia; sweating. *META:* Alteration of glucose metabolism; masking of hypoglycemia; increased triglycerides, uric acid, potassium. *OTHER:* Joint pain; muscle cramps.

Precautions

Pregnancy: Category C. *Lactation:* Excreted in breast milk. *Children:* Safety and efficacy not established. *Abrupt withdrawal:* Has been associated with increased angina and MI; gradually decrease dose over 1-2 wk. *Anaphylaxis:* Deaths have occurred; aggressive therapy may be required. *Bronchospasm:* Oral and ophthalmic forms may precipitate bronchospasm in susceptible patients. *CHF:* Administer drug with caution to patients with CHF controlled by digitalis and diuretics. Notify physician at first sign or symptom of CHF or of unexplained respiratory symptoms in any patient. *Diabetic patients:* Drug may mask signs and symptoms of hypoglycemia, eg, tachycardia, BP changes. Drug may potentiate insulin-induced hypoglycemia. *Peripheral vascular disease:* Drug may precipitate or aggravate symptoms of arterial insufficiency. *Renal/hepatic impairment:* Dosage reduction may be required. *Thyrotoxicosis:* Drug may mask clinical signs, eg, tachycardia, of developing or continuing hyperthyroidism. Abrupt withdrawal may exacerbate symptoms of hyperthyroidism, including thyroid storm.

NURSING CONSIDERATIONS

Administration/Storage

- Administer tablets orally with meals and at bedtime. Administer ophthalmic solutions via dropper provided.
- Tablets may be crushed or swallowed whole.
- Store tablets at room temperature, away from moisture and sunlight.
- Store ophthalmic solution at room temperature away from sunlight. Do *not* freeze.
- Discard ophthalmic solution if brown, cloudy or if contains particles.

Assessment/Interventions

- Obtain patient history, including drug history and any known allergies.
- Monitor and record BP, especially that of renal dialysis patients (report

hypotension); pulse (report tachycardia); blood glucose of diabetic patients on regular basis (report hypoglycemia).

- Assess apical/radial pulse before administration. Notify physician of any changes.
- Assess and document muscle strength of myasthenia gravis patients, and report increased weakness.
- Contact physician immediately if patient shows signs of cardiac failure.
- Have available isoproterenol, dopamine, dobutamine or norepinephrine to reverse effects in emergency.
- Use ophthalmic solution cautiously if patient is taking oral beta-blockers, because solution may be absorbed systemically and create an additive effect.
- If drug is for migraine prevention, monitor effectiveness and consult physician if satisfactory response is not obtained after 6-8 wk of maximum daily dose.
- Monitor I&O and weight daily. Monitor hydration status.
- Assess for edema in feet and legs daily.

OVERDOSAGE: SIGNS & SYMPTOMS

Severe bradycardia, severe hypotension, bronchospasm, acute cardiac failure

Patient/Family Education

- Explain that eye drops commonly produce transient stinging or discomfort and to notify physician if symptoms are severe.
- Teach patient how to instill eye drops: Shake once before using. Wash hands; do not allow dropper to touch eye. Tilt head back, look up; pull lower eyelid down; instill prescribed number of drops. Close eye for 1-2 min and apply gentle pressure over bridge of nose. Do not rub eye.
- Explain that if using eye drops, physician may need to monitor eye pressure at regular intervals and at different times of day.
- Tell patient to consult physician before using otc cough, cold or allergy medications, including nasal decongestants.
- Encourage diabetic patient to use glucometer regularly. This drug may increase chances of hypoglycemic reactions to insulin or may mask signs and symptoms of hypoglycemia.
- Inform patient to notify physician immediately of shortness of breath (especially if lying down), feet swelling, night cough and slow pulse rate.
- Tell patient to notify physician of skin rash, fever, lightheadedness, confusion, depression, sore throat, unusual bleeding or bruising, jaundice and changes in urination.
- Explain ways to avoid sudden changes in posture, and caution against hot baths or showers, especially if dizziness is experienced.
- Tell patient that if nausea, vomiting or diarrhea develops to contact physician quickly. Dehydration may occur and may lower BP severely. Physician may decrease dose during episode.
- Explain need to be cautious when driving or participating in activities needing coordination. This drug may produce drowsiness, dizziness, lightheadedness or blurred vision, especially during first days of therapy or when dose is increased.
- Tell patient that before any surgery, physician should be informed that this drug is being used (even as eye drops). Physician may wish to discontinue drugs temporarily.
- Explain to patient that abrupt withdrawal of the drug is dangerous and dose is generally tapered according to physician's instructions.
- Encourage patient to wear support hose.
- Instruct patient to avoid alcohol, smoking and sodium intake.
- Teach patient to take pulse at home and when to notify physician.

See Patient Guide, pp. 601-602.

Tobramycin

(TOE-bruh-MY-sin)
Nebcin, Tobrex
Class: Antibiotic/aminoglycoside

Action Inhibits bacterial protein synthesis, causing cell death.

Indications Treatment of serious infections caused by susceptible strains of gram-negative bacteria; treatment of serious susceptible staphylococcal infections when other, less toxic drugs are contraindicated. *Ophthalmic use:* Treatment of superficial ocular infections.

Contraindications Previous reactions to aminoglycosides. *Ophthalmic use:* Epithelial herpes simplex keratitis; vaccinia; varicella; mycobacterial infections of eye; fungal infections.

Route/Dosage
ADULTS: **IM/IV** 3-5 mg/kg/day in 3-4 equal doses. **Ophthalmic** 1.25 cm ribbon of ointment bid-tid (q 3-4 hr for severe infections) *or* 1-2 gtt 4-6 times/day (for severe infections, q hr until improvement; then frequency of administration is reduced). CHILDREN: **IM/IV** 6-7.5 mg/kg/day in 3-4 equally divided doses. **Ophthalmic** 1.25 cm ribbon of ointment bid-tid (q 3-4 hr for severe infections) *or* 1-2 gtt 4-6 times/day (for severe infections, q hr until improvement; then frequency of administration is reduced). PREMATURE OR FULL-TERM NEONATES ≤ 1 WK: **IM/IV** Up to 4 mg/kg/day in 2 divided doses.

Interactions
Depolarizing and nondepolarizing muscle relaxants: May enhance neuromuscular blocking effects. Protracted respiratory depression may occur. *Loop diuretics:* May increase auditory toxicity. *Nephrotoxic drugs (eg, amphotericin B, cephalosporins, enflurane, methoxyflurane, vancomycin):* May increase risk of nephrotoxicity. *Penicillins:* Penicillins, particularly carbenicillin and ticarcillin, can inactivate tobramycin in admixture, assay procedures, or patients with renal failure. *Polypeptide antibiotics:* May increase risk of respiratory paralysis and renal dysfunction. INCOMPATIBILITIES: Do not mix with other drugs.

Lab Test Interferences
None well documented.

Adverse Reactions
RESP: Apnea. *CNS:* Headache; fever; confusion; lethargy; disorientation; delirium. *EENT:* Tinnitus; vertigo; dizziness; hearing loss. With ophthalmic preparation: Localized ocular toxicity and hypersensitivity; lid itching; lid swelling; conjunctival erythema. *GI:* Nausea; vomiting; diarrhea. *GU:* Oliguria; proteinuria; increased serum creatinine and BUN. *HEMA:* Anemia; leukopenia; leukocytosis; eosinophilia. *DERM:* Rash; urticaria; itching; pain and irritation at injection site. *META:* Decreased serum calcium, sodium, potassium, or magnesium; increased LFT results.

Precautions
Pregnancy: Category D (parenteral); Category B (ophthalmic). *Lactation:* Undetermined. *Children:* Use parenteral form cautiously in premature infants and neonates due to renal immaturity. *Burn patients:* Pharmacokinetics may be altered; serum levels are important for determining appropriate dosing. *Hypomagnesia:* Occurs often, especially in those with restricted diets or who eat poorly. *Long-term therapy:* Generally not indicated; greatly increases risk of toxic reactions. *Neuromuscular blockade:* Potential curare-like effects may aggravate muscle weakness or cause neurotoxicity. Use drug with caution in patients with neuromuscular disorders, hypomagnesemia, hypocalcemia or hypokalemia; with anesthesia or muscle relaxants, and in neonates whose mothers received magnesium sulfate. *Ophthalmic ointment:* May retard corneal healing. *Toxicity:* Drug is associated with signifi-

cant nephrotoxicity and ototoxicity (both auditory and vestibular). Use drug with particular caution in patients with renal impairment or previous hearing loss and in elderly patients.

NURSING CONSIDERATIONS

Administration/Storage

- Administer separately. Do not mix with other drugs.
- For intravenous administration dilute in 50-100 ml of 0.9% Sodium Chloride Injection or 5% Dextrose Injection. Use less diluent for children. Administer over ≥ 20 min-60 min.
- Administer IM injection deep into large muscle.
- For ophthalmic preparations, wash hands before and after instillation. Have patient tilt head back; place medication in conjunctival sac and have patient close eyes. Apply light finger pressure on lacrimal duct for 1 min following instillation. Do not touch tip of container to any surface.
- Store ophthalmic preparations at room temperature away from sunlight. Do not freeze.
- Discard if solution is brown or cloudy or contains particles.

Assessment/Interventions

- Obtain culture and susceptibility before initiating drug therapy. Treatment can be initiated before results are obtained.
- Obtain patient history, including drug history and any known allergies. Determine if patient has renal impairment, hearing loss, neuromuscular disorders, muscle weakness, Parkinson's disease, myasthenia gravis, mycobacterial infections or fungal infections.
- If patient may be intubated or ventilated, inform anesthetist that patient is taking this drug. Neuromuscular effects may be enhanced with succinylcholine or other neuromuscular blocking agent.
- Do not administer to neonates if mother received magnesium sulfate.
- Monitor and record respiratory status.
- Schedule hearing test prior to administration. Periodically test hearing throughout treatment and 1 mo after treatment is discontinued. Deafness may occur after drug has been discontinued, especially if treated > 10 days.
- Monitor renal function (especially in elderly patients), creatinine clearance rate and BUN. Report any changes from baseline to physician.
- Request periodic urine studies.
- Monitor peak and trough drug levels, especially in elderly patients, and use to guide dosing. Obtain these values within 48 hr of start of therapy and every 3-4 days.
- Monitor for signs of superinfection.
- Monitor I&O and report imbalances to physician.
- Monitor magnesium, sodium, calcium and potassium blood levels. Report low levels to physician.
- Monitor neurologic status and function of cranial nerve VIII. Report tinnitus, vertigo, numbness, tingling, muscle twitching or weakness and convulsions to physician.
- Keep patient well hydrated.
- If toxicity is detected, immediately notify physician. Discontinuation of drug or adjustment of dose or dosing interval may be required.

OVERDOSAGE: SIGNS & SYMPTOMS

Nephrotoxicity, neuromuscular blockade, respiratory paralysis, ototoxicity *With ophthalmic preparation (topical overdose)*: Punctate keratitis, erythema, increased lacrimination, edema, lid itching

Patient/Family Education

- Instruct patient how to administer ophthalmic preparation, including need for careful handwashing.
- Encourage patient to drink plenty of fluids while taking drug.
- Instruct patient to notify physician of

headache, fever, confusion, nausea, vomiting, diarrhea, rashes, itching, pain at injection site, ringing or roaring in ears, dizziness or hearing loss.

- Advise patient to consult with physician before taking any other otc or prescription medications.
- Inform patient that physician will want follow-up blood studies and audiograms.
- Inform patient that ophthalmic preparations may cause temporary blurring of vision or stinging and instruct patient to report excessive stinging, burning, persistent or increased pain, tearing, lid itching, swelling or redness of eyes to physician.
- Instruct patient not to wear contact lenses during treatment.
- For patient using ophthalmic solution, stress need for compliance with complete course of therapy.

See Patient Guide, p. 603.

Tocainide HCl

(TOE-cane-ide HIGH-droe-KLOR-ide)

Tonocard

Class: Antiarrhythmic

Action Produces dose-dependent decreases in sodium and potassium conductance resulting in decrease in myocardial cell excitability.

Indications Treatment of life-threatening ventricular arrhythmias. **Unlabeled uses:** Treatment of myotonic dystrophy and trigeminal neuralgia.

Contraindications Hypersensitivity to tocainide or amide-type local anesthetics; second- or third-degree atrioventricular block in absence of artificial ventricular pacemaker.

Route/Dosage

ADULTS: **PO** 400 mg q 8 hr initially. Maintenance: 1200-1800 mg/day in 3 divided doses.

Interactions

Cimetidine: May decrease tocainide bioavailability and peak concentration. *Rifampin:* May decrease tocainide bioavailability and elimination half-life; may increase tocainide oral clearance.

Lab Test Interferences

None well documented.

Adverse Reactions

CV: Increased ventricular arrhythmias; PVCs; CHF and progression of CHF; tachycardia; hypotension; bradycardia; palpitations; chest pain; conduction disorders. *RESP:* Respiratory arrest; pulmonary fibrosis; pulmonary edema; dyspnea. *CNS:* Dizziness; vertigo; paresthesias; tremor; nervousness; anxiety; confusion; headache; seizures. *EENT:* Visual disturbances; nystagmus; tinnitus; hearing loss. *GI:* Nausea; vomiting; anorexia; diarrhea. *HEMA:* Anemia; leukopenia; thrombocytopenia; aplastic anemia; agranulocytosis. *HEPA:* Increased LFT result; hepatitis; jaundice. *DERM:* Diaphoresis; systemic lupus erythematosus; rash; skin lesion. *OTHER:* Arthritis or arthralgia; myalgia; increased creatine phosphokinase.

Precautions

Pregnancy: Category C. *Lactation:* Excreted in breast milk. *Children:* Safety and efficacy not established. *Blood dyscrasias:* Have occurred, with some fatalities. Blood tests are required weekly for first 3 mo, and frequently thereafter. *Cardiac effects:* Use drug with caution and in lower doses in patients with CHF or reduced cardiac output. *Hypokalemia:* Should be corrected prior to initiation of tocainide therapy to ensure efficacy. *Proarrhythmia:* Tocainide has proarrhythmic effect. *Pulmonary fibrosis:* Has occurred, as have other pulmonary complications. Promptly report any pulmonary symptoms. *Renal or hepatic impairment:* Use drug with caution in patients with renal or hepatic impairment. Dosage reduction and modified dosing intervals may be required.

NURSING CONSIDERATIONS

Administration/Storage

- Administer orally and preferably with food to avoid GI upset.
- Check with physician regarding early adverse effects. In some cases they can be decreased by administering medication with food or in smaller, more frequent doses.
- Store at room temperature away from sunlight and moisture.

Assessment/Interventions

- Obtain patient history, including drug history and any known allergies.
- Monitor and record CBC, including WBC with differential and platelets and LFTs weekly for first 3 mo and frequently thereafter.
- Assess pulmonary function, and report cough, dyspnea, wheezing or rales.
- Assess neurologic status, and report paresthesia or tremor.
- Review blood studies. Report hypokalemia to physician.
- Monitor vital signs, especially pulse and BP and report changes.
- Monitor I&O, and report urinary retention.
- Assess ECG prior to and during therapy.

OVERDOSAGE: SIGNS & SYMPTOMS

Paresthesias, tremors, seizures, arrhythmias, decreased cardiac function, cardiac arrest, nausea, vomiting

Patient/Family Education

- Advise patient that physician may require blood tests weekly for first 3 wk of treatment and frequently thereafter; caution against skipping appointments.
- Tell patient to report persistent or severe nausea, vomiting, diarrhea or loss of appetite immediately.
- Explain that patient may experience tiredness, or hot/cold feelings, taste and smell perversions, joint or muscle aches, dizziness, anxiety or headache and to report symptoms if severe or persistent.
- Tell patient to report signs of infection immediately (chills, fever, sore throat, sore mouth, earache, cough, wheezing, difficulty breathing).
- Tell patient to report changes in heart rate, chest pain, tremors, confusion, visual disturbances, ringing or roaring in ears, profuse sweating, rash, numbness or tingling, slurred speech, dry mouth, yellow skin or whites of eyes, unusual bruising or bleeding or double vision.
- Explain that if dose is missed to take as soon as remembered. If close to next dose, skip dose. If more than one dose is missed, tell patient to contact physician.
- Tell patient not to store medication in bathroom.
- Advise patient that drug may cause drowsiness and dizziness and to use caution while driving or performing other tasks requiring mental alertness.

See Patient Guide, p. 604.

Tolazamide

(tole-AZE-uh-mid)

Tolinase

Class: Antidiabetic/sulfonylurea

Action Decreases blood glucose by stimulating release of insulin from pancreas.

Indications Adjunct to diet to lower blood glucose in patients with non-insulin-dependent diabetes mellitus (type II) whose hyperglycemia cannot be controlled by diet alone. **Unlabeled use:** Temporary adjunct to insulin therapy in selected patients with non-insulin-dependent diabetes mellitus to improve diabetic control.

Contraindications Hypersensitivity to sulfonylureas; diabetes complicated by ketoacidosis, with or without coma; sole therapy of insulin-dependent (type I) diabetes mellitus; gestational diabetes.

Route/Dosage

ADULTS: **PO** 100-250 mg/day with breakfast or first main meal. If fasting blood sugar (FBS) is < 200 mg/dl, initial dose is 100 mg/day or if FBS is > 200 mg/dl, initial dose is 250 mg/day. In malnourished, underweight, elderly patients use 100 mg/day. May adjust dose by 100-250 mg/wk as needed to maximum 1000 mg/day. If > 500 mg/day is required, give in divided doses twice daily. Doses > 1 g/day are not likely to improve control.

Interactions

Androgens, anticoagulants, chloramphenicol, clofibrate, fenfluramine, fluconazole, gemfibrozil, histamine H_2 antagonists, magnesium salts, methyldopa, MAO *inhibitors, phenylbutazone, probenecid, salicylates, sulfinpyrazone, sulfonamides, tricyclic antidepressants, urinary acidifiers:* Increased hypoglycemic effect. *Beta-blockers, cholestyramine, diazoxide, hydantoins, rifampin, thiazide diuretics, urinary alkalinizers:* Decreased hypoglycemic effect.

Lab Test Interferences

None well documented.

Adverse Reactions

CV: Increased risk of cardiovascular mortality. *CNS:* Dizziness; vertigo. *GI:* Nausea; epigastric fullness; heartburn; cholestatic jaundice. *GU:* Mild diuresis. *HEMA:* Leukopenia; thrombocytopenia; aplastic anemia; agranulocytosis; hemolytic anemia; pancytopenia; hepatic porphyria. *DERM:* Allergic skin reactions; eczema; pruritus; erythema; urticaria; morbilliform or maculopapular eruptions; lichenoid reactions. *META:* Hypoglycemia. *OTHER:* Disulfuram-like reaction; weakness; paresthesia; fatigue; malaise.

Precautions

Pregnancy: Category C. *Lactation:* Undetermined. *Children:* Safety and efficacy in children not established. *Elderly and debilitated patients:* Elderly and debilitated patients are particularly susceptible to hypoglycemic action of sulfonylureas. *Hypoglycemia:* Tolazamide may produce severe hypoglycemia, which may be more difficult to recognize in elderly or in patients receiving beta-blockers. *Disulfuram-like syndrome:* Administration with alcohol may include facial flushing reaction and occasional breathlessness. This reaction has been reported more commonly with other sulfonylureas. *Hepatic and renal impairment:* Use drug with caution and monitor liver and renal function frequently. *Hyperglycemia:* Hyperglycemia is major risk factor in development of diabetic complications. Measurement of glycosylated hemoglobin and self-monitoring of blood glucose are useful. *Loss of blood glucose control:* Stress (including fever, trauma, infection or surgery) or secondary failure (wherein drug's effectiveness in lowering blood glucose diminishes over time) may precipitate loss of blood glucose control.

NURSING CONSIDERATIONS

Administration/Storage

- Give with breakfast or with first meal of day.
- Crush tablet if patient unable to swallow tablet whole.

Assessment/Interventions

- Obtain patient history, including drug history and any known allergies.
- Closely monitor glucose control in

elderly patients and promptly adjust dose if hypoglycemia is noted.

- Initially monitor blood glucose and urine ketones three times a day. Once glucose control is established monitor less often in type II diabetic patients.

OVERDOSAGE: SIGNS & SYMPTOMS

Hypoglycemia including symptoms of: tingling of lips and tongue, nausea, lethargy, confusion, agitation, nervousness, tachycardia, sweating, tremor, hunger, convulsions, stupor, coma

Patient/Family Education

- Teach signs and symptoms of hypoglycemia (profuse sweating, excessive hunger, weakness, dizziness, tremor, tachycardia, anxiety, numbness of extremities) and of hyperglycemia (excessive thirst or urination, urinary glucose or ketones, fever, sore throat, unusual bleeding or rash). Remind patient to keep source of quick-acting sugar available at all times.
- When adjusting the dose, tell patient to check urine for ketones and blood for glucose three times a day; 1-2 times a day after stable control is established. Tell patient to notify physician if planning surgery or experiencing vomiting, injury, infection or fever.
- Demonstrate correct technique for performing blood glucose and urine glucose and ketone tests, and ensure correct return demonstrations.
- Tell patient to report repeated abnormal glucose or ketone results to physician.
- Emphasize importance of continuing diet restrictions and exercise regimen.
- Caution about disulfiram-like syndrome (facial flushing, abdominal cramping, nausea) when consuming alcohol. Advise patient to avoid alcohol.
- Inform patient that therapy will not cure disease.

See Patient Guide, p. 605.

Tolbutamide

(tole-BYOO-tuh-mide)

Orinase, Orinase Diagnostic,
♣ *Mobenol*

Class: Antidiabetic/sulfonylurea

Action Decreases blood glucose by stimulating release of insulin from pancreas.

Indications

Oral form: Adjunct to diet to lower blood glucose in patients with non-insulin-dependent diabetes mellitus (type II) whose hyperglycemia cannot be controlled by diet alone. *IV form (tolbutamide sodium):* Aid in diagnosis of pancreatic islet cell adenoma.

Contraindications Hypersensitivity to sulfonylureas; diabetes complicated by ketoacidosis with or without coma; sole therapy of insulin-dependent (type I) diabetes mellitus; diabetes occurring during pregnancy.

Route/Dosage

ADULTS: **PO** Usually 1-2 g/day (range, 0.25-3 g) in 1-2 divided doses.

For Diagnostic Purposes

ADULTS: **IV** 1 g over 2-3 min.

Interactions

Androgens, chloramphenicol, clofibrate, dicumarol, fenfluramine, fluconazole, gemfibrozil, histamine H_2 antagonists, magnesium salts, methyldopa, MAO *inhibitors, phenylbutazone, probenecid, salicylates, sulfinpyrazone, sulfonamides, tricyclic antidepressants, urinary acidifiers:* May increase hypoglycemic effect. *Beta-blockers, cholestyramine, diazoxide, hydantoins, rifampin, thiazide diuretics, urinary alkalinizers:* May decrease hypoglycemic effect. *Digoxin:* May cause increased digoxin serum concentrations. *Ethanol:* May cause disulfiram-like reaction.

Lab Test Interferences

Drug may cause false-positive reaction for albumin with acidificationafter-boiling test; no interference occurs with sulfosalicyclic acid test. Elevated LFTs and elevations in BUN and creatinine may occur.

Adverse Reactions

CV: Increased risk of cardiovascular mortality. *CNS*: Dizziness; vertigo. *EENT*: Tinnitus. *GI*: Nausea; epigastric fullness; heartburn. *HEMA*: Leukopenia; thrombocytopenia; aplastic anemia; agranulocytosis; hemolytic anemia; pancytopenia. *HEPA*: Cholestatic jaundice. *DERM*: Allergic skin reactions; eczema; pruritus; erythema; urticaria; morbilliform or maculopapular eruptions; lichenoid reactions; porphyria; photosensitivity. *META*: Hypoglycemia; SIADH with water retention and dilutional hyponatremia, especially in patients with CHF or hepatic cirrhosis. *OTHER*: Disulfiram-like reaction; weakness; paresthesia; fatigue; malaise; slight burning sensation along course of vein during IV injection; thrombophlebitis with thrombosis of injected vein.

Precautions

Pregnancy: Category C. Insulin is recommended to control elevated blood glucose levels during pregnancy. *Lactation*: Excreted into breast milk. *Children*: Safety and efficacy have not been established. *Elderly or debilitated patients*: Particularly susceptible to hypoglycemic action. Hypoglycemia may be difficult to recognize in elderly. *Disulfiram-like syndrome*: Administration of drug with alcohol may induce facial flushing and breathlessness. *Hepatic and renal impairment*: Use drug with caution.

NURSING CONSIDERATIONS

Administration/Storage

- Administer 30 min prior to meal. May administer with food if GI upset occurs.
- May administer total dose in morning or give in divided doses to decrease GI upset or to decrease blood glucose fluctuation.
- Inject at constant rate over 2-3 min.
- Refer to manufacturer's product information for specific test methodology and interpretation of test results.
- Use within 1 hr of reconstitution but only if solution is complete and clear.

Assessment/Interventions

- Obtain patient history, including drug history and any known allergies. Note diabetes complicated by ketoacidosis, decreased renal or hepatic function or sensitivity to sulfa drugs.
- If renal or hepatic function is diminished, use cautiously and monitor function.
- Monitor elderly closely for hypoglycemic effects.
- Monitor vital signs, blood sugar, weight and I&O daily.
- If jaundice occurs, discontinue drug and notify physician.

OVERDOSAGE: SIGNS & SYMPTOMS

Hypoglycemia including symptoms of: tingling of lips and tongue, nausea, lethargy, confusion, agitation, nervousness, tachycardia, sweating, tremor, hunger, convulsions, stupor, coma

Patient/Family Education

- Instruct patient to follow the diet and exercise regimen prescribed by physician.
- Inform patient of symptoms of and treatment for low blood sugar and advise patient to carry source of sugar at all times.
- Instruct patient to avoid alcohol. Inform patient that alcohol may react with tolbutamide and cause antabuse-like reaction (flushing, headache, dizziness, high BP).
- Instruct patient to monitor weight and to inform physician if steady weight gain occurs.
- Inform patient that surgery, illness or trauma may require temporary use of insulin.

- Instruct patient to alert physician to following problems: nausea, vomiting, GI distress, diarrhea, fever, sore throat, rash, itching, weakness, unusual bruising or bleeding, spilling of glucose or ketones in urine.
- Caution patient to avoid exposure to sunlight and to use sunscreen or wear protective clothing to avoid photosensitivity reaction.
- Recommended that patient carry identification card (eg, Medi-Alert) indicating condition and drug therapy.

See Patient Guide, p. 606.

Tolmetin Sodium

(TOLE-mee-tin SO-dee-uhm)

Tolectin, Tolectin DS

Class: Analgesic/NSAID

Action Decreases inflammation, pain and fever, probably through inhibition of cyclooxygenase activity and prostaglandin synthesis.

Indications Treatment of chronic and acute rheumatoid and osteoarthritis and juvenile rheumatoid arthritis. **Unlabeled use:** Treatment of sunburn.

Contraindications Hypersensitivity to aspirin, iodides or any NSAID.

Route/Dosage

Osteoarthritis/Rheumatoid Arthritis

ADULTS: **PO** 400 mg tid initially; titrate to 600-1600 mg/day for osteoarthritic patients or 600-1800 mg/day in divided doses for rheumatoid arthritis patients. Daily doses exceeding 1800 mg/day are not recommended.

Juvenile Rheumatoid Arthritis

CHILDREN > 2 YR: **PO** 20 mg/kg/day in 3-4 divided doses initially; titrate to 15-30 mg/kg/day (maximum 30 mg/kg/day).

Interactions

Anticoagulants: May increase effect of anticoagulants due to decreased plasma protein binding. May increase risk of gastric erosion and bleeding. *Cyclosporine:* May potentiate nephrotoxicity of both agents. *Methotrexate:* May increase methotrexate levels.

Lab Test Interferences

May prolong bleeding time. May produce false-positive test result for proteinuria using sulfosalicylic acid. Increases in serum uric acid, liver function tests, serum creatinine, BUN.

Adverse Reactions

CV: Edema; sodium retention; hypertension; CHF. *RESP:* Bronchospasm; laryngeal edema, rhinitis, dyspnea, pharyngitis; hemoptysis; shortness of breath. *CNS:* Dizziness; drowsiness; lightheadedness; confusion; increased sweating; vertigo; headaches; nervousness; migraine; anxiety; aggravated Parkinson's disease or epilepsy; paresthesia; peripheral neuropathy; myalgia; fatigue. *EENT:* Blurred vision; tinnitus. *GI:* Nausea; dyspepsia; abdominal pain or discomfort; flatulence; diarrhea; constipation; vomiting; gastritis; anorexia; glossitis; stomatitis; mouth ulcers. *GU:* Hematuria; proteinuria; dysuria; elevations in BUN; acute renal insufficiency; interstitial nephritis; hyperkalemia; hyponatremia; renal papillary necrosis; UTIs. *HEMA:* Increased bleeding time; anemia; decreases in Hgb or Hct; leukopenia; thrombocytopenia; hemolytic anemia. *HEPA:* Hepatitis; increased LFT results. *DERM:* Rash; pruritus; urticaria; purpura; erythema multiforme; skin irritation; sweating.

Precautions

Pregnancy: Category C. *Lactation:* Excreted in breast milk. *Children:* Safety and efficacy not established in children < 2 yr. *Elderly patients:* Increased risk of adverse reactions. *GI effects:* Serious GI toxicity (eg, bleeding, ulceration, perforation) can occur at any time with or without warning symptoms. *Renal impairment:* Use drug with caution in patients with compromised cardiac function, hypertension or other conditions predisposing to fluid retention.

NURSING CONSIDERATIONS

Administration/Storage

- Administer capsules or tablets orally tid with schedule including morning dose and evening dose.
- Do *not* administer with food, milk or sodium bicarbonate.
- If GI distress occurs, give with antacids that do not contain sodium bicarbonate.
- Store at room temperature. Do not expose to sunlight or moisture.

Assessment/Interventions

- Obtain patient history, including drug history and any known allergies.
- Assess renal function before and during therapy, especially in patients with renal impairment.
- Monitor serum uric acid, serum creatinine and BUN and report if increased.
- Monitor periodic urine tests for blood and protein and report positive results to physician. Be aware when testing for proteinuria that using sulfosalicylic acid may cause false-positive results. Use dye-impregnated reagent strips.
- Monitor results of LFTs and report dyscrasias to physician.
- Monitor serum potassium (report hyperkalemia) and sodium (report hyponatremia).
- Monitor Hgb and Hct and notify physician of decrease.
- Obtain periodic occult blood test in stool if patient is receiving long-term therapy.
- Monitor BP and I&O throughout therapy.
- Notify physician of any shortness of breath or other signs of edema.
- Assess visual acuity and hearing with periodic exams for patients on prolonged therapy, especially if patient experiences blurred vision or changes in color vision.

OVERDOSAGE: SIGNS & SYMPTOMS

Drowsiness, dizziness, mental confusion, paresthesia, vomiting, abdominal pain, intense headache, tinnitus, sweating, convulsions, visual disturbances, elevated serum creatinine and BUN levels, hypotension

Patient/Family Education

- Explain that product should not be taken with aspirin or other NSAIDs without consulting physician.
- Explain that full antirheumatic action may not occur for up to 7 days and may not reach maximum effect for up to 1 mo after starting therapy.
- Tell patient to avoid taking with food or milk or immediately after meal. If medication causes stomach upset tell patient to take with antacids that do not contain sodium bicarbonate. Instruct patient to call physician if pain continues.
- Tell patient to avoid smoking or drinking alcohol while taking this drug.
- Explain that dizziness or black stools should be reported to physician immediately.
- Explain that if drowsiness, dizziness or blurred vision occurs, patient should observe caution while driving or performing other tasks requiring alertness.
- Explain that photosensitivity may occur and to use sunscreens and protective clothing when exposed to ultraviolet or sunlight until tolerance is determined.
- Identify potential clinically important adverse reactions: drowsiness, blurred vision, edema, headache,

lightheadedness, confusion, fatigue, swelling feet, ringing of ears, nausea, vomiting, mouth ulcers, unusual bleeding or bruising, rash, itching or skin irritation. Tell patient to notify physician if persistent or severe.

- Tell patient not to store drug in bathroom but in cool, dry place.

See Patient Guide, p. 607.

Tolnaftate

(tahl-NAFF-tate)

Absorbine Antifungal, Absorbine Jr. Antifungal, Aftate for Athlete's Foot, Aftate for Jock Itch, Desenex, Genaspor, NP-27, Quinsana Plus, Tinactin, Tinactin for Jock Itch, Ting, Zeasorb-AF, ♣ *Pitrex Cream, Tinactin Plus*

Class: Topical/antifungal

Action Distorts hyphae and inhibits mycelial growth in susceptible fungi.

Indications Treatment and prophylaxis of tinea pedia (athlete's foot); treatment of tinea cruris (jock itch) or tinea corporis (ringworm) caused by specific fungi; treatment of onchomycosis, chronic scalp infections, palm and sole infections with kerion formation; treatment of tinea versicolor.

Contraindications Standard considerations.

Route/Dosage

ADULTS & CHILDREN: **Topical** Apply small amount of ointment, cream or powder or 1-3 gtt of solution to affected area bid for 2-3 wk (6 wk if skin is thickened); continue treatment to maintain remission. Reserve powder for mild infections.

Interactions None well documented.

Lab Test Interferences

None well documented.

Adverse Reactions

DERM: Sensitization; mild irritation; pruritus; contact dermatitis; stinging.

Precautions

Pregnancy: Pregnancy category undetermined. *Lactation:* Undetermined. *External use only:* Avoid contact with eyes. *Nail and scalp infections:* Do not use drug except as adjunct to systemic treatment. *Sensitization or irritation:* Discontinue treatment if this occurs.

NURSING CONSIDERATIONS

Administration/Storage

- Cleanse skin with soap and water and dry thoroughly before applying.
- Apply small quantities of ointment, cream, solution, spray liquid, gel as primary therapy.
- Use powder or powder aerosol as adjunctive therapy or prophylaxis for athlete's foot. Use as primary therapy only in very mild conditions.
- Consult physician if no improvement after 10 days.
- To prevent recurrence, continue treatment for 2 wk beyond disappearance of symptoms.
- Store at room temperature. Avoid moisture and sunlight. Keep powders from getting wet or damp.

Assessment/Interventions

- Obtain patient history, including drug history and any known allergies.
- Monitor for sensitization, irritation, pruritus, rash, stinging.

Patient/Family Education

- Tell patient to cleanse skin with soap and water and dry thoroughly before applying.
- Emphasize to use only externally in

small amounts massaged well into affected area and surrounding skin.

- Instruct patient to wash hands before and after applying medication.
- Tell patient to avoid contact with eyes.
- Advise patient to wear well-fitting, ventilated shoes and to change shoes and socks at least daily.
- Tell patient not to cover treated site with bandages unless ordered specifically by physician.
- Instruct patient to notify physician if no apparent improvement after 10 days of treatment.
- Emphasize that product should not be used on nail and scalp infections unless using in addition to internal medication prescribed by physician.
- Tell patient to store at room temperature and not in bathroom (especially powders).
- Instruct patient to report these symptoms to physician: persistent or severe irritation, itching, rash, stinging.

See Patient Guide, p. 608.

Torsemide

(TORE-suh-MIDE)

Demadex

Class: Loop diuretic

Action Inhibits sodium/potassium/chloride carrier system in ascending loop of Henle, resulting in increased urinary excretion of sodium, chloride and water. Does not significantly alter glomerular filtration rate, renal plasma flow or acid-base balance.

Indications Management of edema associated with CHF, hepatic cirrhosis and renal disease; treatment of hypertension.

Contraindications Hypersensitivity to sulfonylureas; anuria; severe electrolyte depletion.

Route/Dosage

ADULTS: **PO/IV** 5-20 mg once daily. Titrate dose upward until desired response is obtained. Single doses > 200 mg have not been studied.

Interactions

Aminoglycosides: May increase ototoxicity. *Anticoagulants:* May enhance anticoagulant activity. *Cisplatin:* May cause additive ototoxicity. *Digitalis glycosides:* Electrolyte disturbances may predispose to digitalis-induced arrhythmias. *Lithium:* May increase plasma lithium levels and toxicity. *Nondepolarizing muscle relaxants:* May antagonize or potentiate response to muscle relaxants. *NSAIDs:* May decrease effects of torsemide. *Probenecid:* May reduce action of torsemide. *Salicylates:* May impair diuretic response in patients with cirrhosis and ascites. *Sulfonylureas:* May decrease glucose tolerance, resulting in need for increased sulfonylurea dose. *Thiazide diuretics:* May cause synergistic effects that may result in profound diuresis and serious electrolyte abnormalities.

Lab Test Interferences

None well documented.

Adverse Reactions

CV: ECG abnormality; chest pain; atrial fibrillation; orthostatic hypotension; ventricular tachycardia; shunt thrombosis. *RESP:* Rhinitis; cough increase. *CNS:* Headache; dizziness; asthenia; insomnia; nervousness; syncope. *EENT:* Hearing loss; sore throat. *GI:* Diarrhea; constipation; nausea; dyspepsia; GI hemorrhage; rectal bleeding. *GU:* Excessive urination. *DERM:* Rash; pruritus. *META:* Hyperglycemia; hyperuricemia; hypomagnesemia; hypokalemia; hypocalcemia; hyponatremia; hypochloremia; hypovolemia. *OTHER:* Arthralgia; myalgia.

Precautions

Pregnancy: Category B. *Lactation:* Unknown. *Children:* Safety and efficacy not established. *Hepatic cirrhosis and ascites:* Sudden alterations of electrolyte balance may precipitate hepatic encephalopathy and coma. *Hypersensi-*

tivity. Patients with known sulfonamide sensitivity may show allergic reactions to torsemide. *Hyperuricemia:* Asymptomatic hyperuricemia or gout may occur. *Lipids:* Increases in LDL, total cholesterol and triglycerides with decreases in HDL cholesterol may occur. *Ototoxicity:* Associated with rapid injection or very large doses. *Photosensitivity:* Photosensitization may occur.

NURSING CONSIDERATIONS

Administration/Storage

- Administer oral form with or without food.
- Administer IV form once daily via slow (over 2 min) infusion.
- Store in dry area away from sunlight.

Assessment/Interventions

- Obtain patient history, including drug history and any known allergies. Note whether patient has lupus erythematosus, kidney dysfunction or cirrhosis.
- Assess gross hearing acuity before administration and periodically during drug therapy, especially if drug is being given at high doses or concurrently with another ototoxic drug.
- Monitor lying and standing BP before drug administration. Consult with physician if patient is hypotensive.
- Monitor I&O and body weight.
- Monitor electrolytes. Notify physician of electrolyte imbalances, especially hypokalemia.
- Monitor hepatic and renal function.

OVERDOSAGE: SIGNS & SYMPTOMS

Dehydration, arrhythmias, decreased renal function, blood volume and electrolyte depletion, weakness, dizziness, mental confusion, anorexia, lethargy, vomiting, cramps, circulatory collapse, vascular thrombosis and embolism

Patient/Family Education

- Instruct patient to inform physician of all otc or prescription drugs being taken, especially NSAIDs, digitalis or lithium.
- Advise hypertensive patient to avoid foods or medications that may increase BP, including otc drugs for appetite suppression or cold symptoms, otc drugs to help to keep awake and excessive consumption of coffee or other substances containing caffeine.
- Instruct patient to eat potassium-rich foods daily. These foods include banana, cantaloupe and potatoes.
- Advise patient not to store drug in bathroom, but in a cool, dry place.
- Inform patient that drug may raise blood sugar levels. Instruct diabetic patients to monitor blood glucose regularly and report patterns of hyperglycemia.
- Advise patient that this drug increases urination. Advise patient to take medication early in morning to avoid disrupted sleep.
- Caution patient to notify physician immediately if vomiting and diarrhea occur or if signs of excessive potassium loss (cramps, muscle weakness, nausea, dizziness) are noted.
- Instruct patient to report these symptoms to physician: chest pain, dizziness, rapid heart beat, headache, nausea, increased swelling of feet, black stools, rectal bleeding, rash, face rash, fatigue or hearing loss.
- Caution patient to avoid sudden position changes to prevent dizziness or fainting.
- Advise patient that drug may cause dizziness and to use caution while driving or performing other tasks requiring mental alertness.
- Caution patient to avoid exposure to sunlight and to use sunscreen or wear protective clothing to avoid photosensitivity reaction.

See Patient Guide, p. 609.

Tramadol Hydrochloride

(TRAM-uh-dole HIGH-droe-KLOR-ide)
Ultram
Class: Analgesic

Action Binds to certain opioid receptors and inhibits reuptake of norepinephrine and serotonin; exact mechanism of action unknown.

Indications Relief of moderate to moderately severe pain.

Contraindications Acute intoxication with alcohol, hypnotics, centrally acting analgesics, opioids or psychotropic agents.

Route/Dosage
ADULTS & CHILDREN ≥ 16 YR: **PO** 50-100 mg every 4-6 hr; maximum daily dose 400 mg. ELDERLY PATIENTS > 75 YR: **PO** 50-100 mg every 4-6 hr, maximum daily dose 300 mg. RENAL IMPAIRMENT: CrU < 30 ml/min. **PO** 50-100 mg every 12 hr (maximum 200 mg/day). CIRRHOSIS: 50 mg every 12 hours (maximum 100 mg/day).

Interactions
Carbamazepine: May reduce serum tramadol levels, leading to decreased effectiveness. MAO *inhibitors:* Risk of seizures may be increased.

Lab Test Interferences
None well documented.

Adverse Reactions
CV: Vasodilation. *CNS:* Dizziness/vertigo; headache; somnolence; stimulation; anxiety; confusion; coordination disturbances; euphoria; nervousness; sleep disorder; seizures. *EENT:* Visual disturbances; dry mouth. *GI:* Nausea; diarrhea; constipation; vomiting; dyspepsia; abdominal pain; anorexia; flatulence. *GU:* Urinary retention/frequency; menopausal symptoms; increased creatinine; proteinuria. *HEMA:* Decreased hemoglobin. *HEPA:* Elevated liver enzymes. *DERM:* Pruritus; sweating; rash. *OTHER:* Asthenia; hypertonia.

Precautions
Pregnancy: Category C. *Lactation:* Excreted in breast milk. *Children:* Not recommended for children < 16 yr. *Elderly:* Patients > 75 yr-concentrations may be slightly elevated; may have less ability to tolerate adverse effects; use reduced dosage. *Head trauma:* Use with caution in patients with increased intracranial pressure or head trauma. *Hepatic disease:* Dosage adjustments may be required in patients with cirrhosis. *Renal impairment:* Dosage adjustments may be required. *CNS depressants:* Use with caution and in reduced dosage when administering to patients receiving CNS depressants. *Opioid dependence:* Not recommended for patients who are opioid-dependent; use caution when administering to patients who have recently received substantial amounts of opioids.

NURSING CONSIDERATIONS

Administration/Storage

- Can be taken without regard to meals.
- Administer medication before pain becomes severe.
- Store at room temperature, in a tightly closed container.

Assessment/Interventions

- Obtain patient history.
- Assess degree, location and characteristics of pain before administering.
- Assess vital signs before administering medication. If patient is hypotensive or dyspneic, notify physician before administering.
- Monitor I&O and check for urinary retention.
- Assess the effectiveness of the medication in relieving pain.

OVERDOSAGE: SIGNS & SYMPTOMS

Respiratory depression, seizures, vomiting

Patient/Family Education

- Instruct patient to take the prescribed dose at the recommended intervals.
- Inform patient to check with his/her healthcare provider first before taking any over-the-counter or prescription medications, including analgesics.
- Have patient report any serious side effects to the healthcare provider.
- Advise patient not to wait until pain level is high to self-medicate, because drug will not be as effective.
- Advise patient to avoid taking alcohol or other CNS depressants (eg, sleeping pills).
- Advise the patient that this medication may cause drowsiness and to use caution while driving or using heavy equipment or performing other tasks requiring mental alertness.
- Advise patient to notify the healthcare provider if the pain is not relieved by the medication at the prescribed dosage.

See Patient Guide, p. 610.

Tranylcypromine Sulfate

(tran-ill-SIP-row-meen SULL-fate)

Parnate

Class: Antidepressant/MAO inhibitor

Action Tranylcypromine blocks activity of enzyme MAO, thereby increasing monoamine (eg, epinephrine, norepinephrine, serotonin) concentrations in CNS.

Indications Treatment of reactive depression. **Unlabeled uses:** Bulimia; treatment of panic disorders with associated agoraphobia.

Contraindications Hypersensitivity to MAO inhibitors; pheochromocytoma; CHF; abnormal liver function; history of liver disease; severe renal impairment; cerebrovascular defect; concurrent use of another MAO inhibitor, tricyclic or SSRI antidepressants, dextromethorphan or CNS depressants (eg, alcohol), meperidine, sympathomimetic drugs (eg, amphetamines, dopamine, pseudoephedrine) or related drugs (eg, methyldopa, levodopa), buspirone, cheese or food with high tyramine content; cardiovascular disease; hypertension; history of headache; patients > 60 yr (possibility of cerebral sclerosis).

Route/Dosage

ADULTS: PO 10 mg tid initially; if no improvement after 2 weeks, titrate up to 60 mg daily in 10 mg/day increments at intervals of 1-3 weeks.

Interactions

Amine-containing foods: May cause severe hypertension or hemorrhagic strokes. *Anorexiants:* May cause exaggerated pharmacologic effects (eg, severe headaches, hypertension, hyperpyrexia) of anorexiants (eg, amphetamines and related compounds). *CNS depressants:* May enhance CNS effects. *Dextromethorphan:* Concurrent use has been associated with severe reactions (hyperpyrexia, hypotension, death). *Fluoxetine, fluvoxamine, nefazodone, paroxetine, sertraline, trazodone, venlafaxine:* Although data are limited, interactions comparable to those of tricyclic antidepressants and tranylcypromine may occur. *Guanethidine:* MAO inhibitors may antagonize antihypertensive effect. *Insulin, sulfonylureas:* May enhance hypoglycemic action. *Levodopa:* May cause hypertensive reactions. *Meperidine:* May lead to severe reactions, including agitation, convulsions, diaphoresis, fever, respiratory depression and vascular collapse. *Sympathomimetics:* May cause severe headache, hypertensive crisis and hyperpyrexia. *Tricyclic antidepressants, busipirone, carbamazepine, CNS stimulants, cyclobenzaprine, maprotiline, tyramine:* May lead to potentially fatal reactions, including seizures and hypertensive crisis, mental status changes, hyperthermia.

Lab Test Interferences

None well documented.

Adverse Reactions

CV: Orthostatic hypotension; edema; hypertensive crisis; palpitations; tachycardia. *CNS:* Dizziness; headache; sleep disturbances; tremors; hyperreflexion; manic symptoms; muscle twitching; convulsions; vertigo; confusion; memory impairment; toxic delirium; hypomania; coma. *EENT:* Blurred vision; glaucoma; dry mouth. *GI:* Constipation; nausea; diarrhea; anorexia; abdominal pain. *GU:* Sexual dysfunction; urinary retention; incontinence. *HEMA:* Anemia; leukopenia; agranulocytosis; thrombocytopenia. *HEPA:* Fatal progressive necrotizing hepatocellular damage; elevated serum transaminases; hepatitis. *DERM:* Rash; sweating; photosensitivity. *META:* Weight gain; hypermetabolic syndrome (eg, fever, tachycardia, rapid breathing, rigidity, metabolism, acidosis, coma); hypernatremia.

Precautions

Pregnancy: Category undetermined. *Lactation:* Excreted in breast milk. *Children:* Not recommended for patients < 16 yr. *Elderly:* Use with caution; older patients may suffer more morbidity than younger patients. *Diabetes:* May alter glucose control. *Epilepsy:* May lower seizure threshold. *Depression:* May aggravate coexisting symptoms such as anxiety and agitation. *Hyperthyroidism:* Use with caution because of increased sensitivity to pressor amines. *Suicidal patients:* Strict supervision may be necessary in patients at risk.

NURSING CONSIDERATIONS

Administration/Storage

- Tablets may be crushed before administration and taken with food or fluids if patient has difficulty swallowing pills.
- Avoid administering medication in the evening due to the possibility of insomnia.
- Do not administer unless the patient has been on a tyramine-free diet for at least 2-3 days. Continue this diet for 2 weeks after discontinuing medication.
- Do not administer other antidepressants and MAO inhibitors for at least 2 weeks after discontinuing.
- Store tablets at room temperature in a tightly closed container.

Assessment/Interventions

- Obtain complete patient history. Note history of liver and cardiac disease, cerebrovascular disorders, hypertension, renal disorders, pheochromocytoma or severe headaches.
- Monitor blood pressure both lying and standing before initiating therapy. Monitor BP frequently during initial therapy and periodically thereafter. Tranylcypromine produces hypertensive reactions more frequently than other MAO inhibitors.
- Obtain baseline liver function, CBC and renal function tests prior to initiating therapy. Monitor periodically during treatment with this medication.
- Observe for onset of desired effects (improved mood, improved sleep patterns, better socialization, improved personal hygiene, lower suicidal potential). These should occur with 7-14 days with maximal response in 6 weeks.
- Monitor for signs of hypertensive crisis (severe headache, chest pain, palpitations, diaphoresis, nausea, vomiting, dilated pupils, photophobia and elevated BP).

OVERDOSAGE: SIGNS & SYMPTOMS

Excitement, hypotension, dizziness, movement disorders, irritability, insomnia, weakness, severe headache, anxiety, restlessness, drowsiness, coma, convulsions, flushing, hypertension, sweating, tachypnea, acidosis, hyperpyrexia, tachycardia, cardiorespiratory arrest, incoherence, agitation, mental confusion, shock

Patient/Family Education

- Advise patient that antidepressants restore depressed people to normal moods.
- Inform patient and family that it may be 3-4 weeks before a noticeable improvement in mood is noted.
- Instruct patient to take the medication at the same time every day.
- Advise patient not to take any other medications, including over-the-counter or prescription medications without checking with their healthcare provider first. This medication interacts with a large number of other medications.
- Teach patient to avoid sudden position changes to prevent orthostatic hypotension.
- Instruct patient and family on how to take BP. If the BP is markedly higher than normal, they should notify the healthcare provider.
- Warn patient that eating foods that contain tyramine or tryptophan while taking this medication can produce hypertensive crisis which is potentially fatal. These foods include, but are not limited to, protein foods that are aged or fermented such as cheeses, pickled herring, liver, hard sausage, pods of broad beans, beer, red wine, yeast extract, yogurt, ginseng, soy sauce, bananas, raisins and avocados. Arrange for a consultation with a dietitian.
- Instruct patient to ingest caffeine and chocolate only in small amounts.
- Inform patient to avoid the use of alcohol and other recreational drugs.
- Advise patient to use caution while driving or performing other tasks requiring mental alertness until effect is determined.
- Instruct patient to stop taking the medication and notify the healthcare provider IMMEDIATELY if any of the following occurs: severe headache, chest pain, rapid heart beat, eye pain or photophobia, severe sweating, stiff neck, nausea or vomiting.

See Patient Guide, p. 611.

Trazodone HCl

(TRAY-zoe-dohn HIGH-droe-KLOR-ide)

Desyrel, Desyrel Dividose

Class: Antidepressant

Action Undetermined; may affect serotonin uptake at presynaptic neuronal membrane.

Indications Treatment of depression. **Unlabeled uses:** Treatment of neurogenic pain, aggression, panic disorder, cocaine withdrawal.

Contraindications Standard considerations.

Route/Dosage

ADULTS: **PO** 150 mg/day in divided doses initially; increase in 50 mg increments up to maximum of 400 mg per day (outpatients) or 600 mg per day (inpatients). ELDERLY PATIENTS: **PO** Start with 75 mg/day in divided doses.

Interactions

Alcohol, CNS depressants: CNS depressant effects may be additive. *Fluoxetine:* May increase trazodone serum levels. *Hypotensive agents:* May cause additive hypotensive effects. MAO *inhibitors:* It is unknown whether interactions may take place. Initiate trazodone therapy cautiously if patient is currently taking or has recently stopped taking MAO inhibitors.

Lab Test Interferences

None well documented.

Adverse Reactions

CV: Hypertension; orthostatic hypotension; shortness of breath; syncope; tachycardia; palpitations; chest pain; MI; arrhythmias; sinus bradycardia; conduction block; cardiac arrest. *CNS:* Anger; hostility; nightmares/vivid dreams; confusion; disorientation; decreased concentration; dizziness; drowsiness; excitement; fatigue; headache; insomnia; impaired memory; nervousness; tingling; tremors; convulsions. *EENT:* Blurred vision; "red eyes"; ringing in ears; nasal or sinus congestion. *GI:* Abdominal/gastric disorders; unpleasant taste; dry mouth; nausea; vomiting; diarrhea; constipation. *GU:* Altered libido; impotence; priapism; urinary retention. *HEMA:* Anemia; hemolytic anemia; decreased WBC. *HEPA:* Jaundice; increased LFTs. *OTHER:* Hypersensitivity reaction (eg, skin conditions, edema, rash, itching, purpura); muscle aches and pains; decreased appetite; sweating; changes in weight; malaise.

Precautions

Pregnancy: Category C. *Lactation:* Excreted in breast milk. *Children:* Safety and efficacy in children < 18 yr not established. *Cardiac disease:* Not recommended for patients in acute recovery from MI. Trazodone may also cause arrhythmias; patients with preexisting cardiac disease should be closely monitored. *Lab tests:* Patients who develop fever, sore throat or other signs of infection during therapy should have white blood cell count and differential taken, because trazodone may lower WBC and neutrophil counts. *Priapism:* Priapism (prolonged, painful inappropriate penile erection) has been reported. Condition may require surgical intervention. Any patient experiencing inappropriate or prolonged erection should stop taking trazodone immediately and notify physician. *Suicide:* Patients at risk should be closely monitored and not be given access to excessive quantities.

NURSING CONSIDERATIONS

Administration/Storage

- Administer with meals or with light snack.
- Increase dosage gradually; drowsiness may require administration of bedtime dosage or reduced dosage.
- Assess for initial improvement in 1 wk, with optimal effect evident within 2-4 wk of therapy.
- Store in tight, light-resistant container at room temperature.

Assessment/Interventions

- Obtain patient history, including drug history and any known allergies.
- Obtain blood studies (CBC, differential) and hepatic studies in patients undergoing long-term therapy.
- Assess mood and mental status before and during therapy.
- Check to be sure oral medication is taken.
- Implement oral hygiene measures in presence of dry mouth or unpleasant taste.
- Implement safety precautions to prevent injury, especially during initial therapy until effect is known. Assist with ambulation.
- Monitor patient for urinary retention.
- Monitor BP and pulse throughout therapy.
- Monitor ECG in patients with cardiac disorders.
- Monitor weight weekly.
- Monitor for side effects, particularly drowsiness, dizziness, lightheadedness, changes in blood pressure or pulse, dry mouth, GI disturbances, altered libido.
- Assess for hypotension, particularly

when used concurrently with antihypertensives and nitrates.

OVERDOSAGE: SIGNS & SYMPTOMS

Priapism, respiratory arrest, seizures, ECG changes, death, drowsiness, vomiting

Patient/Family Education

- Tell patient that maximal effect may not be evident for up to 4 wk.
- Instruct family to monitor mood during therapy. Observe for suicidal tendencies.
- Advise patient to check weight weekly because appetite may increase with drug.
- Tell patient taking antihypertensives or nitrates about potential for additive hypotensive effect.
- Instruct patient to report these symptoms to physician: shortness of breath, chest pain, confusion, convulsions, impotence.
- Advise patient to take sips of water frequently, suck on ice chips or sugarless hard candy or chew sugarless gum to prevent dry mouth or unpleasant tastes.
- Instruct patient to avoid intake of alcoholic beverages, sedatives/hypnotics or other CNS depressants.
- Advise patient to use caution while driving or performing other tasks requiring mental alertness until effect is determined.

See Patient Guide, p. 612.

Tretinoin (*trans*-Retinoic Acid, Vitamin A Acid)

(TREH-tih-NO-in)

Retin-A, ✤ *Stieva-A, Vitamin A Acid*

Class: Topical/acne

Action Decreases cohesiveness and stimulates mitotic activity and turnover of follicular epithelial cells, resulting in decreased formation and increased extrusion of comedones.

Indications Topical treatment of acne vulgaris. **Unlabeled uses:** Treatment of skin cancer, various dermatologic conditions including lamellar ichthyosis, warts and Darier's disease; improvement of photoaged skin, especially wrinkles and liver spots.

Contraindications Standard considerations.

Route/Dosage

ADULTS & CHILDREN: **Topical** Apply lightly to affected area once daily before bedtime. May reduce interval to once q 2-3 days if severe irritation occurs.

Interactions

Benzoyl peroxide, cosmetics with drying effects, resorcinol, salicylic acid, soaps or sulfur: May result in significant skin irritation.

Lab Test Interferences

None well documented.

Adverse Reactions

DERM: Temporary hyperpigmentation or hypopigmentation; photosensitivity; red, edematous, blistered or crusted skin; transient warmth or stinging at site of injection.

Precautions

Pregnancy: Category C. *Lactation:* Undetermined. *External use only:* Keep tretinoin away from eyes, mouth, angles of nose, mucous membranes and open wounds. *Irritation:* May cause severe local irritation. May need to use less often or discontinue temporarily or completely. *Photosensitivity:* Tumorigenic potential of ultraviolet radiation may be accelerated. Photosensitization may occur.

NURSING CONSIDERATIONS

Administration/Storage

- Wash hands and cleanse affected area thoroughly and dry completely before application.
- Apply lightly to affected area using gauze pad, cotton swab or fingertip at bedtime. Wash hands immediately after application.
- Avoid application around eyes, mouth, angles of nose, mucous membranes and open wounds.
- Do not apply other topical acne products at same time as tretinoin. In some cases, different medication may be applied at other times of day.

Assessment/Interventions

- Obtain patient history, including drug history and any known allergies.
- Assess and document skin condition before initial application and throughout treatment.
- Monitor for side effects, including red, irritated, blistered or crusted skin.
- Assess for photosensitivity reactions.

> **OVERDOSAGE: SIGNS & SYMPTOMS**
>
> Topical overdose may cause redness, pain, blistering and cracking of the skin

Patient/Family Education

- Inform patient that therapeutic response should be seen after 2-3 wk, but may not be optimal for 6 wk.
- Advise patient that acne symptoms may worsen initially, but that therapy should not be discontinued.
- Tell patient to thoroughly cleanse area before application; to avoid application around eyes, mouth, angles of nose, mucous membranes, and open wounds and to wash hands thoroughly immediately after application.
- Explain that normal use of cosmetics is allowed but instruct patient to avoid oil-based cosmetics.
- Tell patient not to apply other acne products at the same time as tretinoin, and not to apply tretinoin more than once daily.
- Instruct patient that medicated soaps and cosmetics that have strong drying effect and products with high concentration of alcohol, astringents, spices or lime (eg, shaving lotion) may worsen dry skin.
- Identify potential side effects, including photosensitivity. Teach importance of protective measures such as sunscreen, avoidance of ultraviolet light and use of protective clothing.
- Explain that temporary hypopigmentation or hyperpigmentation may occur.

See Patient Guide, p. 613.

Triamcinolone

(TRY-am-SIN-oh-lone)

Triamcinolone

Aristocort, Atolone, Kenacort

Triamcinolone Acetonide

Aristocort, Aristocort A, Azmacort, Delta-Tritex, Flutex, Kenaject-40, Kenalog, Kenalog-H, Kenonei, Tac-3, Tac-40, Triacet, Triam-A, Triamonide 40, Triderm, Tri-Kort, Trilog, ♣ *Oracort, Triaderm*

Triamcinolone Diacetate

Amcort, Aristocort Forte, Aristospan Intralesional, Articulose L.A., Triam Forte, Triamolone 40, Trilone, Tristoject, ♣ *Aristocort Parenteral, Aristocort Syrup*

Triamcinolone Hexacetonide

Aristospan Intra-articular, Aristospan Intralesional

Class: Corticosteroid

Action Anti-inflammatory effect by depressing formation, release and activity of endogenous mediators of inflammation including prostaglandins, kinins, histamine, liposomal enzymes and complement system. Also modifies body's immune response.

Indications

Oral/IM/IV administration: Replacement therapy in endocrine disorders; adjunctive therapy for short-term administration in rheumatic disorders; maintenance therapy or control of exacerbation of collagen diseases; treatment of dermatologic diseases; control of allergic states; management of allergic and inflammatory ophthalmic processes; treatment of respiratory diseases including pulmonary emphysema and diffuse interstitial pulmonary fibrosis; treatment of selected hematologic disorders; palliative management of selective neoplastic diseases; induction of diuresis in edematous states caused by nephrotic syndrome, refractory CHF and in ascites caused by cirrhosis of liver; control of exacerbation in selected GI diseases (eg, inflammatory bowel disease); control of exacerbation of multiple sclerosis; adjunctive treatment of tuberculous meningitis; treatment of trichinosis with neurologic or myocardial involvement; management of postoperative dental inflammatory reactions. *Intra-articular or soft tissue administration:* Short-term adjunctive therapy in synovitis of osteoarthritis, rheumatoid arthritis, bursitis, acute gouty arthritis, epicondylitis, acute nonspecific tenosynovitis, posttraumatic osteoarthritis. *Intralesional administration:* Management of keloids; treatment of localized hypertrophic, infiltrated, inflammatory lesions of lichen planus, psoriatic plaques, granuloma annulare, lichen simplex chronicus; treatment of discoid lupus erythematosus, necrobiosis lipoidica diabeticorum, alopecia areata, cystic tumors of aponeurosis or tendon. *Topical application:* Relief of inflammatory and pruritic manifestations of corticosteroid-responsive dermatoses. *Oral inhalation:* Control of bronchial asthma or corticosteroid-responsive bronchospastic states. *Intranasal administration:* Relief of seasonal and perennial allergic rhinitis symptoms.

Contraindications Systemic fungal infections; IM use in idiopathic thrombocytopenic purpura; administration of live virus vaccines; topical monotherapy in primary bacterial infections; topical use on face, groin or axilla; oral inhalation as primary treatment for status asthmaticus or other acute episodes of asthma; intranasal administration in untreated localized infections involving nasal mucosa.

Route/Dosage

Triamcinolone

ADULTS: **PO** 4-100 mg/day. CHILDREN: **PO** 0.117-1.66 mg/kg/day.

Triamcinolone Acetonide

ADULTS & CHILDREN > 12 YR: **IM** 2.5-60 mg/day. **Intra-articular/intrasynovial/soft tissue** 2.5-40 mg prn. **Intradermal** 1 mg/intradermal injection site. **Inhalation** 2 inhalations tid-qid (maximum 16 inhalations/day). **Intranasal** 1-4 sprays in each nostril daily. CHILDREN 6-12 YR: **IM** 0.03-0.2 mg/kg q 1-7 days. **Inhalation** 1-2 inhalations tid-qid (maximum 12 inhalations/day). ADULTS & CHILDREN: **Topical** Apply sparingly bid-qid.

Triamcinolone Diacetate

ADULTS: **IM** 40 mg/wk. **Intra-articular/intrasynovial/soft tissue** 2-40 mg prn. **Intradermal** 5-48 mg (no more than 12.5 mg per injection site) prn.

Triamcinolone Hexacetamide

ADULTS: **Intra-articular** 2-20 mg prn. **Intradermal** ≤ 0.5 mg/square inch of affected area.

Interactions

Anticholinesterases: May antagonize anticholinesterase effects in myasthenia gravis. *Barbiturates:* May decrease pharmacologic effect of systemically administered triamcinolone. *Hydantoins, rifampin:* May increase clearance and decrease efficacy of systemically administered triamcinolone. *Salicylates:* Systemic administration may reduce serum levels and efficacy of salicylates. *Somatrem:* May inhibit growth-promoting effects of somatrem. *Troleandomycin:* May increase triamcinolone effects.

Lab Test Interferences

Uptake of thyroid I^{131} may be decreased. False-negative results with nitroblue-tetrazolium test may occur. Skin test reactions may be suppressed.

Adverse Reactions

CV: Edema; thromboembolism or fat embolism; thrombophlebitis; necrotizing angiitis; cardiac arrhythmias or ECG changes; syncopal episodes; hypertension; myocardial rupture; CHF. *RESP: With oral inhalation:* Wheezing. *CNS:* Convulsions; pseudotumor cerebri; vertigo; headache; neuritis; paresthesias; psychosis. *EENT:* Posterior subcapsular cataracts; increased intraocular pressure; glaucoma; exophthalmos. *With oral inhalation:* Throat irritation; hoarseness; dysphonia; coughing; thrush; dry mouth. *With intranasal use:* Nasal irritation; burning; stinging; dryness; epistaxis or bloody mucus; congestion; occasional sneezing attacks; rhinorrhea; anosmia; loss of sense of taste; throat discomfort. *GI:* Pancreatitis; nausea; vomiting; increased appetite and weight gain; peptic ulcer; bowel perforation. *HEMA:* Leukocytosis. *DERM:* Impaired wound healing; thin fragile skin; petechiae and ecchymoses; erythema; lupus erythematosus–like lesions; subcutaneous fat atrophy; striae; hirsutism; acneiform eruptions; allergic dermatitis; urticaria; angioneurotic edema; perineal irritation; hyperpigmentation or hypopigmentation (injection). *With topical application:* Burning; itching; irritation; erythema; dryness; folliculitis; hypertrichosis; perioral dermatitis; allergic contact dermatitis; stinging, cracking and tightening of skin; secondary infections; miliaria; telangiectasia. *META:* Sodium and fluid retention; hypokalemia; hypokalemic metabolic alkalosis; hypocalcemia. *OTHER:* Musculoskeletal effects (eg, weakness, myopathy, muscle mass loss, osteoporosis, spontaneous fractures); endocrine abnormalities (eg, menstrual irregularities, cushingoid state, growth suppression in children, sweating, decreased carbohydrate tolerance or hyperglycemia, glycosuria, increased insulin or sulfonylurea requirements in diabetic patients, hirsutism); anaphylactoid or hypersensitivity reactions; aggravation or masking of infections. *With intra-articular use:* Osteonecrosis; tendon rupture; infection; skin atrophy; postinjection flare; hypersensitivity; facial flushing. *With topical use:* May cause adverse effects similar to systemic use because of absorption.

Precautions

Pregnancy: Pregnancy category undetermined. Nasal and topical: Category C. *Lactation:* Excreted in breast milk. *Children:* May be more susceptible to adverse effects from topical use. Monitor growth and development of infants and children on prolonged therapy. Aerosol form not recommended for children < 6 yr. Intranasal form not recommended in children < 12 yr. *Elderly patients:* May require lower doses. *Acute asthma:* Oral inhalation is not indicated for rapid relief of bronchospasm. *Adrenal suppression:* Prolonged therapy may lead to hypothalamic-pituitary-adrenal suppression. *Cardiovascular effects:* Use drug with great caution after recent MI. *Hepatitis:* Drug may be harmful in chronic active hepatitis positive for hepatitis B surface antigen. *Hypersensitivity:* Reactions including anaphylaxis may occur. *Immunosuppression:* Do not administer live virus vaccines while patient is on therapy. *Infections:* Drug may mask signs of infection and may decrease host-defense mechanisms to prevent dissemination of infection. *Ocular effects:* Use drug with caution in ocular herpes simplex because of possible corneal perforation. *Peptic ulcer:* Drug may contribute to peptic ulceration, especially in large doses. *Renal impairment:* Use drug with caution. *Repository injections:* Do not inject subcutaneously. Avoid injection into deltoid muscle and repeated IM injection into same site. *Stress:* Increased dosage of rapidly acting corticosteroid may be needed before, during and after stressful situations. *Tartrazine sensitivity:* Some oral dosage forms of these products contain tartrazine, which may cause allergic-type reactions in susceptible individuals. *Withdrawal:* Abrupt discontinuation may result in adrenal insufficiency.

NURSING CONSIDERATIONS

Administration/Storage

Oral Administration

- Administer with meals or snacks.
- If drug is to be taken only once daily, administer early in morning.
- Administer multiple doses at evenly spaced intervals throughout day.
- When large doses are given, consider administering antacids between meals to help to prevent peptic ulcers.
- Store at room temperature.
- Avoid freezing of oral solution and suspension.
- Protect from light.

Intramuscular Administration

- Shake vial well before withdrawing drug from vial.
- Inject deeply into well-developed muscle.
- Rotate injection sites.
- Avoid injection into deltoid muscle.
- Store at room temperature.

Oral Inhalation

- Open inhaler so that medication canister is vertical and locked into position on built-in spacer.
- Thoroughly shake inhaler. Have patient take drink of water to moisten throat. Place adapter mouthpiece in mouth and gently seal with lips. Have patient tilt head back slightly, activate inhaler into spacer and take slow, deep breath for 3-5 sec while inhaler is activiated. Have patient hold breath for 10 sec and breathe out slowly. Allow at least 1 min between inhalations. Have patient rinse mouth with water or mouthwash after each use.

Intranasal Administration

- Clear nasal passages of secretions prior to use. If patient is conjested, use topical, short-acting decongestant just before administration to ensure adequate penetration of spray.
- Shake canister, place nasal adapter into one nares, gently close other nares with finger. While inhaling from nostril, activate canister. Repeat process on other side.
- Do not blow nose immediately after administration.

Topical Application

- To increase drug penetration, wash or soak area before application.
- May use occlusive dressing such as plastic wrap to increase skin penetration. However, do not use occlusive dressings > 12 hr/day.
- Apply cream/ointment or lotion sparingly in light film; rub in gently.
- Do not place bandages, dressings, cosmetics or other skin products over treated area unless directed by physician.
- Avoid contact with eyes.

Assessment/Interventions

- Obtain patient history, including drug history and any known allergies.
- Obtain periodic electrolyte and renal function tests if systemic preparations are used long-term.
- In patients taking large doses, restrict sodium intake and monitor BP.
- In prolonged use with children, plot growth pattern. Notify physician if abnormalities are evident.
- Monitor weight monthly.

OVERDOSAGE: SIGNS & SYMPTOMS

Excessive or long-term use: moonface, central obesity, striae, hirsutism, acne, ecchymoses, hypertension, osteoporosis, myopathy, sexual dysfunction, hyperglycemia, hyperlipidemia, peptic ulcer, electrolyte and fluid imbalance

Patient/Family Education

- Advise patient to follow dosage guidelines carefully. Do not discontinue or change dose unless directed by physician.

- Instruct patient on long-term steroid therapy to carry identification (eg, Medi-Alert) indicating condition and drug therapy.
- Advise patient to notify physician of stressful events/illnesses that may make dose adjustments necessary.
- Remind patient to use caution when exercising joints that have been recently medicated.
- Inform patient that nasal inhaler is for preventive therapy only and should be used on a daily basis.
- Recommend that patient have eyes examined periodically.
- Stress that oral inhalation is for preventive therapy only, should be used on a daily basis and should not be used to abort acute asthmatic attack. Instruct patient to notify physician if sore throat or sore mouth occur.
- Inform diabetic patient that sugar level in blood will probably be increased during systemic use of steroid and to monitor blood sugar more frequently.
- Remind patient that disease symptoms may reappear even after medication has been discontinued.
- Advise patient to notify physician promptly of signs of adrenal insufficiency: fever, myalgia, arthralgia, malaise, anorexia, nausea, vomiting, dizziness, fainting, diarrhea, low blood sugar.
- Instruct patient to report these symptoms to physician: unusual weight gain, swelling of lower extremities, muscle weakness, black tarry stools, vomiting of blood, puffing of face, menstrual irregularities, prolonged sore throat, fever, cold or infection.

See Patient Guide, pp. 614-617.

Triamterene

(try-AM-tur-een)

Dyrenium

Class: Potassium-sparing diuretic

Action Interferes with sodium reabsorption at distal renal tubule, resulting in increased excretion of sodium and water and decreased excretion of potassium.

Indications Treatment of edema associated with CHF, hepatic cirrhosis and nephrotic syndrome; treatment of steroid-induced edema, idiopathic edema and edema caused by secondary hyperaldosteronism; management of hypertension in patient with diuretic-induced hypokalemia or at risk of hypokalemia.

Contraindications Treatment with spironolactone or amiloride; anuria; severe hepatic disease; hyperkalemia; severe or progressive kidney disease or dysfunction, with exception of nephrosis.

Route/Dosage
ADULTS: **PO** 100 mg bid after meals (maximum 300 mg/day). CHILDREN: **PO** 2-4 mg/kg/day given in one dose or 2 divided doses (maximum 300 mg/day).

Interactions
ACE *inhibitors*: May result in severely elevated serum potassium levels. *Indomethacin*: May cause rapid progression into acute renal failure. *Potassium preparations and salt substitutes*: May severely increase serum potassium levels, possibly resulting in cardiac arrhythmias or cardiac arrest. Do not take with potassium preparations.

Lab Test Interferences
May interfere with fluorometry such as quinidine serum levels and LDH determination.

Adverse Reactions
CV: Hypotension. *CNS*: Weakness; fatigue; dizziness; headache. *GI*: Diarrhea; nausea; vomiting; dry mouth. *HEPA*: Jaundice; liver enzyme abnormalities. *GU*: Azotemia; elevated BUN

and creatinine; renal stones; bluish discoloration to urine; interstitial nephritis. *HEMA:* Thrombocytopenia; megaloblastic anemia. *DERM:* Photosensitivity; rash. *META:* Hyponatremia; hyperchloremic metabolic acidosis; hyperkalemia. *OTHER:* Anaphylaxis; muscle cramps.

Precautions

Pregnancy: Category B. *Lactation:* Undetermined. *Adult-onset diabetes mellitus:* Blood glucose levels may be increased; dosage adjustments of hypoglycemic agents may be needed. *Concurrent diuretic therapy:* Dosage reduction may be necessary. *Electrolyte imbalances and BUN increase:* Hyperkalemia (serum potassium > 5.5 mEq/l), hyponatremia, hyperchloremia and increases in BUN may occur. Monitor serum electrolytes and BUN levels. *Hematologic effects:* Triamterene is weak folic acid antagonist and may contribute to appearance of megaloblastosis. *Metabolic acidosis:* May decrease alkali reserve with possibility of metabolic acidosis. *Renal impairment:* Use drug with caution; monitor renal function. *Renal stones:* Triamterene has been found in renal stones. Use drug with caution in patients with history of stone formation.

NURSING CONSIDERATIONS

Administration/Storage

- Administer after meals.
- Administer once daily dose in morning to avoid disturbing sleep.
- Open capsules and mix with food or fluids if appropriate for patient needs.
- Store at room temperature in tight, light resistent container.

Assessment/Interventions

- Obtain patient history, including drug history and any known allergies.
- Assess renal status, BUN and creatinine levels and fluid and electrolyte status.
- Assess I&O, body weight and hydration status.
- Assess lung sounds and peripheral edema.
- Assess vital signs, especially BP.
- Institute safety precautions to prevent falls, particularly with initial doses.
- Monitor for signs and symptoms of hyperkalemia, especially with diabetic patients.
- Monitor for signs and symptoms of side effects, ie, hyperkalemia, GI disturbances, weakness, dizziness, unusual bleeding or bruising.
- Monitor patient for signs of metabolic acidosis; hyperventilation, drowsiness, restlessness.

OVERDOSAGE: SIGNS & SYMPTOMS

Hypotension, hyperkalemia, metabolic acidosis, nausea, vomiting, weakness, acute renal failure

Patient/Family Education

- Tell patient to avoid salt substitute and limit potassium-rich foods.
- Inform patients taking antihypertensives that additive effects are possible; identify signs and symptoms of hypotension and precautions to be taken.
- Advise patient that medication may cause urine to become blue tinged.
- Explain potential GI side effects and to take medication after meals.
- Tell patient that drug may cause weakness, headache, nausea, vomiting or dry mouth and to notify physician if they become severe or persistent.
- Instruct patient to report these symptoms to physician: fever, sore throat, mouth sores or unusual bleeding or bruising.
- Caution patient to avoid intake of alcoholic beverages or other CNS depressants.
- Advise patient to use caution while driving or performing other tasks requiring mental alertness.
- Caution patient to avoid exposure to

sunlight or ultraviolet light and to use sunscreen or wear protective clothing to prevent photosensitivity reaction.

See Patient Guide, p. 618.

Triazolam

(try-AZE-oh-lam)

Halcion, ♣ *APO-Triazo, Novo-Triolam, Nu-Triazo*

Class: Sedative and hypnotic/ benzodiazepine

Action Potentiates action of GABA (gamma-aminobutyric acid), an inhibitory neurotransmitter, resulting in increased neuronal inhibition and CNS depression, especially in limbic system and reticular formation.

Indications Treatment of insomnia.

Contraindications Hypersensitivity to benzodiazepines; pregnancy.

Route/Dosage

ADULTS: **PO** 0.125-0.5 mg at bedtime. ELDERLY OR DEBILITATED PATIENTS: Initiate with 0.125 mg until individual response is determined.

Interactions

Alcohol, CNS depressants (eg, narcotic sedatives): May cause additive CNS depressant effects. *Cimetidine, disulfiram, omeprazole, oral contraceptives:* Triazolam effects may increase. *Digoxin:* Serum digoxin concentrations may be increased. *Theophylline:* May antagonize sedative effects.

Lab Test Interferences

None well documented.

Adverse Reactions

CNS: Anterograde amnesia; headache; nervousness; drowsiness; confusion; talkativeness; apprehension; irritability; euphoria; weakness; tremor; incoordination; memory impairment; depression; ataxia; dizziness; dreaming/nightmares; hallucinations; paradoxical reactions (eg, anger, hostility, mania, muscle spasms). *EENT:* Visual or auditory disturbances; depressed hearing; taste disturbances. *GI:* Heartburn; nausea; vomiting; diarrhea; constipation; dry mouth; anorexia. *HEMA:* Blood dyscrasias including agranulocytosis; anemia; thrombocytopenia; leukopenia; neutropenia. *HEPA:* Hepatic dysfunction including hepatitis and jaundice. *DERM:* Rash; photosensitivity. *OTHER:* Dependence/withdrawal syndrome (eg, confusion; abnormal perception of movement; depersonalization; muscle twitching; psychosis; paranoid delusions; seizures). Rebound sleep disorder (recurrence of insomnia worse than before treatment) may occur during first 3 nights after abrupt discontinuation.

Precautions

Pregnancy: Category X. *Lactation:* Undetermined. *Children:* Not for use in children < 18 yr. *Special risk patients:* Use drug with caution in elderly patients and patients with renal or hepatic impairment, depression or suicidal tendencies, drug abuse and dependence, chronic pulmonary insufficiency or apnea, seizure disorder. *Dependence:* Prolonged use (> 1-2 wk) can lead to dependence. Withdrawal syndrome may occur; taper dose gradually.

NURSING CONSIDERATIONS

Administration/Storage

- Administer at bedtime with full glass of water.
- Administer with food if GI upset occurs.
- Administer lowest dosage until response is determined.
- If patient exhibits possible suicidal tendencies, ensure that patient swallows drug and that patient does not have access to large quantities.

- Store at room temperature in a tight, light-resistant container.

Assessment/Interventions

- Obtain patient history, including drug history and any known allergies. Identify potential for abuse and underlying depression.
- Assess usual sleep patterns and define type of sleep alteration, ie, insomnia. Assess for modifiable causes of sleep disturbance, such as environmental noise, daytime sleeping and caffeine use.
- Assess therapeutic response to therapy throughout usage.
- Implement safety precautions to prevent injury (eg, assist with ambulation), particularly during initial treatment until individual response is determined.
- Utilize general comfort measures to encourage sleep.
- Implement environmental control measures when appropriate to enhance sleep.
- Monitor for side effects, such as dizziness, drowsiness, headache, change in mood or mental status, GI disturbance, paradoxical excitation.
- Monitor for daytime drowsiness or lethargy.
- Assess for signs of dependence.

OVERDOSAGE: SIGNS & SYMPTOMS

Somnolence, confusion, delirium, lack of coordination, ataxia, slurred speech, respiratory depression, coma, seizures

Patient/Family Education

- Caution patient that this medication must not be taken during pregnancy or when pregnancy is possible. Advise patient to use reliable form of birth control while taking this drug.
- Remind patient that medication should not be abruptly discontinued.
- Review with patient and family other general sleep promotion measures, as well as what to avoid, such as caffeine and excessive exercise at bedtime.
- Explain that medication may cause morning drowsiness or tiredness.
- Caution patient regarding dependence potential.
- Explain potential side effects and what to report to physician (confusion, paradoxical excitement, headache, bleeding, recurrent sleep disorder).
- Instruct patient to avoid intake of alcoholic beverages or other CNS depressants.
- Advise patient to use caution while driving or performing other tasks requiring mental alertness.
- Instruct patient not to take otc medications without consulting physician.

See Patient Guide, p. 619.

Trifluoperazine HCl

(try-flew-oh-PURR-uh-zeen HIGH-droe-KLOR-ide)

Stelazine, Stelazine Concentrate

Class: Antipsychotic/phenothiazine

Action Effects apparently related to dopamine receptor blocking in CNS.

Indications Managemnent of psychotic disorders, short-term treatment (< 12 wk) of nonpsychotic anxiety.

Contraindications Sensitivity to phenothiazines; comatose or severely depressed states; presence of large amount of other CNS depressants; bone marrow depression or blood dyscrasias; liver disease; cerebral arteriosclerosis; coronary artery disease; severe hypotension or hypertension; subcortical brain damage.

Route/Dosage

Individualize dose.

Psychotic Disorder

ADULTS: **PO** 2-5 mg bid initially. Maintenance: 15-20 mg/day in single or divided doses. Few patients may require ≥ 40 mg/day. **IM** 1-2 mg by deep injection q 4-6 hr prn. More than 6 mg in 24 hr is rarely needed. CHILDREN: Individualize dosage based on weight of child and severity of symptoms. CHILDREN 6-12 YR: **PO** 1 mg qd or bid initially. Maintenance: Rarely > 15 mg/day in single or divided doses. **IM** 1 mg daily or bid.

Nonpsychotic Anxiety

ADULTS: **PO** 1-2 mg bid (maximum 6 mg/day).

Interactions

Alcohol and other CNS depressants (eg, narcotics, sedatives): May result in increased CNS depression and may precipitate dystonic reactions. *Anticholinergics:* May reduce therapeutic effects of trifluoperazine and worsen anticholinergic effects of trifluoperazine. May lead to tardive dyskinesia. *Barbiturate anesthetics:* May increase frequency and severity of neuromuscular excitation and hypotension. *Guanethidine:* May inhibit hypotensive action of guanethidine. *Metrizamide:* Possibility of seizure may be increased when subarachnoid metrizamide injection is used.

Lab Test Interferences

Drug may discolor urine pink to red-brown. False-positive pregnancy tests may occur but are less likely to occur with serum test. Increases in protein-bound iodine have been reported.

Adverse Reactions

CV: Orthostatic hypotension; tachycardia; syncope; cardiac arrest; circulatory collapse; lightheadedness; faintness; ECG changes. *RESP:* Laryngospasm; bronchospasm; shortness of breath. *CNS:* Headache; weakness; tremor; fatigue; slurring of speech; insomnia; sedation; vertigo; seizures; twitching; ataxia; tardive dyskinesia; drowsiness; lethargy; paradoxical excitement; pseudoparkinsonism; motor restlessness; oculogyric crises; opisthotonos; hyperreflexia; tardive dyskinesia. *EENT:* Pigmentary retinopathy; glaucoma; photophobia; blurred vision; miosis; mydriasis; increased intraocular pressure; dry mouth or throat; nasal congestion. *GI:* Dyspepsia; constipation; adynamic ileus (may result in death). *GU:* Urinary hesitancy or retention; impotence; sexual dysfunction; menstrual irregularities. *HEPA:* Cholestatic jaundice. *HEMA:* Agranulocytosis; eosinophilia; leukopenia; hemolytic anemia; thrombocytopenic purpura. *DERM:* Photosensitivity; skin pigmentation; dry skin; exfoliative dermatitis; urticarial rash; maculopapular hypersensitivity reaction; seborrhea; contact dermatitis. *META:* Decreased cholesterol. *OTHER:* Increases in appetite and weight; polydipsia; breast enlargement; galactorrhea; heat-illness; neuroleptic malignant syndrome.

Precautions

Pregnancy: Pregnancy category undetermined. *Lactation:* Excreted in breast milk. *Children:* In general, not recommended for children < 12 yr. When drug is used in children with acute illnesses (eg, chickenpox, measles, gastroenteritis or dehydration), they are more susceptible to neuromuscular reactions than adults. Avoid use of drug in children and adolescents with signs and symptoms suggestive of Reye's syndrome. *Elderly, debilitated or emaciated patients:* More susceptible to hypotensive and neuromuscular effects. Require lower initial dosage and more gradual increase in dosage. *Special risk patients:* Use drug with caution in patients with cardiovascular disease or mitral insufficiency, history of glaucoma, EEG abnormalities or seizure disorders, prior brain damage, hepatic or renal impairment. *CNS effects:* Drug may impair mental or physical abilities, especially during first few days of therapy. *Hepatic effects:* Jaundice usually occurs between second and fourth weeks of treatment and is considered hypersensitivity reaction. Usually reversible. *Neuroleptic malignant syndrome:* Has occurred with agents in this class and is potentially fatal. Signs and symptoms are hyperpyrexia, muscle rigidity, altered mental status, irregular pulse, irregular BP, tachycardia and diaphoresis. *Pulmonary effects:* Cases of bronchopneumonia, some fatal, have occurred. *Renal impairment:* Use with caution, lower dose may be necessary. *Sudden death:* Has been reported. Predisposing factors may be seizures or previous brain damage. Flare-ups of psychotic behavior may precede death. *Sulfite sensitivity:* Some of these products contain sulfites, which may cause allergic-type reactions including anaphylactic symptoms and life-threatening or less severe asthmatic episodes in certain susceptible persons.

NURSING CONSIDERATIONS

Administration/Storage

- Administer at bedtime to minimize effects of sedation and orthostatic hypotension.
- Ensure that patient swallows medication and is not hoarding it.
- For IM administration, inject deeply into well-developed muscle.
- For concentrate, dilute just prior to administration. Add desired dose to 60 ml or more of following diluents: tomato or fruit juice, milk, simple syrup, orange syrup, carbonated beverages, decaffeinated coffee or tea or water. May also add dose to semisolid foods such as soups or puddings.
- Store liquid concentrates in amber bottles at room temperature and protect from light.
- Store tablets and injection at room temperature protected from light.
- Avoid freezing oral concentrate and injection.
- Slight yellowish discoloration of injection will not affect potency or efficacy.
- Do not use injection if markedly discolored.

Assessment/Interventions

- Obtain patient history, including drug history and any known allergies.
- Assess for high-risk factors (cardiac history, hepatic or renal impairment, neurologic damage).
- Inquire about patient's alcohol intake.
- Assess efficacy of antipsychotic response during initial dosing.
- Take BP measurements after IM injections of medication.
- Monitor patient carefully for acute neurologic changes after drug administration.
- Monitor for extrapyramidal symptoms.
- Periodically monitor hepatic function.
- Monitor renal function at start of therapy and periodically during therapy. If creatinine is abnormal, notify physician. Dosage adjustment may be necessary.
- Monitor WBC periodically. If significant drop in granulocytes occurs, dosage decrease or discontinuation of therapy may be necessary.
- If fever with flu-like symptoms occurs, obtain LFTs.

OVERDOSAGE: SIGNS & SYMPTOMS

CNS depression (somnolence to coma), hypotension, extrapyramidal symptoms, agitation, restlessness, seizures, fever, hypothermia, hyperthermia, autonomic reactions, ECG changes, cardiac arrhythmias

Patient/Family Education

- Advise patient not to change dose unless instructed by physician.
- Instruct patient not to discontinue medication abruptly.
- Inform patient that urine may change to pink or red-brownish color.
- Advise female patients of possibility

of false-positive urine pregnancy test results.

- Inform patient of possibility of yellowing of skin after several weeks of drug therapy.
- Instruct patient to report these symptoms to physician: abnormal movements, involuntary muscle twitching or jaundice.
- Caution patient to avoid sudden position changes to prevent orthostatic hypotension.
- Instruct patient to avoid intake of alcoholic beverages.
- Advise patient that drug may cause drowsiness and to use caution while driving or performing other tasks requiring mental alertness.
- Caution patient to minimize exposure to sunlight and to use sunscreen or wear protective clothing to avoid photosensitivity reaction.

See Patient Guide, p. 620.

Trihexyphenidyl HCl

(try-hex-ee-FEN-in-dill HIGH-droe-KLOR-ide)

Artane, Artane Sequels, Trihexy-2, Trihexy-5, ♣ *APO-Trihex*

Class: Antiparkinson/anticholinergic

Action Exerts direct inhibitory effect on parasympathetic nervous system by inhibiting actions of acetylcholine; has relaxing effect on smooth musculature.

Indications Adjunct in treatment of all forms of parkinsonism (postencephalitic, arteriosclerotic and idiopathic); adjuvant therapy with levodopa for control of drug-induced extrapyramidal disorders. *Sustained release:* Maintenance therapy after patients have been stabilized on tablets or elixir.

Contraindications Standard considerations.

Route/Dosage

Parkinsonism

ADULTS: PO 1 or 2 mg first day; increase by 2 mg increments at intervals of 3-5 days, until 6-10 mg given daily in divided doses. Some postencephalitic patients may require total daily dose of 12-15 mg. Usually given tid at mealtimes. High doses may be taken qid, at mealtimes and at bedtime.

Concomitant Use with Other Anticholinergics

Gradually initiate trihexyphenidyl with progessive reduction of other anticholinergic.

Drug-Induced Extrapyramidal Disorders

Amount and frequency is individualized. Start with single 1 mg dose. If symptoms are not controlled in few hours, progressively increase until controlled. Daily dosage usually ranges 5-15 mg in divided doses.

Sustained Release

Not for initial therapy. Once patient is stabilized, may switch on equipotent daily basis. Give as single dose after breakfast or in bid doses 12 hr apart.

Interactions

Haloperidol: Schizophrenic symptoms may worsen; haloperidol levels may decrease and tardive dyskinesia may develop. *Phenothiazines:* Actions of phenothiazines may be decreased.

Lab Test Interferences

None well documented.

Adverse Reactions

CV: Tachycardia; palpitations; hypotension. *CNS:* Dizziness; nervousness; psychiatric manifestations such as delusions or hallucinations; mental confusion; agitation; disturbed behavior. *EENT:* Blurred vision; angle-closure glaucoma; difficulty swallowing. *GI:* Dry mouth; nausea; vomiting; constipation; suppurative parotitis; dilation of colon; paralytic ileus. *GU:* Urinary retention; urinary hesitancy; impotence.

DERM: Rash. *OTHER*: Fever; flushing; decreased sweating; heat illness.

Precautions

Pregnancy: Category C. *Lactation:* Undetermined. *Children:* Safety and efficacy not established. *Elderly patients:* More susceptible to adverse effects. *Special risk patients:* Use drug with caution in patients with tachycardia, arrhythmias, hypertension, hypotension, prostatic hypertrophy, liver or kidney disorders, obstructive disease of GI tract. *Anticholinergic effect:* Concomitant use of other drugs with anticholinergic effects will have additive effects. *Heat illness:* Give with caution during hot weather. Severe anhidrosis and fatal hyperthermia may occur. *Ophthalmic:* Incipient narrow-angle glaucoma may be precipitated by drug use; therefore closely monitor patient for symptoms and evaluate intraocular pressure at regular, periodic intervals.

NURSING CONSIDERATIONS

Administration/Storage

- Do not crush sustained release product or allow patient to chew.
- Store at room temperature in light-resistant container. Avoid freezing the elixir.

Assessment/Interventions

- Obtain patient history, including drug history and any known allergies.
- Assess Parkinson's symptoms prior to and throughout therapy.
- Implement safety precautions to prevent injury, particularly during initial therapy until individual response is determined.
- Encourage frequent oral hygiene.
- Implement measures to prevent constipation, ie, fluids, activity, dietary bulk.
- Monitor for side effects: dry mouth, nausea, dizziness, nervousness, blurred vision. If dry mouth occurs, provide patient with ice chips or sugarless hard candy or sugarless gum for comfort.
- Monitor for other anticholinergic side effects: constipation, difficulty voiding. If these effects are noted, increase patient's fluid intake and notify physician if problematic.
- Monitor vital signs per routine and more frequently when increasing dose.
- Monitor frequency of bowel movements, I&O.
- If patient complains of sudden onset of eye pain and blurred vision, discontinue drug and notify physician.
- Assess for behavioral changes, particularly in individuals with history of mental disorder.

OVERDOSAGE: SIGNS & SYMPTOMS

CNS depression, dry skin, dry mucous membranes, fever, dilated, sluggish pupils, respiratory depression, circulatory collapse, coma

Patient/Family Education

- Advise patient to take as directed and not to change dose unless advised by physician.
- Tell patient to be cautious during hot weather to prevent heat-related illness.
- Explain measures to prevent constipation.
- Encourage frequent oral hygiene and use of ice chips and sugarless gum or sugarless hard candy if dry mouth is experienced.
- Identify types of measuring devices that will ensure accurate dosage of elixir.
- Advise patient that therapeutic effect may not be immediately evident.
- Explain rationale for tapering of other anticholinergic drugs on initiation of therapy.
- Instruct patient not to stop taking drug abruptly.
- Explain potential side effects and what should be reported to physician.
- Advise patient that drug may cause

drowsiness and dizziness and to use caution while driving or performing tasks requiring mental alertness.

- Instruct patient not to take otc medications without consulting physician.

See Patient Guide, p. 621.

Trimethobenzamide HCl

(try-meth-oh-BEN-zuh-mide HIGH-droe-KLOR-ide)

Arrestin, T-Gen, Tebamide, Ticon, Tigan, Tiject-20, Trimazide

Class: Antiemetic and antivertigo/anticholinergic

Action Believed to directly affect medullary chemoreceptor trigger zone to inhibit nausea.

Indications Prevention and treatment of nausea and vomiting.

Contraindications Hypersensitivity to benzocaine or other local anesthetics. Suppositories contraindicated in neonates or premature infants; parenteral use contraindicated in children.

Route/Dosage
ADULTS: **PO** 250 mg tid-qid. **PR** 200 mg tid-qid. **IM** 200 mg tid-qid. CHILDREN 14-41 KG: **PO** 100-200 mg tid-qid. **PR** 100-200 mg tid-qid. CHILDREN < 14 KG: **PR** 100 mg tid-qid.

Interactions None well documented.

Lab Test Interferences
None well documented.

Adverse Reactions
CV: Hypotension (after injection). *CNS:* Mood depression; disorientation; headache; drowsiness; opisthotonos; dizziness; seizures; coma; Parkinson-like symptoms. *EENT:* Blurred vision. *GI:* Diarrhea. *HEMA:* Blood dyscrasias. *HEPA:* Jaundice. *OTHER:* Local pain, burning, stinging, redness and swelling (after injection); hypersensitivity reactions; muscle cramps.

Precautions
Pregnancy: Safety not established. *Lactation:* Undetermined. *Hypersensitivity:* Has been reported; discontinue use of drug at first signs of sensitivity.

NURSING CONSIDERATIONS

Administration/Storage

- Do not use oral route with vomiting.
- If necessary, open capsule and mix with food or liquids for administration.
- Use Z-track technique for IM administration.
- Avoid exposure to light; store at room temperature.
- Avoid freezing injectable.

Assessment/Interventions

- Obtain patient history, including drug history and any known allergies.
- Assess bowel sounds and severity of nausea and vomiting.
- Implement safety precautions, particularly during initial therapy until individual response is determined.
- Implement general comfort measures.
- Monitor response to therapy.
- Monitor I&O.
- Monitor vital signs, particularly BP.
- Monitor for potential side effects, particularly drowsiness and hypotension.

Patient/Family Education

- Instruct patient that when used for motion sickness, medication should be taken 30 min before exposure to motion.
- Advise patient to report these symptoms to physician: dizziness, yellowing of skin or eyes, muscle cramps or abnormal movements.
- Instruct patient to avoid intake of

alcoholic beverages or other CNS depressants.

- Advise patient that drug may cause drowsiness or dizziness and to use caution while driving or performing tasks requiring mental alertness.

See Patient Guide, p. 622.

Trimethoprim/ Sulfamethoxazole (Co-trimoxazole; TMP-SMZ)

(try-METH-oh-prim/suhl-fuh-meth-OX-uh-zole)

Bactrim, Cotrim, Septra, Sulfamethoprim, Sulfatrim DS, Sulfatrim, Uroplus SS, ♣ *APO-Sulfatrim, Coptin, Coptin 1, Novo-Trimel, Nu-Cotrimox, Roubac*

Class: Anti-infective

Action Sulfamethoxazole (SMZ) inhibits bacterial synthesis of dihydrofolic acid by competing with PABA. Trimethoprim (TMP) blocks production of tetrahydrofolic acid by inhibiting the enzyme dihydrofolate reductase. This combination blocks two consecutive steps in bacterial biosynthesis of essential nucleic acids and proteins and is usually bactericidal.

Indications

Oral/parenteral: Treatment of UTIs caused by susceptible strains of bacteria, shigellosis enteritis and *Pneumocystis carinii* pneumonitis. *Oral:* Treatment of acute otitis media and acute exacerbations of chronic bronchitis; treatment of traveler's diarrhea. **Unlabeled uses:** Treatment of cholera, salmonella-type infections and nocardiosis; prevention of recurrent UTIs in women; prophylaxis of bacterial infections in susceptible patients; treatment of prostatitis; prophylaxis of *Pneumocystis carinii* pneumonitis.

Contraindications Hypersensitivity to sulfonamides; megaloblastic anemia caused by folate deficiency; pregnancy at term; lactation; infants < 2 mo of age.

Route/Dosage

UTIs, Shigellosis, Acute Otitis Media

ADULTS: **PO** 160 mg TMP/800 mg SMZ q 12 hr for 10-14 days and 5 days for shigellosis. **IV** 8-10 mg/kg/day (based on TMP) in 2-4 divided doses q 6-12 hr for up to 14 days for severe UTIs and 5 days for shigellosis. CHILDREN > 2 MO: **PO** 8 mg/kg TMP/40 mg/kg SMZ daily in 2 divided doses q 12 hr for 10 days and 5 days for shigellosis.

Pneumocystis Carinii Pneumonitis

ADULTS: **PO** 20 mg/kg TMP/100 mg/kg SMZ daily in divided doses q 6 hr for 14 days. **IV** 15-20 mg/kg/day (based on TMP) in 3-4 divided doses for up to 14 days.

Traveler's Diarrhea

ADULTS: **PO** 160 mg TMP/800 mg SMZ q 12 hr for 5 days.

Exacerbation of Chronic Bronchitis

ADULTS: **PO** 160 mg TMP/800 mg SMZ q 12 hr for 14 days.

Interactions

Cyclosporine: May cause decrease in therapeutic effect of cyclosporine and increased risk of nephrotoxicity. *Methotrexate:* May displace methotrexate from protein-binding sites, thus increasing free methotrexate levels. *Phenytoin:* Trimethoprim may inhibit metabolism of phenytoin or other hydantoins. *Procainamide:* Trimethoprim may inhibit renal elimination of procainamide and its metabolites. *Sulfonylureas:* May increase hypoglycemic response to sulfonylureas because of displacement from protein-binding sites or inhibition of hepatic metabolism. *Warfarin:* May cause prolonged PT. INCOMPATIBILITIES: Do not mix with other drugs or solutions other than D5W.

Lab Test Interferences

Can interfere with serum methotrexate assay as determined by competitive binding protein technique when bacterial dihydrofolate reductase is used as binding protein. May interfere with Jaffe alkaline picrate reaction assay for creatinine, resulting in overestimations.

Adverse Reactions

CV: Allergic myocarditis. *RESP:* Pulmonary infiltrates; cough; shortness of breath. *CNS:* Headache; depression; seizures; aseptic meningitis; insomnia; hallucinations. *EENT:* Glossitis; stomatitis. *GI:* Nausea; vomiting; anorexia; abdominal pain; diarrhea; pseudomembranous enterocolitis; pancreatitis; esophageal ulcers. *GU:* Renal failure; interstitial nephritis; toxic nephrosis with oliguria or anuria; crystalluria. *HEPA:* Hepatitis; hepatic necrosis. *HEMA:* Agranulocytosis; aplastic, hemolytic or megaloblastic anemia; thrombocytopenia; leukopenia; neutropenia; hypoprothrombinemia; eosinophilia; methemoglobinemia. *DERM:* Local reaction, pain, and irritation on IV administration; hypersensitivity reactions including rash; urticaria; photosensitization; generalized skin eruptions. *OTHER:* Arthralgia; myalgia; hypersensitivity reactions including erythema multiforme, Stevens-Johnson syndrome, toxic epidermal necrolysis, exfoliative dermatitis, serum sickness, anaphylactoid reactions, angiodema, drug fever, chills, systemic lupus erythematosus, periarteritis nodosa; conjunctival and scleral injection.

Precautions

Pregnancy: Category C. Do not use at term because of risk of neonatal kernicterus. *Lactation:* Undetermined. Not recommended during nursing because sulfonamides are excreted in breast milk and may cause kernicterus. Premature infants and infants with hyperbilirubinemia or G-6-PD deficiency are also at risk for adverse effects. *Children:* Not recommended for infants < 2 mo. *Elderly patients:* Are at increased risk of severe adverse reactions. *Special risk patients:* Use drug with caution in patients with possible folate deficiency (eg, elderly patients, chronic alcoholics, patients undergoing anticonvulsant therapy, patients with malabsorption syndromes or malnutrition), patients with severe allergy or bronchial asthma, patients who have sulfite sensitivity and G-6-PD–deficient individuals. *Ulceration:* Take tablets with water or food to prevent lodging in esophagus and subsequent ulceration. *Hematologic effects:* Sulfonamide-associated deaths, although rare, have occurred from hypersensitivity of respiratory tract, Stevens-Johnson syndrome, toxic epidermal necrolysis, fulminant hepatic necrosis, agranulocytosis, aplastic anemia and other blood dyscrasias. Both components can interfere with hematopoiesis. IV use at high doses for extended periods of time may cause bone marrow depression. *Patients with AIDS:* Incidence of side effects, especially rash, fever and leukopenia, is greatly increased. *Renal and hepatic impairment:* Use drug with caution. Dosage adjustment may be required. *Streptococcal pharyngitis:* Do not use for streptococcal pharyngitis. *Sulfonamides:* Are chemically similar to some goitrogens, diuretics (acetazolamide and the thiazides) and oral hypoglycemic agents. Goiter production, diuresis, and hypoglycemia occur rarely in patients receiving sulfonamides. Cross-sensitivity may occur.

NURSING CONSIDERATIONS

Administration/Storage

- Administer with full glass of water.
- May administer with food if GI upset occurs.
- For IV infusion, must dilute in 75 or 125 ml of D5W only. Administer each dose over 60-90 min. Flush IV line after infusion. Do not use IV

solution if cloudy or precipitates are noted.

- If local irritation or inflammation because of extravascular infiltration occurs, discontinue infusion and restart at another site.
- Avoid rapid or direct IV injection. Do not inject IM.
- Shake oral suspension well before use.
- Store IV solution at room temperature. Do not refrigerate. Discard prepared IV solution if not used within 2 hr (75 ml) or 6 hr (125 ml).
- Store tablets or suspension at room temperature in a tight, light-resistant container.

Assessment/Interventions

- Obtain patient history, including drug history and any known allergies. Note decreased renal or hepatic function and sensitivity to sulfonamides (including sulfonylureas, or thiazide diuretics) and trimethoprim.
- Obtain culture and sensitivity before beginning drug therapy.
- Monitor I&O.
- Encourage fluid intake.
- Monitor renal function during prolonged treatment.
- Notify physician of GI upset, fever, chills, headache, rash, decreased urine output, wheezing, shortness of breath, dizziness, sore throat, unusual bleeding or bruising or arthralgia.

OVERDOSAGE: SIGNS & SYMPTOMS

Anorexia, colic, nausea, vomiting, dizziness, headache, drowsiness, depression, confusion, altered mental status, fever, hematuria, crystalluria, blood dyscrasias, jaundice, bone marrow depression

Patient/Family Education

- Advise patient to complete full course of therapy.
- Encourage patient to maintain adequate fluid intake.
- Advise patient to take tablet with full glass of water.
- Educate patient and family to report any signs of superinfection such as fever, vaginitis, oral candidiasis and fatigue.
- Instruct patient to report these symptoms to physician: skin rash, sore throat, fever, or unusual bruising or bleeding.
- Caution patient to avoid exposure to sunlight and to use sunscreen or wear protective clothing to avoid photosensitivity reaction.

See Patient Guide, pp. 623-624.

Trimetrexate Glucuronate

(TRY-meh-TREK-sate glue-CURE-uh-nate)

Neutrexin

Class: Anti-infective/antiprotozoal

Action Inhibits dihydrofolate reductase necessary for DNA, RNA and protein synthesis, leading to cell death.

Indications As alternative therapy, with concurrent leucovorin administration, for treatment of moderate-to-severe *Pneumocystis carinii* pneumonia in immunocompromised patients in whom trimethoprim-sulfamethoxazole cannot be used. **Unlabeled uses:** Treatment of non–small cell lung, prostate and colorectal cancer.

Contraindications Clinically significant sensitivity to trimetrexate, leucovorin or methotrexate.

Route/Dosage

ADULTS: **IV** 45 mg/m^2 q/day by IV infusion over 60-90 min for 21 days. Leucovorin may be administered IV at dose of 20 mg/m^2 over 5-10 min q 6 hrs for total daily dose of 80 mg/m^2 or **PO** at dose of 20 mg/m^2 q 6 hr for 24 days. Adjust dose of trimetrexate and leucovorin according to hematologic toxicity. Interruption of therapy may be necessary for hematologic, hepatic, renal or mucosal toxicity or for uncontrolled fever.

Interactions

Acetaminophen, cimetidine, clotrimazole, erythromycin, fluconazole, ketoconazole, miconazole, rifabutin, rifampin: May alter trimetrexate levels. *Zidovudine:* Zidovudine should be discontinued during trimetrexate therapy to allow for full therapeutic doses of trimetrexate. INCOMPATIBILITIES: Do not mix with solutions containing either chloride ion (eg, sodium chloride) or leucovorin, because precipitation occurs instantly.

Lab Test Interferences

None well documented.

Adverse Reactions

CNS: Confusion; fatigue. *GI:* Nausea; vomiting; increased serum transaminases; increased alkaline phosphatase; increased bilirubin. *GU:* Increased serum creatinine. *HEMA:* Neutropenia; thrombocytopenia; anemia. *DERM:* Rash; pruritus. *META:* Hyponatremia; hypocalcemia. *OTHER:* Fever.

Precautions

Pregnancy: Category D. *Lactation:* Undetermined. *Children:* Safety and efficacy not established in children < 18 yr. Under Compassionate Use Protocol, younger children have been treated. *Special risk patients:* Use drug with caution in patients with impaired hematologic, renal or hepatic function and in patients who require concomitant therapy with nephrotoxic, myelosuppressive or hepatotoxic drugs. *Concurrent leucovorin:* Trimetrexate must be used with concurrent leucovorin to avoid potentially serious or life-threatening complications including bone marrow suppression, oral and GI mucosal ulceration and renal and hepatic dysfunction.

NURSING CONSIDERATIONS

Administration/Storage

- Administer IV trimetrexate and leucovorin solutions separately. Leucovorin solution may be administered prior to or after trimetrexate. In either case flush IV line thoroughly with at least 10 ml of 5% Dextrose Injection between infusions.
- Avoid contact with skin or mucosa. If trimetrexate contacts skin or mucosa, immediately and thoroughly wash with soap and water.
- Reconstitute with 2 ml of 5% Dextrose for Injection or Sterile Water to yield concentration of 12.5 mg/ml. Do not reconstitute with solutions containing either chloride ion or leucovorin, because precipitation will occur instantly.
- Observe solution, which should dissolve product completely approximately 30 sec after dilution. Reconstituted solution will appear as pale greenish-yellow solution. Do not use if cloudiness or particulate matter is observed.
- Filter solution (0.22 µm) prior to dilution.
- Further dilute reconstituted solution with 5% Dextrose Injection to yield final concentration of 0.25-2 mg/ml.
- Administer diluted solution by IV infusion over 60-90 min.
- Flush IV line with at least 10 ml of 5% Dextrose Injection before and after administering trimetrexate.
- Store vials at controlled room temperature and protect from exposure to light.
- After reconstitution, retain solution at room temperature or under refrigeration for no longer than 24 hours. Do not freeze reconstituted solution.
- Use cytotoxic drug precautions for proper disposal.

Assessment/Interventions

- Obtain patient history, including drug history and any known allergies.
- Assess integrity of IV site prior to infusion.
- Assess for signs and symptoms of oral and GI mucosal ulceration, changes

in mental status, fatigue and signs and symptoms of infection.

- Implement safety precautions until individual response is determined.
- Implement measures to prevent infection.
- Monitor for side effects, including bone marrow suppression and renal and hepatic dysfunction throughout therapy.
- Monitor vital signs, renal and hepatic function, hematologic studies, I&O, body weight and stools for occult blood.
- Consider termination of treatment if fever (oral temperature ≥ 105° F) cannot be controlled by antipyretics.
- Consider discontinuation of therapy if serum creatinine is > 2.5 mg/dl or if transaminase or alkaline phosphatase levels become > 5 times normal.

OVERDOSAGE: SIGNS & SYMPTOMS

Severe neutropenia, severe thrombocytopenia, severe anemia, nausea, vomiting

Patient/Family Education

- Explain that continued, frequent monitoring by physician is necessary.
- Inform patient that blood test must be performed at least twice weekly.
- Explain that leucovorin therapy must be continued for 72 hr after last dose of trimetrexate.
- Describe potential side effects, and what should be reported to physician: fever, mucosal toxicity, etc.
- Explain measures to prevent infection.
- Advise patient to use caution while driving or performing other tasks requiring mental alertness.

See Patient Guide, p. 625.

Triprolidine HCl

(try-PRO-lih-deen HIGH-droe-KLOR-ide)

Actidil, Myidyl

Class: Antihistamine/alkylamine

Action Competitively blocks histamine at H_2 receptor sites.

Indications Symptomatic relief of perennial and seasonal allergic rhinitis, vasomotor rhinitis, allergic conjunctivitis; temporary relief of runny nose and sneezing caused by common cold; management of allergic and non-allergic pruritic symptoms, mild uncomplicated urticaria and angioedema; amelioration of allergic reactions to blood or plasma; treatment of dermatographism; adjunctive therapy in anaphylactic reactions.

Contraindications Hypersensitivity to antihistamines; newborn or premature infants; nursing mothers; narrow-angle glaucoma; stenosing peptic ulcer; symptomatic prostatic hypertrophy; asthmatic attack; bladder neck obstruction; pyloroduodenal obstruction; MAO therapy.

Route/Dosage

ADULTS & CHILDREN ≥ 12 YR: **PO** 2.5 mg q 4-6 hr (maximum 10 mg/24 hr). CHILDREN 6-12 YR: **PO** 1.25 mg q 4-6 hr (maximum 5 mg/24 hr). CHILDREN < 6 YR: Consult physician. Do not exceed 4 doses in 24 hr.

Interactions

Alcohol, CNS depressants (eg, narcotics, sedatives): Additive CNS depression possible. MAO *inhibitors*: Anticholinergic effects may increase.

Lab Test Interferences

In skin testing procedures, may prevent or diminish otherwise positive reaction to dermal reactivity indicators.

Adverse Reactions

CV: Orthstatic hypotension; palpitations; tachycardia; faintness. *RESP*: Thickening of bronchial secretions. *CNS*: Drowsiness (often transient); sedation; dizziness; faintness; disturbed coordination; excitation. *EENT:* Blurred vision; nasal stuffiness; dry mouth, nose and throat; sore throat. *GI:* Epigastric distress; nausea; vomiting; diarrhea; constipation; change in bowel habits. *META:* Increased appetite, weight gain. *OTHER:* Hypersensitivity reactions; photosensitivity.

Precautions

Pregnancy: Category C. *Lactation:* Undetermined. *Children:* Overdosage may cause hallucinations, convulsions and death. Antihistamines may diminish mental alertness. In young child, may produce paradoxical excitation. *Elderly patients:* Greater likelihood of dizziness, excessive sedation, syncope, toxic confusional states and hypotension in patients > 60 yr. Dosage reduction may be required. *Special risk patients:* Use drug with caution in patients with predisposition to urinary retention, history of bronchial asthma, increased intraocular pressure, hyperthyroidism, sleep apnea, cardiovascular disease or hypertension. *Respiratory disease:* Generally not recommended to treat lower respiratory tract symptoms including asthma.

NURSING CONSIDERATIONS

Administration/Storage

- Give with food.
- Store tablets and oral solution at room temperature in a tight, light-resistant container. Do not freeze oral solution.

Assessment/Interventions

- Obtain patient history, including drug history and any known allergies.
- Monitor for potential neurologic side effects especially in elderly and young.
- Obtain CBC if signs of blood dyscrasias are noted.
- Assess LFT results and BUN and serum creatinine as indicated.

OVERDOSAGE: SIGNS & SYMPTOMS

CNS depression, CNS stimulation, hypotension, respiratory depression, coma, seizures

Patient/Family Education

- Explain potential side effects and adverse reactions, and identify problems that should be reported to physician.
- Tell patient not to take within 4 days before skin testing procedures.
- Advise patient to take sips of water frequently, suck on ice chips or sugarless hard candy or chew sugarless chewing gum if dry mouth occurs.
- Instruct patient to avoid alcohol and other CNS depressants.
- Advise patient that drug may cause drowsiness or dizziness and to use caution while driving or performing other tasks requiring mental alertness.

See Patient Guide, p. 626.

Tuberculin, Purified Protein Derivative (PPD)

(too-BURR-kyoo-lin)

Tuberculin PPD Multiple Puncture Device

Aplitest, Tine Test PPD

Tuberculin Purified Protein Derivative

Aplisol, Tubersol

Class: Diagnostic skin test

Action Contains soluble products from mycobacterium, which react with lymphocytes to release mediators of cellular hypersensitivity. Some of these mediators induce inflammatory response. Positive reaction is consistent with previous or current tuberculosis infection or previous BCG vaccination.

Indications Detection of delayed hypersensitivity to *Mycobacterium tuberculosis;* aid in diagnosis of infection with *M. tuberculosis;* routine testing for tuberculosis; testing individuals suspected of having contact with active tuberculosis; follow-up verification testing in individuals who have had reactions to tuberculin multipuncture devices used as screening test.

Contraindications Persons known to be tuberculin-positive reactors.

Route/Dosage
ADULTS & CHILDREN: **Intradermal** 0.1 ml of 5 TU/0.1 ml concentration (Mantoux test) or multiple puncture device. HIGHLY SENSITIZED PERSONS: **Intradermal** 0.1 ml of 1 TU/0.1 ml concentration. INDIVIDUALS WHO FAIL TO REACT TO PREVIOUS INJECTION OF 5 TU: **Intradermal** 0.1 ml of 250 TU/0.1 ml concentration.

Routine Tuberculin Screening
CHILDREN: Perform at 12 mo, 4-6 yr and 14-16 yr.

Interactions
BCG vaccine, previous: May result in positive PPD test (see Precautions). *Corticosteroids or other immunosuppressive drugs:* May suppress reactivity to any tuberculin test. *Recent immunization with live virus vaccines (including influenza, measles, mumps, rubella, polio virus, smallpox, yellow fever):* May suppress reactivity to any tuberculin test. If tuberculin skin testing is indicated, perform it either before or simultaneous with immunization or 4 to 6 wk after immunization.

Lab Test Interferences
None well documented.

Adverse Reactions
DERM: Immediate erythematous reactions, vesiculation, pain, ulceration, necrosis or scarring at administration site; bleeding at puncture site (tine test).

Precautions
Pregnancy: Category C. Use if needed. Unrecognized tuberculosis places infant in grave danger of tuberculosis and tuberculous meningitis. No adverse effects on fetus from tuberculin have been reported. *Lactation:* Undetermined. *Children:* A child who has been exposed to tuberculosis must not be judged free of infection until there is negative tuberculin reaction at least 10 wk after ending contact with tuberculous person. *Elderly patients:* Skin-test responsiveness may be delayed or reduced in magnitude among older persons. Two-step testing is especially important in persons ≥ 35 yr. Reactions may peak after 72 hr. *BCG vaccine:* Persons previously immunized with BCG vaccine may test positive to tuberculin skin test. Tuberculin reactions caused by BCG cannot reliably be distinguished from reactions caused by natural mycobacterial infections. Tuberculin reactivity in BCG vaccinees does not reliably predict protection against *M. tuberculosis*. *Bioequivalency:* The various PPD solutions are generically equivalent but differ from PPD multipuncture devices and from old tuberculin (OT) products. *Immunodeficiency:* Skin-test responsiveness may be suppressed during or for as much as 6 wk after viral infection, live viral vaccination, miliary or pulmonary tuberculosis infection, bacterial infection, severe febrile illness, malnutrition, sarcoidosis, malignancy or immunosuppression (eg, corticosteroids or other immunosuppressive pharmacotherapy). In most patients who are very sick with tuberculosis, a previously negative tuberculin test becomes positive after a few weeks of chemotherapy. *Interpretation of test results:* Positive PPD reaction indicates hypersensitivity to tuberculin and implies past or present infection with *M. tuberculosis*. Positive reactions do not necessarily signify active disease. Further diagnostic procedures (eg, chest radiograph, microbiological examination of sputum) must be conducted before a

diagnosis of tuberculosis can be made. *Multipuncture devices:* Multipuncture devices are screening tools that aid in determining tuberculin hypersensitivity. They may contain either PPD or OT. These devices are comparable to 5 TU of PPD but may yield false-positive reactions because quantity of tuberculin deposited into skin cannot be precisely controlled. Positive reactions to multipuncture devices must be confirmed with intradermal injection of PPD solution. OT cross-reacts with other mycobacteria (eg, *Mycobacterium avium*). Multipuncture devices are useful in persons who object to use of needle and syringe (eg, children). *Repeated testing of uninfected individuals:* Does not sensitize to tuberculin.

NURSING CONSIDERATIONS

Administration/Storage

- Cleanse site with 70% isopropyl alcohol, acetone, ether or soap and water and allow to dry before test injection.
- Avoid areas with rash, hairy areas, scars, pimples, moles and other marks.
- Use fresh solution for injection.
- For intradermal injection, use 26- or 27-gauge ½-inch needle to administer intradermal injection into flexor or dorsal surface of forearm, creating white bleb 6-10 mm in diameter. No dressing is required.
- For multiple puncture device, apply unit firmly and without twisting to volar surface of upper ⅓ of forearm for 1 sec. Make sure all four tines penetrate skin.
- If performing retest, perform on opposite forearm.
- Do not use 250 TU/0.1 ml concentration for initial testing.
- PPD multi-puncture devices should be stored at room temperature.
- PPD solution should be stored in refrigerator.

Assessment/Interventions

- Obtain patient history, including prior PPD test results, BCG vaccination, drug history and any known allergies. Individuals who may have received BCG vaccination will likely exhibit false-positive reactions.
- Assess appropriate timing of testing; viral febrile illnesses, liver virus vaccination, malnutrition or immunosuppression may suppress results. Tuberculin skin testing cannot be performed until 4-6 wk after immunization with live virus vaccines.
- Obtain history of exposure to tuberculous persons prior to skin testing.
- Assess for hypersensitivity, especially in patients with high risk of disease. Have epinephrine readily available.
- Assess ability of patient to accurately read test results.
- Interpret results 48-72 hr after administration. Delayed hypersensitivity reactions begin within 5-6 hr and peak after 48-72 hr. Reactions in elderly persons and those never before tested may peak sometime after 72 hr.
- Measure induration along transverse diameter at right angle to long axis of forearm.
- Detect induration by gently palpating double skinfold between thumb and forefinger, starting in normal area around test site and moving toward test site until thickened area is felt. Consider only induration in interpreting test. If erythema > 10 mm in diameter occurs without induration, injection may have been made too deeply; retest patient.

Interpretation

- Induration < 5 mm in diameter are classified as negative. This indicates lack of hypersensitivity to tuberculin and implies that tuberculous infection is highly unlikely.
- Reactions to PPD with induration ≥ 5 mm diameter are classified as positive in (1) persons with HIV infection or risk factors for HIV infection (including IV drug use) whose HIV status is

unknown, (2) persons with close recent contact with infectious tuberculosis cases and (3) persons with chest radiographs consistent with old healed tuberculosis.

- Induration ≥ 10 mm diameter are classified as positive in (1) foreign-born persons from high-prevalence countries in Asia, Africa or Latin America; (2) HIV-negative IV drug users; (3) medically underserved low-income populations (eg, high-risk racial or ethnic minority populations); (4) residents of long-term care facilities (eg, correctional institutions, nursing homes, institutions for disabled persons); (5) persons with conditions that increase risk of tuberculosis (eg, silicosis, gastrectomy, jejunoileal bypass, body weight ≥ 10% below ideal weight, chronic renal failure, diabetes mellitus, immunosuppressive therapy, leukemias, lymphomas, or other malignancies); (6) other high-risk populations defined locally.
- Induration ≥ 15 mm diameter are classified as positive in all other persons not listed above, especially in persons > 35 yr.
- Reactions to either OT or PPD multipuncture devices with induration ≥ 2 mm in diameter or presence of any vesiculation at application site are classified as positive. Positive response indicates hypersensitivity to tuberculin and implies past or present infection with *M. tuberculosis*. Retesting with PPD solution is necessary in patients who exhibit positive responses (any size induration) to multipuncture devices.
- If patient is BCG positive, use alternative measurement for accuracy of results.
- Apply cold packs or topical corticosteroid preparations to administration site for symptomatic relief of associated pain, pruritus and discomfort.
- If patient is considered at risk for immunodeficiency, PPD should be applied with other skin tests (eg, mumps, candida) to evaluate cell-mediated immunity. Skin tests should be at least 5-10 cm apart.

OVERDOSAGE: SIGNS & SYMPTOMS
Vesiculation, ulceration, necrosis

Patient/Family Education

- Inform patient to return in 48-72 hr for test interpretation or explain how to interpret skin results. Provide card for interpretation.
- Advise patient of significance of test results and stress importance of reporting results.
- If test results are positive, provide information on where patient can obtain further evaluation.

No patient monograph available.

Uracil Mustard

(YOU-ruh-sill mustard)

Available as generic only

Class: Antineoplastic/alkylating

Action Acts as polyfunctional alkylating agent to interfere with DNA replication and transcription of RNA, resulting in disruption of nucleic acid synthesis.

Indications Palliative treatment of symptomatic chronic lymphocytic leukemia, histiocytic or lymphocytic type non-Hodgkin's lymphoma, chronic myelogenous leukemia, early stages of polycythemia vera and mycosis fungoides.

Contraindications Severe leukopenia or thrombocytopenia.

Route/Dosage
ADULTS: **PO** Single weekly dose of 0.15 mg/kg for 4 wk. CHILDREN: **PO** Single weekly dose of 0.3 mg/kg for 4 wk. If response occurs, continue same weekly dose until relapse.

Interactions None well documented.

Lab Test Interferences
None well documented.

Adverse Reactions
CNS: Nervousness; irritability; depression. *GI:* Nausea; vomiting, diarrhea (all dose related). *HEMA:* Dose-related bone marrow depression; leukopenia; thrombocytopenia; anemia. *DERM:* Pruritus; dermatitis; hair loss. *OTHER:* Amenorrhea; azoospermia.

Precautions
Pregnancy: Pregnancy category undetermined. If possible, avoid use. *Lactation:* Undetermined. *Fertility impairment:* May cause amenorrhea and impaired spermatogenesis. *Hematologic effects:* Bone marrow suppression is cumulative and may be delayed. Monitor blood counts, including platelets once or twice weekly. *Malignant infiltration of bone marrow.* Use with caution. *Previous radiation or cytotoxic drug therapy.* Do not administer uracil until 2-3 wk after maximum effect of previous treatment has been obtained. *Tartrazine sensitivity:* This product contains tartrazine, which may induce allergic reactions (eg, bronchial asthma) in susceptible people. Higher risk is associated with prior aspirin hypersensitivity.

NURSING CONSIDERATIONS

Administration/Storage

- Give by mouth only.
- Administer at bedtime to minimize GI side effects.
- Give antacid and antiemetic 30 min before drug administration.
- Store at room temperature in tight container.

Assessment/Interventions

- Obtain patient history, including drug history and any known allergies.
- Calculate cumulative dosage each administration, and document in medical record.
- Administer biologic agents (G-CSF, GM-CSF, EPO) if ordered.
- Monitor CBC and differential prior to drug administration and prior to each dose.
- Monitor liver function tests monthly.
- Withhold drug and notify physician if persistent and severe thrombocytopenia, anemia or leukopenia occurs.
- Assess for nausea or vomiting after each dose, and monitor for signs of dehydration related to vomiting.
- Note changes in neurologic status (increased nervousness, irritability or depression).
- Assess for pruritus or dermatitis.
- Assess patient for evidence of infection and unusual bleeding.
- Monitor need for and efficacy of antiemetics if given.
- Rehydrate with IV fluids if vomiting is excessive.

OVERDOSAGE: SIGNS & SYMPTOMS

Hemorrhage, severe leukopenia, severe thrombocytopenia, severe nausea, severe vomiting, severe diarrhea

Patient/Family Education

- Caution patients that pregnancy should be avoided. Advise use of reliable form of birth control during therapy for both men and women.
- Explain neutropenic precautions.
- Instruct patient to avoid foods with citric acid, hot foods, and foods with rough texture.
- Advise patient to avoid use of razors and to use soft toothbrushes.
- Inform patient of need to maintain hydration, especially if vomiting.
- Provide information on skin care if pruritus is present.
- Teach patient signs and symptoms of thrombocytopenia and anemia: fatigue, faintness.
- Inform patient that hair loss is side effect of medication.

- Instruct patient to report these symptoms to physician immediately: fever, sore throat or other signs of infection, unusual bleeding or bruising, lethargy, or excessive vomiting.
- Instruct patient not to take otc medications without consulting physician.

See Patient Guide, p. 627.

Urokinase

(YUR-oh-KIN-ace)

Abbokinase, Abbokinase Open-Cath

Class: Thrombolytic enzyme

Action Converts plasminogen to plasmin, which then degrades fibrin clots and fibrinogen.

Indications Management/dissolution of pulmonary emboli, coronary artery thrombosis; IV catheter clearance.

Contraindications Active internal bleeding; recent (within 2 months) cerebrovascular accident; intracranial or intraspinal surgery; intracranial neoplasm.

Route/Dosage

Pulmonary Embolus

ADULTS: **IV** Priming dose of 4400 units/kg over 10 min, followed by continuous infusion of 4400 units/kg/hr for 12 hrs.

Lysis of Coronary Artery Thrombi

ADULTS: **IV** 4 ml/min (6000 units/min) for up to 2 hours; administer bolus dose of heparin prior to using urokinase.

IV Catheter Clearance

ADULTS: Inject 5000 U/ml solution, equal to volume of catheter, into occluded catheter. Attempt aspiration q 5 min. If unopened after 30 min, cap catheter, wait 30-60 min and attempt aspiration. If unsuccessful, a second injection can be used.

Interactions *Anticoagulants, antiplatelet agents:* Bleeding complications may occur.

Lab Test Interferences None well documented.

Adverse Reactions *CV:* Bleeding. *OTHER:* Allergic reactions (eg, bronchospasm, skin rash); fever.

Precautions *Pregnancy:* Category B. *Lactation:* Undetermined. *Children:* Safety and efficacy not established. *Arrhythmias:* Rapid lysis of coronary thrombi may cause atrial or ventricular dysrhythmias. *Bleeding:* Can be either superficial (surface) bleeding or internal bleeding. Minor bleeding occurs often; several fatalities because of cerebral and other serious internal hemorrhages have occurred. *High risk patients:* Recent (within 10 days) major surgery or puncture of noncompressible blood vessel, obstetrical delivery, organ biopsy or serious GI bleeding; recent trauma including CPR; severe uncontrolled arterial hypertension; subacute bacterial endocarditis; hemostatic defects; pregnancy; age > 75 yr; cerebrovascular disease; diabetic hemorrhagic retinopathy; septic thrombophlebitis; other conditions in which bleeding may be hazardous. *IV catheter clearance:* Drug is not effective if catheter is occluded by substances other than fibrin clots.

NURSING CONSIDERATIONS

Administration/Storage

- Do not give via IM injection.
- Refrigerate vials of powder for injection. Store powder for solution at room temperature.
- Reconstitute powder for injection with Sterile Water for Injection.
- Further dilute powder for injection with 0.9% Sodium Chloride or D5W to prepare IV infusion solution. Do

not use Bacteriostatic Water for Injection.
- Do not shake during reconstitution. Roll or tilt vial to enhance reconstitution.
- Filter through 0.45 micron or smaller cellulose membrane filter, as indicated.
- Do not add other medications to solution.
- Use immediately after reconstitution, and discard unused portion.
- Reconstituted catheter-clearing solution is stable for 24 hours at room temperature or under refrigeration.
- Administer with infusion control device. Use infusion pump for IV administration.

Assessment/Interventions
- Obtain patient history, including drug history and any known allergies.
- Before therapy, determine hematocrit, platelet count, thrombin time (TT), activated partial thromboplastin time (APTT), prothrombin time (PT), and fibrinogen levels. TT or APTT should be less than twice the normal control value before therapy.
- Determine TT, PT, APTT or fibrinogen level 4 hr after starting infusion.
- Limit blood drawing as much as possible. Do not perform arterial puncture.
- During IV infusion, monitor vital signs q 4 hr.
- Do not take BP in lower extremities.
- Do not implement invasive procedures during infusion.
- Do not give with heparin.
- Monitor for allergic reactions (fever, bronchospasm, skin rash).
- Monitor for signs of internal or frank bleeding. Access mucous membranes, urine and feces for blood.
- Monitor vital signs q 4 hours.
- Check urine, stools and body secretions for occult blood.
- Assess skin for ecchymosis, edema, itching, rash and bruising.
- Report chest pain to physician.
- Control minor bleeding with pressure for 30 minutes; then apply pressure dressing; do not reduce dose.
- With uncontrollable bleeding, discontinue infusion.

OVERDOSAGE: SIGNS & SYMPTOMS
Bleeding, hypotension

Patient/Family Education
- Explain symptoms of internal and external bleeding.
- Teach application of pressure dressing for minor external bleeding.

No patient monograph available.

Valacyclovir Hydrochloride

(val-lay-SIGH-kloe-vihr HIGH-droe-KLOR-ide)

Valtrex

Class: Anti-infective/antiviral

Action Converted to acyclovir, which then inhibits viral DNA replication by interfering with viral DNA polymerase.

Indications Treatment of herpes zoster (shingles) in immunocompetent adults.

Contraindications Hypersensitivity or intolerance to valacyclovir, acyclovir or any component of the formulation.

Route/Dosage
ADULTS: **PO** 1 g tid for 7 days (initiate therapy within 48 hours of onset of rash).

Interactions
Cimetidine, probenecid: Increased acyclovir serum concentrations.

Lab Test Interferences
None well documented.

Adverse Reactions *CNS*: Headache; dizziness. *GI*: Nausea; vomiting; diarrhea; constipation; abdominal pain; anorexia. *OTHER*: Asthenia.

Precautions *Pregnancy:* Category B. *Lactation:* Undetermined (acyclovir is excreted in breast milk). *Children:* Safety and efficacy not established. *Elderly:* Dosage reduction may be necessary, depending on underlying renal status. *Renal impairment:* Dosage reduction may be necessary; exercise caution when giving valacyclovir to patients with renal impairment or those receiving potentially nephrotoxic drugs. *Immunocompromised:* Valacyclovir is not indicated for use in immunocompromised patients.

NURSING CONSIDERATIONS

Administration/Storage

- May be taken without regard to meals.
- Store at room temperature.

Assessment/Interventions

- Obtain patient history.
- Assess for history of present illness and time of rash onset. Should be started no later than 72 hours after rash onset.
- Monitor for effectiveness of treatment: crusting and disappearance of hepatic lesions; pain relief.

OVERDOSAGE: SIGNS & SYMPTOMS
Acute renal failure, anuria

Patient/Family Education

- Advise patient to initiate treatment as soon as possible after diagnosis of herpes zoster and no later than 72 hr after onset of zoster rash.
- Instruct patient to take medication exactly as prescribed.
- Instruct patient not to alter dose or discontinue medication without consulting healthcare provider.
- Instruct patient not to take any other medications, including over-the-counter medications, without checking with healthcare provider first.
- Instruct patient to notify healthcare provider if there is no reduction in severity of lesions within 7 days.
- Inform patient to report any serious side effects to healthcare provider, including: syncope, dizziness, nausea, vomiting, diarrhea, headache, abdominal pain and anorexia.

See Patient Guide, p. 628.

Valproic Acid and Derivatives (Sodium valproate, Divalproex sodium)

(VAL-pro-ik acid)

Sodium Valproate
Depakene

Divalproex Sodium
Depakote

Class: Anticonvulsant

Action Believed to work by increasing brain levels of GABA. It may also inhibit catabolism of GABA, potentiate postsynaptic GABA responses and affect potassium channels or directly stabilize membranes.

Indications Sole and adjunctive therapy in simple (petit mal) and complex absence seizures. Adjunctive therapy in multiple seizure types including absence seizures. Divalproex sodium is used for manic episodes associated with bipolar disorder. **Unlabeled uses:** Treatment of atypical absence, myoclonic and tonic-clonic (grand mal) seizures and atonic, complex partial, elementary partial and infantile spasm seizures; prevention of recurrent pediatric febrile seizures; intractable status epilepticus in patients who have not responded to other therapies; treatment of minor incontinence after ileoanal anastomosis (subchronic administration); migraine prophylaxis; management of anxiety disorders and panic attacks.

Contraindications Hepatic disease or significant hepatic dysfunction.

Route/Dosage

Epilepsy

ADULTS & CHILDREN: **PO** 15 mg/kg/day in divided doses if total dose > 250 mg/day; increase at 1 wk intervals by 5-10 mg/kg/day until seizures are controlled; side effects preclude further increases or a maximum dose of 60 mg/kg/day. Titrate and individualize based on outcomes or side effects.

Mania (Divalproex Sodium)

ADULTS: **PO** 750 mg/day in divided doses. Increase as rapidly as possible to achieve the lowest therapeutic dose that produces the desired clinical effect. Maximum dosage 60 mg/kg/day.

Interactions

Alcohol, CNS depressants: Enhanced CNS depression. *Barbiturates:* May increase barbiturate levels and actions. *Carbamazepine, hydantoins:* May result in increased levels of these drugs and reduced efficacy of valproic acid. *Charcoal:* May reduce absorption of valproic acid. *Chlorpromazines, cimetidine, salicylates:* May increase valproic acid levels. *Felbamate:* Increased valproic acid levels. *Lamotrigine:* Decreased valproic acid levels; increased lamotrigine levels. *Zidovudine:* Increased AUC of valproic acid.

Lab Test Interferences

Valproic acid may yield false-positive results on urine ketone tests; altered thyroid function tests.

Adverse Reactions

CNS: Sedation; tremor; ataxia; headache; dysarthria; emotional upset; depression; dizziness; coma; psychosis; aggression; hyperactivity; behavioral deterioration; incoordination. *EENT:* Nystagmus; diplopia; asterixis; "spots before eyes." *GI:* Nausea; vomiting; indigestion; diarrhea; abdominal cramps; constipation; anorexia with weight loss; increased appetite with weight gain. *GU:* Irregular menses; enuresis; secondary amenorrhea. *HEMA:* Reduced platelet aggregation; hematoma formation; macrocytosis; acute intermittent porphyria; altered bleeding time; thrombocytopenia; bruising; hemorrhage; lymphocytosis; hypofibrinogenemia; leukopenia; eosinophilia; anemia; bone marrow suppression or toxicity (suggestive of myelodysplastic syndrome). *HEPA:* Minor elevations of AST, ALT and LDH; increase in serum bilirubin; abnormal liver function test results; severe hepatotoxicity and possibly death. *DERM:* Transient hair loss; skin rash; petechiae; erythema multiforme; photosensitivity; generalized pruritus; Stevens-Johnson syndrome. *META:* Abnormal thyroid function test results; hyponatremia; inappropriate ADH secretion; Fanconi's syndrome; hypocarnitinaemia; parotid gland swelling; breast enlargement; galactorrhea; hyperammonemia; hyperglycemia. *OTHER:* Extremity edema; weakness; acute pancreatitis; lupus erythematosus; fever.

Mania: *Body as a whole:* Chest pain; chills; chills with fever; cyst; fever; infection; neck pain; neck rigidity. *Cardiovascular:* Hypertension; hypotension; palpitations; posturual hypotension; tachycardia; vascular anomaly; vasodilation. *CNS:* Abnormal dreams; abnormal gait; agitation; ataxia; catatonic reaction; confusion; depression; somnolence; diplopia; dysarthria; hallucinations; hypertonia; hypokinesia; thinking abnormalities; vertigo; insomnia; paresthesia; reflexes increased; tardive dyskinesia. *DERM:* Alopecia; discoid lupus erythematosis; dry skin; furunculosis; maculopapular rash; seborrhea. *GI:* Anorexia; fecal incontinence; flatulence; gastroenteritis; glossitis; periodontal abcess. *GU:* Dysmenorhea; dysuria; urinary incontinence. *HEMA:* Ecchymosis. *META:* Edema; peripheral edema; *Musculoskeletal:* Arthralgia; arthrosis; leg cramps; twitching. *RESP:*

Dyspnea; rhinitis. *Special senses:* Abnormal vision; amblyopia; conjunctivitis; deafness; dry eyes; ear disorder; ear pain; eye pain; tinnitus; accidental injury.

Precautions

Pregnancy: Category D. Risk of neural tube defects may be increased during first trimester. *Lactation:* Excreted in breast milk. *Children:* In children < 2 yr, use drug with extreme caution. This patient group is at considerably increased risk of developing fatal hepatotoxicity. Safety and efficacy of divalproex sodium for treatment of acute mania have not been studied in patients <18 years of age. Safety and efficacy of long-term use (> 3 weeks) have not been systematically evaluated. If used for extended period, continually reevaluate the drug's usefulness. Younger children, especially if receiving enzyme-inducing drugs, will require larger maintenance doses to reach targeted drug concentrations. *Elderly:* Reduce starting dose and base therapeutic dose on clinical response. *Bioavailability:* Bioavailability problems may occur when converting to generic forms. *Concurrent anticonvulsant use:* Valproic acid may interact with other anticonvulsant medications. *GI irritation:* Sustained release divalproex sodium may be less irritating to GI system than valproic acid. *Hematologic effects:* Drug may cause bleeding disorders. *Hepatotoxicity:* Hepatic failure resulting in fatalities has occurred. Reactions usually occur within first 6 mo of therapy preceded by symptoms such as lost seizure control, malaise, weakness, lethargy, facial edema, anorexia, jaundice and vomiting. Use drug with caution in patients with prior history of liver disease. Monitor results of LFTs frequently. *Hyperammonemia:* May occur with or without lethargy and coma and may contribute to hepatotoxicity. *Dose-related adverse reactions:* Frequency of adverse reactions (particularly elevated liver enzymes, thrombocytopenia) may be dose-related. *Mania:* Clinical data from long-term studies are not available.

NURSING CONSIDERATIONS

Administration/Storage

- Administer orally with food if GI upset occurs.
- Instruct patient to swallow tablets or capsules whole and not to chew or crush them.
- Give once a day at bedtime to reduce effects of CNS depression.
- For sprinkle capsule administration, have patient swallow whole or sprinkle on 1 teaspoon of semisolid food (eg, applesauce) and have patient swallow immediately without chewing. Discard unused portion.
- Do not administer oral syrup in carbonated drinks (unpleasant taste, local irritation results).
- Store at room temperature in tight container. Do not freeze syrup.

Assessment/Interventions

- Obtain patient history, including drug history and any known allergies. Note sensitivity to anticonvulsant drugs and history of seizures.
- Observe for development of side effects (eg, GI intolerance, CNS changes, abnormal bleeding or bruising, hair loss).
- Determine platelet counts and bleeding times before therapy, periodically during therapy and before surgery.
- Immediately notify physician of symptoms of hepatotoxicity: lethargy, coma, jaundice.
- Report symptoms of bleeding disorders or abnormal platelet count or bleeding times to physician. Dosage reduction or withdrawal of therapy may be required.
- When drug is administered concomitantly with other anticonvulsant medication, determine drug serum levels before therapy and periodically during treatment.
- Perform LFTs prior to therapy and at

frequent intervals thereafter, especially during first 6 mo of therapy.
- Monitor BP, pulse and respirations.
- Maintain adequate fluid intake.

OVERDOSAGE: SIGNS & SYMPTOMS

Motor restlessness, somnolence, heart block, visual hallucinations, asterixis, deep coma, death

Patient/Family Education
- Advise patient to take with food if GI upset occurs.
- Instruct patient to take once-a-day dose at bedtime to reduce CNS depression.
- Advise patient not to chew tablets or capsules but to swallow them whole.
- When patient has been prescribed sprinkle capsules, inform patient that capsules may be swallowed whole or sprinkled on 1 teaspoon of semisolid food and swallowed immediately without chewing. Instruct patient to discard unused portion.
- Advise patient to carry identification (Medi-Alert) indicating condition and medication regimen.
- Caution patient to avoid intake of alcoholic beverages and other CNS depressants.
- Inform diabetic patient that drug may cause false-positive results for urine ketones.
- Instruct patient not to take otc or prescription medications, especially those containing aspirin, without consulting physician.
- Instruct patient to report these symptoms to physician: unusual bruising or bleeding, skin eruptions, jaundice, lethargy, nausea, vomiting and diarrhea.
- Advise patient that drug may cause drowsiness and to use caution while driving or performing other tasks requiring mental alertness.

See Patient Guide, p. 629.

Vancomycin

(van-koe-MY-sin)

Lyphocin, Vancocin, Vancoled
Class: Anti-infective/antibiotic

Action Inhibits bacterial cell-wall synthesis and alters cell-membrane permeability and RNA synthesis.

Indications
Parenteral: Treatment of serious or severe infections due to susceptible bacteria not treatable with other antimicrobials (eg, staphylococcus). *Oral:* Treatment of pseudomembranous colitis caused by *Clostriduim difficile*; treatment of staphylococcal enterocolitis. **Unlabeled use:** IV prophylaxis against bacterial endocarditis in penicillin-allergic patients.

Contraindications Standard considerations.

Route/Dosage
ADULTS: **PO** 500 mg-2 g/day in 3 or 4 divided doses for 7-10 days. CHILDREN: **PO** 40 mg/kg/day (up to 2 gm/day) in 3 or 4 divided doses for 7-10 days. NEONATES: **PO** 10 mg/kg/day in divided doses. ADULTS: **IV** 500 mg by IV infusion q 6 hr or 1 g q 12 hr. CHILDREN: **IV** 10 mg/kg/dose q 6 hr. INFANTS & NEONATES: **IV** 15 mg/kg initially, followed by 10 mg/kg q 12 hr for neonates in first week of life, and q 8 hr for ages up to 1 month.

Interactions
Aminoglycosides: May increase risk of nephrotoxicity. *Neurotoxic and nephrotoxic agents:* May give additive toxicity. *Nondepolarizing muscle relaxants:* Neuromuscular blockade may be enhanced. INCOMPATIBILITIES: IV solution is incompatible with alkaline injections.

Lab Test Interferences
None well documented.

Adverse Reactions
CV: Hypotension. *RESP:*

Wheezing; dyspnea. *EENT:* Hearing loss. *GI:* Nausea. *GU:* Increased serum creatinine and BUN; renal failure. *HEMA:* Neutropenia; eosinophilia. *DERM:* Rash; urticaria; pruritus; inflammation at site of injection. *OTHER:* Anaphylaxis; drug fever; chills; Red Man Syndrome (hypotension with or without rash over face, neck, upper chest and extremities).

Precautions

Pregnancy: Category C. *Lactation:* Excreted in breast milk. *Children:* Confirming serum levels may be appropriate in neonates. Use of vancomycin with anesthetics may cause erythema and flushing. *Special risk patients:* Use with caution in patients with pre-existing hearing loss, patients receiving ototoxic or nephrotoxic drugs, patients receiving drugs that cause neutropenia; patients with renal impairment; elderly; and neonates. *Hypotension:* Too rapid IV infusion or bolus administration may be associated with exaggerated hypotension, including shock and cardiac arrest, with or without maculopapular rash over face, neck, upper chest and extremities (Red Man or Redneck syndrome). Reaction has been rarely associated with slow infusion or oral or intraperitoneal administration. *Reversible neutropenia:* May occur after total dose of 25 g. *Tissue irritation, thrombophlebitis:* Give by secure IV route. May minimize thrombophlebitis by giving slowly as dilute infusion.

NURSING CONSIDERATIONS

Administration/Storage

- Prepare oral solution by adding 115 ml of water to 10 gm vial or 20 ml of water to 1 gm vial. Further dilute prepared oral solution dose with 30 ml of water or flavoring syrups may be used with oral solution.
- May give oral solution via nasogastric tube as indicated or ordered.
- Reconstitute parenteral form with Sterile Water for Injection.
- Further dilute parenteral medication with compatible solution, eg, 5% Dextrose Injection, 0.9% Sodium Chloride, Lactated Ringer's.
- Parenteral form may be administered by oral route.
- Reconstituted oral solution may be stored in refrigerator for 2 wk after bottle is opened.
- Dilute to minimum dilution of 2.5-5 mg/ml and infuse parenteral solution over at least 60 min. Intermittent infusion preferred.
- Pretreat with antihistamine if patient has previously experienced Red Man Syndrome.
- Dosage or dosage interval may be changed based upon vancomycin serum levels.
- Reconstituted powder for injection is stable at room temperature for 2 wk.
- Dilute solutions (sodium chloride or D5W) are stable at room temperature for 24 hr.

Assessment/Interventions

- Obtain patient history, including drug history and any known allergies.
- Assess results of culture and sensitivity to determine sensitivity.
- Assess hearing acuity before and after therapy. Anticipate ototoxicity.
- Monitor for signs of superinfection.
- Monitor skin for Red Man Syndrome with each dose infused.
- Notify physician of elevated BUN and creatinine, which indicate nephrotoxicity.
- Document hematuria and notify physician.
- Monitor I&O, BP for hypotension and respirations for wheezing or dyspnea.
- Maintain adequate fluid intake.
- Obtain blood levels, new order or protocol. Keep blood levels between 10-20 mcg/ml.
- Ensure that resuscitation equipment is available.

OVERDOSAGE: SIGNS & SYMPTOMS

Increase serum creatinine, increase BUN, hearing loss, ringing in ears, vertigo

Patient/Family Education

- Explain that IV medication is given at regular intervals to maintain blood levels.
- Tell patient to report hearing loss, ringing in ears or vertigo to physician.
- Explain signs of superinfection, eg, vaginitis.
- Identify symptoms of potential adverse reactions.
- Tell patient to maintain adequate fluid intake.

See Patient Guide, pp. 630-631.

Vasopressin (8-Arginine-Vasopressin)

(VAY-so-PRESS-in)

Pitressin Synthetic, ♣ *Pressyn*

Class: Posterior pituitary hormone

Action Promotes resorption of water through kidney. At high doses, stimulates contraction of smooth muscle causing vasoconstriction, increased peri-staltic activity and gallbladder contractions.

Indications Treatment of neurogenic diabetes insipidus; prevention and treatment of postoperative abdominal distention; facilitation of abdominal roentgenography. **Unlabeled use:** Treatment of bleeding esophageal varices.

Contraindications Standard considerations.

Route/Dosage

Diabetes Insipidus

ADULTS & CHILDREN: **IM/SC** 2.5-10 units 2-4 times daily as needed.

Abdominal Distention

ADULTS: **IM** 5 units initially; subsequent injections q 3-4 hr prn. May increase the dose to 10 units if necessary.

Abdominal Roentgenography

ADULTS: **IM/SC** 2 injections of 10 units each administered 2 hr and 30 min before films are exposed.

Bleeding Esophageal Varices

ADULTS: **IV** Infuse initially at 0.2-0.4 U/min and increase to 0.9 U/min if necessary.

Interactions

Carbamazepine, chlorpropamide: May potentiate antidiuretic effect of vasopressin.

Lab Test Interferences

None well documented.

Adverse Reactions

CV: Angina. *GI:* Abdominal cramps; nausea; vomiting; gas. *OTHER:* Gangrene; ischemic colitis; tissue necrosis (with extravasation); allergic reaction (cardiac arrest, tremor, vertigo, sweating).

Precautions

Pregnancy: Category C. *Lactation:* Undetermined. *Special risk patients:* Use drug with caution in patients with epilepsy, migraine, asthma, heart failure or any condition where a rapid rise in extracellular water may result in further compromise. *Chronic nephritis with nitrogen retention:* Contraindicates use until reasonable nitrogen blood levels have been attained. *Extravasation:* Severe vasoconstriction and local tissue necrosis may result if drug extravasates during IV infusion. *Hypersensitivity:* Local or systemic reactions, including anaphylaxis, may occur. *Vascular disease:* Use extreme caution in patients with vascular disease. *Water intoxication:* May occur. Early signs include confusion, drowsiness, listlessness and headache.

NURSING CONSIDERATIONS

Administration/Storage

- Store at room temperature. Do not freeze.
- Give 1-2 glasses of water with dose to prevent skin blanching, abdominal cramps and nausea.
- If administering via IV infusion, 0.9% Normal Saline or D5W to a concentration of 0.1-1 U/ml. Insure patency of venous access and use infusion control device.

Assessment/Interventions

- Obtain patient history, including drug history and any known allergies.
- Monitor for allergic reactions, including tremor, sweating, vertigo, circumoral pallor, "pounding in head," abdominal cramps, flatus, nausea, vomiting, urticaria, bronchial constriction.
- Monitor I&O, and weigh daily.
- Monitor urine specific gravity and osmolarity.
- Monitor vital signs.
- Monitor ECG and fluid and electrolyte status at frequent intervals during prolonged therapy.
- Monitor patient for evidence of water intoxication (confusion, drowsiness, listlessness, headache). Report to physician immediately if noted.
- Monitor for therapeutic response: decreased urine output; decreased thirst.
- Assess reduction of thirst.
- In abdominal distention, assess bowel sounds and presence or absence of flatus.

OVERDOSAGE: SIGNS & SYMPTOMS

Confusion, lethargy, drowsiness, listlessness, headache

Patient/Family Education

- Tell patient to take with 1-2 glasses of water to prevent skin blanching, nausea, abdominal cramping.
- Caution patient to withhold medication and to notify physician of chest pain.
- Tell patient to report drowsiness, listlessness and headache to physician and to restrict water intake.
- Explain that urine output should decrease after use.
- Tell patient to monitor weight daily.
- Instruct patient to avoid alcohol intake during therapy.
- Remind patients with diabetes insipidus to carry appropriate medical identification.

See Patient Guide, p. 632.

Vecuronium Bromide

(veh-CUE-row-nee-uhm BROE-mide)

Norcuron

Class: Nondepolarizing neuromuscular blocker/muscle relaxant; anesthetic adjunct

Action Causes paralysis of skeletal muscles by binding competitively to cholinergic receptors on motor end-plate to antagonize action of acetylcholine, resulting in block of neuromuscular transmission.

Indications Adjunct to general anesthesia to facilitate endotracheal intubation and provide skeletal muscle relaxation during surgery or mechanical ventilation.

Contraindications Hypersensitivity to vecuronium or bromides.

Route/Dosage

ADULTS & CHILDREN > 10 YR: **IV** Initial dose: for inhalation 0.08-0.1 mg/kg. Reduce initial dose by 15% (0.06-0.85 mg/kg) if inhalation agents are already in use. If intubation is performed using succinylcholine, reduce initial dose to 0.04-0.06 mg/kg with inhalation anesthesia and 0.05-0.06 mg/kg with balanced anesthesia. Maintenance: IV bolus 0.01-0.015 mg/kg within 25-40 min of initial dose, then q 12-15 min. IV infusion: 1 mg/kg/min initially beginning 20-40 min after IV bolus. Titrate to desired clinical response. CHILDREN 1-10 YR: **IV** Slightly higher initial doses and more frequent supplementation. INFANTS 7 WK-1 YR: **IV** Slightly lower doses and 1.5 times less frequent.

Interactions

Aminoglycosides, verapamil, inhalation anesthetics (eg, enflurane, isoflurane), lincosamides (eg, clindamycin, lincomycin), magnesium salts, polypeptide antibiotics (eg, bacitracin, polymyxin B): May enhance action of vecuronium (eg, respiratory depression). *Hydantoins, carbamazepine:* May cause vecuronium to have shorter duration or decreased effectiveness. *Quinidine, quinine:* Recurrent paralysis may occur with injection of quinidine during recovery from use of other muscle relaxants. *Theophyllines:* Dose-dependent reversal of neuromuscular blockade is possible. *Thiopurines (eg, mercaptopurine):* May decrease or reverse vecuronium action. *Trimethaphan:* May cause prolonged apnea.

Lab Test Interferences

None well documented.

Adverse Reactions

RESP: Respiratory insufficiency; apnea. *OTHER:* Skeletal muscle weakness; profound and prolonged skeletal muscle paralysis.

Precautions

Pregnancy: Category C. *Lactation:* Undetermined. *Children:* Infants are moderately more sensitive and take longer to recover. Not recommended in neonates; diluent contains benzyl alcohol (fetal-gasping syndrome). *Elderly or debilitated patients:* May experience delayed onset of action. *Circulatory disease (eg, cardiovascular disease, elderly or edematous states):* May cause delayed onset of action, do not increase dosage. *Consciousness:* Vecuronium has no known effect on consciousness, pain threshold or cerebration. Administration of this drug should be accompanied by adequate anesthesia. *Electrolyte imbalance:* Neuromuscular blockade may be altered depending on nature of imbalance. *Hepatic/renal/biliary disease:* Prolonged neuromuscular blockade may occur due to reduced elimination. Higher doses may be needed due to increased volume of distribution. *Malignant hyperthermia:* Monitor patient closely. *Myasthenia gravis:* Small doses may have profound effects; administer test dose in monitoring response to muscle relaxants. *Severe obesity or neuromuscular disease:* May pose airway or ventilation problems requiring special care before, during or after vecuronium.

NURSING CONSIDERATIONS

Administration/Storage

- Administer IV only. Not for IM administration.
- Administer only if intubation, artificial respiration, oxygen and reversal agents are immediately available.
- Reconstitute with 0.9% Sodium Chloride, 5% Dextrose, 5% Dextrose in Saline, Lactated Ringer's Solution or Sterile Water for Injection.
- May reconstitute with Bacteriostatic Water for Injection. When this diluent is used, however, solution contains benzyl alcohol and is contraindicated in newborns.
- Store unopened vial at room temperature. Protect from light.
- Following reconstitution, refrigerate. Use within 8 hr.
- Intended for single use only. Discard unused portions.

Assessment/Interventions

- Obtain patient history, including drug history and any known allergies.
- In patients with myasthenia gravis, perform test dose.
- Observe for histamine-release symptoms, bronchospasm, flushing, redness, hypotension and tachycardia.

- Monitor respirations and be prepared to assist or control respiration.
- Monitor BP and pulse.
- Assess skeletal muscle tone.
- Monitor I&O.
- Check for urinary retention.
- Monitor carefully for signs of increased or decreased efficacy and pharmacologic activity (eg, muscle twitch response to peripheral nerve stimulation).

OVERDOSAGE: SIGNS & SYMPTOMS

Skeletal muscle weakness, neuromuscular block beyond time needed, hypotension, decreased respiratory reserve, low tidal volume, apnea

Patient/Family Education

- Explain to patient and family that patient will recover from anesthesia in 25-40 min.
- Inform patient and family that patient may have difficulty speaking when recovering postoperatively but that speech will improve as effects of medication wear off.
- Inform patient that postoperative urinary retention is possible.

No patient monograph available.

Venlafaxine

(VEN-luh-fax-EEN)

Effexor

Class: Antidepressant

Action Potentiates norepinephrine, serotonin and dopamine neurotransmitter activity in CNS.

Indications Treatment of depression.

Contraindications Concomitant use with MAO inhibitors.

Route/Dosage

ADULTS: **PO** 75 mg/day bid-tid; titrate to clinical effect, adding up to 75 mg/day at intervals of ≥ 4 days (maximum 375 mg/day).

Interactions

MAO inhibitors: MAO inhibitors have produced serious even fatal reactions when given concomitantly with venlafaxine. Do not use venlafaxine together with MAO inhibitors or within 14 days of MAO inhibitor use. Wait at least 7 days after stopping venlafaxine before using MAO inhibitors.

Lab Test Interferences

None well documented.

Adverse Reactions

CV: Hypertension; migraine. *RESP:* Dyspnea. *CNS:* Insomnia; somnolence; anxiety; headache; dizziness; nervousness; tremor; asthenia; abnormal dreams. *EENT:* Blurred vision. *GI:* Nausea; anorexia; dry mouth; constipation; dysphagia. *GU:* Abnormal ejaculation or orgasm; dysuria; hematuria; increased BUN; vaginitis. *HEMA:* Ecchymosis. *HEPA:* Increased LFT results and bilirubin. *META:* Peripheral edema; weight gain. *OTHER:* Sweating.

Precautions

Pregnancy: Category C. *Lactation:* Undetermined. *Children:* Safety and efficacy in patients < 18 yr not established. *Elderly patients:* Take extra care when increasing dose in elderly patients. *Special risk patients:* Use drug with caution in patients with history of seizure, mania, suicidal tendencies, drug abuse or dependence. *Hepatic or renal impairment:* Reduction of dose may be necessary. Use drug with caution. *Hypertension:* Regular monitoring of BP is recommended. Venlafaxine is associated with sustained but small increases in BP (usually associated with doses > 300 mg/day). *Discontinuation:* After 1 wk of therapy, dosage requires tapering if discontinuing; after 6 wk of treatment, taper over 2-wk period.

NURSING CONSIDERATIONS

Administration/Storage

- Administer with meals.
- Store at room temperature in tight container.

Assessment/Interventions

- Obtain patient history, including drug history and any known allergies.
- Establish baseline weight.
- Establish baseline serum cholesterol level.
- After 4-6 wk of therapy, reevaluate long-term usefulness.
- Monitor BP at least twice a week.

OVERDOSAGE: SIGNS & SYMPTOMS

Somnolence, sinus tachycardia

Patient/Family Education

- Advise patient to avoid intake of alcoholic beverages and other CNS depressants.
- Tell patient to report any rash or hives.
- Advise patient to report to physician any other prescription or otc drugs that may be taken.
- Advise patient to take sips of water frequently or to suck on ice chips, sugarless hard candy or sugarless chewing gum if dry mouth occurs.
- Instruct patient to use caution when driving or performing other tasks that require mental alertness or coordination.

See Patient Guide, p. 633.

Verapamil HCl

(veh-RAP-uh-mill HIGH-droe-KLOR-ide)

Calan, Calan SR, Isoptin, Isoptin SR, Verelan, ♣ *APO-Verap, Novo-Veramil, Nu-Verap*

Class: Calcium channel blocker

Action Inhibits movement of calcium ions across cell membrane resulting in depression of mechanical contraction of myocardial and vascular smooth muscle and depression of both impulse formation (automaticity) and conduction velocity.

Indications *Oral:* Treatment of vasospastic (Prinzmetal's variant), chronic stable (classic effort-associated) and unstable (crescendo, preinfarction) angina; adjunctive treatment with digitalis to control ventricular rate in atrial flutter or fibrillation; prophylaxis of repetitive paroxysmal supraventricular tachycardia; management of essential hypertension. Sustained release form is approved only for management of essential hypertension. *Parenteral:* Temporary control of rapid ventricular rate in atrial flutter or fibrillation. **Unlabeled uses:** Treatment of migraine and cluster headaches; treatment of hypertrophic cardiomyopathy.

Contraindications Hypersensitivity to verapamil; sick sinus syndrome or second- or third-degree atrioventricular (AV) block except with functioning pacemaker; hypotension (< 90 mm Hg systolic); severe left ventricular dysfunction; cardiogenic shock and severe CHF, unless secondary to supraventricular tachycardia amenable to verapamil; patients with atrial flutter or fibrillation and accessory bypass tract. IV verapamil should not be used concomitantly (within few hours) of IV beta-adrenergic blocking agents or in ventricular tachycardia.

Route/Dosage ADULTS: **PO** 40-160 mg tid. Do not exceed 480 mg/day. *Sustained release:* **PO** 120-480 mg daily. Lower doses are given once daily, larger doses divided into 2 doses. ADULTS: **IV** 5-10 mg bolus over 2 min. May repeat with 10 mg 30 min after first dose. Give slower (over at least 3 min) in older patients. CHILDREN 1-15 YR: **IV** 0.1 to 0.3 mg/kg (not to exceed 5 mg) over 2 min. May repeat in 30 min. CHILDREN

< 1 YR: **IV** 0.1-0.2 mg/kg (usual range 0.75-2 mg) bolus over 2 min with continuous ECG monitoring.

Interactions

Other antihypertensive agents: Additive hypotension. *Beta blockers:* May result in increased hypotension and adverse effects due to additive depressant effects on myocardial contractility or AV conduction. *Calcium salts:* Clinical effects and toxicities of verapamil may be reversed. *Carbamazepine:* Increased carbamazepine serum levels. *Cyclosporine:* Increased cyclosporine levels may result. *Digitalis glycosides:* Increased serum digoxin or digitoxin levels may occur. *Disopyramide:* Do not use 48 hr before or 24 hr after verapamil. *Flecainide:* May prolong AV conduction. *Nondepolarizing muscle relaxants:* Enhanced muscle relaxant effects and prolonged respiratory depression may occur. *Prazosin:* Increased prazosin serum levels may result. *Quinidine:* Hypotension, bradycardia, ventricular tachycardia, AV block, and pulmonary edema may occur. *Rifampin:* Loss of effectiveness of oral verapamil may occur. IV INCOMPATIBILITIES: Do not mix with sodium lactate in polyvinyl chloride bags, albumin, amphotericin B, hydralazine, aminophylline, sodium bicarbonate, nafcillin or trimethoprim-sulfamethoxazole. Do not mix in solution with pH > 6.

Lab Test Interferences

None well documented.

Adverse Reactions

CV: Peripheral edema; hypotension; AV block; bradycardia; CHF; pulmonary edema; cerebrovascular accident. *RESP:* Shortness of breath; dyspnea; wheezing. *CNS:* Dizziness; lightheadedness; headache; asthenia. *GI:* Nausea; constipation. *HEPA:* Increased transaminases; hepatitis. *DERM:* Dermatitis; rash; sweating; gingival hyperplasia.

Precautions

Pregnancy: Category C. *Lactation:* Excreted in breast milk. *Children:* Children < 6 mo may not respond to IV use. Rare severe hemodynamic side effects have occurred in neonates and infants after IV use. *Elderly:* May have greater hypotensive effects in elderly. Elderly may respond to lower doses. *Antiplatelet effects:* Calcium channel blockers may inhibit platelet function. *Cardiac conduction:* May be associated with variety of cardiac conduction abnormalities including first-, second-, or third-degree AV block; bradycardia; asystole; severe hypotension; nodal escape rhythms; PR prolongation; and ventricular tachycardia in patients with atrial flutter/fibrillation and W-P-W syndrome due to antegrade conduction. *CHF:* Use verapamil with caution in patients with congestive heart failure. *Duchenne's muscular dystrophy:* May decrease neuromuscular transmission in patients with Duchenne's muscular dystrophy and prolong recovery from neuromuscular blocking agent vecuronium. *Hepatic impairment:* Hepatic cirrhosis can significantly alter pharmacokinetics of verapamil. *Hypertrophic cardiomyopathy (IHSS):* Serious adverse effects were seen in patients with hypertrophic cardiomyopathy who received oral verapamil. *Hypotension:* Hypotension may occur during initial therapy or with dosage increases and is more likely in patients taking beta blockers. *Increased intracranial pressure:* IV verapamil has increased intracranial pressure in patients with supratentorial tumors at time of anesthesia induction. *Premature ventricular contractions (PVCs):* May occur after IV use; consider possibility with oral use. *Renal impairment:* Use caution.

NURSING CONSIDERATIONS

Administration/Storage

- Administer with milk or meals if GI upset or intolerance occurs.
- Give IV slowly over 2 min.
- Implement cardiac monitor when administering drug IV and monitor BP.
- Do not give concomitantly with IV beta-adrenergic blockers (within few hr).
- Store injection at room temperature protected from light. Avoid freezing.
- Store oral form at room temperature in tight, light-resistant container.

Assessment/Interventions

- Obtain patient history, including drug history and any known allergies.
- Report any cardiovascular changes to physician.
- Report any chest pain to physician.
- If drug is to be discontinued, aid in gradual reduction of dosage.

> **OVERDOSAGE: SIGNS & SYMPTOMS**
>
> Hypotension, bradycardia, AV block, asystole

Patient/Family Education

- Tell patient if dose is missed to take as soon as possible. If several hours have passed or if it is nearing time for next dose, tell patient not to double dose to catch up unless advised by physician.
- If more than one dose is missed, tell patient to contact physician.
- Caution patient not to change dose unless directed by physician.
- Advise patient not to suddenly stop taking medication.
- Remind patient to brush and floss teeth and see dentist regularly.
- Instruct patient to report any irregular heart beat, shortness of breath, swelling of hands and feet, pronounced dizziness, constipation, nausea or hypotension.
- Advise patient to avoid use of alcohol and otc medications without consulting physician.
- Instruct patient to limit caffeine consumption.
- Advise patient that drug may cause dizziness and to use caution while driving or performing other tasks requiring mental alertness until effects of drug have stabilized.
- Stress to patient the importance of compliance in all areas of treatment regimen: diet, exercise, stress reduction, drug therapy.

See Patient Guide, pp. 634-636.

Vinblastine Sulfate (VLB)

(vin-BLAST-een SULL-fate)

Velban, Velsar, Alkaban-AQ, ♣ *Velbe*

Class: Antineoplastic/mitotic inhibitor

Action Prevents cell division at metaphase stage by binding microtubular protein of the mitotic spindle.

Indications Palliative treatment of Hodgkin's disease, lymphocytic lymphoma, histiocytic lymphoma, mycosis fungoides, testicular carcinoma, Kaposi's sarcoma, Letterer-Siwe disease, (histiocytosis X), choriocarcinoma and breast cancer.

Contraindications Leukopenia; presence of uncontrolled bacterial infection; significant granulocytopenia not associated with disease being treated.

Route/Dosage

ADULTS: **IV** Initial dose: 3.7 mg/m^2. Dosage is increased by 1.8 mg/m^2 at weekly intervals until desired therapeutic response is obtained, leukocyte count decreases to 3000/mm^3 or a maximum weekly dose of 18.5 mg/m^2 is being administered. Maintenance: 1.8 mg/m^2 less than dose required to produce leukopenia. CHILDREN: **IV** Initial dose: 2.5 mg/m^2. Dosage is increased by 1.25 mg/m^2 at weekly intervals until desired therapeutic response is obtained, leukocyte count decreases to 3000/mm^3 or a maximum weekly dose of 12.5 mg/m^2 is being administered. Maintenance: 1.25 mg/m^2 less than dose required to produce leukopenia. Dosing adjustment for hepatic function impairment: Direct serum bilirubin < 3 mg/dl: Use 50% of normal dose. INCOMPATIBILITIES: Mix vinblastine only with normal saline or 5% glucose in water. Do not dilute in solutions that raise or lower pH outside range of 3.5-5.

Interactions

Hydantoins: May decrease plasma hydantoin levels.

Lab Test Interferences

None well documented.

Adverse Reactions

CV: Hypertension. *RESP:* Acute shortness of breath; bronchospasm. *CNS:* Numbness of digits; paresthesias; peripheral neuritis; dizziness; mental depression; loss of reflexes; headache; convulsions. *GI:* Nausea; vomiting; mucositis; abdominal pain; ileus; diarrhea; constipation; anorexia; GI bleeding. *HEMA:* Bone marrow depression (leukopenia [granulocytopenia], anemia, thrombocytopenia). *GU:* Aspermia; amenorrhea. *DERM:* Alopecia; vesiculation; cellulitis following extravasation. *OTHER:* Malaise; tumor site pain; bone and jaw pain; syndrome of inappropriate antidiuretic hormone secretion (SIADH).

Precautions

Pregnancy: Category D. *Lactation:* Undetermined. *Hematologic effects:* Leukopenia is expected; thrombocytopenia and anemia may occur; risk of infection and bleeding is increased. *Hepatic function impairment:* May increase risk of toxicity. Dosage reduction may be necessary. *Eye contamination:* Severe irritation and corneal ulceration may result; thoroughly wash eyes immediately. *Pulmonary reactions:* Acute shortness of breath and bronchospasm may occur; greatest risk with combination therapy including mitomycin-C; onset can be immediate or delayed (up to 2 weeks following mitomycin dose). *For IV use only:* Do not administer by any other route. *Dosage frequency:* Given at intervals of at least 7 days; if leucopenic, delay dose until leukocyte count has returned to at least 4000/mm^3. *Thrombosis:* Do not inject into extremity in which circulation is impaired or potentially impaired (increased risk of thrombosis).

NURSING CONSIDERATIONS

Administration/Storage

- For IV administration only. Do not administer more than once weekly.
- To reconstitute powder, add 10 ml of normal saline (with preservative) to vial for concentration of 1 mg/ml. Preservative-containing diluent is unnecessary if unused portion is discarded immediately.
- Dilute with Normal Saline or D5W only.
- Refrigerate remaining solution up to 30 days.
- Implement appropriate procedures for handling and disposal of drug.
- Inject into tubing of running IV or directly into vein over 1 min. Take caution to prevent extravasation.
- If extravasation occurs, discontinue injection immediately and notify physician. Give remaining dose in another vein. Inject hyaluronidase locally and apply heat to affected area if ordered by physician.
- Do not inject into extremity in which circulation is impaired or potentially impaired (increased risk of thrombosis).
- Store powder for reconstitution and solution for injection in refrigerator. Protect from light.

Assessment/Interventions

- Obtain patient history, includ-

ing drug history and any known allergies.
- Obtain baseline CBC and platelet count.
- Monitor I&O throughout therapy. Encourage fluid intake.
- Monitor for neurotoxicity.
- Monitor for symptoms of gout.
- Administer antiemetics as necessary.

OVERDOSAGE: SIGNS & SYMPTOMS

Neurotoxicity, bone marrow depression, SIADH, death

Patient/Family Education

- Instruct patient to avoid crowds and persons with known infection.
- Advise patient to use soft toothbrush and electric razor.
- Caution patient not to drink alcohol or take aspirin-containing preparations.
- Instruct patient not to receive any vaccines without consulting physician.
- Explain importance of periodic laboratory testing.
- Instruct patient to report any bleeding or unusual bruising, sore throat, fever, chills or sore mouth to physician immediately.
- Explain that hair loss will occur but that hair regrows during maintenance therapy.
- Tell patient to report malaise, weakness, dizziness, pain in tumor site, bone and jaw pain.
- Explain ways to avoid constipation (eg, increased fluid and fiber intake).

See Patient Guide, p. 637.

Vincristine Sulfate (VCR; LCR)

(vin-KRISS-teen SULL-fate)

Oncovin, Vincasar PFS

Class: Antineoplastic/mitotic inhibitor

Action Prevents cell division at metaphase stage by binding microtubular proteins of the mitotic spindle.

Indications Treatment of acute leukemia; combination therapy in Hodgkin's disease, non-Hodgkin's lymphomas, rhabdomyosarcoma, neuroblastoma and Wilms' tumor. **Unlabeled Uses:** Treatment of idiopathic thrombocytopenic purpura, Kaposi's sarcoma, breast and bladder cancer.

Contraindications Demyelinating Charcot-Marie-Tooth syndrome.

Route/Dosage

ADULTS: **IV** 1.4 mg/m^2 at weekly intervals. CHILDREN (> 10 KG OR BODY SURFACE AREA ≥ 1 M^2): **IV** 2 mg/m^2 at weekly intervals. CHILDREN (≤ 10 KG OR BODY SURFACE AREA < 1 M^2): **IV** 0.05 mg/kg once/week. Dosing adjustment for hepatic function impairment: Direct serum bilirubin > 3 mg/dl: Use 50% of normal dose.

Interactions

Digoxin: Combination chemotherapy including vincristine may decrease plasma digoxin levels. *L-asparaginase:* May increase vincristine levels; give vincristine 12-24 hr before L-asparaginase to minimize toxicity. *Mitomycin-C:* Acute pulmonary reactions may occur from concomitant use. *Phenytoin:* Combination chemotherapy including vincristine may decrease plasma phenytoin levels. INCOMPATIBILITIES: Mix vincristine with normal saline or D5W only. Do not dilute in solutions that raise or lower pH outside range of 3.5-5.5.

Lab Test Interferences

None well documented.

Adverse Reactions

CV: Hypertension; hypotension. *RESP:* Acute shortness of breath; bronchospasm. *CNS:* Generalized sensorimotor dysfunction; neuromuscular difficulties; loss of reflexes; paralysis; isolated cranial nerve manifestations; seizures; headache. *EENT:* Optic atrophy with blindness; transient cortical blindness; ptosis; diplopia; photophobia. *GI:* Mucositis; abdominal cramps; nausea; vomiting; diarrhea; constipation; anorexia; intestinal necrosis or perforation; paralytic ileus. *GU:* Polyuria; dysuria; urinary retention; azoospermia; amenorrhea; uric acid nephropathy. *HEMA:* Bone marrow depression (anemia, leukopenia, granulocytopenia, thrombocytopenia). *DERM:* Alopecia. *OTHER:* Syndrome of inappropriate antidiuretic hormone secretion (SIADH) (rare), tissue damage from extravasation; fever. *Hypersensitivity:* Anaphylaxis; rash; edema.

Precautions

Pregnancy: Category D. *Lactation:* Undetermined. *Hypersensitivity:* Acute allergic reactions have occurred. *Acute uric acid nephropathy:* Monitor serum uric acid levels frequently. *Concomitant radiation therapy:* Do not give to patients receiving radiation therapy through ports that include liver. *IV use only:* Do not administer by any other route. Intrathecal injection invariably produces death. *CNS leukemia:* If diagnosed, additional agents may be required. *Eye contamination:* Severe irritation and corneal ulceration may result; thoroughly wash eyes immediately. *Monitoring:* Frequently evaluate for neurotoxicity; perform complete blood count before each dose. *Neurotoxicity:* Dose-related neuropathy may occur; can initially cause sensory impairment and paresthesias, then neuritic pain and motor difficulties; patients with neuromuscular disease or receiving other neurotoxic drugs have greatest risk; dosage adjustment may be necessary. *Pulmonary reactions:* Acute shortness of breath and bronchospasm may occur; greatest risk with combination therapy including mitomycin-C; onset can be immediate or delayed (up to 2 wk following mitomycin dose).

NURSING CONSIDERATIONS

Administration/Storage

- For IV administration only.
- Utilize gloves, gown and mask when handling.
- Mix only with normal saline or dextrose in water.
- Assure that IV site is properly positioned before administration.
- Administer antiemetic as ordered prior to IV injection.
- Administer dose direct IV or into running IV infusion over about 1 min.
- Discontinue administration immediately if infiltration is detected. Notify physician. Give remaining dose in another vein. Locally inject hyaluronidase and apply moderate heat to affected area if ordered by physician.
- Discard IV equipment in designated container.
- Store in refrigerator and protect from light.

Assessment/Interventions

- Obtain patient history, including drug history and any known allergies.
- Obtain baseline CBC and monitor levels throughout therapy.
- Assess integrity of IV site prior to injection.
- Assess for signs and symptoms of infiltration and/or phlebitis throughout therapy.
- Assess for side effects, particularly nausea and vomiting, neurotoxicity, alteration in BP, bone marrow depression.
- Assess bowel sounds.
- Assess nutritional status. Increase patient's fluid intake.
- Assess for alteration in body image, self-esteem.
- Monitor I&O throughout therapy. Encourage fluid intake.
- Monitor effectiveness of antiemetics.
- Modify dietary intake as indicated.

- Monitor liver and renal function throughout therapy.

OVERDOSAGE: SIGNS & SYMPTOMS

Neurotoxicity, bone marrow depression, SIADH, death

Patient/Family Education

- Instruct patient to report any bleeding, unusual bruising, sore throat, fever, chills, sore mouth, stumbling, numbness or "funny feelings" in fingers or toes, neuritic pain or constipation to physician immediately.
- Explain precautions against infection.
- Instruct patient and family in techniques for and importance of frequent handwashing.
- Advise patient to increase fluid intake, follow high-fiber diet and exercise regularly to minimize constipation.
- Explain that alopecia is side effect; inform of alternatives.
- Instruct patient not to receive any vaccinations without advise of physician.
- Emphasize importance of periodic laboratory testing.

See Patient Guide, p. 638.

Warfarin

(WORE-fuh-rin)

Coumadin, Panwarfin, Sofarin, ✤ *Warfilone*

Class: Anticoagulant

Action Interferes with hepatic synthesis of vitamin K–dependent clotting factors, resulting in in vivo depletion of clotting factors, II, VII, IX and X.

Indications Prophylaxis and treatment of venous thrombosis and its extension; prophylaxis and treatment of atrial fibrillation with embolization; prophylaxis and treatment of pulmonary embolism; adjunct in prophylaxis of systemic embolism after MI. **Unlabeled uses:** Prevention of recurrent transient ischemic attacks and reduction of risk of recurrent MI; adjunctive treatment of small cell carcinoma of lung.

Contraindications Pregnancy; hemorrhagic tendencies; hemophilia; thrombocytopenic purpura; leukemia; recent or contemplated surgery of eye or CNS, major regional lumbar block anesthesia, or surgery resulting in large, open surfaces; patients bleeding from GI, respiratory or GU tract; threatened abortion; aneursym; ascorbic acid deficiency; history of bleeding diathesis; prostatectomy; continuous tube drainage of small intestine; polyarthritis; diverticulitis; emaciation; malnutrition; cerebrovascular hemorrhage; eclampsia and preeclampsia; blood dyscrasias; severe uncontrolled or malignant hypertension; severe renal or hepatic disease; pericarditis and pericardial effusion; subacute bacterial endocarditis; visceral carcinoma; following spinal puncture and other diagnostic or therapeutic procedures (eg, IUD insertion) with potential for uncontrollable bleeding; history of warfarin-induced necrosis.

Route/Dosage

ADULTS: **PO** 10 mg/day for 2-4 days; adjust daily dose according to prothrombin time (PT) or international normalization ratio (INR) determinations. Usual maintenance dose is **PO** 2-10 mg daily. ELDERLY PATIENTS: Lower dosages are recommended.

Interactions

Aminoglutethimide, azathioprine, barbiturates, carbamazepine, cholestyramine, ethchlorvynol, glutethimide, griseofulvin, mercaptopurine, rifabutin, rifampin, trazodone and vitamin K: Decreased anticoagulant effect of warfarin. *Androgens, amiodarone, cefamandole, cefazolin, cefoperazone, cefotetan, cefoxi-*

tin, ceftriaxone, chloramphenicol, cimetidine, clofibrate, dextrothyroxine, disulfiram, erythromycin, fluconazole, glucagon, methimazole, metronidazole, miconazole, moxalactam, nalidixic acid, nonsteroidal anti-inflammatory agents, phenylbutazone, propylthiouracil, quinidine, quinine, salicylates, sulfinpyrazone, sulfonamides, thyroid hormones, tricyclic antidepressants and vitamin E: Increased anticoagulant effect of warfarin. *Hydantoins:* Serum hydantoin concentration may be elevated, increasing risk of toxicity.

Lab Test Interferences

Oral anticoagulants may cause red-orange discoloration of alkaline urine, interfering with some laboratory tests.

Adverse Reactions

EENT: Mouth ulcers. *GI:* Nausea; vomiting; diarrhea; paralytic ileus; intestinal obstruction; anorexia; abdominal cramps. *HEMA:* Hemorrhage; leukopenia. *HEPA:* Hepatotoxicity; cholestatic jaundice. *GU:* Red-orange urine. *DERM:* Skin necrosis; gangrene; exfoliative dermatitis; urticaria; alopecia. *OTHER:* Fever; cholesterol microembolization (purple toe syndrome); hypersensitivity.

Precautions

Pregnancy: Category X. *Lactation:* Excreted in breast milk. *Children:* Safety and efficacy not established in children < 18 yr. *Elderly patients:* May be more sensitive to effects. *Special risk patients:* There is increased risk associated with using warfarin in patients with trauma, infection, renal insufficiency, dietary insufficiency, uncontrolled hypertension, polycythemia vera, vasculitis, indwelling catheters. Evaluate benefits of therapy vs. risks. *Adrenal hemorrhage:* Discontinue therapy if patient develops signs and symptoms of adrenal insufficiency. *Hemorrhage/necrosis:* Most serious risks of therapy; may result in death. *Hepatic impairment:* Use cautiously. *Hypersensitivity:* Reactions range from mild to life-threatening. Symptoms may be dermatologic (eg, erythema, eczematous rash, exfoliative dermatitis, exudative erythema multiforme, alopecia), hematologic (eg, eosinophilia, leukopenia, thrombocytopenia), renal, (eg, nephropathy, nephritis, oliguria), gastrointestinal (eg, enanthema, severe stomatitis) or hepatic (eg, mixed hepatocellular damage, cholestasis, jaundice). If signs or symptoms occur, discontinue therapy and notify physician. *Monitoring/prothrombin time:* Individualize treatment based on PT or INR. *Protein C deficiency:* Hereditary, familial or clinical protein C deficiency has been associated with necrosis following warfarin therapy. If warfarin is suspected cause of necrosis, administration should be discontinued. *Purple toe syndrome:* Systemic cholesterol microembolization from release of atheromatous plaque emboli. Discontinue therapy. *Surgical/dental procedures:* Adjust dose to maintain PT or INR at low end of therapeutic range for patients who must be anticoagulated during dental or surgical procedures.

NURSING CONSIDERATIONS

Administration/Storage

- Do not give large loading dose.
- Do not switch brands.
- Administer at same time each day.
- Store at room temperature in tight, light-resistant container.

Assessment/Interventions

- Obtain patient history, including drug history and any known allergies.
- Use care in determining cooperation of patient to ensure compliance.
- Monitor PT or INR.
- Test urine, stool and drainage for occult blood.
- Observe for low back pain and GI symptoms.

- Avoid IM injection and venipuncture if possible.
- If "purple toe syndrome," tissue necrosis or signs of adrenal insufficiency (fever, myalgia, arthralgia, anorexia, nausea, diarrhea) are observed, stop drug and report to physician immediately.
- If bleeding occurs, report to physician immediately.

OVERDOSAGE: SIGNS & SYMPTOMS

Hematuria, excessive menstrual bleeding, melena, petechiae, oozing from superficial injuries

Patient/Family Education

- Caution patient that this medication must not be taken during pregnancy or when pregnancy is possible. Advise patient to use reliable form of birth control while taking this drug.
- Advise patient not to change dose unless advised by physician.
- Advise patient not to drastically change diet or consume alcohol.
- Advise patient not to change brands of medicine.
- Advise patient to limit intake of vitamin K–rich foods, including avocados, bananas, broccoli, dried fruits, grapefruit, lima beans, nuts, oranges, peaches, potatoes, sunflower seeds, spinach, tomatoes.
- Instruct patient to report any GI upset, pink or red discoloration of urine, red or tar-black stools or diarrhea, skin rash, yellowish tint of skin or eyes, unusual bleeding (eg, heavier than normal menstrual flow) or bruising.
- Caution patient not to take aspirin or other salicylates without consulting physician.
- Instruct patient in safety practices: use of soft toothbrush, electric razor, nightlights and avoidance of activities that could result in bruising or bleeding.
- Tell patient not to take any otc or prescription medications without consulting physician.
- Remind patient to wear Medi-Alert identification bracelet.

See Patient Guide, p. 639.

Zalcitabine (Dideoxycytidine; ddC)

(zal-SITE-uh-BEAN)

Hivid

Class: Anti-infective/antiviral

Action Inhibits replication of DNA in HIV.

Indications

Monotherapy: Treatment of HIV infection in adults with advanced HIV disease who are either intolerant to zidovudine or who have disease progression while receiving zidovudine. *Combination therapy*: For the treatment of selected patients with advanced HIV infection.

Contraindications Standard considerations.

Route/Dosage

Monotherapy

ADULTS: **PO** 0.75 mg q 8 hr, 2.25 mg daily dose.

Combination therapy

ADULTS & ADOLESCENTS > 13 YR: **PO** 0.75 mg (administered concomitantly with zidovudine 200 mg) q 8 hr (total daily dose 2.25 mg zalcitabine).

Interactions

Amphotericin, foscarnet, aminoglycosides: May increase risk of peripheral neuropathy and other zalcitabine toxicities due to decreased clearance of zalcitabine. *Chloramphenicol, cisplatin, dapsone, disulfiram, ethionamide, glutethimide, gold, hydralazine, iodoquinol, isoniazid, metronidazole, nitrofurantoin, phenytoin, ribavirin, vincristine*: May increase risk of peripheral neuropathy. *Drugs associated with pan-*

creatitis (eg, pentamidine): Fatal pancreatitis has occurred, possibly related to zalcitabine and IV pentamidine given concurrently.

Lab Test Interferences
None well documented.

Adverse Reactions
CV: Chest pain; cardiomyopathy; CHF. *CNS*: Headache; dizziness; confusion; impaired concentration; peripheral neuropathy. *EENT*: Pharyngitis. *GI*: Pancreatitis; oral ulcers; nausea; dysphagia; anorexia; abdominal pain; vomiting; diarrhea; dry mouth; esophageal ulcers; dyspepsia; glossitis. *DERM*: Rash; pruritus; dermatitis. *META*: Weight decrease; weight gain; increased amylase; hyperglycemia; hyponatremia; hypoglycemia; loss of appetite. *RESP*: Nasal discharge; cough; respiratory distress. *OTHER*: Myalgia; arthralgia; foot pain; fatigue; anaphylactoid reaction; abnormat GGT.

Precautions
Pregnancy: Category C. *Lactation*: Undetermined. It is recommended that HIV-positive women do not breastfeed. *Children*: Safety and efficacy in children < 13 yr not established. *Anaphylactoid reaction*: Has occurred. Urticaria has occurred without other signs of anaphylaxis. *Cardiomyopathy/CHF*: May develop. Use drug with caution in patients with history of cardiomyopathy or CHF. *Esophageal ulcers*: Have occurred. *Hepatic impairment*: In patients with history of liver disease or alcoholism, zalcitabine may exacerbate hepatic dysfunction. Dosage reduction or interruption of therapy may be needed. *HIV infection complications*: Patients receiving zalcitabine or any other antiretroviral therapy may continue to develop opportunistic infections and other complications of HIV infection. *Pancreatitis*: Fatal pancreatitis has occurred. *Peripheral neuropathy*: Most common major toxicity. May be clinically disabling and require reduction of dose or discontinuation of drug. *Renal impairment*: Patients with renal impairment (creatinine clearance < 55 ml/min) may be at greater risk of toxicity due to decreased drug clearance. Dosage reduction may be needed.

NURSING CONSIDERATIONS

Administration/Storage

- Administer on empty stomach 1 hr before or 2 hr after meals for maximum absorption.
- Administer q 8 hr around clock.
- If creatinine clearance is decreased, reduced dose (0.75 mg) may be given q 12 hr (creatinine clearance 10-40 ml/min) or q 24 hr (creatinine clearance < 10 ml/min).
- Store at room temperature in tight containers.

Assessment/Interventions

- Obtain patient history, including drug history and any known allergies. Note cardiac, hepatic and renal dysfunction; peripheral neuropathy; and pancreatitis.
- Perform clinical chemistry tests before and periodically during therapy. Monitor CBC, renal function studies (BUN, serum uric acid, urine creatinine clearance), liver function tests (bilirubin, AST, ALT, alkaline phosphatase) and baseline serum amylase and triglyceride levels in patients with prior history of pancreatitis, increased amylase or ethanol abuse and those on parenteral nutrition.
- Prior to therapy and throughout treatment, assess for signs of peripheral neuropathy: tingling, burning or pain in distal extremities. In patients with moderate symptoms of peripheral neuropathy, drug is discontinued then may be reintroduced at 50% of initial dose only if neuropathy symptoms have improved to mild. Use of drug may be discontinued permanently if severe discomfort due to neuropathy or moderate discomfort progresses ≥ 1 wk.

- Assess for pancreatitis: abdominal pain, nausea, vomiting, elevated liver enzymes. Withhold zalcitabine and zidovudine and notify physician of these symptoms immediately.
- Observe for signs of infection; monitor temperature q 4 hr. Antibiotics may be ordered prophylactically.
- Frequently monitor hematologic indices to detect serious anemia or granulocytopenia. Development of anemia (hemoglobin < 7.5/dl or reduction > 25% of baseline) or granulocytopenia (granulocyte count < 750/min^3 or reduction > 50% of baseline) may require interruption of treatment with both zalcitabine and zidovudine until marrow recovers. Transfusion may be needed.
- In patients developing hematologic toxicity, decreases in hemoglobin may occur as early as 2-4 wk after therapy begins and granulocytopenia may occur after 6-8 wk of therapy.
- Reduction of dose is not required for patients weighing ≥ 30 kg.

OVERDOSAGE: SIGNS & SYMPTOMS
Rash, fever, peripheral neuropathy

Patient/Family Education

- Advise patient to take around the clock as prescribed and not to increase the dose.
- Advise patient not to share the drug with others.
- Inform patient and family that patient may continue to develop opportunistic infections and other complications of HIV infection and should remain under close medical supervision.
- Explain that zalcitabine is not a cure but may offer symptomatic improvement.
- Reinforce fact that zalcitabine does not decrease risk of transmission of HIV through sexual contact or blood contamination.
- Instruct patient to notify physician immediately of signs of peripheral neuropathy (numbness and burning feeling in arms and legs) or pancreatitis (abdominal pain, nausea, vomiting).
- Encourage patient to report all changes in conditions to physician.
- Inform patient that long-term effects of this drug alone and in combination with zidovudine are unknown.

See Patient Guide, p. 640.

Zidovudine (Azidothymidine; AZT; Compound S)

(zid-OH-vue-deen)

Retrovir, ♣ *APO-Zidovudine, Novo-AZT*

Class: Anti-infective/antiviral

Action Inhibits replication of retroviruses including HIV.

Indications
Oral form: Treatment of HIV infection in adults with impaired immunity and children > 3 mo with HIV-related symptoms or laboratory evidence of immunosuppression; prevention of maternal-fetal HIV transmission; treatment of selected patients with advanced HIV disease in combination with zalcitabine. *IV form:* Adult patients with symptomatic HIV infection (AIDS and advanced ARC) with *Pneumocystic carinii* pneumonia or absolute CD4 lymphocyte count of < 200/mm^3 in peripheral blood.

Contraindications Life-threatening hypersensitivity to any component.

Route/Dosage
ORAL

Monotherapy

Symptomatic HIV Infection
ADULTS: **PO** 100 mg (one 100 mg capsule or 2 teaspoonfuls [10 ml] syrup) q 4 hr around the clock initially (600 mg daily dose).

Asymptomatic HIV Infection
ADULTS: **PO** 100 mg q 4 hr while awake (500 mg/day). CHILDREN 3 MO-12 YR: **PO** 180 mg/m^2 q 6 hr initially (720 mg/m^2 day, maximum 200 mg q 6 hr). Dosage adjustment needed due to hematologic toxicity. ADULTS: **IV** 1-2 mg/kg infused over 1 hr at constant rate; administer q 4 hr around clock (6 times daily). Do not give IM.

Maternal-Fetal HIV Transmission
MATERNAL DOSING: >14 weeks of pregnancy-100 mg orally 5 times per day until the start of labor. During labor and delivery, administer IV zidovudine at 2 mg/kg over 1 hour followed by a continuous IV infusion of 1 mg/kg/hr until clamping of the umbilical cord. INFANT DOSING: 2 mg/kg orally every 6 hours starting within 12 hours after birth and continuing through 6 weeks of age. Infants unable to receive oral dosing may be given zidovudine IV at 1.5 mg/kg, infused over 30 minutes, every 6 hours.

Combination therapy with zalcitabine
ADULTS: Zidovudine 200 mg orally with zalcitabine 0.75 mg every 8 hours.

Interactions
Acyclovir: Possible increased risk of neurotoxicity (lethargy or seizure). *Dapsone, pentamidine, amphotericin B, flucytosine, vincristine, vinblastine, adriamycin, interferon:* May increase risk of toxicity, including nephrotoxicity, cytotoxicity or hematologic toxicity. *Experimental nucleoside analogs:* May affect RBC/WBC counts or function and may increase potential for hematologic toxicity. *Ganciclovir:* Life-threatening hematologic toxicity may occur. *Probenecid, acetaminophen, aspirin, indomethacin:* May inhibit metabolism or decrease clearance of zidovudine, causing increase in its serum concentration and potential toxicity.

Lab Test Interferences
None well documented.

Adverse Reactions
CV: ECG abnormality; vasodilation; syncope; cardiomyopathy; CHF. *RESP:* Dyspnea; cough; epistaxis; pharyngitis; rhinitis; sinusitis; hoarseness. *CNS:* Headache; dizziness; insomnia; paresthesia; malaise; asthenia; decreased reflexes; nervousness or irritability. *EENT:* Taste perversion; hearing loss. *GI:* Anorexia; constipation; dyspepsia; nausea; vomiting; dysphagia; flatuence; bleeding of the gums; rectal hemorrhage; mouth ulcers; edema of the tongue; eructation; abdominal pain. *HEMA:* Anemia; granulocytopenia; pancytopenia. *DERM:* Rash; acne. *INFANTS:* Anemia; neutropenia. *OTHER:* Fever, diaphoresis; myalgia; arthralgia; muscle spasm; body odor; chills; edema of the lip; flu syndrome; hyperalgesia; abdominal/back/chest pain; hypersensitivity reaction.

Precautions
Pregnancy: Category C. *Lactation:* Undetermined. *Children:* Dosing regimen not established in children < 3 mo. *Hematologic effects:* Significant anemia and granulocytopenia has occurred. Use with extreme caution in patients with bone marrow compromise (Hgb < 9.5 g/dl or granulocyte count < 1000/mm^3). *Hypersensitivity:* Sensitization reactions, including anaphylaxis, have occurred. *Renal/hepatic impairment:* May have greater risk of toxicity.

NURSING CONSIDERATIONS

Administration/Storage
- Use syrup or capsule form for oral administration according to patient needs. Do *not* interchange between syrup and capsules. Syrup form absorbs faster than capsule form.
- Dilute IV preparation prior to administration. Remove calculate dose from vial; add to 5% Dextrose to achieve concentration of ≤ 4 mg/ml.
- Do *not* mix with biologic or colloidal fluids (eg, blood products or protein solutions).
- Infuse over 1 hr at constant rate. Avoid rapid infusion or bolus.
- Awake patient to administer around

clock unless otherwise instructed by physician.

- Do *not* administer with probenecid, acetaminophen, aspirin or indomethacin (may inhibit metabolism or decrease clearance of zidovudine; serum concentrations may increase to potentially toxic levels).
- Store capsules at room temperature in a tight, light-resistant container. Protect from heat and moisture.
- Store syrup at room temperature. Protect from light.
- After dilution the solution is physically and chemically stable for 24 hours at room temperature and 48 hours if refrigerated. As an additional precaution, administer the diluted solution within 8 hours if stored at room temperature or 24 hours if refrigerated to minimize the potential administration of a microbially contaminated solution. Store undiluted vials at room temperature and protect from light.

Assessment/Interventions

- Obtain patient history, including drug history and any known allergies.
- Assess periodic ECGs.
- Monitor and record WBC and differential q 2 wks (report decreased WBC, especially granulocytes immediately).
- Assess skin for signs of sensitization reactions (report rash).
- Assess Hct and Hgb q 2 wk (severe anemia may require immediate blood transfusion).
- Monitor respiratory and cardiac status (report dyspnea, edema, other signs of CHF).
- Monitor results of liver and renal function studies.

OVERDOSAGE: SIGNS & SYMPTOMS

Nausea, vomiting, hematologic changes

Patient/Family Education

- Advise patient to take exactly as prescribed.
- Advise patient not to share medication and not to exceed the recommended dose.
- Inform patient that fever, sore throat, shortness of breath and dizziness require immediate attention by physician. These may be signs of severe anemia or decreased WBCs and may indicate need for blood transfusion.
- Explain that physician will request follow-up blood and/or urine studies; do not skip appointments.
- Tell patient to notify physician of headache, insomnia, nausea, muscle aches, dyspnea, numbness or tingling, nervousness, loss of appetite, diarrhea, GI pain, vomiting, rash, excessive sweating, swelling of feet and legs, taste perversions.
- Explain that drug does not prevent transmission of disease.
- Caution patient not to take **any** other drugs without consulting physician. This especially includes acetaminophen *(Tylenol)*, aspirin, indomethacin and acyclovir.
- Instruct patient to increase fluid intake to 2-3 L daily.
- Advise patient to weigh self daily and record weight.
- Tell patient to protect medication from light during storage.
- Advise patient that drug may cause drowsiness and to use caution while driving or performing other tasks requiring mental alertness.
- Explain that long-term effects of drug are not known at this time.
- Advise patient that zidovudine therapy has not been shown to reduce the risk of transmission of HIV to others through sexual contact or blood contamination.
- Advise pregnant women considering use of the drug to prevent maternal-fetal transmission of HIV that transmission may still occur in some cases despite therapy. Long-term consequences of in utero and infant exposure are unknown.

See Patient Guide, p. 641.

Zinc Sulfate

(zink SULL-fate)

Eye-Sed, Orazinc, Verazinc, Zinca-Pak, Zincate, ♣ *PMS-Egozinc*

Class: Mineral

Action Acts as integral part of several enzymes important to protein and carbohydrate metabolism, wound healing, maintenance of normal growth and skin hydration, and senses of taste and smell.

Indications Dietary supplementation; supplement to IV solutions given for TPN; treatment or prevention of zinc deficiencies. Ophthalmic solution used as mild astringent for relief of eye irritation. **Unlabeled uses:** Treatment of acrodermatitis enteropathica and delayed wound healing associated with zinc deficiency; treatment of acne, rheumatoid arthritis, Wilson's disease.

Contraindications Direct injection of undiluted solution into peripheral vein.

Route/Dosage

Dietary Supplement

ADULTS: **PO** 25-50 mg/day.

Supplement to IV Solutions

METABOLICALLY STABLE ADULTS: **IV** 2.5-4 mg/day. Add 2 mg/day for acute catabolic state. STABLE ADULTS WITH FLUID LOSS FROM SMALL BOWEL: **IV** Increase dose by 12.2 mg/L TPN or 17.1 mg/kg loose stool or ileostomy output. FULL-TERM INFANTS & CHILDREN < 5 YR: **IV** 100 mcg/kg/day. PREMATURE INFANTS < 3 KG: **IV** 300 mcg/kg/day.

Astringent

ADULTS: **Ophthalmic:** 1-2 gtt into eye(s) up to 4 times daily.

Interactions

Fluoroquinolones; tetracyclines: Absorption of these agents may be decreased.

Lab Test Interferences

None well documented.

Adverse Reactions

GI: Nausea; vomiting (especially in large oral doses).

Precautions

Pregnancy: Category C. Routine supplementation during pregnancy is not recommended. *Lactation:* Excreted in breast milk. *Excessive intake:* In healthy persons may be harmful. *Benzyl alcohol:* Some of these products contain benzyl alcohol, which has been associated with a fetal "gasping" syndrome in premature infants. *Renal impairment:* Dosage reduction may be required in patients with renal dysfunction. *IV products:* Some contain benzyl alcohol, which is associated with fatal "gasping syndrome" in infants.

NURSING CONSIDERATIONS

Administration/Storage

- If GI upset occurs, administer oral form with food but not with dairy products, bran or foods containing caffeine.
- Dilute IV solutions prior to administration.
- To prevent contamination of ophthalmic solution, avoid contacting tip of container with any other surface and tightly close container after use.
- Do not use ophthalmic solution if becomes discolored or cloudy.

Assessment/Interventions

- Obtain patient history, including drug history and any known allergies.
- If eye irritation persists or increases or pain or vision change occurs, consult physician.

OVERDOSAGE: SIGNS & SYMPTOMS

Nausea, vomiting, dehydration, restlessness, sideroblastic anemia, profuse sweating, hyperamylasemia

Patient/Family Education

- Tell patient to contact physician if nausea, severe vomiting, dehydration or restlessness occurs.
- Identify food sources of zinc (seafood, organ meats and wheat germ).
- Inform patient that sense of taste and smell, skin hydration and wound healing should improve.
- Instruct patient to follow RDA guidelines and limitations in terms of vitamin and mineral supplementation.
- Tell patient to take with food if GI upset occurs but to avoid foods high in calcium, phosphorus and phytate. Inform patient that bran, caffeine and dairy products may decrease absorption.
- Tell patient to notify physician if change in vision occurs or if eye irritation or pain persists or increases while using ophthalmic form.
- Teach patient proper administration technique for eye drops.

See Patient Guide, pp. 642-644.

Antibiotic Combinations

These antibiotic combinations are used for the treatment of superficial ocular infections involving the conjunctiva or cornea (eg, conjunctivitis, keratitis, keratoconjunctivitis, corneal ulcers, blepharitis, blepharoconjunctivitis, acute meibomianitis and dacryocystitis) due to strains of micro-organisms susceptible to antibiotics.

Combination Antibiotic Products		
Trade Name	***Strength/Ingredient***	***Average Dose***
AK-Spore Ointment, Neosporin Ophthalmic Ointment, Ocutricin Ointment	10,000 units/g polymyxin B sulfate, 3.5 mg/g neomycin sulfate, 400 units/g bacitracin zinc	Varies for individual products, refer to manufacturer's insert
AK-Spore Solution, Neosporin Ophthalmic Solution	10,000 units/ml polymyxin B sulfate, 1.75 mg/ml neomycin sulfate, 0.025 mg/ml gramicidin	Varies for individual products, refer to manufacturer's insert
AK-Poly-Bac Ointment, Polysporin Ophthalmic Ointment	10,000 units/g polymyxin B sulfate, 500 units/g bacitracin zinc	Varies for individual products, refer to manufacturer's insert
Terak Ointment, Terramycin w/Polymyxin B Ointment	10,000 units/g polymyxin B sulfate, 5 mg/g oxytetracycline HCl	Varies for individual products, refer to manufacturer's insert
Polytrim Ophthalmic Solution	10,000 units/ml polymyxin B sulfate, 1 mg/ml trimethoprim	Varies for individual products, refer to manufacturer's insert

Gastrointestinal Anticholinergic Combinations

Gastrointestinal anticholinergic agents are used primarily to decrease motility (smooth muscle tone) in the GI, biliary and urinary tracts and for their antisecretory effects.

Combination anticholinergic preparations may include the following components:

Barbiturates, *prochlorperazine*, *hydroxyzine*, *meprobamate*, *chlordiazepoxide:* used as sedatives and antianxiety agents.

Ergotamine tartrate: provides inhibition of the sympathetic nervous system.

Antihistamines: used for their antihistaminic effects, sedative or anticholinergic side effects.

Kaolin: used for its adsorbent properties.

Anticholinergic Combinations		
Trade Name	***Strength/Ingredient***	***Average Dose***
Barbidonna No. 2 Tablets	0.025 mg atropine sulfate, 0.0074 mg scopolamine HBr, 0.1286 mg hyoscyamine HBr or SO_4, 32 mg phenobarbital	3 tablets/day
Barbidonna Tablets	0.025 mg atropine sulfate, 0.0074 mg scopolamine HBr, 0.1286 mg hyoscyamine HBr or SO_4, 16 mg phenobarbital	3 to 6 tablets/day
Donnatal Capsules and Tablets, Hyosophen Tablets, Malatal Tablets, Spasmolin Tablets	0.0194 mg atropine sulfate, 0.0065 mg scopolamine HBr, 0.1037 mg hyoscyamine HBr or SO_4, 16.2 mg phenobarbital	3 to 8 capsules or tablets/day
Butibel Tablets	15 mg belladonna extract, 15 mg butabarbital sodium	4 to 8 tablets/day
Chardonna-2 Tablets	15 mg belladonna extract, 15 mg phenobarbital	3 to 8 tablets/day
Belladenal Tablets	0.25 mg l-alkaloids of belladonna, 50 mg phenobarbital	2 to 4 tablets/day
Bellacane, Levsin w/Phenobarbital Tablets	0.125 mg l-hyoscyamine sulfate, 15 mg phenobarbital	3 to 8 tablets/day
Clindex Capsules, Librax Capsules	2.5 mg clidinium, 5 mg chlordiazepoxide HCl	3 to 8 capsules/day
Donnatal Extentabs	0.0582 mg atropine sulfate, 0.0195 mg scopolamine HBr, 0.3111 mg hyoscyamine sulfate, 48.6 mg phenobarbital	2 to 3 tablets/day
Belladenal-S Tablets	0.25 mg l-alkaloids of belladonna, 50 mg phenobarbital, tartrazine	2 tablets/day

Anticholinergic Combinations		
Trade Name	***Strength/Ingredient***	***Average Dose***
Bellacane SR Tablets, Bellergal-S Tablets, Bel-Phen-Ergot SR Tablets, Phenerbel-S Tablets	0.2 mg l-alkaloids of belladonna, 40 mg phenobarbital, 0.6 mg ergotamine tartrate	2 to 3 tablets/day
Bellacane Elixir, Donnatal Elixir[1], Hyosophen Elixir, Susano Elixir[2]	0.0194 mg atropine sulfate, 0.0065 mg scopolamine HBr, 0.1037 mg hyoscyamine HBr or SO_4, 16.2 mg phenobarbital per 5 ml, 23% alcohol	15 to 40 ml/day
Butibel Elixir	15 mg belladonna extract, 15 mg butabarbital sodium per 5 ml, 7% alcohol, saccharin	20 to 40 ml/day
Antrocol Elixir	0.195 mg atropine sulfate, 16 mg phenobarbital per 5 ml, 20% alcohol	Children: 0.5 ml per 15 lbs every 4 to 6 hours
Levsin-PB Drops	0.125 mg hyoscyamine sulfate, 15 mg phenobarbital per ml, 5% alcohol	1 to 2 ml/day Children: 0.5 to 1 ml/day

[1]Contains saccharin. [2]Contains tartrazine.

Nonnarcotic Analgesic Combinations

Components of these combinations include:

Nonnarcotic analgesics: acetaminophen, salicylates, salsalate, salicylamide.

Barbiturates, meprobamate, antihistamines: are used for their sedative effects.

Antacids: are used to minimize gastric upset from salicylates.

Caffeine: a traditional component of many analgesic formulations, may be beneficial in certain vascular headaches.

Belladonna alkaloids: are used as antispasmodics.

Pamabrom: is used as a diuretic.

Cinnamedrine: a sympathomimetic amine, claimed to have a relaxant effect in the uterus, is used in products for premenstrual syndrome. Its real value has not been established.

Aminobenzoate: retards the conjugation of salicylic acid and prolongs the action of salicylates.

Other components listed, but not contributing to the analgesic properties of these products include: calcium gluconate, ipecac and camphor.

Nonnarcotic Analgesic Combinations

Trade Name	***Strength/Ingredient***	***Average Dose***
Equagesic Tablets[1], Micrainin Tablets	325 mg aspirin, 200 mg meprobamate	1 or 2 tablets every 2 to 6 hours
Magsal Tablets	600 mg magnesium salicylate, 25 mg phenyltoloxamine citrate	1 or 2 tablets every 2 to 6 hours
Bancap Capsules, Phrenilin Tablets, Triaprin Capsules	325 mg acetaminophen, 50 mg butalbital	1 or 2 tablets or capsules every 2 to 6 hours
Phrenilin Forte Capsules, Sedapap-10 Tablets	650 mg acetaminophen, 50 mg butalbital	1 or 2 tablets or capsules every 2 to 6 hours
Axotal Tablets	650 mg aspirin, 50 mg butalbital	1 or 2 tablets every 2 to 6 hours

[1]Contains tartrazine.

Narcotic Analgesic Combinations

Components of these combinations include:

Narcotic analgesics: codeine, hydrocodone bitartrate, dihydrocodeine bitartrate, opium, oxycodone HCl, oxycodone terephthalate, meperidine HCl, propoxyphene HCl, propoxyphene napsylate.

Nonnarcotic analgesics: acetaminophen, salicylates, salicylamide.

Caffeine: a traditional component of many analgesic formulations, may be beneficial to certain vascular headaches.

Magnesium-aluminum hydroxides and *calcium carbonate:* are used as buffers.

Barbiturates, *acetylcarbromal*, *carbromal* and *bromisovalum:* are used for their sedative effects.

Promethazine HCl (a phenothiazine derivative with antihistaminic properties), used for its sedative effect.

Belladonna alkaloids: used as antispasmodics.

Narcotic Analgesic Combinations		
Trade Name	***Strength/Ingredient***	***Average Dose***
Rid-A-Pain w/Codeine Tablets	1 mg codeine phosphate, 97.2 mg acetaminophen, 226.8 mg aspirin, 32.4 mg caffeine, 32.4 mg salicylamide	1 or 2 q 4 h
Azdone Tablets, Damason-P Tablets, Lortab ASA Tablets, Panasal 5/500 Tablets	5 mg hydrocodone bitartrate, 500 mg aspirin	1 or 2 q 4 to 6 h up to 8/day
Synalgos-DC Capsules	16 mg dihydrocodeine bitartrate, 356.4 mg aspirin, 30 mg caffeine	2 q 4 h
Percodan-Demi Tablets	2.25 mg oxycodone HCl and 0.19 mg oxycodone terephthalate, 325 mg aspirin	1 or 2 q 6 h
Percodan Tablets, Rox-iprin Tablets	4.5 mg oxycodone HCl and 0.38 mg oxycodone terephthalate, 325 mg/aspirin	1 q 6 h
Mepergan Injection	25 mg meperidine HCl, 25 mg promethazine HCl	1 to 2 ml q 3 to 4 hr
Mepergan Fortis Capsules	50 mg meperidine HCl, 25 mg promethazine HCl	1 q 4 to 6 hr
E-Lor Tablets, Wygesic Tablets	65 mg propoxyphene HCl, 650 mg acetamino-phen	1 q 4 h
Darvon Compound-65 Pulvules	65 mg propoxyphene, 389 mg aspirin, 32.4 mg caffeine	1 q 4 h

Narcotic Analgesic Combinations		
Trade Name	***Strength/Ingredient***	***Average Dose***
B & O Supprettes No. 15A Suppositories	30 mg powdered opium, 16.2 mg powdered belladonna extract, polyethylene glycol base	1 or 2/day
B & O Supprettes No. 16A Suppositories	60 mg powdered opium, 16.2 mg powdered belladonna extract, polyethylene glycol base	1 or 2/day

Antihypertensive Combinations

Effective management of many hypertensive patients frequently requires concomitant administration of two or more antihypertensive agents when a single drug does not achieve adequate control. Synergistic effects are achieved by administration of antihypertensive drugs that act by different mechanisms; therefore, dose-related side effects may be minimized.

The following fixed-combination drugs are not indicated for initial therapy of hypertension. Establish proper therapy by adjusting the dosage of each agent to patient response. Periodically re-evaluate antihypertensive therapy as conditions in each patient warrant. If a fixed combination product represents a satisfactory dosage determined for the patient, its use may be more convenient.

Antihypertensive Combinations		
Trade Name	***Strength/Ingredient***	***Average Dose***
Renese-R Tablets[1]	2 mg polythiazide, 0.25 mg reserpine	Varies for individual products, refer to manufacturer's insert
Regroton Tablets	50 mg chlorthalidone, 0.25 reserpine	Varies for individual products, refer to manufacturer's insert
Diupress-500 Tablets[1]	500 mg chlorothiazide, 0.125 mg reserpine	Varies for individual products, refer to manufacturer's insert
Chloroserpine Tablets, Diupress-250 Tablets[1]	250 mg chlorothiazide, 0.125 mg reserpine	Varies for individual products, refer to manufacturer's insert
Hydropres 50 Tablets[1], Hydro-Serp Tablets, Hydroserpine #2 Tablets	50 mg hydrochlorothiazide, 0.125 mg reserpine	Varies for individual products, refer to manufacturer's insert
Hydropres 25 Tablets[1], Hydroserpine #1 Tablets	25 mg hydrochlorothiazide, 0.125 mg reserpine	Varies for individual products, refer to manufacturer's insert
Salutensin Tablets[1,2]	50 mg hydroflumethiazide, 0.125 mg reserpine	Varies for individual products, refer to manufacturer's insert
Demi-Regroton Tablets[1]	25 mg chlorthalidone, 0.125 mg reserpine	Varies for individual products, refer to manufacturer's insert
Diutensen-R Tablets	2.5 mg methyclothiazide, 0.1 mg reserpine	Varies for individual products, refer to manufacturer's insert
Metatensin #4 Tablets	4 mg trichlormethiazide, 0.1 mg reserpine	Varies for individual products, refer to manufacturer's insert
Metatensin #2 Tablets	2 mg trichlormethiazide, 0.1 mg reserpine	Varies for individual products, refer to manufacturer's insert
Rauzide Tablets	4 mg bendroflumethiazide, 50 mg powdered rauwolfia serpentina	Varies for individual products, refer to manufacturer's insert

[1]Contains lactose. [2]Contains sucrose.

Antihypertensive Combinations		
Trade Name	***Strength/Ingredient***	***Average Dose***
Enduronyl Forte Tablets	5 mg methyclothiazide, 0.5 mg deserpidine	Varies for individual products, refer to manufacturer's insert
Oreticyl Forte Tablets	25 mg methyclothiazide, 0.25 mg deserpidine	Varies for individual products, refer to manufacturer's insert
Enduronyl Tablets	5 mg methyclothiazide, 0.25 mg deserpidine	Varies for individual products, refer to manufacturer's insert
Hydrap-ES Tablets, Marpres Tablets, Ser-Ap-Es Tablets[1,2], Tri-Hydroserpine Tablets, Unipres Tablets[1]	15 mg hydrochlorothiazide, 0.1 mg reserpine, 25 mg hydralazine HCl	Varies for individual products, refer to manufacturer's insert
Apresazide 100/50 Capsules[3]	50 mg hydrochlorothiazide, 100 mg hydralazine HCl	Varies for individual products, refer to manufacturer's insert
Apresazide 50/50 Capsules[3]	50 mg hydrochlorothiazide, 50 mg hydralazine HCl	Varies for individual products, refer to manufacturer's insert
Apresazide 25/25 Capsules[3]	25 mg hydrochlorothiazide, 25 mg hydralazine HCl	Varies for individual products, refer to manufacturer's insert
Tenoretic 100 Tablets	25 mg chlorthalidone, 100 mg atenolol	Varies for individual products, refer to manufacturer's insert
Tenoretic 50 Tablets	25 mg chlorthalidone, 50 mg atenolol	Varies for individual products, refer to manufacturer's insert
Corzide Tablets 80/5	5 mg bendroflumethiazide, 80 mg nadolol, lactose	Varies for individual products, refer to manufacturer's insert
Corzide Tablets 40/5	5 mg bendroflumethiazide, 40 mg nadolol, lactose	Varies for individual products, refer to manufacturer's insert
Ziac Tablets	6.25 mg hydrochlorothiazide, 2.5 mg bisoprolol fumarate	
Ziac Tablets	6.25 mg hydrochlorothiazide, 5 mg bisoprolol fumarate	
Ziac Tablets	6.25 mg hydrochlorothiazide, 10 mg bisoprolol fumarate	
Timolide 10-25 Tablets	25 mg hydrochlorothiazide, 10 mg timolol maleate	Varies for individual products, refer to manufacturer's insert
Inderide LA 160/50 Tablets[1]	50 mg hydrochlorothiazide, 160 mg propranolol HCl	Varies for individual products, refer to manufacturer's insert

[1]Contains lactose. [3]Contains parabens.
[2]Contains sucrose.

Antihypertensive Combinations		
Trade Name	***Strength/Ingredient***	***Average Dose***
Inderide LA 120/50 Tablets[1]	50 mg hydrochlorothiazide, 120 mg propranolol HCl	Varies for individual products, refer to manufacturer's insert
Inderide LA 80/50 Tablets[1]	50 mg hydrochlorothiazide, 80 mg propranolol HCl	Varies for individual products, refer to manufacturer's insert
Inderide 80/25 Tablets[1]	25 mg hydrochlorothiazide, 80 mg propranolol HCl	Varies for individual products, refer to manufacturer's insert
Inderide 40/25 Tablets[1]	25 mg hydrochlorothiazide, 40 mg propranolol HCl	Varies for individual products, refer to manufacturer's insert
Aldoril D50 Tablets	50 mg hydrochlorothiazide, 500 mg methyldopa, EDTA	Varies for individual products, refer to manufacturer's insert
Aldoril D30 Tablets	30 mg hydrochlorothiazide, 500 mg methyldopa, EDTA	Varies for individual products, refer to manufacturer's insert
Aldoclor-250 Tablets	250 mg chlorothiazide, 250 mg methyldopa	Varies for individual products, refer to manufacturer's insert
Aldoclor-150 Tablets	150 mg hydrochlorothiazide, 250 mg methyldopa	Varies for individual products, refer to manufacturer's insert
Aldoril-25 Tablets	25 mg hydrochlorothiazide, 250 methyldopa, EDTA	Varies for individual products, refer to manufacturer's insert
Aldoril-15 Tablets	15 mg hydrochlorothiazide, 250 mg methyldopa, EDTA	Varies for individual products, refer to manufacturer's insert
Lopressor HCT 100/50 Tablets	50 mg hydrochlorothiazide, 100 mg metoprolol tartrate	Varies for individual products, refer to manufacturer's insert
Lopressor HCT 100/25 Tablets[1,2]	25 mg hydrochlorothiazide, 100 mg metoprolol tartrate	Varies for individual products, refer to manufacturer's insert
Lopressor HCT 50/25 Tablets[1,2]	25 mg hydrochlorothiazide, 50 mg metoprolol tartrate	Varies for individual products, refer to manufacturer's insert
Capozide 50/25 Tablets[1]	25 mg hydrochlorothiazide, 50 mg captopril	Varies for individual products, refer to manufacturer's insert
Capozide 25/25 Tablets[1]	25 mg hydrochlorothiazide, 25 mg captopril	Varies for individual products, refer to manufacturer's insert
Capozide 50/15[1]	15 mg hydrochlorothiazide, 50 mg captopril	Varies for individual products, refer to manufacturer's insert
Capozide 25/15[1]	15 mg hydrochlorothiazide, 25 mg captopril	Varies for individual products, refer to manufacturer's insert

[1]Contains lactose. [2]Contains sucrose.

Antihypertensive Combinations		
Trade Name	***Strength/Ingredient***	***Average Dose***
Lotensin HCT Tablets 5/6.25[1]	6.25 mg hydrochlorothiazide, 5 mg benazepril	Varies for individual products, refer to manufacturer's insert
Lotensin HCT Tablets 10/12.5[1]	12.5 mg hydrochlorothiazide, 10 mg benazepril	Varies for individual products, refer to manufacturer's insert
Lotensin HCT Tablets 20/12.5[1]	12.5 mg hydrochlorothiazide, 20 mg benazepril	Varies for individual products, refer to manufacturer's insert
Lotensin HCT Tablets 20/25[1]	25 mg hydrochlorothiazide, 20 mg benazepril	Varies for individual products, refer to manufacturer's insert
Prinzide 25 Tablets, Zestoretic Tablets	25 mg hydrochlorothiazide, 20 mg lisinopril	Varies for individual products, refer to manufacturer's insert
Prinzide 12.5 Tablets, Zestoretic Tablets	12.5 mg hydrochlorothiazide, 20 mg lisinopril	Varies for individual products, refer to manufacturer's insert
Combipres 0.3 Tablets[1,3]	15 mg chlorthalidone, 0.3 mg clonidine HCl	Varies for individual products, refer to manufacturer's insert
Combipres 0.2 Tablets[1,3]	15 mg chlorthalidone, 0.2 mg clonidine HCl	Varies for individual products, refer to manufacturer's insert
Combipres 0.1 Tablets[1,3]	15 mg chlorthalidone, 0.1 mg clonidine HCl	Varies for individual products, refer to manufacturer's insert
Minizide 5 Capsules[2]	0.5 mg polythiazide, 5 mg prazosin HCl	Varies for individual products, refer to manufacturer's insert
Minizide 2 Capsules[2]	0.5 mg polythiazide, 2 mg prazosin HCl	Varies for individual products, refer to manufacturer's insert
Minizide 1 Capsules[2]	0.5 mg polythiazide, 1 mg prazosin HCl	Varies for individual products, refer to manufacturer's insert
Esimil Tablets[1,2]	25 mg hydrochlorothiazide, 10 mg guanethidine monosulfate	Varies for individual products, refer to manufacturer's insert

[1]Contains lactose.
[2]Contains sucrose.
[3]Contains parabens.

Migraine Combinations

Ergotamine tartrate is used for its specific action against migraine.

Caffeine, a cranial vasoconstrictor, is added to ergotamine to enhance vasoconstrictive effects. It may enhance the absorption of ergotamine.

Barbiturates are used for sedation.

Belladonna alkaloids are used for their anticholinergic and antiemetic effects in individuals experiencing excessive nausea and vomiting during attacks.

Migraine Combinations

Trade Name	***Strength/Ingredient***	***Average Dose***
Cafergot Tablets, Ercaf Tablets, Wigraine Tablets	1 mg ergotamine tartrate, 100 mg caffeine	2 tablets at first sign of an attack; follow with 1 tablet every ½ hour, if needed. Maximum dose is 6 tablets/attack. Do not exceed 10 tablets/wk.
Cafatine-PB Tablets	1 mg ergotamine tartrate, 100 mg caffeine, 0.125 mg l-alkaloids of belladonna, 30 mg sodium pentobarbital	2 tablets at first sign of attack; follow with 1 tablet every ½ hour, if needed. Maximum dose is 6 tablets/attack. Do not exceed 10 tablets/wk.
Cafatine Suppository, Cafetrate Suppository	2 mg ergotamine tartrate, 100 mg caffeine	Maximum dose is 2/attack.
Wigraine Suppository	2 mg ergotamine tartrate, 100 mg caffeine, 21.5 mg tartaric acid	Maximum dose is 2/attack.

Diuretic Combinations

Fixed-dose combination drugs are not indicated for initial therapy of edema or hypertension; they require therapy titrated to the individual patient. If the fixed combination represents the determined dosage, its use may be more convenient in patient management. The treatment of hypertension and edema is not static; re-evaluate as conditions in each patient warrant.

The combination of a thiazide and a potassium-sparing diuretic provides additive diuretic activity and antihypertensive effects through different mechanisms of action and also minimizes the potassium depletion characteristic of thiazides.

Triamterene/Hydrochlorothiazide:

Bioavailability: Use caution when changing a patient to another triamterene/ hydrochlorothiazide combination product. Combination products are not equivalent.

Diuretic Combinations		
Trade Name	***Strength/Ingredient***	***Average Dose***
Moduretic Tablets	5 mg amiloride HCl, 50 mg hydrochlorothiazide	1 to 2 tablets daily, with meals
Aldactazide Tablets	25 mg spironolactone, 25 mg hydrochlorothiazide	1 to 8 tablets daily
Aldactazide Tablets	50 mg spironolactone, 50 mg hydrochlorothiazide	1 to 4 tablets daily

Respiratory Combination Products

These combination products are presented in groups based on the components of their formulations.

Antiasthmatic Combinations contain xanthine derivatives and sympathomimetics for bronchodilation. Many products also contain expectorants to facilitate mobilization of mucus.

Upper Respiratory Combinations are used primarily for relief of symptoms associated with colds, upper respiratory infections and allergic conditions (eg, acute rhinitis, sinusitis).

Ingredients:

Antihistamines are used for symptomatic relief from allergic rhinitis (hay fever) including runny nose, sneezing, itching of the nose or throat, and itchy and watery eyes. The anticholinergic effects of antihistamines may cause a thickening of bronchial secretions; therefore, these agents may be counterproductive in respiratory conditions characterized by congestion. Antihistamines may cause drowsiness.

Xanthines, primarily theophylline, relieve bronchial spasm by direct action on the bronchial smooth muscle in bronchospastic conditions such as asthma and chronic bronchitis. Some xanthine-containing combination products are available over-the-counter, but asthmatic patients should use them only under physician supervision.

Sympathomimetics are used for their vasoconstrictor/decongestant or bronchodilator effects.

Decongestants: Used for temporary relief of nasal congestion due to colds or allergy. Given orally, they are less effective than topical nasal decongestants, and they have a potential for systemic side effects. Frequent or prolonged topical use may lead to local irritation and rebound congestion.

Bronchodilators: Ephedrine is common in these combinations; however, it stimulates cardiac (β_1) receptors. Bronchodilation is weaker than with the catecholamines; α-adrenergic effects may decrease congestion of mucous membranes. Other β-active agents are effective bronchodilators, but pseudoephedrine is not.

Analgesics (eg, acetaminophen, aspirin, ibuprofen, sodium salicylate) are frequently included for symptoms of headache, fever, muscle aches and pain.

Anticholinergics are included for their drying effects on mucous secretions. This action may be beneficial in acute rhinorrhea; however, drying of respiratory secretions may lead to obstruction. Traditionally, anticholinergics have been avoided in patients with asthma or chronic obstructive pulmonary disease (COPD); however, some patients respond well to these agents. Caution is still advised in this group.

An anticholinergic for oral inhalation is available as a bronchodilator for maintenance of bronchospasm associated with COPD, including chronic bronchitis and emphysema.

Papaverine HCl relaxes the smooth muscle of the bronchial tree.

Barbiturates are included for their sedative effects as "correctives" in combination with xanthines or sympathomimetics, which may cause CNS stimulation. The sedative efficacy of low doses (eg, 8 mg phenobarbital) is questionable.

Caffeine is included in some combinations for CNS stimulation to counteract antihistamine depression and to enhance concomitant analgesics.

Antiasthmatic Combinations		
Trade Name	***Strength/Ingredient***	***Average Dose***
Quibron-300 Capsules	300 mg theophylline, 180 mg guaifenesin	16 mg/kg/day or 400 mg/day in divided doses, q 6 to 8 h
Bronchial Capsules, Quibron Capsules	150 mg theophylline, 90 mg guaifenesin	16 mg/kg/day or 400 mg/day, in divided doses, q 6 to 8 h
Glyceryl-T Capsules	150 mg theophylline, 90 mg guaifenesin	1 or 2 bid or tid
Slo-Phyllin GG Capsules[1,2]	150 mg theophylline, 90 mg guaifenesin	3 mg/kg/day q 6 to 8 h
Asbron G Inlay-Tabs[3]	150 mg theophylline, (300 mg theophylline sodium glycinate), 100 mg guaifenesin	1 or 2 tid or qid
Mudrane GG-2 Tablets	111 mg theophylline, (130 mg aminophylline anhydrous), 100 mg guaifenesin	1 tid or qid
Dilor-G Tablets	200 mg dyphylline, 200 mg guaifenesin	1 tid or qid
Dyflex-G Tablets	200 mg dyphylline, 200 mg guaifenesin	1 or 2 qid
Dyline G.G. Tablets	200 mg dyphylline, 200 mg guaifenesin	1 tid or qid
Lufyllin-GG Tablets	200 mg dyphylline, 200 mg guaifenesin	1 qid
Glyceryl-T Liquid, Theolate Liquid	150 mg theophylline, 90 mg guaifenesin per 15 ml	15 ml q 6 to 8 h
Slo-Phyllin GG Syrup[1,3,5]	150 mg theophylline, 90 mg guaifenesin per 15 ml	3 mg/kg/day q 6 to 8 h
Asbron G Elixir[1,3,5]	150 mg theophylline, (300 mg theophylline sodium glycinate), 100 mg guaifenesin, 15% alcohol per 15 ml	3 mg/kg q 6 to 8 h
Synophylate-GG Syrup[1,3,5]	150 mg theophylline, (300 mg theophylline sodium glycinate), 100 mg guaifenesin, 10% alcohol per 15 ml	3 mg/kg q 8 h
Elixophyllin GG Liquid[1]	100 mg theophylline, 100 mg guaifenesin per 15 ml	3 mg/kg q 8 h
Theophylline KI Elixir	80 mg theophylline, 130 mg potassium iodide per 15 ml, alcohol	3 mg/kg q 8 h

[1]Contains sorbitol. [2]Contains parabens. [3]Contains sucrose. [5]Contains saccharin.

Antiasthmatic Combinations		
Trade Name	***Strength/Ingredient***	***Average Dose***
Elixophyllin-KI Elixir[3,5]	80 mg theophylline, 130 mg potassium iodide per 15 ml, 10% alcohol, sodium bisulfite, anise oil	3 mg/kg q 8 h
Iophylline Elixir	120 mg theophylline, 30 mg iodinated glycerol per 15 ml	15 to 30 ml tid
Dilor-G Liquid[1,3,5], Dyline-GG Liquid[1,3,5]	300 mg dyphylline, 300 mg guaifenesin per 15 ml	5 or 10 ml tid or qid
Lufyllin-GG Elixir[3,5]	100 mg dyphylline, 100 mg guaifenesin per 15 ml, 17% alcohol	30 ml qid
Brondelate Elixir	192 mg theophylline (300 mg oxtriphylline), 150 mg guaifenesin per 15 ml, alcohol	10 ml qid
Hydrophed Tablets, Marax Tablets	130 mg theophylline, 25 mg ephedrine sulfate, 10 mg hydroxyzine HCl	1 bid to qid
Mudrane GG Tablets	111 mg theophylline (130 mg aminophylline anhydrous), 16 mg ephedrine HCl, 100 mg guaifenesin, 8 mg phenobarbital	1 tid or qid
Mudrane Tablets	111 mg theophylline (130 mg aminophylline anhydrous), 16 mg ephedrine HCl, 195 mg guaifenesin, 8 mg phenobarbital	1 tid or qid
Quadrinal Tablets	65 mg theophylline (130 mg theophylline calcium salicylate), 24 mg ephedrine HCl, 320 mg potassium iodide, 24 mg phenobarbital	1 tid or qid
Lufylline-EPG Tablets[4]	100 mg dyphylline, 16 mg ephedrine HCl, 200 mg guaifenesin, 16 mg phenobarbital	1 to 2 q 6 h
Lufyllin-EPG Elixir[3,5]	150 mg dyphylline, 24 mg ephedrine HCl, 300 mg guaifenesin, 24 mg phenobarbital per 15 ml, 5.5% alcohol, methylparaben	10 to 20 ml q 6 h
Theomax DF Syrup	97.5 mg theophylline, 18.75 ephedrine, 7.5 mg hydroxyzine HCl per 15 ml, 5% alcohol	Children (> 5 yrs): 5 ml tid or qid; (2 to 5 yrs): 2.5 to 5 ml tid or qid
Marax-DF Syrup[3]	97.5 mg theophylline, 18.75 mg ephedrine, 7.5 mg hydroxyzine HCl per 15 ml, alcohol	Children (> 5 yrs): 5 ml tid or qid; (2 to 5 yrs): 2.5 to 5 ml tid or qid

[1]Contains sorbitol. [3]Contains sucrose. [5]Contains saccharin.
[2]Contains parabens. [4]Contains lactose.

Upper Respiratory Combinations		
Trade Name	***Strength/Ingredient***	***Average Dose***
Cophene No. 2 Capsules, Rescon Capsules	120 mg pseudoephedrine HCl, 12 mg chlorpheniramine maleate	1 q 12 hr
Anamine T.D. Capsules	120 mg pseudoephedrine HCl, 8 mg chlorpheniramine maleate	1 q 8 to 12 h
Brexin L.A. Capsules, Chlorafed Timecelles, Chlordrine S.R. Capsules, Chlorphedrine SR Capsules, Codimal-L.A. Capsules, Colfed-A Capsules, Deconamine SR Capsules, Deconamed SR Capsules, Duralex Capsules, Fedahist Timecaps Capsules, Klerist-D Capsules, Kronofed-A Capsules, N D Clear Capsules, Novafed A Capsules, Pseudo-Chlor Capsules, Rescon-ED Capsules, Rinade B.I.D. Capsules, Time-Hist Capsules	120 mg pseudoephedrine HCl, 8 mg chlorpheniramine maleate	1 q 12 hr
Fedahist Gyrocaps	65 mg pseudoephedrine HCl, 10 mg chlorpheniramine maleate	1 q 12 h
Chlorafed HS Timecelles, Codimal-L.A. Half Capsules	60 mg pseudoephedrine HCl, 4 mg chlorpheniramine maleate	1 or 2 q 12 h
Ed A-Hist Tablets, Prehist Capsules	20 mg phenylephrine HCl, 8 mg chlorpheniramine maleate	1 q 12 g
Allent Capsules, Bromfed Capsules, Endafed Capsules, Iofed Capsules, Ultrabrom Capsules	120 mg pseudoephedrine HCl, 12 mg brompheniramine maleate	1 q 12 h
Biohist-LA Tablets, Carbiset-TR Tabs, Carbodec TR Tabs, Rondec-TR Tablets	120 mg pseudoephedrine HCl, 8 mg carbinoxamine maleate	1 q 12 h
Trinalin Repetabs	120 mg pseudoephedrine HCl, 1 mg azatadine maleate	1 bid
Seldane-D Tablets	120 mg pseudoephedrine HCl, 60 mg terfenadine	1 q AM and at bedtime
Lodrane LD Capsules, Respahist Capsules, Touro A & H Capsules	60 mg pseudoephedrine HCl, 6 mg brompheniramine maleate	1 or 2 q 12 h
Bromfed Tablets	60 mg pseudoephedrine HCl, 4 mg brompheniramine maleate	1 q 4 h
Deconamine Tablets, Klerist-D Tablets	60 mg pseudoephedrine HCl, 4 mg chlorpheniramine maleate	1 tid or qid

Upper Respiratory Combinations		
Trade Name	***Strength/Ingredient***	***Average Dose***
Semprex-D Capsules	60 mg pseudoephedrine HCl, 8 mg acrivastine	1 q 4 to 6 h up to 4/day
Disobrom Tablets, Dexaphen-S.A. Tablets	120 mg pseudoephedrine sulfate, 6 mg dexbrompheniramine maleate	1 q 12 h
Claritin-D Tablets	120 mg pseudoephedrine sulfate, 5 mg loratadine	
Drize Capsules, Ornade Spansules Capsules, Resaid Capsules, Rhinolar-EX 12 Capsules	75 mg phenylpropranolamine HCl, 12 mg chlorpheniramine maleate	1 q 12 h
Dura-Vent/A Capsules	75 mg phenylpropranolamine HCl, 10 mg chlorpheniramine maleate	1 q 12 h
Rhinolar-EX Capsules	75 mg phenylpropranolamine HCl, 8 mg chlorpheniramine maleate	1 q 12 h
E.N.T. Tablets	75 mg phenylpropanolamine HCl, 12 mg brompheniramine maleate	1 q 12 h
Comhist LA Capsules	20 mg phenylephrine HCl, 4 mg chlorpheniramine maleate, 50 mg phenyltoloxamine citrate	1 q 8 to 12 hr
Nolamine Tablets	50 mg phenylpropanolamine HCl, 4 mg chlorpheniramine maleate, 24 mg phenindamine tartrate	1 q 8 to 12 h
Poly-Histine-D Capsules	50 mg phenylpropanolamine HCl, 16 mg phenyltoloxamine citrate, 16 mg pyrilamine maleate, 16 mg pheniramine maleate	1 q 8 to 12 h
Bromophen T.D. Tablets, Tamine S.R. Tablets	15 mg phenylpropanolamine HCl, 15 mg phenylephrine HCl, 12 mg brompheniramine maleate	1 q 8 to 12 h
Decongestabs Tablets, Decongestant Tablets, Naldecon Tablets, Nalgest Tablets, Tri-Phen-Chlor Tablets, Uni-Decon Tablets	40 mg phenylpropanolamine HCl, 10 mg phenylephrine HCl, 5 mg chlorpheniramine maleate, 15 mg phenyltoloxamine citrate	1 tid
Dura-Tap/PD Capsules, Kronofed-A Jr. Capsules, Rescon JR Capsules	60 mg pseudoephedrine HCl, 4 mg chlorpheniramine maleate	Children (6 to 12 years): 1 q 12 h
Atrohist Pediatric Capsules	60 mg pseudoephedrine HCl, 4 mg chlorpheniramine maleate	Children (6 to 12 years): 1 to 2 q 12 h
Bromfed-PD Capsules, Dallergy-JR Capsules, ULTRAbrom PD Capsules	60 mg pseudoephedrine HCl, 6 mg brompheniramine maleate	Children (6 to 12 years): 1 q 12 h

Upper Respiratory Combinations		
Trade Name	***Strength/Ingredient***	***Average Dose***
Poly-Histine D Ped Caps	25 mg phenylpropanolamine HCl, 8 mg phenyltoloxamine citrate, 8 mg pyrilamine maleate, 8 mg pheniramine maleate	Children (6 to 12 years): 1 q 8 to 12 h
Carbiset Tablets, Carbodec Tablets, Rondec Tablet	60 mg pseudoephedrine HCl, 4 mg carbinoxamine maleate	1 qid
Comhist Tablets	10 mg phenylephrine HCl, 2 mg chlorpheniramine maleate, 25 mg phenyltoloxamine citrate	1 or 2 tid q 8 h
R-Tannate Tablets, Rhinatate Tablets, R-Tannamine Tablets, Rynatan Tablets, Tanoral Tablets, Triotann Tablets, Tri-Tannate Tablets	25 mg phenylephrine tannate, 8 mg chlorpheniramine tannate, 25 mg pyrilamine tannate	1 or 2 q 12 h
Hista-Vadrin Tablets	40 mg phenylpropanolamine HCl, 5 mg phenylephrine HCl, 6 mg chlorpheniramine maleate	1 q 6 h
Histalet Forte Tablets, Vanex Forte Caplets	50 mg phenylpropanolamine HCl, 10 mg phenylephrine HCl, 4 mg chlorpheniramine maleate, 25 mg pyrilamine maleate	1 bid or tid
Tanafed Suspension	75 mg pseudoephedrine tannate, 4.5 mg chlorpheniramine tannate	10 to 20 ml q 12 h
Brofed Elixir	30 mg pseudoephedrine HCl, 4 mg brompheniramine maleate per 5 ml	10 ml tid or qid
Ed-A-Hist Liquid	10 mg phenylephrine HCl, 4 mg chlorpheniramine maleate per 5 ml, 5% alcohol	5 ml tid or qid
Histor-D Syrup	5 mg phenylephrine HCl, 2 mg chlorpheniramine maleate per 5 ml, 2% alcohol	5 to 10 ml q 4 to 6 h
Prometh VC Plain Liquid	5 mg phenylephrine HCl, 6.25 mg promethazine per 5 ml, alcohol	5 ml q 4 to 6 h
Phenergan VC Syrup[3]	5 mg phenylephrine HCl, 6.25 mg promethazine per 5 ml, 7% alcohol	5 ml q 4 to 6 h
Carbodec Syrup, Cardec-S Syrup, Rondec Syrup	60 mg pseudoephedrine HCl, 4 mg carbinoxamine per 5 ml	5 ml qid

[1]Contains sorbitol.
[2]Contains sugar.
[3]Contains saccharin.
[4]Contains methylparaben.
[5]Contains sucrose.
[6]Contains lactose.

Upper Respiratory Combinations		
Trade Name	***Strength/Ingredient***	***Average Dose***
Histalet Syrup	45 mg pseudoephedrine HCl, 3 mg chlorphenir-amine maleate per 5 ml	10 ml qid
Anamine Syrup, Anaplex Liquid	30 mg pseudoephedrine HCl, 2 mg chlorphenir-amine maleate per 5 ml	10 ml q 4 to 6 h
Deconamine Syrup	30 mg d-pseudoephed-rine HCl, 2 mg chlor-pheniramine maleate per 5 ml	5 to 10 ml tid or qid
Liqui-Histine-D Elixir, Poly-Histine-D Elixir	12.5 mg phenylpropanol-amine HCl, 4 mg pyrilamine maleate, 4 mg phenyltoloxamine citrate, 4 mg pheniramine maleate per 5 ml, 4% alcohol	10 ml q 4 h
Naldelate Syrup, Nalgest Syrup[1], Naldecon Syrup, Tri-Phen-Chlor Syrup	20 mg phenylpropanol-amine HCl, 5 mg phenylephrine HCl, 2.5 mg chlorpheniramine maleate,7.5 mg phenyltoloxamine citrate	5 ml q 3 to 4 h up to 20 ml/day
Rondec Oral Drops	25 mg pseudoephedrine HCl, 2 mg carbinoxamine maleate per ml	Infants: 0.25 to 1 ml qid
Atrohist Pediatric Sus-pension, R-Tannamine Pediatric Suspension, R-Tannate Pediatric Sus-pension[3,4,5], Rynatan Pediatric Suspension[3,4,5], Rynatan-S Pediatric Sus-pension[3,4,5], Tri-Tannate Pediatric Suspension[3,4,5]	5 mg phenylephrine tannate, 2 mg chlorphen-iramine tannate, 12.5 mg pyrilamine tannate per 5 ml	Children (> 6 yrs): 5 to 10 ml q 12 h; (2 to 6 yrs): 2.5 to 5 ml q 12 h
Triaminic Oral Infant Drops[1,3,5]	20 mg phenylpropanol-amine HCl, 10 mg pyrilamine maleate, 10 mg pheniramine maleate per ml	Infants: 1 drop/2 lbs qid
Naldelate Pediatric Syrup, Naldecon Pediatric Syrup[1], Nalgest Pediatric Syrup[1], Tri-Phen-Mine Pediatric Syrup, Tri-Phen-Chlor Pediatric Syrup[1]	5 mg phenylpropanol-amine HCl, 1.25 mg phenylephrine HCl, 0.5 mg chlorpheniramine maleate, 2 mg phenyltol-oxamine citrate per 5 ml	Children (6 to 12 mos): 2.5 ml q 3 to 4 h up to 10 ml/day; (1 to 6 yrs): 5 ml q 3 to 4 h up to 20 ml/day; (6 to 12 yrs): 10 ml q 3 to 4 h up to 40 ml/day
Naldecon Pediatric Drops[1], Nalgest Pediatric Drops, Tri-Phen-Mine Pe-diatric Drops, Tri-Phen-Chlor Pediatric Drops	5 mg phenylpropanol-amine HCl, 1.25 mg phenylephrine HCl, 0.5 mg chlorpheniramine maleate, 2 mg phenyltoloxamine citrate per ml	Children (3 to 6 mos): 0.25 ml q 3 to 4 h; (6 to 12 mos): 0.5 ml q 3 to 4 h; (1 to 6 yrs): 1 ml q 3 to 4 h up to 4 doses/day

[1]Ccntains sorbitol. [3]Contains saccharin. [5]Contains sucrose.
[2]Contains sugar. [4]Contains methylparaben. [6]Contains lactose.

Upper Respiratory Combinations		
Trade Name	***Strength/Ingredient***	***Average Dose***
Norel Plus Capsules[6]	25 mg phenylpropanolamine HCl, 4 mg chlorpheniramine maleate, 25 mg phenyltoloxamine dihydrogen citrate, 325 mg acetaminophen	1 q 3 to 4 h up to 6/day
Rhinolar Capsules	75 mg phenylpropanolamine HCl, 8 mg chlorpheniramine maleate, 2.5 mg methscopolamine nitrate	1 q 12 h
Dallergy Capsules, Dura-Vent/DA Tablets, Extendryl SR Capsules, OMNhist L.A. Tablets, Prehist D Capsules and Tablets	20 mg phenylephrine HCl, 8 mg chlorpheniramine, 2.5 mg methscopolamine nitrate	1 q 12 h
Atrohist Plus Tablets, Phenclor S.H.A. Tablets, Ru-Tuss Tablets, Stahist Tablets, Phenahist-TR Tablets	50 mg phenylpropanolamine HCl, 25 mg phenylephrine HCl, 8 mg chlorpheniramine maleate, 0.19 mg hyoscyamine sulfate, 0.04 mg atropine sulfate, 0.01 mg scopolamine HBr	1 q 12 hr
Mescolor Tablets	120 mg pseudoephedrine HCl, 8 mg chlorpheniramine maleate, 2.5 mg methscopolamine nitrate	1 q 12 h
Dallergy Tablets	10 mg phenylephrine HCl, 4 mg chlorpheniramine maleate, 1.25 mg methscopolamine nitrate	1 q 4 to 6 h
AH-chew Tablets, D.A. Chewable Tablets, Extendryl Chewable Tablets	10 mg phenylephrine HCl, 2 mg chlorpheniramine maleate, 1.25 mg methscopolamine nitrate	1 or 2 q 4 h
Extendryl Syrup	10 mg phenylephrine HCl, 2 mg chlorpheniramine maleate, 1.25 mg methscopolamine nitrate	5 or 10 ml q 3 or 4 h qid
Dallergy Syrup	10 mg phenylephrine HCl, 2 mg chlorpheniramine maleate, 0.625 mg methscopolamine nitrate	10 ml q 4 to 6 h up to 4 doses/day
Extendryl JR Capsules	10 mg phenylephrine HCl, 4 mg chlorpheniramine maleate, 1.25 mg methscopolamine nitrate	Children (6 to 12 yrs): 1 q 12 h

[1]Contains sorbitol. [2]Contains sugar. [3]Contains saccharin. [4]Contains methylparaben. [5]Contains sucrose. [6]Contains lactose.

Orphan Drugs

The Orphan Drug Act defines an orphan drug as a drug or biological product for the diagnosis, treatment or prevention of a rare disease or condition. A rare disease is one which affects < 200,000 persons in the US or one which affects > 200,000 persons but for which there is no reasonable expectation that the cost of developing the drug and making it available will be recovered from sales of that drug in the US.

The FDA Office of Orphan Products Development (OPD) provides an information package that includes an overview of the FDA's orphan drug program, a brief description of the orphan products grant program and a current list of designated orphan products. OPD's information package also contains a directory sheet listing sources of information about the treatment of rare diseases, patient organizations and availability of orphan drugs. Requests for the Rare Disease Information Directory, or the entire orphan drugs information package, may be made by contacting OPD:

Office of Orphan Products Development (HF-35)
5600 Fishers Lane
Rockville, MD 20857
(301) 443-2043

Drug (Trade name)	***Proposed use***	***Sponsor***
Acetylcysteine *(Mucomyst, Mucomyst 10 IV)*	IV for moderate to severe acetaminophen overdose	Apothecon
Acid implant (intravitreal, ganciclovir-free) *(Vitrasert Implant)*	Cytomegalovirus retinitis	Chiron Vision
Aconiazide	Tuberculosis	Lincoln Diagnostics
Adeno-associated viral-based vector cystic fibrosis gene therapy	Cystic fibrosis	Targeted Genetics
Aerosol talc (sterile)	Malignant pleural effusion	Bryan
AI-RSA	Autoimmune uveitis	Autoimmune, Inc.
Albendazole	Hydatid cyst disease (cystic echinococcosis due to *E granulosus* larvae or alveolar echinococcosis due to *E multilocularis* larvae); neurocysticercosis due to Taenia solium as chemotherapy of parenchymal, subarachnoidal and racemose (cysts in spinal fluid) neurocysticercosis in symptomatic cases; prophylaxis of epilepsy and other sequelae in asymptomatic neurocysticercosis.	SmithKline Beecham Pharm
Aldesleukin *(Proleukin)*	Metastatic renal cell carcinoma[1]; primary immunodeficiency disease associated with T-cell defects	Chiron Cetus

[1]Approved for marketing.

Drug (Trade name)	Proposed use	Sponsor
Alglucerase Injection *(Ceredase)*	Replacement therapy in Gaucher's disease type 1[1]	Genzyme
Allopurinol sodium *(Zyloprim for Injection)*	Management of leukemia, lymphoma and solid tumor malignancies in patients who cannot tolerate oral therapy and are receiving cancer therapy that causes elevations of serum and urinary uric acid levels	Glaxo Wellcome
Alpha-galactosidase A *(FABRase)* *(CC-Galactosidase)*	Fabry's disease	Robert J. Desnick, MD David H. Calhoun, PhD
Alpha-1-antitrypsin (recombinant DNA origin)	Supplementation therapy for alpha-1-antitrypsin deficiency in the ZZ phenotype population	Cooper Development
Alpha-1-proteinase inhibitor *(Prolastin)*	Replacement therapy in the alpha-1-proteinase inhibitor congenital deficiency state[1]	Cutter Biological
Alprostadil *(Vasoprost)*	Severe peripheral arterial occlusive disease (critical limb ischemia) in patients where other procedures, grafts or angioplasty, are not indicated	Schwarz Pharma
Altretamine *(Hexalen)*	Advanced ovarian adenocarcinoma[1]	U.S. Bioscience
Amifostine *(Ethyol)*	Chemoprotective agent for: Cisplatin in metastatic melanoma and advanced ovarian carcinoma; cyclophosphamide in advanced ovarian carcinoma	U.S. Bioscience
Amiloride HCL solution for inhalation	Cystic fibrosis	Glaxo Wellcome
Aminocaproic acid	Topical treatment of traumatic hyphema of the eye	Orphan Medical
Aminosalicylate sodium	Crohn's disease	Syncom
Aminosalicylic acid *(Pasar Granules)*	Tuberculosis infections	Jacobus
4-Aminosalicylic acid (*Pamisyl* [Parke-Davis]; *Rezipas* [Squibb])	Mild to moderate ulcerative colitis in patients intolerant to sulfasalazine	Warren Beeken, MD
Aminosidine *(Gabbromicina)* *(Paromomycin)*	*Mycobacterium avium* complex; Visceral leishmaniasis (KALA-AZAR)	Thomas P. Kanyok, PharmD
Amiodarone *(Amio-Aqueous)* *(Cordarone)*	Incessant ventricular tachycardia[1]; acute treatment[1] and prophylaxis of life-threatening ventricular tachycardia or ventricular fibrillation	Academic Pharm Wyeth-Ayerst
Ammonium tetrathiomolybdate	Wilson's disease	George J. Brewer, MD
Amphotericin B lipid complex	Cryptococcal meningitis	Liposome Co.

[1]Approved for marketing.

Drug (Trade name)	Proposed use	Sponsor
Anagrelide	Polycythemia vera; essential thrombocythemia; thrombocytosis in chronic myelogenous leukemia	Roberts Pharm
Ananain, Comosain *(Vainain)*	For enzymatic debridement of severe burns	Genzyme
Anaritide acetate *(Auriculin)*	Improvement of early renal allograft function following renal transplantation; acute renal failure	Scios Nova
Ancrod *(Arvin)*	Antithrombotic in patients with heparin-induced thrombocytopenia or thrombosis who require immediate and continued anticoagulation	Knoll Pharm
Antiepilepsirine	Drug-resistant generalized tonic-clonic epilepsy in children and adults	Children's Hospital, Columbus, OH
Antihemophilic factor, human *(Humate P)*	Von Willebrand's disease	Behringwerke Aktiengesellschaft
Antihemophilic factor (recombinant) *(Kogenate)*	Prophylaxis/treatment of bleeding in hemophilia A[1]; for prophylaxis when surgery is required in these patients[1]	Miles
Anti-Tac, humanized	Prevention of acute renal allograft rejection; prevention of acute graft-vs-host disease following bone marrow transplantation	Hoffmann-LaRoche
Antithrombin III Concentrate IV *(Kybernin)*	Prophylaxis/treatment of thromboembolic episodes in genetic AT-III deficiency	Hoechst-Marion Roussel
Antithrombin III human *(Thrombate III)* *(ATnativ)*	Hereditary antithrombin III deficiency in connection with surgical or obstetrical procedures or thromboembolism[1]; replacement therapy in congenital deficiency of AT-III to prevent and treat thrombosis and pulmonary emboli[1]; to prevent/arrest episodes of thrombosis in patients with congenital AT-III deficiency or to prevent the occurrence of thrombosis in patients with AT-III deficiency who have undergone trauma or are about to undergo surgery or parturition	Red Cross Miles Kabivitrum
Anti-thymocyte serum *(Nashville Rabbit Anti-thymocyte serum)*	Allograft rejection, including kidney, liver, heart, lung, pancreas and bone marrow transplantation	Applied Medical Research
Antivenin, polyvalent crotalid (Ovine) Fab *(Crotab)*	Treatment of the envenomations inflicted by North American crotalid snakes[1]	Therapeutic Antibodies
Antivenom (Crotalidae) Purified (Avain)	Treatment of envenomation by poisonous snakes belonging to the crotalidae family[1]	Ophidian
APL 400-200	Cutaneous t-cell lymphoma	Apollon

[1]Approved for marketing.

Drug (Trade name)	***Proposed use***	***Sponsor***
Apomorphine HCl	Treatment of the on-off fluctuations associated with late-stage Parkinson's disease	Forum Products
Aprotonin *(Trasylol)*	Prophylaxis to reduce perioperative blood loss and the homologous blood transfusion requirement in patients undergoing repeat coronary artery bypass graft (CABG) surgery, and in selected cases of primary CABG surgery when the risk of bleeding is especially high or where transfusion is unavailable or unacceptable[1]	Miles
Arginine Butyrate	Beta-hemoglobinopathies and beta-thalassemia; sickle cell disease and beta-thalassemia	Susan P. Perrine, MD Vertex Pharm
Atoquavone *(Mepron)*	AIDS-associated *Pneumocystis carinii* pneumonia (PCP)[1]; prevention of PCP in high-risk, HIV-infected patients (defined by one or more episodes of PCP or a peripheral CD4+ lymphocyte count $\leq 200/mm^3$); treatment/suppression of *Toxoplasma gondii* encephalitis; primary prophylaxis of HIV-infected persons at high risk for developing *T gondii* encephalitis	Glaxo Wellcome
Autolymphocyte therapy; ALT	Renal cell carcinoma; renal cancer	Cellcor
Bacitracin *(Altracin)*	Antibiotic-associated pseudomembranous enterocolitis caused by toxins A and B elaborated by *C difficile*	A.L. Labs
Baclofen *(Lioresal intrathecal)*	Intractable spasticity caused by spinal cord injury/multiple sclerosis and other spinal diseases (ie, spinal ischemia, spinal tumor, cerebral palsy, transverse myelitis, cervical spondylosis and degenerative myelopathy)[1]	Medtronic
Benzoate and phenylacetate *(Ucephan)*	Adjunctive therapy to prevent/treat hyperammonemia in patients with urea cycle enzymopathy due to carbamylphosphate synthetase, ornithine, transcarbamylase or arginosuccinate synthetase deficiency[1]	Kendall McGaw
Benzylpenicillin, benzylpenicilloic, benzylpenilloic acid *(Pre-Pen/MDM)*	To assess risk of penicillin use when it is the preferred drug in adults who previously received penicillin and have a history of sensitivity	Kremers-Urban

[1]Approved for marketing.

Drug (Trade name)	Proposed use	Sponsor
Beractant *(Survanta Intratracheal Suspension)*	To prevent/treat neonatal respiratory distress syndrome[1]; full-term newborns with respiratory failure caused by meconium aspiration syndrome; persistent pulmonary hypertension of the newborn; or pneumonia and sepsis	Ross
Betaine	Homocystinuria	Orphan Medical
Bispecific antibody 520C9x22	In vivo serotherapy of ovarian cancer	Medarex
Bleomycin sulfate *(Blenoxane)*	Malignant pleural effusion	Bristol-Myers Squibb
Botulinum toxin type A *(Botox)* *(Dysport)*	Blepharospasm and strabismus associated with dystonia in adults (≥ 12 years old)[1]; cervical dystonia; dynamic muscle contracture in pediatric cerebral palsy; essential blepharospasm; synkinetic closure of the eyelid associated with VIII cranial nerve aberrant regeneration	Associated Synapse Biologics Allergan Porton
Botulinum toxin type B	Cervical dystonia	Athena Neurosciences
Botulinum toxin type F	Spasmodic torticollis (cervical dystonia); essential blepharospasm	Porton
Botulism immune globulin	Infant botulism	CA Dept. Health Service
Bovine colostrum	AIDS-related diarrhea	Donald Hastings, DVM
Bovine whey protein concentrate *(Immuno-C)*	Cryptosporidiosis caused by *Cryptosporidium parvum* in the GI tract of patients who are immunodeficient/immunocompromised or immunocompetent	Biomune Systems
Branched chain amino acids	Amyotrophic lateral sclerosis	Mount Sinai Medical Center
Bromhexine	Mild/moderate keratoconjunctivitis sicca in Sjogren's syndrome	Boehringer Ingelheim
Bromodeoxyuridine	Radiation sensitizer in the treatment of primary brain tumors	NeoPharm
Buprenorphine HCl	With naloxone or alone for treatment of opiate addictions	Reckitt and Coleman
Busulfan	Preparative therapy for malignancies treated with bone marrow transplantation	Sparta Orphan Medical
Butyrylcholinesterase	Reduction and clearance of toxic blood levels of cocaine in overdose; post-surgical apnea	Pharmavene
C1-Esterase-inhibitor, human, pasteurized	Prevention/treatment of acute attacks of hereditary angioedema	Behringwerke Aktiengesellschaft

[1]Approved for marketing.

Drug (Trade name)	Proposed use	Sponsor
C1 inhibitor *(C1-Inhibitor (human) Vapor Heated, Immuno)*	Treatment of acute attacks of angioedema; prevention of acute attacks of angioedema, including short-term prophylaxis for patients requiring dental or other surgical procedures	Immuno
Caffeine *(Neocaf)*	Apnea of prematurity	O.P.R. Development, L.P.
Calcitonin-human for injection *(Cibacalcin)*	Symptomatic Paget's disease of bone (osteitis deformans)[1]	Ciba-Geigy
Calcium acetate *(Phos-Lo)*	Hyperphosphatemia in end-stage renal failure/disease[1]	Pharmedic Braintree
Calcium carbonate *(R&D Calcium Carbonate/600)*	Hyperphosphatemia in end-stage renal disease	R & D
Calcium gluconate gel *(H-F Gel)* *(Calcium gluconate gel 2.5%)*	Emergency topical treatment of hydrogen fluoride (hydrofluoric acid) burns	LTR Pharm Paddock
Carbovir	AIDS; symptomatic HIV infection and CD4 count < 200/mm^3	Glaxo Wellcome
Cascara sagrada fluid extract	For oral drug overdosage to speed lower bowel evacuation	Intramed
CCD 1042	Infantile spasms	Cocensys, Inc.
CD4 immunoglobulin G, recombinant human	AIDS resulting from HIV-1 infection	Genentech
CD4, recombinant soluble human (rCD4) *(Receptin)*	AIDS, including patients infected with HIV	Genentech Biogen
CD5-T lymphocyte immunotoxin *(Xomazyme-H65)*	Graft-vs-host disease or rejection in bone marrow transplants	Xoma
Ceramide trihexosidease/alpha-galactosidase A	Fabry's disease	Genzyme
Chenodiol *(Chenix)*	For radiolucent stones in well opacifying gallbladders, where elective surgery would be undertaken except for presence of increased surgical risk due to systemic disease or age[1]	Solvay
Chimeric A2 (human-murine) IgG monoclonal anti-TNF antibody (cA2)	Crohn's disease	Centocor
Chimeric M-T412 (human-murine) IgG monoclonal anti-CD4	Multiple sclerosis	Centocor
Chimeric (murine variable, human constant) Mab (C2B8) to CD20	Non-Hodgkin's B-cell lymphoma	Idec Pharm

[1]Approved for marketing.

Drug (Trade name)	*Proposed use*	*Sponsor*
Chlorhexidine gluconate mouthrinse *(Peridex)*	Amelioration of oral mucositis associated with cytoreductive therapy for conditioning patients for bone marrow transplantation	Procter & Gamble
2-Chlorodeoxyade-nosine	Acute myeloid leukemia	RW Johnson Res
Choline chloride	Choline deficiency, specifically the choline deficiency, hepatic steatosis, and cholestasis, associ-ated with long-term parenteral nutrition	Alan Buchman, MD
Chondroitinase	Patients undergoing vitrectomy	Storz Ophthalmics
Ciliary neutrotrophic factor	Amyotrophic lateral sclerosis	Regeneron Pharm
Ciliary neutrotrophic factor (recombinant human)	Spinal muscular atrophies; motor neuron disease (including amyo-trophic lateral sclerosis, progres-sive muscular atrophy, progressive bulbar palsy and primary lateral sclerosis)	Syntex-Synergen
Citric acid, glucono-delta-lactone and mag carbonate *(Renacidin Irrigation)*	Renal and bladder calculi of the apatite or struvite variety[1]	United-Guardian
Cladribine *(Leustatin Injection)*	Hairy-cell[1] and chronic lympho-cytic leukemias; non-Hodgkin's lymphoma; chronic multiple sclerosis	RW Johnson Res
Clindamycin *(Cleocin)*	Treatment/prevention of *Pneumo-cystis carinii* pneumonia associ-ated with AIDS	Upjohn
Clofazimine *(Lamprene)*	Lepromatous leprosy, including dapsone-resistant lepromatous leprosy and lepromatous leprosy complicated by erythema nodosum leprosum[1]	Ciba-Geigy
Clonazepam *(Klonopin)*	Hyperekplexia (startle disease)	Hoffman-La Roche
Clonidine	Epidural use for pain in cancer patients tolerant/unresponsive to intraspinal opiates	Fujisawa
Clotrimidazole	Sickle cell disease	Carlo Brugnara, MD
Coagulation factor IX *(Mononine)*	Replacement/prophylaxis of hemorrhagic complications of hemophilia B[1]	Armour Pharm
Coagulation factor IX (human) *(AlphaNine)*	Replacement therapy in hemo-philia B for prevention and control of bleeding episodes; during surgery to correct defective hemostasis[1]	Alpha Therapeutic
Coagulation factor IX (recombinant)	Hemophilia B	Genetics Institute

[1]Approved for marketing.

Drug (Trade name)	*Proposed use*	*Sponsor*
Colchicine	Arresting progression of neurologic disability due to chronic progressive multiple sclerosis	PharmaControl
Colfosceril palmitate, cetyl alcohol, tyloxapol *(Exosurf Neonatal for Intratracheal Suspension) (Exosurf)*	To prevent hyaline membrane disease (respiratory distress syndrome) in infants born at ≤ 32 weeks gestation[1]; to treat established hyaline membrane disease at all gestational ages[1]; adult respiratory distress syndrome	Glaxo Wellcome
Collagen (Purified Type II) *(Colloral)*	Juvenile rheumatoid arthritis	AutoImmune
Collagenase (lyophilized) for injection *(Plaquase)*	Peyronie's disease	Advance Biofactures
Copolymer 1 *(Copaxone)*	Multiple sclerosis	Lemmon
Corticorelin Ovine Triflutate *(Acthrel)*	To differentiate between pituitary and ectopic production of ACTH in ACTH-dependent Cushing's syndrome	Ferring
Coumarin *(Oncostate)*	Renal cell carcinoma	Schaper and Brummer GmbH & Co.
Cromolyn sodium *(Gastrocrom)*	Mastocytosis[1]	Fisons
Cromolyn sodium 4% ophthalmic solution *(Opticrom)*	Vernal keratoconjunctivitis[1]	Fisons
Cryptosporidium hyperimmune bovine colostrum IgG concentrate	Diarrhea in AIDS patients caused by infection with *Cryptosporidium parvum*	Immucell
Cryptosporidium parvum bovine immunoglobulin concentrate *(Sporidin-G)*	Treatment/symptomatic relief of *Cryptosporidium parvum* infection of the GI tract in immunocompromised patients	Galagen
CY-1503	Post-ischemic pulmonary reperfusion edema following surgical treatment for chronic thromboembolic pulmonary hypertension	Cytel
CY-1899	Chronic active hepatitis B infection in HLA-A2 positive patients	Cytel
Cyclosporine ophthalmic *(Optimmune)*	Severe keratoconjunctivitis sicca with Sjogren's syndrome	University of Georgia
Cyclosporine 2% ophthalmic ointment	Treatment of patients at high risk of graft rejection following penetrating keratoplasty; corneal melting syndromes of known or presumed immunologic etiopathogenesis, including Mooren's ulcer	Allergan

[1]Approved for marketing.

Drug (Trade name)	Proposed use	Sponsor
Cysteamine *(Cystagon)*	Nephropathic cystinosis	Jess Thoene, MD Mylan
Cystic fibrosis gene, lipid/DNA human	Cystic fibrosis	Genzyme
Cystic fibrosis gene therapy	Cystic fibrosis	Genzyme
Cystic fibrosis transmembrane conductance regulator	Cystic fibrosis transmembrane conductance regulator protein replacement therapy in cystic fibrosis patients	Genzyme
Cystic fibrosis transmembrane conductance regulator gene	Cystic fibrosis	Genetic Therapy
Cystic Fibrosis Tr gene therapy (recombinant adenovirus) *(AdGVCFTR.10)*	Cystic fibrosis	Genvac
Cytarabine, depofoam encapsulated	Neoplastic meningitis	Kim Sinil, MD
Cytomegalovirus immune globulin (human)	Prevention or attenuation of primary cytomegalovirus disease in immunosuppressed recipients of organ transplants[1]	MA Public Health Bio Labs
Cytomegalovirus immune globulin IV (human)	With ganciclovir sodium for the treatment of CMV pneumonia in bone marrow transplant patients	Miles
Cytomegalovirus monoclonal antibody (human)	Prophylaxis of cytomegalovirus disease in patients undergoing solid organ transplantation; treatment of cytomegalovirus retinitis in patients with AIDS	Protein Design Labs
Dapsone	Prophylaxis of toxoplasmosis in severely immunocompromised patients with CD4 counts < 100	Jacobus Pharm
Dapsone, USP	Prophylaxis of *Pneumocystis carinii* pneumonia; with trimethoprim for treatment of PCP	Jacobus Pharm
Daunorubicin, liposomal *(Daunoxome)*	Treatment of patients with advanced HIV-associated Kaposi's sarcoma	Vestar
Defibrotide	Thrombotic thrombocytopenic purpura	Crinos International
Dehydrex	Recurrent corneal erosion unresponsive to conventional therapy	Holles Labs
Dehydroepiandrosterone	Systemic lupus erythematosus (SLE) and reduction of steroid use in SLE patients	Genelabs
Deoxycytidine, 5-aza-2′	Acute leukemia	Pharmachemie U.S.A.
Deslorelin *(Somagard)*	Central precocious puberty	Roberts Pharm
Desmopressin acetate	Mild hemophilia A and von Willebrand's disease[1]	Rhone-Poulenc Rorer

[1]Approved for marketing.

Drug (Trade name)	*Proposed use*	*Sponsor*
Dexrazoxane *(Zinecard)*	Prevention of cardiomyopathy associated with doxorubicin administration	Adria
Dextran and deferoxamine *(Bio-Rescue)*	Acute iron poisoning	Biomedical Frontiers
Dextran sulfate, (inhaled, aerosolized) *(Uendex)*	As an adjunct to the treatment of cystic fibrosis	Kennedy & Hoidal, MDs
Dextran sulfate sodium	AIDS	Ueno Fine Chemicals
3,4-Diaminopyridine	Lambert-Eaton myasthenic syndrome	Jacobus Pharm
Dianeal peritoneal dialysis soln with 1.1% amino acid *(Nutrineal [Peritoneal Dialysis Soln with 1.1% Amino Acid])*	Nutritional supplement for malnourishment in patients undergoing continuous ambulatory peritoneal dialysis	Baxter Healthcare
Diazepam viscous rectal solution	Rectal administration for acute repetitive seizures	Athena
Dibromodulcitol	Recurrent invasive or metastatic squamous cervical carcinoma	Biopharmaceutics
Diethyldithiocarbomate *(Imuthiol)*	AIDS	Connaught
Digoxin Immune fab (ovine) *(Digibind)* *(Digidote)*	Treatment of potentially life-threatening digitalis intoxication in patients refractory to management by conventional therapy[1]; life-threatening acute cardiac glycoside intoxication manifested by conduction disorders, ectopic ventricular activity and sometimes hyperkalemia	Glaxo Wellcome Boehringer Mannheim
5,6-dihydro-5-azacytidine	Malignant mesothelioma	ILEX Oncology
Dihydrotestosterone *(Androgel-DHT)*	Weight loss in AIDS patients with HIV-associated wasting	Unimed Pharm
24,25 Dihydroxycholecalciferol	Uremic osteodystrophy	Lemmon
Dimethyl Sulfoxide	Increased intracranial pressure in patients with severe, closed-head injury for whom no other effective treatment is available	Pharma 21
Dipalmitoylphosphatidylcholine/ phosphatidylglycerol *(ALEC)*	Prevention/treatment of neonatal respiratory distress syndrome	Forum Products
Disaccharide tripeptide glycerol dipalmitoyl *(Immther)*	Pulmonary and hepatic metastases in colorectal adenocarcinoma	Immuno Therapeutics
Disodium clodronate	Hypercalcemia of malignancy	Discovery Experimental & Development

[1]Approved for marketing.

Drug (Trade name)	Proposed use	Sponsor
Disodium clodronate tetrahydrate *(Bonefos)*	Increased bone resorption due to malignancy	Leiras Pharm
Disodium silibinin dihemisuccinate *(Legalon)*	Hepatic intoxication by *Amanita phalloides* (mushroom poisoning)	Pharmaquest
Dornase alfa *(Pulmozyme)*	Reduces mucous viscosity and enables the clearance of airway secretions in cystic fibrosis[1]	Genentech
Dronabinol *(Marinol)*	For the stimulation of appetite and prevention of weight loss in patients with a confirmed diagnosis of AIDS[1]	Unimed
Dynamine	Lambert-Eaton myasthenic syndrome; hereditary motor and sensory neuropathy type I (Charcot-Marie-Tooth disease)	Mayo Foundation
Eflornithine HCl *(Ornidyl)*	*Trypanosoma brucei gambiense* (sleeping sickness)[1]	Hoechst-Marion Roussel
Elcatonin	Intrathecal treatment of intractable pain	Innapharma
Elliot's B Solution	Acute lymphatic leukemias and acute lymphoblastic lymphomas	Orphan Medical
Epidermal growth factor (human)	Acceleration of corneal epithelial regeneration and healing of stromal tissue in non-healing corneal defects	Chiron
Epoetin alfa *(Epogen)* *(Procrit)*	Anemia associated with end-stage renal disease, or HIV infection or treatment[1]; myelodysplastic syndrome	RW Johnson Res Amgen
Epoetin beta *(Marogen)*	Anemia associated with end-stage renal disease	Chugai-USA
Epoprostenol *(Flolan)*	Primary pulmonary hypertension; replacement of heparin in patients requiring hemodialysis at increased risk of hemorrhage	Glaxo Wellcome
Erwinia L-asparaginase *(Erwinase)*	Acute lymphocytic leukemia	Porton
Erythropoietin (recombinant human)	Anemia related to HIV infection or treatment; anemia associated with end-stage renal disease[1]; anemia of premature infants	McDonnell Douglas RW Johnson Res
Ethanolamine oleate *(Ethamolin)*	Esophageal varices that have recently bled, to prevent rebleeding[1]	Block
Ethinyl estradiol, USP	Turner's syndrome	Bio-Technology
Etidronate disodium *(Didronel)*	Hypercalcemia of malignancy inadequately managed by dietary modification or oral hydration[1]	MGI
Etiocholanedione	Aplastic anemia	SuperGen
Exemestane	Hormonal therapy of metastatic carcinoma of the breast	Pharmacia

[1]Approved for marketing.

Drug (Trade name)	*Proposed use*	*Sponsor*
Factor VII-a (recombinant, DNA origin)	Hemophilia A and B with and without antibodies against Factors VIII/IX; von Willebrand's disease	Novo Nordisk
Factor XIII (placenta-derived) *(Fibrogammin P)*	Congenital Factor XIII deficiency	Hoechst-Marion Roussel
Fampridine *(Neurelan)*	Relief of symptoms of multiple sclerosis	Elan Pharm Res
Felbamate *(Felbatol)*	Lennox-Gastaut syndrome	Wallace
FGN-1	For suppression and control of colonic adematous polyps in adenomatous polyposis coli	Cell Pathways
FIAU	Adjunctive treatment of chronic active hepatitis B	Oclassen
Fibrinogen (human)	Control of bleeding and prophylactic treatment of patients deficient in fibrinogen	Alpha Therapeutic
Fibronectin (human plasma derived)	Non-healing corneal ulcers or epithelial defects unresponsive to conventional therapy (underlying cause has been eliminated)	New York Blood Center
Filgrastim *(Neupogen)*	Myelodysplastic syndrome; severe chronic neutropenia (absolute neutrophil count < $500/mm^3$); neutropenia associated with bone marrow transplants; AIDS patients with CMV retinitis being treated with ganciclovir	Amgen
Fire ant venom, allergenic extract, imported	For skin testing of victims of fire ant stings to confirm fire ant sensitivity and if positive, for use as immunotherapy for the prevention of IgE-mediated anaphylactic reactions	ALK Lab
Fludarabine phosphate *(Fludara)*	Treatment/management of non-Hodgkin's lymphoma; chronic lymphocytic leukemia (CLL) including refractory CLL[1]	Berlex
Flumecinol *(Zixoryn)*	Hyperbilirubinemia in newborns unresponsive to phototherapy	Farmacon
Flunarizine *(Sibelium)*	Alternating hemiplegia	Janssen
Flourouracil *(Adrucil)*	With interferon alpha-2a esophageal/advanced colorectal carcinoma; with leucovorin for metastatic adenocarcinoma of the colon and rectum	Hoffman-LaRoche Lederle
Fomepizole *(Antizol)*	Methanol or ethylene glycol poisoning	Orphan Medical
Fosphenytoin	Acute treatment of patients with status epilepticus of the grand mal type	Warner-Lambert
Gabapentin *(Neurontin)*	Amyotrophic lateral sclerosis	Warner-Lambert

[1]Approved for marketing.

Drug (Trade name)	*Proposed use*	*Sponsor*
Gallium nitrate injection *(Ganite)*	Hypercalcemia of malignancy[1]	Fujisawa
Gamma-hydroxybutyrate	Narcolepsy	Orphan Medical
Gammalinolenic acid	Juvenile rheumatoid arthritis	Robert B. Zurier, MD
Gelsolin, recombinant human	Respiratory symptoms of cystic fibrosis; treatment of acute and chronic respiratory symptoms of bronchiectasis	Biogen
Gentamicin impregnated PMMA beads on surgical wire *(Septopal)*	Chronic osteomyelitis of posttraumatic, postoperative or hematogenous origin	EM
Gentamicin liposome injection *(Maitec)*	Disseminated *Mycobacterium avium*-intracellulare infection	Liposome Company
Glucocerebrosidase, recombinant retroviral vector	Enzyme replacement therapy for types I, II or III Gaucher's Disease	Genetic Therapy
Glutamine	With human growth hormone in treatment of short bowel syndrome (nutrient malabsorption from the GI tract resulting from an inadequate absorptive surface)	Research Triangle Pharm
Glyceryl trioleate and glyceryl trierucate	Adrenoleukodystrophy	Hugo W. Moser, MD
Gonadorelin acetate *(Lutrepulse)*	Ovulation induction in women with hypothalamic amenorrhea due to a deficiency or absence in quantity or pulse pattern of endogenous Gn-RH secretion[1]	RW Johnson Res
Gossypol	Cancer of the adrenal cortex	Marcus M Reidenberg, MD
Growth hormone releasing factor	Long-term treatment of children who have growth failure due to a lack of adequate endogenous growth hormone secretion	ICN Pharm
Guanethidine monosulfate *(Ismelin)*	Moderate/severe reflex sympathetic dystrophy and causalgia	Ciba-Geigy
Halofantrine *(Halfan)*	Mild to moderate acute malaria caused by susceptible strains of *Plasmodium falciparum* and *P vivax*[1]	SmithKline Beecham
Heme arginate *(Normosang)*	Symptomatic stage of acute porphyria; myelodysplastic syndromes	Leiras
Hemin *(Panhematin)*	Amelioration of recurrent attacks of acute intermittent porphyria (AIP) temporarily related to menstrual cycle and similar symptoms which occur in other patients with AIP, *porphyria variegata* and *heredita coproporphyria*[1]	Abbott

[1]Approved for marketing.

Drug (Trade name)	*Proposed use*	*Sponsor*
Hemin and zinc mesoporphyrin *(Hemex)*	Acute porphyric syndromes	Herbert L. Bonkovsky, MD
Heparin, 2-0-desulfated *(Aeropin)*	Cystic fibrosis	Kennedy & Hoidal, MDs
Hepatitis B immune globulin IV *(H-BIGIV)*	Prophylaxis against hepatitis B virus reinfection in liver transplant patients	North American Biologics
Herpes simplex virus gene	Primary and metastatic brain tumors	Genetic Therapy, Inc.
Histrelin	Treatment of acute intermittent porphyria, hereditary copro-porphyria, and variegate porphyria	Karl E. Anderson, MD
Histrelin acetate *(Supprelin Injection)*	Central precocious puberty[1]	Roberts
HIV-neutralizing anti-bodies *(Immupath)*	AIDS	Hemacare
Human growth hormone	With glutamine in the treatment of short bowel syndrome (nutrient malabsorption from the GI tract resulting from an inadequate absorptive surface)	Research Triangle Pharm
Human immunodefi-ciency virus immune globulin *(Hivig)*	AIDS; HIV-infected pregnant women and infants of HIV-infected mothers; HIV-infected pediatric patients	North American Biologicals
Hydrox-ocobalamin/sodium thiosulfate	Severe acute cyanide poisoning	Michael A. Yamin, PhD
Hydroyurea *(Hydrea)*	Treatment of patients with sickle cell anemia as shown by the presence of hemoglobin S	Bristol-Myers Squibb
I-131 radiolabeled B1 monoclonal antibody	Non-Hodgkin's B-cell lymphoma	Coulter Corp.
Idarubicin HCl *(Idamycin)*	Myelodysplastic syndromes; chronic myelogenous leukemia; acute myelogenous leukemia (acute nonlymphocytic leukemia)[1]; acute lymphoblastic leukemia in pediatric patients	Adria
Idoxuridine	Nonparenchymatous sarcomas.	NeoPharm
Ifosfamide *(Ifex)*	With other antineoplastics for third-line chemotherapy in the treatment of germ-cell testicular cancer[1]; bone sarcomas; soft tissue sarcomas	Bristol-Myers Squibb
Imciromab pentetate *(Myosinct)*	Detecting early necrosis as an indication of rejection of orthotopic cardiac transplants	Centocor
Imiglucerase *(Cerezyme)*	Replacement therapy in patients with types I, II and III Gaucher's disease	Genzyme

[1]Approved for marketing.

Drug (Trade name)	Proposed use	Sponsor
Immune globulin IV (human) *(Iveegam, Immuno)* *(Gamimune N)* *(Immune Globulin Intravenous (human) Immuno)*	Juvenile rheumatoid arthritis; polymyositis/dermatomyositis; infection prophylaxis in pediatric patients with HIV; acute myocarditis	Immuno Miles
In-111 murine Mab (2b8-mx-dtpa) & Y-90 murine Mab (2b8-mxdtpa) *(Melimmune)*	B-cell non-Hodgkin's lymphoma	Idec
Indium in 111 altumomab pentetate *(Hybri-ceaker)*	Detection of suspected and previously unidentified tumor foci of recurrent colorectal carcinoma	Hybritech
Indium in 111 murine monoclonal antibody Fab to myosin *(Myosinct)*	Aid in diagnosis of myocarditis	Centocor
Inosine pranobex *(Isoprinosine)*	Subacute sclerosing panencephalitis	Newport
Insulin-like growth factor-1 *(Myotrophin)*	Amyotrophic lateral sclerosis	Cephalon
Insulin-like growth factor-1 (recombinant human) *(IGF-1)*	Growth hormone receptor deficiency; antibody-mediated growth hormone resistance in patients with isolated growth hormone deficiency Ia; post-poliomyelitis syndrome	Pharmacia Cephalon
Interferon alfa-2a (recombinant) *(Roferon A)*	Chronic myelogenous leukemia; with fluorouracil for advanced colorectal cancer and esophageal carcinoma; with teceleukin for metastatic malignant melanoma and renal-cell carcinoma; AIDS-related Kaposi's sarcoma[1]; renal-cell carcinoma	Hoffman-LaRoche
Interferon alfa-2b (recombinant) *(Intron A)*	AIDS-related Kaposi's sarcoma[1]; acute hepatitis B; chronic myelogenous leukemia	Schering
Interferon alfa-nl *(Wellferon)*	AIDS-related Kaposi's sarcoma; human papillomavirus in severe resistant/recurrent respiratory (laryngeal) papillomatosis	Glaxo Wellcome
Interferon beta (recombinant human)	Primary brain tumors; AIDS; acute non-A, non-B hepatitis	Biogen Berlex Chiron
Interferon beta (recombinant) *(R-IFN-beta)* *(Rebif)*	Systemic treatment of cutaneous T-cell lymphoma, cutaneous malignant melanoma and metastatic renal-cell carcinoma; intralesional/systemic treatment of AIDS-related Kaposi's sarcoma; symptomatic patients with AIDS (including CD4 T-cell counts < 200 cells/mm^3)	Biogen Serono

[1]Approved for marketing.

Drug (Trade name)	Proposed use	Sponsor
Interferon beta-1b *(Betaseron)*	Multiple sclerosis[1]	Chiron & Berlex Labs
Interferon gamma 1-b *(Actimmune)*	Chronic granulomatous disease[1]	Genentech
Interleukin-1 receptor antagonist, (recombinant human) *(Antril)*	Juvenile rheumatoid arthritis; prevention/treatment of graft-vs-host disease in transplant recipients	Synergen
Interleukin-2 *(Teceleukin)*	Alone and with interferon alfa-2a for metastatic renal-cell carcinoma and metastatic malignant melanoma	Hoffmann-LaRoche
Interleukin-2, recombinant liposome encapsulated	Cancers of the kidney, renal pelvis; brain and CNS tumors	Oncotherapeutics
Iobenguane Sulfate I 131	Diagnostic adjunct in patients with pheochromocytoma[1]	CIS-US
Iodine I^{123} murine monoclonal antibody to alpha-fetoprotein	Detects hepatocellular carcinoma and hepatoblastoma and alpha-fetoprotein-producing germ-cell tumors	Immunomedics
Iodine I^{123} murine monoclonal antibody to hCG	Detection of hCG-producing tumors (eg, germ-cell/trophoblastic-cell tumors)	Immunomedics
Iodine I^{131} 6B-iodomethyl-19-norcholesterol	Adrenal cortical imaging	William Beierwaltes, MD
Iodine I^{131} murine monoclonal antibody to alpha-fetoprotein	Hepatocellular carcinoma and hepatoblastoma; alpha-fetoprotein-producing germ-cell tumors	Immunomedics
Iodine I^{131} murine monoclonal antibody to hCG	hCG-producing tumors (ie, germ-cell and trophoblastic-cell tumors)	Immunomedics
Iodine I^{131} murine monoclonal antibody IgG2a to B cell *(Immurait; L^{12}-I^{131})*	B-cell lymphoma and B-cell leukemia	Immunomedics
Isobutyramide *(Isobutyramide oral solution)*	Sickle cell disease and beta-thalassemia Beta-hemoglobinopathies and beta-thalassemia syndromes	Vertex Susan P. Perrine, MD
KL4-surfactant	Acute respiratory distress syndrome in adults; respiratory distress syndrome in premature infants	RW Johnson Res Charles G. Cochrane, MD
Lactobin	AIDS-associated diarrhea unresponsive to initial antidiarrheal therapy	Roxane
Lamotrigine *(Lamictal)*	Lennox-Gastaut syndrome	Glaxo Wellcome

[1]Approved for marketing.

Drug (Trade name)	Proposed use	Sponsor
L-Baclofen *(Neuralgon)*	Intractable spasticity from spinal cord injury or multiple sclerosis[1]; intractable spasticity in children with cerebral palsy; trigeminal neuralgia	Gerhard Fromm, MD WTD, Inc.
L-Cycloserine	Gaucher's disease	Meir Lev, MD
L-Cysteine	Prevention and lessening of photosensitivity in erythropoietic protoporphyria	Tyson & Assoc
Leucovorin *(Leukovorin Calcium)* *(Wellcovorin)*	With 5-fluorouracil for metastatic colorectal cancer[1]; rescue use after high-dose methotrexate therapy in the treatment of osteosarcoma[1]	Lederle Glaxo Wellcome
Leukocyte protease inhibitor, recombinant secretory	Congenital alpha-1 antitrypsin deficiency; cystic fibrosis	Synergen
Leukocyte protease inhibitor, secretory	Bronchopulmonary dysplasia	Synergen
Leupeptin	As an adjunct to microsurgical peripheral nerve repair	Research Triangle Pharm
Leuprolide acetate *(Lupron)*	Central precocious puberty[1]	TAP Pharm
Leutinizing hormone (recombinant human)	With recombinant human follicle stimulating hormone for chronic anovulation due to hypogonadotropic hypogonadism	Serano Labs
Levocarnitine *(Vitacarn, Carnitor)*	Genetic carnitine deficiency[1]; treatment of manifestations of carnitine deficiency in patients with end-stage renal disease who require dialysis; primary and secondary carnitine deficiency of genetic origin[1]; prevention/treatment of secondary carnitine deficiency in valproic acid toxicity; pediatric cardiomyopathy	Sigma-Tau
Levomethadyl acetate HCl *(Orlaam)*	Treatment of heroin addicts suitable for maintenance on opiate agonists[1]	Biodevelopment Corp.
L-5 hydroxytryptophan	Postanoxic intention myoclonus	Circa Pharm
L-Glutathione *(Cachexon)*	AIDS-associated cachexia	Telluride Pharm
Lidocaine patch 5% *(Lidoderm Patch)*	Post-herpetic neuralgia resulting from Herpes zoster infection	Hind Health Care
Liothyronine sodium injection *(Triostat)*	Myxedema coma/precoma[1]	SmithKline-Beecham
Liposomal prostaglandin E1 injection	Acute respiratory distress syndrome	The Liposome Co.

[1]Approved for marketing.

Drug (Trade name)	Proposed use	Sponsor
L-Leucovorin *(Isovorin)*	With high-dose methotrexate in the treatment of osteosarcoma; in combination chemotherapy with the approved agent 5-fluorouracil in the palliative treatment of metastatic adenocarcinoma of the colon and rectum	Lederle
Lodoxamide tromethamine *(Alomide ophthalmic solution)*	Vernal keratoconjunctivitis[1]	Alcon
L-Threonine *(Threostat)*	Spasticity associated with familial spastic paraparesis; amyotrophic lateral sclerosis	Interneuron Tyson
L-2-oxothiazolidine-4-carboxylic acid *(Procysteine)*	Adult respiratory distress syndrome	Free Radical Sciences
Mafenide acetate solution *(Sulfamylon Solution)*	Prevention of graft loss of meshed autografts on excised burn wounds	Dow B. Hickam
Matrix metal-loproteinase inhibitor *(Galardin)*	Corneal ulcers	Glycomed
Mazindol *(Sanorex)*	Duchenne muscular dystrophy	Platon J. Collipp, MD
Mecasermin	Growth hormone insufficiency syndrome	Genentech
Mefloquine HCl *(Mephaquin) (Lariam)*	Treat/prevent chloroquine-resistant falciparum malaria[1]; acute malaria due to *Plasmodium falciparum* and *P vivax*[1]; prophylaxis of resistant *P falciparum*[1]	Mepha AG Hoffman-LaRoche
Megestrol acetate *(Megace)*	Anorexia, cachexia or significant weight loss (≥ 10% of body weight) with confirmed diagnosis of AIDS	Bristol-Myers Squibb
Melanoma cell vaccine	Invasive melanoma	Morton, Donald L. M.D.
Melanoma vaccine *(Melacine)*	Stage III-IV melanoma	Ribi Immunochem Research
Melatonin	Circadian rhythm sleep disorders in blind people with no light perception	Robert Sack, MD
Melphalan *(Alkeran for Injection)*	Multiple myeloma when oral therapy is inappropriate[1]; hyperthermic regional limb perfusion to treat metastatic melanoma of the extremity	Glaxo Wellcome
Mesna *(Mesnex)*	Prophylactic in reducing incidence of ifosfamide-induced hemorrhagic cystitis[1]; inhibition of the urotoxic effects induced by oxazaphosphorine compounds (eg, cyclophosphamide)	Degussa Corp. Asta

[1]Approved for marketing.

Drug (Trade name)	*Proposed use*	*Sponsor*
Methionyl human stem cell factor (recombinant)	With filgrastim to decrease the number of phereses required to collect peripheral blood progenitor cells capable of providing rapid multi-lineage hematopoietic reconstitution following myelosuppressive or myeloablative therapy; primary bone marrow failure	Amgen
Methionyl neurotrophic factor (brain-derived, recombinant)	Amyotrophic lateral sclerosis	Amgen
Methotrexate *(Rheumatrex)*	Juvenile rheumatoid arthritis	Lederle
Methotrexate sodium	Osteogenic sarcoma[1]	Lederle
Methotrexate with laurocapram *(Methotrexate/Azone)*	Topical treatment of *Mycosis fungoides*	Discovery Therapeutics
8-Methoxsalen *(Uvadex)*	In conjunction with the UVAR photopheresis to treat diffuse systemic sclerosis; prevention of acute rejection of cardiac allografts	Therakos, Inc.
Metronidazole (topical) *(Flagyl)* *(Metrogel)*	Grade III and IV, anaerobically infected, decubitus ulcers; acne rosacea[1]; perioral dermatitis	Searle Galderma Curatek
Microbubble contrast agent *(Filmix Neurosonographic Contrast Agent)*	Intraoperative aid in the identification and localization of intracranial tumors	CAV-CON
Midodrine HCl *(Amatine)*	Idiopathic orthostatic hypotension	Roberts
Mitoguazone	Treatment of diffuse non-Hodgkin's lymphoma, including AIDS-related diffuse non-Hodgkin's lymphoma	CTRC Research
Mitolactol	Adjuvant therapy in the treatment of primary brain tumors	Biopharmaceutics
Mitomycin-C	Refractory glaucoma as an adjunct to ab externo glaucoma surgery	IOP
Mitoxantrone HCl *(Novantrone)*	Acute myelogenous leukemia (acute nonlymphocytic leukemia)[1]	Lederle
Modafinil	Excessive daytime sleepiness in narcolepsy	Cephalon
Monoclonal Ab (murine) anti-idiotype melanoma associated antigen *(Melimmune)*	Invasive cutaneous melanoma	Idec
Monoclonal antibodies PM-81	Adjunctive treatment of acute myelogenous leukemia	Medarex

[1]Approved for marketing.

Drug (Trade name)	*Proposed use*	*Sponsor*
Monoclonal antibodies PM-81 and AML-2-23	For the exogenous depletion of CD14 and CD15 positive acute myeloid leukemic bone marrow transplantation	Medarex
Monoclonal antibody 17-1A *(Panorex)*	Pancreatic cancer	Centocor
Monoclonal antibody to CD4, 5a8	Post-exposure prophylaxis for occupational exposure to HIV	Biogen
Monoclonal antibody (human) to hepatitis B virus	Prophylaxis of hepatitis B reinfection in patients undergoing liver transplantation secondary to end-stage chronic hepatitis B infection	Protein Design Labs
Monoclonal antibody for lupus nephritis	Immunization against lupus nephritis	Medclone
Monolaurin *(Glylorin)*	Congenital primary ichthyosis	Cellegy Pharm
Monomercapto-undecahydro-closo-dodecaborate sodium *(Borocelli)*	For use in boron neutron capture therapy in the treatment of glioblastoma multiforme	Neutron Tech Corp. and Neutron R & D
Monoctanoin *(Moctanin)*	Dissolution of cholesterol gall-stones retained in the common bile duct[1]	Ethitek
Morphine sulfate concentrate (preservative-free) *(Infumorph)*	For use in microinfusion devices for intraspinal administration for intractable chronic pain[1]	Elkins-Sinn
Multi-vitamin infusion (neonatal formula)	Establishment/maintenance of total parenteral nutrition in very low birth weight infants	Astra
Mycobacterium avium sensitin RS-10	Diagnosis of invasive *Mycobacterium avium* disease in immunocompetent individuals	Statens Seruminstitut
Myelin	Multiple sclerosis	Autoimmune
Nafarelin acetate *(Synarel Nasal Solution)*	Central precocious puberty[1]	Syntex (USA)
Naltrexone HCl *(Trexan)*	Blockade of exogenous opioid effects as adjunct to maintenance of detoxified, formerly opioid-dependent, individuals[1]	Du Pont Pharm
Nebacumab *(Centoxin)*	Gram-negative bacteremia which has progressed to endotoxin shock	Centocor
Neurotropin-1	Motor neuron disease/amyotrophic lateral sclerosis	Arthur Dale Ericsson, MD
NG-29 *(Somatrel)*	Diagnostic measure of the capacity of the pituitary gland to release growth hormone	Ferring Labs
Nifedipine	Interstitial cystitis	Jonathan Fleischmann, MD
9-(3-pydidylmethyl)-9-deazaguanine	Cutaneous T-cell lymphoma	Briocryst Pharm

[1]Approved for marketing.

Drug (Trade name)	*Proposed use*	*Sponsor*
Nitazoxanide	Cryptosporidiosis in HIV-positive and AIDS patients	Unimed Pharm
Nitric oxide	Primary pulmonary hypertension in the newborn	Ohmeda
NTBC	Tyrosinemia type 1	Swedish Orphan Ab
N-trifluoroacetyladriamycin-14-valerate	Carcinoma in situ of the urinary bladder	Anthra Pharm
Ofloxacin *(Ocuflox Ophthalmic Solution)*	Bacterial corneal ulcers	Allergan, Inc
OM 401 *(Drepanol)*	Prophylactic treatment of sickle cell disease	Omex International
Omega-3 (n-3) polyunsaturated fatty acid with all double bonds in the cis configuration	Prevention of organ graft rejection	Research Triangle Pharm
Oncorad OV103	Ovarian cancer	Cytogen
Orgotein for Injection	Familial amyotrophic lateral sclerosis associated with a mutation of the gene (chromosome 21q) for copper, zinc superoxide dismutase	Oxis
Oxaliplatin	Ovarian cancer	Axion
Oxandrolone *(Oxandrin)* *(Hepandrin)*	Short stature associated with Turner's syndrome; constitutional delay of growth and puberty; adjunctive therapy for AIDS patients with HIV-wasting syndrome; moderate/severe acute alcoholic hepatitis and moderate protein calorie malnutrition	Bio-Technology
Oxymorphone HCl *(Numorphan H.P.)*	Relief of severe intractable pain in narcotic-tolerant patients	Du Pont Merck
Pegademase bovine *(Adagen)*	Enzyme replacement in ADA deficiency in patients with severe combined immunodeficiency (SCID)[1]	Enzon
Pegaspargase *(Oncaspar)*	Acute lymphocytic leukemia[1]	Enzon
PEG-glucocerebrosidase	Chronic enzyme replacement therapy in Gaucher's disease patients who are deficient in glucocerebrosidase	Enzon
Peg-interleukin-2	Primary immunodeficiencies associated with T-cell defects	Chiron
Pentamidine isethionate *(Pentam 300), (NebuPent)*	Treatment of *Pneumocystis carinii* pneumonia (PCP)[1]; PCP prevention in high-risk patients[1]	Rhone-Poulenc Rorer Fujisawa
Pentamidine isethionate (inhalation) *(Pneumopent)*	PCP prevention in high-risk patients	Fisons

[1]Approved for marketing.

Drug (Trade name)	Proposed use	Sponsor
Pentastarch *(Pentaspan)*	Adjunct in leukapheresis to improve the harvesting and increase the yield of leukocytes by centrifugal means[1]	Du Pont
Pentosan sodium polysulphate *(Elmiron)*	Interstitial cystitis	Baker Norton
Pentostatin	Chronic lymphocytic leukemia	Warner-Lambert
Pentostatin Injection *(Nipent)*	Hairy-cell leukemia[1]	Warner-Lambert
Phenylalanine ammonia-lyase *(Phenylase)*	Hyperphenylalaninemia	Ibex
Phosphocysteamine	Cystinosis	Medea Research
Physostigmine salicylate *(Antilirium)*	Friedreich's and other inherited ataxias	Forest
Pilocarpine HCl *(Salagen)*	Xerostomia and keratoconjunctivitis sicca in Sjogren's syndrome patients; xerostomia induced by radiation therapy for head and neck cancer[1]	MGI Pharma
Piracetum *(Nootropil)*	Myoclonus	UCB Secteur
Polifeprosan 20 with carmustine *(Gliadel)*	Localized placement in the brain for the treatment of recurrent malignant glioma	Guilford Pharm
Poloxamer 188 *(Rheothrx Copolymer)*	Sickle cell crisis; severe burns requiring hospitalization	Glaxo Wellcome
Poloxamer 331 *(Protox)*	Initial therapy of toxoplasmosis in AIDS patients	CytRx Corporation
Poly I: Poly C12U *(Ampligen)*	AIDS; renal-cell carcinoma; chronic fatigue syndrome; invasive metastatic melanoma (stage IIB, III, IV)	HEM Pharm
Polymeric oxygen	Sickle cell anemia	Capmed USA
Porcine Islet preparation, Encapsulated *(BetaRx)*	Type I diabetic patients who are already on immunosuppression	VivoRx
Porfimer sodium *(Photofrin)*	Photodynamic therapy in patients with transitional cell carcinoma in situ of urinary bladder and patients with primary or recurrent obstructing (either partially or completely) esophageal carcinoma	QLT Phototherapeutics
Porfiromycin	Head and neck cancer	OncoRx
Potassium citrate *(Urocit K)*	Prevention of uric acid nephrolithiasis[1]; prevention of calcium renal stones in patients with hypocitraturia[1]; avoidance of the complication of calcium stone formation in uric lithiasis[1]	Univ. of Texas Health Sciences
Prednimustine *(Sterecyt)*	Malignant non-Hodgkin's lymphomas	Kabi Pharmacia
Primaquine phosphate	With clindamycin in the treatment of PCP associated with AIDS	Sanofi Winthrop

[1]Approved for marketing.

Drug (Trade name)	*Proposed use*	*Sponsor*
Progesterone	Establishment and maintenance of pregnancy in women undergoing in vitro fertilization or embryo transplant procedures	Gynopharma
Propamidine isethionate 0.1% ophthalmic soln *(Brolene)*	Acanthamoeba keratitis	Bausch & Lomb
Protein C concentrate *(Protein C concentrate [human] vapor heated, immuno)*	For replacement therapy in patients with congenital or acquired protein C deficiency for the prevention and treatment of: Warfarin-induced skin necrosis during oral anticoagulation, thrombosis, pulmonary emboli and purpura fulminans; prevention/treatment of purpura fulminans in meningococcemia	Immuno
Protirelin	Prevention of infant respiratory distress syndrome associated with prematurity	UCB Pharm
Pseudomonas hyperimmune globulin (mucoid exploysaccharide) *(MEPIG)*	Treatment/prevention of pulmonary *Pseudomonas aeruginosa* infections in cystic fibrosis	Univax
Pulmonary surfactant replacement	Prevention/treatment of infant respiratory distress syndrome	Scios Nova
Pulmonary surfactant replacement, porcine *(Curosurf)*	Prevention/treatment of respiratory distress syndrome in premature infants	Dey Labs
RII Retinamide	Myelodysplastic syndromes	Sparta
R-VIII SQ *(REFACTO)*	Long-term or hospital treatment of hemophilia A or treatment of hemophilia A in connection with surgical procedures	Pharmacia
Recombinant vaccinia (human papillomavirus) *(TA-HPV)*	Cervial cancer	Cantab Pharm
Relaxin (recombinant, human)	Progressive systemic sclerosis	Connective Therapeutics
Respiratory syncytial virus immune globulin (Human) *(Hypermune RSV)* *(Respigam)*	Prophylaxis of respiratory syncytial virus lower respiratory tract infections in infants and young children, especially ones at high risk of RSV disease; treatment of RSV lower respiratory tract infections in hospitalized infants and young children	Medimmune
Retinoic acid, 9-CIS	Acute promyelocytic leukemia	Ligand
Retinoin	Squamous metaplasia of the occular surface epithelia (conjunctiva and/or cornea) with mucus deficiency and keratinization	Hannan Ophthalmic Marketing
RGG0853, E1A lipid complex	Advanced ovarian cancer that overexpresses the HER/neu oncogene	RGene Therapeutics

[1]Approved for marketing.

Drug (Trade name)	Proposed use	Sponsor
Rho (D) immune globulin intravenous (human) *(WinRho SD)*	Immune thrombocytopenic purpura[1]	Rh Pharm
Ribavirin *(Virazole)*	Hemorrhagic fever with renal syndrome	ICN
Ricin (blocked) conjugated murine MCA (anti-B4)	B-cell leukemia and B-cell lymphoma; ex vivo purging of leukemic cells from bone marrow of non-T-cell ALL patients in complete remission	Immunogen
Ricin (blocked) conjugated murine MCA (anti-MY9)	Ex vivo treatment of autologous bone marrow and subsequent reinfusion in acute myelogenous leukemia; myeloid leukemia, including AML, and blast crisis of CML	Immunogen
Ricin (blocked) conjugated murine MCA (N901)	Small-cell lung cancer	Immunogen
Ricin (blocked) conjugated murine moab (CD6)	Cutaneous T-cell lymphomas, acute T-cell leukemia-lymphoma, and related mature T-cell malignancies	Immunogen
Rifabutin *(Mycobutin)*	Treatment of disseminated *Mycobacterium avium* complex disease; prevention of disseminated MAC disease in advanced HIV infection[1]	Adria
Rifampin *(Rifadin I.V.)*	Antituberculosis treatment when oral doseform is not feasible[1]	Hoechst-Marion Roussel
Rifampin, isoniazid, pyrazinamide *(Rifater II)*	Short course treatment of tuberculosis	Hoechst-Marion Roussel
Rifapentine	Pulmonary tuberculosis; *Mycobacterium avium* in patients with AIDS; prophylaxis of *M avium* complex in patients with AIDS and a CD4+ count ≤ to 75/mm	Hoechst-Marion Roussel
Riluzole	Amyotrophic lateral sclerosis	Rhone-Poulenc Rorer
Roquinimex *(Linomide)*	Prolongs time to relapse in leukemia patients who have undergone autologous bone marrow transplantation	Kabi Pharmacia
Sargramostim *(Leukine)*	Neutropenia associated with bone marrow transplant, graft failure and delay of engraftment, and for the promotion of early engraftment[1]; reduction of neutropenia and leukopenia and decrease the incidence of death due to infection in patients with acute myelogenous leukemia	Immunex
Satumomab pendetide *(Oncosinct CR/OV)*	Detection of ovarian carcinoma[1]	Cytogen

[1]Approved for marketing.

Drug (Trade name)	*Proposed use*	*Sponsor*
Secalciferol *(Osteo-D)*	Familial hypophosphatemic rickets	Lemmon
Selegiline HCl *(Eldepryl)*	Adjuvant to levodopa/carbidopa in idiopathic Parkinson's disease (paralysis agitans), postencephalitic parkinsonism/symptomatic parkinsonism[1]	Somerset
Sermorelin acetate *(Geref)*	Idiopathic or organic growth hormone deficiency in children with growth failure; adjunct to gonadotropin in ovulation induction in anovulatory or oligoovulatory infertility after treatment with clomiphene or gonadotropin alone; AIDS-associated cachexia	Serono
Serratia marcescens extract (polyribosomes) *(Imuvert)*	Primary brain malignancies	Cell Technology
Short chain fatty acid solution	Active phase of ulcerative colitis with involvement restricted to the left side of the colon	Orphan Medical
Sodium benzoate/sodium phenylacetate	Treatment of urea cycle disorders: Carbamylphosphate synthetase deficiency, ornithine transcarbamylase deficiency and argininosuccinic acid synthetase deficiency	Saul W. Brusilow, MD
Sodium dichloroacetate	Congenital lactic acidosis; lactic acidosis in patients with severe malaria; homozygous familial hypercholesterolemia	Peter W. Stacpoole, PhD, MD
Sodium/Gamma hydroxybutyrate	Narcolepsy and auxiliary symptoms of cataplexy, sleep paralysis, hypnagogic hallucinations and automatic behavior	Biocraft
Sodium phenylbutyrate	Sickling disorders that include S-S, S-C and S-thalassemia hemiglobinopathy; urea cycle disorders: Carbamylphosphate synthetase deficiency, ornithine transcarbamylase deficiency and arginiosuccinic acid synthetase deficiency	Saul W. Brusilow, MD
Sodium tetradecyl sulfate *(Sotradecol)*	Bleeding esophageal varices	Elkins-Sinn
Soluble complement receptor (recombinant human) type 1	Prevention or reduction of adult respiratory distress syndrome	T Cell Sciences, Inc.
Somatostatin	Bleeding esophageal varices	UCB Pharm
Somatrem for Injection *(Protropin)*	Short stature associated with Turner's Syndrome; long-term treatment of children who have growth failure due to lack of adequate endogenous growth hormone secretion[1]	Genentech

[1]Approved for marketing.

Drug (Trade name)	Proposed use	Sponsor
Somatropin *(Biotropin)* *(Humatrope)* *(Norditropin)* *(Nutropin)* *(Saizen)* *(Genotropin/ Genotonorm)* *(Serostim)*	Idiopathic or organic growth hormone deficiency in children with growth failure; AIDS-associated cachexia; long-term treatment of children who have growth failure due to inadequate secretion of endogenous growth hormone[1]; short stature associated with Turner's syndrome; enhancement of nitrogen retention in hospitalized severely burned patients; growth retardation associated with chronic renal failure; AIDS-associated catabolism/weight loss; adults with growth hormone deficiency; children with AIDS-associated failure-to-thrive including AIDS-associated wasting	Bio-Technology Lilly Novo Nordisk Genentech Serono Pharmacia
Sorivudine *(BRAVADIR)*	Herpes zoster (shingles) in immunocompromised patients	Bristol-Meyers Squibb
Sotalol HCl *(Betapace)*	Treatment[1]/prevention of life-threatening ventricular tachyarrhythmias	Berlex
Streptococcus immune globulin group B	Disseminated Group B streptococcal infection in neonates	Univax
ST1-RTA immunotoxin (SR 44163)	B-chronic lymphocytic leukemia; prevention of acute graft-vs-host disease in bone marrow transplantation	Sanofi
SU-101	Malignant glioma; ovarian cancer	Sugen
Succimer *(Chemet)*	Mercury intoxication; lead poisoning in children[1]; prevention of cystine kidney stones in patients with homozygous cystinuria who are prone to stone development	McNeil-CPC
Sucralfate	Oral mucositis and stomatitis following radiation for head and neck cancer	Fuisz Technologies
Sucralfate Suspension	Oral ulcerations and dysphagia in patients with epidermolysis bullosa; oral complications of chemotherapy in bone marrow transplant	Darby
Sucrase (yeast-derived) *(Sacarasa)*	Congenital sucrase-isomaltase deficiency	William R. Treem, MD
Sulfadiazine	With pyrimethamine for *Toxoplasma gondii*[1] encephalitis in patients with and without AIDS	EON Labs
Sulfapyridine	Dermatitis herpetiformis	Jacobus

[1]Approved for marketing.

Patient Drug Information Index Supplement

Please affix this index supplement to pg. 671. To avoid inaccurate entries, use these references prior to checking the main index.

Trade names appear in italics.

Drug (Trade name)	*Proposed use*	*Sponsor*
Superoxide dismutase (human)	Protection of donor organ tissue from damage or injury during the necessary periods of ischemia (hypoxia, anoxia), and especially reperfusion, associated with the operative procedure	Pharmacia-Chiron Partnership
Superoxide dis-mutase (recombinant human)	Prevention of reperfusion injury to donor organ tissue; broncho-pulmonary dysplasia in premature infants < 1500 mg	Bio-Technology General Corp
Surface active ex-tract of saline lavage of bovine lungs *(Infasurf)*	To treat/prevent respiratory failure due to pulmonary surfactant deficiency in preterm infants	Ony
Synsorb Pk	Verocytotoxogenic *E. coli* infec-tions	Synsorb Biotech
T4 endonuclease V, liposome encapsu-lated	Prevent cutaneous neoplasms and other skin abnormalities in xeroderma pigmentosum	Applied Genetics
Technetium TC-99M antimelanoma murine monoclonal antibody *(Oncotrac Melanoma Imaging Kit)*	Detecting, by imaging, metastases of malignant melanoma	Neorx
Technetium Tc-99M murine monoclonal antibody to hCG *(ImmuRAID, hCG-Tc-99m)*	Detection of hCG-producing tumors such as germ-cell and trophoblastic cell tumors	Immunomedics
Technetium Tc-99M murine monoclonal antibody to human AFP *(ImmuRAID, AFP-Tc-99m)*	Detection of hepatocellular carci-noma and hepatoblastoma; detec-tion of alpha-fetoprotein-producing germ-cell tumors	Immunomedics
Technetium Tc-99M murine monoclonal antibody (IgG2a) to B cell *(LymphoScan)*	Diagnostic imaging in the evaluation of the extent of disease in patients with histologically confirmed non-Hodgkin's B-cell lymphoma, acute B-cell lympho-blastic leukemia and chronic B-cell lymphocytic leukemia	Immunomedics
Teniposide *(Vumon Injection)*	Refractory childhood acute lymphocytic leukemia[1]	Bristol-Myers Squibb
Teriparatide *(Parathar)*	Diagnostic agent for patients with clinical/laboratory evidence of hypocalcemia due to hypoparathy-roidism or pseudohypoparathy-roidism[1]	Rhone-Poulenc Rorer
Terlipressin *(Glypressin)*	Bleeding esophageal varices	Ferring
Testosterone *(Androgel)*	Weight loss in AIDS patients with HIV-associated wasting	Unimed Pharm
Testosterone propionate ointment 2%	Vulvar dystrophies	Star

[1]Approved for marketing.

Drug (Trade name)	Proposed use	Sponsor
Testosterone sublingual	Constitutional delay of growth and puberty in boys	Bio-Technology General
Thalidomide *(Synovir)*	Prevent/treat graft-vs-host disease in bone marrow transplantation; treatment/maintenance of reactional lepromatous leprosy; clinical manifestations of mycobacterial infection caused by *Mycobacterium tuberculosis* and nontuberculous mycobacteria; severe recurrent aphthous stomatitis and treatment/prevention of recurrent aphthous ulcers in severely, terminally immunocompromised patients; erythema nodosum leprosum; HIV-associated wasting syndrome	Pediatric Pharm Andrulis Calgene
Thymosin alpha-1	Adjunctive treatment of chronic active hepatitis B	Alpha 1 Biomedicals
Thyroid stimulating hormone (TSH) *(Thyrogen)*	Adjunct in the diagnosis of thyroid cancer	Genzyme
Tiopronin *(Thiola)*	Prevention of cystine nephrolithiasis in patients with homozygous cystinuria[1]	Charles Y.C. Pak, MD
Tiratricol *(Triacana)*	With levothyroxine to suppress TSH in patients with well differentiated thyroid cancer intolerant of adequate doses of levothyroxine alone	Marcofina Labs
Tizanidine HCl *(Zanaflex)*	Spasticity associated with multiple sclerosis and spinal cord injury	Athena
T-lymphotrophic virus type III gp 160 antigens *(Vaxsyn HIV-1)*	AIDS	Microgenesys
Tobramycin for inhalation	Bronchopulmonary infections of *pseudomonas aeruginosa* in cystic fibrosis patients	Pathogenesis Corp.
Topiramate *(Topamax)*	Lennox-Gastaut syndrome	RW Johnson Res
Toremifene	Hormonal therapy of metastatic breast carcinoma; desmoid tumors	Orion
Transforming growth factor-beta 2	Full thickness macular holes	Celtrix
Treosulfan *(Ovastat)*	Ovarian cancer	Medac
Tretinoin *(Vesanoid)* *(Tretinoin LF, IV)*	Acute promyelocytic leukemia[1]; acute and chronic leukemia	Hoffman-La Roche Argus
Trientine HCl *(Cuprid)*	Wilson's disease intolerant of or not responsive to penicillamine[1]	Merck

[1]Approved for marketing.

Drug (Trade name)	Proposed use	Sponsor
Trimetrexate glucuronate *(Neutrexin)*	Advanced non-small cell carcinoma of the lung; *Pneumocystis carinii* pneumonia (PCP) in AIDS patients[1]; metastatic carcinoma of head and neck; metastatic colorectal adenocarcinoma; pancreatic adenocarcinoma	U.S. Bioscience
Trisaccharides A and B *(Biosyniect)*	Moderate/severe forms of hemolytic disease of the newborn from placental transfer of antibodies against blood groups A and B; ABO-incompatible solid organ transplantation including kidney, heart, liver, pancreas; prevention of AB hemolytic reactions arising from ABO-incompatible bone marrow transplantation	Chembiomed
Trisodium citrate concentration *(Hemocitrate)*	Use in leukapheresis procedures	Hemotec Medical Products
Troleandomycin	Severe steroid-requiring asthma	Stanley M. Szefler, MD
Tumor necrosis factor-binding protein I and II	Symptomatic patients with AIDS including CD4 counts < 200 cells/mm^3	Serono
Tyloxapol	Cystic Fibrosis	Kennedy & Hoidal, MDs
Uridine 5′-triphosphate	Cystic fibrosis	Inspire Pharm
Urofollitropin *(Metrodin)*	Ovulation induction in patients with polycystic ovarian disease who have an elevated LH/FSH ratio and who have failed to respond to adequate clomiphene citrate therapy[1]	Serono
Urogastrone	Acceleration of corneal epithelial regeneration and healing of stromal incisions (corneal transplant surgery)	Chiron Vision
Ursodeoxycholic acid *(Ursofalk)*	Primary biliary cirrhosis	Axcan
Ursodiol *(Actigall)*	Management of primary biliary cirrhosis	Ciba-Geigy
Valine, isoleucine and leucine *(VIL)*	Hyperphenylalaninemia	Leas Res Products
Vasoactive intestinal polypeptide	Acute esophageal food impaction	Research Triangle Pharm
Zalcitabine *(Hivid)*	AIDS[1]	National Cancer Inst. Hoffman-La Roche
Zidovudine *(Retrovir)*	AIDS and AIDS-related complex[1]	Glaxo Wellcome
Zinc acetate	Wilson's disease	Lemmon

[1]Approved for marketing.

Investigational Agents

Acecainide HCl *(Napa)* – Antiarrhythmic agent

Pharmacology: Acecainide (also known as N-acetylprocainamide, NAPA and acetylprocainamide) is an antiarrhythmic agent which was first identified as the major active metabolite produced by N-acetylation of procainamide (eg, *Pronestyl, Procan SR*). The drug has distinct electrophysiologic and pharmacologic effects which differ from the parent compound.

Acecainide is classified as a Type III (Vaughn-Williams classification) antiarrhythmic agent, along with amiodarone *(Cordarone)* and bretylium (eg, *Bretylol*), because of its ability to prolong atrial and ventricular action potential durations and refractory periods. This occurs without significant depression of conduction velocity. Sinus cycle length, sinus node recovery time, atrioventricular (AV) node refractory period and conduction intervals (eg, atrio-His, His-ventricular) are also not affected by therapeutic concentrations of the drug. Electrocardiographically, the PR interval and QRS duration show no significant changes during acecainide therapy. However, the rate corrected QT interval (QTc) is significantly increased at concentrations of the drug which produce arrhythmia suppression (12 to 35 mcg/ml).

Blood pressure and heart rate may be reduced, but this effect is not consistently seen. There is no significant effect on cardiac output or pulmonary artery wedge pressure. Several studies have shown that acecainide increases myocardial contractility.

Pharmacokinetics: Acecainide is well absorbed after oral administration, with bioavailability values ranging from 82% to 100% using capsule and tablet dosage formulations. Peak levels occur within 1 to 3 hours after oral administration. Protein binding averages 10% and is independent of plasma concentration.

Metabolism of acecainide is limited. A small amount (2% to 5%) is deacetylated back to the parent compound, procainamide, or converted to desethyl N-acetylprocainamide (< 1%). The majority of the drug (59% to 87%) is excreted unchanged in the urine, and there appears to be a strong correlation between renal clearance and creatinine clearance. Additional metabolic or excretion pathways are presumed to exist since approximately 10% to 15% of an administered dose cannot be accounted for in present studies.

The half-life ranges from 4 to 13 hours in patients with normal renal function to as long as 42 hours in functionally anephric patients. Elderly patients show a reduction in acecainide clearance which may reflect both age-related decrease in renal function and reduced renal tubular secretion of the drug.

Hemodialysis and continuous arteriovenous hemofiltration enhance clearance.

Clinical trials: The fact that acecainide produces electrophysiologic effects which are distinctly different from procainamide requires that the drug be evaluated separately. A positive response to procainamide is not necessarily predictive of a positive response to acecainide.

Acecainide has been used to suppress premature ventricular complexes (PVCs) and refractory ventricular arrhythmias. About 50% of patients with at least one PVC/minute achieved 50% suppression of arrhythmia; 40% achieved 75% suppression at plasma levels which averaged 22 mcg/ml. In the only published long-term trial of acecainide in drug refractory ventricular arrhythmias, 63% of patients were effectively controlled at 12 months.

Animal studies suggest acecainide may be useful in converting atrial flutter to sinus rhythm.

Side effects: Side effects are common, ≈ 45%. Discontinuation of therapy due to side effects, however, is only required in ≈ 10% of patients. Gastrointestinal disturbances are the most common (nausea, vomiting), followed by neurologic symptoms such as dizziness, lightheadedness, blurred vision, numbness and tingling.

Acecainide has little tendency to cause a drug-induced lupus-like syndrome which frequently limits the usefulness of procainamide. This reaction appears to be caused by the parent compound; however, a small amount of administered acecainide is converted back to procainamide. Like all antiarrhythmics, acecainide may have a proarrhythmic effect. Although not systematically studied in humans, reports of acecainide-induced torsade de pointes have been recorded.

Summary: Acecainide appears to be a potentially useful antiarrhythmic. The fact that it has little tendency to induce the lupus-like syndrome frequently associated with procainamide is of interest, but other alternatives to procainamide also exist. Additional studies are necessary to compare the efficacy of this drug to currently available agents and further define its place in therapy.

On December 10, 1993, Medco announced that development of acecainide has been discontinued since it appears to offer no increased benefit over currently available antiarrhythmic agents.

Acetorphan – Enkephalinase inhibitor

Pharmacology: Acetorphan is a lipophilic inhibitor of enkephalinase, a peptidase present in the gastrointestinal tract and the central nervous system. By inhibiting enkephalinase, endogenous enkephalin concentrations increase, giving acetorphan varied therapeutic indications.

Acetorphan is used for symptomatic treatment of acute diarrhea in adults. Treatment should not last more than 7 days. Acetorphan administration does not obviate the need for hydration when relevant.

Pharmacokinetics: Available pharmacokinetic data in humans is limited to the dosing information included below.

Clinical trials: A double-blind cross-over design evaluated the ability of acetorphan to prevent diarrhea in patients receiving castor oil. Acetorphan was administered 45 minutes after the castor oil. Castor oil was selected to induce an experimental "secretory diarrhea." Six subjects were studied. Prophylactic acetorphan significantly reduced the mean number of stools during the following 24 hours by 50% and the stool weight by 37%. No side effects other than nausea and discomfort, which were noted in all subjects, were reported.

One hundred ninety-nine patients randomly received acetorphan or placebo after being diagnosed with infectious diarrhea. Patients took two capsules (100 mg each) on enrollment into the study and one capsule after each unformed stool for a maximum of 10 days. No other therapies were initiated during the trial, with the exception of acetaminophen as needed. Patients receiving acetorphan experienced a significantly shorter duration of diarrhea. Of the patients still experiencing diarrhea on day 10, 7% received acetorphan and 24% received placebo. Side effects were similar between the two groups.

One study compared the efficacy of acetorphan (100 mg three times daily) and loperamide (eg, *Imodium A-D*; 1.33 mg three times daily) in the treatment of infectious diarrhea. Therapy continued until resolution of diarrhea or for a maximum of 7 days. Thirty-seven patients received acetorphan, and 32 patients received loperamide. The mean duration of diarrhea did not differ between the two groups. Abdominal distension and constipation, however, were significantly more common in the loperamide group.

Another study compared the efficacy of acetorphan and clonidine (eg, *Catapres*) in suppressing opiate withdrawal symptoms. Nineteen heroin or synthetic opiate addicts were treated with 50 mg IV acetorphan twice daily or clonidine 0.075 mg five times daily if they displayed opioid withdrawal syndrome within 24 hours after a hospital admission. Changes in the overall Opiate Withdrawal Scale did not differ between the two groups; however, diarrhea and lacrimation were more improved in the acetorphan group. No side effects were noted in the acetorphan group; one clonidine patient experienced severe hypotension.

Published studies evaluating analgesic activity are only in the animal model. The potential for a new analgesic mechanism of action makes acetorphan a promising agent. Acetorphan has been shown to have minimal abuse potential and withdrawal is not precipitated upon abrupt discontinuation of the drug in animals.

Finally, a possible role in the treatment of gastroesophageal reflux disease (GERD) has been suggested based on the results of a study evaluating the drug's effects on the lower esophageal sphincter.

Side effects: No side effects significantly different from placebo have been identified in the clinical trials.

Summary: Acetorphan is not commercially available in the US, but it is available in France as 100 mg capsules. Recent research, however, suggests it will provide a novel antidiarrheal agent with minimal side effects. Several potential additional indications are currently being investigated, such as the treatment of opioid withdrawal, GERD and analgesia.

Amifloxacin – Fluoroquinolone antibiotic

Pharmacology: Amifloxacin is a fluorinated quinolone-carboxylic acid that is structurally related to nalidixic acid (*NegGram*) and cinoxacin (eg, *Cinobac*). It has a broad spectrum of activity against many gram-positive and gram-negative organisms including *Escherichia coli*, *Klebsiella pneumoniae*, *Proteus vulgaris*, *Citrobacter freundii*, *Pseudomonas aeruginosa* and *Serratia marcescens*. Because of its high degree of renal excretion, it may be effective for the treatment of urinary tract infections.

Pharmacokinetics: The pharmacokinetic parameters of multiple oral dosing of amifloxacin were evaluated in 48 men randomized to receive amifloxacin every 12 hours (200, 400 or 600 mg) or every 8 hours (400, 600 or 800 mg) orally for 10 days. Amifloxacin was rapidly absorbed with a T_{max} of 0.98 hours. Steady-state concentrations in the urine were > 100 mcg/ml for all doses except for the 200 mg every 12 hour regimen (where the concentration was > 40 mcg/ml). The half-life ranged from 4.25 to 5.78 hours, and the renal clearance ranged from 128 to 73 ml/hr/kg with the 200 mg every 12 hour and 800 mg every 8 hour regimens, respectively. The major route of elimination was renal with ≈ 54% of the administered dose excreted in the urine. Amifloxacin exhibited concentration-dependent pharmacokinetics. Pharmacokinetic parameters were comparable to those of other quinolones.

A single oral dose of amifloxacin 200 mg was evaluated in 10 elderly subjects (aged 65 to 79 years). The time to maximum concentration was 1.6 hours, the half-life was 5.37 hours for men and 4.47 hours for women and 42% was excreted renally. Dose adjustment of amifloxacin in the elderly is probably not necessary.

Clinical trials: The in vitro activity of amifloxacin was compared with that of ciprofloxacin *(Cipro)* and ofloxacin *(Floxin)*against 500 isolates of gram-positive and gram-negative bacteria. Overall, amifloxacin had high in vitro activity against a wide range of organisms, especially *Enterobacteriaceae*.

In another trial, the in vitro activity of amifloxacin against *Staphylococcus saprophyticus* and *E coli* was compared with that of other standard antibiotics used for the treatment of acute urinary tract infections. The drugs evaluated included amifloxacin, gentamicin (eg, *Garamycin*), amoxicillin (eg, *Amoxil*), cephalexin (eg, *Keflex*), trimethoprim (TMP; eg, *Trimpex*), trimethoprim-sulfamethoxazole (TMP-SMZ; eg, *Septra*) and cinoxacin (eg, *Cinobac*). Overall, the isolates were more susceptible to TMP-SMZ, TMP and amifloxacin than to the other drugs tested.

The in vitro activity of seven different quinolone antibiotics (ciprofloxacin, ofloxacin, amifloxacin, enoxacin, norfloxacin and two investigational agents) against 115 strains of MRSA was evaluated; all of the agents were effectively bactericidal.

In vivo trials with amifloxacin that have been published to date are limited. In one trial, the safety and efficacy of oral amifloxacin was compared with that of SMZ/TMP for the treatment of uncomplicated urinary tract infections in women (n = 153) with signs and symptoms of a UTI and bacteria in the urine. Patients received amifloxacin 200 mg every 12 hours (n = 52) or 400 mg every 12 hours (n = 54) or TMP 160 mg/SMZ 800 mg every 12 hours (n = 47) for 10 days. The outcomes were defined as bacteriologic cure, failure or superinfection, and clinical cure or improvement. There was no significant difference in bacteriologic cure rates at 5 to 9 days post-therapy between the two drugs. All evaluable patients showed clinical improvement or cure at the 5 to 9 day visit. Persistent cure was seen in almost all cases at the 4 to 6 week follow-up visit.

Side effects: In clinical trials the adverse effects seen with amifloxacin were mild and self-limited. In the multiple dose study, four patients required discontinuation of therapy due to amifloxacin; one developed pruritus and three experienced a 5- to 8-fold increase in serum ALT (above upper normal limits) that was asymptomatic and resolved spontaneously once the drug was discontinued. The primary adverse effects noted were nausea (15%), abdominal pain (8.3%), dyspepsia (6.7%), headache (8.3%), insomnia (3.3%), tinnitus (3.3%) and pruritus (5%). The renal (asymptomatic crystalluria) and hepatic adverse effects were seen in subjects receiving > 1200 mg daily. Doses < 1200 mg daily were well tolerated.

Summary: Amifloxacin is a fluoroquinolone antibiotic with activity and pharmacokinetics similar to other commercially available quinolones. Because it is primarily renally eliminated, it may be effective for the treatment of urinary tract infections. Overall, it appears to be well tolerated with the major side effects being GI in nature.

Amifloxacin, which is in late clinical trials, will be available from Sterling Winthrop. An anticipated approval date for amifloxacin is unknown.

Cabergoline – Antiparkinson agent

Pharmacology: Cabergoline, a synthetic ergoline, is a dopamine agonist that has high specificity and affinity for the D_2 receptor. The continuous stimulation of dopamine receptors may make cabergoline useful for the treatment of motor fluctuations associated with Parkinson's disease (PD). It has also been used for the treatment of hyperprolactinemia, inhibitions of lactation, prolactinomas and acromegaly.

Pharmacokinetics: Cabergoline is well absorbed after oral administration. Administration with food does not affect the absorption or disposition of cabergoline. Peak plasma levels are seen between 0.5 and 4 hours. Once absorbed, cabergoline is widely distributed to well perfused organs and is approximately 41% plasma protein bound. Cabergoline is extensively metabolized after oral administration to a number of inactive metabolites. Fecal excretion is the major route of elimination. There is no fecal excretion within 24 hours suggesting biliary excretion and enterohepatic recycling. Urinary excretion of unchanged drug accounts for < 14% of the administered dose. The estimated half-life in healthy volunteers is 63 to 68 hours.

Clinical trials: Initial treatment of PD with levodopa produces a dramatic response, but disease progression results in a shortening of response duration with clinical fluctuations. To date, bromocriptine *(Parlodel)* and pergolide *(Permax)*, direct-acting dopamine agonists, have helped alleviate this change in clinical response. However, they have a short duration of action requiring multiple daily doses. Cabergoline has the advantages of increased potency and a very long half-life allowing for once daily dosing.

The efficacy of cabergoline was studied in a randomized, double-blind study of 61 patients (44 males, 17 females) with PD who were stabilized on levodopa/carbidopa *(Sinemet)* but had response fluctuations. Cabergoline was initiated at 0.5 mg daily and increased by 0.5 mg per week for 5 weeks until there were 12 patients in each dose group (0.5, 1, 1.5, 2, 2.5 mg/day). If patients improved by at least 25% on activities of daily living (ADL) and motor score on the Unified Rating Scale for PD (URSPD), then they continued on the assigned dose for an additional 8 weeks. If not, the dose was increased by 0.5 mg per week until a 25% improvement occurred or a dose of 5 mg was reached. At the end of 5 weeks, the mean ADL on the URSPD decreased by 22%. Twenty-three patients (38%) had at least 25% improvement; 37 required a further dose adjustment. At week 13, the mean ADL decreased by 35%, and the percent "off" time decreased by 31%. Four patients withdrew early due to adverse effects (confusion, angina, heart failure, increased dyskinesias); not all of these were cabergoline-related.

In an open-label trial, 36 patients (27 males, 9 females) with PD stabilized on levodopa/carbidopa received cabergoline 0.5 to 1 mg initially with dose increases every 7 to 14 days until there was the best control of "off" periods. After 3 months of cabergoline (mean dose 9.2 mg), "off" time significantly decreased. A reduction in "off" hours continued after a mean period of 14.2 months of treatment. There was also a significant decrease in daily levodopa dose. Response was dramatic in 10 patients, moderate in 23 patients and 3 patients were considered treatment failures.

In a recent trial with a similar study design to those previously described (5 week double-blind dose escalation followed by 8 week evaluation), 41 patients with PD (mean duration, 9 years) were evaluated. Three patients dropped out of the trial, 2 due to cardiac conditions not related to cabergoline and 1 due to medication-related confusion. The mean cabergoline dose was 2.8 mg. There was an 18% reduction in mean total levodopa dose. Mean Parkinson motor score, timed finger tapping score and timed walking test scores all significantly improved. There was a 42% reduction in "off" time (6.2 vs 3.6 hr/day). When patients self-rated their response to therapy, 14 showed marked improvement, 7 moderate improvement and 6 mild improvement. Physician ratings showed 9 marked, 21 moderate and 6 mild improvements. No patients deteriorated during the trial.

Side effects: Cabergoline appears to be well tolerated with side effects similar to those seen with other dopamine agonists. In clinical trials involving patients with PD, the major adverse effects noted were mild and transient and included dizziness/vertigo, somnolence, headache, nausea, symptomatic orthostatic hypotension, vivid dreams, visual hallucinations, confusion, increased dyskinesias and nasal stuffiness. One case of pleuropulmonary disease has been reported in a PD patient receiving cabergoline.

Summary: Cabergoline is a dopamine agonist that is more potent and has a longer half-life than either bromocriptine or pergolide. These two features make it an attractive alternative for the treatment of response fluctuations in patients with PD. Clinical trials to date have shown promising results, and the drug has been well tolerated. Its major limiting adverse effect is hypotension. An anticipated approval date for cabergoline, which will be available from Adria, is unknown.

Carprofen *(Rimadyl)* – Nonsteroidal anti-inflammatory agent

Pharmacology: Carprofen [(D,L)-6-chloro-alpha-methylcarbazole-2-acetic acid] is a member of the arylpropionic acid class of nonsteroidal anti-inflammatory drugs (NSAIDs) which includes ibuprofen (eg, *Motrin*), naproxen (eg, *Naprosyn*) and others. The drug also possesses analgesic and antipyretic activity.

Although the site and exact mechanism of action of the NSAIDs has not been fully elucidated, most investigators agree that these drugs owe their analgesic and anti-inflammatory activity, as well as their gastric irritant properties, to their ability to inhibit prostaglandin synthetase. Carprofen is considered to be a less potent inhibitor of prostaglandin biosynthesis than naproxen or ibuprofen, and is only 1% to 4% as potent as indomethacin (eg, *Indocin*).

Considerable evidence suggests that the anti-inflammatory activity of carprofen is due primarily to the D-isomer; the L-isomer is only about one-seventh as potent.

Pharmacokinetics:

Absorption/Distribution – Carprofen is rapidly and extensively absorbed after oral administration. Peak concentrations of approximately 6 to 12 mcg/ml are achieved in 1 to 3 hours; absolute bioavailability is approximately 90%. Ingestion of food results in a slight reduction in the rate of absorption as well as the peak plasma concentration. However, the total amount of the drug absorbed is not reduced. Peak plasma concentrations may be higher in the elderly. Carprofen is highly protein bound (> 98%). In patients with osteoarthritis (OA) or rheumatoid arthritis (RA), the drug enters the synovial fluid rapidly, where it may achieve concentrations in excess of plasma concentrations.

Metabolism–Approximately 65% to 70% of an administered dose is metabolized by direct conjugation to an ester glucuronide. The elimination half-life ($t½$) is between 13 to 25 hours. Despite the extensive hepatic metabolism, no difference has been observed in pharmacokinetics between cirrhotics and normal volunteers. Thus, dosage adjustments are unnecessary in patients with renal or hepatic insufficiency.

Excretion–Most of an orally administered dose of carprofen (65% to 70%) is eliminated in the urine as the glucuronide metabolite; only 3% to 12% of a dose is excreted unchanged. The remainder of the drug is excreted in the feces after undergoing extensive enterohepatic recycling.

Clinical trials: Carprofen is effective in a variety of clinical settings including treatment of rheumatoid arthritis, osteoarthritis, ankylosing spondylitis, extra-articular inflammatory processes (eg, tendonitis, bursitis), acute pain syndromes (eg, dental and post-traumatic pain) and acute gouty arthritis. Dosages have ranged from 150 to 600 mg/day in two or three divided doses. The few available comparative studies have usually shown carprofen to be equal to, or superior to, aspirin up to 3600 mg/day. Comparisons with indomethacin 75 to 150 mg/day have usually shown the lower doses (up to 300 mg/day) of carprofen to be slightly less effective but better tolerated than indomethacin. Larger doses of carprofen (400 to 600 mg/day) have been used in the treatment of OA; however, the use of larger doses may not produce any additional response over lower doses.

Side effects: *Gastrointestinal* effects have occurred in approximately 15% of patients. Pain, nausea, heartburn and dyspepsia are most common, while diarrhea is uncommon (approximately 1%). More serious GI side effects such as peptic ulceration are rare. Carprofen has been used along with antacids in patients with active peptic ulcer disease and has been well tolerated.

Renal or urinary adverse reactions including urinary frequency, dysuria, burning, hematuria, nephritis, proteinuria and acute renal failure occurred in 3.4% of 1521 patients in premarketing clinical trials.

Cutaneous reactions such as eczema, skin rash, urticaria and photosensitivity have occurred in 6% to 10% of patients.

Hepatic enzyme elevation occurred in 1.4% of patients in European trials and in as many as 14% of patients in large American trials. These enzyme elevations are usually asymptomatic.

Summary: Carprofen appears to be an effective NSAID which offers convenient twice daily dosing. Despite a low incidence of serious GI side effects, the drug does not appear superior to currently available agents.

Carprofen was approved by the FDA December 31, 1987. However, Roche has made a decision not to market carprofen at this time.

Celiprolol HCl *(Selecor)* – Cardioselective beta-adrenergic blocking agent

Pharmacology: Celiprolol is a third-generation, cardioselective, hydrophilic beta-adrenoreceptor blocking agent. It possesses weak vasodilating and bronchodilating effects attributed to partial, selective β_2-adrenoreceptor agonist activity and, possibly, direct papaverine-like smooth muscle relaxation. There is evidence for intrinsic sympathomimetic activity (ISA) at the β_2-receptor. The drug is devoid of membrane stabilizing activity (MSA, or quinidine-like effect). Weak alpha$_2$-antagonist properties are also present but are not considered clinically significant at therapeutic doses.

At therapeutic doses, celiprolol reduces heart rate and blood pressure. While the drug does not generally produce any ECG changes, it can increase the AV nodal functional refractory period. Celiprolol does not appear to alter pulmonary function, nor inhibit bronchodilation induced by agents such as aminophylline (eg, *Phyllocontin*), albuterol (eg, *Proventil*) and ipratropium (*Atrovent*). Triglycerides, LDL cholesterol and total cholesterol are decreased in some patients while HDL is increased; it appears that total lipid levels are not increased. A reduction in fibrinogen levels has occurred, which may be of some benefit in hypertensive patients with hypercoagulability.

Pharmacokinetics: Following oral administration, absorption is non-linear and dose-dependent. Bioavailability ranges from 30% to 70% following a single 100 mg dose and averages 74% after a 400 mg dose. Single-dose bioavailability is reduced by chlorthalidone (eg, *Hygroton*), hydrochlorothiazide (eg, *Esidrix*) and theophylline (eg, *Theo-Dur*). Food has also reduced bioavailability in some studies, but data are conflicting. Peak plasma concentrations and pharmacodynamic activity are seen 2 to 4 hours after oral administration; pharmacodynamic activity persists for 24 hours. Protein binding is ≈ 25% and the drug follows a hydrophilic pattern of distribution.

Celiprolol is largely unmetabolized and is excreted unchanged in urine and feces. It does not undergo first-pass hepatic metabolism and there are no significant active metabolites. Approximately 15% (range, 3% to 22%) of an oral dose and 50% of an IV dose is recovered in the urine within 3 days, the rest being excreted in the feces. Steady-state concentrations are achieved after 2 to 3 days. The predominant mode of excretion of active drug is renal; renal dysfunction may cause a reduction in systemic clearance and the need for dose reduction. Bioavailability is decreased and the extent of renal elimination increased in patients with cirrhosis. The pharmacokinetics are not significantly different in the elderly. The elimination half-life averages 4 to 5 hours. Placental transfer averages 3% at steady state compared to 18% for propranolol (eg, *Inderal*) and 6% for atenolol (*Tenormin*).

Clinical trials: Celiprolol is a safe and effective drug for treatment of hypertension and angina. In doses of 200 to 500 mg once daily in the morning, celiprolol reduces blood pressure to comparable levels seen with other β-blockers, calcium blockers and ACE inhibitors. In comparative trials in patients with mild to moderate hypertension, a 200 to 600 mg dose was similar in efficacy to 80 to 160 mg/day propranolol or 100 mg/day atenolol. In patients with angina, celiprolol 300 to 600 mg daily was as effective as propranolol 80 to 160 mg/day or atenolol 50 to 100 mg/day in improving exercise performance, reducing the number of angina attacks and nitroglycerin requirements, and increasing the time to, or reducing the degree of, ST segment depression. The addition of a diuretic to doses of 200 to 400 mg/day may be more effective at controlling blood pressure than the use of celiprolol monotherapy in doses of 300 to 600 mg/day.

Side effects: In a study of > 2300 patients, side effects were mild. GI symptoms (eg, nausea, abdominal discomfort, diarrhea), the most frequently reported complaints, were responsible for drug discontinuation in 13 patients. Cardiovascular symptoms included development of a modest degree of CHF, AV nodal block and bradycardia. Other side effects included: Headache (6%); fatigue (4%); dizziness (3%); insomnia (1%); Raynaud's phenomenon; orthostatic hypotension; bronchial obstruction; tremor; rash; muscle cramps; impotence.

Summary: Celiprolol appears to be well tolerated and effective for the treatment of hypertension and angina. Its combination of cardioselectivity, β_2-agonist activity, hydrophilicity and long duration of action make it unique among currently available drugs in this class. Whether these properties will be useful in the myriad of other applications for which β-blockers have been used (eg, post-MI prophylaxis, migraine, selected arrhythmias) will require additional experience. The NDA for celiprolol was filed by Rhone-Poulenc Rorer in June 1987 for long-term use in controlling hypertension and angina. The drug will be co-marketed by Upjohn under the name *Selecor*. A 1995 approval is expected.

Cetirizine *(Reactine)* – Antihistamine

Pharmacology: Cetirizine is a carboxylated metabolite of hydroxyzine (eg, *Vistaril*) which acts as a potent H_1-receptor antagonist. The H_1-receptors are distributed in those areas most closely related to the IgE-mediated allergic response. Cetirizine inhibits both histamine release and eosinophil chemotaxis during the secondary phase of the allergic response. It reduces inflammatory cell infiltration (ie, eosinophils, neutrophils, basophils) by 75% during the late-phase response. However, it is not cytolytic for eosinophils already present. The drug also inhibits the release of cytotoxic mediators from platelets. Platelets have specific IgE receptors which, when stimulated, can release cytotoxic substances which may contribute to the mediation of the inflammatory response. Cetirizine has less affinity than hydroxyzine or terfenadine *(Seldane)* for calcium, adrenergic α_1, dopaminergic D_2, serotonergic 5-HT and muscarinic receptors. It has little effect on mast cells and the release of mediators of immediate hypersensitivity reactions. After oral administration of a 10 mg dose, suppression of the histamine-induced wheal and flare response occurs within 1 hour and persists for 24 hours. Cetirizine 10 mg is more potent than terfenadine 60 mg, loratadine *(Claritin)* 10 mg and chlorpheniramine (eg, *Chlor-Trimeton*) 6 mg, and equal in potency to diphenhydramine (eg, *Benadryl*) 50 mg, hydroxyzine 25 mg and terfenadine 180 mg.

Neither subjective nor objective assessments of cognition and task performance were significantly altered by cetirizine 10 mg.

Pharmacokinetics: Cetirizine is rapidly absorbed after oral administration; peak plasma levels are reached within 1 hour. Food does not affect the extent of absorption but may decrease the rate. Cetirizine is widely distributed (Vd 30 to 40 L) but does not appear to cross the blood-brain barrier to any significant extent. Protein binding averages 93%. The elimination half-life is 7 to 10 hours in adults, 6 to 7 hours in children, and 18 to 21 hours in patients with renal dysfunction. Normal adult clearance is 0.04 to 0.05 L/hr/kg. After oral administration of a 10 mg dose, 70% of the drug is excreted unchanged in the urine within 72 hours and 10% is excreted in the feces. The drug is not removed by hemodialysis to any significant degree.

Clinical trials: Comparative trials have shown cetirizine to be safe and as effective as chlorpheniramine, hydroxyzine and terfenadine in the treatment of seasonal and perennial allergic rhinitis and chronic idiopathic urticaria. Tachyphylaxis was not reported, even with long-term treatment. Cetirizine has also shown promise in the treatment of pollen-associated asthma in atopic individuals, angioedema, atopic dermatitis, and certain types of physical urticaria such as delayed-pressure urticaria, dermatographia and cold urticaria.

Side effects: As with other drugs of this class, the most common side effects are somnolence and sedation. A reported incidence of 5% to 20% is similar to that seen with terfenadine and astemizole *(Hismanal)*. In placebo controlled trials, there was no significant difference between cetirizine and placebo in anticholinergic and cardiovascular effects, GI disturbances, headache or dizziness. Conflicting data have been published about whether cetirizine enhances the sedative effects of alcohol. There is no evidence that second-generation H_1-receptor antagonists like cetirizine cause fetal anomalies in humans.

Drug interactions: Data are currently being studied regarding the potential for an interaction between cetirizine and erythromycin (eg, *E-Mycin*) and ketoconazole *(Nizoral)*. However, since cetirizine excretion is primarily renal, the potential for an interaction is minimized.

Summary: Cetirizine appears to be a safe and effective alternative to presently available antihistamines. Further studies are required to determine whether it offers any significant advantages over other second-generation antihistamines.

The NDA for cetirizine has been pending since July 1988. On April 7, 1993 an FDA advisory committee recommended approval for once-daily treatment of seasonal and perennial allergic rhinitis and chronic idiopathic urticaria at doses of 5, 10 and 20 mg/day; however, they also agreed that the sedative effect requires further study. Cetirizine, which is currently available in Canada, will be available as *Reactine* from Pfizer. A 1994 or early 1995 approval is anticipated.

Cifenline Succinate *(Cipralan)* – Antiarrhythmic agent

Pharmacology: Cifenline succinate (formerly cibenzoline) is a new antiarrhythmic agent. It is an imidazoline derivative, structurally unrelated to any other currently available antiarrhythmic.

Cifenline's primary electrophysiologic effects are similar to those produced by quinidine (eg, *Duraquin*, *Quinidex*). The drug acts predominantly on the fast sodium current, reducing the rate of rise of phase 0 of the action potential and prolonging the effective refractory period. These effects are characteristic of Class IA (Vaughn-Williams classification) agents such as quinidine, procainamide (eg, *Pronestyl*, *Procan SR*) and disopyramide (eg, *Norpace*).

The drug has also been shown to increase the action potential duration, a property of Class III agents, and may produce blockade of the slow inward calcium channel similar to the Class IV agents. The contribution of these secondary effects to the drug's clinical usefulness has not been clearly delineated.

The drug produces a plasma concentration-dependent prolongation of the QRS duration. Prolongation of the PR interval and the rate-corrected QT interval have not been consistently observed, but these effects are compatible with the drug's known electrophysiologic effects and may be seen at higher doses or in patients with underlying conduction disturbances.

Pharmacokinetics: Cifenline is well absorbed after oral administration. Absolute bioavailability is approximately 85%, with peak plasma concentrations occurring approximately 1.5 hours after administration. Coadministration with food slightly decreases the rate, but not the extent, of absorption. Approximately 55% of the drug is bound to plasma proteins, primarily albumin.

Following multiple doses, the elimination half-life of the drug is approximately 12 hours (range, 8 to 12 hours). As much as 60% of a dose is excreted unchanged in the urine, and total body clearance correlates closely with creatinine clearance. Therefore, in patients with chronic renal failure, dosage should be reduced. Older patients also clear the drug more slowly, probably as a result of age-related reductions in renal function. The plasma concentrations of unchanged drug are apparently responsible for its antiarrhythmic effect. Studies have shown that the antiarrhythmic response following twice-daily administration of cifenline is equivalent to a 4 times a day regimen.

Clinical trials: Cifenline is effective in suppressing a variety of ventricular arrhythmias, including complex PVCs and nonsustained ventricular tachycardia. In these applications, the drug has produced response rates similar to or higher than those for quinidine, procainamide, disopyramide and tocainide *(Tonocard)*. Data for patients with sustained ventricular tachycardia resistent to conventional therapy is limited; however, response rates of 25% have occurred. Long-term follow-up studies (12 to

24 months) have reported sustained therapeutic efficacy in 36% to 80% of initial responders.

Side effects: Cifenline appears to be well tolerated, especially when compared to the other Class IA antiarrhythmics. Gastrointestinal intolerance is the most common reason cited for discontinuation of therapy due to side effects. Other adverse effects reported include: Lightheadedness, dizziness, nervousness, tremulousness, blurred vision and dry mouth.

Worsening of preexisting left ventricular dysfunction has occurred. The drug should be used with caution in patients with CHF, especially if baseline ejection fraction is less than 30%. The proarrhythmic effect that may occur (as with all antiarrhythmic agents) has occurred in 10% to 15% of patients receiving cifenline.

No serious hematologic or laboratory abnormalities have been reported.

Summary: Cifenline is a unique antiarrhythmic agent which may offer similar efficacy with a more favorable side effect profile than currently available Class IA agents. The long half-life which permits twice-daily dosing may also be considered an advantage. Cifenline will be co-marketed as *Cipralan* by Roche and Glaxo. The NDA has been pending since December 1985. The official generic name was recently changed from cibenzoline to cifenline.

Cilazapril *(Inhibace)* – Non-sulfhydryl-containing ACE inhibitor

Pharmacology: Cilazapril is a potent, structurally new, non-sulfhydryl-containing orally active angiotensin-converting enzyme (ACE) inhibitor prodrug under investigation for use in patients with hypertension and CHF. Following oral administration, cilazapril is de-esterified in the liver and other tissues to the active diacid form, cilazaprilat. Cilazaprilat is ≈ 10 times more potent than captopril *(Capoten)* and 5 times more potent than enalaprilat, the active form of enalapril *(Vasotec)*.

ACE inhibitors block the enzymatic conversion of angiotensin I to the potent vasoconstrictor angiotensin II. While this inhibition also results in reduced metabolism of bradykinin, alterations in the prostaglandin system and reductions in plasma aldosterone and antidiuretic hormone, these responses do not appear to be responsible for the primary therapeutic effects of these agents. Blockade of angiotensin II production reduces supine and standing blood pressure in hypertensive patients. In patients with CHF, the vasodilatory response reduces afterload, leading to an increase in cardiac output. These beneficial responses may be facilitated by the responses mentioned above.

After administration of cilazapril, ACE activity, angiotensin II and plasma aldosterone concentrations, total peripheral resistance, blood pressure (systolic, diastolic and mean), and the response to exogenous angiotension I are all reduced, while heart rate, baroreceptor reflex sensitivity, cardiovascular reflexes and glomerular filtration rate are usually unchanged.

Pharmacokinetics: Cilazapril is rapidly absorbed after oral administration, with peak levels of the parent compound achieved at ≈ 1 hour. Conversion to cilazaprilat, the active form, is rapid and extensive, with peak levels attained at ≈ 1.8 hours with 57% absolute bioavailability of the active compound. In contrast to some other ACEIs, the bioavailability is not significantly reduced by food. After single doses of 0.5, 1, 2.5 and 5 mg, peak plasma levels of cilazaprilat were 5.4, 12.4, 37.7 and 94.2 ng/ml, respectively, indicating that greater than proportional increases in the active compound are achieved over this dose range. The elimination of cilazaprilat is biphasic, with an initial half-life of 1 to 2 hours controlled by the rate of conversion to this active form, followed by a prolonged terminal elimination half-life of 30 to 50 hours. The volume of distribution is ≈ 20 L.

Clearance of cilazaprilat is almost exclusively renal. Patients with severe renal or hepatic impairment may require smaller or less frequent doses. One study suggests that hypertensive patients undergoing hemodialysis can be controlled on 0.5 mg cilazapril post-dialysis. Presence of CHF or advanced age has not been shown to significantly alter pharmacokinetic parameters.

Clinical trials: Clinical trials in > 4500 hypertensive patients have evaluated the efficacy of cilazapril. Single daily doses of 2.5 to 5 mg are as effective as single daily doses of: Hydrochlorothiazide (HCTZ; eg, *Esidrix*) 25 to 50 mg; atenolol *(Tenormin)* 50 to 100 mg; sustained release propranolol (eg, *Inderal LA*) 80 to 160 mg; and enalapril 10 to 20 mg. In patients with mild to moderate hypertension, a 5 mg cilazapril dose produces a maximal effect, which can be enhanced by the addition of 12.5 to 25 mg HCTZ. In patients with severe hypertension, including patients with left ventricular hypertrophy, the mean effective dose was 10 mg in combination with 12.5 to 25 mg of HCTZ daily.

Side effects: Cilazapril appears to be well tolerated. In controlled trials of cilazapril monotherapy in > 3500 patients, the most frequently reported side effects were: Headache (4.5%); dizziness (3.3%); fatigue (1.7%); cough (1.6%); chest pain (0.8%); rash, somnolence (0.6%). In patients ≥ 65 years of age, cough, dizziness, palpitations and somnolence occurred slightly more frequently than in younger patients. The addition of HCTZ in an additional 1000 patients resulted in a slightly higher incidence of dizziness, cough and somnolence, while the incidence of other side effects was comparable to cilazapril monotherapy.

Drug interactions: Indomethacin (eg, *Indocin*) considerably attenuates the antihypertensive activity of cilazapril. This attenuation was most pronounced when cilazapril was added to indomethacin, while the addition of indomethacin to a stable cilazapril regimen resulted in a degree of attenuation of effect which was considered to be clinically insignificant. Thus, the significance of this interaction appears to be dependent on the order of drug administration.

Summary: Cilazapril is a long-acting, potent ACE inhibitor. It appears to be well tolerated, while offering the advantage of once-daily dosing; this property may make it a useful addition to a class of drugs whose safety and efficacy continue to be confirmed in a variety of disease states. An NDA for cilazapril was filed in September 1989 for hypertension. Roche and Glaxo will comarket cilazapril as *Inhibace*.On August 13, 1992, the FDA classified cilazapril as "approvable". A 1995 approval is expected.

Clobazam *(Frisium)* – Benzodiazepine

Clobazam and nitrazepam are investigational benzodiazepine derivatives. The profile of these agents parallels those of approved benzodiazepines; subtle differences account for individual product distinction.

Clobazam is structurally and pharmacologically related to approved benzodiazepines. Antianxiety and anticonvulsant properties are similar to diazepam; the usual adult dose is 20 to 30 mg daily. Initially, clobazam is effective against all varieties of epilepsy; however, efficacy decreases within a few days to a few weeks in approximately one-third of patients. Success has also been demonstrated in cyclic exacerbations of epilepsy associated with menstruation. Clobazam is a weak hypnotic agent.

The pharmacokinetics are independent of dose and concentration. Oral clobazam is 87% absorbed. Concomitant administration with alcohol increases clobazam's bioavailability by 50%. Food may slow the rate, but does not alter total absorption. Absorption is not influenced by age or sex. Clobazam is 85% bound to human serum protein; peak serum concentrations occur 1 to 4 hours after ingestion. It is metabolized via dealkylation and hydroxylation to a pharmacologically active metabolite, N – desmethylclobazam, and several inactive metabolites. The mean half-life of the unchanged drug is 18 hours, and up to 77 hours for metabolites. Clobazam is 81% to 97% excreted in the urine; accumulation is expected in impaired renal function.

The most frequent (10% to 44%) side effects include: Drowsiness, hangover effects, dizziness, weakness and lightheadedness. Less frequent (5% to 10%) adverse reactions include: Weight gain, orthostatic hypotension, syncope, headache, dry mouth and incoordination.

Dilevalol *(Unicard)* – β-adrenergic blocking agent

Pharmacology: Dilevalol, a noncardioselective β-adrenergic blocking agent, is the R,R-isomer of labetalol *(Normodyne, Trandate)*, one of four optical isomers of the drug. Although dilevalol is virtually devoid of α_1-blocking activity, having only one-fourth to one-third the activity of labetalol, it has ≈ 7 times the vasodilatory effect. However, this effect appears to be mediated via a β_2-agonist effect as opposed to an α_1-blocking effect. Dilevalol also has ≈ 4 times the β-blocking (β_1 and β_2) effect of labetalol. The degree of β_1 receptor blockade appears to be similar to propranolol (eg, *Inderal*).

The β-agonist activity of dilevalol appears to be selective for β_2 receptors. The vasodilatory response is blocked by propranolol, but not metoprolol *(Lopressor)* pretreatment, indicating the vasodilatory actions are mediated by β_2 receptor stimulation. Pindolol *(Visken)*, which has significant intrinsic sympathomimetic activity (ISA), differs from dilevalol in that its agonist activity is not β_2 selective.

Dilevalol appears to decrease peripheral vascular resistance with no effect on cardiac output. The reflex increase in heart rate that might be expected with vasodilation is counteracted by the drug's β-blocking activity. In one study of 29 patients, heart rate actually decreased by 8 beats per minute compared to placebo. Dilevalol slightly decreased plasma renin activity in one study. In a study comparing dilevalol and metoprolol on the lipid profile of 309 patients, dilevalol increased HDL cholesterol and slightly decreased LDL cholesterol, a finding that is opposite that seen with other agents in this class besides pindolol and acebutolol *(Sectral)*.

Pharmacokinetics:

Absorption/Distribution – Dilevalol is rapidly absorbed following oral administration, reaching peak levels within 1 hour. Following absorption, it is rapidly distributed in the extravascular system. In 12 volunteers, the mean maximum concentration was 62 ng/ml. Plasma levels appear to increase in a dose-related manner.

Metabolsim/Excretion – Dilevalol undergoes extensive first-pass metabolism (85% to 95%), resulting in an absolute bioavailability of 11% to 14%. The half-life is ≈ 8 hours following oral administration, and 12 hours following IV, indicating dilevalol need only be given once daily. The metabolites are conjugated with glucuronides and are excreted in urine. Approximately 3% of the drug was excreted unchanged after an IV dose in 12 volunteers.

Plasma concentrations do not appear altered in severe renal impairment. In a study of six volunteers, only 0.007% (mean, 27 mcg) of a dose was excreted in breast milk over 48 hours.

Clinical trials: Dilevalol, in once-daily doses of 100 to 800 mg, is effective in the treatment of mild to moderate hypertension. Because of its vasodilatory effects, it may be more useful than other agents of this class in hypertensive patients with compromised myocardial function or peripheral vascular insufficiency. Since it does not affect glomerular filtration rate, renal plasma flow, renal blood flow or renal vascular resistance, it may be useful in patients with renal insufficiency. Some studies also indicate a possible benefit in black patients. It is effective when administered orally and IV. In several studies, dilevalol was equal to or greater than labetalol, metoprolol and atenolol *(Tenormin)* in antihypertensive efficacy, with less side effects. In one study comparing dilevalol with atenolol, patients receiving dilevalol showed a greater and longer-lasting decrease in mean arterial pressure.

Although only reported in two patients, dilevalol may be useful for the treatment of pheochromocytoma. It may also be useful, administered IV, in the management of severe hypertension. Further studies are needed.

Side effects: Dilevalol appears to be well tolerated. It has a relatively low incidence of CNS side effects, despite its lipid solubility. When compared to placebo, the most common side effects associated with dilevalol were dizziness, somnolence and nausea.

Drug interactions: In one study involving nine healthy subjects, cimetidine *(Tagamet)* slightly increased dilevalol's bioavailability. The clinical significance was not determined.

Summary: Dilevalol, an isomer of labetalol, is a noncardioselective β-adrenergic blocking agent with significant vasodilatory (β_2 agonist) activity; therefore, it may have advantages over other agents in this class in certain hypertensive patients with altered cardiac conduction. Black patients and patients with renal insufficiency may also benefit. It also appears to be well tolerated, with minimal side effects reported. It is usually administered once daily, and can be given orally or IV.

An NDA for the oral form was filed in 1986. In January 1990, the FDA's Cardio-Renal Advisory Committee recommended approval for dilevalol. However, due to an increasing incidence of hepatotoxicity, the manufacturer decided to withdraw the NDA and discontinue the worldwide marketing of the drug.

Dirithromycin *(Dynabac)* – Macrolide antibiotic

Pharmacology: Dirithromycin, an erythromycin analog, is an oral macrolide antibiotic. A modification in structure gives dirithromycin greater stability in an acidic environment. It also offers the advantages of increased tissue concentrations and a longer half-life allowing for once daily dosing. Therefore, the limitations with erythromycin such as decomposition in gastric acid, erratic absorption and a pharmacokinetic profile that requires dosing every 6 to 8 hours, are potentially eliminated with dirithromycin.

Dirithromycin reversibly binds to the 23S component of the 50S ribosomal unit thereby impairing transpeptidation or translocation. The net result is that it inhibits RNA-dependent protein synthesis. Its spectrum is similar to that of erythromycin including gram positive organisms, *Legionella*, *Helicobacter pylori* and *Chlamydia trachomatis*. It is not effective for *Listeria monocytogenes*, *L pneumophilia*, *H influenzae*, *N gonorrhoeae*, *Pseudomonas* or methicillin-resistant *S aureus* or *S epidermidis*.

Pharmacokinetics: Following a 500 mg oral dose, the mean peak plasma concentration (C_{max}) was 0.48 mg/L, with a mean time to peak concentration (T_{max}) of 4 hours and a mean plasma concentration vs time curve (AUC) of 3.37 mg • hr/L. While administration with food may increase T_{max} (3.7 vs 5.5 hr) and the AUC (1.43 vs 1.67 mg • hr/L), no change in C_{max} was noted. Therefore, dirithromycin may be taken without regard to meals.

Dirithromycin achieves relatively high tissue concentrations within 4 to 24 hours after dosing. Due to its lipid solubility and low ionization, it is able to cross biological membranes better than erythromycin. Plasma protein binding ranges between 15% to 32%. Dirithromycin has good tissue penetration into the lower respiratory tract, upper respiratory tract and prostate.

After oral administration, dirithromycin undergoes rapid, nonenzymatic hydrolysis to erythromycylamine which is an active metabolite. The primary route of elimination is fecal and hepatic elimination. Only 1% to 3% is eliminated in the urine compared to 81% to 97% in the stool. The plasma half-life is about 44 hours, allowing for once daily dosing.

Clinical trials: Patients with skin and skin structure infections were randomized to receive dirithromycin 500 mg daily or erythromycin base 250 mg 4 times daily for 7 days; 71.8% of patients receiving dirithromycin were cured and 21.8% improved. Similar results were seen with erythromycin (74% cured, 19.1% improved). There were no significant differences in clinical or bacteriological outcome in any trials.

The efficacy of dirithromycin 500 mg daily was compared to that of erythromycin 250 mg 4 times daily for 10 days in 389 patients with pharyngitis or tonsillitis caused by group A beta-hemolytic streptococci. Of patients receiving dirithromycin, 80.4% were cured and 11.3% improved vs 82.8% cured and 11.1% improved with erythromycin. In another similar study, an overall favorable clinical response was seen in 94% of patients in each treatment group.

Patients with acute bacterial exacerbation of chronic bronchitis were randomized to receive dirithromycin 500 mg daily or erythromycin 250 mg 4 times daily for a minimum of 7 days. There were no significant differences in overall favorable response (77.9% vs 80.9%, respectively).

Dirithromycin 500 mg daily was compared to erythromycin 250 mg 4 times daily for the treatment of community-acquired pneumonia (n = 571) or bacterial lobar or bronchopneumonia (n = 591). A favorable response (cure or improvement) was seen in > 90% of patients in both groups.

Side effects: The side effect profile of dirithromycin is similar to that of erythromycin. The most common complaints were GI in nature (abdominal pain, 5.6%; diarrhea, 5%; nausea, 4.9%). Headache (4.5%) was also commonly reported.

Drug interactions: Dirithromycin appears to have less potential to interact with the cytochrome P450 system than does erythromycin. With concomitant dirithromycin and theophylline therapy, there was an increase in theophylline clearance resulting in decreases in the trough concentration (18%) and C_{max} (26%) of theophylline. The concomitant administration of dirithromycin with antacids and H_2-receptor antagonists has resulted in increased and faster absorption.

Summary: Dirithromycin is a macrolide antibiotic that offers several advantages over erythromycin in that it has a more favorable pharmacokinetic profile allowing once daily dosing, increased tissue penetration and fewer drug interactions.

Dirithromycin *(Dynabac)* was approved by the FDA in August 1995 for patients ≥ 12 years of age with acute bacterial exacerbations of chronic bronchitis or secondary bacterial infection of acute bronchitis due to M *catarrhalis* or S *pneumoniae*. Recommended dosing is 500 mg once daily for 7 to 14 days. It will be available as 250 mg enteric-coated tablets.

Domperidone *(Motilium)* – Antiemetic

Pharmacology: Acute nausea and vomiting induced by cytotoxic chemotherapy are frequent and serious toxicities distressful to cancer patients. Symptoms can be so pronounced and refractory that they interfere with therapeutic measures and patient nutrition. Available antiemetics block the chemoreceptor trigger zone (CTZ) (neuroleptics), sedate the vomiting centers (antihistamines), block afferent impulses at the vomiting center (anticholinergics), act peripherally and in the CNS (metoclopramide), or by less defined central mechanisms (cannabinoids). These agents are effective in most patients; however, side effects (eg, drowsiness, dry mouth, hypotension, extrapyramidal effects) are limitations. Domperidone, an investigational antiemetic, appears to act with minimum adverse effects.

Domperidone is chemically unrelated to the butyrophenones, phenothiazines or metoclopramide; however, it shares pharmacological properties with these agents. In the medulla it produces a direct blocking effect of dopamine receptors in the CTZ. Like metoclopramide and haloperidol, domperidone is a peripheral dopamine antagonist; however, it contrasts in that it does not cross the blood-brain barrier and produce CNS effects. It selectively blocks peripheral dopamine receptors in the gastrointestinal wall, thus enhancing normal synchronized GI peristalsis and motility in the proximal portion of the GI tract; it may also counteract anticholinergic-induced relaxation of the lower esophageal sphincter (LES).

Pharmacokinetics: Peak plasma levels are achieved within 30 minutes following IM or oral administration and between 1 to 4 hours after rectal administration. Approximately 40% of a dose is rapidly distributed into peripheral compartments. It is metabolized in the liver and eliminated in the urine, primarily as conjugates. Less than 1% appears in the urine as unchanged drug. Excretion is almost complete within 4 days. The duration of activity is between 2 and 4 hours following IV administration.

Clinical trials: The effectiveness of domperidone in the treatment of nausea and vomiting associated with cytotoxic chemotherapy has been evaluated. Several double-blind studies were conducted in patients with Hodgkin's disease. Domperidone 16 mg IV was preferred and superior to placebo; it was effective and well tolerated, and decreased the duration of nausea and vomiting by greater than ⅓ when injected 1 hour before the start of cytostatic treatment. Domperidone, 1 to 40 mg IV daily, was administered with chemotherapy infusion in 172 patients. Vomiting induced by agents considered to be moderate emetics (eg, cyclophosphamide, 5-fluorouracil, vinblastine) was reduced; however, patients with emesis induced by doxorubicin or mechlorethamine did not respond as well. The higher dosages of domperidone did not achieve a proportionally augmented response rate. In another study, domperidone 4 mg IV produced excellent or good response in 72% of patients receiving varied chemotherapy; poor responses occurred in patients receiving dacarbazine. When domperidone 12 mg IV was compared to metoclopramide 10 mg IV, both drugs produced a good or excellent response in 70% of patients; however, metoclopramide had a higher incidence of side effects. Domperidone 1 mg/kg IV or metoclopramide 0.5 mg/kg IV was used to prevent chemotherapy-induced nausea and vomiting in children. In the random crossover trial, domperidone decreased nausea and vomiting to a significantly greater extent than metoclopramide.

Domperidone has been compared favorably to cimetidine in 20 gastric ulcer patients; it may also have value in treating symptoms of gastroesophageal reflux and post-operative- or bromocriptine-induced nausea and vomiting.

Side effects: Domperidone does not appear to produce significant side effects or toxicities. Doses of 40 mg IV or 100 mg orally have not been reported to produce CNS or cardiovascular side effects, only facial flushing, headache, slight somnolence and dry mouth. Unlike metoclopramide, domperidone does not cross the blood-brain barrier; therefore, the incidence of extrapyramidal or psychotropic effects should be low. Yet there have been isolated reports of idiosyncratic extrapyramidal reactions. Domperidone does not stimulate aldosterone secretion.

Summary: Domperidone selectively blocks peripheral dopamine receptors both in the GI wall and in the CTZ. Its major advantage appears to be the lack of significant side effects; it may be an effective alternative to available antiemetics, including metoclopramide. Domperidone, like other antiemetics, produces variable effects on cytotoxic chemotherapy-induced nausea and vomiting, depending on the agent administered. There is limited or no data available comparing domperidone to more standard antiemetic agents other than metoclopramide. Domperidone was developed in Belgium by Janssen Pharmaceutica; it is available in Europe. Clinical trials are still in progress in the US; a New Drug Application (NDA) was filed in 1985.

Dothiepin HCl *(Prothiaden)* – Tricyclic antidepressant

Pharmacology: Dothiepin, a thio analog of amitriptyline (eg, *Elavil*), is a tricyclic antidepressant (TCA) used for the treatment of depression. It is also structurally related to doxepin (eg, *Sinequan*). The efficacy of dothiepin does not appear to differ significantly from other available TCAs, and it appears comparable in efficacy to other antidepressants including fluoxetine *(Prozac)* and trazodone (eg, *Desyrel*). The anticholinergic effects may be less than with amitriptyline, although the sedative and anxiolytic activity appears to be similar.

Dothiepin and its metabolites inhibit the neuronal uptake of norepinephrine in vitro, thereby facilitating noradrenergic neurotransmission. The drug may also enhance serotonergic neurotransmission by inhibiting serotonin uptake. In vitro, dothiepin is a potent antagonist of histamine H_1-receptors, an effect common with other antidepressants. As with other TCAs, the therapeutic effects may not occur for 2 to 4 weeks following initiation of therapy.

Pharmacokinetics: Following oral administration, dothiepin is rapidly and completely absorbed. Peak plasma concentrations are achieved in 2 to 4 hours, and reach steady-state concentrations within 12 days (1 or 3 times daily administration).

Dothiepin undergoes extensive hepatic metabolism resulting from N-demethylation and S-oxidation. Following the first-pass effect, oral bioavailability is ≈ 30%. In one study in healthy volunteers, peak plasma concentrations and AUC of dothiepin-S-oxide were higher than the parent drug; the peak plasma concentrations of the other two metabolites were lower. It is not known if the metabolites contribute to the therapeutic efficacy of the drug. The terminal elimination half-lives of dothiepin and its metabolites are: Dothiepin 14.4 to 23.9 hrs; dothiepin-S-oxide 22.7 to 25.5 hrs; northiaden 34.7 to 45.7 hrs; northiaden-S-oxide 24.2 to 33.5 hrs. In two subjects, within 96 hours of administration, ≈ 56% of a dothiepin dose was recovered in the urine, and 15% in the feces. Unchanged dothiepin accounted for only 0.5% of the dose.

In elderly subjects, the time to peak plasma concentration, elimination half-life and AUC of dothiepin are increased, and the absorption rate constant, volume of distribution and plasma clearance are decreased. Dothiepin also appears in the breast milk in a concentration of ≥ 1 mcg/dl (dose: 75 mg/day).

Clinical trials: In several noncomparative studies using dothiepin (75 to 300 mg/day for 4 to 24 weeks), a marked improvement in symptoms of depression occurred in a large percentage of patients. However, results are difficult to assess due to lack of controls and short duration of therapy in some cases. Although one study showed the efficacy of dothiepin (75 to 225 mg/day) to be greater with a single dose at night vs a 3 times daily regimen, others reported no significant difference in efficacy.

In randomized double-blind studies of amitriptyline and dothiepin (50 to 300 mg/day) for 4 to 12 weeks, no significant difference in efficacy was noted, although dothiepin may have a faster onset of action. Dothiepin is also comparable in efficacy to doxepin, imipramine (eg, *Tofranil*), maprotiline (*Ludiomil*), fluoxetine and trazodone. In patients with mixed depression and anxiety symptoms, dothiepin is equally effective as alprazolam (*Xanax*), and equal or superior to chlordiazepoxide (eg, *Librium*).

Dothiepin also appears to have significant analgesic activity and may be useful in patients with idiopathic fibromyalgia syndrome (eg, generalized musculoskeletal aching, multiple tender points, fatigue, stiffness, sleep disturbances), rheumatoid arthritis or psychogenic facial pain.

Side effects: The adverse effects are similar to those seen with other TCAs. The following occurred in data pooled from 12 studies (n = 5755): Dry mouth (24%); drowsiness (16.8%); GI disorders (10.8%); dizziness (10.3%); tremor (8.5%); sweating, insomnia (5.7%); blurred vision (4.5%); weight gain (3.5%); palpitations (2.8%); hypotension, headache (1.9%); cardiac dysrhythmias (0.1%). Approximately 5% of patients withdrew from treatment due to side effects. Dothiepin appears to produce a lower incidence of anticholinergic, cardiac and sedative effects than amitriptyline; tolerability is similar to doxepin and imipramine.

Summary: Dothiepin is a TCA that is effective in the treatment of depression but appears to offer no significant advantage over existing agents. The lower incidence of anticholinergic effects compared to amitriptyline may make it more useful in elderly patients. The initial dosage appears to be 75 mg/day either divided 3 times daily or as a single nighttime dose. Dosage range appears to be 75 to 300 mg/day.

The NDA for dothiepin was originally submitted in 1979 by Boots licensee Marion. In 1982 the drug was recommended for approval by an FDA advisory committee; however, in 1987 the FDA requested additional safety information for the higher dosage ranges (200 to 300 mg) ≈ 6 months after Boots reacquired rights to the drug. A 1994 approval is expected. Dothiepin will be marketed as *Prothiaden*.

Fenoterol HBr *(Berotec)* – β_2 agonist

Pharmacology: Fenoterol HBr is a β_2-adrenergic agonist undergoing investigation in the US as a bronchodilating agent. It has been available outside the US since the early 1970s as a metered dose inhaler (MDI), a solution for nebulization, a powder for inhalation and an oral dosage form.

Stimulation of β_2-adrenoreceptors activates adenyl cyclase which converts adenosine triphosphate into cAMP. Increased levels of cAMP inhibit mediator release and produce bronchodilation. Although controversial, an increase in mucociliary transport may also occur. In addition, β_2 stimulation causes vasodilatation of peripheral blood vessels. This effect can result in a baroreceptor-mediated reflex-positive chronotropic response (increase in heart rate) and stimulation of skeletal muscle, leading to tremor. Fenoterol has greater β_2 selectivity than metaproterenol, but it is approximately equal in selectivity to albuterol and terbutaline. Bronchoselectivity is enhanced by administering fenoterol by inhalation; this allows for use of a lower dose to achieve a therapeutic effect and reduce dose-related side effects.

Usual therapeutic doses (200 to 400 mcg) of inhaled fenoterol do not significantly affect the cardiovascular system; however, marked cardiovascular effects have been observed after oral, SC, IM or IV administration. Fenoterol prevents immediate antigen-induced bronchospasm but does not prevent delayed allergic reactions. A transient reduction in serum potassium levels (representing the uptake of potassium into the intracellular space), and an increase in serum glucose levels have been observed, but the clinical significance remains unclear.

Pharmacokinetics: Approximately 60% of an oral dose is absorbed, with peak plasma levels reached in 2 hours. After inhalation, fenoterol appears to undergo a two-stage absorption process; the first stage is independent of dose, while the second is similar to that seen after oral administration. This is consistent with the observation that, when a drug is administered by inhalation, as much as 90% of the dose is swallowed. Fenoterol undergoes extensive first-pass metabolism. The half-life of total radioactive-labelled drug is 7 hours; however, this does not represent a true half-life for the parent compound. Although maximum effect of inhaled fenoterol is not achieved for 1 to 2 hours, 60% of the maximal response is seen within the first few minutes. The duration of action is ≈ 4 to 6 hours. However, since the lower therapeutic dose produces near maximal bronchodilatation, increasing the dose to near maximal effective concentrations will increase the duration of action without affecting the intensity of the peak response. After oral administration, < 2% of the dose is eliminated unchanged in the urine; the balance is excreted as acid conjugates in the urine and feces (40%).

Clinical trials: Clinical trials have established the efficacy of fenoterol for maintenance therapy in patients with moderate to severe asthma, therapy of chronic obstructive pulmonary disease (COPD), protection against exercise-induced asthma and treatment of acute asthma attacks. It is difficult to evaluate many of the studies because they are single-dose studies, or because they do not compare equipotent doses when evaluated against albuterol and terbutaline. However, at equipotent doses (1 puff fenoterol [200 mcg/puff] = 2 puffs albuterol [100 mcg/puff] = 2 puffs terbutaline [250 mcg/puff]), there appears to be no clinically significant difference in duration of action, bronchoselectivity or therapeutic efficacy among the three agents. The dose of fenoterol used to treat an acute asthma attack is 200 mcg (1 puff) repeated once in 5 minutes for children, and 1 to 3 puffs for adults. Maintenance therapy is 1 to 2 puffs 2 to 4 times daily for adults; give 1 puff twice daily to children. Increasing an inhaled dose of fenoterol to > 600 mcg (3 puffs) does not appear to increase the therapeutic response but may increase the incidence of side effects. In one study, an 800 mcg dose increased the heart rate 10% with a slow return to baseline over 2 hours. Although inhaled bronchodilators have many advantages, as many as 10% of the patients may not receive maximal therapeutic benefit due to improper MDI use.

Side effects: After inhalation of therapeutic doses of fenoterol, side effects are rare. After oral therapy, skeletal muscle tremor, tachycardia, palpitations and nervousness occur occasionally. Fenoterol is not recommended for use in patients with hyperthyroidism. Use with caution in patients with cardiovascular disease, diabetes mellitus and hepatic or renal dysfunction.

Summary: Fenoterol by inhalation appears to be a safe and effective treatment for prophylaxis of exercise-induced bronchospasm, acute attacks of mild to moderate asthma and maintenance therapy for chronic asthma or COPD. However, no apparent advantage of fenoterol over equipotent doses of the currently available β_2-selective agonists, albuterol or terbutaline, has yet been demonstrated. A New Drug Application (NDA) is pending. Fenoterol will be marketed as *Berotec* from Boehringer Ingelheim.

Flupirtine Maleate – Nonnarcotic analgesic

Pharmacology: Flupirtine maleate, a triaminopyridine derivative, is a nonnarcotic analgesic structurally unrelated to other analgesic agents. Although its exact mechanism of action is not known, flupirtine lacks affinity for any type of opiate receptor and therefore, has a mechanism that differs from the opiates. Flupirtine also appears to lack some of the side effects of the opiates including constipation, respiratory depression, withdrawal phenomena, development of tolerance and abuse potential. It is suggested that flupirtine is a medium to strong analgesic; its duration of action is comparable to codeine, and it is up to three times as potent as codeine and propoxyphene (eg, *Darvon*), up to twice as potent as meperidine (eg, *Demerol*) and approximately ten times as potent as acetaminophen (eg, *Tylenol*).

Pharmacokinetics: The pharmacokinetics of flupirtine have not been well defined. The drug appears to have linear kinetics. A dosage of 100 mg 3 times daily achieves average steady-state blood levels equivalent to the peak for a single 200 mg dose. In one study of 55 patients, the analgesic effect occurred within 45 minutes to 2 hours; the duration of action was 4 to 6 hours. The half-life of flupirtine appears to be 7 to 10 hours.

In 13 elderly patients receiving flupirtine 100 mg 3 times daily for 12 days, the mean elimination half-life was higher than in healthy young subjects (mean, 18.6 hours on day 12 vs 6.5 hours). This was associated with an increased maximum serum concentration and reduced clearance in the elderly subjects.

In 12 patients with renal impairment, the half-life of flupirtine was higher compared to healthy subjects (mean, 9.8 hours vs 6.5 hours) following a single oral 100 mg dose.

Flupirtine peak levels and area under the curve may be higher in patients with primary biliary cirrhosis. In a study of ten patients, flupirtine did not induce hepatic microsomal enzymes.

Clinical trials: Flupirtine is effective in the treatment of pain resulting from various procedures or conditions including episiotomy, cancer, and postoperative and dental pain. Dosages used have ranged from 100 to 600 mg/day; the most common dosages were 100 mg once daily or 100 mg 3 times daily. Capsules were used in most studies although the suppository form was also used. Analgesic efficacy of flupirtine was judged to be as effective as other analgesics used in the studies including acetaminophen, codeine, pentazocine *(Talwin NX)*, oxycodone plus acetaminophen (eg, *Percocet*), naproxen (eg, *Naprosyn*) and diclofenac *(Voltaren)*. Flupirtine appears to have no tolerance or addiction potential. In one study, the average number of capsules taken per month remained constant for 12 months, as did the analgesic effect.

Flupirtine significantly reduced seizure frequency in eight of nine patients with minimal side effects; however, since other derivatives of the drug may have greater activity, no further studies in the treatment of epilepsy are planned at this time.

Side effects: Flupirtine does not appear to share the common side effects of the opiates such as respiratory depression and constipation. The drug is generally well tolerated. In a study of 55 patients, the most common adverse effects were dizziness (11%), drowsiness (9% to 10%), pruritis (9%) and dry mouth (5%). Other side effects that occurred included: Pain in forehead; sensation of excessive fullness in stomach; muscular tremor; nausea; other GI disturbances (eg, vomiting, abdominal discomfort).

Summary: Flupirtine is a nonnarcotic analgesic that compares favorably in efficacy with other available analgesics. At this time, however, it offers no clear advantage over the nonsteroidal anti-inflammatory agents except perhaps in the GI and CNS side effect profile. It does offer an advantage over the opiates in side effect profile, abuse potential, withdrawal phenomena and development of tolerance. The average dose appears to be 100 mg 1 to 3 times daily. It has been used in both a capsule and suppository formulation.

An NDA was filed for flupirtine by Carter-Wallace in April 1986. At one time, a 1989 approval was anticipated; however, there has been no recent projected approval date. The company is also working with a combination product of flupirtine with codeine.

Gepirone HCl – Anxiolytic and antidepressant

Pharmacology: Gepirone, an azapirone, is chemically related to buspirone (*Buspar*) but unrelated to the benzodiazepines in structure or pharmacology. Gepirone does not directly or indirectly interact with the benzodiazepine-GABA receptor-chloride ion channel complex. Differing from buspirone, gepirone does not interact with dopamine receptors. Its principle effect relates to its action on brain serotonin activity.

The biochemical basis of psychiatric disorders of anxiety and depression may be viewed as a dynamic serotonergic continuum with anxiety representing a relative serotonin (5-HT) excess disease and depression a relative 5-HT deficit disease. Gepirone acts as a *total* agonist on presynaptic 5-HT_1A autoreceptors (inhibit neuronal firing and decrease 5-HT synthesis) and as a *partial* agonist at postsynaptic 5-HT_1A receptors (linked to cyclic-AMP and probably modulate signal transfer).

Partial agonists recognize and bind to receptors, but exert less activity than the *full* agonist. In the absence of the endogenous full agonist (serotonin), gepirone would exert its agonist effects. However, when full agonists are also present, partial agonists compete for receptors. When partial agonists (which have less intrinsic activity) displace full agonists from receptor sites, they decrease synaptic neurotransmission relative to what would have been achieved by the full agonist alone, and thus essentially act as functional antagonists. Therefore, the effects that 5-HT partial agonists (eg, buspirone, gepirone) ultimately exert on 5-HT neurotransmission depend on the serotonergic tone of the synapse in which the drug is working.

In the 5-HT excess state of anxiety, gepirone would act as an agonist on presynaptic 5-HT_1A receptors to decrease 5-HT synthesis and neuronal firing and on the post-synaptic 5-HT_1A receptor as a functional antagonist, resulting in a reduction of hyperserotonergic tone in the brain and an amelioration of anxiety symptomatology. However, effects of gepirone in the relative serotonin deficit disease of depression would be quite different. Gepirone would bind to presynaptic

$5\text{-}HT_1A$ receptors and exert its agonist effects to decrease neuron activity. In the 5-HT-deficit state of depression, this action would allow 5-HT depleted neurons to replenish their serotonin stores and thus serve 5-HT homeostasis. Gepirone would also bind to postsynaptic $5\text{-}HT_1A$ receptors, but in the 5-HT-deficient state it would express its agonist effects thus causing normosensitization of postsynaptic $5\text{-}HT_1A$ receptors and restoration of postsynaptic serotonergic activity. This normalization of hyposerotonergic tone in depression would produce antidepressant effects and improvement of depressive symptoms.

Pharmacokinetics: Gepirone is rapidly absorbed after oral administration, reaching peak levels in about 1 hour. It undergoes extensive first-pass metabolism by the liver and has an oral bioavailability of only 15%. Both it and buspirone are hepatically metabolized to the major active metabolite 1-(2-pyrimidinyl) piperazine (1-PP). The plasma half-life of gepirone is 2 to 3 hours. No change in dosing would be anticipated in patients with renal insufficiency or failure.

Clinical trials: Gepirone 30 to 60 mg/day and placebo were compared in a 6 week double-blind trial in 30 outpatients with generalized anxiety disorder. According to various scales, gepirone was significantly superior to placebo and produced improvement in both somatic and psychic anxiety. Significant improvement was delayed and occurred after 2 to 3 weeks of treatment. Predictors of clinical improvement included high levels of baseline anxiety and length of time off anxiolytic therapy (ie, the longer the time off benzodiazepines, etc, the more likely a positive response).

Both a single blind study using doses of 25 to 75 mg/day and a double-blind, placebo controlled study using doses ranging from 5 to 90 mg/day found gepirone exerted significant antidepressant effects in patients with major depression.

Side effects: Gepirone is well tolerated with most side effects reported as mild to moderate. The most frequently reported adverse effects were dizziness, nausea, headache, drowsiness and weakness. Gepirone does not impair memory, verbal fluency or psychomotor performance. Like buspirone, gepirone does not appear to have a potential for causing physical dependence or addiction in humans, and it is expected that gepirone will not interact with alcohol or sedative/hypnotic drugs.

Summary: Gepirone is a nonbenzodiazepine drug similar in structure to buspirone. It lacks the sedative and adverse psychomotor and memory impairment effects of the benzodiazepines and does not appear to have the potential for causing physical dependence or addiction. Gepirone selectively affects the serotonergic system, targeting specifically the serotonin $5\text{-}HT_1A$ receptor subtype. Clinical studies indicate that it possesses both antianxiety and antidepressant properties and is well tolerated.

Gepirone is currently in Phase II/III clinical trials and will be available from Bristol-Myers Squibb. An anticipated approval date is unknown.

Halofantrine HCl *(Halfan)* – Antimalarial

Pharmacology: Halofantrine, an antimalarial agent developed by the US Army Antimalarial Program, is active against multi-drug resistant *Plasmodium falciparum* malaria. It is a phenanthrenemethanol, structurally related to mefloquine *(Lariam)*. Halofantrine and its active metabolite, N-desbutylhalofantrine (DHF), are blood schizontocides active against the erythrocyte stages of *Plasmodium* sp. The mechanism of action has not been fully elucidated, but may be similar to other blood schizontocides or involve inhibition of a proton pump at the host-parasite interface.

In vitro and clinical data suggest that cross-resistance occurs with mefloquine-resistant strains.

Pharmacokinetics: Following oral administration, absorption is erratic and variable, with a high degree of intra- and intersubject variability. Influencing factors appear to include dietary fat content and the presence or absence of active disease. Racial and genetic factors may also play a role. Since the cure rate appears to be influenced by plasma concentration, irregular absorption and variable peak drug concentrations may be responsible for some treatment failures.

The lack of an IV formulation due to poor solubility precludes accurate bioavailability data. However, the maximum plasma concentration (C_{max}) and area under the plasma concentration-time curve (AUC) of both the parent and active metabolite are significantly increased (up to 6 fold) following administration with a high fat meal. AUC and C_{max} are proportionally related to dose in the range of 250 to 500 mg, but do not increase proportionally when the dose is increased from 500 to 1000 mg. This may explain why single doses of 1.5 g are associated with a high relapse rate. In healthy subjects, half-lives of halofantrine and DHF are approximately 2 and 10 days (range, 4 to 13), respectively. In patients with active disease, the half-life for both compounds is approximately 4 days.

The drug is widely distributed in most tissues and is excreted mainly in the feces as unchanged drug.

Clinical trials: The risk of mortality associated with inadequately treated malaria and the documented efficacy of agents such as chloroquine (eg, *Aralen*) precludes the use of placebo controlled trials and limits comparative trials with halofantrine.

Non-comparative trials, using oral doses of 500 mg every 6 hours for 3 doses in adults and children > 40 kg (8 mg/kg in smaller children), have shown the drug to be both safe and effective in the treatment of *P falciparum* infections. A second course of therapy, administered 7 days after initial treatment, is recommended for patients such as non-immune travelers or young children with no previous (or minimal) exposure to malaria.

Cure rates of 83% to 100% have been recorded in areas with high rates of *P falciparum* malaria resistant to chloroquine and sulfonamide/pyrimethamine (eg, *Fansidar*). Following treatment, many symptoms improve within the first day. Fever usually decreases within 18 to 100 hours while parasitemia clears within 34 to 78 hours in most cases. Resolution of splenomegaly and hepatomegaly occurs in approximately 75% of treated patients. A relapse rate of 5.8% has been reported, but it was noted that some of these cases may have represented reinfection. Experience in treatment of *P ovale* and *P malariae* is too limited to be conclusive. Present trials do not support halofantrine's use for prophylaxis.

Side effects: Abdominal pain, vomiting and diarrhea have occurred in 15% to 25% of treated patients. Whether these represent drug- or disease-related events is difficult to distinguish. Pruritus occurs in 2.3% of patients and represents an advantage for African populations, in which chloroquine-induced pruritus is intolerable in 8% to 20% of patients. The pruritus has been characterized as a generalized burning sensation, most pronounced on the soles of the feet, scalp and perineal areas. Onset is usually within the first 14 hours with resolution after 20 hours. Headache and rash have occurred. Anecdotal reports of neuromuscular spasm, mouth ulcers, seizures, ventricular ectopy (PVCs) and intravascular hemolysis have been attributed to halofantrine; cause and effect have not been established.

Summary: Halofantrine appears to be a safe and effective alternative to current therapy for *Plasmodium falciparum* malaria. Additional studies are needed to delineate the role of true drug resistance versus bioavailability factors as causes for treatment failures. Its role in the treatment of *P ovale*, *P vivax* and *P malariae* has not been determined. Halofantrine was approved by the FDA on July 24, 1992; however, it is not yet commercially available. A release date is unknown at this time.

Hexoprenaline Sulfate *(Delaprem)* – Tocolytic agent

Pharmacology: Hexoprenaline sulfate is a β_2-selective adrenergic agonist. Structurally, it is two norepinephrine molecules joined through their amino groups by a hexamethylene bridge. This compound, while retaining the catechol moiety, has a longer duration of action than classic catecholamines (eg, isoproterenol [eg, *Isuprel*]), and is orally active. Stimulation of uterine β_2-receptors results in a decrease in the frequency and intensity of uterine smooth muscle contractions, believed to be due to a decrease in myometrial cellular calcium. These local effects, as well as the systemic effects, are mediated by adenyl cyclase and cyclic adenosine 3′-5′-monophosate (cAMP) and are antagonized by β-blocking compounds. Uterine activity and the frequency and intensity of uterine contractions following an IV bolus of 7.5 mcg are reduced by 70%, 40% and 50%, respectively; further reductions can be achieved with repeat boluses or administration of a continuous infusion. IV administration is associated with a dose-dependent increase in heart rate (> 20 to 30 beats/minute) and systolic blood pressure (mean, +13 mm Hg), and a reduction in diastolic blood pressure (mean, -21 mm Hg), producing a widening of the pulse pressure. At equivalent tocolytic doses, the increase in heart rate and systolic blood pressure is reported to be less than that seen with ritodrine (*Yutopar*). Maternal glucose, insulin, glucagon and free fatty acid levels increase while serum potassium levels and pH may decrease.

Pharmacokinetics: A lack of published data in humans precludes an accurate description of the pharmacokinetic profile of hexoprenaline. However, certain characteristics may be inferred from available clinical trials. Following administration of an IV bolus of 7.5 mcg, the mean time to onset of stable uterine activity was 12.9 ± 6.9 minutes, with return to baseline activity at 33.7 ± 17.8 minutes. Similar values (34.9 ± 12.7 minutes) were reported for the time required for the heart rate to return to baseline. Return to uterine activity and heart rate baselines was similar following discontinuation of a continuous infusion of 0.38 mcg/min for 20 minutes (37.3 ± 13 minutes and 35.3 ± 13 minutes, respectively). In rats, two methylated metabolites have been identified, one of which is active.

Clinical trials: In available, published clinical trials, hexoprenaline is an effective tocolytic. When compared to ritodrine, equivalent tocolytic doses produced less maternal tachycardia and elevation of systolic blood pressure. It has also been used, as an IV bolus or bolus plus infusion, to control contraction-related fetal heart rate abnormalities, a marker of fetal distress. In this latter setting, the desired increase in fetal heart rate was attributed to control of uterine contractions and, possibly, an increase in placental blood flow, since < 1% of hexoprenaline was shown to cross the placenta in rabbits and in an in vitro model.

Side effects: Hexoprenaline shares the side effect profile of the β_2-agonists such as tremor, tachycardia (maternal and fetal), arrhythmias (supraventricular and ventricular), myocardial ischemia, hypotension, hyperglycemia and hypokalemia. However, available data suggest that the frequency and severity of these adverse effects is less than that seen with β_2-agonist tocolytics currently in clinical use (eg, ritodrine, terbutaline [*Brethine*, *Bricanyl*]) and are usually only seen in the higher dose ranges. A recent report also describes non-cardiac pulmonary edema, a recognized complication of this form of therapy but not previously reported with hexoprenaline. As with the other β_2-agonist tocolytics, preexisting myocardial dysfunction, iatrogenic fluid overload and the concomitant administration of glucocorticoids appear to increase the risk of this complication.

Summary: Hexoprenaline appears to be a safe and effective agent for the treatment of premature uterine contractions. Limited available data suggest that, at doses that produce effective tocolysis, side effects, particularly maternal tachycardia, are less frequent or severe than those seen with currently used β_2-agonist tocolytics. Additional data are required to determine its relative place in therapy. An NDA has been filed by Altana and is currently pending. On February 2, 1990, the FDA's Fertility and Maternal Health Drugs Advisory Committee recommended approval for hexoprenaline for suppression of uterine contractions during premature labor. Hexoprenaline, which will be available as *Delaprem*, is currently available in several other countries.

Indecainide HCl *(Decabid)* – Antiarrhythmic agent

Pharmacology: Indecainide is a class IC antiarrhythmic agent that is structurally similar to the investigational agent aprindine. Other available class IC antiarrhythmics are encainide *(Enkaid)* and flecainide *(Tambocor)*. This class of drugs markedly suppresses premature ventricular complexes (PVCs) and depresses intramyocardial conduction. Indecainide prolongs the PR and QRS intervals, significantly increasing intraventricular conduction time without significantly affecting atrial or ventricular refractoriness. There appear to be no significant hemodynamic effects.

Pharmacokinetics: Indecainide is completely absorbed following oral administration. In animals, the half-life is 3 to 5 hours; however, the half-life in patients is considerably longer (9 to 10 hours), suggesting that twice-daily dosing may be effective in some patients. Indecainide is metabolized in the liver to desisopropyl indecainide. This metabolite appears to have a longer half-life than the parent drug, although the plasma levels of the metabolite are only approximately 10% those of indecainide. It is not known if desisopropyl indecainide possesses any antiarrhythmic effects.

Approximately 63% of indecainide is recovered in the urine with < 10% recovered as the metabolite. In one study, there was no correlation between percent suppression of ventricular ectopic depolarizations and plasma levels or half-life of either indecainide or the metabolite.

Clinical trials: Clinical information regarding the efficacy of indecainide is available only through several studies using small patient populations. Antiarrhythmic efficacy appears similar to encainide and flecainide. Efficacy was maintained in some patients for up to 2 years. Indecainide orally or IV markedly suppresses the frequency of PVCs, particularly repetitive forms. In one study, 63% to 82% of patients had suppression of PVCs, 60% to 82% had more than a 95% elimination of couplets, and 56% to 74% had complete elimination of ventricular tachycardia. The average suppression of PVCs with most available antiarrhythmics ranges from 50% to 75%. The degree of suppression was comparable to encainide and flecainide. Other studies have reported a 90% reduction in PVCs in approximately 85% of patients, and elimination of ventricular tachycardia in approximately 86% of patients. In a study involving 231 patients, indecainide reduced PVCs by 93%, while disopyramide reduced PVCs by 80%; suppression of runs of ventricular tachycardia were equivalent for both drugs. In a study of 11 patients, indecainide suppressed ventricular premature beats in 90% of patients, but suppression of ventricular tachycardia was achieved in only 45% of patients.

In data from five clinical trials through the manufacturer involving 792 patients, 70% receiving indecainide responded to ≤ 200 mg/day, and 90% responded to 300 mg/day.

Side effects: In clinical trials, the following side effects were noted: Dizziness (18% with the 200 mg dose, 12% with 150 mg and 9% with 100 mg); proarrhythmias (14.8%); congestive heart failure (3.9%). Each effect appeared to be dose-related. Other adverse reactions reported in the smaller patient population studies included headache, blurry vision, impotence, lightheadedness, confusion, thought disorders, nausea and constipation. Most reactions appear mild and may respond to dosage adjustment.

Drug interactions: In five patients receiving concurrent indecainide and digoxin, the digoxin concentration increased (range, 47% to 300%) in three of the five patients. The digoxin concentration decreased significantly when indecainide was discontinued. The clinical significance of this pharmacokinetic interaction was not determined.

Summary: Indecainide is an effective class IC antiarrhythmic agent that may offer an alternative for the patients who cannot tolerate the GI side effects of quinidine or the CNS effects of the other class IC agents. Lilly is recommending a dosage of 100 to 200 mg/day, and they plan to market only the twice-daily formulation (an immediate release form for 4 times daily administration was also tested in clinical trials).

Because of the recent findings of the Cardiac Arrhythmia Suppression Trial (CAST), which reduced the indications for encainide and flecainide to treatment of life-threatening arrhythmias only, Lilly is reviewing the CAST study data to determine if there is any potential relevance to indecainide.

In November, 1988, the FDA's Cardio-Renal Drugs Advisory committee unanimously recommended approval for indecainide for sustained ventricular tachycardia, ventricular fibrillation, nonsustained ventricular and chronic benign PVCs. Indecainide was approved by the FDA in December, 1989. However, Lilly has made a decision not to market the drug at this time.

Inosiplex *(Isoprinosine)* – Immunomodulating agent

Pharmacology: Inosiplex (inosine pranobex, BAN) is a synthetic complex formed from the p-acetamidobenzoic acid salt of N – N dimethylamino-2-propanol and inosine in a 3:1 molar ratio. Early studies examined inosiplex as an antiviral agent. However, recent research has focused on its immunomodulating properties and suggests that its anti-viral activity involves enhancement of host defenses rather than direct inhibition of viral replication. Inosiplex may be more appropriately classed with those agents that regulate immunity, eg, levamisole.

Inosiplex augments immunological events triggered by such agents as mitogens, antigens, phagocyte stimulants or lymphokines. Inosiplex alone does not appear to affect lymphocytes or macrophages. In the presence of triggering agents, it results in an increase in mitogen responses, T– lymphocyte differentiation, total rosette-forming T– cells, lymphotoxin production, virus-induced lymphoproliferative responses, lymphocyte cytotoxicity to viral-infected target cells and skin test responses. This augmentation of responses occurs at inosiplex levels of 0.1 to > 100 mcg/ml with a biphasic profile. Such a profile suggests action on more than one cell population or, more likely, a dual action on a single cell population which is concentration-dependent. Exactly how the drug acts on the lymphocyte to alter the magnitude of triggered responses is unclear. It may involve one or several cell surfaces and nuclear metabolic events linked to RNA metabolism, cyclic nucleotide levels or calcium ion flux. Inosiplex also potentiates interferon activity through mechanisms which remain unclear.

Pharmacokinetics: Inosiplex is rapidly metabolized after both oral and IV administration. The half-life of the inosine portion of the parent complex is 3 minutes after IV administration and 50 minutes after oral administration. In animal models, 90% of the inosine moiety is excreted in the urine as allantoin and uric acid, along with small amounts of hypoxanthine, xanthine and adenine. The p-acetamidobenzoic acid moiety and the N – N-dimethylamino-2-propanol moiety are excreted in the urine after glucuronidation and oxidation, respectively.

Clinical trials examining the use of inosiplex in a variety of viral disorders (eg, herpes zoster, herpes simplex, rhinovirus, influenza A and subacute sclerosing panencephalitis), rheumatoid arthritis and solid tumors have not been able to establish definite efficacy of the drug in any of these disorders. A preliminary study involving four patients with a pre-Acquired Immune Deficiency Syndrome (AIDS) complex (a prodrome of AIDS) and five patients with AIDS given 4 g inosiplex per day for 4 weeks showed enhancement of mitogen-induced lymphocyte proliferative responses in two patients with the pre-AIDS complex. These results agreed with data from an in vitro study of inosiplex's effect on lymphocytes from pre-AIDS patients, patients with AIDS and healthy heterosexual controls which demonstrated that inosiplex could partially restore some of the depressed lymphocyte functions associated with AIDS. The data also suggested, however, that this effect was likely to have clinical significance only in those patients with the milder, pre-AIDS condition. After examination of the combined preliminary results of three studies (unpublished data), Newport Pharmaceuticals reported to FDA officials that there appeared to be a trend toward a delay in the development of fully developed AIDS in pre-AIDS patients treated with inosiplex for 28 days. A multicenter study is in progress to evaluate the use of inosiplex in pre-AIDS patients.

Side effects: In tolerance studies involving healthy volunteers and in clinical trials involving various patient groups, no serious side effects were reported after continuous inosiplex administration for 1 week to 7 years at doses of 1 to 8 g/day. Occasional transient nausea was associated with the ingestion of large numbers of tablets; a transient rise in serum and urinary uric acid, related to the metabolism of the drug, occurred in a small number of patients. Initiate concomitant administration of drugs that increase uric acid levels with caution, since potential for additive effects has not been studied.

Summary: Inosiplex is a new immunomodulating agent. Preliminary data indicate that the compound may improve the immunologic status of some pre-AIDS patients and may delay progression of pre-AIDS to AIDS. Inosiplex could presumably be used long-term in these patients, since it is administered orally and has not been associated with serious side effects. However, more extensive clinical trials are needed to establish the safety and efficacy of the agent. Newport Pharmaceuticals submitted a New Drug Application (NDA) September 3, 1985, requesting approval of inosiplex (*Isoprinosine*) for immunorestoration in pre-AIDS patients, but it was rejected by the FDA in February 1986. Research continues.

Isoxicam *(Maxicam)* – Nonsteroidal anti-inflammatory drug

Pharmacology: Isoxicam, like piroxicam (*Feldene*), is a member of the oxicam class of drugs. It is about one-tenth as potent (on a weight basis) as piroxicam and has a long duration of action which permits once-daily dosing. Clinical studies show it to be as effective as or superior to other NSAIDs. Isoxicam is well tolerated; GI disturbance is the most common side effect.

Rheumatoid arthritis (RA) and degenerative joint disease (DJD) are common chronic rheumatic disorders which cause considerable human suffering and disability. The NSAIDs are first-line agents for pain relief in both disorders and for the reduction of inflammation in RA. Salicylates have long been established as analgesic anti-inflammatory drugs and are usually drugs of first choice. However, since therapeutic failure and side effects are frequent, newer agents are steadily being introduced as alternatives.

Isoxicam has potent and prolonged antipyretic, analgesic and anti-inflammatory activity. It inhibits the synthesis of prostaglandins which may contribute to the development of the cardinal signs/symptoms of inflammation. It is also a potent inhibitor of platelet aggregation. This effect likely underlies its potentiation of sodium warfarin's anticoagulant action (see below).

Pharmacokinetics: Isoxicam is well absorbed orally and generally reaches peak plasma concentration 4 to 8 hours after administration. Both its rate and extent of absorption increase when given with meals.

Isoxicam is 95% to 98% protein bound. It is extensively metabolized with only 1% to 2% of the dose appearing in the urine as unchanged drug. This suggests that the drug's dose need not be changed in patients with renal dysfunction. Isoxicam has a half-life of approximately 31 hours (range, 21 to 70 hours) which permits once-daily dosing. Because of its long half-life, steady-state levels occur after 1 to 2 weeks of daily administration. As a result, a continual increase in response is expected until steady state is achieved.

Clinical trials: In a placebo controlled multicenter study, isoxicam was superior to placebo for the treatment of patients with RA or DJD. Morning stiffness was reduced by more than 60% in the isoxicam group, compared to 19% for patients in the placebo group; 52% of patients in the placebo group withdrew from the study because of lack of treatment efficacy, compared to 18% withdrawal in the isoxicam group.

An aspirin (3.6 g/day) and placebo controlled study of isoxicam (200 mg/day) in the treatment of RA found isoxicam superior to aspirin and placebo. Patient withdrawal rates for insufficient efficacy were 17.1%, 31.1% and 58.5% for isoxicam, aspirin and placebo, respectively.

In comparative studies of isoxicam (200 mg/day) vs naproxen (750 mg/day) and ibuprofen (1200 mg/day) in patients with RA, no significant efficacy differences were observed. In similar studies involving patients with DJD, isoxicam (200 mg/day) was as effective as naproxen (750 mg/day) and indomethacin (150 mg/day) in relieving pain and improving articular function. Patients on isoxicam experienced significantly fewer adverse effects than those on indomethacin.

Side effects: Isoxicam has so far been well tolerated and has caused few problems other than gastrointestinal effects. Other less commonly reported adverse effects include headache, dizziness and tinnitus. A higher than anticipated rate of skin reactions has occurred in foreign countries where isoxicam is available.

Drug interactions: The use of aspirin with NSAIDs is not generally recommended because of aspirin-induced reductions of NSAID blood levels and a lack of therapeutic advantage with concomitant use. However, the use of aspirin with isoxicam does not appear to lower plasma isoxicam levels, but the combination increases GI blood loss. It remains to be determined whether an isoxicam-aspirin combination offers any therapeutic advantage. When used with sodium warfarin, isoxicam potentiates warfarin's anticoagulant effect. Monitor the prothrombin time in patients on both agents more frequently and adjust the sodium warfarin dosage if needed. No interaction occurs between cimetidine and isoxicam.

Summary: Isoxicam is a novel NSAID of the oxicam class. It appears to be as effective as or superior to aspirin and nonaspirin agents for the treatment of common rheumatic disorders. The ability to administer isoxicam once a day is an important advantage. Parke-Davis (Warner-Lambert) submitted an NDA for isoxicam in August 1983, to be marketed under the name *Maxicam*. The drug was withdrawn from the European market in October 1985 following reports of adverse skin reactions during which time the NDA was pending in the US. In 1987, Warner-Lambert asked the FDA to reactivate the NDA since the skin reactions were apparently due to a manufacturing byproduct.

Ketotifen *(Zaditen)* – Antiasthmatic agent

Pharmacology: Asthma is a chronic respiratory disease characterized by episodes of reversible airway obstruction due to bronchospasms. Although a variety of effective agents are available for the prophylaxis and treatment of asthmatic conditions, both the incidence of side effects and inconvenience of administration by inhalation encourage the search for new modes of therapy. Ketotifen is an orally active agent with significant antihistamine and antianaphylactic properties which may prove useful in asthma prophylaxis.

The factors responsible for intrinsic asthma are poorly understood. Extrinsic allergic asthma results from a series of events triggered by an allergen (antigen) which activates the release of chemical mediators of bronchoconstriction (histamine and the slow-reacting substance of anaphylaxis) from sensitized mast cells. Bronchodilators (beta-adrenergic agonists or theophylline) counteract these bronchoconstrictor effects. Antihistamines are somewhat useful in blocking the effects of histamine. The introduction of cromolyn sodium was the advent of a true prophylactic measure for allergic asthma. Although not effective during an acute asthma episode, chronic therapy with cromolyn stabilizes the mast cell membrane and inhibits the release of histamine and slow-reacting substance of anaphylaxis.

Ketotifen appears to act by the same pharmacological mechanism as cromolyn; however, it has the advantage of being active on oral administration. Ketotifen is a benzocycloheptathiophene derivative with antihistaminic and antianaphylactic activity. It is well absorbed orally; effects are sustained for up to 12 hours. As with cromolyn, the onset of its prophylactic activity is slow; 4 to 6 weeks are required to achieve full prophylactic value. Therapeutic serum levels range between 1 and 4 mcg/ml.

Clinical studies: Ketotifen, 1 mg orally, twice daily was found to be equivalent to 20 mg sodium cromolyn 4 times daily (via spinhaler). No statistically significant differences were demonstrated between the two drugs for daily peak respiratory flow rates and spirometry during the 3 months that each drug was administered to 35 skin test positive (allergic) asthmatic adults. Ketotifen prevented histamine-induced bronchoconstriction in 24 patients with mild to moderate extrinsic (allergic) asthma. Histamine challenge was used to evaluate bronchial reactivity following 1 week of treatment with theophylline and salbutamol spray. Ketotifen, 1 mg twice daily, was then added to the regimen. Patients were rechallenged with histamine after 4, 8 and 12 weeks of ketotifen therapy. Decrease in bronchial reactivity to histamine was noted at 4 weeks and maintained for 12 weeks.

In a double-blind study of 50 patients with allergic asthma, ketotifen, 1 or 2 mg twice daily, was added to existing inhalation therapy of salbutamol or corticosteroid. Ketotifen, 2 mg twice daily, slightly decreased the number of puffs per week of salbutamol and improved breathing. No improvement was noted in patients using inhaled corticosteroids. Ketotifen, 1 mg twice daily, failed to provide prophylaxis in adults with intrinsic (nonallergic) asthma; however, there was no deterioration of the condition.

In a double-blind study in 23 children with asthma, 0.5 to 0.94 mg/kg ketotifen failed to provide protection against bronchoconstriction. Ketotifen 1 mg twice daily for 3 days was compared to cromolyn 20 mg administered 15 minutes prior to exercise. Ketotifen was ineffective in preventing exercise-induced bronchospasm, while cromolyn was effective.

Side effects: The most frequently reported side effects, sedation and drowsiness, may require dosage reduction or discontinuation if the severity does not decrease with continued therapy. Alcohol may potentiate these adverse reactions. Weight gain, dry mouth, headache, dizziness and giddiness have also been reported. In addition, symptoms of overdosage have included: Mild abdominal pain, confusion, hyperexcitability, bradycardia, tachycardia, dyspnea, tachypnea, cyanosis, convulsions and unconsciousness.

Summary: Ketotifen appears to be a potential alternative in the prophylaxis of asthma; however, it is unlikely to replace established drugs. Several weeks of administration are required to produce maximum prophylactic effects; additionally, it frequently produces marked drowsiness. Ketotifen is long-acting and offers the convenience of oral administration which may be useful in individuals who develop bronchospasms following inhalation of other products. Ketotifen is available in Britain and Europe; Sandoz filed a New Drug Application (NDA) in November 1982 which is pending, and plans to market the drug under the name *Zaditen*.

Lacidipine *(Lacipil)* – Dihydropyridine calcium antagonist

Pharmacology: Lacidipine, a 1,4 dihydropyridine calcium channel blocker, is a selective vasodilator which exerts little effect on myocardial contractility. The dose required to impair cardiac function is approximately 50 times greater than that needed for significant blood pressure reduction. Electrocardiographic studies indicate that it has no effect on SA node function or AV node conduction. Lacidipine effectively reduces blood pressure and decreases systemic vascular resistance by dilating peripheral and coronary arteries. This may lead to reflex tachycardia during the early stages of therapy. In addition to its cardiovascular effects, lacidipine has been shown in animal studies to have mild diuretic and natriuretic effects. In vitro studies have also demonstrated anti-oxidant activity and a possible tissue protective effect. As with other calcium channel blockers, there is some evidence to suggest activity toward inhibiting atherosclerosis. Lacidipine has been shown via a rat model to decrease infarct size following cerebral artery occlusion. The drug does not appear to affect carbohydrate or lipid metabolism.

Pharmacokinetics: Lacidipine is rapidly absorbed after oral administration and undergoes extensive first-pass metabolism. Virtually no parent drug is excreted in the urine or feces. Of the two primary metabolites, neither possesses pharmacologic activity. Due to the first-pass effect, the absolute bioavailability of lacidipine is < 20%. Its high lipophilicity results in a prolonged pharmacologic effect, thus facilitating a single daily dose regimen. The elimination half-life ranges from 2 to 10 hours after a single dose, but increases to 12 to 15 hours at steady state. Plasma protein binding exceeds 90%. Volume of distribution after a single dose is ≈ 1 to 2 L/kg.

Metabolism of lacidipine is decreased in elderly patients and in those with liver impairment. The elimination of the drug appears to be unaffected by renal function.

Clinical trials: Dose titration studies involving over 400 patients with mild to moderate hypertension demonstrate a minimum response rate of 77%, as defined by the achievement of a diastolic blood pressure (DBP) ≤ 90 mm Hg or a reduction in DBP of ≥ 15 mm Hg. Doses of lacidipine ranged from 2 to 8 mg, administered once daily. One study treated 96 hypertensive patients with lacidipine, starting at a dose of 4 mg for 1 month. If DBP was not controlled after 1 month, the dose was increased to 8 mg. If DBP was not controlled after the second month, a beta blocker was added to the regimen. At 2 months, mean values for DBP and systolic blood pressure (SBP) dropped significantly. After 5 months, 87% of the patients were controlled: 63% on 4 mg, 21% on 8 mg and 3% with combination therapy.

Studies have compared lacidipine 2 to 6 mg/day to hydrochlorothiazide (eg, *Esidrix*) 25 to 50 mg/day, atenolol (eg, *Tenormin*) 50 to 100 mg/day, sustained release nifedipine (eg, *Procardia XL*) 20 to 40 mg twice daily and enalapril (*Vasotec*) 10 to 20 mg/day. In all cases, the difference in mean decrease for both SBP and DBP were not significantly different. In studies comparing lacidipine 4 mg/day to other long-acting dihydropyridine calcium antagonists, lacidipine showed greater antihypertensive effect than amlodipine (*Norvasc*) 10 mg/day and similar efficacy to that of isradipine 5 mg/day; further study is needed to clarify this issue.

Side effects: Adverse effects for lacidipine correspond to those expected for the dihydropyridine calcium antagonists, due mostly to the vasodilatory properties of these drugs: Headache (15%); flushing (10%); edema (8%); dizziness (6%); palpitations (5%); fatigue (4%); gastric irritation (3%). Generally, the side effects are mild and diminish over time. In most cases, they appear to be dose-related. Less common effects include paresthesia, sexual impotence and changes in liver function tests. The tolerability of lacidipine compares favorably to nifedipine; further study is needed to compare lacidipine to newer long-acting drugs in the class (eg, amlodipine).

Summary: Lacidipine appears to be a safe, effective agent for first-line treatment of mild to moderate hypertension. The recommended starting dose is 2 to 4 mg, titrated as needed up to 8 mg/day. Elderly patients and those with liver impairment should be started at 2 mg daily. Future clinical trials may elucidate additional beneficial effects of lacidipine and perhaps define new therapeutic roles for the drug.

Lacidipine is marketed as an antihypertensive drug in Italy and Portugal by Glaxo. It is also available under license to Boehringer Ingelheim in both England and France. It can be found under a variety of trade names, including *Lacipil*, *Viapres*, *Lacirex*, and *Motens*. Future marketing plans in the US are uncertain, largely because lacidipine would compete with Sandoz's isradipine (*DynaCirc*), for which Glaxo also holds the marketing rights. Despite considerable use and investigation of lacidipine in other countries, it may be quite some time before it appears in the US.

L-5-Hydroxytryptophan (L-5HTP) – Agent for myoclonus

Pharmacology: L-5HTP is available as an "orphan" drug for the treatment of post-anoxic intention myoclonus. Myoclonus is an uncommon neuromuscular movement disorder characterized by involuntary, irregular muscle contraction; it is associated with a variety of brain lesions. There is evidence that at least some of these disorders are related to brain neurotransmitter levels or function, specifically serotonin. L-5HTP is an aromatic amino acid, the immediate precursor of serotonin.

L-5HTP is administered with carbidopa (see individual monograph), a peripheral dopa-decarboxylase inhibitor that decreases the conversion of L-5HTP to serotonin in the extracerebral tissues. This permits the administration of lower doses of L-5HTP and reduces the peripheral GI side effects such as diarrhea and nausea.

Pharmacokinetics: When administered orally with carbidopa (which produces a 5 to 15 fold increase in plasma L-5HTP), the systemic availability of L-5HTP is 47% to 84%; peak plasma concentrations of L-5HTP are reached at 1 to 3 hours. The biological half-life of L-5HTP, after pretreatment with carbidopa, is 2 to 7 hours. The major metabolic pathway of L-5HTP is decarboxylation to serotonin by L-aromatic amino acid decarboxylase; the highest activity is in the kidney, liver and small intestine. However, carbidopa-decarboxylase inhibition is incomplete; this may account for the GI side effects.

Indications: L-5HTP in combination with carbidopa is effective in the therapy of post-anoxic intention myoclonus. In 41 patients, 65% experienced a 50% or more improvement. However, patients with intention myoclonus associated with head trauma and methyl bromide toxicity, progressive myoclonus epilepsy, essential myoclonus and palatal myoclonus also show improvement. In addition, L-5HTP has shown some success in treating depression and in migraine prophylaxis.

Contraindications: L-5HTP/carbidopa is contraindicated in patients with renal disease, peptic ulcer, platelet disorders, scleroderma and Parkinson's disease.

Drug interactions: Do not give **monoamine oxidase inhibitors** or **reserpine** concurrently with L-5HTP/carbidopa. Discontinue these drugs at least 2 weeks prior to initiating treatment with L-5HTP/carbidopa.

Discontinue **tricyclic antidepressants** with a major serotonin reuptake inhibition mechanism (ie, imipramine) prior to L-5HTP/carbidopa therapy. Also, avoid serotonin receptor antagonists like **methysergide** or **cyproheptadine,** which may reduce the therapeutic effects of L-5HTP/carbidopa.

Fenfluramine releases brain serotonin from serotonergic nerve terminals and may potentiate L-5HTP/carbidopa.

Precautions: Use L-5HTP/carbidopa with caution in patients with severe emotional or psychiatric disorders because of occasional mental side effects. Mental depression has improved in some patients.

Adverse reactions:

Most common (GI) — Anorexia, nausea, diarrhea and vomiting. These can usually be avoided or minimized by gradual increases of L-5HTP dosage; they rapidly disappear when the dose is reduced or discontinued. The diarrhea will respond to therapy with diphenoxylate; the other GI symptoms respond to treatment with prochlorperazine or trimethobenzamide. These side effects eventually disappear or diminish.

Other adverse effects include mental changes (ie, euphoria) which may progress to hypomania, restlessness, rapid speech, anxiety, insomnia, aggressiveness and agitation; mydriasis, lightheadedness, sleepiness, blurring of vision and bradycardia. Dyspnea, sometimes accompanied by hyperventilation and lightheadedness, is rare. L-5HTP/carbidopa might unmask subclinical scleroderma in patients with an abnormality in kynurenine metabolism.

Overdosage of L-5HTP/carbidopa can produce respiratory difficulties and hypotension.

Administration and dosage: Begin with 25 mg L-5HTP 4 times daily; increase by 100 mg/day every 3 to 5 days if there are no significant side effects. If significant GI side effects develop, reduce the rate of increase to every 1 to 2 weeks. A reduction in myoclonus is usually first observed at 600 to 1000 mg/day (with carbidopa); the usual optimal dose of L-5HTP is between 1000 and 2000 mg/day in 4 divided doses.

Summary: L-5HTP is available through a treatment IND under the FDA's orphan drug program from Bolar Pharmaceuticals, Inc., 130 Lincoln Street, Copiague, NY 11726; (516) 842-8383. The drug will be beneficial to a small number of patients; further research may elucidate additional uses as we increase our understanding of the brain's complex chemistry. Carbidopa may be obtained for use with L-5HTP by contacting Audrey A. Geist, MD, Professional Information, MSD, West Point, PA 19486; (215) 661-7300.

Meropenem *(Merrem) – Broad-spectrum antibiotic.*

Pharmacology: Meropenem is a parenteral carbapenem antibiotic similar in structure to imipenem. Because it is more stable than imipenem against inactivation by renal dehydropeptidase-1 (DHP-1), meropenem does not require concomitant administration with a DHP-1 inhibitor like cilastatin, as in the case of imipenem/cilastatin (*Primaxin*). The bactericidal activity of meropenem results from a high affinity for binding to penicillin binding proteins and stability against beta-lactamase enzymes.

In vitro studies demonstrate an extremely broad range of antibacterial activity. Meropenem is more active than imipenem against gram-negative *Enterobacteriaceae*, *Haemophilus influenzae* and *Neisseria gonorrhoeae*, with MIC_{90} values well below 1 mg/L. *Pseudomonas aeruginosa*, though usually susceptible, is not as sensitive, with an MIC_{90} in the range of 2 to 8 mg/L. Meropenem is active against gram-positive aerobes, including penicillin-resistant strains of *Streptococcus pneumoniae*, but is not active against methicillin-resistant strains of *Staphylococcus aureus*. Most strains of *Enterococcus faecalis* are susceptible, but strains of E *faecium* are generally resistant. MIC_{90} values for meropenem against gram-positive organisms are quite low, only slightly higher than for imipenem. Meropenem is highly active against anaerobes, including *Bacteroides fragilis*, with MIC_{90}s below 1 mg/L, except for *Clostridium difficile*, which demonstrates sensitivity with an MIC_{90} of about 2 mg/L.

Pharmacokinetics: Meropenem can be administered by IV infusion over 30 minutes, IV push over 5 minutes or by IM injection. After IV infusion, meropenem achieves peak plasma concentrations > 50 mg/L with a 1 g dose and 100 mg/L with a 2 g dose. The volume of distribution is about 0.25 L/kg and protein binding is < 20%. More than 70% of meropenem elimination results from renal excretion of unchanged drug, mostly via glomerular filtration. Up to 30% of a dose is metabolized to a microbiologically inactive metabolite, then eliminated renally. Only 2% is excreted in the feces. The elimination half-life is 1 hour, assuming normal renal function, but dosing adjustments are needed when creatinine clearance (Ccr) falls below 50 ml/min. The standard dose is usually 500 mg or 1 g every 8 hours. If the Ccr is 26 to 50 ml/min, the interval is 12 hours; if Ccr is 10 to 25 ml/min, half the standard dose is given every 12 hours; if the Ccr is < 10 ml/min, half the standard dose is given every 24 hours. Meropenem distributes into virtually all body tissues and fluids, including the CSF. Though tissue concentrations are characteristically low, as with other lactam antibiotics, concentrations are usually well above the MIC_{90} for common pathogens.

Clinical trials: Meropenem has been studied in > 3000 patients, covering a full range of infection sites and pathogens. The majority of controlled studies compared meropenem as monotherapy against a cephalosporin, such as ceftazidime (eg, *Fortaz*), cefotaxime (*Claforan*) or ceftriaxone (*Rocephin*), or a cephalosporin in combination with either an aminoglycoside, clindamycin (*Cleocin*) or metronidazole (eg, *Flagyl*). Some studies also included imipenem/cilastatin. Meropenem has demonstrated bacteriological and clinical efficacy comparable to standard antibiotic treatment regimens for intra-abdominal infections, febrile episodes in neutropenic patients, meningitis in both children and adults, lower respiratory tract infections including cystic fibrosis patients, urinary tract infections, skin and soft tissue infections, obstetric/gynecological infections and septicemia.

Pediatric clinical trials have been conducted with both neonates and children, at dosages ranging from 10 to 20 mg/kg 3 times daily (40 mg/kg for meningitis), with documented efficacy. Results suggest that meropenem provides effective monotherapy for moderate to severe infections, including meningitis, especially against resistant strains of *S pneumoniae*, *H influenzae* and other beta-lactamase producing gram-negative organisms.

Side effects: Trials indicate that meropenem is safer and better tolerated than imipenem/cilastatin. It does not seem to have the same propensity for causing seizures in patients with underlying neurological conditions or renal insufficiency. Commonly reported adverse effects include: Diarrhea, nausea (4%); rash, inflammation at injection site, headache (2%); pruritus (1%). Mild alterations in lab values have also been reported: Thrombocytosis (2%); eosinophilia (1%); liver enzyme elevations (ALT [7%] and AST [6%]). These laboratory changes were found to be reversible and not clinically significant. Adverse effects caused the withdrawal of therapy in 1.4% of patients.

Summary: Meropenem is a carbapenem antibiotic that seems to have empiric monotherapy use for a wide range of infections, including meningitis. It is not currently available in the US. Zeneca filed an NDA for *Merrem* in 1993, and it remains under review. Recently published literature suggests that this drug might eventually play a useful role as part of the armamentarium of antibiotics.

Mifepristone *(RU 486)* – Antiprogesterone

Pharmacology: Mifepristone is a synthetic progesterone and glucocorticosteroid receptor antagonist.

Mifepristone's antagonist activity at the glucocorticosteroid receptor disrupts the negative pituitary feedback resulting from the normal morning rise in cortisol level.

When used as an abortifacient, mifepristone acts as an antagonist at progesterone receptors in the endometrium and the trophoblast, allowing prostaglandins to stimulate uterine contractions and causing the conceptus to detach from the uterine wall. Various vascular changes are produced which may decrease placental viability as well as decrease glandular secretory activity, accelerate degenerative changes, and increase stromal but not glandular mitotic activity in the endometrium causing sloughing of the endometrium.

Pharmacokinetics: Mifepristone is rapidly absorbed after oral administration. After a single dose of 25 mg and up to 25 mg/kg, peak plasma levels of 3.5 to 7.5 mcmol/L have been reported at 1 to 3 hours after administration. The drug is 94% bound to protein, with the majority (91%) bound to albumin. The volume of distribution is ≈ 1.5 L/kg. Cerebrospinal fluid levels equal to 4% of the plasma concentration have occurred. The half-life is 20 or 54 hours, depending on the method of pharmacokinetic analysis used in the study. Three active metabolites have been identified. Less than 0.5% of the drug is excreted in the urine.

Mifepristone also crosses the placental barrier, achieving levels equal to one-third of the maternal plasma levels in the fetal circulation.

Clinical trials: Clinical trials have demonstrated that mifepristone is an effective abortifacient in early pregnancy (< 56 days of amenorrhea). A variety of dosing regimens have been successful. Dosages from 25 mg twice daily for 4 days to 50 mg 3 times daily for 4 days have resulted in success rates of 61% to 85%. Once-daily administration of 50 to 100 mg for 7 days was successful in 50% to 73% of cases. A single 600 mg dose has a success rate of 72% to 100%. Menses typically begins within 5 days of initiation of therapy and continues for 1 to 2 weeks. Preliminary evidence suggests that the combination of a single dose of mifepristone followed within 48 hours by the administration of gemeprost, an investigational synthetic prostaglandin in vaginal suppository form, may improve the success rate by stimulating myometrial contraction, cervical softening and dilation. Patients are treated as outpatients unless complications occur.

Preliminary data suggest that the antiglucocorticosteroid action of mifepristone 20 mg/kg/day is useful in the treatment of Cushing's syndrome in some patients.

Mifepristone has also been used in patients with tamoxifen (*Nolvadex*) resistant breast cancer who have evidence of progesterone receptors. A dose of 200 mg/day resulted in a response rate of 18% at 3 months in one study.

Other uses under investigation are treatment of open-angle glaucoma, postcoital contraception (600 mg single dose within 72 hours of unprotected intercourse) and induction of labor. Due to the transplacental passage of mifepristone, the latter application requires further clarification of the drug's effect on a viable fetus.

Side effects: The most common side effect of mifepristone used as an abortifacient is heavy bleeding. Dilation and curettage or transfusion may be required to manage this side effect in some cases. The severity of bleeding is directly related to the use of higher doses (> 800 mg) and a longer duration of gestation before therapy.

Other common side effects include abdominal pain (80%), mild to moderate nausea and vomiting (43%), mild to moderate uterine pain (26%), headache (15%) and diarrhea (7.5%). These can usually be controlled with mild analgesics and antiemetic agents.

Summary: Mifepristone appears to be a safe and effective alternative to presently available forms of abortion. Efficacy is increased when used concurrently with a prostaglandin. It also shows promise in several disease states, such as Cushing's syndrome and breast cancer, which may respond to its specific receptor antagonist effects.

Mifepristone is currently marketed in France as *Mifegyne* by Roussel-Uclaf, and it also is approved in Sweden and the UK. On April 20, 1993, Roussel-Uclaf licensed the drug to the Population Council; this US research group will conduct large-scale clinical trials of the drug starting in October 1994 and establish selection criteria for a US firm to manufacture the product following FDA approval. Companies potentially interested in marketing mifepristone include Gynex, Cabot Medical and Adeza Biomedical. Roussel-Uclaf's parent company, Hoechst AG, will not allow them to manufacture the drug for the US market. The FDA is willing to accept foreign clinical trial data as evidence of safety and efficacy to speed the approval process.

Nitrazepam *(Mogadon)* – Benzodiazepine

Nitrazepam has been widely used for many years in Europe and Canada as a sedative/hypnotic in doses of 2.5 to 10 mg, and in the management of myoclonic seizures of childhood epilepsy. Its structure and clinical effects are also analogous to other benzodiazepines.

Nitrazepam is 80% bioavailable following oral administration. Absorption is rapid: 0.5 to 5 hours to peak concentration; concomitant administration with food decreases peak levels by 30%. Nitrazepam is lipophilic and is widely distributed in the body; 10% to 15% is found in the cerebrospinal fluid; 85% to 90% is plasma protein bound. It crosses the placenta and is found in breast milk (50% and about 50% to 100% of maternal plasma concentration, respectively). Metabolism is extensive and excretion is urinary, primarily as inactive metabolites; only 1% is excreted as the unchanged drug. The elimination half-life is approximately 30 hours.

The frequency of adverse reactions increases with age and dosage, and parallels those of other benzodiazepines. The most common include: Fatigue, dizziness, lightheadedness, drowsiness, lethargy, mental confusion, staggering, ataxia and falling. Nightmares, insomnia, agitation, rash, pruritus, headache and GI disturbances have also been reported. The hangover effect is also common and may be a function of nitrazepam's long half-life.

Summary: Nitrazepam and clobazam appear to be safe and effective agents with antianxiety, anticonvulsant and hypnotic properties. These agents have long elimination half-lives; this enhances the potential for drug accumulation and increases the potential for residual side effects. These agents are unlikely to replace established benzodiazepine derivatives; however, they may provide viable therapeutic alternatives.

Nitrendipine *(Baypress)* – Type II calcium channel blocking agent

Pharmacology: Nitrendipine is a 1,4-dihydropyridine derivative calcium entry blocker, structurally similar to nifedipine. It is further classified as a Type II calcium antagonist because, at usual doses and concentrations, it is devoid of electrophysiologic effects, but is a potent peripheral vasodilator. Relaxation of peripheral vascular smooth muscle occurs as a result of inhibition of calcium influx across cellular membranes.

Nitrendipine causes a decrease in both systolic and diastolic blood pressure, primarily due to arteriolar dilatation. Significant peripheral venodilation is unlikely, since postural hypotension is usually not seen. Reflex increases in heart rate, AV nodal conduction and myocardial contractility occur frequently at therapeutic doses and may precipitate myocardial ischemia in patients with coronary artery disease. Plasma renin activity and catecholamine concentrations increase during therapy with nitrendipine; however, the fact that it reduces the pressor response to norepinephrine but affects no change in responses to angiotensin II may explain its greater effectiveness in the treatment of low-renin hypertension. Nitrendipine does not alter glomerular filtration rate (GFR), renal blood flow or plasma aldosterone levels. A short-term, modest diuretic and natriuretic effect has been observed on initiation of therapy.

The dose/response relationship for this effect appears to be flat; a 10 mg dose produces maximum diuresis. It is unlikely that this has any therapeutic implications during long-term therapy. Preliminary data suggest that nitrendipine has no effect on blood glucose, total cholesterol, triglyceride or uric acid levels.

Pharmacokinetics: Available pharmacokinetic data are based on experience with small numbers of patients using assays of varying sensitivity; data vary.

Nitrendipine appears to be well absorbed after oral administration. Peak serum concentrations are seen at 1 to 2 hours; peak effect is seen at approximately 4 hours. The distribution half-life ($t½$-α) is approximately 1 hour. Beta elimination half-life ($t½$-β) averages 8 to 11 hours. Nitrendipine is metabolized by the liver to an inactive pyridine analog and to several more polar metabolites that are excreted in the urine. Dosage adjustments appear to be necessary in patients with hepatic dysfunction, but specific guidelines are not established. A single-dose study in 16 patients with various degrees of renal dysfunction found no alterations in any kinetic parameters; dosage adjustments appear unnecessary in renal patients.

Clinical trials: Nitrendipine is effective in the treatment of mild to moderate hypertension (diastolic blood pressure 90 to 114 mm Hg). Initial data suggest that the drug is particularly useful in low-renin hypertension, which accounts for 20% to 30% of the hypertensive population. Doses of 10 to 80 mg/day have been used, administered as a single dose or in 2 to 3 divided doses per day. Although a single daily dose will decrease blood pressure for 24 hours, most patients require twice-daily dosing for optimal blood pressure control. Due to reflex increases in heart rate and contractility, concomitant β-blocker therapy may be required in some patients. It has not been determined whether nitrendipine, like verapamil and nifedipine, tends to be more effective in older patients.

Side effects: Nitrendipine has a side effect profile similar to nifedipine. The side effect reported most frequently is headache. Fatigue, peripheral edema, flushing, palpitations, dizziness, polyuria and mild elevations in liver function (in two patients) have also occurred.

Summary: Nitrendipine is a potent vasodilator which effectively reduces blood pressure when given 1 to 3 times daily. The drug appears most useful in low-renin hypertensives. Biochemical abnormalities common to other currently used antihypertensives (eg, hypokalemia, hyperglycemia, increased uric acid and lipids) are not seen with this class of drugs and may represent an advantage over β-blockers and diuretics. Although most patients will require twice-daily dosing, the only other available dihydropyridine (nifedipine) usually requires dosing 3 to 4 times a day.

A New Drug Application (NDA) is pending with the FDA for an antihypertensive indication. Nitrendipine will be co-marketed by Miles and Roche.

Penciclovir – Antiherpes virus agent

Pharmacology: Penciclovir is a potent, selective antiherpes virus agent that has activity in vitro against herpes simplex virus (HSV) type 1 and 2 and varicella-zoster virus (VZV). Its spectrum of antiviral activity is similar to that of acyclovir (*Zovirax*), but it has the advantage of a longer duration of effect.

Both acyclovir and penciclovir are efficient inhibitors of viral DNA replication. They are initially phosphorylated to the monophosphate salt, a reaction that is catalyzed by virus-induced thymidine kinase. There is then subsequent phosphorylation to the triphosphate ester (TPE) by cellular enzymes. In in vitro studies, both penciclovir and acyclovir were phosphorylated to the TPE in HSV-1, HSV-2 and VZV infected cells; only very low concentrations of the ester were noted in uninfected cells. The concentration of the TPE was much greater and was maintained for a longer period of time in all three viral strains treated with penciclovir vs acyclovir. The half-lives of the penciclovir-TPE were 10, 20 and 7 hours in HSV-1, HSV-2 and VZV infected cells, respectively, compared to approximately 1 hour for acyclovir. It is thought that the TPE of acyclovir is rapidly metabolized to the acylonucleoside which then diffuses out of the cell. In contrast, penciclovir maintains its activity even when blood levels decrease since this diffusion is not observed with its ester. It is the TPE of both agents that is an efficient inhibitor of viral replication. Unlike acyclovir, penciclovir is not an obligate DNA chain terminator. Inhibition of viral DNA polymerase is effective due to the high concentration of penciclovir in infected cells.

Pharmacokinetics: The pharmacokinetic parameters of penciclovir were studied in 15 healthy male subjects. A single dose was administered as a 60 minute infusion at doses of 10, 15 or 20 mg/kg. There were 5 subjects for each dosing level and escalation to the next dose only occurred if subjects tolerated the previous dose level. Penciclovir exhibited a linear pharmacokinetic profile in the dose range studied. The C_{max} was 12.1, 19.6 and 22.7 mcg/ml for doses of 10, 15 and 20 mg/kg, respectively. It is believed that penciclovir distributes into tissues because the volume of distribution for all three dose levels exceeded 100 L. Elimination was primarily renal with > 70% of the drug being recovered in the urine after 72 hours. Penciclovir has shown limited oral absorption in animal trials, so there have been a variety of prodrugs developed to facilitate oral administration. One such drug that is already commercially available is famciclovir (*Famvir*); > 50% of an oral dose of famciclovir is absorbed and is then rapidly converted to penciclovir. Famciclovir (125, 250, 500 and 750 mg) was administered to 20 healthy male subjects; at all four dose levels penciclovir was the major metabolite detected 15 to 30 minutes after oral administration. The C_{max} occurred at 0.5 to 0.75 hours after the dose was administered. Approximately 60% of the oral famciclovir dose was excreted as penciclovir in the urine within 24 hours.

Clinical trials: In vitro, penciclovir decreased HSV yield with a shorter period of exposure compared to acyclovir. In addition, HSV replication remained inhibited for several days after removal of penciclovir from the medium. This same effect has not been seen with acyclovir. In one trial, 20 isolates each of HSV-1 and HSV-2 were treated with acyclovir and penciclovir; the drugs had similar activity against both strains of HSV. One isolate of HSV-1 was intermediate to acyclovir but sensitive to penciclovir. Seven isolates of each HSV-1 and HSV-2 were then studied for the effect of in vitro pulse therapy; penciclovir was better than acyclovir at inhibiting viral replication. The activity of penciclovir has also been studied against 23 isolates of HSV that were either acyclovir-sensitive or -resistant. The activity of penciclovir paralleled that of acyclovir; isolates highly resistant to acyclovir were also highly resistant to penciclovir. Therefore, penciclovir does not show promise for the treatment of acyclovir-resistant strains of HSV. In vivo trials with penciclovir have not been published to date.

Side effects: In the dose-escalation, pharmacokinetic trial described above there were no significant adverse drug effects observed with penciclovir administration. One subject developed a mild headache 1 hour after dosing that lasted for 9 hours. There was a slight decrease in supine diastolic blood pressure 1 hour after the infusion and standing diastolic blood pressure 2 hours after the 20 mg/kg dose and a slight increase in creatinine clearance was also noted; however, the effects were not clinically significant.

Summary: Penciclovir is a new antiviral agent with similar activity to acyclovir. However, because it is able to achieve higher levels of the TPE within the viral cell and to sustain the levels for a longer period of time, it may offer the advantages of treatment with lower doses at less frequent intervals compared to acyclovir. Because of poor oral absorption, oral administration will require the use of prodrugs. In vivo clinical trials evaluating its efficacy are currently in progress. SmithKline Beecham planned to file an NDA for penciclovir in 1995. An anticipated approval date is unknown.

Phenformin – Antidiabetic agent (Available under IND exemption)

The biguanide hypoglycemic agent, phenformin, was removed from the US market on October 23, 1977, as a result of concern over the unacceptably high risk of lactic acidosis associated with its use. Phenformin is now available only through an Investigational New Drug (IND) Application which must be filed with the US Food and Drug Administration. Use of phenformin is restricted to specific clearly defined situations and requires registration and reporting to the FDA. Complete information on use of phenformin, physician sponsor applications, patient consent forms and request forms for ordering phenformin tablets or capsules are available from:

Center for Drug Evaluation and Research
Division of Metabolism and Endocrine
Drug Products (HFD-510)
Room 14B03
5600 Fishers Lane
Rockville, Maryland 20857
301-443-3510

Indications: May be used only in adult-onset, nonketotic diabetics who meet all of the following criteria: In addition to elevated blood glucose, have symptoms such as polydipsia; symptoms are not controlled with diet and sulfonylureas or cannot take sulfonylureas because of nontolerance or allergy; symptoms are controlled by phenformin; no underlying risk factors which contraindicate the use; (a) occupation is such that the risk of hypoglycemia from insulin would threaten their jobs or be a hazard to them or others, or (b) cannot take insulin because of disability and have no practical way to receive assistance.

Phenformin is also available under a separate IND for a dermatological condition called atrophie blanche or livedo vasculitis.

Contraindications: Although there is no absolute way to predict the population at risk for lactic acidosis, the following are recognized contraindications: Insulin-dependent diabetes; hypersensitivity to phenformin; renal disease with even mild degrees of impaired renal function; liver disease; history of lactic acidosis; alcohol abuse; any acute medical situation such as cardiovascular collapse (shock), congestive heart failure, myocardial infarction, surgery or septicemia; disease states that may be associated with hypoxemia; complications of diabetes such as metabolic acidosis, coma, infection or gangrene; acute gastrointestinal disturbances (vomiting or diarrhea) which are likely to result in dehydration and prerenal azotemia.

Lactic acidosis in patients taking phenformin has been estimated to occur in 0.25 to 4 cases per 1000 phenformin treatment years. Lactic acidosis is characterized by elevated lactate levels, increased lactate-to-pyruvate ratio and decreased blood pH. In many of the reported cases, azotemia ranging from mild to severe was present.

Nausea, vomiting, hyperventilation, malaise or abdominal pain may herald the onset of lactic acidosis. Instruct the patient to discontinue phenformin and notify the physician immediately if any of these symptoms occur.

Warn patients against using alcohol while receiving phenformin, since ethanol and phenformin potentiate the tendency of each to cause elevated blood lactate levels.

Conclusions: Although phenformin has been removed from the market because of the potential for adverse effects, a select group of patients may require use of this agent. Careful patient selection is necessary to assure a reasonable risk-benefit ratio. Supplies of phenformin are available to practicing physicians from the FDA under an IND exemption.

Pinacidil *(Pindac)* – Antihypertensive agent

Pharmacology: Pinacidil is a vasodilator under investigation for use as an antihypertensive agent. Pinacidil acts at the level of the precapillary, arteriolar (resistance) vessels, causing direct relaxation of vascular smooth muscle. Its vasodilator effect is not altered by blockade of β-adrenergic, cholinergic or histaminic receptors, or by the presence of prostaglandin inhibitors such as indomethacin.

When compared to other vasodilators with similar sites of action (eg, minoxidil [*Loniten*], guancydine, diazoxide [*Hyperstat*]), pinacidil, at comparable levels of blood pressure reduction, produces quantitatively identical increases in heart rate, reflex sympathetic mediated cardiac contractility and cardiac output. However, when compared to hydralazine (another precapillary arteriolar vasodilator), pinacidil, at doses which produce equivalent reductions in total peripheral resistance, is a more potent blood pressure lowering agent. Since blood pressure is a function of the cardiac output multiplied by the total peripheral resistance, this difference may be explained by the fact that hydralazine appears to have a direct (as well as the indirect) cardiostimulatory effect which offsets some of the blood pressure reduction caused by vasodilation. As would be expected from their differing effects on cardiac output, pinacidil produces less of an increase in myocardial oxygen consumption than hydralazine.

Although an active metabolite has been identified, it does not appear to contribute significantly to the overall antihypertensive activity.

There is a linear correlation between pinacidil drug levels and the fall in mean blood pressure and total peripheral resistance; minimal therapeutic levels are 50 ng/ml.

Pharmacokinetics:

Absorption/Distribution — Available data are complicated by the fact that at least two different oral formulations have been used in clinical trials. However, in general, bioavailability approaches 100% after oral administration, with both peak serum levels and effect occurring at 1 hour. Coadministration of food does not alter bioavailability but slightly delays absorption. Approximately 60% of a dose is protein bound.

Metabolism/Excretion — Pinacidil is metabolized by the liver to a number of metabolites, the most significant being the active metabolite, pinacidil N – oxide. Within the first 24 hours, 55% to 60% of an administered dose appears in the urine as pinacidil or the N – oxide, 20% to 30% is excreted in the urine as other metabolites and 3% is recovered in the feces. The elimination half-life (t½) varies between 1.5 to 3 hours. Average clearance values are 42 ± 5 L/hr.

Although exact dosage guidelines have not been established, patients with liver disease should have therapy initiated slowly, at low doses, and with careful blood pressure monitoring. Eight patients with chronic, stable cirrhosis showed a 50% reduction in clearance, prolongation of the half-life and a decrease in the percentage of parent compound converted to the N – oxide metabolite.

Clinical trials: Only a limited number of clinical studies, each involving only a few patients, have been published. This may reflect that pinacidil is not considered to be a first- or second-line drug in the stepped-care approach.

Pinacidil use has generally been confined to patients with moderate to severe hypertension. It is safe and effective, especially when added to a regimen of a diuretic and β-blocker in patients who failed the initial combination regimen. Pinacidil has been particularly effective in selected patients with renal impairment (both dialysis and nondialysis patients) with drug-resistant, non-volume dependent hypertension.

Although most studies have used doses of 10 to 100 mg twice daily, some clinicians feel that the drug may require 3 times daily dosing. The most effective dose range appears to be 12.5 or 25 mg twice daily.

Side effects: Pinacidil appears to be well tolerated. Only a few reports of mild side effects (eg, dizziness, headache and facial flushing) have been noted.

Edema has occurred in 23.5% to 45.2% of patients on doses of pinacidil alone of 25 to 50 mg. Concomitant diuretics may be required in most patients.

Two patients developed positive anti-nuclear antibody (ANA) titers while receiving pinacidil. Neither had clinical manifestations of a lupus-like syndrome, and a direct cause and effect relationship could not be linked to pinacidil; further studies are necessary to investigate the potential for pinacidil to cause a drug-induced lupus syndrome.

Summary: Pinacidil appears to be a promising alternative agent for the treatment of moderate to severe hypertension. However, further studies are needed to clarify the drug's optimal dosing schedule, long-term side effects and optimal drug combinations.

The FDA's Cardio-Renal Drugs Advisory Committee recommended approval of pinacidil on May 28, 1987, with the stipulation that it be used concomitantly with diuretics. The drug was approved by the FDA in December 1989; however, Lilly has no plans to market pinacidil at this time.

Pirenzepine HCl *(Gastrozepine)* – Antiulcer agent

Pharmacology: Pirenzepine is a tricyclic benzodiazepine antiulcer agent comparable to standard antiulcer agents such as cimetidine and ranitidine. However, its uniqueness and mechanism of action hinge on *selective* antimuscarinic activity for gastric acid secretory cells.

Pirenzepine selectively suppresses both basal and stimulated acid and pepsin secretion with lesser effects on other muscarinic sites (eg, salivary secretion) compared to atropine and other classic anticholinergic agents. Controlled trials show that 50 mg, 2 to 3 times daily, inhibits acid secretion at least up to 4.5 hours after dosing. Higher doses inhibit esophageal and colonic motility and decrease lower esophageal sphincter pressure. Pirenzepine may also have cytoprotective effects; however, this is of questionable significance since it has little or no effect on gastric mucus and endogenous gastric prostaglandin production.

Pharmacokinetics: Pirenzepine is a hydrophilic molecule which has systemic bioavailability after oral dosing of 20% to 30%. Approximately 10% of the drug is protein bound. Little drug is found in the brain; brain to serum concentration is 1 to 10.

At least 80% is renally excreted unchanged. Most metabolites are of a desmethyl variety. The parent molecule has a half-life of about 10 hours.

These data indicate the potential for few CNS effects and the need to adjust dosage in patients with impaired renal function.

Clinical studies: Numerous short-term (1 to 6 weeks) studies have been conducted comparing pirenzepine to placebo and other antiulcer drugs in ulcer patients. In small doses (50 to 75 mg/day) duodenal ulcer healing percentages with pirenzepine are not superior to placebo. Doses of 100 to 150 mg/day produce healing in 70% to 90% of patients. Statistically significant symptomatic improvement (decreased antacid use and pain) occurs with both dosage levels.

Short-term double-blind studies comparing duodenal ulcer healing rates of pirenzepine (100 to 150 mg/day) and cimetidine (1 g/day) produced similar results (60% to 79% for pirenzepine and 53% to 85% for cimetidine). A single study comparing pirenzepine (100 mg/day) to cimetidine (1 g/day) and ranitidine (300 mg/day) found similar rates of ulcer healing. However, pirenzepine showed a slower effect on symptom disappearance.

Fewer studies have been conducted in patients with gastric ulcer. Double-blind studies comparing pirenzepine to placebo show a need to use adequate doses (100 to 150 mg/day). Pirenzepine and cimetidine have produced similar healing rates (50% vs 48%) in patients with gastric ulcer, but more studies are indicated.

Trials were performed comparing maintenance doses of pirenzepine (30 to 50 mg/day) to placebo and cimetidine (400 mg/day) in duodenal ulcer patients for 12 months. Results indicate statistically significant reductions in ulcer recurrences for active treatment groups vs placebo (24% recurrence in active treatment group vs 80% in placebo-treated patients). No difference was demonstrated in recurrence rates between pirenzepine and cimetidine patients.

Combined use of pirenzepine with ranitidine or cimetidine shows more effective inhibition of gastric acid secretion than with use of a single agent. Such combinations may be useful in peptic ulcer conditions resistant to single drug therapy and in the Zollinger-Ellison syndrome.

Side effects: Pirenzepine is well tolerated with few reported adverse effects. Dry mouth is the most common effect, but nausea, vomiting, diarrhea, constipation, increased appetite, anorexia, tiredness and difficulty of accommodation have all occurred. Daily doses of less than 150 mg seem to significantly reduce the incidence of at least some of these problems.

Summary: In clinical studies, pirenzepine is equally effective as cimetidine in the treatment of peptic ulcer disease. Its low incidence of side effects and selective inhibition of muscarinic gastric acid secretion will make it a valuable addition to existing agents used to treat ulcers. Pirenzepine is currently available in some European countries; expected date of availability in the United States is unknown. A New Drug Application (NDA) is pending.

Propiram *(Dirame)* – Opioid analgesic

Pharmacology: Propiram, also known as Bay 4503, is an opioid analgesic with μ receptor partial agonist activities. It acts centrally at the μ receptor and has both agonist and weak antagonistic activities at the receptor.

Pharmacokinetics: Propiram has been studied in oral, rectal and injectable forms. The majority of literature available, however, evaluated the oral tablet formulation, propiram fumarate. Bioavailability of the oral formulation is > 97% with a T_{max} of 1.4 hours. Elimination half-life is 5.17 hours and 24% of an orally administered dose is excreted as the parent drug in the urine within 48 hours of administration, indicating extensive metabolism. Total body clearance is 444 ml/min and the V_d is 2.3 L/kg. Duration of action is 3 to 4 hours.

Clinical trials: Relative potencies between injectable propiram and morphine in a ratio of ≈ 10:1, and oral to injectable propiram of 150 mg to 100 mg were identified. Peak analgesic activity was seen at doses of 100 mg propiram (equivalent to 10 mg injectable morphine).

A limited number of clinical trials have been published, and most have been single-dose studies evaluating the efficacy of propiram in post-operative pain. One non-comparative trial, however, evaluated the efficacy of oral propiram 50 to 100 mg repeated as needed every 4 hours for postoperative ocular pain. Of patients enrolled, 64% received 1 or 2 tablets each day and duration of therapy was 1 to 2 days in 80% of those studied. While 93% of the patients rated their pain relief as excellent or good, the authors do not report the degree of relief the current "standard" analgesic provides.

Several single-dose studies have been performed in patients tolerating oral analgesics. Both 50 and 100 mg of oral propiram were shown to be more effective than codeine 60 mg and placebo for the treatment of episiotomy pain. Aspirin 650 mg orally, however, was more effective than 50 mg oral propiram in the treatment of dental pain post-impaction. Both aspirin and propiram proved to be more effective than 60 mg oral codeine or placebo.

One study found 50 mg oral propiram to be equivalent in analgesic efficacy to 50 mg oral pentazocine (*Talwin*) and 60 mg oral codeine; all therapies provided significantly better analgesia than placebo. A second study reported similar results using the same doses of codeine, propiram and placebo. However, a subset of patients in the second study were evaluable for 6 hours after the analgesic was administered; within this subset 50 mg propiram had a significantly better Pain Intensity Difference score at 5 hours than did 60 mg oral codeine sulfate. The patient populations in both of these trials included post-operative cholecystectomy, hemorrhoidectomy, gynecologic and orthopedic surgery patients.

Much of this literature was published during the 1970s and early 1980s and study design either is not well described or is of questionable scientific design in many of the trials. Questions include whether "randomization" included random order of administration in cross-over design studies; whether solid conclusions can be drawn about analgesia when baseline pain and the number of post-operative days when the patient is enrolled are not standardized; whether the study drugs were actually the first analgisic administered post-operatively; and when a drop-out rate/rate of incomplete data collection is considered high.

Side effects: The side effects of propiram are similar to other opioids and appear to be dose-related. The most common side effect, sedation, is reported to occur between 25% and 31%. Other side effects include nausea (5% to 6%) and dizziness (2.2% to 20%). With long-term administration both constipation and dry mouth are frequent side effects.

Despite statements throughout the literature regarding propiram's lower "abuse potential" than morphine or other μ agonists, use of propiram has resulted in display of drug-seeking behavior in non-tolerant addicts. Also, upon abrupt discontinuation of propiram, a mild withdrawal can be experienced by patients, supporting some degree of the development of physical dependence in patients.

Summary: Propiram, an oral partial agonist, appears to be a safe and effective analgesic and provides pain relief for a longer time period than 60 mg codeine. An anticipated approval date is unknown. It will be available as *Dirame* by Roberts.

Remoxipride *(Roxiam)* – Antipsychotic agent

Pharmacology: Remoxipride, a substituted benzamide, is an atypical antipsychotic agent. It is a weak, but selective, dopamine-2 (D_2) receptor antagonist. D_2 receptors are thought to act in an inhibitory manner on adenylate cyclase, while dopamine-1 (D_1) receptors are associated with adenylate cyclase stimulation. The presynaptic dopamine "autoreceptors", which regulate the synthesis and release of dopamine, appear to be of the D_2 subtype. Many investigators have suggested that it is blockade of the D_2 receptor that mediates the clinical effects of most antipsychotic agents.

Remoxipride has a marked affinity for sigma receptors, which mediate opioid effects; clinical significance is unknown. There is a wide range between the dose that blocks apomorphine-induced hyperactivity and the dose that produces catalepsy, suggesting a favorable separation between the dose associated with antipsychotic effects and that producing extrapyramidal symptoms. The administration of remoxipride causes a significant, transient increase in prolactin release; however, prolonged administration (> 15 days) results in a reduction in this response.

Pharmacokinetics: Remoxipride is almost completely absorbed after oral administration with a bioavailability of 96% for both standard and controlled release (CR) formulations. There is no first-pass metabolism. Plasma levels peak within 1 to 2 hours after administration of standard formulations and within 2 to 6 hours after CR formulations and are linearly related to dose. Volume of distribution averages 0.5 to 0.7 L/kg. Protein binding averages 80%. CSF levels average 6% to 17% of total plasma levels. Breast milk concentrations are ≈ 30% of those in plasma.

Approximately 70% of an administered dose is metabolized in the liver to six inactive oxidized metabolites. Plasma concentrations of unchanged remoxipride are higher in slow debrisoquine metabolizers. Between 10% and 40% of an oral dose is excreted unchanged in the urine. Plasma elimination half-life averages 4 to 7 hours.

Remoxipride is a weak base (pKa 8.9). Urinary elimination is reduced and plasma half-life is prolonged in alkaline urine (pH 7.2). Conversely, acidification of urine (pH 5.2) results in increased urinary elimination and a reduction in half-life. Mean plasma concentrations are increased and the half-life is prolonged in the elderly, in patients with creatinine clearances < 25 ml/min, and in severe liver disease. Most investigators recommend initiating therapy with one-half the usual dose in the elderly.

Clinical trials: Remoxipride is an effective treatment for chronic schizophrenia and acute exacerbations of chronic schizophrenia. Improvement was documented in both positive (eg, thought disturbances, hostility/suspiciousness, hallucinations, delusions) and negative (eg, emotional withdrawal, motor retardation) symptoms. In doses of 150 to 600 mg/day, remoxipride had similar antipsychotic efficacy to haloperidol (eg, *Haldol*) 5 to 45 mg/day and thioridazine (eg, *Mellaril*) 150 to 750 mg/day.

In most clinical trials, therapy was initiated with 300 mg/day. Patients responded to total daily doses of 300 to 450 mg/day (maximum dose, 600 mg/day) during initiation of therapy, and were tapered to usual maintenance doses of 150 to 300 mg/day. Dosage adjustments were made no more frequently than every 3 days and were based on patient response.

Remoxipride may also be effective in the treatment of acute mania.

Side effects: Remoxipride, like other atypical antipsychotic agents (eg, clozapine [*Clozaril*]), causes less frequent extrapyramidal symptoms (EPS) than the classic antipsychotic agents (eg, haloperidol). Long-term, comparative trials reported an EPS incidence of 2% to 15% and 7% to 27% in the remoxipride- and haloperidol-treated groups, respectively. Pooled data from nine comparative trials with haloperidol also showed a lower incidence of insomnia, tiredness/drowsiness, difficulty in concentration and dry mouth in the remoxipride-treated group. Although isolated reports of cardiovascular effects such as postural hypotension are documented, they are not considered to be clinically significant.

Summary: Available data suggests that remoxipride is a safe and effective treatment for schizophrenia. Its favorable side effect profile makes it an important therapeutic option for patients unable to tolerate traditional antipsychotic agents. Additional comparative and long-term studies are necessary to clarify its overall role in the treatment of schizophrenia and evaluate its potential to cause tardive dyskinesia.

An NDA for remoxipride was filed in December 1988. It is currently in phase III clinical trials for the treatment of acute and chronic schizophrenia. However, because of recent reports of aplastic anemia, including one death, in European patients, Astra/Merck notified investigators to discontinue use of the drug. The company has recommended restricting the use of the drug to patients who have failed other antipsychotics. The drug, which will be marketed as *Roxiam* by Astra/Merck, is currently available in the UK, Denmark and Luxembourg.

Ritanserin – Specific central serotonin S_2-antagonist

Pharmacology: Ritanserin is a specific, long-acting central serotonin S_2-antagonist which does not affect norepinephrine, acetylcholine or central dopamine antagonism, but does antagonize peripheral histamine. Ritanserin improves sleep quality, decreases fatigue, increases energy levels, improves depressed mood and anxiety and appears to lack abuse potential. Ritanserin 10 mg twice daily also improves neuroleptic-induced akathisia in patients resistant to traditional therapy (eg, anticholinergics, benzodiazepines, beta-blockers). These actions of ritanserin have caused researchers to investigate its effects in the treatment of anxiety, schizophrenia, alcoholism, drug abuse, depressive disorders and Parkinsonism.

Pharmacokinetics: The oral bioavailability is about 75%. Following oral administration, very little drug is recovered unchanged in the urine after a 5 mg IV dose suggesting that it is extensively metabolized by the liver. In a study involving nine healthy volunteers, peak plasma concentrations occurred within 2.39 hours after oral administration. Steady-state plasma concentrations are achieved within 1 week after initiating dosing and the half-life is ≈ 40 hours. Ritanserin is usually administered with or after a meal to decrease the incidence of transient side effects (eg, dizziness, tiredness, lightheadedness) that have been reported in 10% of patients.

Clinical trials: A trial involving 33 patients was conducted to determine the effectiveness of ritanserin in decreasing the negative symptoms in type II schizophrenia over a 6 week period. Patients initially received 10 mg ritanserin. Doses were increased by 10 mg increments to 30 mg as tolerated. The average total dose at the end of the study was 26 mg. Ritanserin significantly improved several negative symptoms such as facial expressions, global affective flattening and relationships with friends and peers and also caused significant reductions in scores for emotional withdrawal and depressive mood compared to placebo. Three patients in the ritanserin group dropped out of the study because of lack of efficacy and one due to side effects (eg, unrest).

In another study, nine patients with acute schizophrenia received ritanserin 10 mg twice daily for 4 weeks. Five of the nine patients experienced a 50% decrease in comprehensive psychological rating scale scores, and scores for negative symptoms also decreased significantly from baseline. No extrapyramidal side effects or akathisia that could be attributed to ritanserin were reported.

Several studies have examined the ability of ritanserin to affect the motor symptoms of Parkinson's disease. Initial studies demonstrated that ritanserin significantly reduced tremor. In contrast, two recent studies determined that ritanserin (range, 5 to 30 mg/day) had a positive effect on dyskinesias but not tremor.

Ritanserin's effect on dysthymia has been studied compared to placebo, amitriptyline (eg, *Elavil*) and imipramine (eg, *Tofranil*). Ritanserin was superior to placebo and equal to amitriptyline and imipramine for up to 8 weeks (n > 300).

Several studies have determined that ritanserin is effective in relieving anxiety, decreasing fatigue and increasing energy in patients with generalized anxiety disorders compared to placebo, and ritanserin 10 mg appears to have equal efficacy to lorazepam (eg, *Ativan*). The antianxiety effects occurred after 2 to 4 weeks of treatment.

Ritanserin decreases craving for alcohol and cocaine. One study involving 39 patients concluded that ritanserin 5 mg decreased desire and craving for alcohol but did not change the amount of alcohol intake during 14 days of study. Another small study (n = 5) suggested that patients receiving ritanserin 10 mg for 28 days not only had no desire to drink but also demonstrated improvement in mood. Several large scale double-blind studies that will include > 900 patients with various types of alcohol dependence are currently underway.

Slow wave sleep (SWS) patterns were significantly improved in several studies when ritanserin was given to patients with alcoholism and depressive disorders; one study found that ritanserin did not affect SWS in 12 depressed patients.

Side effects: Ritanserin appears to be well tolerated. Observed side effects in clinical trials were minimal, with 10% of patients reporting transient dizziness, tiredness and lightheadedness.

Summary: Although ritanserin shows promise in the treatment of a variety of psychiatric illnesses including anxiety, schizophrenia, alcoholism, drug abuse, depressive disorders and Parkinsonism, it is still undergoing clinical trials and has not been approved by the FDA. The dosing range used in the studies was from 5 to 30 mg per day in adults. Side effects are minimal and mild and there seems to be a lack of clinically significant changes in vital signs, laboratory values, ECGs or mood evaluations. An anticipated approval date for the drug, which will be available from Janssen, is unknown.

Sertindole – Antipsychotic agent

Pharmacology: Sertindole is a new "atypical" antipsychotic agent with unique pharmacologic properties compared to traditional agents. The mechanism of action of sertindole is via its strong antagonism of dopamine D_2, serotonin 5-HT_2 and norepinephrine $alpha_1$ receptors. Sertindole appears to have low extrapyramidal symptoms (EPS) potential, does not cause anticholinergic side effects, does not inhibit cognitive functioning and has potent anxiolytic activity.

Pharmacokinetics:

Immunocompromised patients – Sertindole is slowly absorbed from the GI tract with a peak plasma concentration achieved after 8 to 10 hours. Following a single oral dose, the elimination half-life is approximately 60 hours, but there is great patient variability with 10% of subjects demonstrating half-lives > 100 hours after administration of a single dose. Due to sertindole's long half-life, steady-state concentrations are not reached until after 3 to 4 weeks. The long half-life of sertindole should allow for once-daily dosing. Sertindole is characterized by nonlinear kinetics. Increasing the dose by 20% can increase plasma concentrations by approximately 40%. Sertindole is significantly bound to plasma proteins (> 99%), with only a small amount of the drug being renally excreted; therefore, sertindole will presumably not be eliminated by dialysis. In vitro studies have shown that sertindole is predominately metabolized by the hepatic cytochrome P450 3A4 isoform system and eliminated via the GI tract. Sertindole has two metabolites, norsertindole and Lu 28-092, but the activity of these metabolites has not been established.

Clinical trials: In seven phase I trials, more than 100 healthy patients received sertindole 0.5 to 32 mg as a single dose or in escalating dosing for up to 14 days. These studies demonstrated that, overall, sertindole was safe and well tolerated.

Three phase II studies examined the efficacy of sertindole in doses of 4 to 24 mg/day. The first was a pilot, double-blind, randomized, placebo controlled, multicenter study designed to compare the efficacy of sertindole (n = 27) and placebo (n = 11) in patients diagnosed with schizophrenia or schizoaffective disorder. The study concluded that sertindole was effective in most patients at a dose of 16 or 20 mg/day and this therapy was associated with minimal adverse effects.

The second and third phase II studies were randomized, double-blind, multicentered and placebo controlled with identical study designs except that each study had four different treatment groups: 8, 12 or 20 mg/day of sertindole or placebo in the second trial, and the third study had 4 or 12 mg/day sertindole, placebo or haloperidol (eg, *Haldol*) 8 mg twice daily. All patients taking sertindole were titrated upwards starting with 4 mg/day and increasing by 4 mg every third day until the desired dose was reached. The titration phase lasted 12 days and the maintenance phase period was 28 days. Patients enrolled in both studies had to have a previous response to antipsychotic drugs. There were 205 patients enrolled in the second trial and 109 in the third; 153 patients completed at least 13 of the total 40 days of the second trial and were included in the final analysis (107 completed the entire study). Only the 20 mg sertindole group significantly improved in all efficacy parameters compared to placebo. Sertindole 20 mg was equally efficacious to haloperidol but caused fewer side effects.

In a long term, open-label study, sertindole 4 to 24 mg/day was administered to 170 patients for up to 2 years to determine its safety and efficacy. The mean exposure to sertindole was 121 days (range, 2 to 532 days) and the most common dose administered was 20 mg/day (33%).

Side effects: Adverse effects observed during phase I trials included lethargy, drowsiness, nasal congestion, sexual dysfunction, GI complaints, dizziness, lightheadedness, mild tremor, orthostatic hypotension, syncope, dystonia, postural hypotension and cogwheel rigidity. No patients experienced EPS. The most common adverse effects experienced during phase II trials that occurred more often with sertindole 20 mg/day than with placebo included: Headache (26%); nasal congestion (26%); dry ejaculation (17%); constipation, dizziness, somnolence (11%). Dry ejaculation was the only side effect that was found to be significantly greater than placebo ($p < 0.05$). Adverse effects experienced during the long term study were similar, but incidence rates were higher.

Summary: Sertindole should provide an effective and safe alternative treatment when therapy with traditional antipsychotics have failed due to lack of efficacy or intolerable side effects. Additional trials are necessary to establish the long term safety, especially the incidence of tardive dyskinesia, and efficacy of sertindole. An NDA for sertindole was filed in October, 1995 by Abbott. An anticipated approval date is unknown.

Sibutramine *(Meridia)* – Weight loss agent

Pharmacology: Sibutramine is a novel monoamine reuptake inhibitor antidepressant that is being investigated as a weight loss agent. Its mechanism of action as a weight loss agent has not been explored. However, the mechanism of sibutramine and its desmethylated metabolites for depression is via inhibition of monoamine reuptake (not inhibition of monoamine oxidase), noradrenaline and 5-hydroxytryptamine (5-HT) and possibly inhibition of dopamine uptake. However, sibutramine lacks anticholinergic activity, central depressant effects and is nonsedating. These characteristics may cause sibutramine to have a more favorable side effect profile than other weight control products. In several models, sibutramine was shown to have a more rapid onset of antidepressant action after administration (several hours to 3 days) compared with other antidepressants, which can take several weeks to show an antidepressant effect.

Pharmacokinetics: No published pharmacokinetic information is available.

Clinical trials: Unpublished phase I and II trials from Boots Pharmaceuticals have shown that 15 nonobese volunteers receiving either 2.5 or 5 mg sibutramine per day for 15 weeks lost 3.3% of their initial weight without dieting. Another 15 volunteers in the study who received 5 to 10 mg/day lost 3.7% compared with nine volunteers who received placebo who lost 0.2% of their initial body weight. In another unpublished 6 week trial, 15 healthy nonobese volunteers who received sibutramine 30 mg lost 6% of their initial body weight compared to five patients receiving placebo who gained 0.5%. One last unpublished study involving depressed patients showed that 11 patients who received 2.5 to 5 mg/day lost 1.2% of their initial body weight, 14 patients receiving 5 to 10 mg lost 1.7% and 28 subjects who received 10 to 20 mg lost 2.1% compared to 25 subjects receiving placebo who gained 0.4%.

The only published study was a randomized, double-blind, placebo controlled trial to determine the safety and efficacy of sibutramine 5 and 20 mg administered as adjunctive therapy to caloric restriction (eg, 22 to 25 cal/kg IBW/day), behavior modification and exercise. Following an initial 3 week individualized diet, behavior modification and exercise period, 55 morbidly obese (between 130% and 180% overweight), otherwise healthy subjects received either sibutramine 5 mg (n = 18), sibutramine 20 mg (n = 18) or placebo (n = 19) for 8 weeks and then were followed up 1 week after discontinuing therapy. Sibutramine 5 and 20 mg caused an average weight loss of 2.9 kg (3%) and 5 kg (5.1%), respectively, vs placebo 1.4 kg (1.3%). Sibutramine 20 mg caused a significantly greater weight loss than sibutramine 5 mg and placebo. The authors stated that successful weight loss would include losing between 0.5 to 0.7 kg/week. Patients meeting or exceeding this criteria were as follows in each group: Placebo (n = 2), sibutramine 5 mg (n = 4), sibutramine 20 mg (n = 11). None of the participants receiving sibutramine 20 mg gained weight during the study, and only one subject receiving sibutramine 5 mg gained weight.

Side effects: Adverse effects noted in phase I and II clinical trials included: Insomnia, rapid heartbeat, and periodically, diastolic hypertension. One case of serious, reversible thrombocytopenia has occurred. In the one published trial including only obese, otherwise healthy subjects, sibutramine caused an increase in blood pressure, pulse and heart rate, which appeared similar to placebo, although the statistical significance was not determined. Other side effects noted in this trial included headache, sleep difficulty, irritability, dry mouth, rash or dry skin. Sibutramine users, especially those in the 20 mg group also reported CNS stimulation noted as clearheadedness, increased interest and alertness.

When single-dose sibutramine 30, 45 and 60 mg was compared with amitriptyline (eg, *Elavil*) 50 mg and placebo in six healthy male volunteers, sibutramine 60 mg caused statistically significant increases in heart rate and systolic blood pressure at 1, 2 and 6 hours after administration compared to both amitriptyline and placebo. With sibutramine 30 mg, this difference was only significant at 2 hours. More patients taking amitriptyline reported a decrease in salivation and an increase in drowsiness, whereas patients in the sibutramine group did not. Further studies will be required to determine sibutramine's cardiovascular effects.

Summary: Although only one clinical trial has been published to date, sibutramine shows promise as an adjunctive weight loss therapy to diet and exercise. The weight loss effects of sibutramine may be dose-related. Additional clinical trials are necessary to establish the long-term safety and efficacy of sibutramine as a weight loss agent.

Sibutramine, which will be available as *Meridia* from Knoll, is in late clinical trials for treatment of depression and obesity. Approval is anticipated in 1997.

Teicoplanin *(Targocid)* – Glycopeptide antibiotic

Pharmacology: Teicoplanin (teichomycin A2) is a glycopeptide antibiotic complex structurally related to vancomycin (eg, *Vancocin*). It has a similar spectrum of activity but a longer half-life which allows less frequent dosing. It may be administered by IM and IV injection and brief (30 minute) infusion. Teicoplanin is a mixture of six closely related glycopeptide components designated as teicoplanin-A2 (1 through 5) and teicoplanin-A3. The components of the A2 complex account for 90% to 95% of teicoplanin. The drug interferes with cell wall synthesis in susceptible organisms by inhibiting peptidoglycan polymerization.

Like vancomycin, teicoplanin is active only against gram-positive organisms. It is bactericidal against most susceptible strains, with the possible exception of some coagulase-negative staphylococci (which may show reduced susceptibility), where it may be bacteriostatic. It has equivalent or superior activity (based on MIC data) to vancomycin against staphylococci, including both methicillin-sensitive and -resistant *S aureus*, *S epidermidis*, streptococci (including viridans group, and groups B, C, F and G), enterococci, and many anaerobic gram-positive bacteria, including *Clostridium difficile*, *C perfringens*, *Listeria monocytogenes* and *Corynebacterium jeikeium*. Vancomycin-resistant enterococci may be resistant to teicoplanin.

Teicoplanin is usually synergistic with aminoglycosides and imipenem, and additive with rifampin (eg, *Rifadin*). A post-antibiotic effect of 2.4 to 4.1 hours has been reported with both methicillin-sensitive and -resistant strains of *S aureus*.

Pharmacokinetics: Like vancomycin, teicoplanin is minimally absorbed after oral administration; this route is acceptable only for the treatment of pseudomembranous colitis. Following IM administration of 3 mg/kg, peak levels of 5 to 7 mcg/ml are achieved at 2 to 4 hours; bioavailability is 90%. Peak serum levels after IV administration are dependent on the dose and the method of administration. Following administration of 3 mg/kg, peak levels after a 30 second injection or a 30 minute infusion average 53 and 20 mcg/ml, respectively. Trough (24 hour) levels are not influenced. The drug is widely distributed in most tissues and fluids (with the exception of CSF), although the rate and extent varies. Volume of distribution (Vd) at steady state averages 0.6 to 0.8 L/kg. Protein binding is 90%.

The drug does not appear to undergo metabolism and is excreted in the urine almost entirely by glomerular filtration. The terminal elimination half-life averages 45 to 70 hours. In patients with renal dysfunction and the elderly, the elimination half-life is increased but the Vd is unchanged. Current dosing recommendations for renal impairment state that usual doses be given for the first 3 days. Thereafter, either the dose is reduced or the interval prolonged, based on the degree of renal insufficiency according to the following scheme: Creatinine clearance (Ccr) 40 to 60 ml/min, half the dose or twice the interval; Ccr < 40 ml/min, one-third the dose or triple the interval.

Clinical trials: Reported response rates by type of infection are: Skin and soft tissue (90%); septicemia, bone and joint (89%); endocarditis (83%); respiratory tract (77%). Other applications in which the drug has demonstrated efficacy include: Endocarditis prophylaxis in dental surgery; Hickman catheter and other indwelling device-related infections; neurosurgical shunt ventriculitis; CAPD-related peritonitis (added to dialysate); surgical prophylaxis; presumed gram-positive infections in immunocompromised patients. The usual loading and maintenance doses of 6 mg/kg followed by 3 mg/kg/24 hours may need to be increased in children and in the treatment of *S aureus* endocarditis and septicemia. A reduction in efficacy has been noted in diabetics, immunocompromised patients and when foreign bodies are present.

Side effects: The overall incidence of side effects is 10.3%. Most commonly reported effects include: Non-specific complaints (fatigue, headache, diarrhea) (5.1%); injection site intolerance (pain, redness, phlebitis) (3%); hypersensitivity skin reactions (pruritus, urticaria, maculopapular rash) (2.4%); hematologic abnormalities (eosinophilia, reversible neutropenia, increased platelet count) (2.2%); transient elevation of LFTs (1.7%); nephrotoxicity (0.35% to 0.6%); high-frequency hearing loss which may be irreversible (0.28%); bronchospasm (0.2%); anaphylactoid reactions (0.07%). Teicoplanin does not appear to cause the dose or infusion rate-related histamine release associated with the "red man syndrome", as does vancomycin. Concomitant use of an aminoglycoside appears to increase the incidence of nephrotoxicity.

Summary: Teicoplanin appears to be a safe and effective alternative to vancomycin. Potential advantages appear to be the availability of IM administration, reduced infusion times and volume requirements, the lack of infusion-related reactions and once daily dosing. The NDA for teicoplanin was filed in March 1991. The FDA has given the drug a "1A" priority review rating. Teicoplanin is currently available in 13 countries. It will be available as *Targocid* by Marion Merrell Dow. A 1995 approval is anticipated.

Tenidap *(Enable)* – Anti-inflammatory cytokine inhibitor

Pharmacology: Tenidap sodium is an anti-inflammatory agent being developed for use in the treatment of rheumatoid arthritis and osteoarthritis. Whereas NSAIDs decrease prostaglandin synthesis by inhibiting cyclooxygenase, tenidap appears to inhibit both cyclooxygenase and 5-lipoxygenase, thus impairing production of both prostaglandins and leukotrienes.

Although the exact mechanism of action has not been determined, in vitro studies suggest that tenidap lowers concentrations of interleukin-1, interleukin-6, leukotriene B4, tumor necrosis factor and C-reactive proteins. It also inhibits the release of neutrophil collagenase. The arachidonic acid metabolites inhibited by tenidap are potent inflammatory mediators that profoundly augment leukocyte chemotaxis. The failure of NSAIDs to inhibit the lipoxygenase pathway partially explains their inability to significantly alter the progressive tissue destruction often associated with rheumatoid arthritis. Thus, the unique pharmacology of tenidap provides the drug with a distinct pharmacologic advantage over NSAIDs.

Pharmacokinetics: To date, pharmacokinetic data on tenidap have not been published. It is known that the drug is roughly 99% reversibly bound to albumin, and multiple dosing of 120 mg/day yields a serum concentration of approximately 5 to 15 mg/L.

Clinical trials: A recent report describes four separate studies comparing tenidap to naproxen (eg, *Naprosyn*) or placebo in treating rheumatoid arthritis (RA). Doses of tenidap ranged from 40 to 120 mg/day; naproxen dosage was 500 mg twice daily. Patients were allowed to remain on other medications, such as auranofin *(Ridaura)*, penicillamine *(Cuprimine; Depen)*, hydroxychloroquine *(Plaquenil Sulfate)* and prednisone (eg, *Deltasone*). Durations ranged from 2 weeks to 1 year. All four studies demonstrated a significantly greater reduction in C-reactive protein with tenidap than with naproxen or placebo.

In another study, 374 patients with RA treated previously with only NSAIDs were randomized to receive either tenidap 120 mg/day or auranofin 3 mg twice daily with diclofenac *(Cataflam; Voltaren)* 50 mg 3 times daily. Evaluation included patient and physician assessments of disease activity, number of painful joints, swollen joints and pain. After 9 months, there was no significant difference between the two therapies, though a higher rate of discontinuation was reported for auranofin due to diarrhea.

A similar trial involving 367 RA patients compared 120 mg/day of tenidap to piroxicam (eg, *Feldene*) 20 mg/day, alone and in combination with hydroxychloroquine 400 mg/day, for 2 years. Based on clinical evaluation, results indicated that tenidap therapy was more effective than piroxicam and equally as effective as the combination of piroxicam and hydroxychloroquine.

A 1-year multi-center study of 488 RA patients compared clinical efficacy of treatment with 40, 80 or 120 mg/day tenidap to treatment with 500, 750 or 1000 mg/day naproxen, beginning with the lowest dose and titrating to clinical response. Efficacy of the two treatments was not significantly different during the first 4 weeks, but tenidap became significantly more efficacious by 24 weeks. Reductions in all acute phase reactants were significantly greater in the tenidap-treated group.

Side effects: The most significant side effect reported in tenidap clinical trials has been reversible proteinuria of proximal tubular origin, occurring in ≤ 20% of patients. This has not been associated with renal function impairment. One study reported 24% GI side effects in patients receiving tenidap.

Summary: Studies conducted to date, both in vitro and in vivo, clearly suggest that tenidap is a unique anti-rheumatoid agent with disease modifying potential. Based on clinical and laboratory parameters, tenidap is more efficacious than NSAIDs and comparable to current mainstays of RA therapy. Tenidap appears to hold promise as a major new drug in the management of rheumatoid arthritis and osteoarthritis.

Pfizer filed an NDA with the FDA for tenidap on December 22, 1993. A 1995 approval was anticipated. It will be available as *Enable*.

Terodiline HCl *(Micturin)* – Agent for urinary incontinence

Pharmacology: Terodiline is a secondary amine which has non-selective anticholinergic and calcium blocking effects. Although originally investigated as an antianginal agent, terodiline is presently undergoing evaluation in the treatment of patients with bladder incontinence. Terodiline provides the advantage of both anticholinergic and calcium blocking effects within the same plasma concentration range, with anticholinergic effects predominating at lower plasma concentrations and calcium entry blocking action predominating at higher plasma concentrations.

The motor nerve supply to the bladder and urethra is from the parasympathetic system; the neurotransmitter active in this system is acetylcholine. Therefore, anticholinergic agents have been used to treat incontinence, but side effects often limit their usefulness. In addition to parasympathetic activity, it appears that calcium entry from the extracellular space is important in the contractile activity of urinary tract smooth muscle. Calcium blockers reduce frequency and amplitude of detrusor contractions and improve bladder capacity; however, side effects associated with their use have prevented their use in treating incontinence.

Pharmacokinetics: Terodiline is well absorbed after oral administration with a bioavailability of ≈ 90%. Peak serum levels occur 2 to 8 hours (average, 4 hours) after administration. Although therapeutic levels have not been clearly established, a steady-state concentration of 0.6 mg/L is generally well tolerated. Higher concentrations of 0.8 to 1.1 mg/L can be maintained in some patients without serious adverse effects.

The volume of distribution is 500 L, ≈ 80% to 85% is bound to serum proteins, and the half-life is ≈ 60 hours. Due to the long half-life, maximum clinical effects will not be seen until ≈ 10 days after initiation of therapy.

Terodiline is extensively metabolized in liver. The major metabolite, parahydroxyterodiline, is minimally active compared to the parent. Approximately 15% of the drug can be recovered unchanged in urine.

Major pharmacokinetic changes occurred in patients with an average age of 85 years (eg, prolongation of half-life, decreased unbound drug fraction and body clearance, increased time to reach steady-state plasma concentrations). A 25 mg/day dose achieved similar plasma concentrations as a 37.5 to 50 mg/day dose in younger, healthier patients. This suggests that elderly patients should have therapy initiated at a dose not to exceed 12.5 mg twice daily, and increased doses should not occur prior to 4 weeks post-initiation.

Clinical trials: Terodiline 12.5 to 25 mg twice daily was effective in the treatment of some patients with urge urinary incontinence. Patients treated with terodiline have a decrease in both pre-micturition symptoms such as urgency and in urinary frequency. One study reported a decrease in voluntary micturitions from a mean of 10.8 to 7.9/day after 6 months of treatment. Another group reported a decrease in involuntary micturitions from 2.5 to 1.5/day with greater effects in those patients with higher baseline micturition frequency.

An increase in bladder capacity has been observed in several studies with one group reporting an average increase from 252 to 335 ml after 6 months of therapy.

A preliminary study suggests that terodiline may be effective in children 6 to 14 years of age involved in a bladder training program to correct urgency or urge incontinence.

Side effects: Up to 50% of patients in some studies reported side effects during the first 3 months of therapy vs 35% with placebo. Most side effects were mild, anticholinergic-related and decreased in frequency (34%) between 3 and 6 months of continuous therapy. The most commonly reported effect was dry mouth (27% during first 3 months, 19% between 3 and 6 months). Other side effects reported during the first 3 months include: Blurred vision (15%); tremor (14%); weight gain (11%); tachycardia (4%); ankle edema (2%). The incidence of these effects decreased between 3 and 6 months. One study reported a small increase (2 mm Hg) in resting diastolic blood pressure after 6 months. Other side effects include: Vertigo; headache; nausea; polymorphic ventricular tachycardia (PVT; reported in other countries).

Summary: Studies to date suggest that terodiline is a safe and effective agent for the treatment of urinary incontinence. Its unique combination of both anticholinergic and calcium blocking activity may provide an advantage over presently available treatments. However, further studies are required to clarify long-term safety and to identify those patients most likely to benefit from terodiline therapy. Forest Labs acquired US licensing rights for the oral tablets from KabiPharmacia in December 1987. Kabi temporarily discontinued the sale of terodiline world wide following reports of an association with PVT. Clinical trials in the US have been put on hold at the request of the FDA. Forest submitted an NDA on August 30, 1989. An anticipated approval date for the drug, which will be marketed as *Micturin*, is now unknown.

Tiagabine – Antiepileptic

Pharmacology: Evidence has shown that decreased GABAergic inhibition may be a cause or partial cause of epilepsy. There are several ways of increasing GABAergic inhibition; augmenting the synthesis of GABA (eg, valproic acid [eg, *Depakene*]); by giving drugs that act as GABA agonists; inhibition of GABA metabolism (eg, vigabatrin [*Sabril*; investigational]); stimulating the release of GABA; and inhibiting the uptake of GABA (eg, tiagabine). Tiagabine is a second generation antiepileptic which appears to prolong the action of GABA by increasing brain GABA levels via inhibition of the high-affinity uptake systems into presynaptic neurons and glia.

Pharmacokinetics: The exact bioavailability of tiagabine is not known. Following oral administration approximately 25% of the dose is recovered in the urine and

63% in the feces. Very little drug is recovered unchanged in the urine suggesting that tiagabine is extensively metabolized. The absorption of tiagabine is complete and rapid with peak plasma concentrations occurring within 0.5 to 1 hour after administration. Food reduces the rate, but not the extent of absorption of tiagabine. The elimination half-life of tiagabine is variable with a range from 4.5 to 13.4 hours (mean, 6.7) but does not appear to be dose-related or significantly affected by single or multiple dosing. Tiagabine does not influence hepatic metabolism of other antiepileptic agents but it may be metabolized by the cytochrome P450 system, and therefore its metabolism may be influenced by other antiepileptic agents. A study involving elderly subjects concluded that the pharmacokinetics of tiagabine are similar to younger subjects.

Clinical trials: Single or add-on therapy with traditional antiepileptic agents fails to control seizure frequency in up to 30% of epileptic patients. Studies examining the efficacy of tiagabine were primarily add-on trials in patients with resistant epilepsy. A few of the studies utilized a technique referred to as enrichment (Amery design). This design initially enrolls all subjects under open, dose escalation conditions for 4 to 8 weeks. Only those patients who respond at a preset percent reduction in seizure frequency and do not experience unacceptable adverse effects continue to the double-blind, crossover or parallel phase of the study where tiagabine is compared to placebo for up to 23 weeks. There are both advantages and disadvantages to this design. The main disadvantage is the difficulty in comparing results from this type of study to traditional clinical trials.

Reductions in seizure frequency have been observed in patients with complex partial, simple partial and secondarily generalized tonic-clonic seizures receiving other antiepileptic agents. Tiagabine doses ranged from 8 to 64 mg/day. When combining all clinical trials, 24% to 26% of subjects with complex partial seizures, 37% with simple seizures and 44% to 63% with tonic-clonic seizures involved in the double-blind phase of the studies showed a > 50% decrease in seizure frequency. In all cases, tiagabine was found to reduce seizure frequency significantly more than placebo. One study determined that the minimum effective dose for tiagabine is 32 mg/day.

Side effects: Tiagabine appears to be well tolerated with minimal, mild side effects. It does not cause any significant changes in vital signs or laboratory values. The incidence and severity of adverse effects appear to be dose related. Side effects are mild/moderate when patients are administered 12 mg/day; 24 mg/day leads to a higher incidence. Tiagabine has only been administered as add-on therapy, therefore it is difficult to determine the exact side effect profile. The incidence of side effects with tiagabine add-on therapy are similar to placebo. Data from pooled studies indicate that the most common side effects are: Dizziness; asthenia; headache; somnolence; ataxia; tiredness; poor concentration; abnormal thinking; depression; nervousness; tremor.

Drug interactions: Tiagabine does not influence hepatic metabolism, therefore it should not affect the metabolism of other antiepileptic agents. Several combinations of antiepileptic agents have been shown to affect the metabolism of tiagabine and therefore, adjustments in the dose of tiagabine are probably warranted. Combination administration of carbamazepine (eg, *Tegretol*) and phenytoin (eg, *Dilantin*), primidone (eg, *Mysoline*) or vigabatrin has been shown to induce the metabolism of tiagabine, although valproate has not been shown to cause this effect.

Summary: Tiagabine appears to be effective in the treatment of complex partial, simple partial and secondarily generalized tonic-clonic seizures. The dosing range used in studies was from 8 to 64 mg/day in adults, with a dose of 32 mg/day appearing to be the minimum effective dose.

Tiagabine is currently in late clinical trials. An anticipated approval date is unknown.

Tirilazad *(Freedox)* – 21-aminosteroid antioxidant

Pharmacology: Tirilazad mesylate is a 21-aminosteroid (also referred to as lazaroids) with distinct antioxidant properties. It does not manifest glucocorticoid activity. Tirilazad acts as a cytoprotective agent that oxidizes peroxyl radicals and stabilizes cell membranes. It also helps to preserve the membrane content of vitamin E (alphatocopherol), another important antioxidant. As a result of its ability to prevent lipid peroxidation in cell membranes, tirilazad promotes tissue survival in the vicinity of a CNS injury.

Due to the high content of polyunsaturated lipids in neuronal membranes, the CNS is particularly susceptible to the destructive effects of oxygen radicals. Tissue injury occurring during CNS trauma or a stroke increases oxygen radical production, which in turn leads to damaging lipid peroxidation reactions. Such oxygen radical-mediated processes appear to be involved in posttraumatic brain edema, spinal axonal degeneration and microvascular damage. The progressive secondary tissue destruction which follows the precipitating event may be amenable to therapy with antioxidants.

Pharmacokinetics: Tirilazad is administered in a citrate solution as an IV infusion over not more than 30 minutes. It is a lipophilic substance that distributes extensively to tissue, with a volume of distribution of about 1.7 L/kg. The drug appears to follow a multi-compartment elimination pattern. Following a single dose, the half-life is approximately 3.75 hours. However, upon multiple dosing, a terminal elimination half-life of 35 hours has been observed. Elimination occurs via hepatic metabolism. The clearance of tirilazad is roughly equal to hepatic plasma flow.

Clinical trials: In numerous neurological studies of animal models, tirilazad has shown distinct promise as a useful therapeutic agent for brain and spinal injury, aneurysmal subarachnoid hemorrhage (SAH) and stroke. Phase III clinical trials are currently being conducted in each of these areas.

The second National Acute Spinal Cord Injury Study (NASCIS 2) demonstrated that patients treated with high-dose methylprednisolone (eg, *Solu-Medrol*; 8 to 9 g/day) within 8 hours of injury, experienced significantly greater neurological improvement than those treated with placebo. The efficacy of methylprednisolone in slowing the progression of CNS damage is believed to be due to its antioxidant properties rather than its glucocorticoid activity. For this reason, in NASCIS 3 (an ongoing follow-up study), one of the three treatment arms involves 2 g methylprednisolone bolus, followed by 2.5 mg/kg tirilazad infusion every 6 hours for a total of 48 hours.

To date, most of the clinical efficacy trials conducted with tirilazad have studied its use in SAH. Upjohn has submitted three double-blind, randomized, placebo controlled study results to the FDA in support of an NDA for tirilazad in the treatment of SAH. However, an FDA committee determined that these studies did not confirm efficacy; one study showed an improvement in males, but this was not replicated in another study, and there were no differences in females.

Tirilazad and newer, more potent antioxidants may also be studied in other neurologic conditions in which peroxidative mechanisms have been implicated. These include Alzheimer's disease, Parkinson's disease and multiple sclerosis.

Side effects: Tirilazad has been shown to be safe in elderly patients (average age, 66 years) with acute ischemic stroke at doses up to 6 mg/kg/day for 3 days. In healthy volunteers, tirilazad had no effect on cerebral blood flow or cerebral oxygen metabolism. Studies have failed to show any significant glucocorticoid effect to be caused by the drug. Up to 50% of subjects in one study exhibited a moderate, transient increase in serum alanine transaminase. Thus far, the most noted side effect has been mild to moderate pain at the injection site, occurring in 60% to 80% of patients.

Studies involving tirilazad and both nimodipine *(Nimotop)* and cimetidine (eg, *Tagamet*) have failed to identify a clinically significant drug interaction with either of those drugs.

Summary: Tirilazad is a potent antioxidant, similar in structure to other steroids, but without glucocorticoid activity. Due to its ability to prevent oxygen radical-mediated lipid peroxidation, it may prove to be useful in preventing progressive neuronal degeneration and associated complications following brain and spinal injury, SAH and stroke.

Upjohn submitted a new drug application in June 1994 for tirilazad with the indication of SAH. Due to the lack of serious side effects that have been documented thus far, and the considerable potential benefit that this drug possesses as a therapeutic agent in areas greatly in need of new treatment modalities, approval is anticipated, quite possibly in 1995. However, on September 26, 1994, the FDA's Peripheral and Central Nervous System Drugs Advisory Committee decided that the studies for tirilazad did not confirm efficacy and that further studies would be necessary. A Treatment IND program was discussed as a possibility.

Tizanidine *(Zanaflex)* – Centrally acting α_2 agonist

Pharmacology: Tizanidine is a centrally acting α_2 agonist structurally similar to clonidine (eg, *Catapres*) used for treatment of spasticity in various conditions (eg, multiple sclerosis [MS], spinal cord injury). The antispasmodic activity of tizanidine is thought to be a result of indirect depression of polysynaptic reflexes by antagonizing the excitatory actions of spinal interneurons.

Pharmacokinetics: The pharmacokinetics of tizanidine were evaluated in two separate studies involving MS patients (n = 17) and spinal cord injury patients (n = 10). The researchers identified a linear relationship between dose and antispastic action with oral doses of 2 to 8 mg. Peak serum concentrations occurred between 1 and 2 hours. A difference from baseline spasticity was evident in both populations for 3 to 4 hours post-dose. A weak relationship was identified between subjects and plasma concentrations, indicating high interpatient variability. Elimination half-life is between 2.7 and 4.2 hours. Tizanidine undergoes first-pass effect (80%) and is nearly completely metabolized hepatically to metabolites which are primarily renally eliminated.

Clinical trials:

Spasticity caused by multiple sclerosis – In one study, a greater improvement in muscle tone using the Ashworth Score was seen in the placebo arm of the trial than in the treatment arm (tizanidine) at the end of the titration phase and again at the study endpoint (13 weeks). After the study was completed, it was discovered that no consideration was given to timing of measurement of tonicity in relationship to the treatment. When comparing mean changes from baseline to 3 hours post-dose, a greater improvement was seen in the tizanidine patients. When blindly evaluating global efficacy and tolerability of the two treatments, tizanidine was significantly better than placebo.

In a 12-week study, muscle tone was reduced to a significantly greater extent in the tizanidine group vs placebo. Muscle strength was not affected by either therapy. Spasms and pain decreased in both treatment arms during the study.

One study compared the efficacy and side effects of tizanidine and baclofen (*Lioresal*) in patients with spasticity. Similar efficacy and tolerability of both agents were reported.

Spasticity caused by spinal cord injury – A study compared placebo and escalating doses of tizanidine. The Ashworth Scale and other outcome measures were assessed 1 to 2 hours after the study medication was administered so measurements would coincide with peak blood levels of tizanidine. A significantly greater decrease in muscle tone from baseline was seen in the tizanidine group than in the placebo group. A greater decrease in the frequency of spasms was also seen in the tizanidine-treated patients.

Meta-analysis data – A study reported summary data from 20 short-term studies dating back to 1977. Patients suffered from spasticity due to MS, cerebrovascular disorders and ALS. Analysis of patient-data revealed equal efficacy of tizanidine, baclofen and diazepam (eg, *Valium*) in decreasing muscle tone with significantly better muscle strength in the tizanidine-treated group.

Other – A trial comparing tizanidine with baclofen over a 12 month period found similar effectiveness for the treatment of spasticity in patients with cerebrovascular lesions. In one study, tizanidine was as effective as diazepam in the treatment of cerebral spasticity in patients following a cerebrovascular accident or cranial trauma.

Side effects: Side effects reported in clinical trials are similar to other α_2 agonists. More common or potentially severe side effects include dry mouth (45% to 49%), drowsiness (48% to 54%), asthenia (41%), dizziness (16%), liver function abnormalities (< 1%) and hallucinations (1%). Hypotension and orthostatic hypotension may occur. Side effects have been found to be dose related and often resolve with a decrease in dose. Slow titration of doses appears to decrease the frequency of side effects.

Summary: Tizanidine offers a novel mechanism of action for the treatment of spasticity in multiple sclerosis, spinal cord injury patients and other settings. Efficacy is comparable to baclofen. Although most studies use every 8 hour dosing, as needed dosing would be appropriate in the MS population. Side effects frequently occur and efficacy approaches good to excellent in only 24% and poor to fair in 76% of the population based on self-evaluation by the patient.

Tizanidine has been commercially available in the foreign market since 1984. Athena Neurosciences, Inc. has marketing rights in Canada, the UK and the US. Athena was denied an NDA in March 1995 and is proceeding with the reapplication process. The product will be marketed as an oral agent, *Zanaflex*, available in 4 mg tablets.

Tolrestat *(Alredase)*–Aldose reductase inhibitor

Pharmacology: Tolrestat, a carboxylic acid, is an aldose reductase inhibitor currently undergoing clinical trials to assess its value in controlling the biochemical abnormalities responsible for the late complications of diabetes (eg, diabetic neuropathy and retinopathy).

Diabetic neuropathy, characterized by postural hypotension, diarrhea, pain and tingling in muscle groups, impotence, etc, occurs in about 10% of diabetic patients with good glycemic control and in up to 70% of patients with poorly controlled diabetes. Diabetic retinopathy occurs in approximately 75% of long-standing (up to 20 years) diabetics. These late complications of insulin-dependent diabetes appear to be related to the accumulation of intracellular sorbitol and galactitol which results in cellular damage. A deficit of myo-inositol may also be involved, especially in the diabetic neuropathies.

Aldose reductase is the first enzyme in the sorbitol (polyol) pathway. This pathway is responsible for conversion of glucose to sorbitol, and of galactose to galactitol. Under conditions of hyperglycemia, sorbitol accumulation occurs. By inhibiting aldose reductase, tolrestat prevents the accumulation of intracellular sorbitol.

Pharmacokinetics: Tolrestat is almost completely absorbed after oral administration in healthy subjects. Bioavailability is reduced in diabetic patients, but the difference is not statistically significant. Peak plasma concentrations are achieved in 1 to 2 hours. Maximum decreases in red blood cell (RBC) sorbitol levels occur after 3 days of treatment with 100 mg twice daily. The distribution half-life averages 2 to 3 hours, whereas the elimination half-life averages 10 to 13 hours. Protein binding is extensive (99.5%).

Metabolism of tolrestat is minimal. The drug is excreted primarily by the kidneys as unchanged drug. The need for dosage reductions in patients with compromised renal function has not been established.

Clinical trials: The majority of published data on tolrestat involves animal or in vitro studies. However, a study of 23 diabetic patients receiving tolrestat 25 or 100 mg twice daily showed a dose-dependent reduction of RBC sorbitol levels of 21% and 57%, respectively.

In two unpublished clinical efficacy trials, tolrestat was administered to patients with diabetic neuropathy in a randomized, double-blind placebo controlled fashion. The short-term (8 week) trial in 260 patients compared placebo to 200 mg twice daily or 400 mg once daily; the long-term (1 year) trial in 548 patients compared placebo to 50, 100 or 200 mg once daily or 100 mg twice daily. Compared with placebo, 28% of patients in the long-term study receiving tolrestat 200 mg once daily showed improvement of nerve conduction velocity and paresthesias but not pain. Improvement was seen in both trials with a once-daily dose of 200 or 400 mg, but not when the same dose was given twice daily.

Side effects: The most common side effect reported by the manufacturer in unpublished clinical trials was dizziness, which occurred in 11% of patients receiving 200 mg tolrestat daily. Other adverse effects that have occurred include skin rash and liver enzyme elevations. A clear cause-and-effect relationship between tolrestat therapy and these adverse effects has not been established.

Drug interactions: Studies with warfarin (eg, *Coumadin*) indicated that no drug interaction occurred due to protein binding displacement at therapeutic doses. Salicylates at concentrations of 100 to 200 mcg/ml displace tolrestat (21% and 35%, respectively). Tolbutamide (eg, *Orinase*) also displaces tolrestat (22% displacement at tolbutamide concentrations of 160 mcg/ml).

Summary: Published data, although scant, suggest that tolrestat is safe and well tolerated. The ability of aldose reductase inhibition to decrease RBC sorbitol accumulation has been demonstrated in humans. Despite evidence for a favorable biochemical effect, supporting evidence for a beneficial clinical effect (ie, prevention of late complications of diabetes) has yet to be conclusively established. Furthermore, the groups most likely to benefit from this form of therapy, those with poor glycemic control or long-standing diabetes, present methodologic problems for assessing cause and effect relationships with any form of therapy.

The NDA for tolrestat was filed on April 4, 1986 for diabetic neuropathy. It is in Phase III trials for diabetic retinopathy. Tolrestat will be marketed as *Alredase* by Wyeth-Ayerst.

Topiramate *(Topamax)* – Antiepileptic drug

Pharmacology: Topiramate is a sulfamate-substituted monosaccharide which is structurally unique in comparison to other antiepileptic drugs. It is a weak carbonic anhydrase inhibitor, originally developed in a search for new antidiabetic agents. The presence of the sulfamate moiety, similar to that of acetazolamide (eg, *Diamox*), does not explain its antiepileptic effects. Topiramate appears to act by blocking the spread of seizure activity rather than raising seizure threshold, yet the exact mechanism of action remains to be defined. It does not significantly affect receptor binding or neuronal uptake of any of the major neurotransmitters, but does appear to block voltage-dependent sodium and calcium channels. Electrophysiologic studies suggest that topiramate reduces the frequency of repetitive neuronal firing.

The anticonvulsant profile of topiramate is similar to that of phenytoin (eg, *Dilantin*) and carbamazepine (eg, *Tegretol*). It has demonstrated effectiveness against simple and complex partial and generalized tonic-clonic seizures. It has also proven to be efficacious in treating Lennox-Gastaut syndrome.

Pharmacokinetics: Topiramate is well absorbed after oral administration, with an absolute bioavailability > 75%. When administered with food, the rate of absorption is moderately slowed but extent of absorption is unaffected. Time to peak after an oral dose varies from about 2 to 4 hours. Topiramate is mainly excreted as unchanged drug in the urine; the fraction excreted unchanged ranges from 70% to 97%. The drug demonstrates linear pharmacokinetics over a wide range of doses, with an average elimination half-life of approximately 20 hours. Volume of distribution is 0.6 to 0.8 L/kg, and the extent of binding to serum proteins is only about 15%.

Topiramate does not appear to affect the metabolism of phenytoin, carbamazepine or valproic acid (eg, *Depakene*), although concomitant administration with any of these drugs tends to lower the AUC of topiramate by 15% to 50%. Topiramate increases the clearance of ethinyl estradiol (*Estinyl*) by 15% to 33%. As with carbamazepine, topiramate therapy must be initiated at low doses (about 50 mg/day) and gradually titrated upward, in order to minimize side effects.

Clinical trials: Clinical trials of topiramate have evaluated daily doses ranging from 200 to 1000 mg. Although most literature to date has been published in abstract form, the results of the studies have been impressive. Many such studies have been add-on trials in which patients who were refractory to prior therapy had topiramate added to the drug regimen. A placebo controlled, add-on trial of 356 patients showed at least a 50% reduction in seizure frequency for 58% of patients who received 600 mg. Another study conducted an add-on, double-blind, placebo controlled, parallel, multicenter study with 56 intractable partial seizure patients.

At doses of 200 to 800 mg/day, 50% of the patients showed at least a 50% improvement in seizure frequency.

Two recent US dose-response studies compared doses of 400, 600, 800 and 1000 mg/day. Using a 50% seizure reduction as the definition of a positive response, 400 mg/day appeared to be the optimal dose, with 46.7% of the patients responding. Larger doses did not produce an enhanced therapeutic effect. Placebo response rates of the two studies were 17.8% and 8.5% respectively. A long-term study was conducted of add-on topiramate therapy in 18 patients with refractory partial epilepsy. At a mean daily dose of 500 mg, 13 of the patients responded. Efficacy was maintained over a 2-year period. Another study reported results of topiramate monotherapy in 12 patients. Four showed 75% reduction in seizure frequency, and another four patients became seizure-free.

Side effects: Adverse effects caused by topiramate have been dose-related and reversible. The most common adverse reactions reported during clinical trials include sedation, dizziness/ataxia, paresthesia, visual disturbances, diarrhea, decreased appetite with weight loss and cognitive dysfunction. Most side effects attributed to topiramate have been relatively mild. Cognitive dysfunction, reported to be as high as 83% in one study, appears to be the most limiting adverse effect of the drug. Animal studies suggest that topiramate may be teratogenic.

Summary: Topiramate is a promising anticonvulsant drug that is currently undergoing phase III trials. It appears to have a unique mechanism of action which is as yet unknown, and seems to be most effective in treating partial seizures. The drug has been shown to have a relatively narrow therapeutic range, with the optimal dose being in the vicinity of 400 mg/day. Generally the drug is given in two divided doses. Over a dozen studies are currently in progress.

An NDA for topiramate was filed in December 1994. It will be available as *Topamax* by Ortho-McNeil. An anticipated approval date is unknown.

Trospectomycin *(Spexil)* – Aminocyclitol antibiotic

Pharmacology: Trospectomycin is a water soluble analog of spectinomycin (*Trobicin*) that is 8 to 10 times more potent and has a broader spectrum of activity. It has good gram-positive and gram-negative aerobic and anaerobic activity, including in vitro activity against *Staphylococci*, *Streptococci*, *Peptostreptococci*, *Peptococci*, *Haemophilus*, *Gardnerella*, *Neisseria*, *Bacteroides*, *Chlamydia*, *Mycoplasma* and *Ureaplasma*. It has moderate activity against *Enterobacteriaceae* and no activity against *Pseudomonas*.

Trospectomycin acts by binding to the 30S component of the ribosome unit thereby inhibiting protein synthesis. It has a greater affinity for the 30S ribosome unit than spectinomycin and therefore has higher activity. Cross-resistance to spectinomycin has been observed in vitro.

Pharmacokinetics: Patients (n = 128) were randomized to receive trospectomycin (75 to 1000 mg) by IM injection or by 20 minute IV infusion. The IM product was 100% bio-available. The mean peak plasma concentration and AUC were linear relative to dose, and the half-life was 2.1 hours. Serum concentrations were < 2 mcg/ml 12 hours post-dose, suggesting 2 to 3 times daily dosing as the MIC for most organisms is between 2 to 4 mcg/ml. In another trial, trospectomycin was administered by IV infusion. While almost no drug was found in the feces, 48% to 62% was recovered in the urine during the first 48 hours, suggesting that the drug is slowly released from tissues. The half-life of 2.18 hours did not change with increasing dose.

Clinical trials: The in vitro activity of trospectomycin was compared to that of amikacin (eg, *Amikin*), cephalothin (eg, *Keflin*) and vancomycin (eg, *Vancocin*) against 342 gram-positive organisms. Vancomycin was the most active agent overall, and trospectomycin was better than amikacin, especially for *Staphylococci* and *Streptococci*.

The activity of trospectomycin, clindamycin (eg, *Cleocin*), metronidazole (eg, *Flagyl*), imipenem (*Primaxin*), cefoxitin (*Mefoxin*) and piperacillin (*Pipracil*) was evaluated against 72 strains of *Bacteroides*. Trospectomycin had very good activity and was comparable to imipenem and metronidazole. Its activity was greater than that of piperacillin and cefoxitin. In another trial, trospectomycin was comparable to clindamycin and cefoxitin against *Bacteroides fragilis*, and there was no cross-resistance between the three drugs. Of the organisms tested, 90% to 100% were resistant to ampicillin (eg, *Polycillin*) and cefaclor (eg, *Ceclor*), and > 50% were resistant to doxycycline (eg, *Vibramycin*). None of the organisms tested were resistant to trospectomycin.

The effect of trospectomycin and several other antibiotics was evaluated against *Mycoplasma pneumoniae*, M *hominis* and *Ureaplasma urealyticum*. Trospectomycin and spectinomycin were equivalent to tetracycline (eg, *Achromycin*) against M *pneumoniae* but less active against M *horminis*. It was concluded that trospectomycin is active against *Mycoplasma*-induced respiratory or genital infections.

To date, published in vivo trials with trospectomycin are limited. The efficacy of a single 1 g IM dose was evaluated in 10 men with uncomplicated C *trachomatis* urethritis. All were culture-positive at follow-up on days 4 to 8. On follow-up on days 21 to 28, six of the eight men were still culture-positive. It was concluded that a single IM dose for the treatment of uncomplicated C *trachomatis* urethritis is not effective.

Side effects: In one study, mild, transient and local reactions were seen in 20% of subjects receiving trospectomycin vs 22% with placebo; none of the reactions were thought to be drug-related. Overall, mild and transient side effects were seen in 32 of 64 subjects receiving trospectomycin; 12 had dizziness or lightheadedness and 17 who received > 600 mg had perioral/facial numbness. Results from a similar trial using IM injection were comparable.

In a multiple-dose trial involving 10 healthy males, trospectomycin caused significantly more pain at the injection site. There was also a significant increase in perioral paresthesias with increasing doses (especially at the 500 to 750 mg doses). Perioral paresthesias were mild and transient, were seen shortly after dosing and lasted about 1 to 2 hours. Tolerance did not develop over the 7 days of the study. Clinically significant orthostatic hypotension occurred after the first dose in patients receiving 500 or 750 mg but was not seen with subsequent dosing.

Summary: Trospectomycin is an injectable aminocyclitol aminoglycoside that is structurally related to spectinomycin. It has good gram-positive and gram-negative aerobic and anaerobic activity and may prove to be useful for the treatment of upper respiratory tract infections, bacterial vaginitis, pelvic inflammatory disease and gonorrhea. Overall, it appears to be well tolerated and the major side effects are pain at the injection site and perioral paresthesias.

Trospectomycin is currently in phase III clinical trials. A 1996 approval is anticipated. It will be available as *Spexil* from Upjohn.

Velnacrine *(Mentane)*–Cholinesterase inhibitor for Alzheimer's disease

Pharmacology: Alzheimer's disease is associated with alterations in a number of central neurotransmitters, including norepinephrine, serotonin, somatostatin, corticotropin-releasing factor and acetylcholine. Of these, a disturbance in cholinergic function mediated by a specific deficit of neuronal choline acetyltransferase (an enzyme responsible for the formation of acetylcholine) plays a central role in the etiology of cognitive symptoms in Alzheimer's disease patients. As a result of this association, cholinomimetic compounds such as physostigmine *(Antilirium)* and the investigational agent tacrine (tetrahydroaminoacridine; THA; *Cognex*) have been evaluated with encouraging preliminary results.

Velnacrine (HP 029) is the maleate salt of an alcohol derivative of tacrine. It produces cholinergic-mediated physiological effects and inhibits true- and pseudocholin-esterase. The cholinomimetic effects are not due to release of acetylcholine or to a direct muscarinic agonist effect.

Pharmacokinetics: Velnacrine is rapidly and extensively absorbed after oral administration. Peak plasma concentrations are achieved in approximately 1 hour, are linearly proportional to dose and tend to be slightly higher in the elderly (0.9 to 1.7 hours). There appears to be no correlation between plasma levels and therapeutic or adverse effects in individual patients. The drug undergoes conjugation in the liver; the fate and activity of these metabolites are not known. Approximately 11% to 30% of an administered dose is excreted unchanged in the urine. Renal clearance is markedly reduced in the elderly; however, accumulation has not been detected. The half-life is about 2 hours in younger volunteers and is slightly longer (2.5 to 3 hours) in elderly volunteers. Food appears to delay the rate but not extent of absorption.

Clinical trials: Cholinomimetic agents are most effective at improving memory (a core feature of Alzheimer's disease) and reversing scopolamine-induced dementia in animal models. Limited published data suggest that velnacrine, 150 to 225 mg/day in divided doses, produces modest benefit in cognitive function in up to two-thirds of patients, as judged by performance-based measures. Improvement tends to be greatest during dose titration, suggesting the potential for tolerance or the use of inadequate performance measures.

Current evidence suggests that the predominant neurotransmitter defect may vary from one patient to another. Attempts to identify subsets of patients most likely to benefit from cholinesterase inhibitors have yielded conflicting results. In addition, some patients may require combination therapy with different classes of drugs. Until markers are identified that will help predict response, single-drug efficacy trials in all Alzheimer's disease patients are likely to show only modest results.

Side effects: The side effect profile of velnacrine is similar to other cholinomimetic drugs. Nausea, diarrhea, flushing, headache, dizziness and abnormal cramping are reported most frequently and occur more commonly at the higher dose ranges (150 to 300 mg).

In the largest protocol group reported to date, 78% of the patients discontinuing the drug due to an adverse event did so because of elevated liver enzymes. The hepatotoxicity of velnacrine appears to be dose-related, mild and reversible, usually within 4 weeks of discontinuation. Clinical features of the enzyme elevation were consistent with a biochemical insult (70%), hypersensitivity (10%), or a mixture of both.

Summary: Velnacrine appears to be a promising agent for the treatment of Alzheimer's disease. Additional trials are needed to identify subsets of patients most likely to respond, demonstrate sustained efficacy, and assess its place in combination therapy.

An NDA was filed by Hoechst-Roussel in early 1992 for velnacrine *(Mentane)*. The FDA was considering a treatment IND for velnacrine; however, due to concerns over safety and efficacy, the FDA's Peripheral and Central Nervous System Drugs Advisory Committee unanimously decided not to recommend approval of the drug, even under treatment IND status.

Vesnarinone *(Arkin-Z)*–Inotropic agent for CHF

Pharmacology: Vesnarinone, a quinolinone derivative, is an oral inotropic agent with little to no effect on heart rate or myocardial oxygen consumption. The mechanism of action is largely unknown. It may be related to a slight inhibition of PDE III which causes an increase in cyclic AMP and finally an increase in the inward calcium current. There is also a reduction in the potassium current.

In addition, vesnarinone inhibits the production and release of cytokines such as TNF-alpha, IL-1, IL-2 and IFN-gamma. This inhibition may relate directly to its efficacy as an inotropic agent. Increased concentrations of TNF-alpha are seen in patients with chronic heart failure. These increased concentrations depress myocardial contractility, alter muscle membrane potential, decrease blood pressure and precipitate pulmonary edema. Therefore, reducing the concentration of TNF-alpha is beneficial in patients with heart failure.

Interestingly, vesnarinone also inhibits the replication of HIV-1 in peripheral blood lymphocytes and in chronically infected macrophages, suggesting that it may be useful in treating patients with HIV-1 disease.

Pharmacokinetics: The pharmacokinetic parameters of vesnarinone were evaluated in 21 healthy male volunteers in a two-phase, nonblinded trial. In phase I, subjects received vesnarinone in a sequentially ascending single dose ranging from 7.5 to 240 mg. In phase II, three subjects received vesnarinone 30 mg daily for 15 days. The elimination half-life was 44.7 ± 1.2 hour and the clearance 0.284 ± 0.018 L/hr. The drug was fairly extensively metabolized, with only 11% to 27% (mean, 17.7%) being excreted unchanged in the urine. The authors concluded that elimination of vesnarinone is dose-dependent and that plasma concentrations are proportional to the dose administered.

Clinical trials: In two small, uncontrolled trials, vesnarinone was administered to a total of 20 patients with CHF; significant hemodynamic and functional improvement was seen. In a small, placebo controlled study, eight patients with chronic, stable, moderate CHF received vesnarinone 60 mg/day or placebo for 4 to 8 weeks. Patients were then crossed over to the alternate treatment group. Symptomatic improvement was noted in four patients while receiving vesnarinone. In addition, vesnarinone caused an increase in contractility of the left ventricle. Mild to moderate dyspnea and fatigue on exertion was seen in all patients while receiving placebo. In two placebo controlled double-blind trials, a total of 159 patients with CHF were randomized to receive vesnarinone 60 mg/day or placebo for 12 weeks. In both trials there was an improvement in the quality of life and a reduction in the severity or progression of heart failure in patients receiving vesnarinone.

The long-term use of vesnarinone was evaluated in a double-blind trial involving 477 patients with CHF. Patients were randomized to receive vesnarinone 60 mg/day or placebo for 6 months. Patients receiving vesnarinone experienced an improvement in their quality of life and a reduction in morbidity and mortality when compared to patients receiving placebo. In the initial design of this trial, patients could also be randomized to receive vesnarinone 120 mg/day. However, this treatment group was stopped after the first 253 patients had been enrolled because of a significant increase in mortality. These results suggest that vesnarinone may have a narrow therapeutic window.

Side effects: The primary side effect noted with vesnarinone use is reversible neutropenia seen in 2.5% of patients. Other reported side effects include: Reversible agranulocytosis; palpitations; dyspnea; gastric discomfort; nausea; headache; skin rash.

Summary: Vesnarinone is a new positive inotropic agent that appears to be effective in the management of CHF. Because of its unique mechanism of action involving inhibition of cytokines, vesnarinone may prove to be a useful alternative in the long-term management of this patient population. It appears to be well tolerated with the exception of the relatively high incidence of reversible neutropenia. Because of this potentially serious toxicity, the clinical utility of vesnarinone remains to be determined.

An NDA for vesnarinone is pending. It is currently available in Japan. It will be available as *Arkin-Z* by Otsuka. An anticipated approval date is unknown.

Vigabatrin *(Sabril)*–Anticonvulsant agent

Pharmacology: Vigabatrin is a second generation antiepileptic which appears to exert its mechanism of action via increasing brain GABA levels by inhibition of GABA metabolism. These effects on GABA appear to be dose-related. Vigabatrin has an S(+)-enantiomer that inhibits GABA-T, whereas the R(-)-enantiomer has almost no effect. Vigabatrin's mechanism of action may also be attributed to its ability to decrease excitation-related amino acids, aspartate, glutamate and glutamine concentrations in the brain but these same changes do not occur in the CSF.

Pharmacokinetics: Although the exact bioavailability of vigabatrin is not known, following oral administration about 80% of the dose is recovered in the urine. In healthy volunteers, its absorption was rapid and peak plasma concentrations occurred within the first 2 hours. When vigabatrin was administered with food, its approximate bioavailability was 92% ± 11%. Vigabatrin has a volume of distribution of about 0.8 L/kg, is not bound to plasma proteins and distributes into the CSF. The drug does not appear to be metabolized by the liver, or influence hepatic metabolism. The elimination half-life observed in 24 volunteers was approximately 7 hours and does not appear to be significantly affected by single or multiple dosing, and appears to be similar in both adults and children. Dosing adjustments may be necessary in patients with renal impairment (Ccr less than 60 ml/min) and in the elderly.

Clinical trials: When traditional antiepileptic therapies including add on treatments are used, up to 25% of patients still experience seizures. The studies examining the efficacy of vigabatrin as an antiepileptic medication were primarily add-on trials in patients with resistant epilepsy. Reductions in seizure frequency have been observed in patients with partial and complex partial seizures, but reductions have been observed less frequently with primary generalized seizures, and no reductions (and even worsening) of absence and myoclonic seizures. In a meta-analysis of nine European trials, of the patients with complex partial seizures, 72% showed a > 25% decrease in seizure frequency over a 7 to 12 week period. When combining all clinical trials (including European studies) examining the efficacy of vigabatrin in treatment of resistant partial complex epilepsy, between 33% and 61% of patients experienced a > 50% reduction in seizure frequency at doses between 1 and 4 g/day.

The use of vigabatrin in doses ranging from 50 to 150 mg/kg/day has also been studied as add-on therapy in children with partial, generalized, Lennox-Gaustaut Syndrome and West Syndrome. Results appear similar to those in adults; children with partial seizures appeared to respond better with rates between 38% and 49% of patients experiencing between a 50 to 100 reduction in seizure frequency. Vigabatrin has also been examined in the use of intractable infantile spasms and was found to be effective in reducing spasms > 50% in 30 patients (71%), with complete relief of spasms in 16 patients (38%). Caution should be used in the interpretation of these results since great variability can occur with the incidence of infantile seizures over time.

Side effects: Vigabatrin appears to be well tolerated with minimal side effects and when they do occur, they are mild. In a trial of 254 patients who received vigabatrin from 12 months to > 2 years, up to 75% of patients reported no side effects. Data from pooled studies indicate that the most common side effects are: Somnolence; fatigue; irritability; dizziness; headache; depression; confusion; poor concentration; abdominal pain; anorexia (some trials have reported weight gain). In the studies involving children, the main side effects observed were agitation and insomnia, with a similar number of patients reporting a lack of side effects (79%).

Drug interactions: One of the major advantages of vigabatrin is the fact that it does not appear to be metabolized by the liver, nor influence hepatic metabolism. Therefore, the typical drug interactions observed with traditional anticonvulsants are not seen with vigabatrin. However, vigabatrin was shown to decrease phenytoin (eg, *Dilantin*) levels by 20% to 30% in clinical trials. No mechanism of action could account for the decreased levels; therefore, phenytoin levels should be monitored if vigabatrin is added. Vigabatrin does not appear to interact with phenobarbital, primidone, carbamazepine (eg, *Tegretol*) or valproate (eg, *Depakene*) to any clinically significant degree.

Summary: Vigabatrin appears to be effective in the treatment of complex partial seizures, less effective for primary generalized seizures and not effective (and may even worsen) absence and myoclonic seizures. The dosing range is from 1 to 4 g/day in adults, with 2 to 3 g appearing to be the most optimal and a dose of 50 to 150 mg/kg/day in children. Side effects are minimal and mild and there seems to be a lack of clinically significant drug interactions, except that observed with phenytoin.

Vigabatrin is already available in Europe and is expected to have FDA approval late 1994 or early 1995.

Viloxazine *(Catatrol)*–Bicyclic antidepressant

Pharmacology: Viloxazine is a bicyclic antidepressant agent. It has noradrenergic reuptake blocking properties and acts, in part, as an amphetamine-like central stimulant. Overall sympathomimetic, sedative and anticholinergic activity is less than that seen with the tricyclic antidepressants (eg, imipramine [eg, *Tofranil*]). Conflicting data has been reported on the effects of viloxazine on the seizure threshold, with some reports indicating that seizure risk is greater, while others claiming it is less than that seen with traditional tricyclics. Rapid eye movement (REM) sleep and overall sleep time is markedly reduced with viloxazine. It does not appear to potentiate the effects of alcohol.

Pharmacokinetics: Viloxazine is rapidly and almost completely (85%) absorbed after oral administration in the small intestine. Peak blood levels occur 1 to 4 hours after ingestion; however, no correlation has been established between blood levels and clinical response. Volume of distribution averages 0.78 L/kg. The elimination half-life ranges from 2 to 5 hours. The drug is extensively metabolized by hydroxylation and oxidation to inactive metabolites in the liver. Only 12% to 15% of the parent compound is eliminated unchanged by the kidneys. In patients > 60 years of age, there appears to be a reduction in viloxazine clearance, possibly due to decreased hepatic metabolism. Specific dosage guidelines in the elderly and patients with hepatic dysfunction have not been established.

Clinical trials: Viloxazine was an effective antidepressant in controlled clinical trials of both hospitalized and outpatient populations with depression. Its efficacy appears to be equivalent to imipramine, with a 60% response rate. Published trials have not examined whether efficacy rates vary with specific types of depression. Viloxazine has also been studied in small groups of patients with narcolepsy and cataplexy (a form of narcolepsy characterized by periods of momentary paralysis); this appears to be a potential target population. Fewer sleep attacks were reported during treatment.

Side effects: Nausea is the most commonly reported side effect, with an average incidence of 19%, but some studies have reported an incidence as high as 50%. Nausea progressing to vomiting was reported in 4.7% of patients. These effects may be minimized by initiating therapy with low doses accompanied by slow, upward dose titration. Headache is also commonly reported. Less frequently reported side effects include: Insomnia; taste disturbances; hypomania; mania; dizziness; tachycardia; ataxia; tremor; confusion; restlessness; dry mouth; constipation; drowsiness; difficult micturition; seizures. The anticholinergic-related side effects appear to occur less frequently than with the tricyclic agents.

Drug interactions: Viloxazine decreases the elimination rate of theophylline (eg, *Theo-Dur*), carbamazepine (eg, *Tegretol*) and phenytoin (eg, *Dilantin*), possibly by competing for the same microsomal enzymes. When viloxazine was added to a stable regimen of these drugs, theophylline toxicity was reported (no levels available), carbamazepine levels increased by 55% and those of its active metabolite by 16%, and phenytoin levels increased by an average of 36%.

Summary: Viloxazine is a safe and effective antidepressant with a somewhat different side effect profile than the tricyclic antidepressants, although it is most likely to be used in patients with narcolepsy or cataplexy. Available data has not established whether viloxazine has any advantages over currently available agents. Additional studies in specific populations of patients are needed to establish its place in therapy. Viloxazine currently has orphan drug status for the treatment of cataplexy and narcolepsy. An NDA was filed in July 1987 for viloxazine, which will be available as *Catatrol* by Zeneca.

Vindesine Sulfate *(Eldisine)*–Antineoplastic

Pharmacology: Vindesine sulfate (Lilly 99094, NSC-245467, DAVA, desacetyl vinblastine amide sulfate) is a synthetic vinca alkaloid derived from vinblastine sulfate, but more closely resembling the activity of vincristine.

A large number of studies support its utility in a diverse group of cancer types. Major and dose-limiting toxicities include myelosuppression and neurotoxicity.

The mechanism of vindesine's anticancer action is probably like that of the other vinca alkaloids; it is cell-cycle specific and blocks mitosis with metaphase arrest. Vinca alkaloids bind specifically to cellular microtubules of the mitotic apparatus and disrupt their function. This leads to inability of the dividing cell to correctly segregate chromosomes and ultimately, to cell death.

Pharmacokinetics: Vindesine sulfate appears to have similar pharmacokinetics to vincristine and vinblastine. The triphasic clearance profile of IV vindesine is summarized below:

IV Vindesine Clearance		
Phase	Half-life (minutes)	Volume of distribution (liters)
Alpha (α)	3 ± 1	5 ± 2
Beta (β)	99 ± 45	58 ± 51
Gamma (γ)	1213 ± 493	598 ± 294

Elimination in the urine in the first 24 hours accounts for 13.2% of the total dose administered. The remainder is sequestered in the body or eliminated in the bile.

Clinical trials: Overall, vindesine demonstrates good activity in difficult-to-treat and refractory cancer types. Responses to vindesine in patients who have received vincristine or vinblastine therapy suggest a lack of cross-resistance between these agents. Doses have ranged from 3 to 4.5 mg/m^2 as an IV bolus every 1 to 2 weeks *or* 1 to 2 mg/m^2/day for 2 to 10 days every 2 to 3 weeks. The results of clinical studies are summarized below:

Vindesine Clinical Studies				
		Response rate		
Cancer type	Number of patients treated	Range (%)	Average (%)	Complete No. of patients
Lung	234	17-43	30	10
Esophageal	76	17-55	43	0
Colorectal	33	6	6	1
Metastatic breast	120	0-28	18	0
Lymphoma	61	34-50	41	4
Leukemias	26	15-61	38	4
TOTAL	550	0-61	29	19

Side effects: Major dose-limiting toxicities include myelosuppression and neuropathy. The primary *hematologic* toxicity is leukopenia, which is reversible with dosage reduction or discontinuation. Anemia and thrombocytopenia occur, but are rarely severe. *Neurotoxicity* appears to be a function of cumulative dose. Patients with hepatic dysfunction and those over 60 years old may be at greater risk. Neurotoxic manifestations include peripheral paresthesia, decreased tendon reflexes, muscle weakness and myalgia, headache, parotid and jaw pain, constipation and paralytic ileus.

Other side effects – Nausea; vomiting; stomatitis; hoarseness; transient hepatic dysfunction; inappropriate antidiuretic hormone secretion; fever; skin rash; alopecia; local cellulitis. Vindesine sulfate is a potent vesicant; avoid extravasation into the SC tissues.

Summary: Vindesine sulfate is a vinca alkaloid which demonstrates promise for a wide variety of cancer types; however, its full extent of activity remains to be determined. Its major toxicities are similar to those of its family, myelotoxicity and neurotoxicity. It was recommended for approval by FDA's Oncologic Drugs Advisory Committee in September 1982. A New Drug Application (NDA) is pending.

Zileuton *(Leutrol)*–Potent, selective 5-lipoxygenase inhibitor

Pharmacology: Zileuton is a selective 5-lipoxygenase inhibitor that is being investigated to treat asthma, allergic rhinitis, arthritis, ulcerative colitis (UC) and systemic lupus erythematosus (SLE). 5-lipoxygenase causes the metabolism of arachidonic acid to form products (eg, leukotriene B_4) that have been speculated to cause narrowing of airways observed in asthma. It also exhibits anti-inflammatory activity and inhibits antigen-induced contraction of the trachea and bronchospasm in guinea pigs. Although zileuton inhibits 5-lipoxygenase, it has no influence on myeloperoxidase activity, neutrophil degranulation, mast cell histamine release, cyclo-oxygenase products or phospholipase A_2 activity.

Pharmacokinetics: Zileuton is rapidly absorbed with a T_{max} of about 1.5 to 4.5 hours and a half-life of 1.5 hours. Zileuton is eliminated primarily by hepatic glucuronidation, therefore, dosing adjustments may be warranted in patients with hepatic dysfunction. When zileuton was administered with sulfasalazine in patients with UC, the pharmacokinetic profile of sulfasalazine and its metabolites were not affected.

Clinical trials: A trial involving 139 patients was conducted to assess the efficacy of zileuton 600 mg 4 times daily or 800 mg twice daily in the treatment of mild-to-moderate asthma over a 4 week period. Zileuton 600 mg significantly increased FEV_1 compared with placebo beginning 1 hour after administration and continued to cause improvement throughout the study period. The group receiving 800 mg twice daily also showed improvement in FEV_1 compared with placebo, but this difference failed to reach statistical significance. Patients who received zileuton 2.4 g/day also had significant improvement in FVC, airway function and reported asthma symptoms compared with placebo. Zileuton 2.4 g/day caused a significant decrease (24%) in β-agonist use compared with placebo (7%). In another study involving 8 aspirin-sensitive asthmatics, zileuton 600 mg 4 times daily not only prevented the development of nasal, GI and dermal symptoms associated with aspirin ingestion, but it also curtailed the maximum rise in urinary LTE_4 and averted the fall in FEV_1.

A study involving 8 patients with allergic rhinitis was conducted to assess the effects of zileuton 800 mg after two different nasal challenges. Nasal congestion induced by allergens was significantly decreased in the zileuton patients but prostaglandin D_2, histamine release and sneezing were not.

Zileuton has been studied in the treatment of UC since it has been acknowledged that leukotriene B_4 is a prominent intermediary of mucosal inflammation. A study was conducted to examine the effects of zileuton 800 mg/day in decreasing the symptoms of UC in 11 Hispanic patients with mild to moderately active UC over a 28 day period. Ten patients were allowed to continue sulfasalazine therapy (1.5 to 4.5 g/day) since they were taking a constant dose prior to the start of the study. Eight of the 11 patients (73%) had improvement in the gross appearance in the sigmoidoscopy and 100% of the patients encountered a reduction in discomfort of symptoms of their UC. None of the patients experienced any histologic improvement.

A study was conducted to determine the effects of zileuton 600 mg 4 times daily in

40 patients with mild SLE over an 8 week period. Zileuton significantly improved the symptoms associated with SLE compared with placebo.

A study involving rheumatoid arthritis patients was conducted to determine the effect of zileuton on leukotriene generation and clinical response. At the end of 1 week of study, patients receiving zileuton had a 70% decrease in leukotriene synthesis and an improvement in clinical response.

Side effects: Zileuton appears to be well tolerated. In one clinical trial involving 139 asthma patients, observed side effects included headache (10% receiving 2.4 g/day, 16% receiving 1.6 g/day, 14% receiving placebo). Although one patient experienced hives and abnormal liver function tests 24 hours after initiating zileuton 800 mg twice daily therapy, these symptoms resolved after zileuton was suspended.

Summary: Potential therapeutic uses of zileuton include asthma, allergic rhinitis, arthritis, ulcerative colitis and systemic lupus erythematosus. It shows promise in all of these diseases, but only asthma is currently being sought as an FDA indication.

On April 10, 1995, the Pulmonary-Allergy Drugs Product Advisory Committee voted to recommend the approval of zileuton for the treatment of asthma, provided that liver function tests be routinely monitored. However, on October 19, 1995, Abbott received a "not approvable" letter from the FDA concerning zileuton. The FDA stated that the NDA contained inadequate information pertaining to preclinical toxicity, especially liver test irregularities. Abbott will try to address the FDA's concerns and supply the necessary information.

AIDS Drugs in Development

Acquired Immune Deficiency Syndrome (AIDS) is an immunodeficiency state caused by an infection with the human immunodeficiency virus, HIV. This retrovirus has also been referred to as human T-cell lymphotropic virus, type III (HTLV-III), lymphadenopathy-associated virus (LAV) and the AIDS-related virus. There are several drugs being studied for AIDS, AIDS-Related Complex (ARC), AIDS-associated infections (*Pneumocystis carinii*, *Mycobacterium avium-intracellulare* complex [MAC], cryptosporidiosis, cytomegalovirus) and Kaposi's sarcoma. Listed below are some antiviral, cytokine and immunomodulating drugs currently undergoing clinical trials.

AIDS Drugs in Development

Drug	Drug type	FDA status	Treatment sponsor
141W94	protease inhibitor	Phase I HIV	Glaxo Wellcome
1592U89	antiviral	Phase I/II HIV	Glaxo Wellcome
Acemannan *(Carrisyn)*	antiviral, immunomodulator	Phase I AIDS, ARC	Carrington Laboratories
Acetylcysteine *(Fluimucil)*	immunomodulator	Phase I HIV, ARC, AIDS	Zambon
AD-439	antiviral	Phase II HIV, AIDS	Tanox Biosystems
AD-519	antiviral	Phase II HIV, AIDS	Tanox Biosystems
AIDS vaccine (eg, gp 120, rgp 160, rgp 160 MN, rp 24, *VaxSyn HIV-1)*	antiviral	Phase I to III AIDS, HIV prophylaxis and treatment	MicroGeneSys/ Genentech/Immuno/ Connaught/Virogenetics
AL-721	antiviral	Phase I/II AIDS, ARC, HIV positive	Matrix Laboratories
Aldesleukin[1] (interleukin-2; IL-2; *Proleukin)*	cytokine	Phase II with zidovudine for HIV	Cetus Oncology
Alvircept sudotox (sCD4-PE40)	antiviral	Phase II AIDS	Upjohn
Ampligen	immunomodulator	Phase II/III HIV	HEM Pharmaceutical
AR-121 *(Nystatin-LF I.V.)*	antiviral	Phase I/II HIV	Argus
AS-101	immunomodulator	Phase I/II ARC, AIDS	Wyeth-Ayerst
Atevirdine mesylate	antiviral	Phase II HIV, AIDS	Upjohn
Azidouridine (AzdU)	antiviral	Phase I HIV-positive symptomatic, ARC, AIDS	Berlex
AZT-P-ddI *(Scriptene)*	antiviral	Phase I AIDS	Baker Norton
Bropirimine (ABPP)	immunomodulator	Phase II Kaposi's	Upjohn
CD4, soluble human, recombinant	antiviral	Phase II ARC, AIDS	Biogen
CD4-IgG	antiviral	Phase I Maternal/fetal HIV transfer	Genentech
Cidofovir[1]	antiviral	Phase II ARC	Gilead Sciences

[1]Approved for other indications.

AIDS Drugs in Development			
Drug	Drug type	FDA status	Treatment sponsor
Curdlan sulfate (CRDS)	antiviral	Phase I/II HIV	Lenti-Chemico Pharmaceuticals
Cytomegalovirus IV hyper-immune globulin *(CytoGam)*	antiviral	Phase I ARC	MedImmune
DAB_{389}IL-2 fusion toxin	cytokine	Phase I/II HIV	Seragen
Delavirdine mesylate	antiviral	Phase III HIV, AIDS	Upjohn
Delaverdine mesylate *(Rescriptor)*	antiviral	Phase III HIV, AIDS	Upjohn
Deoxynojirimycin, n-butyl (DNJ)	antiviral	Phase II ARC, AIDS	Searle
Dextran sulfate *(Uendex)*	antiviral	Phase II AIDS, ARC, HIV-positive asymptomatic	Ueno Fine Chemicals Industry Ltd.
Diethyldithiocarbamate *(Imuthiol)*	immunomodulator	Phase II/III AIDS, ARC, HIV, pediatric HIV	Connaught
Fiacitabine (FIAC)	antiviral	Phase I/II HIV, ARC, AIDS	Oclassen
Fialuridine (FIAU)	antiviral	Phase II HIV	Oclassen
Filgrastim[1] (granulocyte colony-stimulating factor; G-CSF; *Neupogen)*	cytokine	Phase III AIDS	Amgen
FK-565	immunomodulator	Phase I HIV	Fujisawa
Fluorothymidine (FLT)	antiviral	Phase II HIV, ARC, AIDS	Lederle
Foscarnet sodium[1] (topical, *Foscavir)*	antiviral	Phase I ARC	Astra
Gem 91	antiviral	Phase I HIV	Hybridon
HBY097 (nonnucleoside reverse transcriptase inhibitor	antiviral	Phase II HIV	Hoechst Marion Roussel
Growth hormone, human recombinant (rhGH) with insulin-like growth factor, human recombinant (rhIGF-1) *(Nutropin)*	cytokine	Phase II AIDS wasting in HIV-1 patients	Genentech
HIV immune globulin *(HIVIG)*	immunomodulator	Phase III Prevention of HIV in infants born to HIV-positive mothers	North American Biologicals
HIV immunotherapeutic	antiviral	Phase I HIV (symptomatic)	Viagene
HIV immunotherapeutic vaccine	antiviral	Phase II/III HIV asymptomatic	Immunization Products Ltd. (joint venture of RPR and Immune Response Corp.)
HIV vaccine (gp 120)	antiviral	Phase I AIDS	Chiron/Ciba-Geigy
Hypericin *(VIMRxyn)*	antiviral	Phase I AIDS, HIV	VIMRx Pharm
Immune globulin IV[1] (IGIV; eg, *Gamimune-N)*	immunomodulator	Phase II/III Pediatric HIV; with zidovudine for AIDS, ARC	Miles

[1]Approved for other indications.

AIDS Drugs in Development			
Drug	Drug type	FDA status	Treatment sponsor
Imreg-1	immunomodulator	Phase III HIV	Imreg
Insulin-like growth factor, human recombinant	cytokine	Phase II AIDS wasting in HIV-1 patients	Genentech
Interferon alfa *(Wellferon)*	cytokine	Phase III with zalcitabine and zidovudine for HIV disease, non-AIDS	Glaxo Wellcome
Interferon, alfa-2a[1] *(Roferon-A)*	cytokine	Phase I ARC	Hoffman-LaRoche
Interferon, alfa-2b[1] *(Intron A)*	cytokine	Phase I/II with zidovudine for AIDS	Schering-Plough
Interferon, alfa-n3[1] *(Alferon N; Alferon LDO* [low-dose oral])	cytokine	Phase I/II ARC, AIDS, asymptomatic AIDS	Interferon Sciences
Interferon, beta *(Betaseron)*	cytokine	Phase II/III Kaposi's, AIDS, ARC	Berlex
Interleukin-1 receptor, soluble	antiviral	Phase I Inhibits HIV replication	Immunex
Interleukin-2 PEG	cytokine	Phase II with zidovudine for AIDS	Chiron
Interleukin-3, recombinant human	cytokine	Phase I HIV with cytopenia	Sandoz
Iscador	antiviral	Phase I HIV, ARC, AIDS	Hiscia
ISIS 2922	antiviral	Phase III ARC	ISIS Pharm.
Isoprinosine (inosine pranobex, inosiplex, methiso-prinol)	antiviral, immunomodulator	Phase III ARC, HIV seropositive asymptomatic; NDA rejected February 1986	Newport Pharmaceuti-cals
KNI-272	antiviral	Phase I HIV	Japan Energy
Lamivudine *(3TC)*	antiviral	Phase II/III HIV	Glaxo Wellcome
Lentinan *(Lentinan-Ajinomoto)*	immunomodulator	Phase II/III with didanosine for AIDS HIV-positive (symptomatic/ asymptomatic), ARC, AIDS, pediatric AIDS	Lenti-Chemico Pharmaceuticals
Lobuvacir	antiviral	Phase I ARC	BM Squibb
MDL 28,574	glucosidase inhibitor	Phase II HIV	Hoechst Marion Roussel
Methionine-enkephalin	immunomodulator	Phase I Stimulation of cellular function in immune deficiency states	TNI Pharmaceuticals
Molgramostim (GM-CSF; *Leucomax)*	cytokine	Phase II/III with zidovudine for AIDS	Sandoz/Genetics Insti-tute/Schering-Plough
Monoclonal antibody (MSL-109; MAb)	antiviral	Phase I AIDS	Sandoz
N-acetylcystein	antiviral	Phase I/II ARC, AIDS	Zambon
Nevirapine	antiviral	Phase II HIV-1 with zidovudine	Boehringer Ingelheim

[1]Approved for other indications.

AIDS Drugs in Development

Drug	Drug type	FDA status	Treatment sponsor
Non-nucleoside reverse transcriptase inhibitor	antiviral	Phase II HIV	Merck
Novapren	antiviral	Phase I HIV inhibitor	Novaferon Labs
Nystatin	antiviral	Phase II	Aronex
Oxandrolone[1] *(Oxandrin)*	cytokine	Phase II/III HIV wasting syndrome	Bio-Technology General
Oxothiazolidine carboxylate *(Procysteine)*	immunomodulator	Phase II Restoration of glutathione depletion in HIV, ARC, AIDS; prevention of inflammation-induced HIV replication	Free Radical Sciences
PMEA *(GS 393)*	antiviral	Phase I/II HIV	Gilead Sciences
RBC-CD4	antiviral	Phase I/II HIV	Sheffield Medical Technologies
Ribavirin[1] *(Virazole)*	antiviral	Phase II/III Asymptomatic HIV positive, ARC; IND denied	Viratek/ICN
Roquinimex *(Linomide)*	immunomodulator	Phase II HIV	Kabi Pharmacia
Sargramostim[1] (granulocyte macrophage colony stimulating factor; GM-CSF; *Leukine)*	cytokine	Phase II HIV	Immunex
Sevirumab	antiviral	Phase II ARC	Protein Design Labs
Sorivudine *(Bravavir)*	antiviral	application submitted ARC	Bristol-Myers Squibb
T30177, AR-177 oligonucleotide	antiviral	Phase I AIDS	Aronex
T4, soluble human, recombinant	antiviral	Phase I/II HIV	Biogen
TAT antagonist	antiviral	Phase I/II HIV	Hoffman LaRoche
Thymic humoral factor	immunomodulator	Phase I HIV-positive	Adria
Thymopentin *(Timunox)*	immunomodulator	Phase III Asymptomatic HIV	Immunobiology Research Institute
Thymostimuline *(TP-1)*	immunomodulator	Phase III AIDS	Serono Laboratories
TI-23	antiviral	Phase I ARC	Teijin America
Trichosanthin *(GLO223;* Compound Q)	antiviral	Phase II ARC, AIDS	Genelabs Technologies
Tucaresol	immunopotentiator	Phase I/II HIV	Glaxo Wellcome
Tumor necrosis factor (TNF)	antiviral	Phase I inhibits HIV replication	Immunex
Veldona	cytokine	Phase I AIDS	Veldona USA
Wellferon	alpha interferon w/zidovudine and zalcitabine	application submitted HIV	Glaxo Wellcome
Zidovudine, controlled released[1] *(Aztec)*	antiviral	Phase III HIV, AIDS	Verax Laboratories

[1]Approved for other indications.

FDA Pregnancy Categories

The rational use of any medication requires a risk versus benefit assessment. Among the myriad of risk factors which complicate this assessment, pregnancy is one of the most perplexing.

The FDA has established five categories to indicate the potential of a systemically absorbed drug for causing birth defects. The key differentiation among the categories rests upon the degree (reliability) of documentation and the risk vs benefit ratio. Pregnancy Category X is particularly notable in that if any data exist that may implicate a drug as a teratogen and the risk vs benefit ratio does not support use of the drug, the drug is contraindicated during pregnancy. These categories are summarized below:

FDA Pregnancy Categories

Pregnancy Category	***Definition***
A	Adequate studies in pregnant women have not demonstrated a risk to the fetus in the first trimester of pregnancy and there is no evidence of risk in later trimesters.
B	Animal studies have not demonstrated a risk to the fetus but there are no adequate studies in pregnant women ... or ... Animal studies have shown an adverse effect, but adequate studies in pregnant women have not demonstrated a risk to the fetus during the first trimester of pregnancy and there is no evidence of risk in later trimesters.
C	Animal studies have shown an adverse effect on the fetus but there are no adequate studies in humans; the benefits from the use of the drug in pregnant women may be acceptable despite its potential risks ... or ... There are no animal reproduction studies and no adequate studies in humans.
D	There is evidence of human fetal risk, but the potential benefits from the use of the drug in pregnant women may be acceptable despite its potential risks.
X	Studies in animals or humans demonstrate fetal abnormalities or adverse reaction reports indicate evidence of fetal risk. The risk of use in a pregnant woman clearly outweighs any possible benefit.

Regardless of the designated Pregnancy Category or presumed safety, no drug should be administered during pregnancy unless it is clearly needed and potential benefits outweigh potential hazards to the fetus.

General Management of Acute Overdosage

Rapid intervention is essential to minimize morbidity and mortality in an acute toxic ingestion. Institute measures to prevent absorption and hasten elimination as soon as possible; however, symptomatic and supportive care takes precedence over other therapy. It is assumed that basic life support measures, ie, cardiopulmonary resuscitation (CPR), have been instituted. Specific antidotes are discussed in the overdosage section of individual drug monographs. The discussion below outlines procedures used in the management of acute overdosage of orally ingested systemic drugs.

Advanced Life Support Measures:

Adequate Airway must be established and maintained, generally via oropharyngeal or endotracheal airways, cricothyrotomy or tracheostomy.

Ventilation may then be performed via mouth-to-mouth insufflation, hand-operated bag (ambu bag) or a mechanical ventilator.

Circulation must be maintained.

- *Hypotension:* If hypotension/hypoperfusion occurs, place the patient in shock position (head lowered, feet elevated); specific therapy may include:

  Establish IV access and initiate IV fluids (eg, normal [0.9%] saline, 0.45% saline, Ringer's lactate, dextrose solutions). A maintenance flow rate is generally 100 to 200 ml/hour; individualize as necessary.

  Plasma, plasma protein fractions, whole blood or plasma expanders may be required.

  Severe hypotension may require judicious use of cardiovascular active agents. The most commonly recommended agents are dopamine, dobutamine and norepinephrine.
- *Arrhythmia* treatment is dictated by the offending drug.
- *Hypertension*, sometimes severe, may occur.

For specific information on individual drugs or drug classes, see individual or group monographs.

Seizures: Simple isolated seizures may require only observation and supportive care. Repetitive seizures or status epilepticus require therapy. Diazepam IV or phenytoin are generally the agents of choice; phenobarbital may also be considered.

Reduction of Drug Absorption:

Gastric emptying is generally recommended as soon as possible; however, this is generally not very effective unless employed within the first 1 to 2 hours after ingestion. Syrup of ipecac and gastric lavage are the two most commonly employed methods.

- *Syrup of ipecac* is the method of choice outside the hospital, but administer only on the advice of a qualified health-care professional.
- *Gastric lavage* is indicated in the comatose patient and for those in whom syrup of ipecac fails to produce emesis. Airway protection via endotracheal intubation is appropriate for the patient without a gag reflex. Position the patient on his left side and use a large bore tube. Instill warm water or saline 37° C (98.6° F), 100 to 300 ml per wash for adults; 10 ml/kg to a maximum of 250 ml for children, until lavage solution returns clear. Instill the fluid over 1 to 2 minutes, leave in place about 1 minute and drain over 3 to 4 minutes.

Adsorption, using activated charcoal after completion of emesis or lavage, is indicated for virtually all significant toxic ingestions. It adsorbs a wide variety of toxins and there are no contraindications. However, it adsorbs many orally administered antidotes as well, so space dosage properly.

Catharsis is sometimes recommended, generally using a saline or osmotic cathartic (eg, magnesium sulfate or citrate or sorbitol) to promote passage of the toxin through the GI tract.

Whole bowel irrigation (WBI) utilizes rapid administration of large volumes of lavage solutions, such as PEG. It may be most useful for removal of iron tablets and cocaine-containing condoms or balloons.

Elimination of Absorbed Drug:

Interruption of enterohepatic circulation by "gastric dialysis" uses scheduled doses of activated charcoal for 1 to 2 days. Gastric dialysis not only interrupts the enterohepatic cycle of some drugs, but also creates an osmotic gradient, drawing drug from the plasma back into the gastrointestinal lumen where it is bound by the charcoal and excreted in the feces.

Diuresis may be effective as identified in the individual drug monographs.

- *Forced diuresis* is occasionally useful. The most common agents employed are furosemide and osmotic diuretics.
- *Alkaline diuresis* is appropriate for certain compounds (eg, phenobarbital, salicylates) and is usually accomplished by the administration of IV sodium bicarbonate.
- *Acid diuresis* may be indicated (eg, in overdose with amphetamines, fenfluramine, quinine) but use with caution in patients with renal or liver disease. It is usually accomplished with oral or IV ascorbic acid or ammonium chloride.

Dialysis is indicated in a minority of severe overdose cases. Drug factors that alter dialysis effectiveness include volume of distribution, drug compartmentalization, protein binding and lipid/water solubility.

- *Peritoneal dialysis* and *hemodialysis* have been the most common methods used. *Charcoal or resin hemoperfusion* is a relatively new procedure with promising clinical potential (eg, with theophylline).

Poison Control Center:

Consultation with a regional poison control center is highly recommended.

Management of Acute Hypersensitivity Reactions

Type I hypersensitivity reactions (immediate hypersensitivity or anaphylaxis) are immunologic responses to a foreign antigen to which a patient has been previously sensitized. Anaphylact*oid* reactions are not immunologically mediated; however, symptoms and treatment are similar.

Signs and Symptoms

Acute hypersensitivity reactions typically begin within 1 to 30 minutes of exposure to the offending antigen. Tingling sensations and a generalized flush may proceed to a fullness in the throat, chest tightness or a "feeling of impending doom." Generalized urticaria and sweating are common. *Severe* reactions include life-threatening involvement of the airway and cardiovascular system.

Treatment:

Appropriate and immediate treatment is imperative. The following general measures are commonly employed:

Epinephrine 1:1000, 0.2 to 0.5 mg (0.2 to 0.5 ml) SC is the primary treatment. In children, administer 0.01 mg/kg or 0.1 mg. Doses may be repeated every 5 to 15 minutes if needed. A succession of small doses is more effective and less dangerous than a single large dose. Additionally, 0.1 mg may be introduced into an injection site where the offending drug was administered. If appropriate, the use of a tourniquet above the site of injection of the causative agent may slow its absorption and distribution. However, remove or loosen the tourniquet every 10 to 15 minutes to maintain circulation.

Epinephrine IV (generally indicated in the presence of hypotension) is often recommended in a 1:10,000 dilution, 0.3 to 0.5 mg over 5 minutes; repeat every 15 minutes, if necessary. In children, inject 0.1 to 0.2 mg or 0.01 mg/kg/dose over 5 minutes; repeat every 30 minutes.

A conservative IV epinephrine protocol includes 0.1 mg of a 1:100,000 dilution (0.1 mg of a 1:1000 dilution mixed in 10 ml normal saline) given over 5 to 10 minutes. If an IV infusion is necessary, administer at a rate of 1 to 4 mcg/min. In children, infuse 0.1 to 1.5 (maximum) mcg/kg/min.

Dilute epinephrine 1:10,000 may be administered through an endotracheal tube, if no other parenteral access is available, directly into the bronchial tree. It is rapidly absorbed there from the capillary bed of the lung.

Airway: Ensure a patent airway via endotracheal intubation or cricothyrotomy (ie, inferior laryngotomy, used prior to tracheotomy) and administer oxygen. Severe respiratory difficulty may respond to IV aminophylline or to other bronchodilators.

Hypotension: The patient should be recumbent with feet elevated. Depending upon the severity, consider the following measures:

- Establish a patent IV catheter in a suitable vein.
- Administer IV fluids (eg, normal saline, lactated Ringer's).
- Administer plasma expanders.
- Administer cardioactive agents (see group and individual monographs). Commonly recommended agents include dopamine, dobutamine, norepinephrine and phenylephrine.

Adjunctive therapy does not alter acute reactions, but may modify an ongoing or slow-onset process and shorten the course of the reaction.

- *Antihistamines: Diphenhydramine* — 50 to 100 mg IM or IV, continued orally at 5 mg/kg/day or 50 mg every 6 hours for 1 to 2 days. For children, give 5 mg/kg/day, maximum 300 mg per day.

  Chlorpheniramine — (adults, 10 to 20 mg; children, 5 to 10 mg) IM or slowly IV.

  Hydroxyzine — 10 to 25 mg orally or 25 to 50 mg IM 3 to 4 times daily.
- *Corticosteroids*, eg, hydrocortisone IV 100 to 1000 mg or equivalent, followed by 7 mg/kg/day IV or oral for 1 to 2 days. The role of corticosteroids is controversial.
- *H_2 antagonists: Cimetidine* — *Children*, 25 to 30 mg/kg/day IV in six divided doses; *adults*, 300 mg every 6 hours. *Ranitidine* — 50 mg IV over 3 to 5 minutes. May be of value in addition to H_1 antihistamines, although this opinion is not universally shared.

Calculations

To calculate milliequivalent weight: $\text{mEq} = \frac{\text{gram molecular weight/valence}}{1000}$

$\text{mEq} = \frac{\text{mg}}{\text{eq wt}}$ equivalent weight or $\text{eq wt} = \frac{\text{gram molecular weight}}{\text{valence}}$

Commonly used mEq weights			
Chloride	35.5 mg = 1 mEq	Magnesium	12 mg = 1 mEq
Sodium	23 mg = 1 mEq	Potassium	39 mg = 1 mEq
Calcium	20 mg = 1 mEq		

To convert temperature °C ↔ °F: $\frac{°C}{°F - 32} = \frac{5}{9}$ or $°C = \frac{5}{9}(°F - 32)$

$°F = 32 + \frac{9}{5}\, °C$

To calculate creatinine clearance (Ccr) from serum creatinine:

Male: $\text{Ccr} = \frac{\text{weight (kg)} \times (140 - \text{age})}{72 \times \text{serum creatinine (mg/dl)}}$ Female: Ccr = 0.85 × calculation for males

To calculate ideal body weight (kg):

Male = 50 kg + 2.3 kg (each inch > 5 ft) Female = 45.5 kg + 2.3 kg (each inch > 5 ft)

To calculate body surface area (BSA) in adults and children:

1) *Dubois method:*

$\text{SA (cm}^2) = \text{wt (kg)}^{0.425} \times \text{ht (cm)}^{0.725} \times 71.84$

$\text{SA (m}^2) = K \times \sqrt[3]{\text{wt}^2}\text{ (kg)}$ (common K value 0.1 for toddlers, 0.103 for neonates)

2) *Simplified method:*

$\text{BSA (m}^2) = \sqrt{\frac{\text{ht (cm)} \times \text{wt (kg)}}{3600}}$

To approximate surface area (m²) of children from weight (kg):

Weight range (kg)	≈ Surface area (m²)
1 to 5	(0.05 x kg) + 0.05
6 to 10	(0.04 x kg) + 0.10
11 to 20	(0.03 x kg) + 0.20
21 to 40	(0.02 x kg) + 0.40

Suggested Weights for Adults

Height*	Weight in pounds†
4′10″	91-119
4′11″	94-124
5′0″	97-128
5′1″	101-132
5′2″	104-137
5′3″	107-141
5′4″	111-146
5′5″	114-150
5′6″	118-155
5′7″	121-160
5′8″	125-164
5′9″	129-169
5′10″	132-174
5′11″	136-179
6′0″	140-184
6′1″	144-189
6′2″	148-195
6′3″	152-200
6′4″	156-205
6′5″	160-211
6′6″	164-216

* Without shoes. † Without clothes.

The higher weights in the ranges generally apply to people with more muscle and bone. Source: Nutrition and Your Health: Dietary Guidelines for Americans, 4th ed, 1995. US Department of Agriculture, US Department of Health and Human Services. At press time, these new guidelines had not been officially released. It is possible some changes to this chart will occur.

International System of Units

The *Systeme international d'unités* (International System of Units) or *SI* is a modernized version of the metric system. The primary goal of the conversion to SI units is to revise the present confused measurement system and to improve test-result communications.

The SI has 7 basic units from which other units are derived:

Base Units of SI		
Physical quantity	Base unit	SI symbol
length	meter	m
mass	kilogram	kg
time	second	s
amount of substance	mole	mol
thermodynamic temperature	kelvin	K
electric current	ampere	A
luminous intensity	candela	cd

Combinations of these base units can express any property although, for simplicity, special names are given to some of these derived units.

Representative Derived Units		
Derived unit	Name and symbol	Derivation from base units
area	square meter	m^2
volume	cubic meter	m^3
force	newton (N)	$kg{\cdot}m{\cdot}s^{-2}$
pressure	pascal (Pa)	$kg{\cdot}m^{-1}{\cdot}s^{-2}$ (N/m^2)
work, energy	joule (J)	$kg{\cdot}m^2{\cdot}s^{-2}$ ($N{\cdot}m$)
mass density	kilogram per cubic meter	kg/m^3
frequency	hertz (Hz)	s^{-1}
temperature degree	Celsius (°C)	°C = °K − 273.15
concentration		
mass	kilogram/liter	kg/L
substance	mole/liter	mol/L
molality	mole/kilogram	mol/kg
density	kilogram/liter	kg/L

Prefixes to the base unit are used in this system to form decimal multiples and submultiples. The preferred multiples and submultiples listed below change the quantity by increments of 10^3 or 10^{-3}. The exceptions to these recommended factors are within the middle rectangle.

Prefixes and Symbols for Decimal Multiples and Submultiples

Factor	Prefix	Symbol
10^{18}	exa	E
10^{15}	peta	P
10^{12}	tera	T
10^{9}	giga	G
10^{6}	mega	M
10^{3}	kilo	k
10^{2}	hecto	h
10^{1}	deka	da
10^{-1}	deci	d
10^{-2}	centi	c
10^{-3}	milli	m
10^{-6}	micro	μ
10^{-9}	nano	n
10^{-12}	pico	p
10^{-15}	femto	f
10^{-18}	atto	a

To convert drug concentrations to or from SI units:

$$\text{Conversion factor (CF)} = \frac{1000}{\text{mol wt}}$$

Conversion *to* SI units: µg/ml × CF = µmol/L

Conversion *from* SI units: µmol/L × CF = µg/ml

Normal Laboratory Values

In the following tables, normal reference values for commonly requested laboratory tests are listed in traditional units and in SI units. The tables are a guideline only. Values are method dependent and "normal values" may vary between laboratories.

Blood, Plasma or Serum		
	Reference Value	
Determination	Conventional Units	SI Units
Ammonia (NH_3)	10-80 µg/dl	5-50 µmol/L
Amylase	≤ 130 U/L	≤ 130 U/L
Antinuclear antibodies	negative at 1:10 dilution of serum	negative at 1:10 dilution of serum
Antithrombin III (AT III)	80%-120%	
Bilirubin: conjugated	≤ 0.2 mg/dl	≤ 4 µmol/L
total	0.1-1 mg/dl	2-18 µmol/L
Calcitonin	< 100 pg/ml	< 100 ng/L
Calcium: female < 50 years old	8.8-10 mg/dl	2.2-2.5 mmol/L
female > 50 years old	8.8-10.2 mg/dl	2.2-2.56 mmol/L
male	8.8-10.3 mg/dl	2.2-2.58 mmol/L
all populations	4.4-5.1 mEq/L	2.2-2.56 mmol/L
Carbon dioxide content	22-28 mEq/L	22-28 mmol/L
Carcinoembryonic antigen	< 3 ng/ml	< 3 µg/L
Chloride	95-105 mEq/L	95-105 mmol/L
Coagulation screen:		
Bleeding time	3-9.5 min	180-570 sec
Prothrombin time	< 2 sec from control	< 2 sec from control
Partial thromboplastin time (activated)	22-37 sec	22-37 s
Protein C	58%-148%	
Protein S	58%-148%	
Copper, total	70-140 µg/dl	11-22 µmol/L
Corticotropin (ACTH)	20-100 pg/ml	4-22 pmol/L
Cortisol: 0800 hr	4-19 µg/dl	110-520 nmol/L
1800 hr	2-15 µg/dl	50-410 nmol/L
2400 hr	< 5 µg/dl	< 140 nmol/L
Creatine phosphokinase, total (CK, CPK)	≤ 150 U/L	≤ 150 U/L
Creatine kinase isoenzymes, MB fraction	> 5% in MI	> 0.05 fraction of 1
Creatinine	0.6-1.2 mg/dl	50-110 µmol/L
Fibrinogen (coagulation factor I)	150-350 mg/dl	1.5-3.5 g/L
Follicle stimulating hormone (FSH):		
female	2-15 mIU/ml	2-15 IU/L
peak production	20-50 mIU/ml	20-50 IU/L
male	1-10 mIU/ml	1-10 IU/L
Glucose, fasting	70-110 mg/dl	3.9-6.1 mmol/L
Haptoglobin	50-220 mg/dl	0.5-2.2 g/L
Hematologic tests:		
Hematocrit (Hct), female	33%-43%	0.33-0.43 fraction of 1
male	39%-49%	0.39-0.49 fraction of 1
Hemoglobin (Hb), female	14-18 g/dl	140-180 g/L
male	11.5-15.5 g/dl	115-155 g/L
Leukocyte count (WBC)	3200-9800/mm^3	3.2-9.8 x 10^9/L
Erythrocyte count (RBC), female	3.5-5 × 10^6/mm^3	3.5-5 x 10^{12}/L
male	4.3-5.9 × 10^6/mm^3	4.3-5.9 x 10^{12}/L
Mean corpuscular volume (MCV)	76-100 µm^3	76-100 fL

Blood, Plasma or Serum		
Determination	Reference Value	
	Conventional Units	SI Units
Mean corpuscular hemoglobin (MCH)	27-33 pg	27-33 pg
Mean corpuscular hemoglobin concentration (MCHC)	33-37 g/dl	330-370 g/L
Erythrocyte sedimentation rate (sedrate, ESR): female	≤ 30 mm/hr	≤ 30 mm/hr
male	≤ 20 mm/hr	≤ 20 mm/hr
Erythrocyte enzymes:		
Glucose-6-phosphate dehydrogenase (G6PD)	5-15 U/g Hb	5-15 U/g Hb
Pyruvate kinase	13-17 U/g Hb	13-17 U/g Hb
Ferritin	18-300 ng/ml	18-300 μg/L
Folic acid: normal	> 3.3 ng/ml	> 7.3 nmol/L
borderline	2.5-3.2 ng/ml	5.75-7.39 nmol/L
Platelet count	130-400 × 10^3/mm^3	130-400 × 10^9/L
Vitamin B_{12}	200-1000 pg/ml	150-750 pmol/L
Iron		
female	60-160 μg/dl	11-29 μmol/L
male	80-180 μ/dl	14-32 μmol/L
Iron binding capacity	250-460 μg/dl	45-82 μmol/L
Lactic acid (lactate)	0.5-2 mEq/L	0.5-2 mmol/L
Lactic dehydrogenase	50-150 U/L	50-150 U/L
Lead	≤ 60 μg/dl	≤ 2.9 μmol/L
Lipids:		
Lipids, total	400-850 mg/dl	4-8.5 g/L
Total cholesterol		
< 29 years old	< 200 mg/dl	< 5.2 mmol/L
30-39 years old	< 225 mg/dl	< 5.85 mmol/L
40-49 years old	< 245 mg/dl	> 6.35 mmol/L
> 50 years old	< 265	< 6.85
LDL	50-190 mg/dl	1.3-4.9 mmol/L
HDL		
female	30-90 mg/dl	0.8-2.35 mmol/L
male	30-70 mg/dl	0.8-1.8 mmol/L
Triglycerides	< 460 mg/dl	< 1.8 g/L
Magnesium	1.6-2.4 mEq/L	0.8-1.2 mmol/L
Osmolality	280-300 mOsm/kg	280-300 mmol/kg
Oxygen saturation (arterial)	96%-100%	0.96-1 fraction of 1
PCO_2, arterial	35-45 mm Hg	4.7-6 kPa
pH, arterial	7.35-7.45	7.35-7.45
PO_2, arterial: Breathing room air[1]	75-100 mm Hg	10-13.3 kPa
On 100% O_2	> 500 mm Hg	
Phosphatase (acid), total:	≤ 3 King-Armstrong units/dl	≤ 5.5 U/L
	≤ 3 Bodansky units/dl	≤ 16.1 U/L
Phosphatase (alkaline)[2]	30-120 U/L	30-120 U/L
Phosphorus, inorganic[3], (phosphate)	2.5-5 mg/dl	0.8-1.6 mmol/L
Potassium	3.5-5 mEq/L	3.5-5 mmol/L
Progesterone		
Follicular phase	< 2 ng/ml	< 6 nmol/L
Luteal phase	2-20 ng/ml	6-64 nmol/L
Prolactin	< 20 ng/ml	< 20 μg/L
Prostate specific antigen	0-4 ng/ml	

Blood, Plasma or Serum		
	Reference Value	
Determination	Conventional Units	SI Units
Protein: Total	6-8 g/dl	60-80 g/L
Albumin	4-6 g/dl	40-60 g/L
Globulin	2.3-3.5 g/dl	23-35 g/L
Rheumatoid factor	< 80 IU/ml	< 80 kIU/L
Sodium	135-147 mEq/L	135-147 mmol/L
Testosterone: female	< 0.6 ng/ml	< 2 nmol/L
male	4-8 ng/ml	14-28 nmol/L
Thyroid Hormone Function Tests:		
Thyroid-stimulating hormone (TSH)	2-11 μU/ml	2-11 mU/L
Thyroxine-binding globulin capacity	12-28 μg/dl	150-360 nmol/L
Total triiodothyronine (T_3)	75-220 ng/dl	1.2-3.4 nmol/L
Total thyroxine by RIA (T_4)	4-11 μg/dl	51-142 nmol/L
T_3 resin uptake	25%-35%	0.25-0.35 fraction of 1
Transaminase, AST (aspartate aminotransferase, SGOT)	≤ 35 U/L	≤ 35 U/L
Transaminase, ALT (alanine aminotransferase, SGPT)	≤ 35 U/L	≤ 35 U/L
Urea nitrogen (BUN)	8-18 mg/dl	3-6.5 mmol/L
Uric acid	2-7 mg/dl	120-420 μmol/L
Vitamin A (retinol)	10-50 μg/dl	0.35-1.75 μmol/L
Zinc	75-120 μg/dl	11.5-18.5 μmol/L

[1] Age-dependent.
[2] Infants and adolescents up to 104 U/L.
[3] Infants in the first year up to 6 mg/dl.

Urine					
		Reference Value			
Determination		Conventional Units		SI Units	
Catecholamines: Epinephrine		< 10 μg/day		< 55 nmol/day	
Norepinephrine		< 100 μg/day		< 590 nmol/day	
Creatinine: female		14-22 mg/kg/24 h		0.12-0.19 mmol/kg/day	
male		20-26 mg/kg/24 h		0.18-0.23 mmol/kg/day	
Potassium (diet-dependent)		25-100 mEq/day		25-100 mmol/day	
Protein, quantitative		< 150 mg/day		< 0.15 g/day	
Steroids:		(mg/day)		(μmol/day)	
	Age (yrs)	male	female	male	female
17-Ketosteroids	10	1-4	1-4	3-14	3-14
	20	6-21	4-16	21-73	14-56
	30	8-26	4-14	28-90	14-49
	50	5-18	3-9	17-62	10-31
	70	2-10	1-7	7-35	3-24
17-Hydroxycorticosteroids (as cortisol):					
female		2-8 mg/day		5-25 μmol/day	
male		3-10 mg/day		10-30 μmol/day	

Drug Determination		Reference Value: Conventional Units	Reference Value: SI Units
Aminoglycosides (peak levels)	Amikacin	16-32 µg/ml	nd
	Gentamicin	4-8 µg/ml	nd
	Kanamycin	15-40 µg/ml	nd
	Netilmicin	6-10 µg/ml	nd
	Streptomycin	20-30 µg/ml	nd
	Tobramycin	4-8 µg/ml	nd
Antiarrhythmics	Amiodarone	0.5-2.5 µg/ml	nd
	Bretylium	0.5-1.5 µg/ml	nd
	Digitoxin	9-25 µg/L	11.8-32.8 nmol/L
	Digoxin	0.5-2.2 ng/ml	0.6-2.8 nmol/L
	Disopyramide	2-8 µg/ml	6-18 µmol/L
	Flecainide	0.2-1 µg/ml	nd
	Lidocaine	1.5-6 µg/ml	4.5-21.5 µmol/L
	Mexiletine	0.5-2 µg/ml	nd
	Procainamide	4-8 µg/ml	17-34 µmol/ml
	Propranolol	50-200 ng/ml	190-770 nmol/L
	Quinidine	2-6 µg/ml	4.6-9.2 µmol/L
	Tocainide	4-10 µg/ml	nd
	Verapamil	0.08-0.3 µg/ml	nd
Anti-convulsants	Carbamazepine	4-12 µg/ml	17-51 µmol/L
	Phenobarbital	15-40 µg/ml	65-172 µmol/L
	Phenytoin	10-20 µg/ml	40-80 µmol/L
	Primidone	5-12 µg/ml	25-46 µmol/L
	Valproic acid	50-100 µg/ml	350-700 µmol/L
Antidepressants	Amitriptyline	110-250 ng/ml	nd
	Amoxapine	200-500 ng/ml	nd
	Bupropion	25-100 ng/ml	nd
	Clomipramine	80-100 ng/ml	nd
	Desipramine	125-300 ng/ml	nd
	Doxepin	100-200 ng/ml	nd
	Imipramine	200-350 ng/ml	nd
	Maprotiline	200-300 ng/ml	nd
	Nortriptyline	50-150 ng/ml	nd
	Protriptyline	100-200 ng/ml	nd
	Trazodone	800-1600 ng/ml	nd
Antipsychotics	Chlorpromazine	30-500 ng/ml	nd
	Fluphenazine	0.13-2.8 ng/ml	nd
	Haloperidol	5-20 ng/ml	nd
	Perphenazine	0.8-1.2 ng/ml	nd
	Thiothixene	2-57 ng/ml	nd
Miscellaneous	Amantadine	300 ng/ml	nd
	Amrinone	3.7 µg/ml	nd
	Chloramphenicol	10-20 µg/ml	31-62 µmol/L
	Cyclosporine[1]	250-800 ng/ml (whole blood, RIA)	nd
		50-300 ng/ml (plasma, RIA)	nd
	Ethanol[2]	0 mg/dl	0 mmol/L
	Hydralazine	100 ng/ml	nd
	Lithium	0.5-1.5 mEq/L	0.5-1.5 mmol/L
	Salicylate	100-200 mg/L	724-1448 µmol/L
	Sulfonamide	5-15 mg/dl	nd
	Terbutaline	0.5-4.1 ng/ml	nd
	Theophylline	10-20 µg/ml	55-110 µmol/L
	Vancomycin (peak)	30-40 ng/ml	nd

Table title: **Drug Levels†**

† The values given are generally accepted as desirable for achieving therapeutic effect without toxicity for most patients. However, exceptions are not uncommon.

[1] 24 hour trough values.

[2] Toxic: 50-100 mg/dl (10.9-21.7 mmol/L).

nd – No data available.

Drug Names That Look Alike And Sound Alike

Dispensing errors can be caused by drug names that look alike (such as *Omnipen* and *Unipen*), sound alike (such as *Nicobid* and *Nitro-Bid*) or both (such as Digoxin and Digitoxin). Familiarity with this list may save the prescriber from making a dispensing error.

A

Accutane	Accurbron
Acetazolamide	Acetophenazine
Achromycin	Aureomycin
Actidil	Actifed
Actinomycin	Achromycin
Actinomycin	Aureomycin
Acutrim	Accutane
Adapin	Atabrine
Aerolone	Aralen
Aerolone	Arlidin
Afrin	Afrinol
Agoral	Argyrol
Albuterol	Albutein
Albuterol	Atenolol
Aldactone	Aldactazide
Aldoril	Aldomet
Ambenyl	Aventyl
Amicar	Amikin
Amitril	Emetrol
Amitriptyline	Aminophylline
Amitriptyline	Nortriptyline
Amoxapine	Amoxicillin
Amoxapine	Amoxil
Amoxil	Amcill
Amrinone	Amiodarone
Anaprox	Anaspaz
Ancobon	Oncovin
Antrenyl	Anturane
Anturane	Artane
Anusol	Aplisol
Anusol	Aquasol
Appedrine	Ephedrine
Apresoline	Apresazide
Apresoline	Priscoline
Ara-A	Ara-C
Ara-C	Eryc
Aralen	Arlidin
Arfonad	Afrin
Arthralgen	Auralgan
Atarax	Ativan
Atarax	Marax
Atenolol	Timolol
Ativan	Avitene
Atromid-S	Clomid
Auralgan	Ophthalgan
Azathioprine	Azulfidine
Azlin	Mezlin

B

Baclofen	Beclovent
Bactocill	Pathocil
Bactrim	Bacitracin
Banthine	Bentyl
Belladonna	Belladenal
Benadryl	Belladenal
Benadryl	Bentyl
Benadryl	Benylin
Benadryl	Caladryl
Benemid	Beminal
Benoxyl	PanOxyl
Bentyl	Aventyl
Bentyl	Bontril
Betalin	Benylin
Betalin	Betadine
Bicillin	V-Cillin
Bicillin	Wycillin
Bontril	Vontrol
Brethine	Banthine
Brethine	Brethaire
Bretylol	Brethaire
Brevital	Bretylol
Brondecon	Bronkotabs
Butabarbital	Butalbital
Butisol	Butazolidin

C

Calan	Colace
Calciparine	Calcidrine
Calcitriol	Calcifediol
Calcitriol	Calciferol
Calcitriol	Calcitonin
Capastat	Cēpastat
Captopril	Capitrol
Catapres	Catarase
Catapres	Diupres
Cefonicid	Cefobid

Cefotaxime .... Ceftizoxime
Cefoxitin .... Cefotaxime
Cefuroxime .... Cefotaxime
Cephalexin .... Cephalothin
Cephalothin .... Cefazolin
Cephapirin .... Cephradine
Chlorambucil .... Chloromycetin
Chloromycetin ..... Chlor-Trimeton
Chlorpromazine .... Chlorpropamide
Chlorpromazine .... Promethazine
Chymex .... Chenix
Chymex .... Chorex
Cleocin .... Clinoril
Clofibrate .... Clorazepate
Clomid .... Clonidine
Clomiphene .... Clonidine
Clonidine .... Quinidine
Clotrimazole .... Co-Trimoxazole
Coactin .... Koate
Codeine .... Cordran
Colestid .... Colistin
Colistin .... Colestipol
Combipres .... Catapres
Cordarone .... Cordran
Cortone .... Cort-Dome
Cyclocort .... Cyclopar
Cyclopar .... Cytosar
Cyclosporine .... Cycloserine
Cytarabine .... Vidarabine
Cytoxan .... Cefoxitin
Cytoxan .... Cytosar

D

Dacarbazine .... Procarbazine
Dactinomycin ...... Daunorubicin
Dalmane .... Demulen
Danocrine .... Dacriose
Dantrium .... Danthron
Daranide .... Daraprim
Daricon .... Darvon
Darvon-N .... Darvocet-N
Daunorubicin .... Doxorubicin
Decadron .... Decaderm
Decadron .... Percodan
Delsym .... Delcid
Demerol .... Demulen
Demerol .... Dicumarol
Demerol .... Dymelor
Demerol .... Pamelor
Deprol .... Demerol
DES .... E.E.S.
Desferal .... Disophrol
Desipramine .... Deserpidine
Desoximetasone .... Dexamethasone
Desoxyn .... Digitoxin
Desyrel .... Delsym
Dextran .... Dexedrine
Dialume .... Dalmane
Dialume .... Diabinese
Diazepam .... Diazoxide
Dicarbosil .... Dacarbazine
Digitoxin .... Digoxin
Digoxin .... Desoxyn
Dilaudid .... Dilantin
Dimacol .... Dimercaprol
Dimetane .... Dimentabs
Dimetane .... Dimetapp
Diphenhydramine Dimenhydrinate
Disipal .... Disophrol
Disophrol .... Isuprel
Disophrol .... Stilphostrol
Disopyramide .... Dipyridamole
Ditropan .... Dithranol
Diuril .... Doriden
Diutensen .... Salutensin
Dobutamine .... Dopamine
Dolene .... Dilone
Donnatal .... Donnagel
Donnazyme .... Entozyme
Dopar .... Dopram
Dopram .... Dopamine
Doriden .... Doxidan
Doryx .... Durrax
Doxorubicin .... Dactinomycin
Doxycycline .... Doxylamine
Drisdol .... Drysol
Dronabinol .... Droperidol
Dyazide .... Thiacide
Dyclone .... Dilone
Dyclonine .... Dicyclomine
Dyrenium .... Pyridium

E

Ecotrin .... Edecrin
Edecrin .... Ethaquin
Elavil .... Aldoril
Elavil .... Equanil
Elavil .... Mellaril
Emetine .... Emetrol
Endecon .... Edecrin
Endecon .... Enduron
Endep .... Depen

Enduron	Empirin
Enduron	Eutron
Enduron	Imuran
Enduronyl	Inderal
Eryc	Emcyt
Ery-Tab	Eryc
Esimil	Estinyl
Esimil	Ismelin
Ethatab	Estratab
Ethionamide	Ethinamate
Eurax	Urex
Euthroid	Thyroid
Eutonyl	Eutron

F

Factrel	Sectral
Feldene	Seldane
Feosol	Feostat
Fer-in-Sol	Feosol
Festal	Feosol
Festal	Festalan
Fiogesic	Wygesic
Flaxedil	Flexeril
Florinef	Fiorinal
Fluocinonide	Fluocinolone
Fostex	pHisoHex
Furacin	Fulvicin

G

Gamastan	Garamycin
Gantrisin	Gantanol
Garamycin	Kanamycin
Garamycin	Terramycin
Gelfoam	Ger-O-Foam
Gentamicin	Kanamycin
Glucagon	Glaucon
Glutethimide	Guanethidine
Guanadrel	Gonadorelin
Guanethidine	Guanidine

H

Halcion	Halcinonide
Haldol	Winstrol
Haldrone	Haldol
Halodrin	Haldrone
Halog	Haldol
Halog	Mycolog
Halotestin	Halothane
Halotex	Halotestin
Healon	Halcion
Hespan	Histaspan
Hexadrol	Hexalol
Hispril	Hiprex
Hycodan	Hycodaphen
Hycodan	Hycomine
Hycodan	Vicodin
Hycomine	Hycodan
Hydralazine	Hydroxyzine
Hydropres	Catapres
Hydropres	Diupres
Hydroxyzine	Hydroxyurea
HyperHep	Hyperstat
HyperHep	Hyper-Tet
Hyperstat	Hyper-Tet
Hyperstat	Nitrostat
Hytone	Vytone

I

Ilosone	Ionosol
Imipramine	Imferon
Imuran	Imferon
Inapsine	Nebcin
Inderal	Imuran
Inderal	Inderide
Inderal	Isordil
Inderal	Medrol
Indocin	Lincocin
Indocin	Minocin
Intropin	Ditropan
Isoptin	Intropin
Isopto Carpine	Isopto Eserine
Isordil	Isuprel
Isuprel	Ismelin

K

Kaon	Kaolin
Keflex	Keflin
Kemadrin	Coumadin
Ketalar	Kenalog
Klonopin	Clonidine
K-Lor	Kaochlor
K-Lor	Klor

L

Larotid	Lomotil
Lasix	Esidrix
Lasix	Lasan
Levophed	Levoprome
Levothyroxine	Liothyronine
Levsinex	Lanoxin
Lidex	Lasix
Lincocin	Cleocin

Liotrix	Klotrix
Lithobid	Lithotabs
Lithostat	Lithotabs
Lotrimin	Otrivin
Luminal	Tuinal
Lupron	Lopurin

M

Maalox	Camalox
Maalox	Maolate
Maalox	Marax
Mandol	Nadolol
Maxzide	Maxidex
Mebaral	Mellaril
Mebaral	Tegretol
Mebendazole	Mazindol
Medrol	Mebaral
Mellaril	Moderil
Mephenytoin	Mesantoin
Mephyton	Mephenytoin
Meprobamate	Mepergan
Meprobamate	Meperidine
Mestinon	Mesantoin
Metandren	Metahydrin
Metatensin	Mesantoin
Metatensin	Mestinon
Methadone	Mephyton
Methenamine	Methionine
Methyldopa	Levodopa
Metoprolol	Metaproterenol
Metyrapone	Metyrosine
Mexate	Mexitil
Mexitil	Mezlin
Milontin	Miltown
Minocin	Lincocin
Minocin	Mithracin
Minocin	Niacin
Mithramycin	Mitomycin
Mitotane	Mitomycin
Mobidin	Moban
Modane	Matulane
Modane	Mudrane
Molindone	Mobidin
Mycelex	Myoflex
Myciguent	Mycitracin
Mydfrin	Midrin
Mylanta	Milontin
Myleran	Mylaxen
Myleran	Mylicon
Mylicon	Modicon

N

Nalfon	Naldecon
Naloxone	Naltrexone
Naprosyn	Meprospan
Nardil	Norinyl
Nebcin	Naprosyn
Nembutal	Myambutol
Nicobid	Nitro-Bid
Nilstat	Nitrostat
Nilstat	Nystatin
Nitroglycerin	Nitroglyn
Nitrospan	Ditropan
Nitrospan	Nitrostat
Nitrospan	Nystatin
Nitrostat	Nystatin
Norlestrin	Novahistine
Norlutin	Norlutate
Norpramin	Imipramine
Norpramin	Norpace
Nortriptyline	Norpramin
Nubain	Navane
Nuprin	Lupron

O

Omnipen	Unipen
Ophthochlor	Ophthocort
Orasone	Oracin
Oretic	Oreton
Orinase	Ornade
Ornex	Orexin
Ornex	Orinase
Ornex	Ornade
Otobiotic	Urobiotic
Ovulen	Ovral
Oxymetholone	Oxymetazoline
Oxymetholone	Oxymorphone

P

Pamelor	Dymelor
Pantopon	Parafon
Pantopon	Protopam
Paramethadione	Paramethasone
Paregoric	Percogesic
Pathocil	Pathilon
Pathocil	Pitocin
Pathocil	Placidyl
Pavulon	Paxipam
Pavulon	Peptavlon
Penicillin	Penicillamine
Penicillin	Polycillin
Pentothal	Pentritol

Percodan .... Percogesic
Percodan .... Percorten
Periactin .... Percodan
Periactin .... Persantine
Periactin .... Taractan
Peritrate .... Lotusate
Peritrate .... Periactin
Permitil .... Persantine
Persantine .... Persistin
Pertofrane .... Persantine
Phenaphen .... Phenergan
Phenelzine .... Phenazine
Phenelzine .... Phenylzin
Phenergan .... Theragran
Phenobarbital ...... Pentobarbital
Phentermine .... Phentolamine
Phospholine .... Phosphaljel
Physostigmine ...... Pyridostigmine
Pindolol .... Panadol
Pitocin .... Pitressin
Ponstel .... Pronestyl
Pramoxine .... Pralidoxime
Prazepam .... Pyrroxate
Prazepam .... Prazosin
Prednisone .... Promethazine
Prednisone .... Prednisolone
Procaine .... Procan
Promazine .... Promethazine
Pronestyl .... Prostaphlin
Prostigmine .... Physostigmine
Protopam .... Protamine
Protropin .... Protamine
Protropin .... Protopam
Pyridium .... Pyridoxine
Pyridoxine .... Pralidoxime

Q

Quarzan .... Questran
Quinidine .... Quinine
Quinora .... Quinidine

R

Ranitidine .... Ritodrine
Reglan .... Regonol
Regroton .... Hygroton
Regroton .... Regonol
Restoril .... Vistaril
Reticulex .... Reticulogen
Ribavirin .... Riboflavin
Rifadin .... Ritalin
Riopan .... Repan
Ritalin .... Ismelin
Ritodrine .... Ritalin

S

Sebutone .... Sebulex
Sectral .... Septra
Ser-Ap-Es .... Catapres
Serax .... Eurax
Serax .... Psorex
Serax .... Xerac
Serentil .... Surital
Simethicone .... Cimetidine
Sinarest .... Allerest
Slow-K .... Slow Fe
Somophyllin .... Slo-Phyllin
Sparine .... Sterane
Sulfamethoxazole .. Sulfamethizole
Surfak .... Surbex
Sustaire .... Sustacal

T

Tace .... Tao
Teractan .... Tinactin
Tedral .... Teldrin
Tegopen .... Tagamet
Tegopen .... Tegretol
Tegopen .... Tegrin
Tegretol .... Tegrin
Temaril .... Demerol
Tenormin .... Ionamin
Tenormin .... Norpramin
Tepanil .... Demerol
Tepanil .... Temaril
Tepanil .... Terfonyl
Tepanil .... Tofranil
Terbutaline .... Tolbutamide
Terfonyl .... Tofranil
Testolactone .... Testosterone
Thiamine .... Thorazine
Thyrar .... Thyrolar
Thyrolar .... Theolair
Tigan .... Ticar
Tobramycin .... Trobicin
Topicort .... Topic
Trandate .... Trental
Trandate .... Trendar
Trendar .... Trental
Trental .... Trientine
Tretinoin .... Trientine
Triamcinolone ...... Triaminicin
Triaminic .... Triaminicin

Triaminicol	Triamcinolone
Triamterene	Trimipramine
Tridil	Tedral
TriHemic	Triaminic
Trimeprazine	Trimipramine
Trimox	Diamox
Trimox	Tylox
Trinalin	Phrenilin
Tronothane	Tronolane
Trophite	Troph-Iron
Tuinal	Tylenol
Tylosterone	Tylenol
Tylox	Tylenol

U

Unipen	Unicap
Unipen	Urispas
Urispas	Urised

V

Valadol	Panadol
Valmid	Valpin
Valmid	Velban
Valpin	Valium
Vansil	Vanceril
Vasodilan	Vasocidin
Vasosulf	Velosef
Velban	Valpin
Versed	VePesid
Vicodin	Hycomine
Vigran	Wigraine
Vincristine	Myochrysine
Vincristine	Vinblastine
Viroptic	Timoptic
Visken	Visidex
Vitron-C	Vicon-C
Vivox	Vivonex
VōSol	Vontrol

W

Wyamine	Wydase
Wycillin	V-Cillin
Wymox	Tylox

Z

Zantac	Zarontin
Zantac	Xanax
Zarontin	Zaroxolyn
Zarontin	Zentron
Zyloprim	ZORprin

Reproduced with permission from Ben Teplitsky, Pharmacy Editor. This article is a revision and update of an article published in *Pharmacy Times*, 1988 (Feb); 99-101.

Oral Dosage Forms That Should Not Be Crushed Or Chewed

Drug Product	Manufacturer	Dosage Form	Reason/Comments
Accutane	Roche	Capsule	Mucous membrane irritant
Actifed 12 Hour	Warner Wellcome	Capsule	Slow release (i)
Acutrim	Ciba Consumer	Tablet	Slow release
Aerolate SR, JR, III	Fleming & Co.	Capsule	Slow release*(i)
Afrinol Repetabs	Schering	Tablet	Slow release
Allerest 12 Hour	Fisons	Caplet	Slow release
Artane Sequels	Lederle	Capsule	Slow release*(i)
Arthritis Bayer Time Release	Bayer	Capsule	Slow release
ASA Enseals	Lilly	Tablet	Enteric-coated
Asbron G Inlay	Sandoz	Tablet	Multiple compressed tablet (i)
Atrohist Plus	Adams	Tablet	Slow release
Atrohist Sprinkle	Adams	Capsule	Slow release*
Azulfidine Entabs	Pharmacia Labs	Tablet	Enteric-coated
Baros	Lafayette	Tablet	Effervescent Tab (d)
Bayer Extra Strength Enteric 500	Bayer	Tablet	Slow Release
Bayer Low Adult 81 mg Strength	Bayer	Tablet	Enteric-coated
Bayer Regular Strength 325 mg Caplet	Bayer	Tablet	Enteric-coated
Betachron E-R	Inwood	Capsule	Slow release
Betapen-VK	Apothecon	Tablet	Taste (c)
Biohist-LA	Wakefield	Tablet	Slow release (h)
Biphetamine	Fisons	Capsule	Slow release
Bisacodyl	(various)	Tablet	Enteric-coated (a)
Bisco Lax	Raway	Tablet	Enteric-coated (a)
Bontril SR	Carnrick	Capsule	Slow release
Breonesin	Sanofi Winthrop	Capsule	Liquid filled (b)
Brexin LA	Savage	Capsule	Slow release
Bromfed	Muro	Capsule	Slow release (i)
Bromfed PD	Muro	Capsule	Slow release (i)
Calan SR	Searle	Tablet	Slow release (h)
Cama Arthritis Pain Reliever	Sandoz Consumer	Tablet	Multiple compressed tablet
Carbiset-TR	Nutripharm	Tablet	Slow release
Cardizem	Hoechst Marion Roussel	Tablet	Slow release
Cardizem CD	Hoechst Marion Roussel	Capsule	Slow release*

For references, see legend page 1217 in this edition.

Drug Product	Manufacturer	Dosage Form	Reason/Comments
Cardizem SR	Hoechst Marion Roussel	Capsule	Slow release*
Carter's Little Pills	Carter-Wallace	Tablet	Enteric-coated
Cefal Filmtab	Abbott	Tablet	Enteric-coated
Charcoal Plus	Kramer	Tablet	Enteric-coated
Chloral Hydrate	(various)	Capsule	Liquid in capsule (i)
Chlorpheniramine Maleate Time Release	(various)	Capsule	Slow release
Chlor-Trimeton Repetab	Schering	Tablet	Slow release (i)
Choledyl SA	Parke-Davis	Tablet	Slow release (i)
Cipro	Bayer	Tablet	Taste (c)
Codimal LA	Central	Capsule	Slow release
Colace	Bristol-Meyers	Capsule	Taste (c)
Comhist LA	Procter & Gamble	Capsule	Slow release*
Compazine Spansule	Smith Kline Beecham	Capsule	Slow release (i)
Congress SR, JR	Fleming & Co.	Capsule	Slow release
Constant T	Geigy	Tablet	Slow release*
Contac	SmithKline Beecham	Capsule	Slow release*
Cotazym S	Organon	Capsule	Enteric-coated*
Creon 10, 20	Solvay	Capsule	Enteric-coated*
Cystospaz-M	Schwartz Pharma	Capsule	Slow release
Cytoxan	Bristol-Myers	Tablet	Drug may be crushed but maker recommends using injection
Dallergy	Laser	Capsule	Slow release
Dallergy-D	Laser	Capsule	Slow release
Dallergy-JR	Laser	Capsule	Slow release
Deconamine SR	Berlex	Capsule	Slow release (i)
Deconsal II	Adams	Tablet	Slow release
Deconsal Sprinkle	Adams	Capsule	Slow release*
Defen-LA	Horizon	Tablet	Slow release (h)
Demazine Repetabs	Schering	Tablet	Slow release (i)
Depakene	Abbott	Capsule	Slow release mucous membrane irritant (i)
Depakote	Abbott	Capsule	Enteric-coated
Desoxyn Gradumets	Abbott	Tablet	Slow release
Desyrel	Bristol Myers	Tablet	Taste (c)
Dexatrim, Max. Strength	Thompson Medical	Tablet	Slow release
Dexedrine Spansule	SmithKline Beecham	Capsule	Slow release
Diamox Sequels	Lederle	Capsule	Slow release

For references, see legend page 1217 in this edition.

Drug Product	Manufacturer	Dosage Form	Reason/Comments
Dilatrate SR	Reed & Carnrick	Capsule	Slow release
Dimetane Extentab	Robins	Tablet	Slow release (i)
Disobrom	Geneva Pharm	Tablet	Slow release
Disophrol Chronotab	Schering	Tablet	Slow release
Dital	UAD	Capsule	Slow release
Donnatal Extentab	Robins	Tablet	Slow release (i)
Donnazyme	Robins	Tablet	Enteric-coated
Drisdol	Sanofi Winthrop	Capsule	Liquid filled (b)
Drixoral	Schering	Tablet	Slow release (i)
Drixoral Allergy Sinus	Schering	Tablet	Slow release
Dulcolax	Boehringer	Tablet	Enteric-coated (a)
Dynabac	Bock Pharmacal	Tablet	Enteric-coated
Easprin	Parke-Davis	Tablet	Enteric-coated
Ecotrin	SmithKline Beecham	Tablet	Enteric-coated
E.E.S. 400	(various)	Tablet	Enteric-coated (i)
E-Mycin	Knoll Pharm	Tablet	Enteric-coated
Endafed	UAD	Capsule	Slow release
Entex LA	Procter & Gamble	Tablet	Slow release (i)
Entozyme	Robins	Tablet	Enteric-coated
Equanil	Wyeth-Ayerst	Tablet	Taste (c)
Ergostat	Parke-Davis	Tablet	Sublingual form (g)
Eryc	Parke-Davis	Capsule	Enteric-coated *
Ery-tab	Abbott	Tablet	Enteric-coated
Erythrocin Stearate	(various)	Tablet	Enteric-coated
Erythromycin Base	(various)	Tablet	Enteric-coated
Eskalith CR	SmithKline Beecham	Tablet	Slow release
Fedahist Timecaps	Schwarz Pharma Kremers-Urban	Capsule	Slow release (i)
Feldene	Pfizer	Capsule	Mucous membrane irritant
Feocyte	Dunhall	Tablet	Slow release
Feosol	SmithKline Beecham	Tablet	Enteric-coated (i)
Feosol	SmithKline Beecham	Capsule	Slow release*(i)
Feratab	Upsher-Smith	Tablet	Enteric-coated (i)
Fergon	Sanofi Winthrop	Capsule	Slow release*
Fero-Grad 500 mg	Abbott	Tablet	Slow release
Fero-Gradumet	Abbott	Tablet	Slow release

For references, see legend page 1217 in this edition.

Drug Product	Manufacturer	Dosage Form	Reason/Comments
Ferralet SR	Mission	Tablet	Slow release
Festal II	Hoechst Marion Roussel	Tablet	Enteric-coated
Feverall Sprinkle Caps	Upsher-Smith	Capsule	Taste*(j)
Fumatinic	Laser	Capsule	Slow release
Gastrocrom	Fisons	Capsule	Dissolve in water (k)
Geocillin	Roerig	Tablet	Taste
Glucotrol XL	Pratt	Tablet	Slow release
Gris-Peg	Allergan Herbert	Tablet	Crushing may precipitate (l)
Guaifed	Muro	Capsule	Slow release
Guaifed-PD	Muro	Capsule	Slow release
Guaifenex LA	Ethex	Tablet	Slow release (h)
Guaifenex PSE 120	Ethex	Tablet	Slow release (h)
Humibid DM	Adams	Tablet	Slow release
Humibid DM Sprinkle	Adams	Capsule	Slow release*
Humibid LA	Adams	Tablet	Slow release
Humibid Sprinkle	Adams	Capsule	Slow release*
Hydergine LC	Sandoz	Capsule	Liquid in capsule (i)
Hydergine Sublingual	Sandoz	Tablet	Sublingual route (i)
Hytakerol	Sanofi Winthrop	Capsule	Liquid filled (b)(i)
Iberet	Abbott	Tablet	Slow release (i)
Iberet 500	Abbott	Tablet	Slow release (i)
ICaps Plus	LaHaye Labs	Tablet	Slow release
ICaps Time Release	LaHaye Labs	Tablet	Slow release
Ilotycin	Dista	Tablet	Enteric-coated
Imdur	Key	Tablet	Slow release (h)
Inderal LA	Wyeth-Ayerst	Capsule	Slow release
Inderide LA	Wyeth-Ayerst	Capsule	Slow release
Indocin SR	Merck	Capsule	Slow release*(i)
Ionamin	Fisons	Capsule	Slow release
Isoclor Timesule	Fisons	Capsule	Slow release (i)
Isoptin SR	Knoll Pharm	Tablet	Slow release
Isordil Sublingual	Wyeth-Ayerst	Tablet	Sublingual form (g)
Isordil Tembid	Wyeth-Ayerst	Tablet	Slow release
Isosorbide Dinitrate Sublingual	(various)	Tablet	Sublingual form (g)
Isosorbide Dinitrate SR	(various)	Tablet	Slow release
Isuprel Glossets	Sanofi Winthrop	Tablet	Sublingual form (g)
K + 8	Alra	Tablet	Slow release (i)
K + 10	Alra	Tablet	Slow release (i)
Kaon CL 6.7 mEq	Pharmacia	Tablet	Slow release (i)
Kaon CL 10	Pharmacia	Tablet	Slow release (i)
K + Care	Alra	Tablet	Effervescent tablet (d)(i)

For references, see legend page 1217 in this edition.

Drug Product	Manufacturer	Dosage Form	Reason/Comments
K-Lease	Pharmacia	Capsule	Slow release*(i)
Klor-Con	Upsher-Smith	Tablet	Slow release (i)
Klor-Con/EF	Upsher-Smith	Tablet	Effervescent tablet (d)(i)
Klorvess	Sandoz	Tablet	Effervescent tablet (d)(i)
Klotrix	Bristol-Meyers	Tablet	Slow release (i)
K-Lyte	Bristol-Meyers	Tablet	Effervescent tablet (d)
K-Lyte CL	Bristol-Meyers	Tablet	Effervescent tablet (d)
K-Tab	Abbott	Tablet	Slow release (i)
Levsinex Timecaps	Schwarz Pharma Kremers-Urban	Capsule	Slow release
Lithobid	Ciba	Tablet	Slow release (i)
Lodrane LD	ECR Pharmaceutical	Capsule	Slow release*
Mag-Tab SR	Niche	Tablet	Slow release
Meprospan	Wallace	Capsule	Slow release*
Mestinon Timespan	ICN	Tablet	Slow release (i)
Mi-Cebrin	Dista	Tablet	Enteric-coated
Mi-Cebrin T	Dista	Tablet	Enteric-coated
Micro K	Robins	Capsule	Slow release*(i)
Motrin	Upjohn	Tablet	Taste (c)
MS Contin	Purdue Frederick	Tablet	Slow release (i)
MSC Triaminic	Sandoz	Tablet	Enteric-coated
Muco-Fen-LA	Wakefield	Tablet	Slow release (h)
Naldecon	Bristol	Tablet	Slow release (i)
Nasatab LA	ECR Pharmaceutical	Tablet	Slow release (h)
Nico 400	Jones Medical	Capsule	Slow release
Nicobid	Rhone-Poulenc Rorer	Capsule	Slow release
Nitro Bid	Hoechst Marion Roussel	Capsule	Slow release*
Nitrocine Timecaps	Schwarz Pharma Kremers-Urban	Capsule	Slow release
Nitroglyn	Kenwood	Capsule	Slow release*
Nitrostat	Parke-Davis	Tablet	Sublingual route (g)
Nitrong	Rhone-Poulenc Rorer	Tablet	Sublingual route (g)
Nitro-Time	Time-Cap Labs	Capsule	Slow release
Nolamine	Carnrick	Tablet	Slow release
Nolex LA	Carnrick	Tablet	Slow release

For references, see legend page 1217 in this edition.

Drug Product	Manufacturer	Dosage Form	Reason/Comments
Norflex	3M Pharmaceuticals	Tablet	Slow release
Norpace CR	Searle	Capsule	Slow release
Novafed	Hoechst Marion Roussel	Capsule	Slow release
Novafed A	Hoechst Marion Roussel	Capsule	Slow release
Ondrox	Unimed	Tablet	Slow release
Optilets 500 filmtab	Abbott	Tablet	Enteric-coated
Optilets M 500 filmtab	Abbott	Tablet	Enteric-coated
Oragrafin	Bracco DXS	Capsule	Liquid in capsule
Oramorph SR	Roxane	Tablet	Slow release (i)
Ornade Spansule	SmithKline Beecham	Capsule	Slow release
Pabalate	Robins	Tablet	Enteric-coated
Pancrease	Ortho McNeil	Capsule	Enteric-coated*
Pancrease MT	Ortho McNeil	Capsule	Enteric-coated*
Panmycin	Upjohn	Capsule	Taste
Papaverine Sustained Action	(various)	Capsule	Slow release
Pathilon	Lederle	Capsule	Slow release*
Pavabid Plateau	Hoechst Marion Roussel	Capsule	Slow release*
PBZ-SR	Geigy	Tablet	Slow release (i)
Perdiem	Rhone-Poulenc Rorer	Granules	Wax coated
Peritrate SA	Parke-Davis	Tablet	Slow release (h)
Permitil Chronotab	Schering	Tablet	Slow release (i)
Phazyme	Reed & Carnrick	Tablet	Slow release
Phazyme 95	Reed & Carnrick	Tablet	Slow release
Phenergan	Wyeth-Ayerst	Tablet	Taste (c)(i)
Phyllocontin	Purdue Frederick	Tablet	Slow release
Plendil	Astra Merck	Tablet	Slow release
Pneumomist	ECR Pharmaceutical	Tablet	Slow release (h)
Polaramine	Schering	Tablet	Slow release (i)
Prelu-2	Boehringer Ingelheim	Capsule	Slow release
Prevacid	TAP Pharmaceutical	Capsule	Slow release
Prilosec	Astra Merck	Capsule	Slow release
Pro-Banthine	SCS	Tablet	Taste
Procainmide HCL SR	(various)	Tablet	Slow release
Procan SR	Parke-Davis	Tablet	Slow release

For references, see legend page 1217 in this edition.

Drug Product	Manufacturer	Dosage Form	Reason/Comments
Procardia	Pfizer	Capsule	Delays absorption (b)(e)
Procardia XL	Pfizer	Tablet	Slow release, AUC is unaffected
Profen II	Wakefield	Tablet	Slow release (h)
Profen-LA	Wakefield	Tablet	Slow release (h)
Pronestyl SR	Bristol-Myers Squibb	Tablet	Slow release
Proventil Repetabs	Schering	Tablet	Slow release (i)
Prozac	Dista	Capsule	Slow release*
Quadra Hist	Schein	Tablet	Slow release
Quibron-T SR	Bristol-Myers Squibb	Tablet	Slow release (i)
Quinaglute Dura Tabs	Berlex	Tablet	Slow release
Quinidex Extentabs	Robins	Tablet	Slow release
Respa-1st	Respa	Tablet	Slow release (h)
Respa-DM	Respa	Tablet	Slow release (h)
Respa-GF	Respa	Tablet	Slow release (h)
Respahist	Respa	Capsule	Slow release*
Respaire SR	Laser	Capsule	Slow release
Respid	Boehringer Ingelheim	Tablet	Slow release
Ritalin SR	Ciba	Tablet	Slow release
Robimycin Robitab	Robins	Tablet	Enteric-coated
Rondec TR	Dura	Tablet	Slow release (i)
Roxanol SR	Roxane	Tablet	Slow release (i)
Ru-Tuss	Knoll Pharm	Tablet	Slow release
Ru-Tuss DE	Knoll Pharm	Tablet	Slow release
Sinemet CR	DuPont Pharm	Tablet	Slow release (h)
Singlet	Hoechst Marion Roussel	Tablet	Slow release
Slo-Bid Gyrocaps	Rhone-Poulenc Rorer	Capsule	Slow release*
Slo-Niacin	Upsher Smith	Tablet	Slow release (h)
Slo-Phyllin GG	Rhone-Poulenc Rorer	Capsule	Slow release (i)
Slo-Phyllin Gyrocaps	Rhone-Poulenc Rorer	Capsule	Slow release*(i)
Slow-FE	Ciba Self-Medication	Tablet	Slow release (i)
Slow-FE with Folic Acid	Ciba Self-Medication	Tablet	Slow release
Slow-K	Summit	Tablet	Slow release (i)
Slow-Mag	Searle	Tablet	Slow release
Sorbitrate SA	Zeneca	Tablet	Slow release
Sorbitrate Sublingual	Zeneca	Tablet	Sublingual route
Sparine	Wyeth-Ayerst	Tablet	Taste (c)

For references, see legend page 1217 in this edition.

Drug Product	Manufacturer	Dosage Form	Reason/Comments
S-P-T	Fleming	Capsule	Liquid gelantin thyroid suspension
Sudafed 12 hour	Warner Wellcome	Capsule	Slow release (i)
Sudex	Atley	Tablet	Slow release (h)
Sustaire	Pfizer	Tablet	Slow release (i)
Syn-RX	Adams Lab	Tablet	Slow release
Tavist-D	Sandoz	Tablet	Multiple compressed tablet
Tedral SA	Parke-Davis	Tablet	Slow release
Teldrin	SmithKline Beecham	Capsule	Slow release*
Tepanil Ten-Tab	3M Pharmaceuticals	Tablet	Slow release
Tessalon Perles	Forest	Capsule	Slow release
Theo-24	Searle	Tablet	Slow release (i)
Theobid Duracaps	Whitby	Capsule	Slow release*(i)
Theobid Jr. Duracaps	Whitby	Capsule	Slow release*(i)
Theoclear LA	Central	Capsule	Slow release (i)
Theochron	(various)	Tablet	Slow release
Theo-Dur	Key	Tablet	Slow release (i)
Theo-Dur Sprinkle	Key	Capsule	Slow release*(i)
Theo-Sav	Savage	Tablet	Slow release (h)
Theovent	Schering	Capsule	Slow release (i)
Theo-X	Carnrick	Tablet	Slow release
Therapy Bayer	Bayer	Caplet	Enteric-coated
Thorazine Spansule	SmithKline Beecham	Capsule	Slow release
T-Phyl	Purdue Frederick	Tablet	Slow release
Trental	Hoechst Marion Roussel	Tablet	Slow release
Triaminic	Sandoz	Tablet	Enteric-coated (i)
Triaminic 12	Sandoz	Tablet	Slow release (i)
Triaminic TR	Sandoz	Tablet	Multiple compressed tablet (i)
Trilafon Repetabs	Schering	Tablet	Slow release (i)
Triptone Caplets	Del Pharm	Tablet	Slow release
Toprol XL	Astra	Tablet	Slow release (h)
Tuss LA	Hyrex	Tablet	Slow release
Tuss Ornade Spansule	SmithKline Beecham	Capsule	Slow release
Tylenol Extended Relief	McNeil	Capsule	Slow release
ULR-LA	Geneva Pharm	Tablet	Slow release
Uniphyl	Purdue Frederick	Tablet	Slow release
Valrelease	Roche	Capsule	Slow release

For references, see legend page 1217 in this edition.

Drug Product	Manufacturer	Dosage Form	Reason/Comments
Verelan	Lederle	Capsule	Slow release*
Volmax	Muro	Tablet	Slow release
Wellbutrin	Burroughs Wellcome	Tablet	Anesthetize mucous membrane
Wygesic	Wyeth-Ayerst	Tablet	Taste
ZORprin	Boots	Tablet	Slow release
Zymase	Organon	Capsule	Enteric-coated

The listing is included to alert the health care practitioner about oral dosage forms that should not be crushed and to serve as an aid in consulting with patients. Revised by John F. Mitchell, Pharm.D., from an article originally appearing in *Hospital Pharmacy*, 31:27-37, 1996.

* Capsule may be opened and the contents taken without crushing or chewing; soft food such as applesauce or pudding may facilitate administration; contents may generally be administered via nasogastric tube using an appropriate fluid provided entire contents are washed down the tube.

(a) Antacids and/or milk may prematurely dissolve the coating of the tablet.
(b) Capsule may be opened and the liquid contents removed for administration.
(c) The taste of this product in a liquid form would likely be unacceptable to the patient; administration via nasogastric tube should be acceptable.
(d) Effervescent tablets must be dissolved in the amount of diluent recommended by the manufacturer.
(e) If the liquid capsule is crushed or the contents expressed, the active ingredient will be, in part, absorbed sublingually.
(f) Acid contents of the stomach may prematurely activate the ingredients.
(g) Tablets are made to disintegrate under the tongue.
(h) Tablet is scored and may be broken in half without affecting release characteristics.
(i) Liquid dosage forms of the product are available; however, dose, frequency of administration, and manufacturers may differ from that of the solid dosage form.
(j) Capsule contents intended to be placed in a teaspoonful of water or soft food.
(k) Contents may be dissolved in water for administration.
(l) Crushing may result in precipitation of larger particles.

Notes

Notes

Notes

Notes

Notes

Notes

Notes

Notes

Notes

Notes

Color Locator

The Color Locator is an aid in identifying tablets and capsules by their appearance. The products pictured include commonly used prescription drug products. Most products pictured have a corresponding drug monograph or are included in the combination tables. The index indicates the page numbers for the drug information and/or the color photograph. Because of the similarity in size, shape and color of products with significantly different ingredients, product identification should be confirmed by identifying imprints.

Organization

Products are arranged by dosage form, color, size, and shape. Every effort has been made to accurately reproduce the color of each product. However, variations will occur and exact reproductions are sometimes not possible. See the Table of Contents below for dosage form arrangement.

Contents

Each product pictured is identified with the product trade name, strength and manufacturer. For products with a product identification code imprint, that imprint is included following the manufacturer's name. Products are also indicated as prescription (℞) or controlled substance (C-II, C-III, C-IV or C-V).

Slight variations of color and ID code may occur. Drug manufacturers are expanding the use of product imprints to identify products by name or ID code. During this transition, various lots of the same product may have differing imprints. The ID code following the manufacturer name may not appear on all products pictured.

Table of Contents

℞

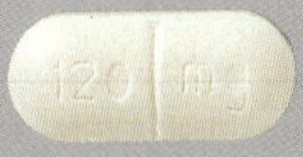

Cardizem 120 mg
Hoechst Marion Roussel 120

℞

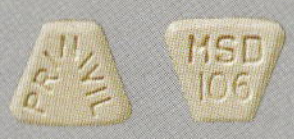

Prinivil 10 mg
Merck MSD 106

C-II

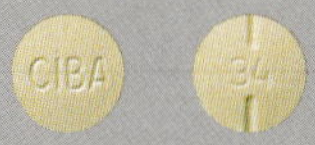

Ritalin 20 mg
Ciba Geneva 34

℞

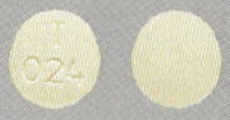

Colchicine 0.6 mg
Trinity T 024

℞

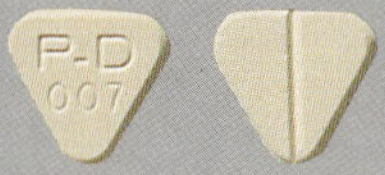

Dilantin Infatab 50 mg
Parke-Davis P-D 007

C-II

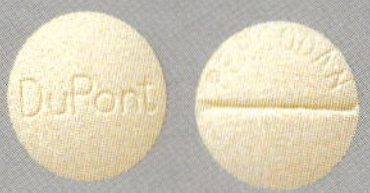

Percodan
DuPont

℞

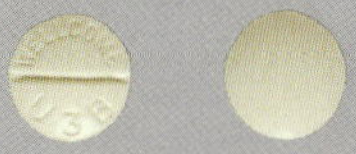

Thioguanine 40 mg
Glaxo Wellcome U3B

℞

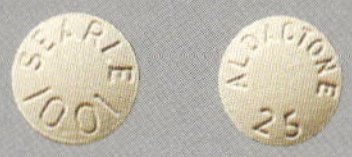

Aldactone 25 mg
Searle 1001 25

℞

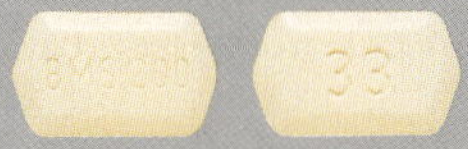

Serzone 200 mg
B-M Squibb BMS 200 33

℞

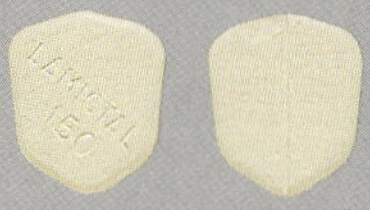

Lamictal 150 mg
Glaxo Wellcome 150

℞

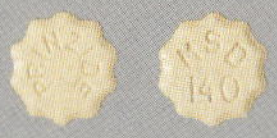

Prinzide 12.5 12.5 mg
Merck MSD 140

℞

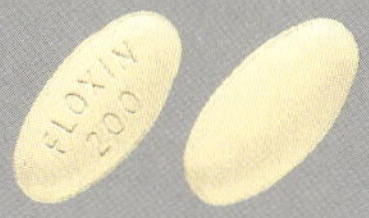

Floxin 200 mg
McNeil 200

℞

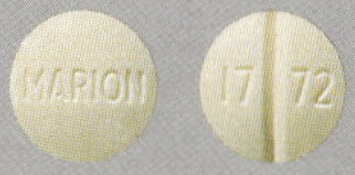

Cardizem 60 mg
Hoechst Marion Roussel 1772

℞

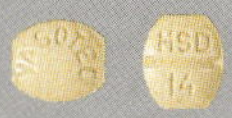

Vasotec 2.5 mg
Merck MSD 14

℞

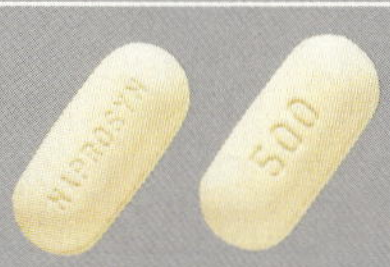

Naprosyn 500 mg
Roche 500

℞

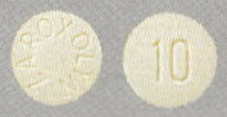

Zaroxolyn 10 mg
Fisons 10

℞

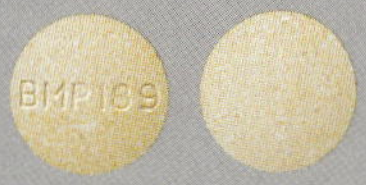

Augmentin ‘125’ Chewable
SmithKline Beecham BMP 189

℞

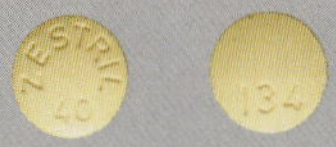

Zestril 40 mg
Zeneca 40 134

℞

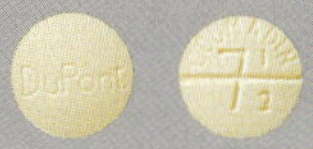

Coumadin 7.5 mg
DuPont 7 1/2

℞

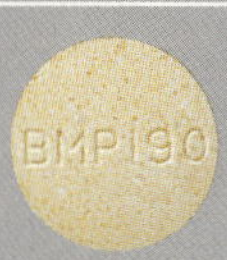

Augmentin ‘250’ Chewable
SmithKline Beecham BMP 190

℞

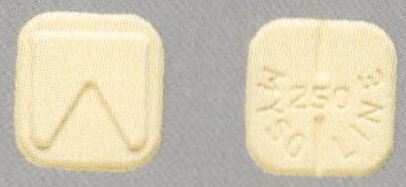

Mysoline 250 mg
Wyeth-Ayerst 250

℞
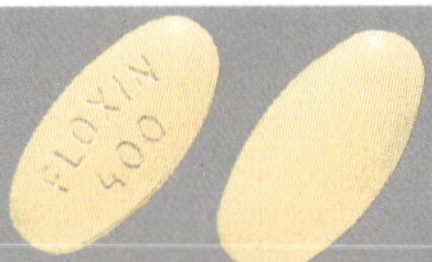

Floxin 400 mg
McNeil 400

℞
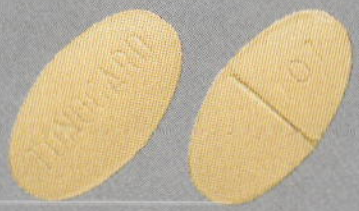
Tonocard 400 mg
Astra Merck 707

℞
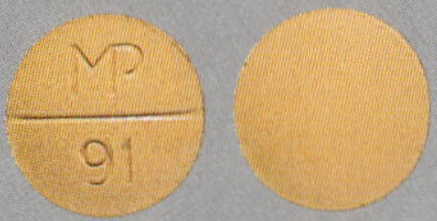

Sulfasalazine 500 mg
Mutual MP 91

℞
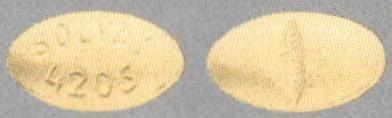
Luvox 50 mg
Solvay 4205

℞

Cardura 2 mg
Roerig 2

℞
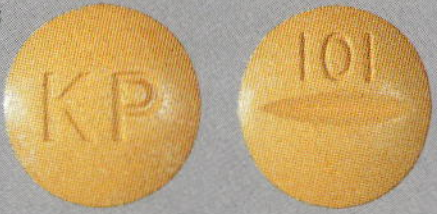

Azulfidine 500 mg
Pharmacia KP 101

℞
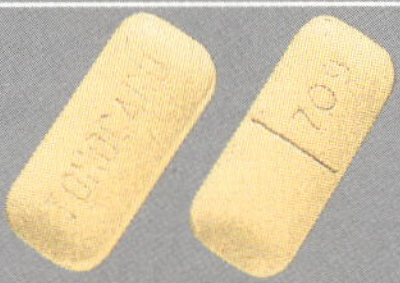
Tonocard 600 mg
Astra Merck 709

℞
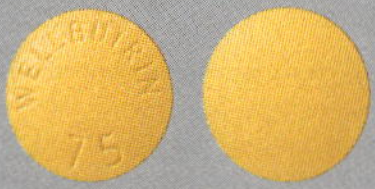

Wellbutrin 75 mg
Glaxo Wellcome 75

℞
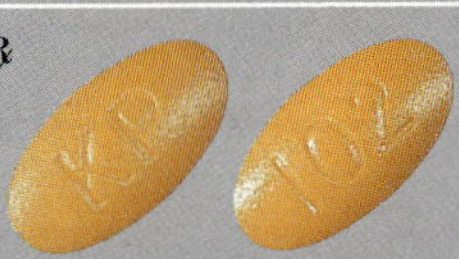

Azulfidine EN-tabs 500 mg
Pharmacia KP 102

℞
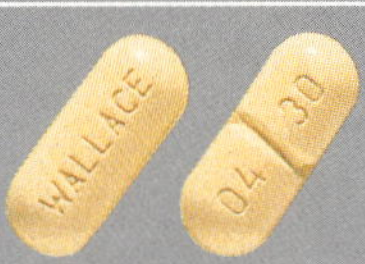

Felbatol 400 mg
Wallace 04 30

℞
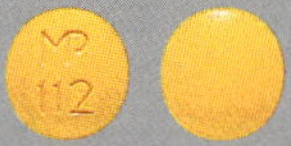

Sulindac 150 mg
Mutual MP 112

℞
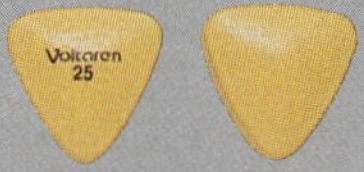

Voltaren 25 mg
Ciba Geneva 25

℞
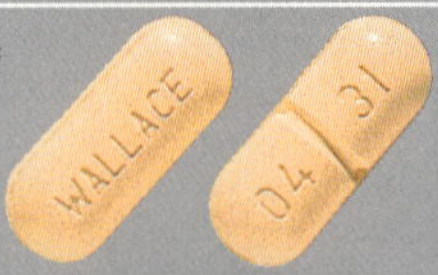

Felbatol 600 mg
Wallace 04 31

℞
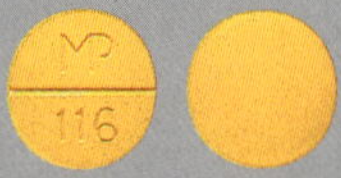

Sulindac 200 mg
Mutual MP 116

℞
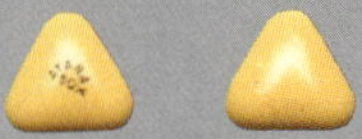
Atarax 50 mg
Roerig 50

℞
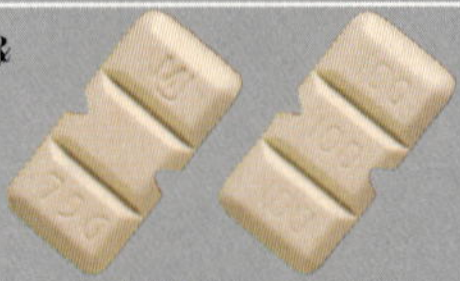
Desyrel Dividose 300 mg
Mead Johnson MJ 796 100

℞
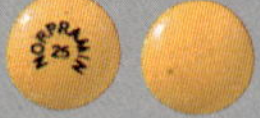

Norpramin 25 mg
Hoechst Marion Roussel 25

℞
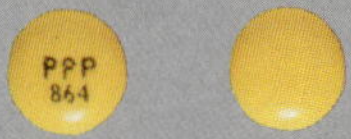

Prolixin 2.5 mg
Apothecon PPP 864

℞
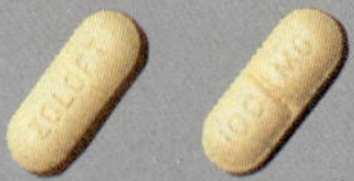
Zoloft 100 mg
Roerig 100

℞
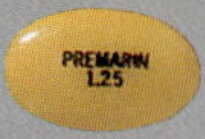

Premarin 1.25 mg
Wyeth-Ayerst 1.25

℞
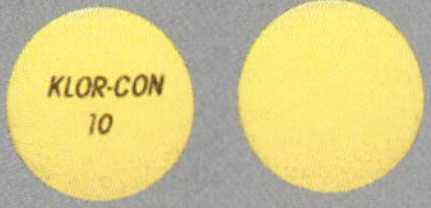

Klor-Con 10 10 mEq
Upsher-Smith 10

℞
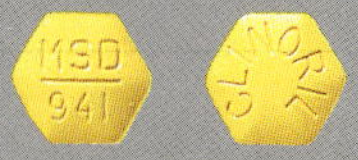

Clinoril 150 mg
Merck MSD 941

℞
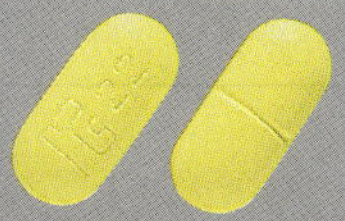
Levatol 20 mg
Schwarz Pharma RC 22

℞
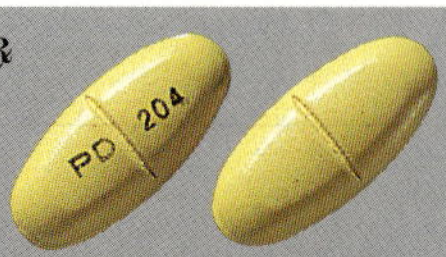

Procan SR 500 mg
Parke-Davis P-D 204

℞
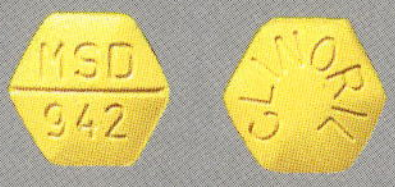

Clinoril 200 mg
Merck MSD 942

℞
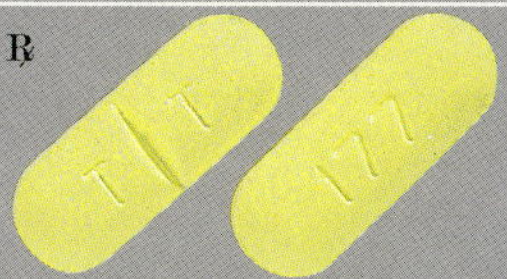
Guaifenesin 600 Pseudoephidrine 120
Trinity TT 177

℞
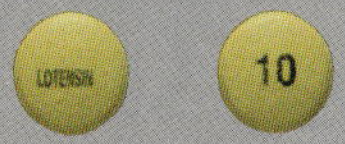

Lotensin 10 mg
Ciba Geneva 10

℞
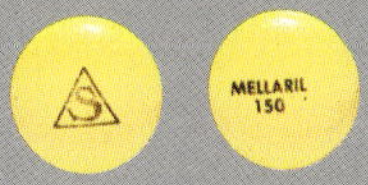

Mellaril 150 mg
Sandoz 150

℞
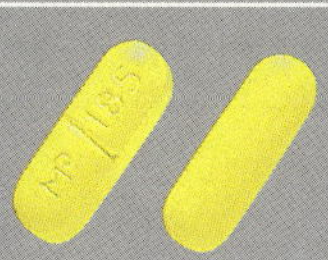
Metoprolol Tartrate 100 mg
Mutual MP 185

℞
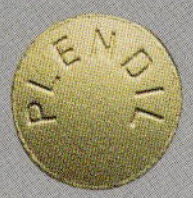

Plendil 2.5 mg
Astra Merck

℞
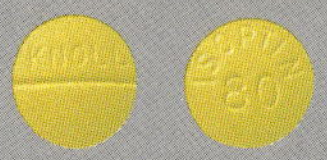
Isoptin 80 mg
Knoll 80

℞
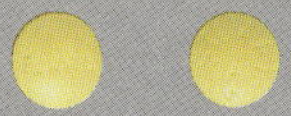
Elavil 25 mg
Zeneca Stuart 45

℞
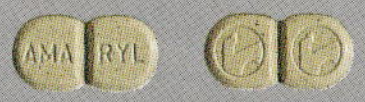

Amaryl 2 mg
Hoechst Marion Roussel

℞
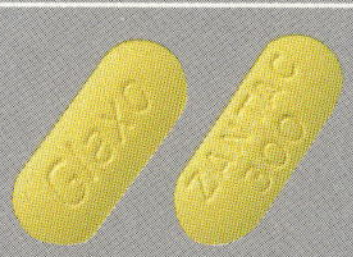

Zantac 300 mg
Glaxo Wellcome 300

℞
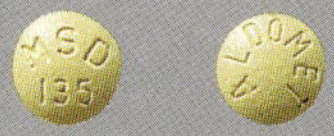

Aldomet 125 mg
Merck MSD 135

℞
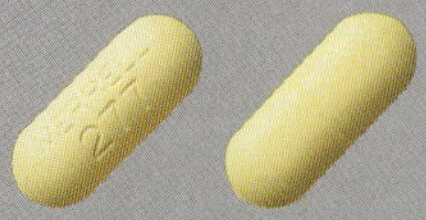
Hiprex 1 g
Hoechst Marion Roussel 277

℞
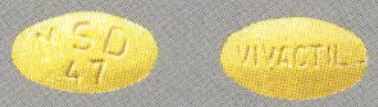
Vivactil 10 mg
Merck MSD 47

℞
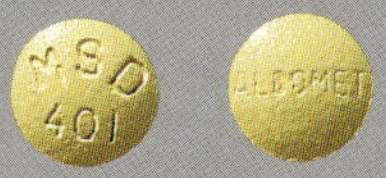

Aldomet 250 mg
Merck MSD 401

℞
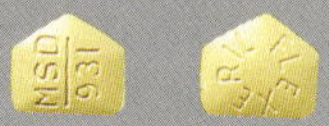
Flexeril 10 mg
Merck MSD 931

℞
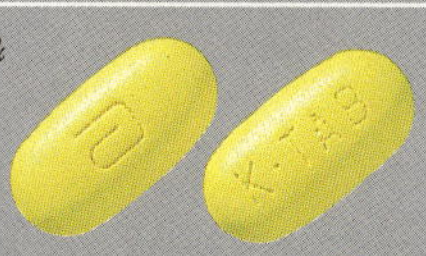
K-Tab 10 mEq
Abbott

℞
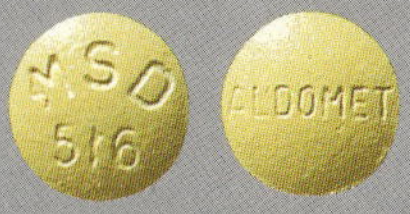

Aldomet 500 mg
Merck MSD 516

℞
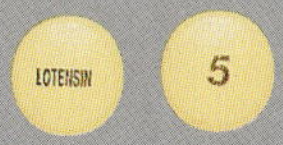

Lotensin 5 mg
Ciba Geneva 5

CL-6

℞
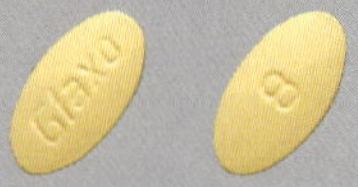

Zofran 8 mg
Glaxo Wellcome 8

℞
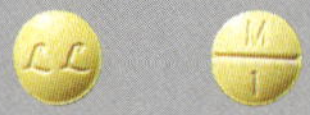

Rheumatrex 2.5 mg
Lederle LL M1

℞
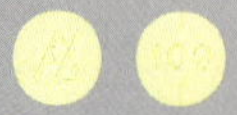

Levothroid 100 mcg
Forest Pharm 100

℞
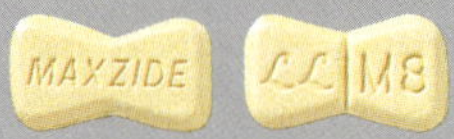

Maxzide 75/50
Lederle LL M8

℞
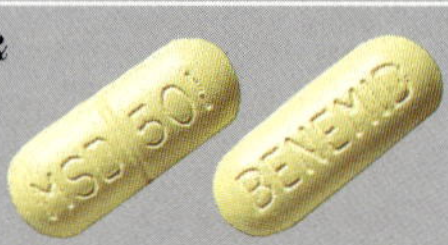

Benemid 0.5 g
Merck MSD 501

℞
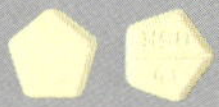

Decadron 0.5 mg
Merck MSD 41

℞
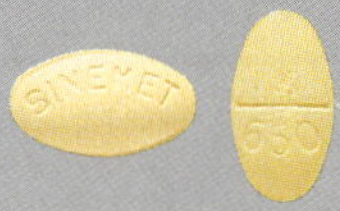

Sinemet-25/100
DuPont 650

℞
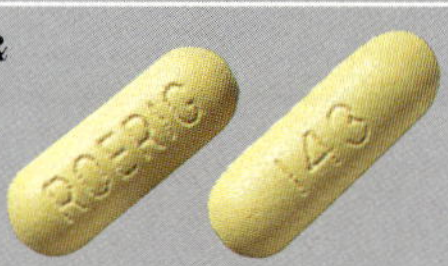

Geocillin 382 mg
Roerig 143

℞
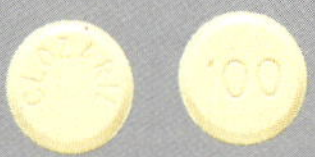

Clozaril 100 mg
Sandoz 100

℞
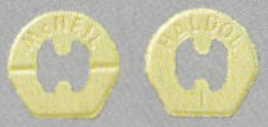

Haldol 1 mg
McNeil 1

℞
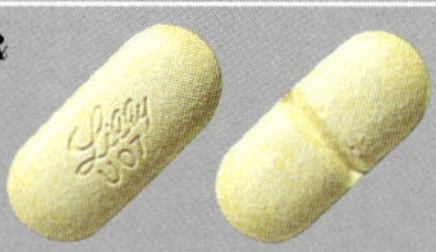

Dymelor 500 mg
Lilly U07

℞
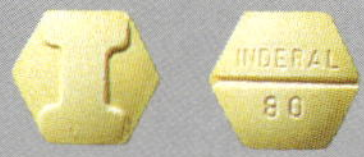

Inderal 80 mg
Wyeth-Ayerst I 80

℞
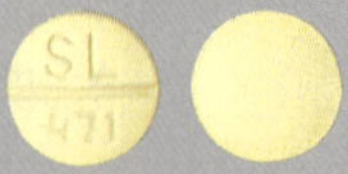

Propranolol 80 mg
Rugby SL 471

℞
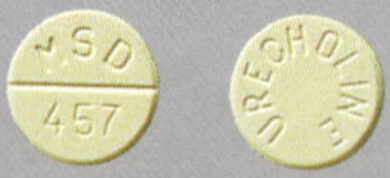

Urecholine 25 mg
Merck MSD 457

℞
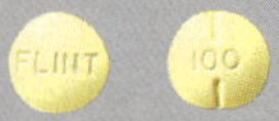

Synthroid 0.1 mg
Knoll Flint 100

℞
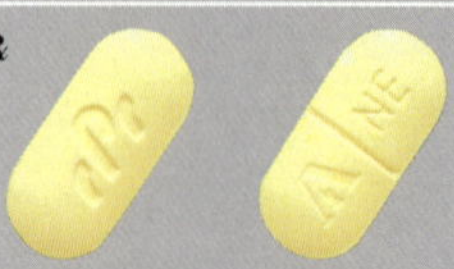

Nicolar 500 mg
Rhone-Poulenc Rorer NE

℞
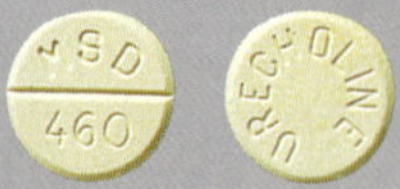

Urecholine 50 mg
Merck MSD 460

℞
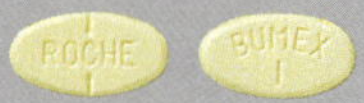

Bumex 1 mg
Roche 1

℞
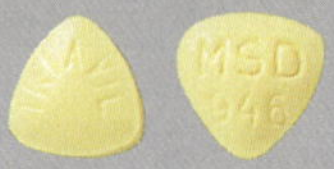

Triavil 4-25
Merck MSD 946

C-IV
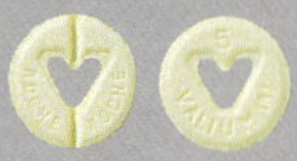

Valium 5 mg
Roche 5

℞
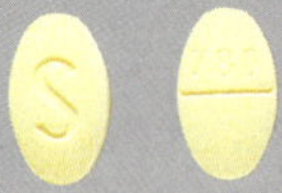

Sorbitrate 10 mg
Zeneca S 780

℞

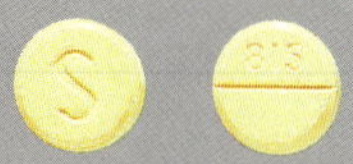

Sorbitrate 10 mg Chewable
Zeneca S 815

℞

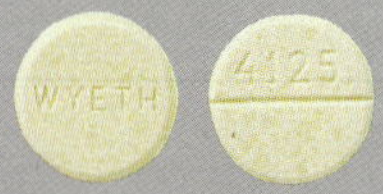

Isordil Tembids 40 mg
Wyeth-Ayerst 4125

℞

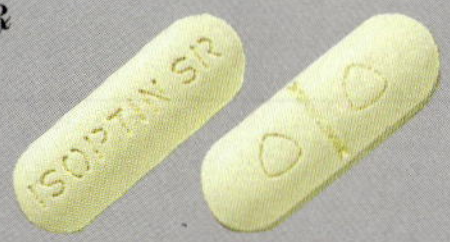

Isoptin SR 240 mg
Knoll SR

℞

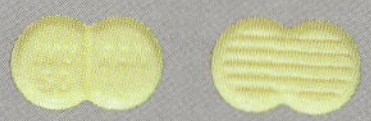

Imuran 50 mg
Glaxo Wellcome 50

℞

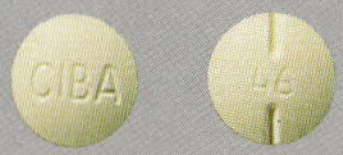

Esidrix 50 mg
Ciba Geneva 46

℞

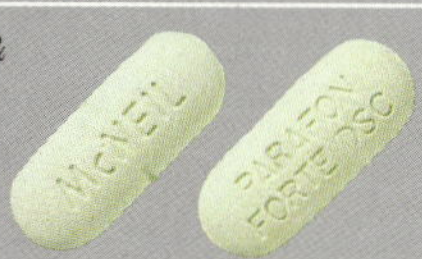

Parafon Forte DSC 500 mg
McNeil DSC

℞

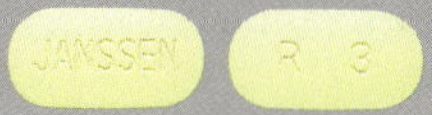

Risperdal 3 mg
Janssen R 3

℞

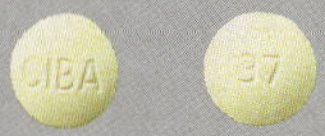

Apresoline 10 mg
Ciba Geneva 37

℞

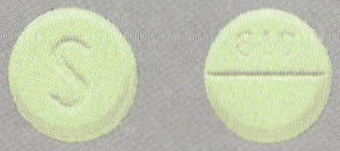

Sorbitrate 5 mg Chewable
Zeneca S 810

C-II

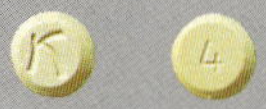

Dilaudid 4 mg
Knoll K 4

℞

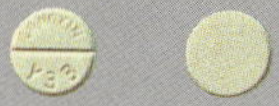

Lanoxin 0.125 mg
Glaxo Wellcome Y3B

℞

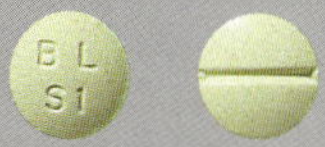

Salutensin
Bristol BL S1

C-IV

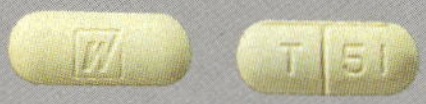

Talwin NX
Sanofi Winthrop W T51

℞

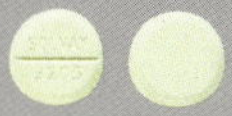

Dexone 0.5 mg
Solvay 3205

℞

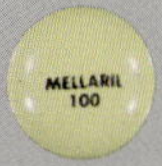

Mellaril 100 mg
Sandoz 100

C-II

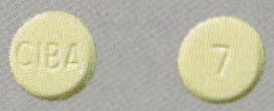

Ritalin 5 mg
Ciba Geneva 7

℞

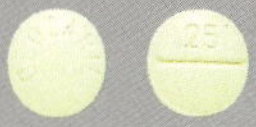

Clozaril 25 mg
Sandoz 25

℞

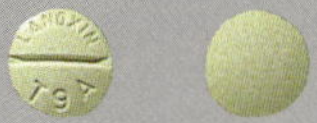

Lanoxin 0.5 mg
Glaxo Wellcome T9A

℞

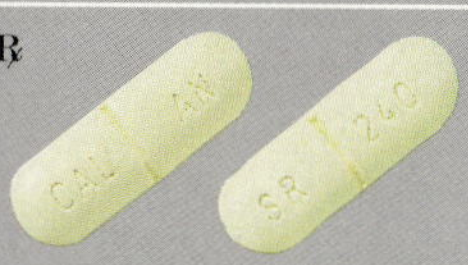

Calan SR 240 mg
Searle SR 240

℞

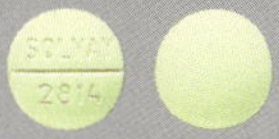

Orasone 20 mg
Solvay 2814

℞

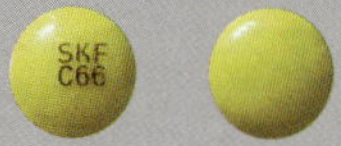

Compazine 5 mg
SmithKline Beecham SKF C66

℞
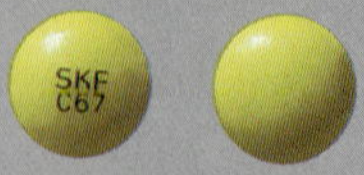

Compazine 10 mg
SmithKline Beecham SKF C67

℞
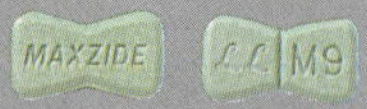

Maxzide-25MG (37.5/25)
Lederle LL M9

℞
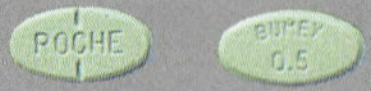

Bumex 0.5 mg
Roche 0.5

℞
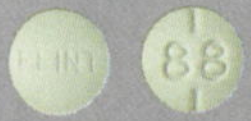

Synthroid 0.088 mg
Knoll Flint 88

℞
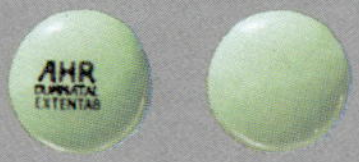

Donnatal Extentabs
Robins AHR

℞
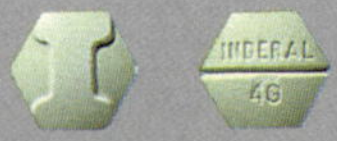

Inderal 40 mg
Wyeth-Ayerst I 40

℞
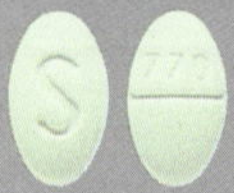

Sorbitrate 5 mg
Zeneca S 770

℞
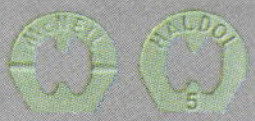

Haldol 5 mg
McNeil 5

℞
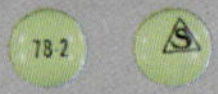

Mellaril 10 mg
Sandoz 78-2

℞
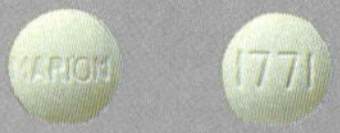

Cardizem 30 mg
Hoechst Marion Roussel 1771

℞
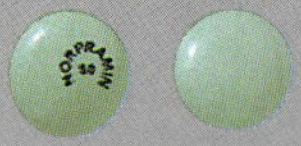

Norpramin 50 mg
Hoechst Marion Roussel 50

℞
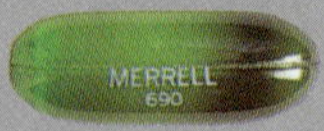

Tace 12 mg
Hoechst Marion Roussel 690

℞
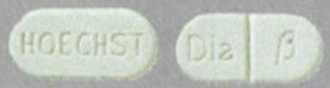

DiaBeta 5 mg
Hoechst Marion Roussel Dia ß

℞
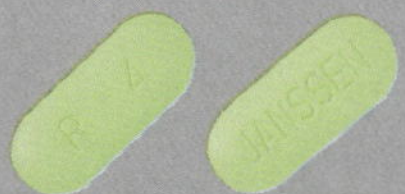

Risperdal 4 mg
Janssen R 4

℞
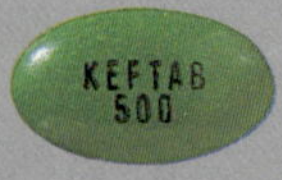

Keftab 500 mg
Dista 500

℞
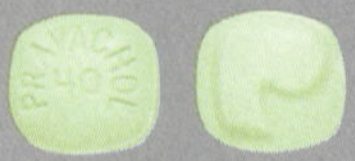

Pravachol 40 mg
B-M Squibb P 40

℞
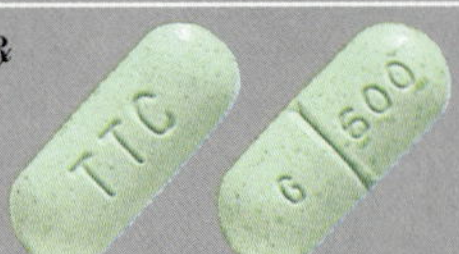

Guaifenesin 600 mg ER
Trinity TTC G 600

℞
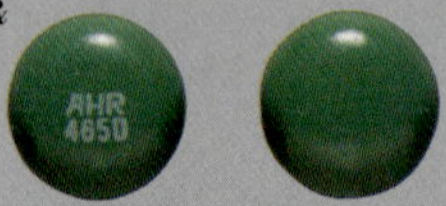

Donnazyme
Robins AHR 4650

℞
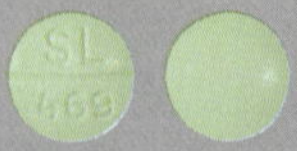

Propranolol 40 mg
Rugby SL 469

℞
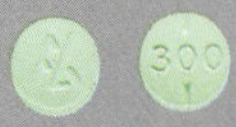

Levothroid 300 mcg
Forest Pharm 300

℞
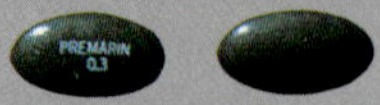

Premarin 0.3 mg
Wyeth-Ayerst 0.3

℞

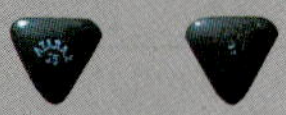

Atarax 25 mg
Roerig 25

℞

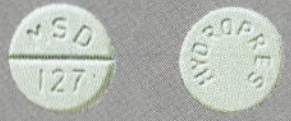

Hydropres-50 50 mg
Merck MSD 127

℞

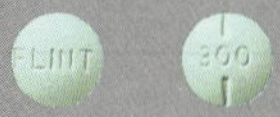

Synthroid 0.3 mg
Knoll Flint 300

C-IV

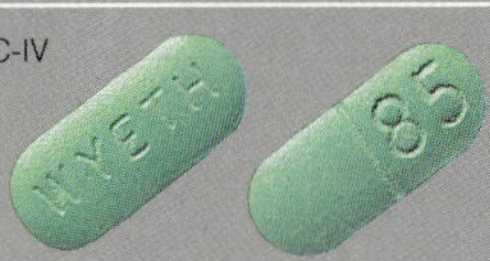

Wygesic
Wyeth-Ayerst 85

℞

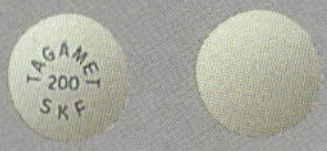

Tagamet 200 mg
SmithKline Beecham SKF 200

℞

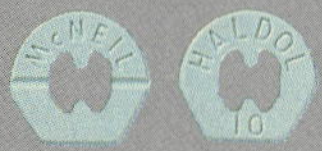

Haldol 10 mg
McNeil 10

℞

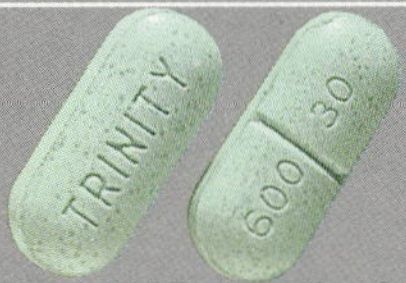

Guaifenesin 600 Dextromethorphan 30
Trinity 600 30

℞

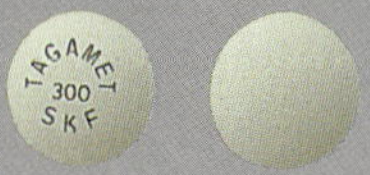

Tagamet 300 mg
SmithKline Beecham SKF 300

℞

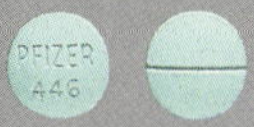

Renese-R
Pfizer 446

℞

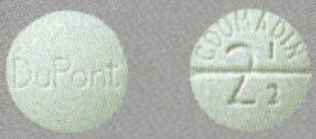

Coumadin 2.5 mg
DuPont 2 1/2

℞

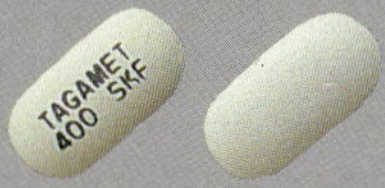

Tagamet 400 mg
SmithKline Beecham 400 SKF

℞

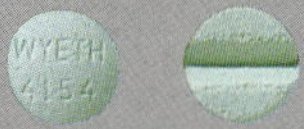

Isordil Titradose 20 mg
Wyeth-Ayerst 4154

℞

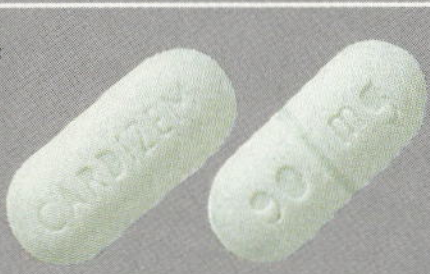

Cardizem 90 mg
Hoechst Marion Roussel 90

℞

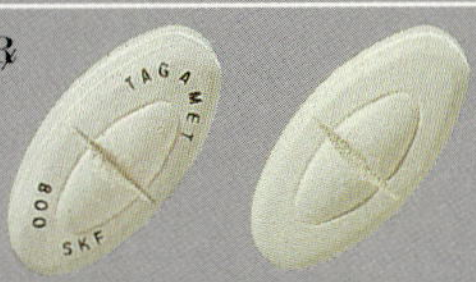

Tagamet 800 mg
SmithKline Beecham 800 SKF

℞

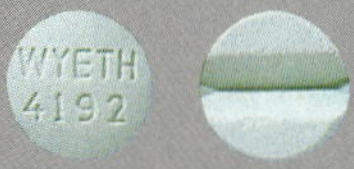

Isordil Titradose 40 mg
Wyeth-Ayerst 4192

℞

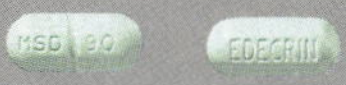

Edecrin 50 mg
Merck MSD 90

℞

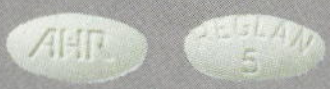

Reglan 5 mg
Robins AHR 5

℞

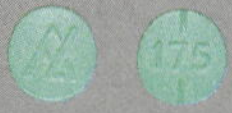

Levothroid 175 mcg
Forest Pharm 175

℞

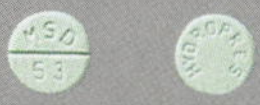

Hydropres-25 25 mg
Merck MSD 53

℞

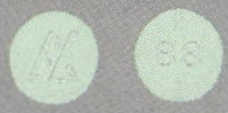

Levothroid 88 mcg
Forest Pharm 88

C-II

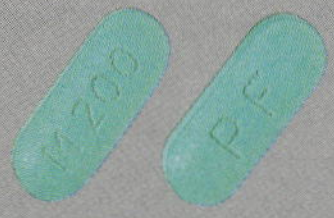

MS Contin 200 mg
Purdue Frederick PF M200

CL-10

℞

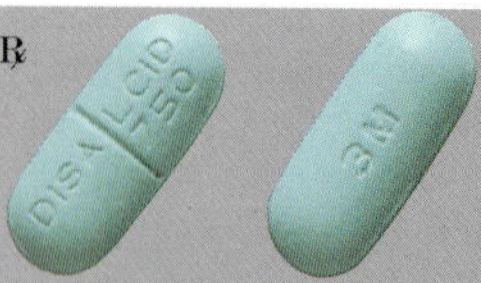

Disalcid 750 mg
3M Pharm 750

℞

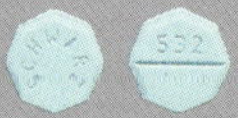

Levsin/SL 0.125 mg
Schwarz Pharma 532

℞

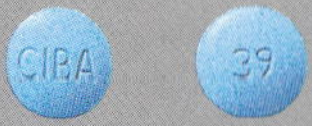

Apresoline 25 mg
Ciba Geneva 39

℞

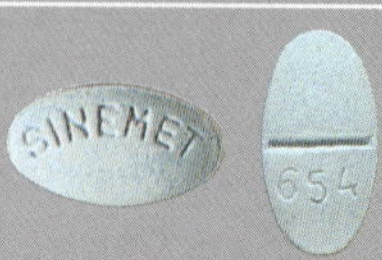

Sinemet-25/250
DuPont 654

C-IV

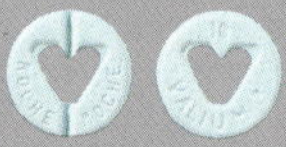

Valium 10 mg
Roche 10

℞

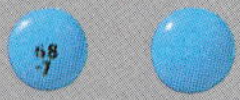

Norpramin 10 mg
Hoechst Marion Roussel 68-7

C-II

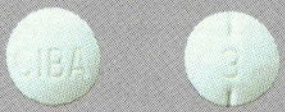

Ritalin 10 mg
Ciba Geneva 3

℞

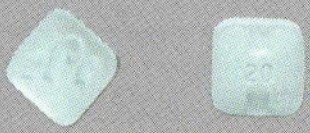

Hygroton 50 mg
Rhone-Poulenc Rorer H 20

℞

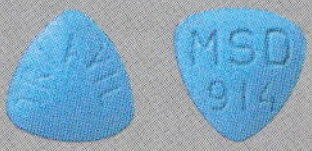

Triavil 2-10
Merck MSD 914

℞

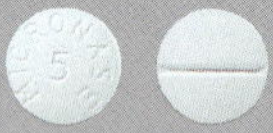

Micronase 5 mg
Upjohn 5

℞

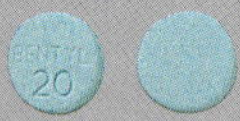

Bentyl 20 mg
Hoechst Marion Roussel 20

℞

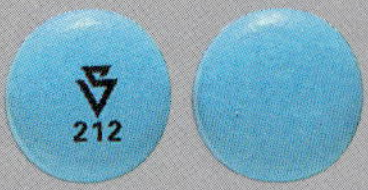

Kaon-CL 8 mEq
Savage 212

℞

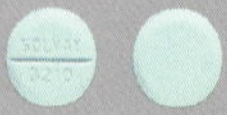

Dexone 0.75 mg
Solvay 3210

℞

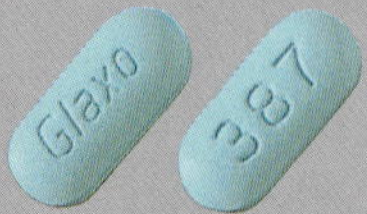

Ceftin 250 mg
Glaxo Wellcome 387

℞

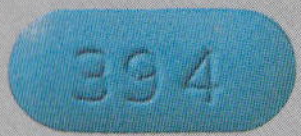

Ceftin 500 mg
Glaxo Wellcome 394

℞

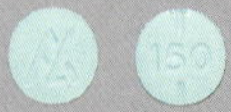

Levothroid 150 mcg
Forest Pharm 150

℞

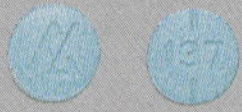

Levothroid 137 mcg
Forest Pharm 137

℞

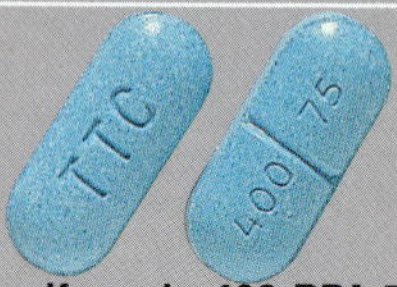

Guaifenesin 400 PPA 75
Trinity TTC 400 75

℞

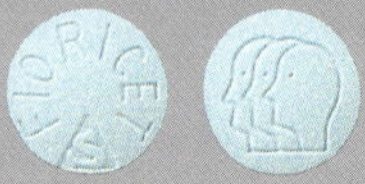

Fioricet
Sandoz S

℞

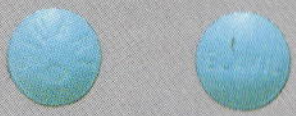

Elavil 10 mg
Zeneca Stuart 40

℞

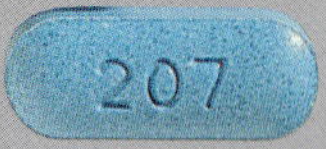

Guaifenesin 600 Pseudoephedrine 60
Trinity TT 207

℞
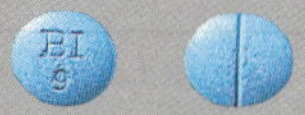

Combipres 0.2 mg
Boehringer Ingelheim BI 9

℞
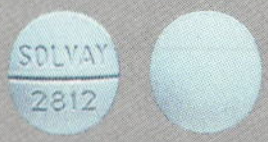

Orasone 10 mg
Solvay 2812

℞
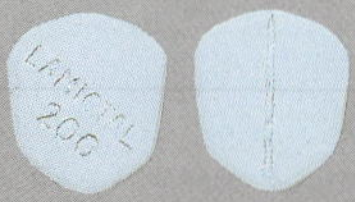

Lamictal 200 mg
Glaxo Wellcome 200

℞
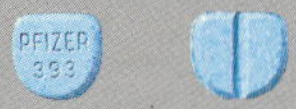

Diabinese 100 mg
Pfizer 393

℞
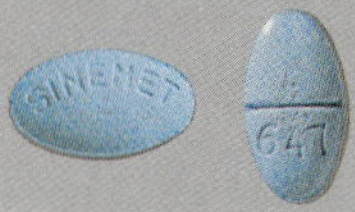

Sinemet-10/100
DuPont 647

℞
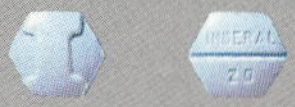
Inderal 20 mg
Wyeth-Ayerst I 20

℞
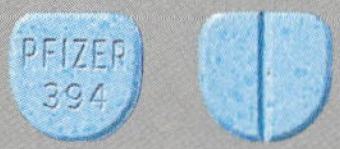

Diabinese 250 mg
Pfizer 394

℞
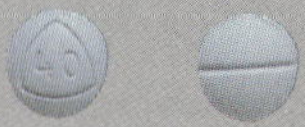

Isoptin 40 mg
Knoll 40

℞
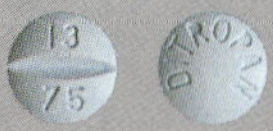

Ditropan 5 mg
Hoechst Marion Roussel 1375

℞
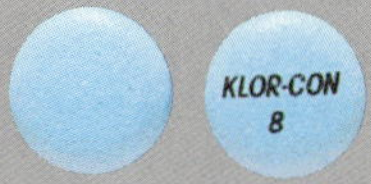

Klor-Con 8 8 mEq
Upsher-Smith 8

℞
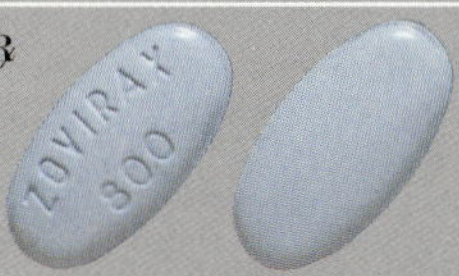

Zovirax 800 mg
Glaxo Wellcome 800

℞
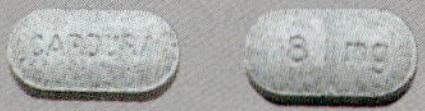

Cardura 8 mg
Roerig 8

℞
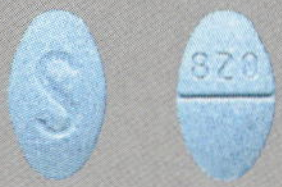

Sorbitrate 20 mg
Zeneca S 820

℞
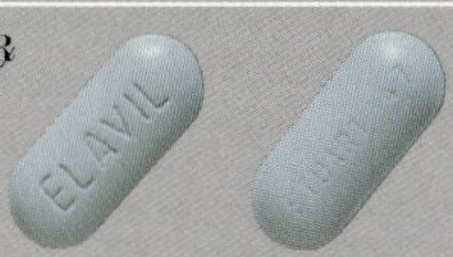

Elavil 150 mg
Zeneca Stuart 47

C-IV
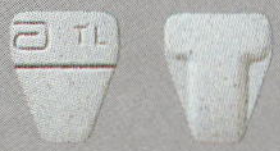

Tranxene 3.75 mg
Abbott TL

℞
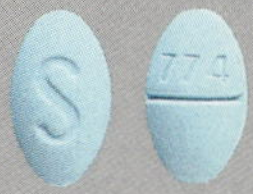

Sorbitrate 40 mg
Zeneca S 774

℞
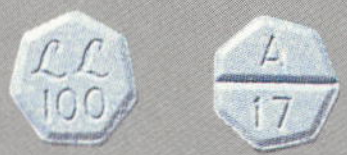

Asendin 100 mg
Lederle LL 100 A17

℞
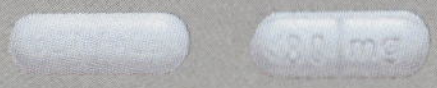
Betapace 80 mg
Berlex 80

℞
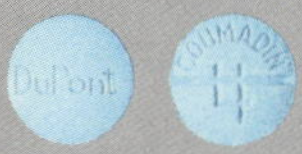

Coumadin 4 mg
DuPont 4

C-IV
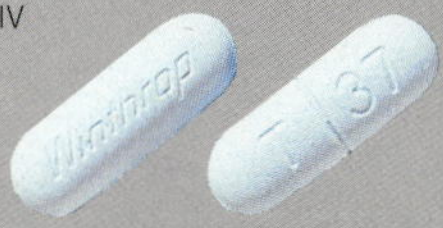

Talacen Caplets
Sanofi Winthrop T37

℞
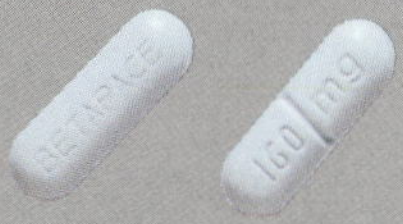

Betapace 160 mg
Berlex 160

℞

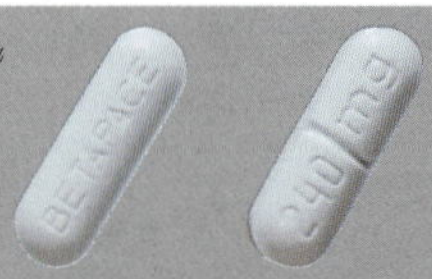

Betapace 240 mg
Berlex 240

℞

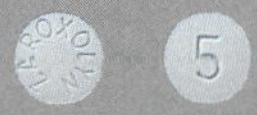

Zaroxolyn 5 mg
Fisons 5

℞

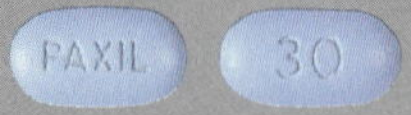

Paxil 30 mg
SmithKline Beecham 30

℞

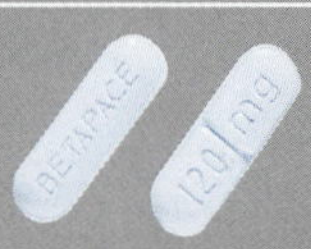

Betapace 120 mg
Berlex 120

℞

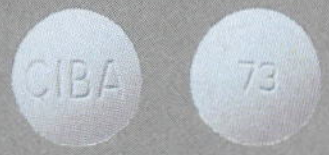

Apresoline 50 mg
Ciba Geneva 73

℞

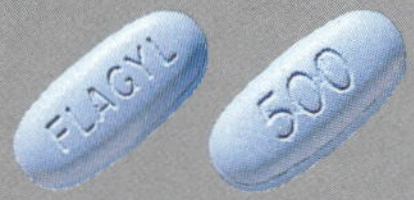

Flagyl 500 mg
Searle 500

℞

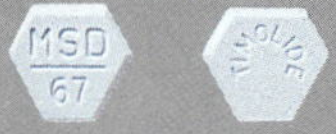

Timolide 10/25
Merck MSD 67

C-IV

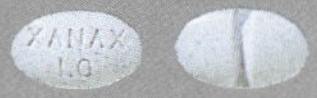

Xanax 1 mg
Upjohn 1.0

℞

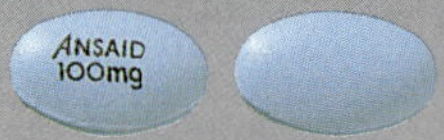

Ansaid 100 mg
Upjohn 100

℞

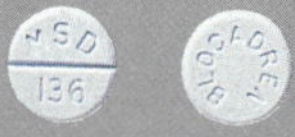

Blocadren 10 mg
Merck MSD 136

℞

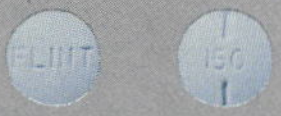

Synthroid 0.15 mg
Knoll Flint 150

℞

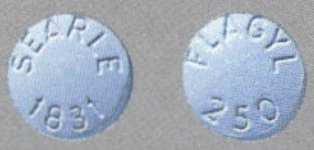

Flagyl 250 mg
Searle 1831 250

℞

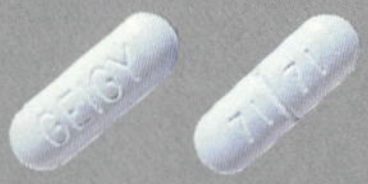

Lopressor 100 mg
Ciba Geneva Geigy 71 71

℞

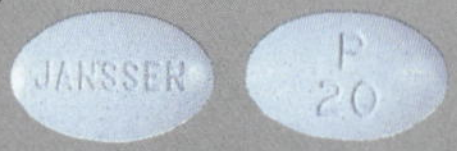

Propulsid 20 mg
Janssen P 20

℞

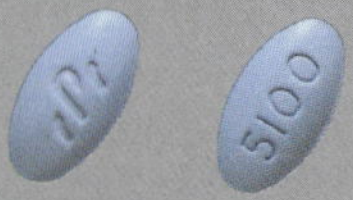

Penetrex 200 mg
Rhone-Poulenc Rorer 5100

℞

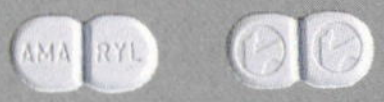

Amaryl 4 mg
Hoechst Marion Roussel

C-IV

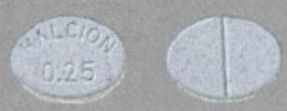

Halcion 0.25 mg
Upjohn 0.25

℞

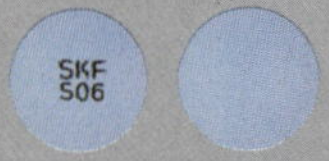

Stelazine 5 mg
SmithKline Beecham SKF S06

℞

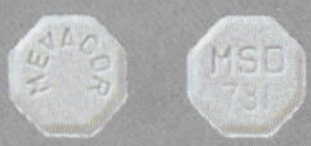

Mevacor 20 mg
Merck MSD 731

℞

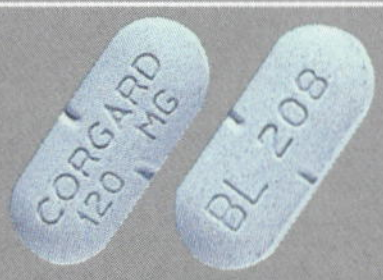

Corgard 120 mg
B-M Squibb 120 BL 208

℞

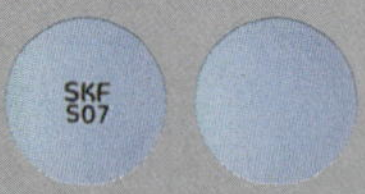

Stelazine 10 mg
SmithKline Beecham SKF S07

℞

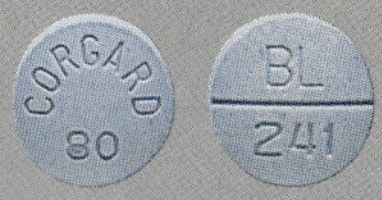

Corgard 80 mg
B-M Squibb 80 BL 241

℞

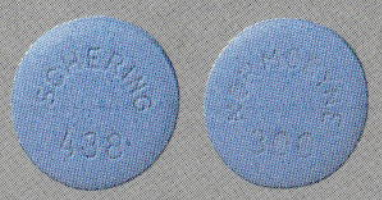

Normodyne 300 mg
Schering 438 300

C-II

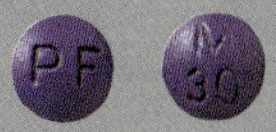

MS Contin 30 mg
Purdue Frederick PF M 30

℞

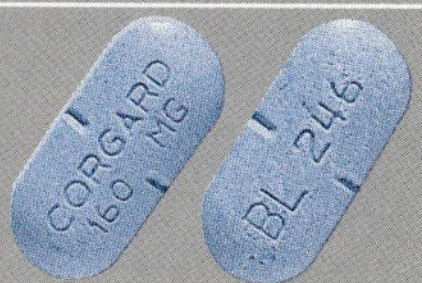

Corgard 160 mg
B-M Squibb 160 BL 246

℞

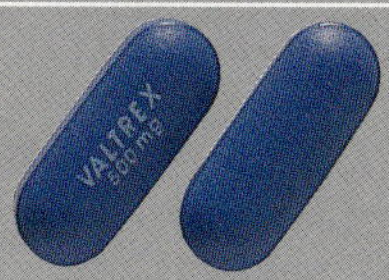

Valtrex 500 mg
Glaxo Wellcome 500

℞

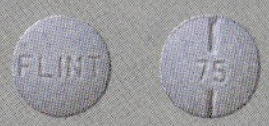

Synthroid 0.075 mg
Knoll Flint 75

℞

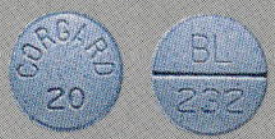

Corgard 20 mg
B-M Squibb 20 BL 232

℞

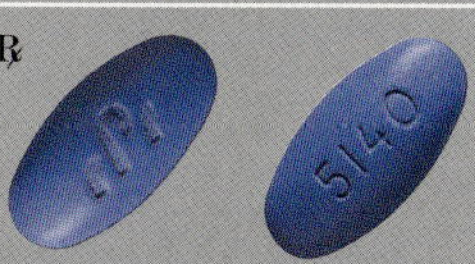

Penetrex 400 mg
Rhone-Poulenc Rorer 5140

℞

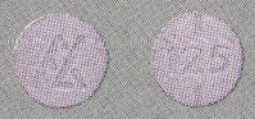

Levothroid 125 mcg
Forest Pharm 125

℞

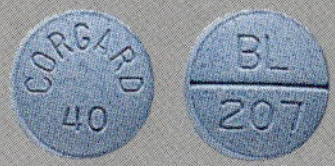

Corgard 40 mg
B-M Squibb 40 BL 207

C-IV

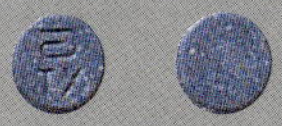

Tranxene-SD 11.25 mg
Abbott TX

℞

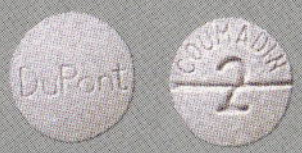

Coumadin 2 mg
DuPont 2

C-II

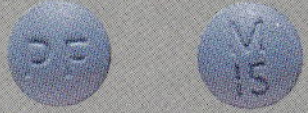

MS Contin 15 mg
Purdue Frederick PF M 15

℞

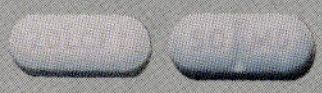

Zoloft 50 mg
Roerig 50

℞

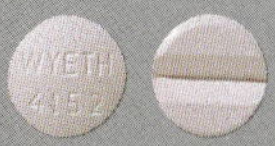

Isordil Titradose 5 mg
Wyeth-Ayerst 4152

℞

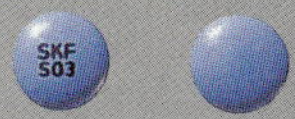

Stelazine 1 mg
SmithKline Beecham SKF S03

℞

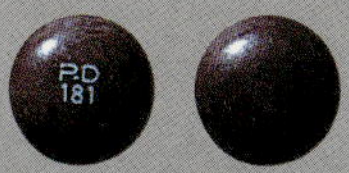

Pyridium 200 mg
Parke-Davis P-D 181

℞

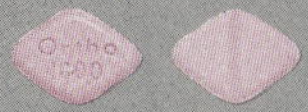

Ortho-Est 1.25 mg
Ortho 1800

℞

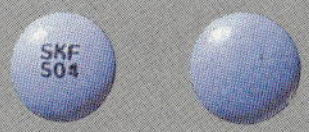

Stelazine 2 mg
SmithKline Beecham SKF S04

℞

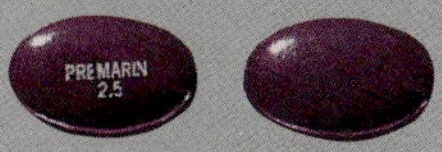

Premarin 2.5 mg
Wyeth-Ayerst 2.5

℞

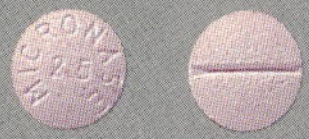

Micronase 2.5 mg
Upjohn 2.5

℞
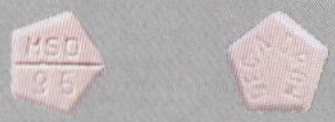

Decadron 1.5 mg
Merck MSD 95

℞
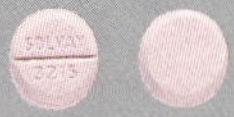

Dexone 1.5 mg
Solvay 3215

℞
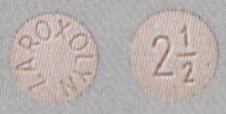

Zaroxolyn 2.5 mg
Fisons 2 1/2

℞
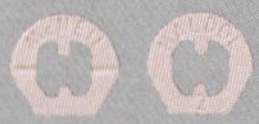

Haldol 2 mg
McNeil 2

℞
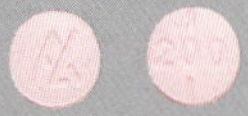

Levothroid 200 mcg
Forest Pharm 200

℞
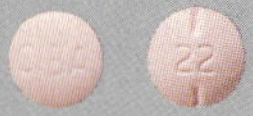

Esidrix 25 mg
Ciba Geneva 22

℞
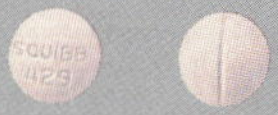

Florinef Acetate 0.1 mg
Apothecon Squibb 429

℞
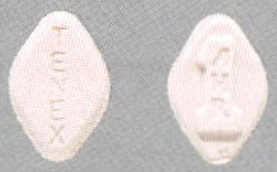

Tenex 1 mg
Robins AHR 1

℞
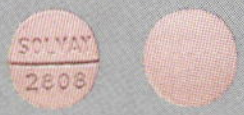

Orasone 1 mg
Solvay 2808

℞
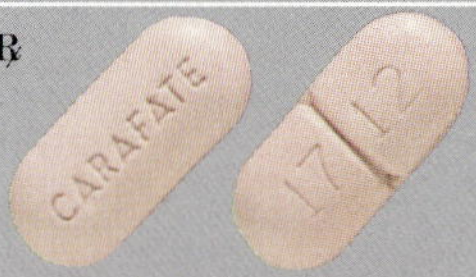

Carafate 1 g
Hoechst Marion Roussel 1712

℞
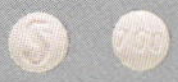

Sorbitrate 5 mg Sublingual
Zeneca S 760

℞
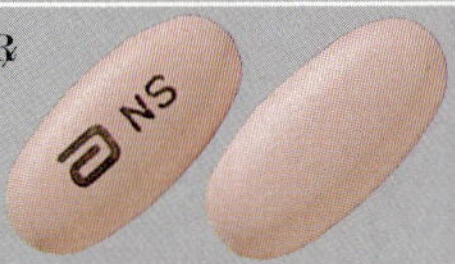

Depakote 500 mg
Abbott NS

℞
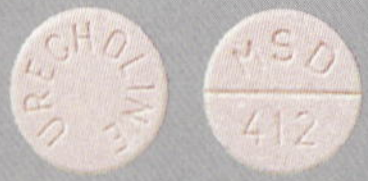

Urecholine 10 mg
Merck MSD 412

℞
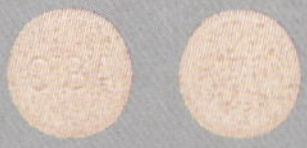

Ser-Ap-Es
Ciba Geneva 71

℞
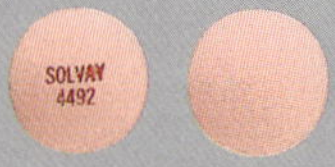

Lithobid Slow-Release 300 mg
Solvay 4492

℞
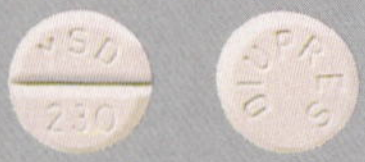

Diupres-250 250 mg
Merck MSD 230

℞
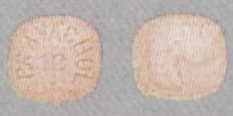

Pravachol 10 mg
B-M Squibb P 10

℞
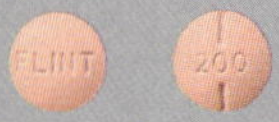

Synthroid 0.2 mg
Knoll Flint 200

℞
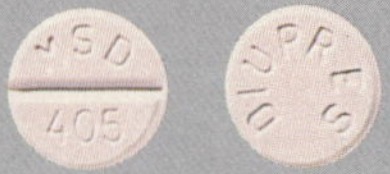

Diupres-500 500 mg
Merck MSD 405

℞
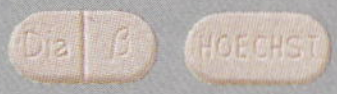

DiaBeta 2.5 mg
Hoechst Marion Roussel Dia ß

℞
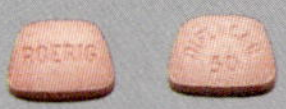

Diflucan 50 mg
Roerig 50

℞ 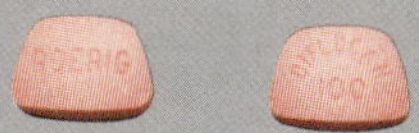 **Diflucan 100 mg** Roerig 100	℞ 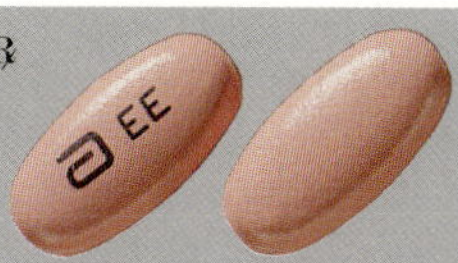 **E.E.S. 400 400 mg** Abbott EE	℞ 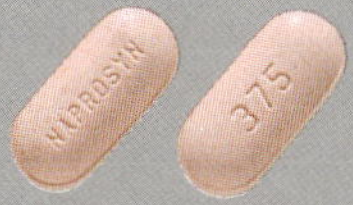 **Naprosyn 375 mg** Roche 375
℞ 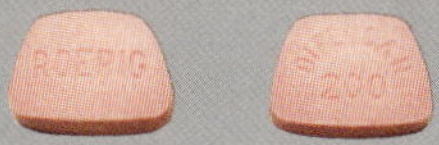 **Diflucan 200 mg** Roerig 200	℞ 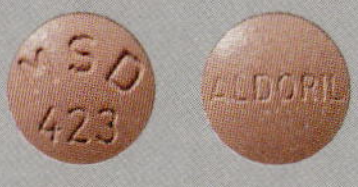 **Aldoril-15** Merck MSD 423	℞ 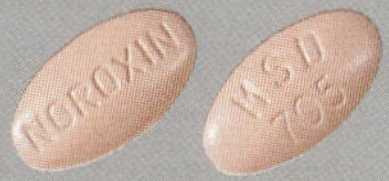 **Noroxin 400 mg** Merck MSD 705
℞ 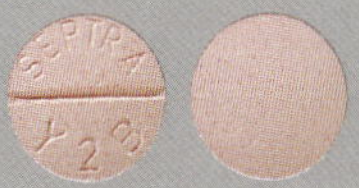 **Septra 80/400** Glaxo Wellcome Y2B	℞ 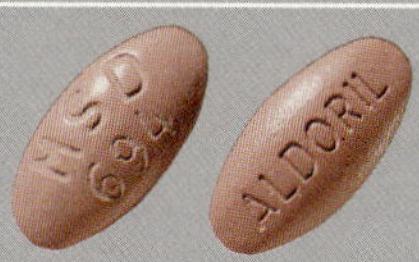 **Aldoril D30** Merck MSD 694	℞ 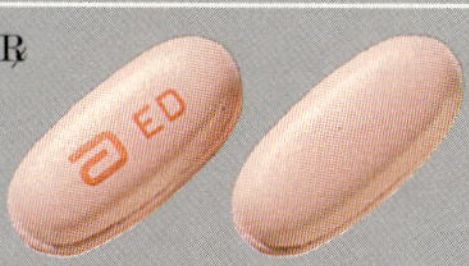 **Ery-Tab 500 mg** Abbott ED
℞ 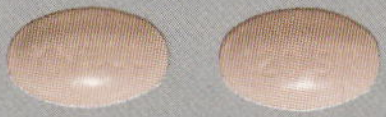 **Isoptin SR 120 mg** Knoll 120 SR	℞ 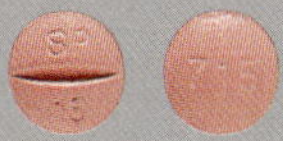 **Univasc 15 mg** Schwarz Pharma SP 15 715	℞ 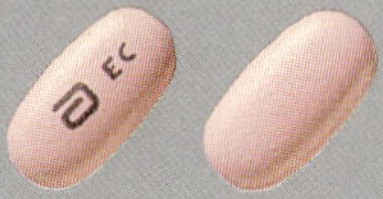 **Ery-Tab 250 mg** Abbott EC
℞ 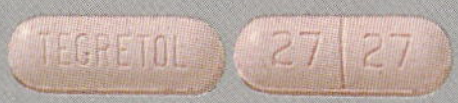 **Tegretol 200 mg** Ciba Geneva 27 27	℞ 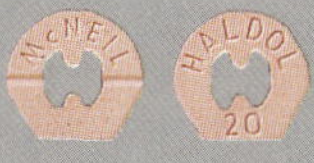 **Haldol 20 mg** McNeil 20	℞ 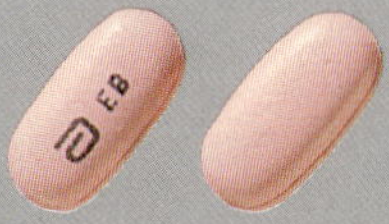 **Erythromycin 250 mg** Abbott EB
℞ 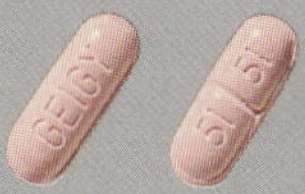 **Lopressor 50 mg** Ciba Geneva 51 51	℞ 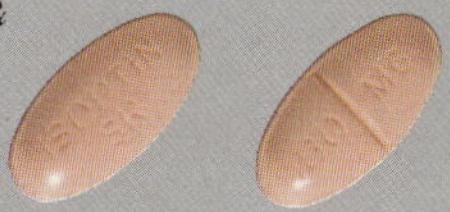 **Isoptin SR 180 mg** Knoll SR 180	℞ 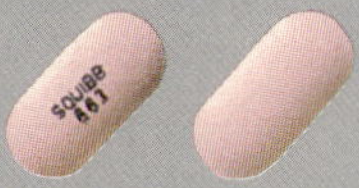 **Sumycin 250 mg** Apothecon Squibb 663
℞ 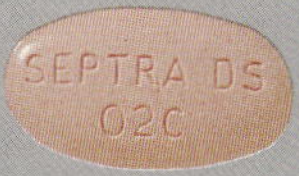 **Septra DS 160/800** Glaxo Wellcome O2C	℞ 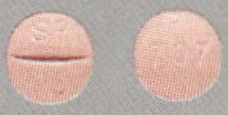 **Univasc 7.5 mg** Schwarz Pharma SP 7.5 707	℞ 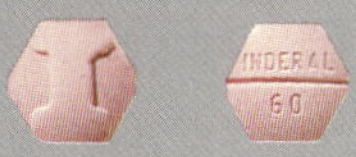 **Inderal 60 mg** Wyeth-Ayerst I 60

℞

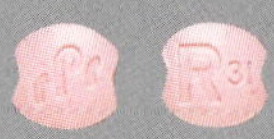

Regroton
Rhone-Poulenc Rorer R31

℞

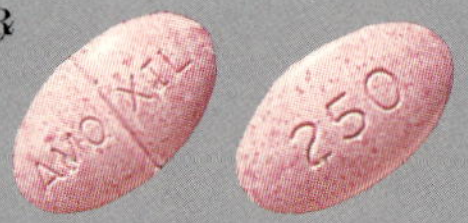

Amoxil 250 mg Chewable
SmithKline Beecham 250

℞

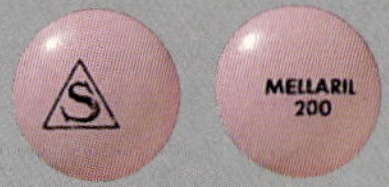

Mellaril 200 mg
Sandoz 200

℞

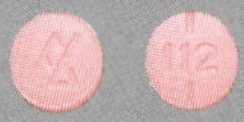

Levothroid 112 mcg
Forest Pharm 112

℞

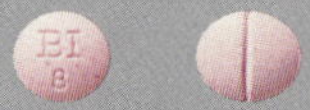

Combipres 0.1 mg
Boehringer Ingelheim BI 8

℞

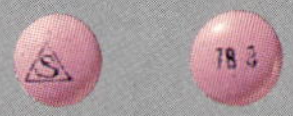

Mellaril 15 mg
Sandoz 78-8

C-IV

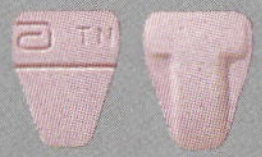

Tranxene 15 mg
Abbott TN

℞

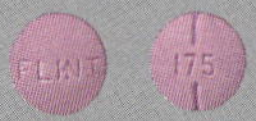

Synthroid 0.175 mg
Knoll Flint 175

℞

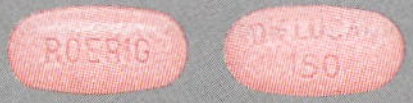

Diflucan 150 mg
Pfizer Roerig 150

℞

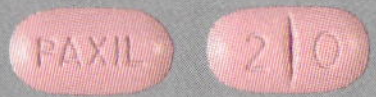

Paxil 20 mg
SmithKline Beecham 20

℞

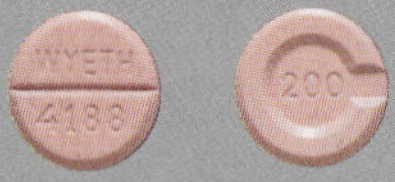

Cordarone 200 mg
Wyeth-Ayerst C 200 4188

℞

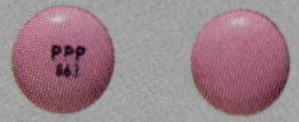

Prolixin 1 mg
Apothecon PPP 863

℞

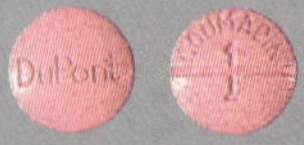

Coumadin 1 mg
DuPont 1

℞

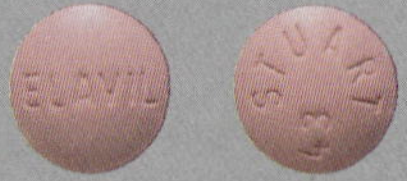

Elavil 100 mg
Zeneca Stuart 43

℞

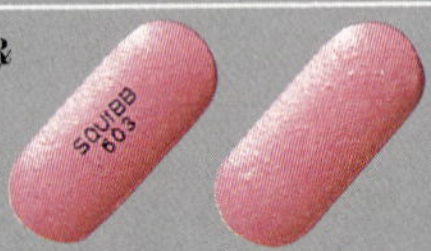

Sumycin 500 mg
Apothecon Squibb 603

℞

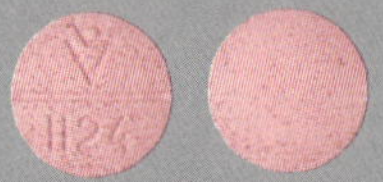

Dilor G
Savage 1124

℞

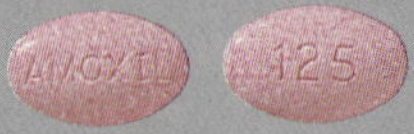

Amoxil 125 mg Chewable
SmithKline Beecham 125

℞

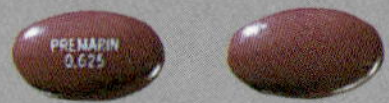

Premarin 0.625 mg
Wyeth-Ayerst 0.625

℞

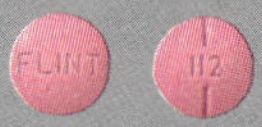

Synthroid 0.112 mg
Knoll Flint 112

℞

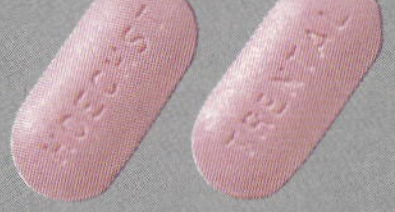

Trental 400 mg
Hoechst Marion Roussel

℞

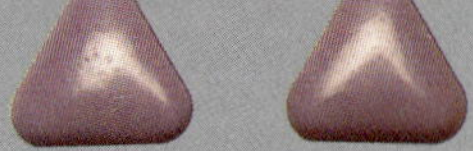

Atarax 100 100 mg
Roerig 100

℞

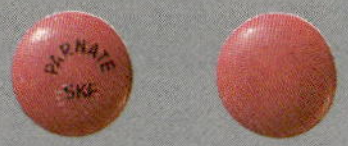

Parnate 10 mg
SmithKline Beecham SKF

℞

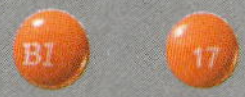

Persantine 25 mg
Boehringer Ingelheim BI 17

C-IV

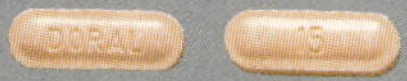

Doral 15 mg
Wallace 15

℞

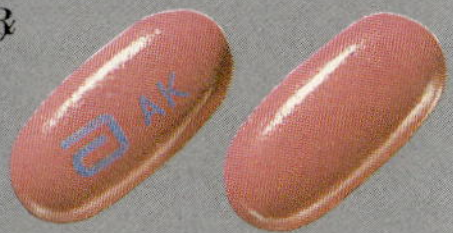

Iberet-Folic-500
Abbott AK

℞

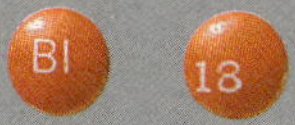

Persantine 50 mg
Boehringer Ingelheim BI 18

C-IV

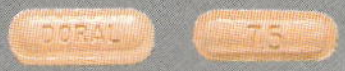

Doral 7.5 mg
Wallace 7.5

℞

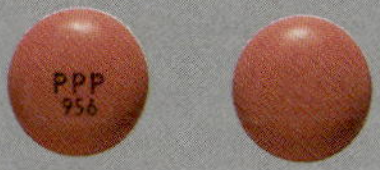

Prolixin 10 mg
Apothecon PPP 956

℞

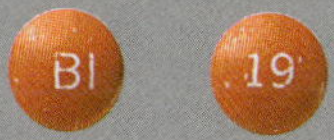

Persantine 75 mg
Boehringer Ingelheim BI 19

℞

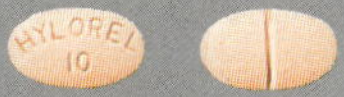

Hylorel 10 mg
Fisons 10

℞

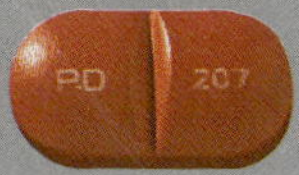

Procan SR 1000 mg
Parke-Davis P-D 207

℞

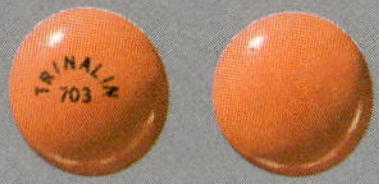

Trinalin Repetabs
Key 703

℞

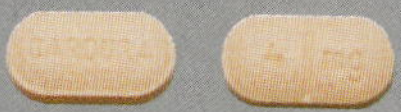

Cardura 4 mg
Roerig 4

℞

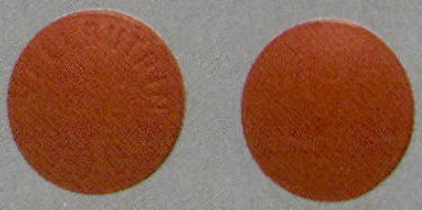

Wellbutrin 100 mg
Glaxo Wellcome 100

℞

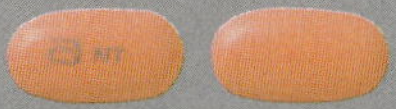

Depakote 125 mg
Abbott NT

℞

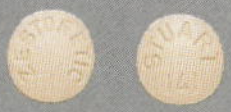

Zestoretic 10/12.5 mg
Zeneca Stuart 141

℞

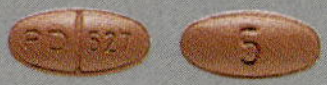

Accupril 5 mg
Parke-Davis PD 527 5

℞

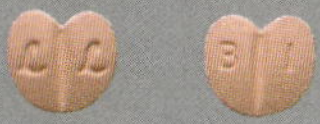

Zebeta 5 mg
Lederle LL B1

℞

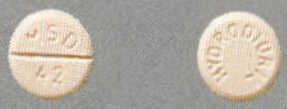

HydroDIURIL 25 mg
Merck MSD 42

C-IV

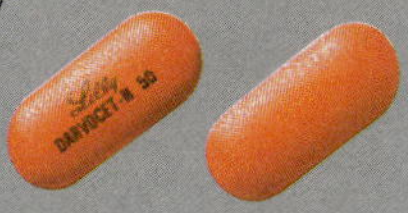

Darvocet-N 50
Lilly 50

℞

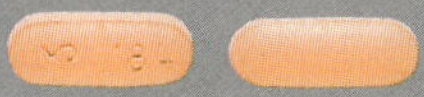

Metoprolol Tartrate 50 mg
Mutual MP 184

℞

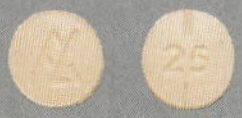

Levothroid 25 mcg
Forest Pharm 25

℞

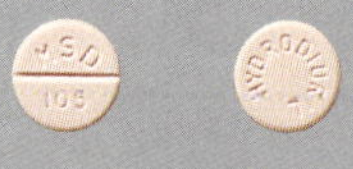

HydroDIURIL 50 mg
Merck MSD 105

℞

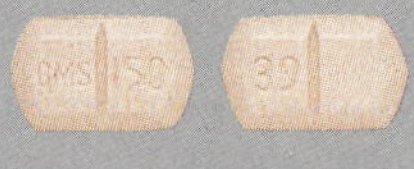

Serzone 150 mg
B-M Squibb BMS 150 39

℞

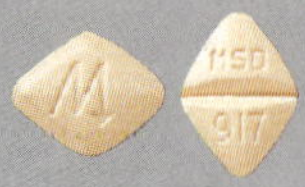

Moduretic
Merck MSD 917

℞

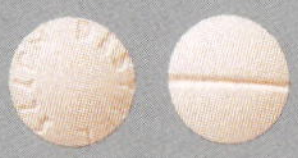

Desyrel 50 mg
Mead Johnson MJ 775

℞

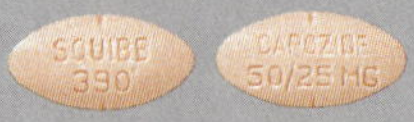

Capozide 50/25
B-M Squibb 390 50/25

℞

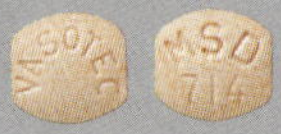

Vasotec 20 mg
Merck MSD 714

℞

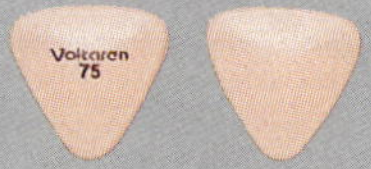

Voltaren 75 mg
Ciba Geneva 75

℞

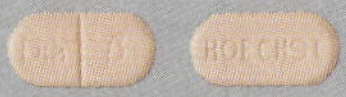

DiaBeta 1.25 mg
Hoechst Marion Roussel Dia ß

℞

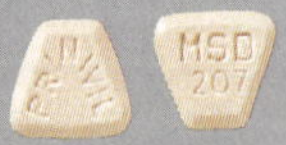

Prinivil 20 mg
Merck MSD 207

℞

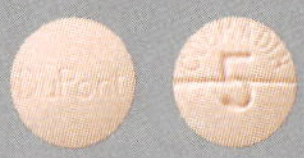

Coumadin 5 mg
DuPont 5

℞

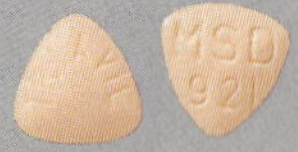

Triavil 2-25
Merck MSD 921

℞

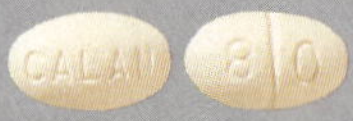

Calan 80 mg
Searle 80

℞

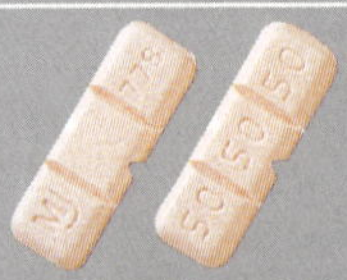

Desyrel Dividose 150 mg
Mead Johnson MJ 778 50

℞

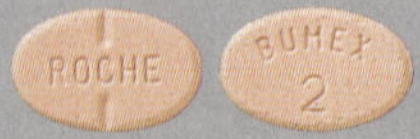

Bumex 2 mg
Roche 2

C-II

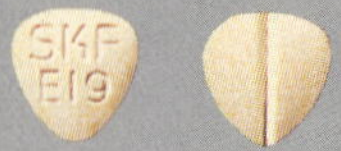

Dexedrine 5 mg
SmithKline Beecham SKF E19

℞

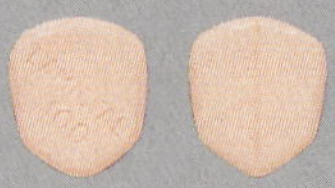

Lamictal 100 mg
Glaxo Wellcome 100

℞

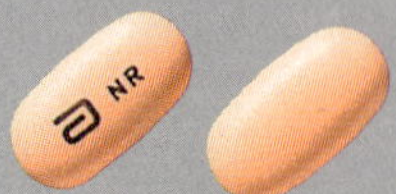

Depakote 250 mg
Abbott NR

℞

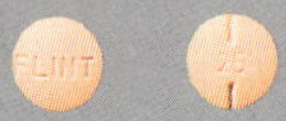

Synthroid 0.025 mg
Knoll Flint 25

℞

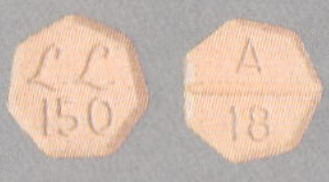

Asendin 150 mg
Lederle LL 150 A18

℞

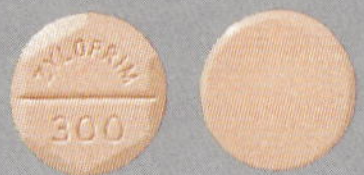

Zyloprim 300 mg
Glaxo Wellcome 300

℞

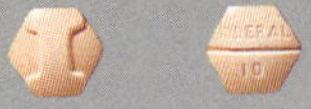

Inderal 10 mg
Wyeth-Ayerst I 10

℞

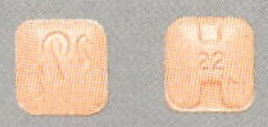

Hygroton 25 mg
Rhone-Poulenc Rorer H 22

℞

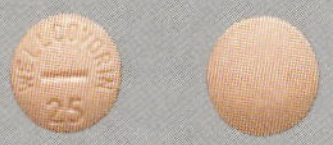

Wellcovorin 25 mg
Glaxo Wellcome 25

℞

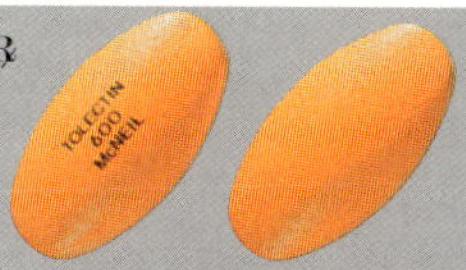

Tolectin 600 600 mg
McNeil 600

℞

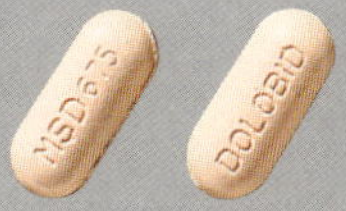

Dolobid 250 mg
Merck MSD 675

℞

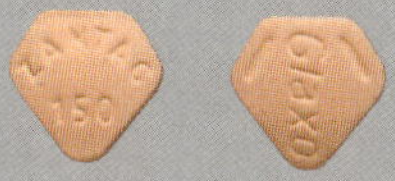

Zantac 150 mg
Glaxo Wellcome 150

C-IV

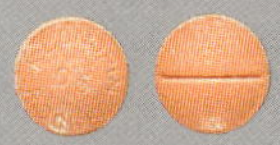

Klonopin 0.5 mg
Roche 0.5

℞

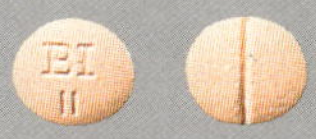

Catapres 0.3 mg
Boehringer Ingelheim BI 11

℞

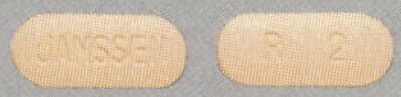

Risperdal 2 mg
Janssen R 2

℞

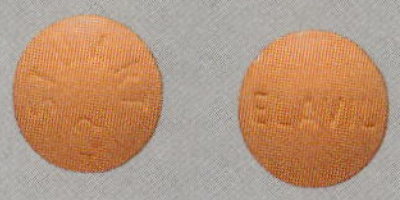

Elavil 75 mg
Zeneca Stuart 42

℞

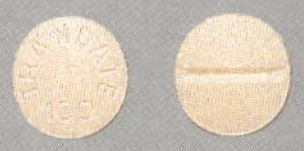

Trandate 100 mg
Glaxo Wellcome 100

℞

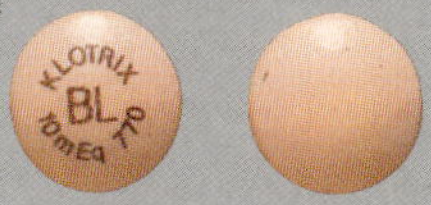

Klotrix 10 mEq
Bristol BL 770

℞

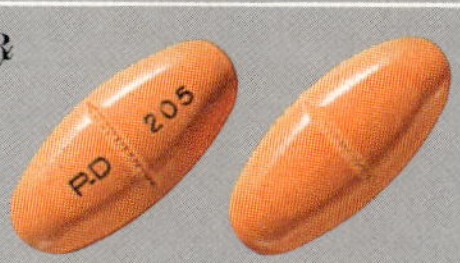

Procan SR 750 mg
Parke-Davis P-D 205

℞

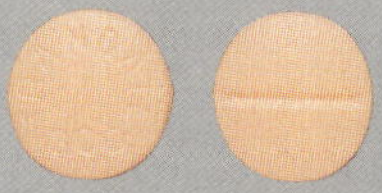

Trandate 300 mg
Glaxo Wellcome 300

C-II

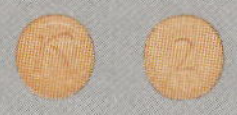

Dilaudid 2 mg
Knoll 2

℞

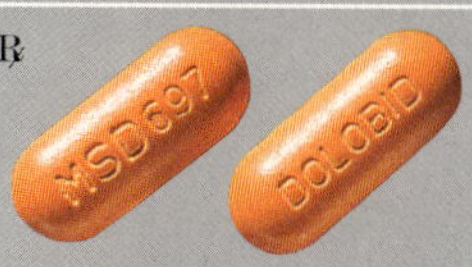

Dolobid 500 mg
Merck MSD 697

℞

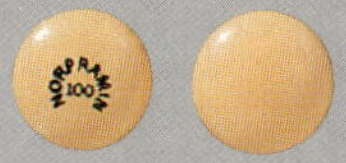

Norpramin 100 mg
Hoechst Marion Roussel 100

℞

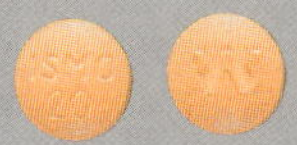

ISMO 20 mg
Wyeth-Ayerst W20

℞

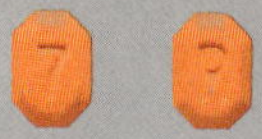

Lozol 1.25 mg
Rhone-Poulenc Rorer 7 R

℞

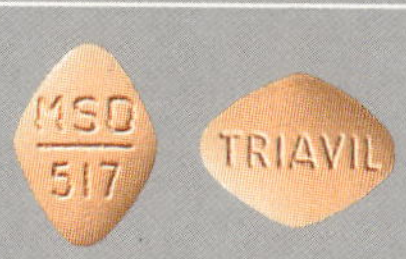

Triavil 4-50
Merck MSD 517

℞

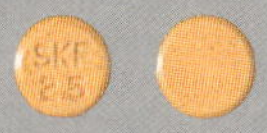

Vontrol 25 mg
SmithKline Beecham SKF 25

℞

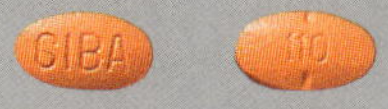

Ludiomil 25 mg
Ciba Geneva 110

℞
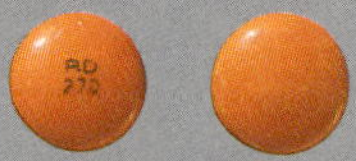

Nardil 15 mg
Parke-Davis P-D 270

℞
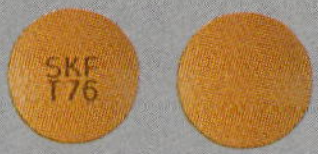

Thorazine 50 mg
SmithKline Beecham SKF T76

℞
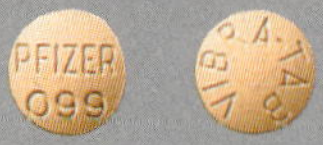

Vibra-Tabs 100 mg
Pfizer 099

℞
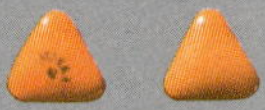

Atarax 10 mg
Roerig 10

℞
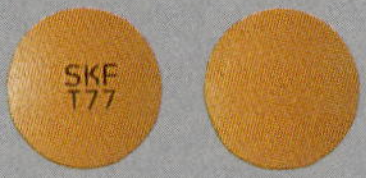

Thorazine 100 mg
SmithKline Beecham SKF T77

℞
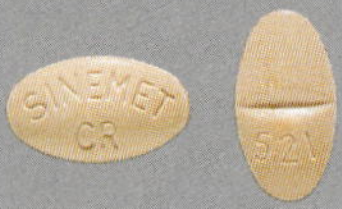

Sinemet CR
DuPont 521

℞
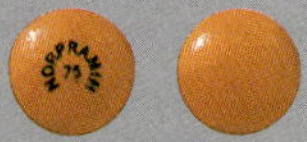

Norpramin 75 mg
Hoechst Marion Roussel 75

℞
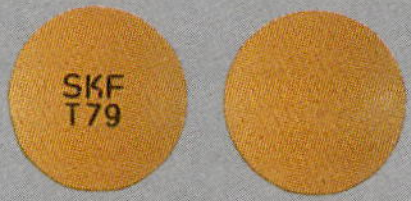

Thorazine 200 mg
SmithKline Beecham SKF T79

C-IV
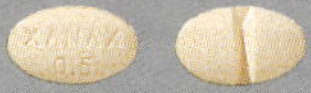

Xanax 0.5 mg
Upjohn 0.5

C-IV
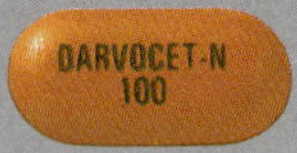

Darvocet-N 100
Lilly 100

℞
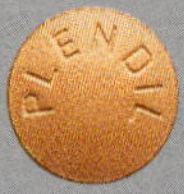

Plendil 10 mg
Astra Merck

℞
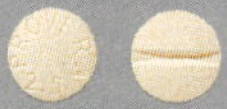

Provera 2.5 mg
Upjohn 2.5

℞
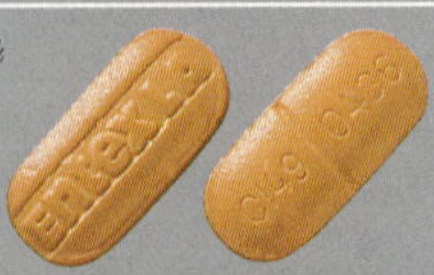

Entex LA
Procter & Gamble 0149 0436

C-II
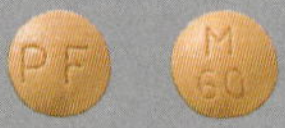

MS Contin 60 mg
Purdue Frederick PF M 60

℞
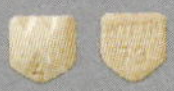

Wytensin 4 mg
Wyeth-Ayerst W4 73

℞
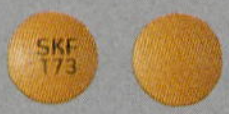

Thorazine 10 mg
SmithKline Beecham SKF T73

℞
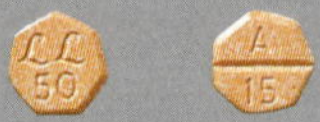

Asendin 50 mg
Lederle LL 50 A15

℞
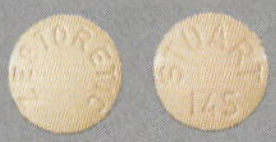

Zestoretic 20/25
Zeneca Stuart 145

℞
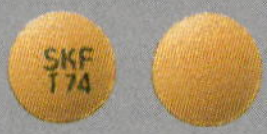

Thorazine 25 mg
SmithKline Beecham SKF T74

℞
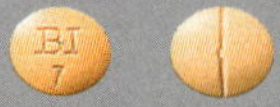

Catapres 0.2 mg
Boehringer Ingelheim BI 7

C-IV
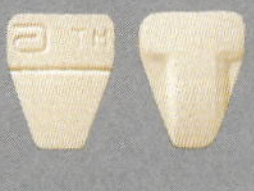

Tranxene 7.5 mg
Abbott TM

℞
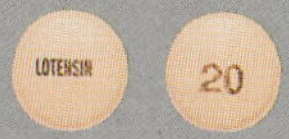

Lotensin 20 mg
Ciba Geneva 20

℞
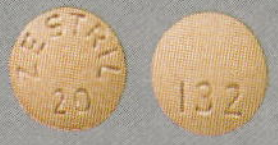

Zestril 20 mg
Zeneca 20 132

℞
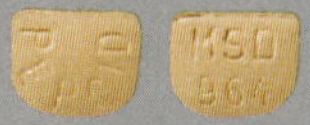

Pepcid 40 mg
Merck MSD 964

℞
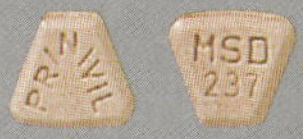

Prinivil 40 mg
Merck MSD 237

℞
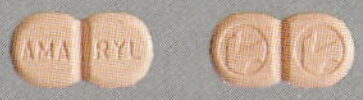

Amaryl 1 mg
Hoechst Marion Roussel

℞
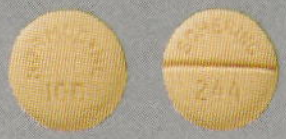

Normodyne 100 mg
Schering 100 244

℞
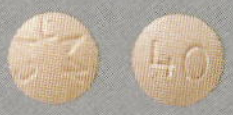

Calan 40 mg
Searle 40

℞
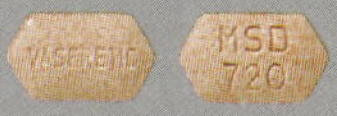

Vaseretic 10-25
Merck MSD 720

℞
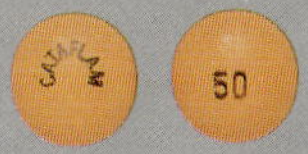

Cataflam 50 mg
Ciba Geneva 50

℞
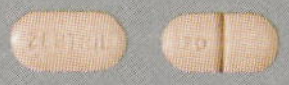

Zestril 5 mg
Zeneca 130

℞
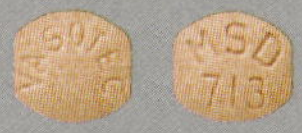

Vasotec 10 mg
Merck MSD 713

℞
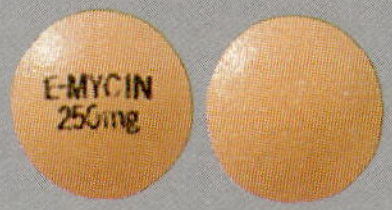

E-Mycin 250 mg
Knoll 250

℞
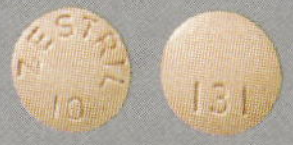

Zestril 10 mg
Zeneca 10 131

℞
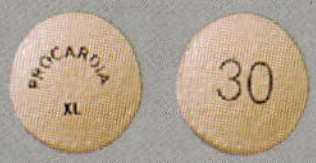

Procardia XL 30 mg
Pratt Pfizer 30

℞
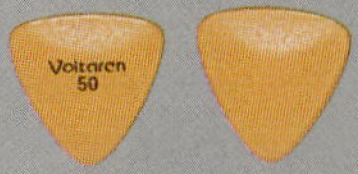

Voltaren 50 mg
Ciba Geneva 50

℞
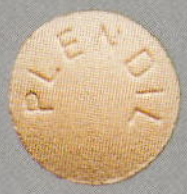

Plendil 5 mg
Astra Merck

℞
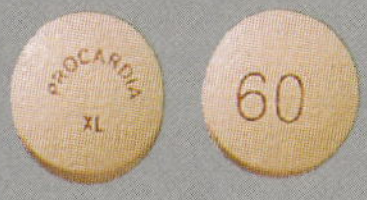

Procardia XL 60 mg
Pratt Pfizer 60

℞
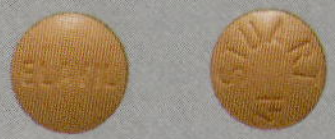

Elavil 50 mg
Zeneca Stuart 41

℞
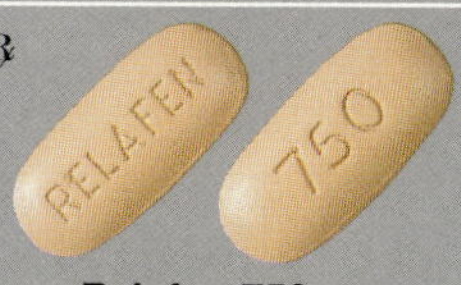

Relafen 750 mg
SmithKline Beecham 750

℞
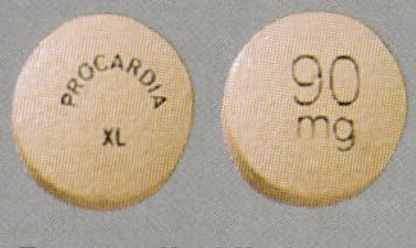

Procardia XL 90 mg
Pratt Pfizer 90

℞
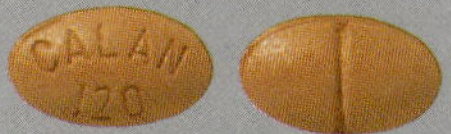

Calan 120 mg
Searle 120

℞

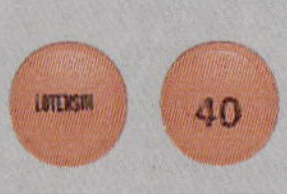

Lotensin 40 mg
Ciba Geneva 40

℞

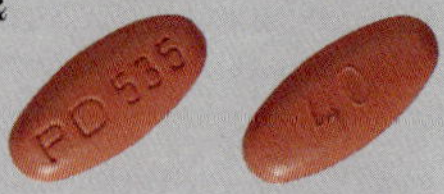

Accupril 40 mg
Parke-Davis P-D 535 40

℞

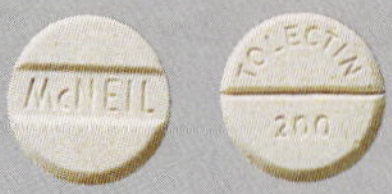

Tolectin 200 200 mg
McNeil 200

℞

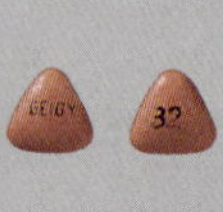

Tofranil 10 mg
Ciba Geneva Geigy 32

℞

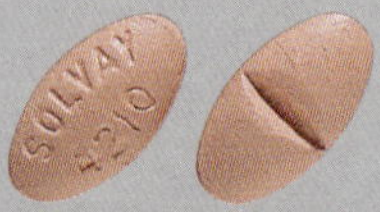

Luvox 100 mg
Solvay 4210

℞

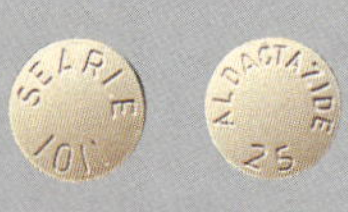

Aldactazide 25/25
Searle 1011 25

℞

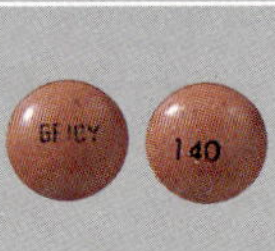

Tofranil 25 mg
Ciba Geneva Geigy 140

℞

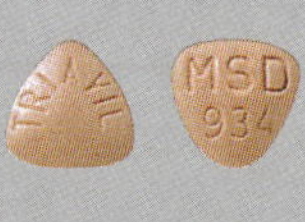

Triavil 4-10
Merck MSD 934

℞

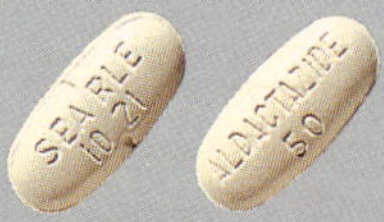

Aldactazide 50/50
Searle 1021 50

℞

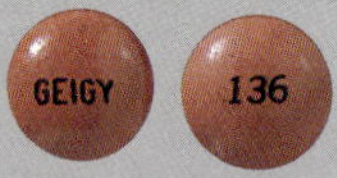

Tofranil 50 mg
Ciba Geneva Geigy 136

℞

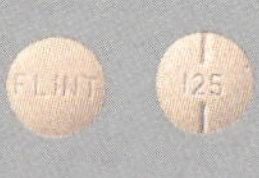

Synthroid 0.125 mg
Knoll Flint 125

℞

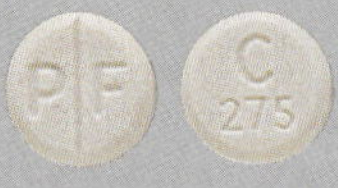

Cardioquin 275 mg
Purdue Frederick PF C275

℞

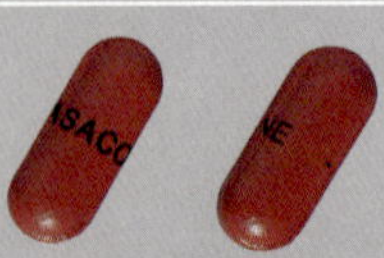

Asacol 400 mg
Procter & Gamble NE

℞

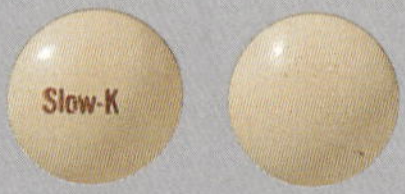

Slow-K 8 mEq
Ciba Geneva

℞

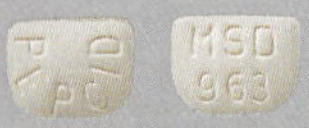

Pepcid 20 mg
Merck MSD 963

℞

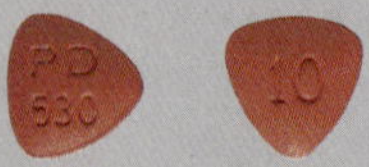

Accupril 10 mg
Parke-Davis P-D 530 10

℞

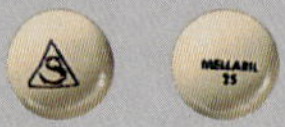

Mellaril 25 mg
Sandoz 25

℞

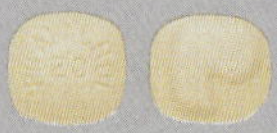

Pravachol 20 mg
B-M Squibb P 20

℞

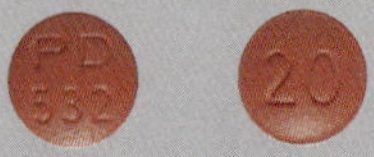

Accupril 20 mg
Parke-Davis P-D 532 20

℞

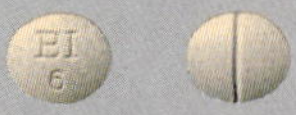

Catapres 0.1 mg
Boehringer Ingelheim BI 6

℞

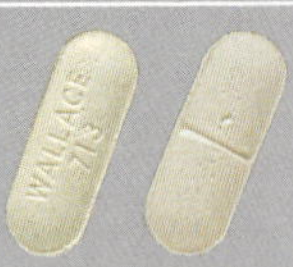

Rynatan
Wallace 713

℞

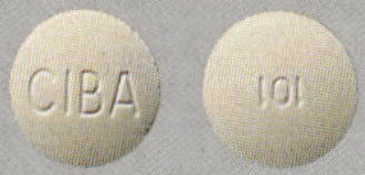

Apresoline 100 mg
Ciba Geneva 101

C-III

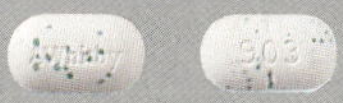

Lortab 7.5/500
Whitby 903

C-III

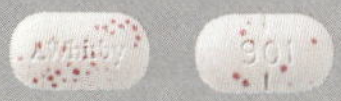

Lortab 2.5/500
Whitby 901

℞

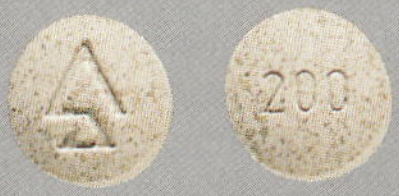

Ilozyme
Savage 200

℞

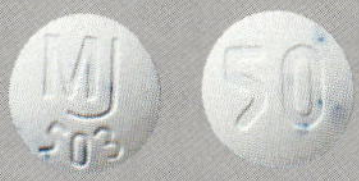

Cytoxan 50 mg
BMSOI MJ 503 50

℞

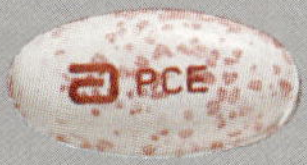

PCE 333 mg
Abbott

℞

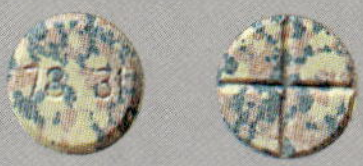

Bellergal-S
Sandoz 78-31

℞

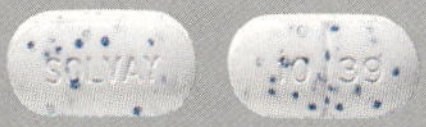

Histalet Forte
Solvay 1039

℞

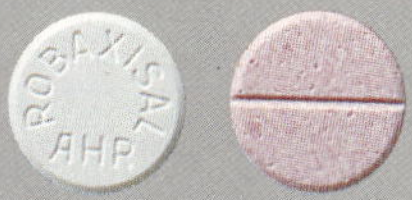

Robaxisal
Robins AHR

℞

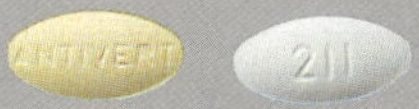

Antivert/25 25 mg
Roerig 211

℞

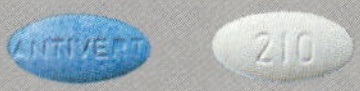

Antivert 12.5 mg
Roerig 210

℞

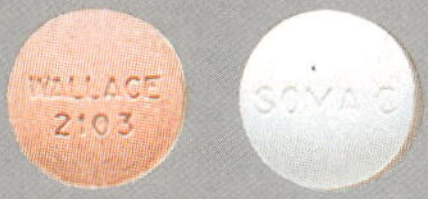

Soma Compound
Wallace 2103

C-III

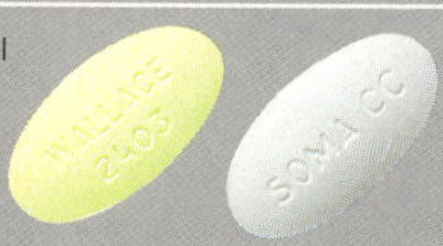

Soma Compound w/ Codeine
Wallace 2403 CC

℞

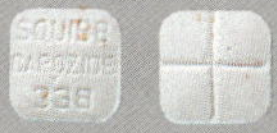

Capozide 25/15
B-M Squibb 338

C-II

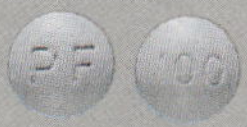

MS Contin 100 mg
Purdue Frederick PF 100

℞

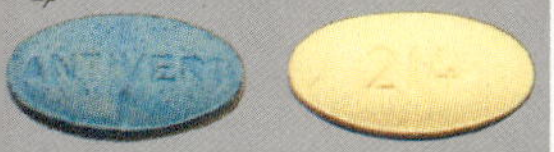

Antivert/50 50 mg
Roerig 214

℞

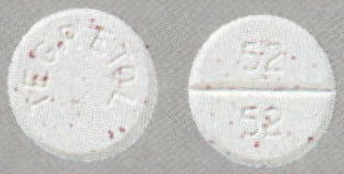

Tegretol 100 mg Chewable
Ciba Geneva 52 52

℞

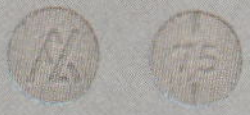

Levothroid 75 mcg
Forest Pharm 75

C-III

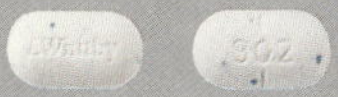

Lortab 5/500
Whitby 902

℞

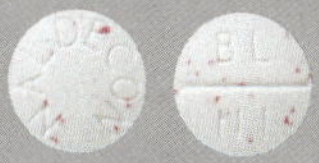

Naldecon
Apothecon BL N1

℞

Nitrostat 0.3 mg
Parke-Davis

℞
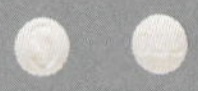
Sorbitrate 2.5 mg Sublingual
Zeneca S 853

℞
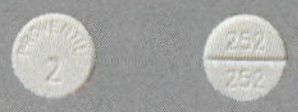
Proventil 2 mg
Schering 2 252

℞
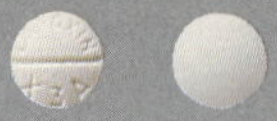
Lanoxin 0.25 mg
Glaxo Wellcome X3A

℞
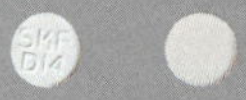
Cytomel 5 mcg
SmithKline Beecham SKF D14

℞
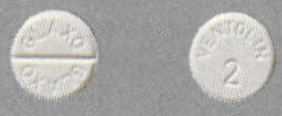
Ventolin 2 mg
Glaxo Wellcome 2

℞
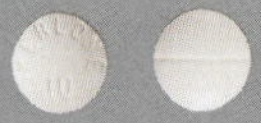
Kerlone 10 mg
Searle 10

C-V
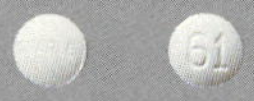
Lomotil
Searle 61

℞
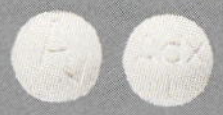
Arimidex 1 mg
Zeneca Adx 1

℞
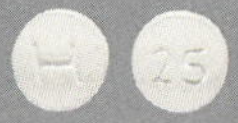
Imitrex 25 mg
Glaxo Wellcome I 25

℞
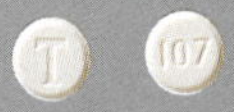
Tenormin 25 mg
Zeneca T 107

℞
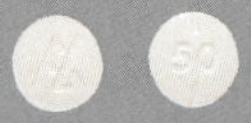
Levothroid 50 mcg
Forest Pharm 50

℞
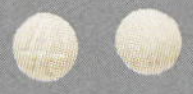
Armour Thyroid 1/4 gr
Forest Pharm A TC

C-II
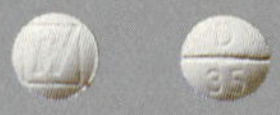
Demerol HCl 50 mg
Sanofi Winthrop WD 35

℞
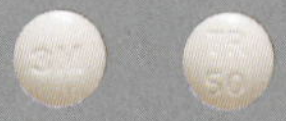
Tambocor 50 mg
3M Pharm TR 50

℞
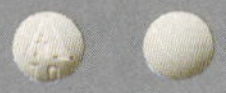
Armour Thyroid 1/2 gr
Forest Pharm A TD

℞
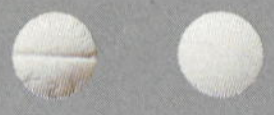
Myleran 2 mg
Glaxo Wellcome K2A

℞
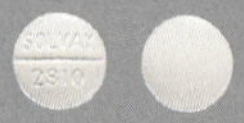
Orasone 5 mg
Solvay 2810

℞
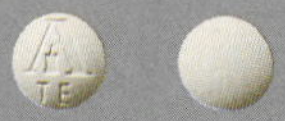
Armour Thyroid 1 gr
Forest Pharm A TE

℞
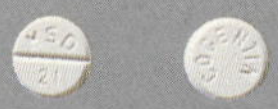
Cogentin 0.5 mg
Merck MSD 21

℞
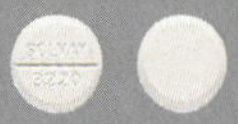
Dexone 4 mg
Solvay 3220

℞
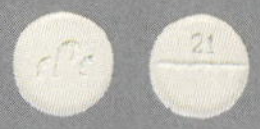
Hygroton 100 mg
Rhone-Poulenc Rorer 21

℞
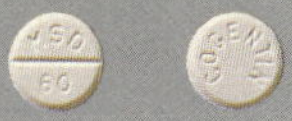
Cogentin 2 mg
Merck MSD 60

℞
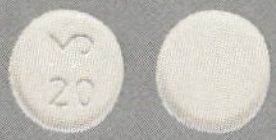
Ergoloid Mesylate 1 mg
Mutual MP 20

℞
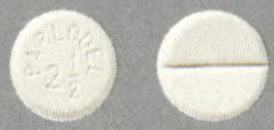
Parlodel 2.5 mg
Sandoz 2 1/2

℞
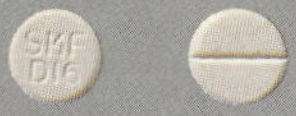
Cytomel 25 mcg
SmithKline Beecham SKF D16

℞
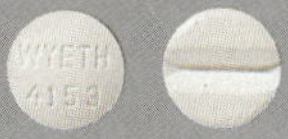
Isordil Titradose 10 mg
Wyeth-Ayerst 4153

℞
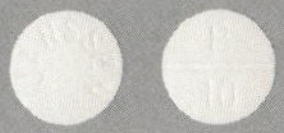
Propulsid 10 mg
Janssen P 10

℞
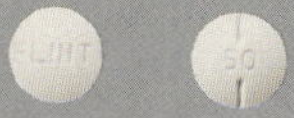
Synthroid 0.05 mg
Knoll Flint 50

℞
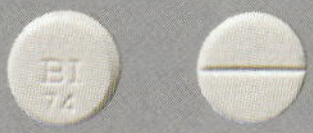
Alupent 10 mg
Boehringer Ingelheim BI 74

℞
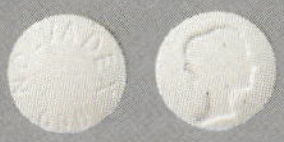
Nolvadex 10 mg
Zeneca 600

℞
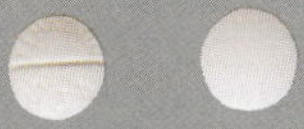
Kemadrin 5 mg
Glaxo Wellcome S3A

℞
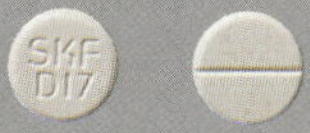
Cytomel 50 mcg
SmithKline Beecham SKF D17

℞
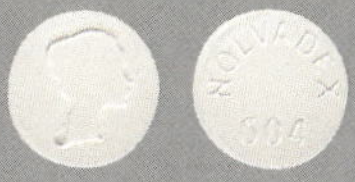
Nolvadex 20 mg
Zeneca 604

℞
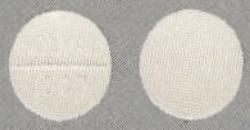
Curretab 10 mg
Solvay 1007

C-IV
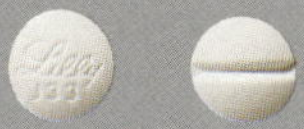
Phenobarbital 100 mg
Lilly J33

℞
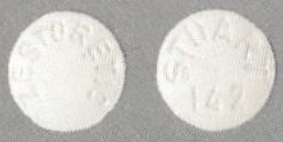
Zestoretic 20/12.5
Zeneca Stuart 142

℞
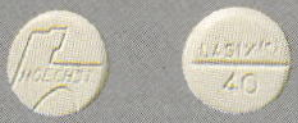
Lasix 40 mg
Hoechst Marion Roussel 40

℞
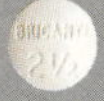
Bricanyl 2.5 mg
Hoechst Marion Roussel 2 1/2

℞
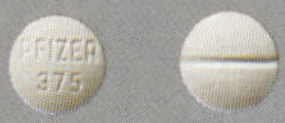
Renese 1 mg
Pfizer 375

℞
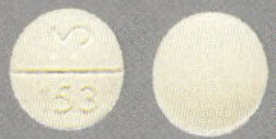
Atenolol/Chlorthalidone 50/25
Mutual MP 153

℞
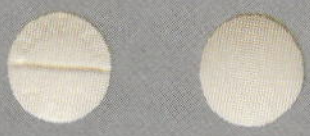
Alkeran 2 mg
Glaxo Wellcome A2A

℞
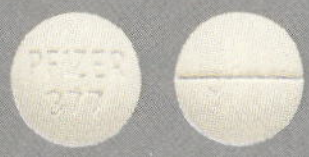
Renese 4 mg
Pfizer 377

℞
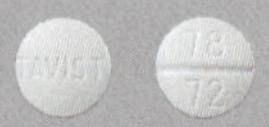

Tavist 2.68 mg
Sandoz 78 72

℞
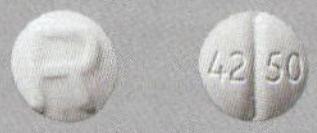

Donnatal
Robins R 4250

℞
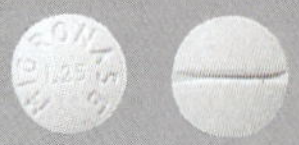
Micronase 1.25 mg
Upjohn 1.25

℞
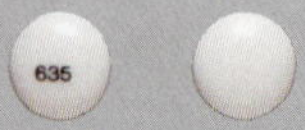

Leukeran 2 mg
Glaxo Wellcome 635

℞
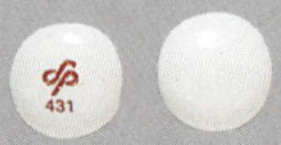

Proventil Repetabs
Schering 431

℞
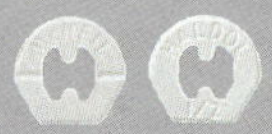
Haldol 0.5 mg
McNeil 1/2

℞
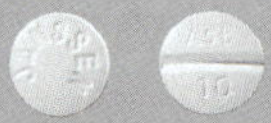
Hismanal 10 mg
Janssen AST 10

C-II
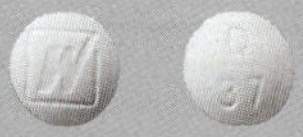
Demerol HCl 100 mg
Sanofi Winthrop WD 37

℞
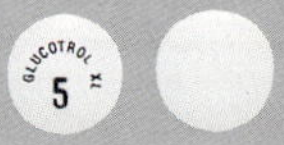

Glucotrol XL 5 mg
Pratt Pfizer 5

℞
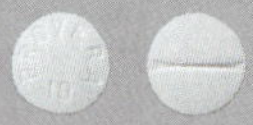
Provera 10 mg
Upjohn 10

℞
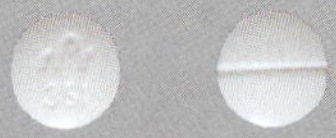
Slo-Phyllin 100 mg
Rhone-Poulenc Rorer 351

℞
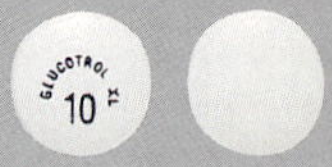

Glucotrol XL 10 mg
Pratt Pfizer 10

℞
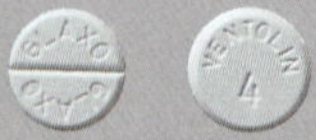

Ventolin 4 mg
Glaxo Wellcome 4

℞
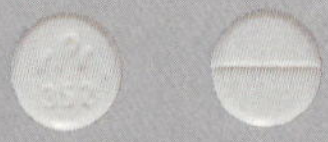
Slo-Phyllin 200 mg
Rhone-Poulenc Rorer 352

℞
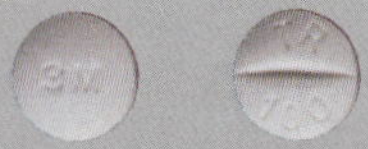
Tambocor 100 mg
3M Pharm TR 100

℞
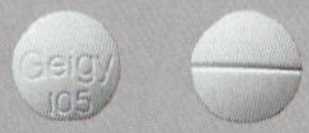

Brethine 5 mg
Ciba Geneva Geigy 105

℞
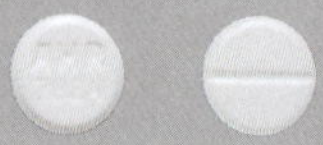
Robinul 1 mg
Robins AHR 7824

℞
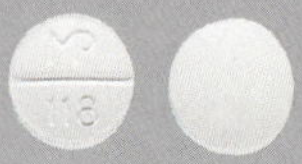
Trazodone HCl 50 mg
Mutual MP 118

℞
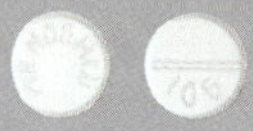
Tenormin 50 mg
Zeneca 105

℞
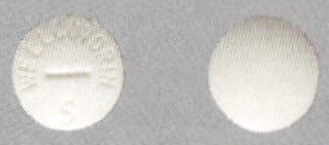
Wellcovorin 5 mg
Glaxo Wellcome 5

℞
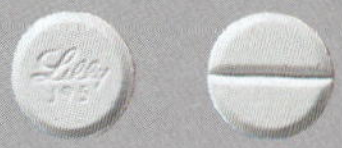
Tapazole 10 mg
Lilly J95

℞

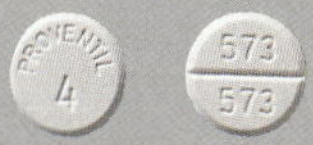

Proventil 4 mg
Schering 4 573

℞

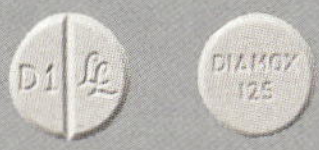

Diamox 125 mg
Lederle D1 LL 125

℞

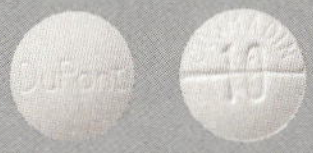

Coumadin 10 mg
DuPont 10

℞

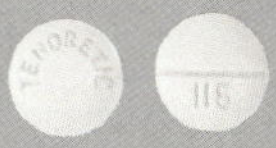

Tenoretic 50
Zeneca 115

℞

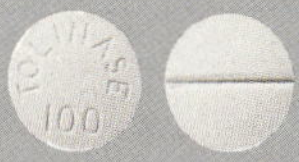

Tolinase 100 mg
Upjohn 100

℞

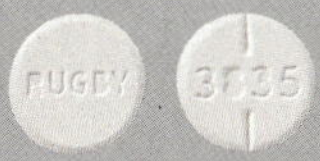

Furosemide 80 mg
Rugby 3835

℞

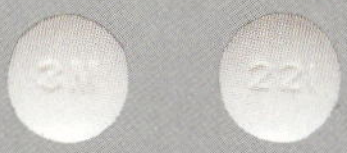

Norflex 100 mg
3M Pharm 221

℞

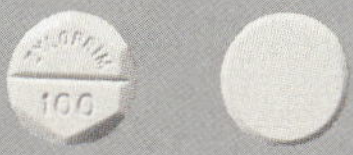

Zyloprim 100 mg
Glaxo Wellcome 100

℞

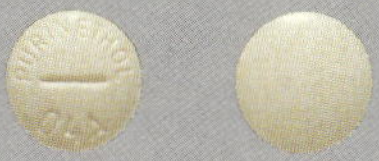

Purinethol 50 mg
Glaxo Wellcome 04A

C-IV

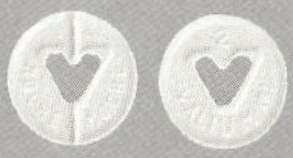

Valium 2 mg
Roche 2

℞

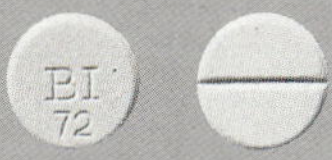

Alupent 20 mg
Boehringer Ingelheim BI 72

℞

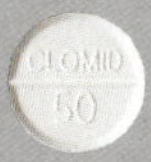

Clomid 50 mg
Hoechst Marion Roussel 50

℞

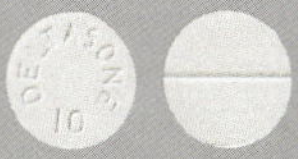

Deltasone 10 mg
Upjohn 10

℞

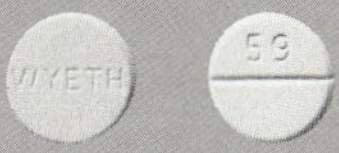

Pen•Vee K 250 mg
Wyeth-Ayerst 59

℞

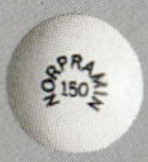

Norpramin 150 mg
Hoechst Marion Roussel 150

℞

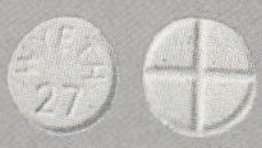

Phenergan 25 mg
Wyeth-Ayerst 27

℞

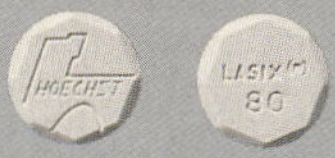

Lasix 80 mg
Hoechst Marion Roussel 80

℞

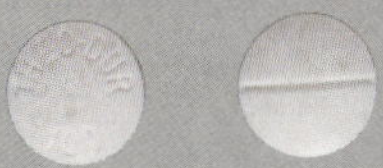

Theo-Dur 100 mg
Key 100

℞

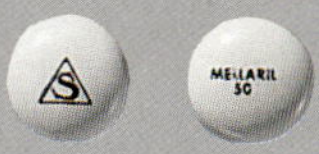

Mellaril 50 mg
Sandoz 50

℞

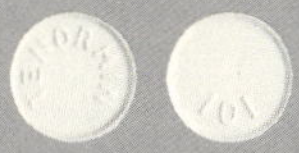

Tenormin 100 mg
Zeneca 101

℞

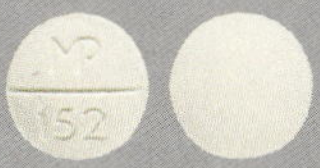

Atenolol/Chlorthalidone 100/25 mg
Mutual MP 152

℞

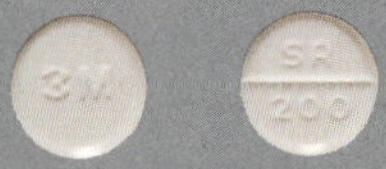

Theolair-SR 200 mg
3M Pharm SR 200

℞

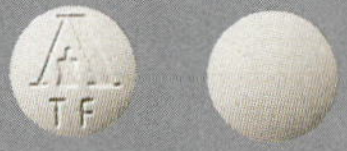

Armour Thyroid 2 gr
Forest Pharm A TF

℞

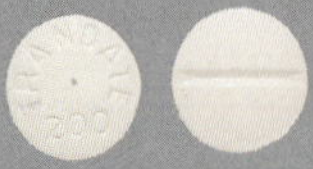

Trandate 200 mg
Glaxo Wellcome 200

℞

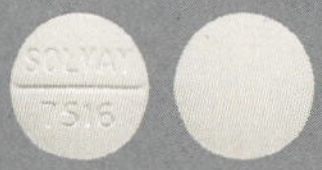

Lithotabs 300 mg
Solvay 7516

℞

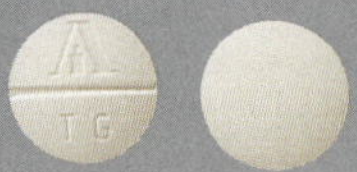

Armour Thyroid 3 gr
Forest Pharm A TG

℞

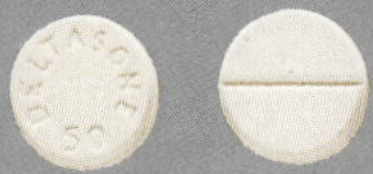

Deltasone 50 mg
Upjohn 50

℞

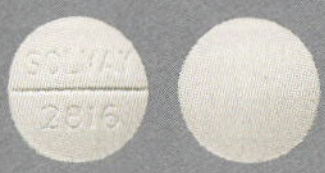

Orasone 50 mg
Solvay 2816

℞

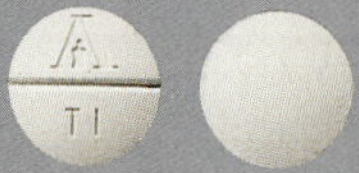

Armour Thyroid 5 gr
Forest Pharm A TI

℞

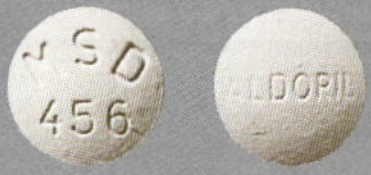

Aldoril-25
Merck MSD 456

℞

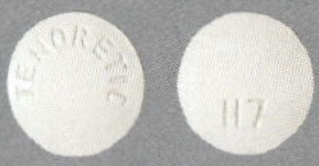

Tenoretic 100
Zeneca 117

℞

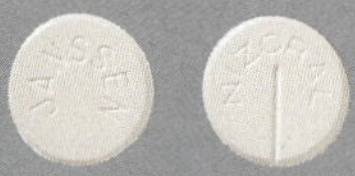

Nizoral 200 mg
Janssen

℞

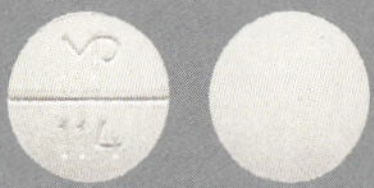

Trazodone HCl 100 mg
Mutual MP 114

℞

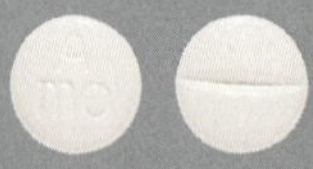

Toprol-XL 50 mg
Astra A MO

℞

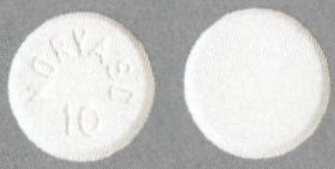

Norvasc 10 mg
Pfizer 10

C-III

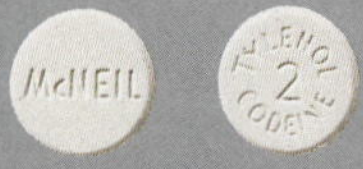

Tylenol w/Codeine No. 2
McNeil 2

℞

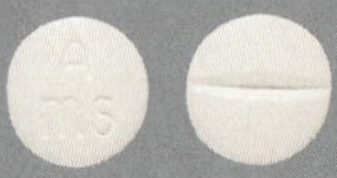

Toprol-XL 100 mg
Astra A MS

℞

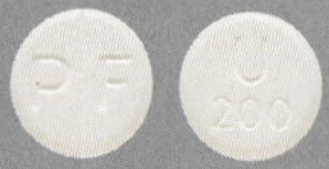

T-Phyl 200 mg
Purdue Frederick PF U200

C-III

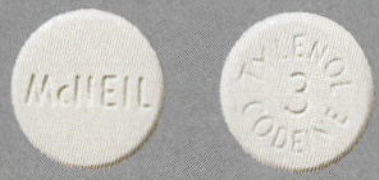

Tylenol w/Codeine No. 3
McNeil 3

℞

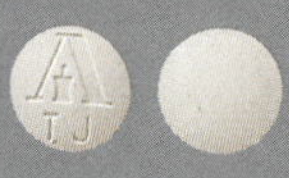

Armour Thyroid 1-1/2 gr
Forest Pharm A TJ

℞

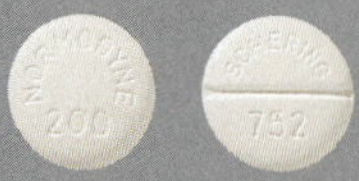

Normodyne 200 mg
Schering 200 752

C-III

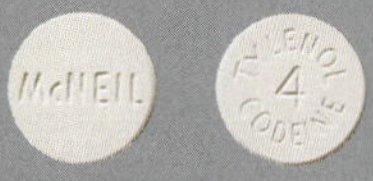

Tylenol w/Codeine No. 4
McNeil 4

℞

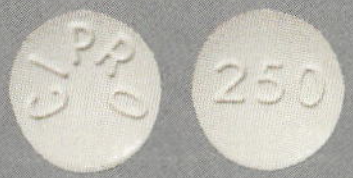

Cipro 250 mg
Bayer Corp 250

℞

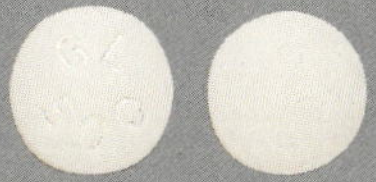

Glucophage 500 mg
B-M Squibb GL 500

℞

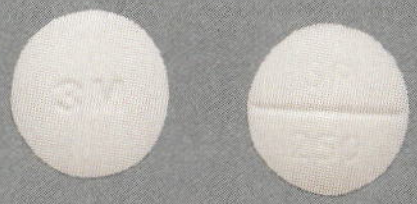

Theolair-SR 250 mg
3M Pharm SR 250

℞

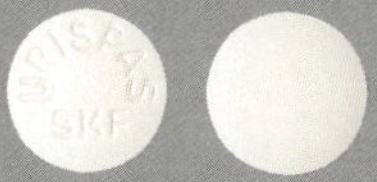

Urispas 100 mg
SmithKline Beecham SKF

℞

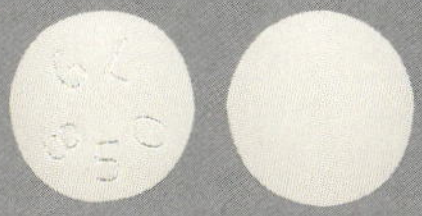

Glucophage 850 mg
B-M Squibb GL 850

℞

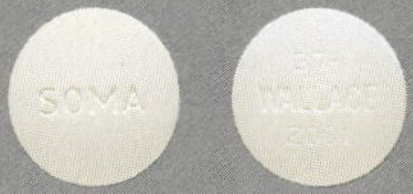

Soma 350 mg
Wallace 37-2001

℞

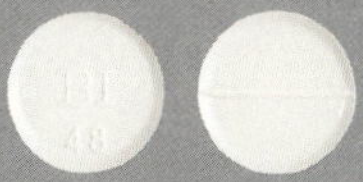

Respbid 250 mg
Boehringer Ingelheim BI 48

℞

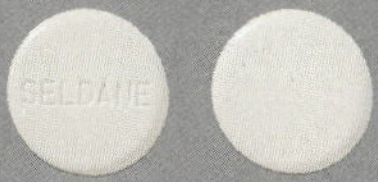

Seldane 60 mg
Hoechst Marion Roussel

℞

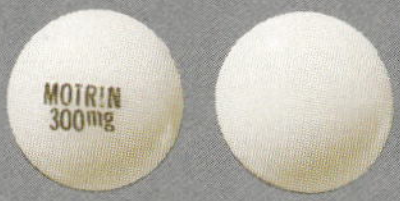

Motrin 300 mg
Upjohn 300

℞

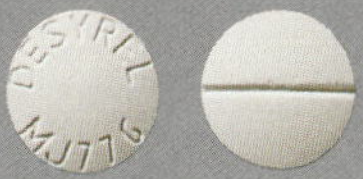

Desyrel 100 mg
Mead Johnson MJ 776

℞

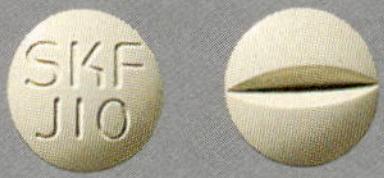

Eskalith CR 450 mg
SmithKline Beecham SKF J10

℞

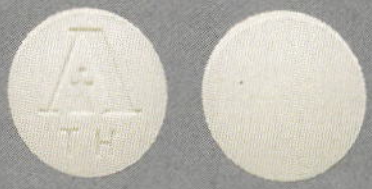

Armour Thyroid 4 gr
Forest Pharm A TH

C-III

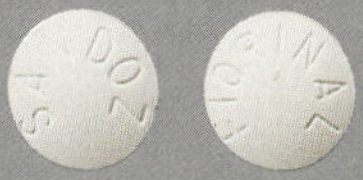

Fiorinal
Sandoz

℞

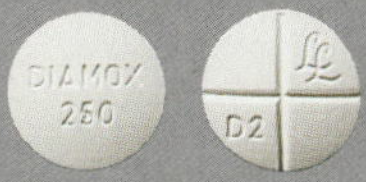

Diamox 250 mg
Lederle 250 D2 LL

℞

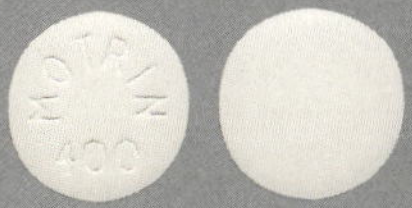

Motrin 400 mg
Upjohn 400

℞

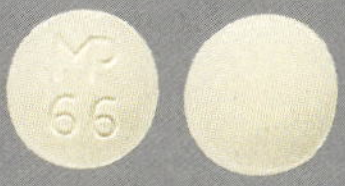

Quinidine Gluconate ER 324 mg
Mutual MP66

℞

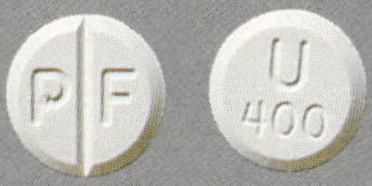

Uniphyl 400 mg
Purdue Frederick PF U400

℞

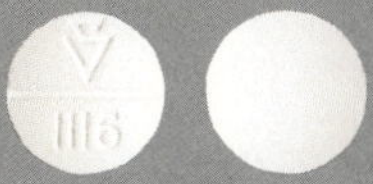

Dilor-400 400 mg
Savage 1115

℞

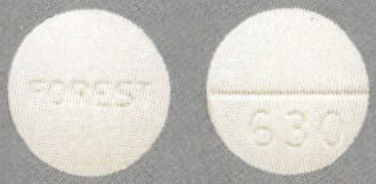

Esgic
Forest Pharm 630

℞

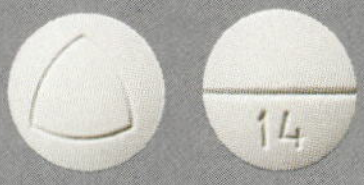

Quadrinal
Knoll 14

℞

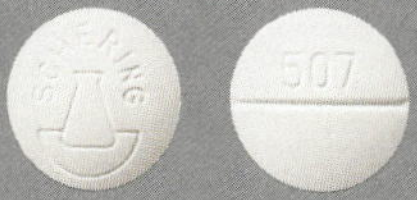

Fulvicin P/G 250 mg
Schering 507

℞
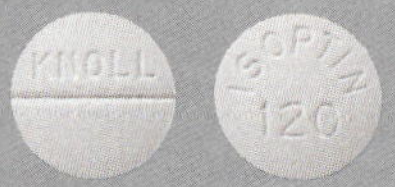

Isoptin 120 mg
Knoll 120

℞
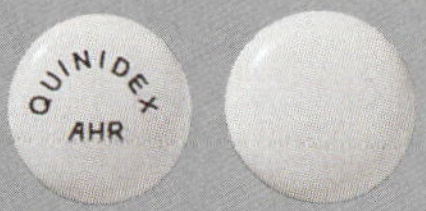

Quinidex Extentabs 300 mg
Robins AHR

C-IV
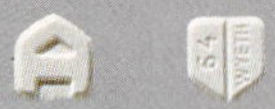
Ativan 1 mg
Wyeth-Ayerst A 64

℞
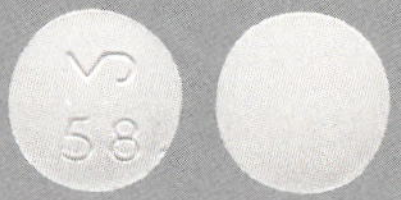

Carisoprodol 350 mg
Mutual MP 58

℞
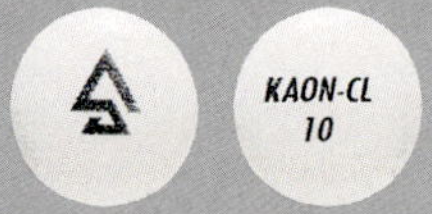

Kaon-CL 10 10 mEq
Savage 10

C-IV
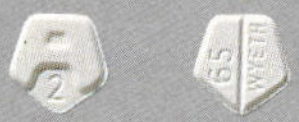
Ativan 2 mg
Wyeth-Ayerst A2 65

℞
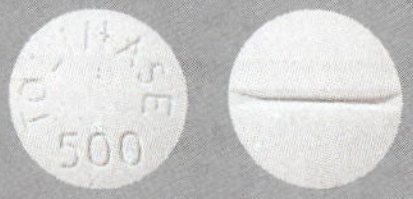

Tolinase 500 mg
Upjohn 500

℞
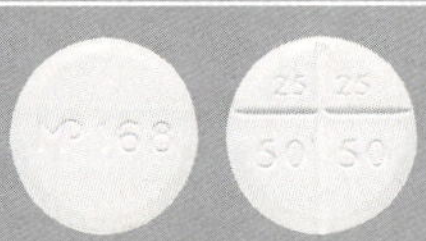
Trazodone HCl 150 mg
Mutual MP 168 25 50

℞
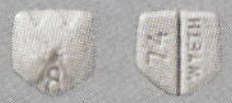
Wytensin 8 mg
Wyeth-Ayerst W8 74

℞
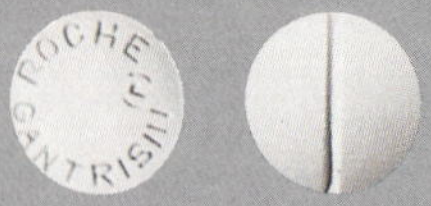

Gantrisin 500 mg
Roche

℞
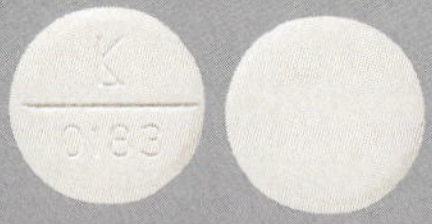
Deconamine Chewable
Kenwood/Bradley K 0183

℞
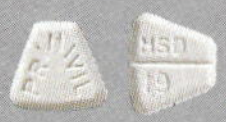
Prinivil 5 mg
Merck MSD 19

℞
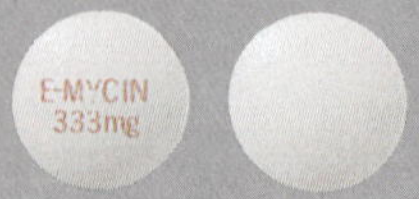

E-Mycin 333 mg
Knoll 333

℞
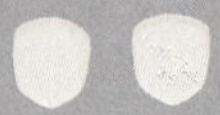
Lamictal 25 mg
Glaxo Wellcome 25

℞
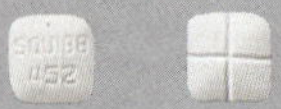
Capoten 25 mg
B-M Squibb 452

C-II
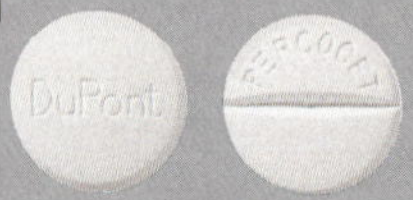

Percocet
DuPont

℞
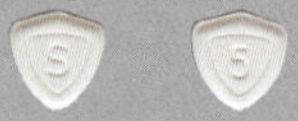
ELDEPRYL 5 mg
Somerset S5

℞
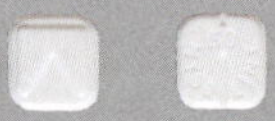
Mysoline 50 mg
Wyeth-Ayerst 50

℞
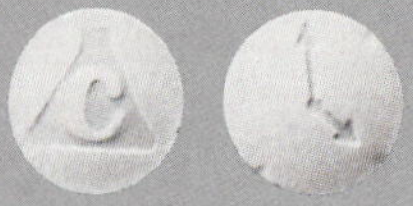
Quinaglute 324 mg SR
Berlex C

C-IV
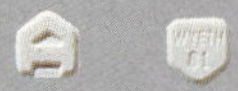
Ativan 0.5 mg
Wyeth-Ayerst A 81

℞
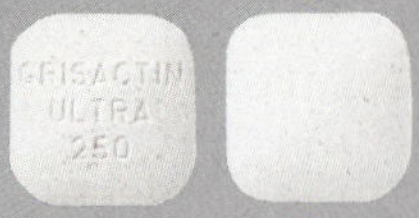

Grisactin Ultra 250 mg
Wyeth-Ayerst 250

℞
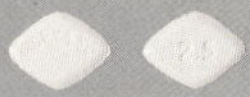
Norvasc 2.5 mg
Pfizer 2.5

℞
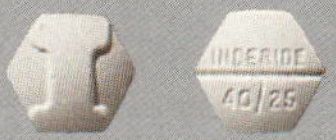
Inderide 40/25
Wyeth-Ayerst I 40/25

℞
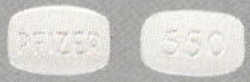
Zyrtec 5 mg
Pfizer 550

℞
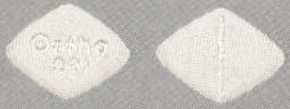
Ortho-Est 0.625 mg
Ortho 1801

℞
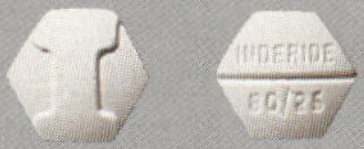
Inderide 80/25
Wyeth-Ayerst I 80/25

℞
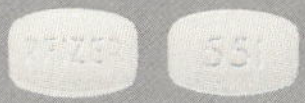
Zyrtec 10 mg
Pfizer 551

℞
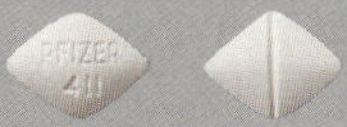
Glucotrol 5 mg
Pratt Pfizer 411

℞
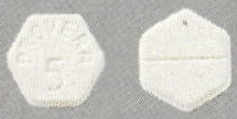
Provera 5 mg
Upjohn 5

℞
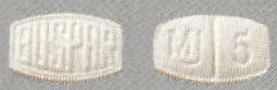
BuSpar 5 mg
B-M Squibb MJ 5

℞
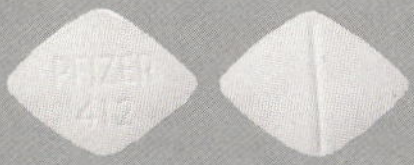
Glucotrol 10 mg
Pratt Pfizer 412

℞
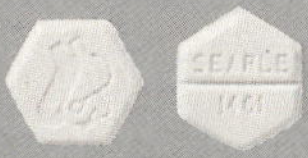
Cytotec 200 mcg
Searle 1461

℞
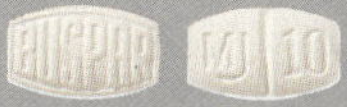
BuSpar 10 mg
B-M Squibb MJ 10

℞
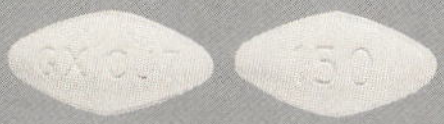
Epivir 150 mg
Glaxo Wellcome GX CJ7 150

℞
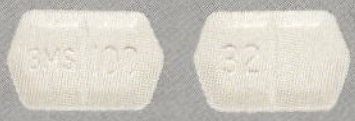
Serzone 100 mg
B-M Squibb BMS 100 32

℞
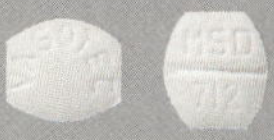
Vasotec 5 mg
Merck MSD 712

℞
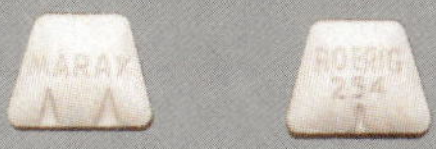
Marax
Roerig 254

℞
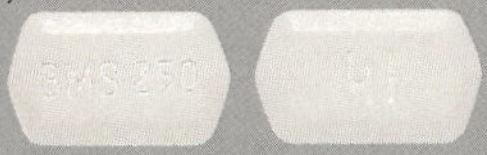
Serzone 250 mg
B-M Squibb BMS 250 41

℞
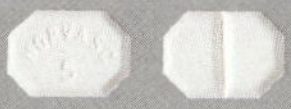
Norvasc 5 mg
Pfizer 5

℞
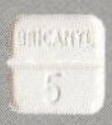
Bricanyl 5 mg
Hoechst Marion Roussel 5

℞
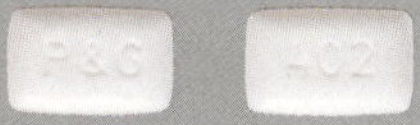
Didronel 200 mg
Procter & Gamble 402

℞
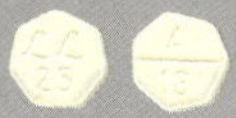
Asendin 25 mg
Lederle LL 25 A13

℞

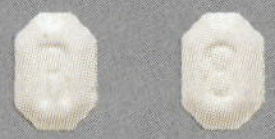

Lozol 2.5 mg
Rhone-Poulenc Rorer R 8

℞

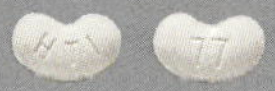

Thalitone 15 mg
Horus Therapeutics HTI 77

℞

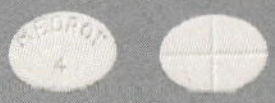

Medrol 4 mg
Upjohn 4

℞

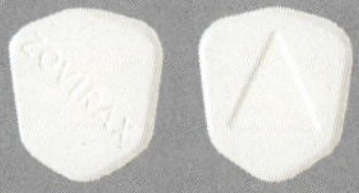

Zovirax 400 mg
Glaxo Wellcome

℞

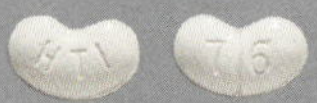

Thalitone 25 mg
Horus Therapeutics HTI 76

℞

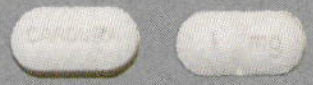

Cardura 1 mg
Roerig 1

℞

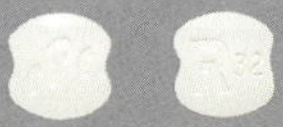

Demi-Regroton
Rhone-Poulenc Rorer R32

℞

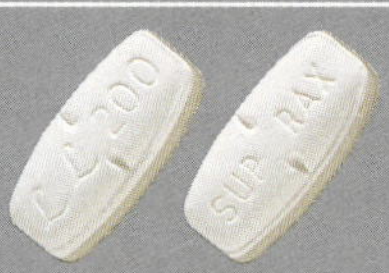

Suprax 200 mg
Lederle LL 200

℞

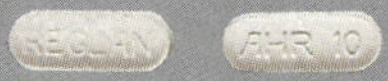

Reglan 10 mg
Robins AHR 10

C-II

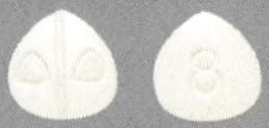

Dilaudid 8 mg
Knoll 8

℞

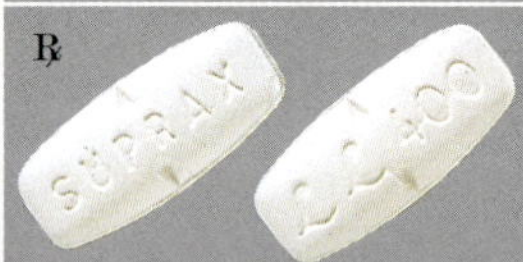

Suprax 400 mg
Lederle LL 400

C-IV

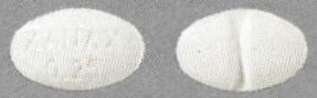

Xanax 0.25 mg
Upjohn 0.25

℞

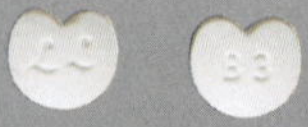

Zebeta 10 mg
Lederle LL B3

℞

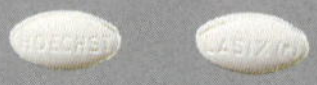

Lasix 20 mg
Hoechst Marion Roussel

℞

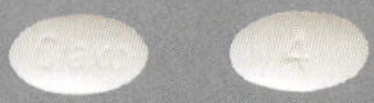

Zofran 4 mg
Glaxo Wellcome 4

℞

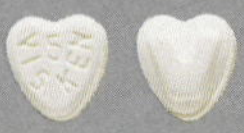

Visken 5 mg
Sandoz 5 V

℞

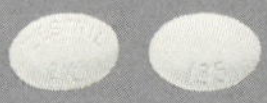

Zestril 2.5 mg
Zeneca 2 1/2 135

℞

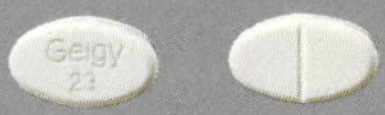

Lioresal 10 mg
Ciba Geneva Geigy 23

℞

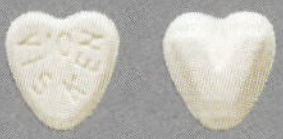

Visken 10 mg
Sandoz 10 V

C-IV

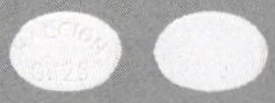

Halcion 0.125 mg
Upjohn 0.125

℞

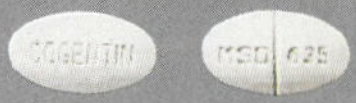

Cogentin 1 mg
Merck MSD 635

℞
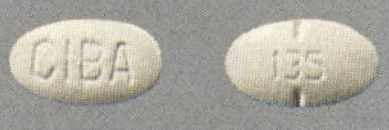

Ludiomil 75 mg
Ciba Geneva 135

℞
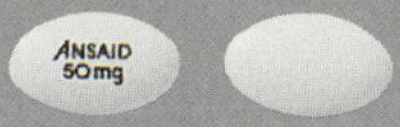

Ansaid 50 mg
Upjohn 50

℞
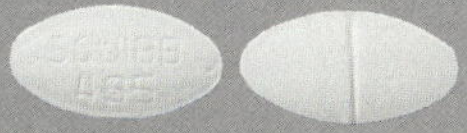
Capoten 100 mg
B-M Squibb 485

℞
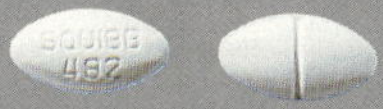
Capoten 50 mg
B-M Squibb 482

℞
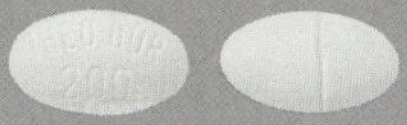
Theo-Dur 200 mg
Key 200

℞
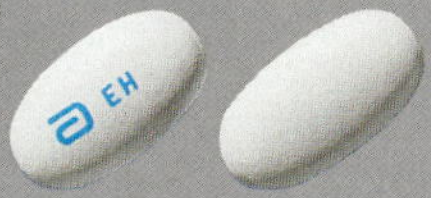

Ery-Tab 333 mg
Abbott EH

℞
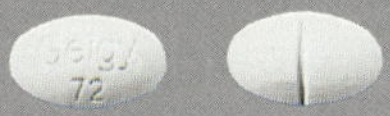
Brethine 2.5 mg
Ciba Geneva Geigy 72

℞
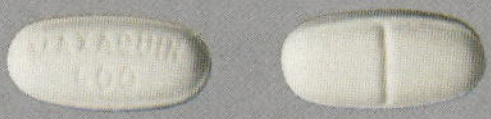
Maxaquin 400 mg
Searle 400

℞
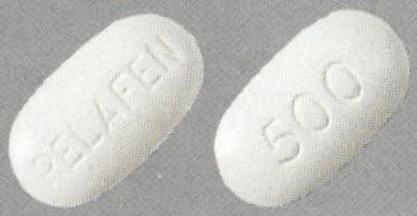

Relafen 500 mg
SmithKline Beecham 500

℞

Hylorel 25 mg
Fisons 25

℞
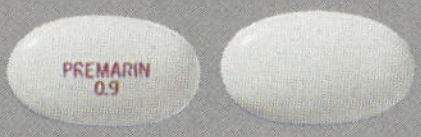

Premarin 0.9 mg
Wyeth-Ayerst 0.9

C-III
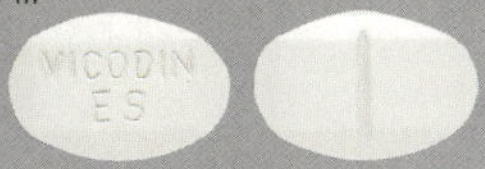

Vicodin ES
Knoll

℞
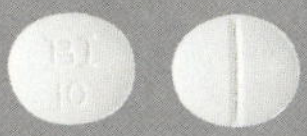
Combipres 0.3 mg
Boehringer Ingelheim BI 10

℞
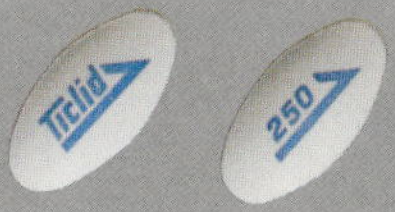

Ticlid 250 mg
Roche 250

℞
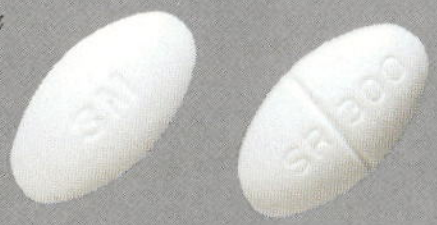
Theolair-SR 300 mg
3M Pharm SR 300

℞
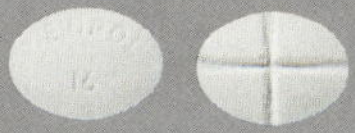
Medrol 16 mg
Upjohn 16

℞
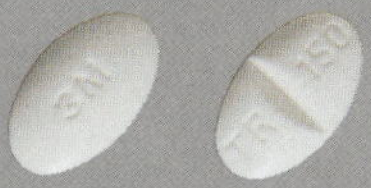
Tambocor 150 mg
3M Pharm TR 150

℞
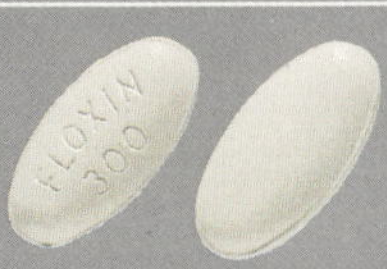

Floxin 300 mg
McNeil 300

℞
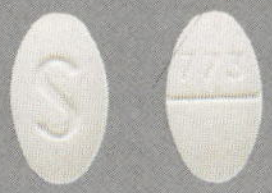
Sorbitrate 30 mg
Zeneca S 773

℞
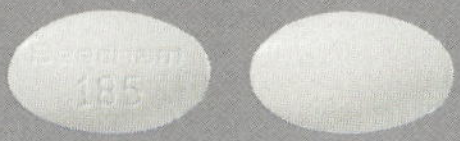
Beepen-VK 250 mg
SmithKline Beecham 185

℞
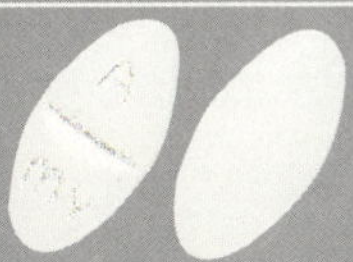
Toprol-XL 200 mg
Astra A MY

℞
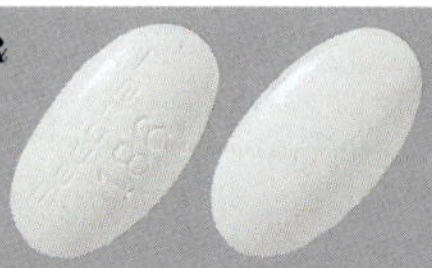
Beepen-VK 500 mg
SmithKline Beecham 186

℞
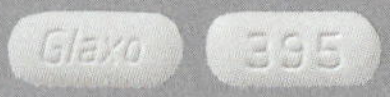

Ceftin 125 mg
Glaxo Wellcome 395

℞
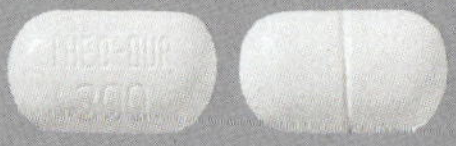
Theo-Dur 300 mg
Key 300

℞
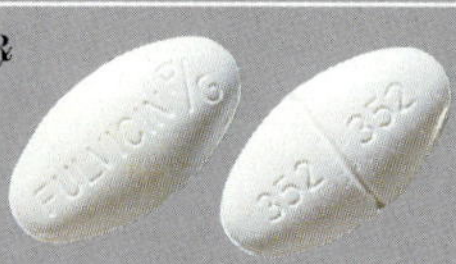

Fulvicin P/G 330 mg
Schering 352

℞
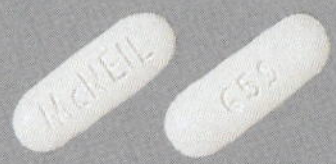
Ultram 50 mg
McNeil 659

℞
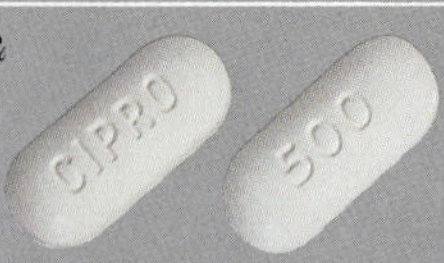

Cipro 500 mg
Bayer Corp 500

℞
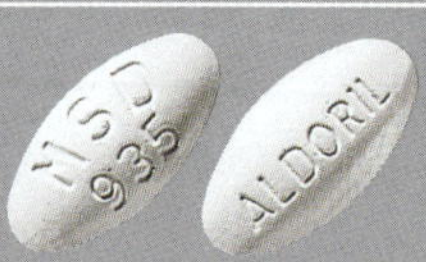

Aldoril D50
Merck MSD 935

℞
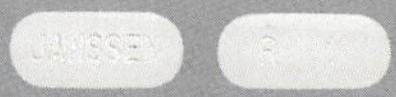
Risperdal 1 mg
Janssen R 1

℞
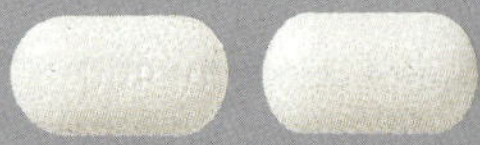
K-Dur 10 10 mEq
Key 10

℞
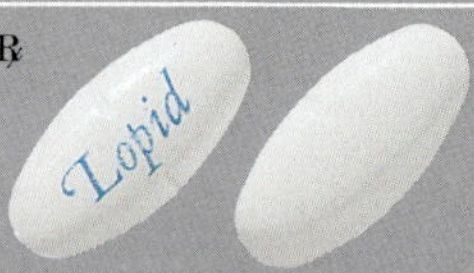

Lopid 600 mg
Parke-Davis

℞
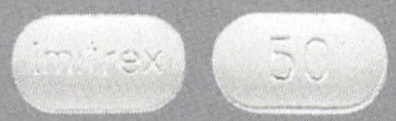

Imitrex 50 mg
Glaxo Wellcome 50

C-III
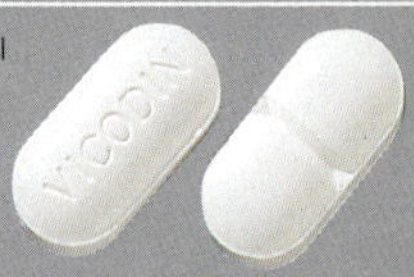

Vicodin
Knoll

℞
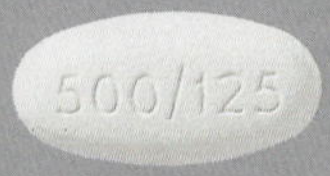

Augmentin '500'
SmithKline Beecham 500/125

℞
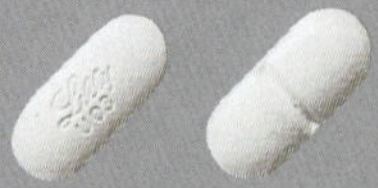
Dymelor 250 mg
Lilly U03

℞
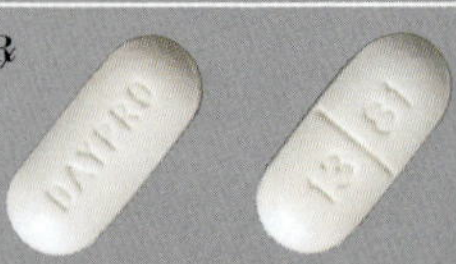

Daypro 600 mg
Searle 1381

℞

Capoten 12.5 mg
B-M Squibb 450

℞
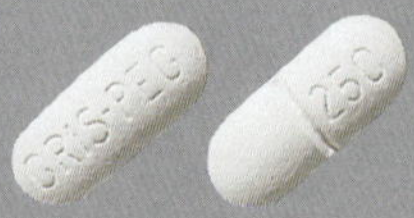

Gris-PEG 250 mg
Allergan Herbert 250

℞
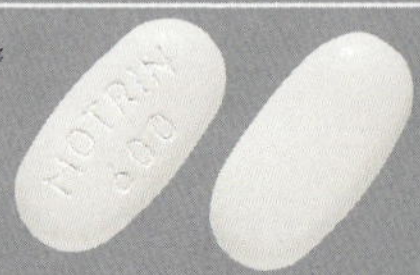
Motrin 600 mg
Upjohn 600

C-II
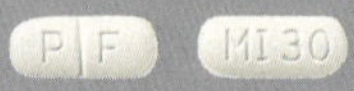

MSIR 30 mg
Purdue Frederick PF MI 30

℞
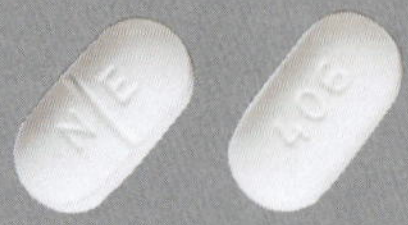

Didronel 400 mg
Procter & Gamble NE 406

℞

Seldane-D
Hoechst Marion Roussel

℞
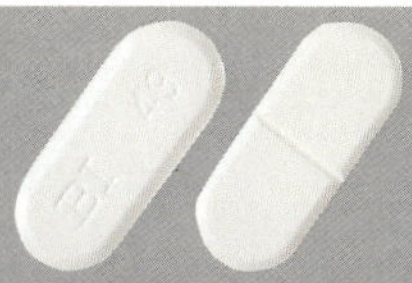

Respbid 500 mg
Boehringer Ingelheim BI 49

℞
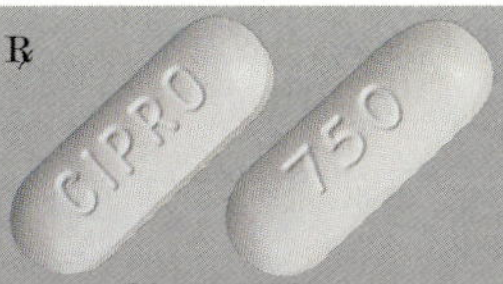

Cipro 750 mg
Bayer Corp 750

℞
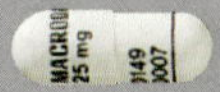

Macrodantin 25 mg
Procter & Gamble 0149 0007

℞
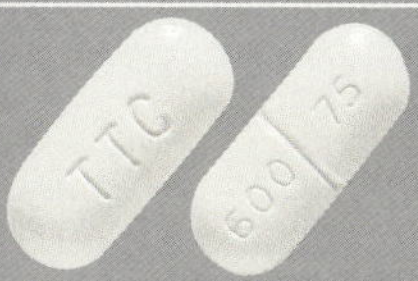

Guaifenesin 600/PPA 75 ER
Trinity TTC 600 75

℞
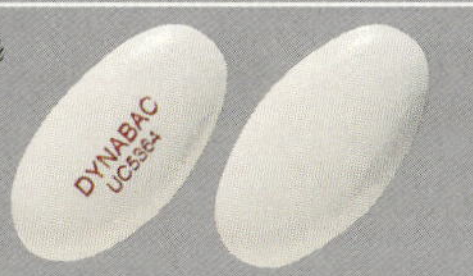

Dynabac 250 mg
Bock UC5364

℞
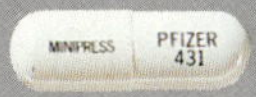

Minipress 1 mg
Pfizer 431

℞
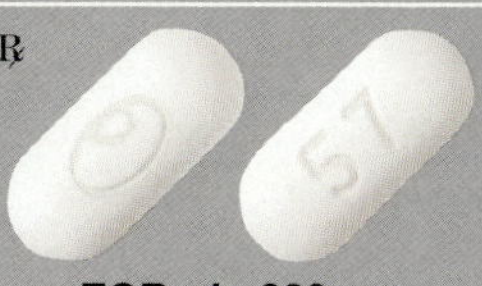

ZORprin 800 mg
Knoll 57

℞
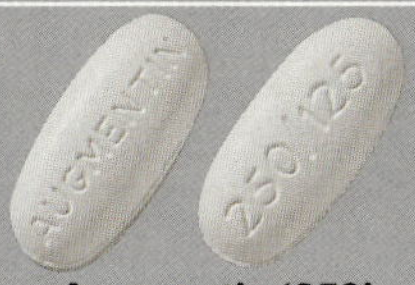

Augmentin ‘250’
SmithKline Beecham 250/125

℞
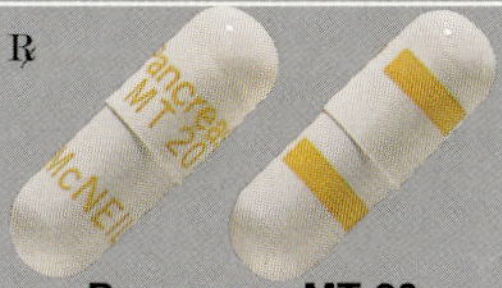

Pancrease MT 20
McNeil MT 20

℞
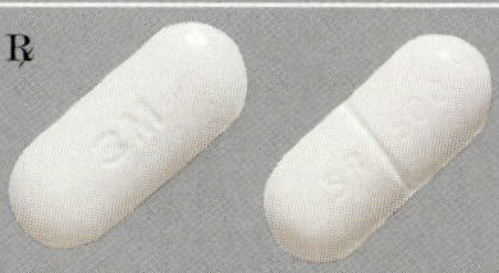

Theolair-SR 500 mg
3M Pharm SR 500

℞
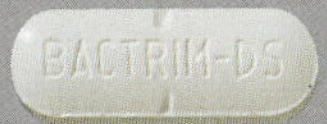

Bactrim DS
Roche 01

℞
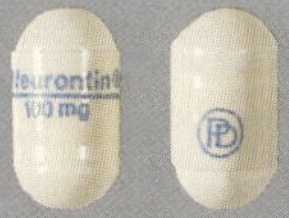

Neurontin 100 mg
Parke-Davis 100

℞
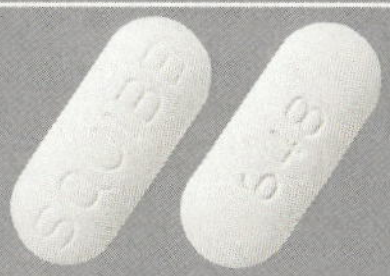

Veetids 500 mg
Apothecon Squibb 648

℞
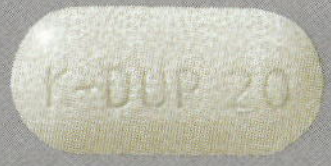

K-Dur 20 20 mEq
Key 20

℞
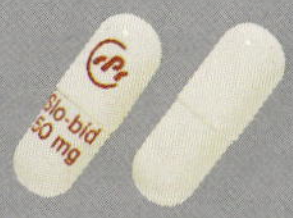

Slo-Bid 50 mg
Rhone-Poulenc Rorer 50

℞
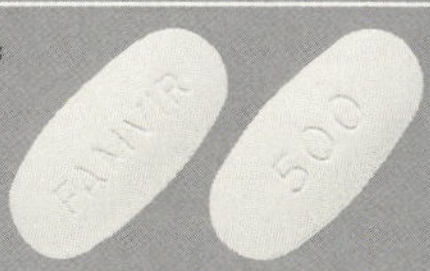

Famvir 500 mg
SmithKline Beecham 500

℞
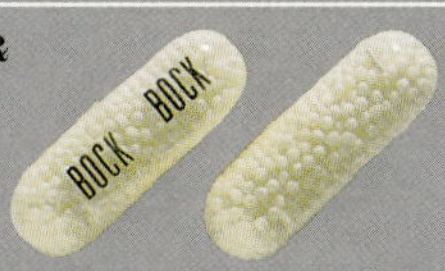

Poly-Histine-D Ped Caps
Bock

℞
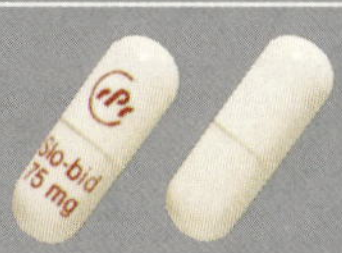

Slo-Bid 75 mg
Rhone-Poulenc Rorer

℞
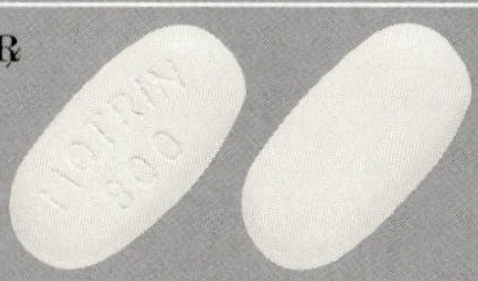

Motrin 800 mg
Upjohn 800

℞
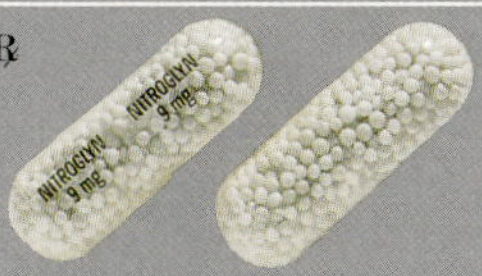

Nitroglyn E-R 9 mg
Kenwood/Bradley 9

℞
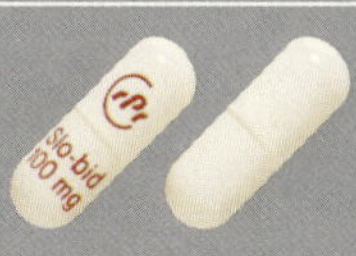

Slo-Bid 100 mg
Rhone-Poulenc Rorer

℞
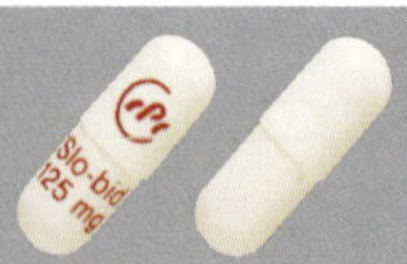

Slo-Bid 125 mg
Rhone-Poulenc Rorer

℞
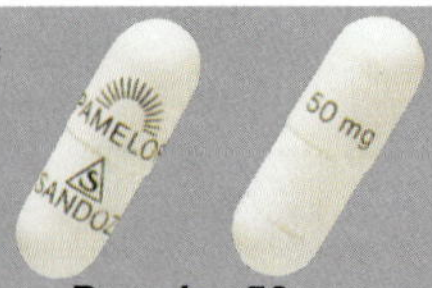

Pamelor 50 mg
Sandoz 50

℞
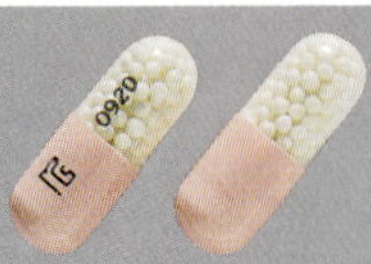

Dilatrate-SR 40 mg
Schwarz Pharma RC 0920

℞
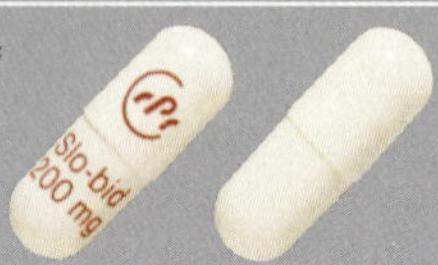

Slo-Bid 200 mg
Rhone-Poulenc Rorer

℞
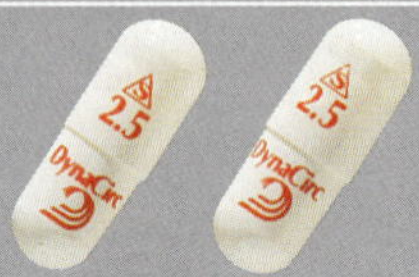

DynaCirc 2.5 mg
Sandoz 2.5

℞
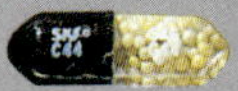
Compazine Spansule 10 mg
SmithKline Beecham SKF C44

℞
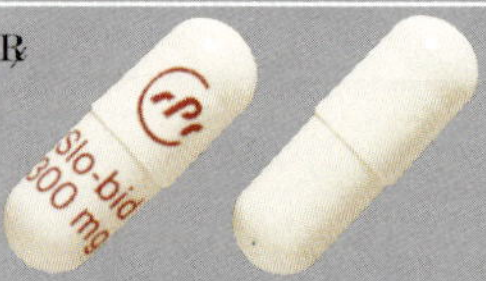

Slo-Bid 300 mg
Rhone-Poulenc Rorer

℞
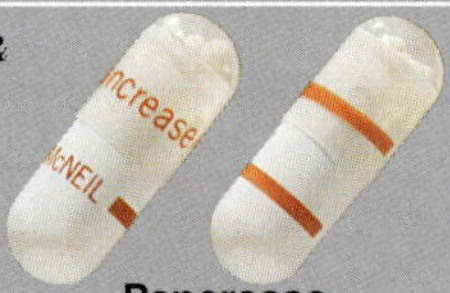

Pancrease
McNeil

℞
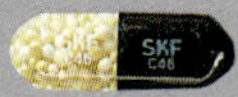

Compazine Spansule 15 mg
SmithKline Beecham SKF C46

℞
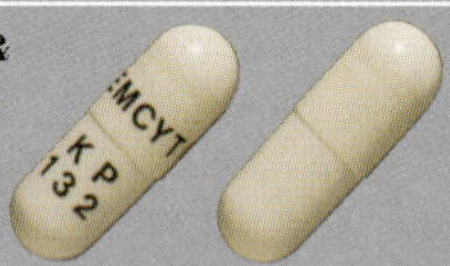

Emcyt
Pharmacia KP 132

℞
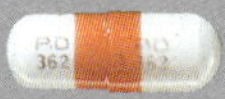
Dilantin 100 mg
Parke-Davis P-D 362

℞
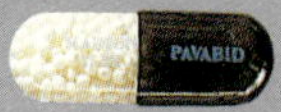

Pavabid 150 mg
Hoechst Marion Roussel 1555

℞
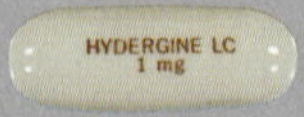

Hydergine LC 1 mg
Sandoz LC 1

℞
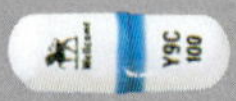

Retrovir 100 mg
Glaxo Wellcome Y9C 100

C-II
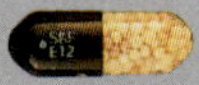
Dexedrine 5 mg
SmithKline Beecham SKF E12

℞
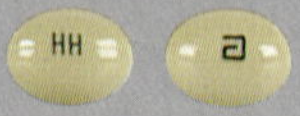

Hytrin 1 mg
Abbott HH

℞
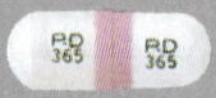

Dilantin Kapseals 30 mg
Parke-Davis P-D 365

C-II
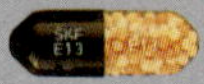
Dexedrine 10 mg
SmithKline Beecham SKF E13

℞
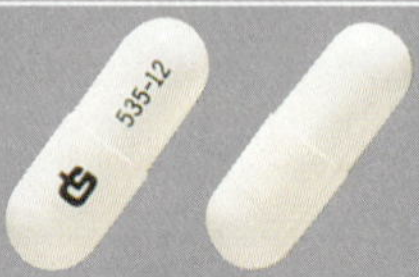

Esgic
Forest Pharm 535-12

℞
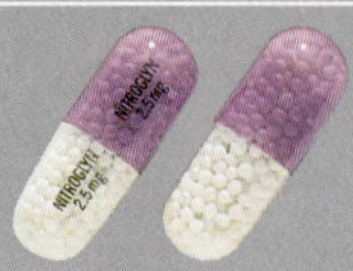
Nitroglyn E-R 2.5 mg
Kenwood/Bradley 2.5

C-II
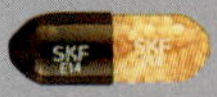

Dexedrine 15 mg
SmithKline Beecham SKF E14

℞
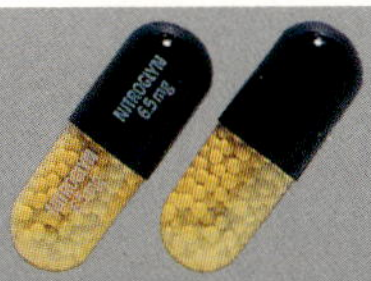

Nitroglyn E-R 6.5 mg
Kenwood/Bradley 6.5

℞
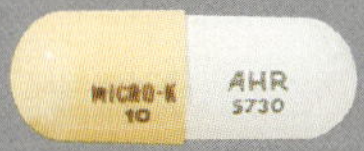

Micro-K 10 Extencaps 10 mEq
Robins 10 AHR 5730

℞
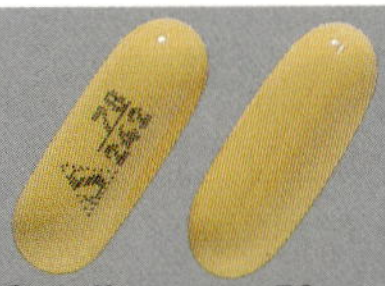

Sandimmune 50 mg
Sandoz 78 242

℞
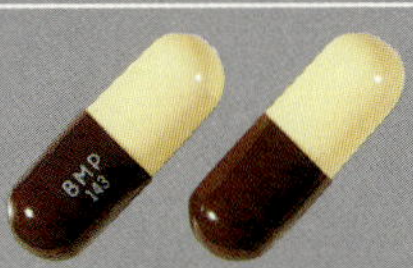

Bactocill 250 mg
SmithKline Beecham BMP 143

℞
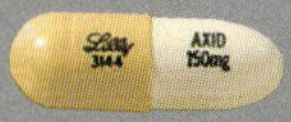

Axid 150 mg
Lilly 3144 150

℞
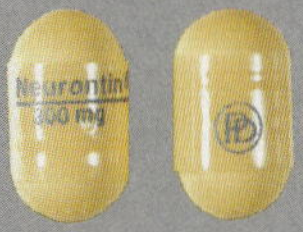

Neurontin 300 mg
Parke-Davis 300

℞
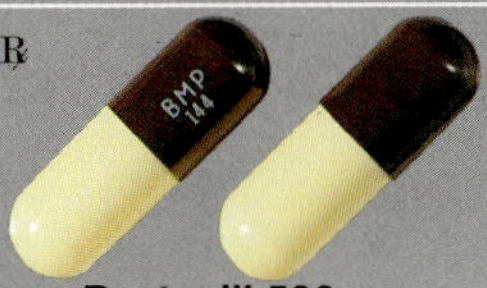

Bactocill 500 mg
SmithKline Beecham BMP 144

℞
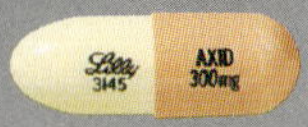

Axid 300 mg
Lilly 3145 300

℞
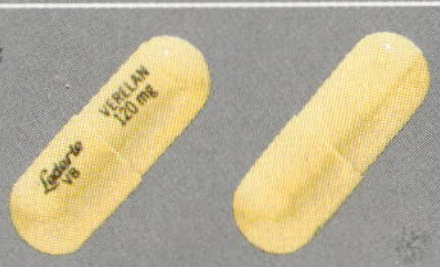

Verelan 120 mg
Lederle V8 120

℞
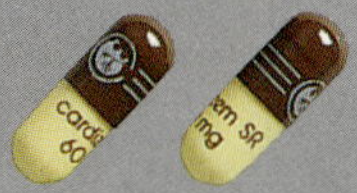

Cardizem SR 60 mg
Hoechst Marion Roussel 60

℞
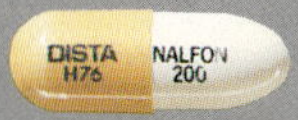

Nalfon 200 mg
Dista H76 200

℞
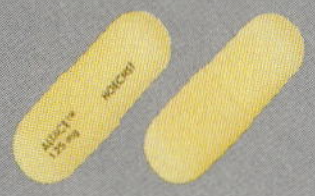

Altace 1.25 mg
Hoechst Marion Roussel 1.25

℞
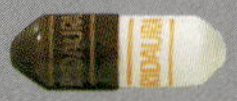

Ridaura 3 mg
SmithKline Beecham

℞
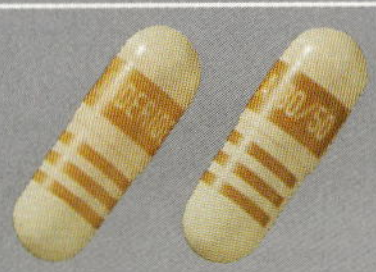

Inderide LA 80/50
Wyeth-Ayerst 80/50

℞
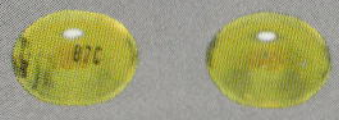

Lanoxicaps 0.1 mg
Glaxo Wellcome B2C

℞
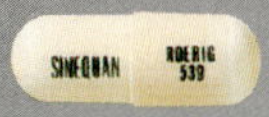

Sinequan 75 mg
Roerig 539

℞
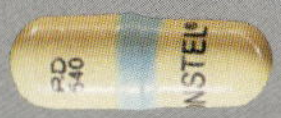

Ponstel 250 mg
Parke-Davis P-D 540

℞
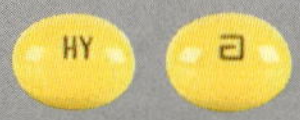

Hytrin 2 mg
Abbott HY

℞
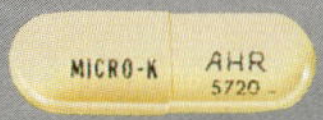

Micro-K Extencaps 8 mEq
Robins AHR 5720

℞
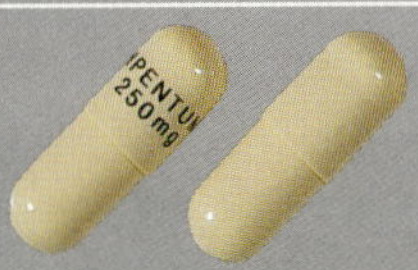

Dipentum 250 mg
Pharmacia 250

℞
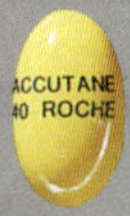

Accutane 40 mg
Roche 40

C-II

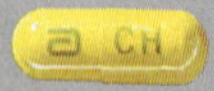

Nembutal Sodium 100 mg
Abbott CH

℞

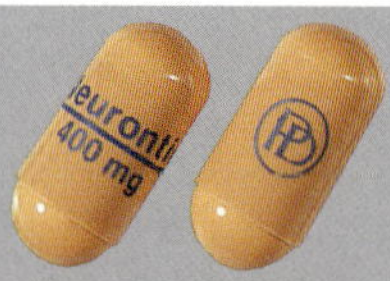

Neurontin 400 mg
Parke-Davis 400

℞

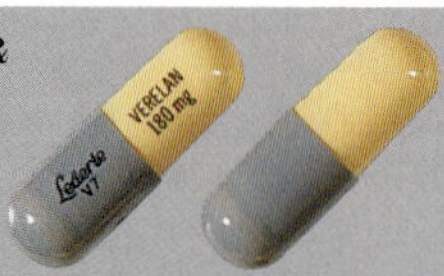

Verelan 180 mg
Lederle V7 180

℞

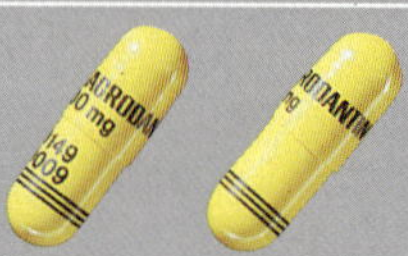

Macrodantin 100 mg
Procter & Gamble 0149 0009

℞

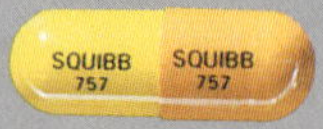

Pronestyl 500 mg
Princeton Squibb 757

℞

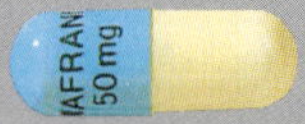

Anafranil 50 mg
Ciba Geneva 50

℞

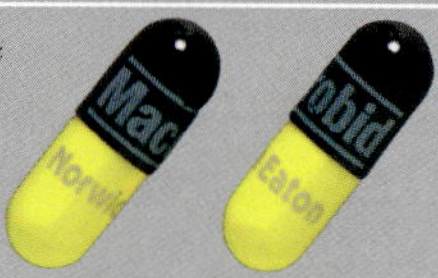

Macrobid 100 mg
Procter & Gamble

C-IV

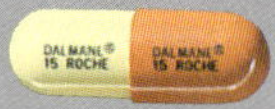

Dalmane 15 mg
Roche 15

℞

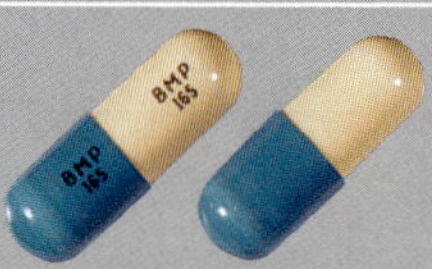

Dycill 250 mg
SmithKline Beecham BMP 165

℞

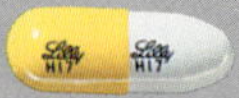

Aventyl HCl 10 mg
Lilly H17

℞

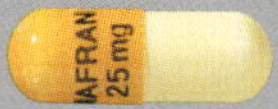

Anafranil 25 mg
Ciba Geneva 25

℞

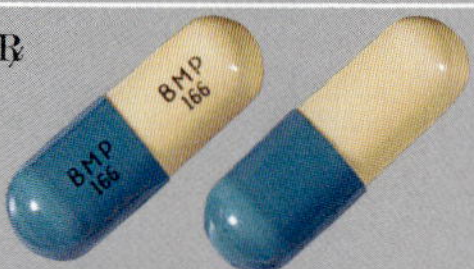

Dycill 500 mg
SmithKline Beecham BMP 166

℞

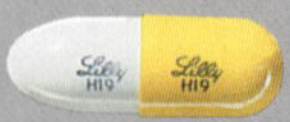

Aventyl HCl 25 mg
Lilly H19

℞

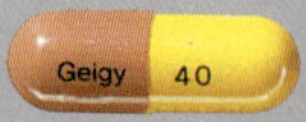

Tofranil-PM 100 mg
Ciba Geneva Geigy 40

℞

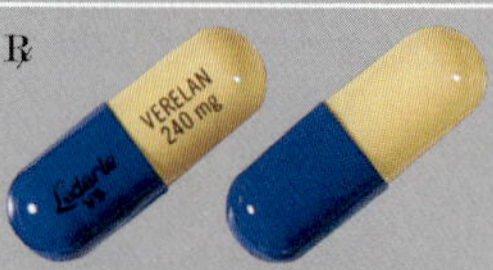

Verelan 240 mg
Lederle V9 240

℞

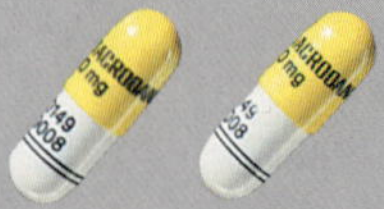

Macrodantin 50 mg
Procter & Gamble 0149 0008

℞

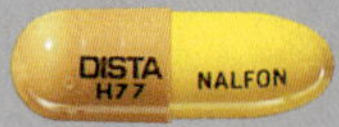

Nalfon 300 mg
Dista H77

C-III

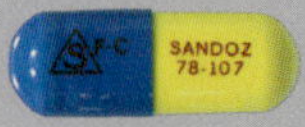

Fiorinal w/Codeine
Sandoz F-C 78-107

℞

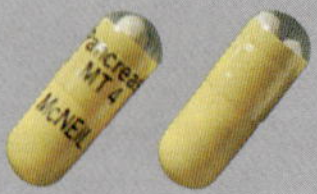

Pancrease MT 4
McNeil MT 4

℞

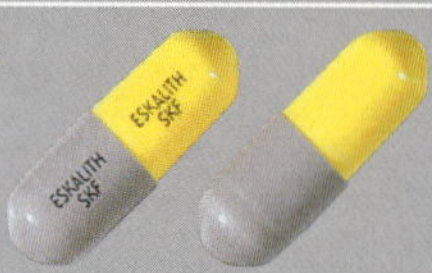

Eskalith 300 mg
SmithKline Beecham SKF

℞

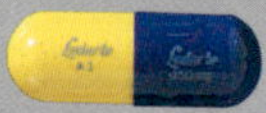

Achromycin V 250 mg
Lederle A3 250

℞

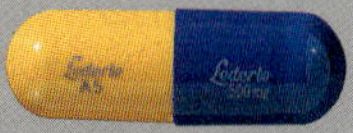

Achromycin V 500 mg
Lederle A5 500

℞

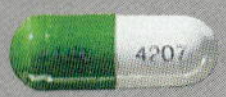

Donnatal
Robins AHR 4207

℞

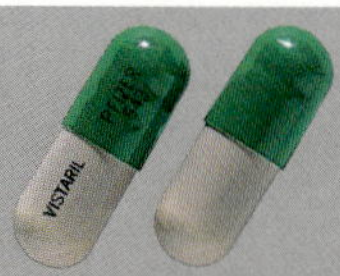

Vistaril 100 mg
Pfizer 543

℞

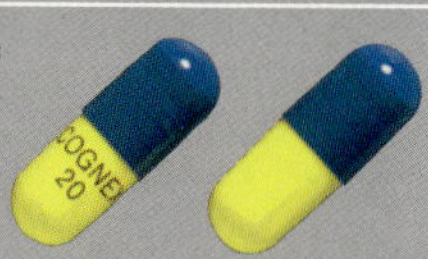

Cognex 20 mg
Parke-Davis 20

℞

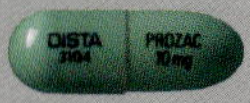

Prozac 10 mg
Dista 3104 10

℞

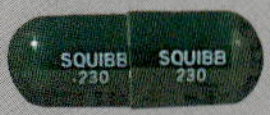

Trimox 250 mg
Apothecon Squibb 230

℞

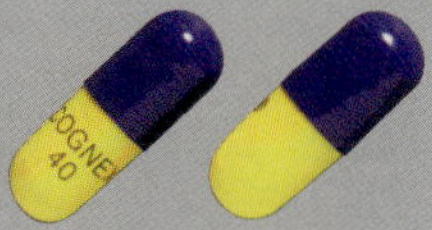

Cognex 40 mg
Parke-Davis 40

℞

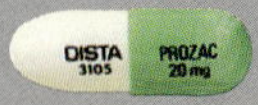

Prozac 20 mg
Dista 3105 20

℞

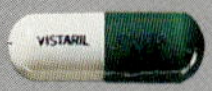

Vistaril 50 mg
Pfizer 542

℞

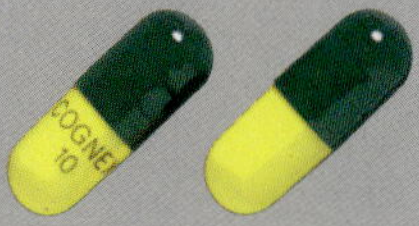

Cognex 10 mg
Parke-Davis 10

C-IV

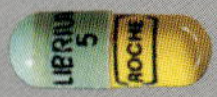

Librium 5 mg
Roche 5

℞

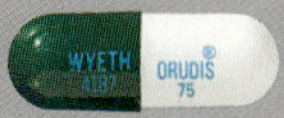

Orudis 75 mg
Wyeth-Ayerst 4187 75

℞

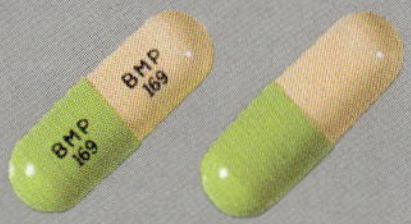

Cloxapen 250 mg
SmithKline Beecham BMP 169

C-IV

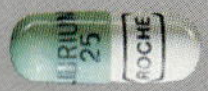

Librium 25 mg
Roche 25

℞

Keflex 250 mg
Dista H69 250

℞

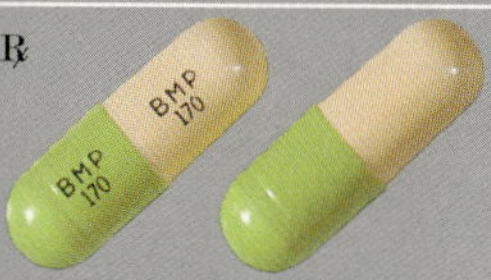

Cloxapen 500 mg
SmithKline Beecham BMP 170

℞

Librax
Roche

℞

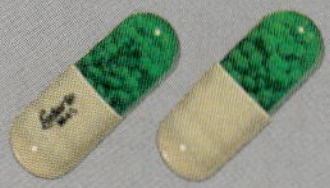

Minocin 50 mg
Lederle M45

℞

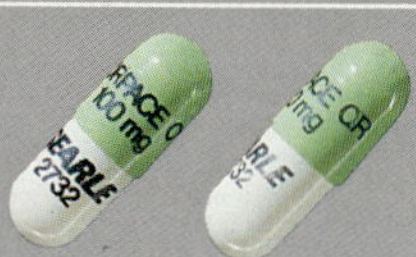

Norpace CR 100 mg
Searle 2732 100

℞

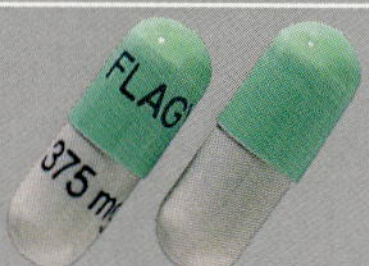

Flagyl 375 mg
Searle 375

℞

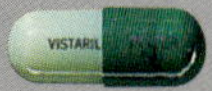

Vistaril 25 mg
Pfizer 541

℞

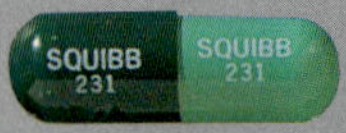

Trimox 500 mg
Apothecon Squibb 231

C-IV

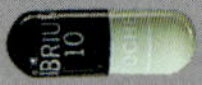

Librium 10 mg
Roche 10

℞

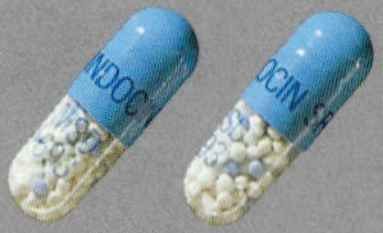

Indocin SR 75 mg
Merck MSD 693

℞

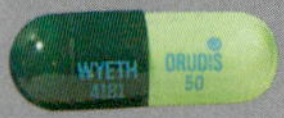

Orudis 50 mg
Wyeth-Ayerst 4181 50

℞

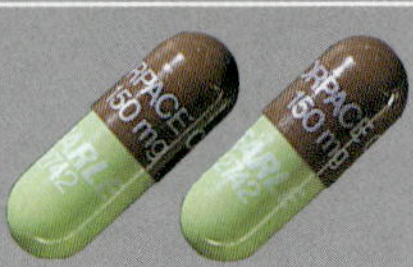

Norpace CR 150 mg
Searle 2742 150

C-IV

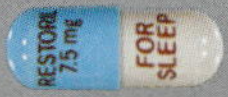

Restoril 7.5 mg
Sandoz 7.5

℞

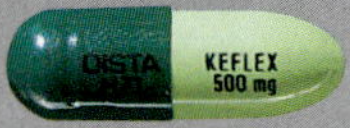

Keflex 500 mg
Dista H71 500

℞

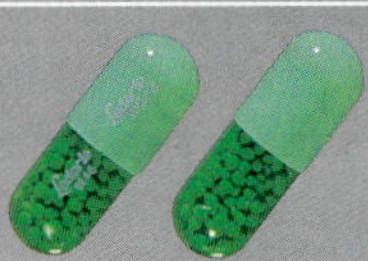

Minocin 100 mg
Lederle M46

℞

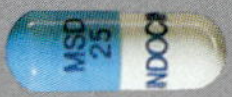

Indocin 25 mg
Merck MSD 25

C-III

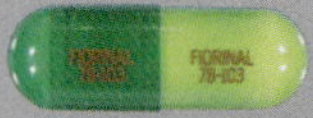

Fiorinal
Sandoz 78-103

℞

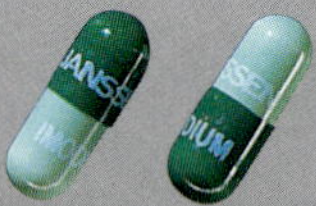

Imodium 2 mg
Janssen

℞

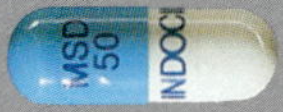

Indocin 50 mg
Merck MSD 50

℞

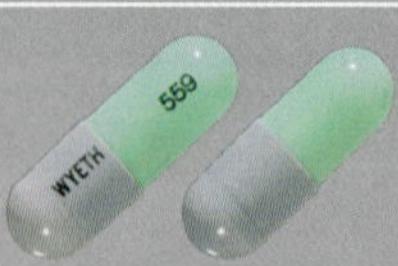

Wymox 250 mg
Wyeth-Ayerst 559

℞

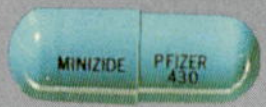

Minizide 1
Pfizer 430

℞

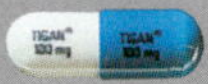

Tigan 100 mg
SmithKline Beecham 100

℞

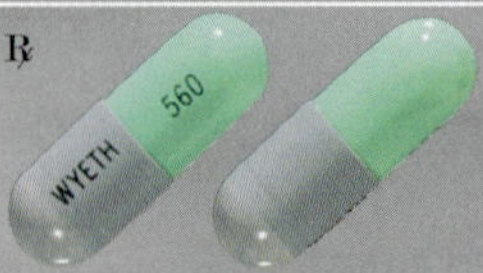

Wymox 500 mg
Wyeth-Ayerst 560

℞

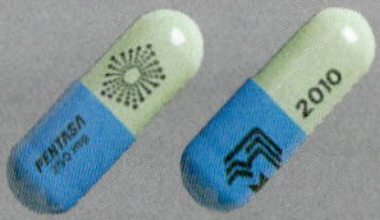

Pentasa 250 mg
Hoechst Marion Roussel 2010

℞

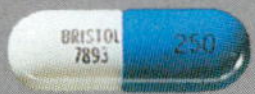

Dynapen 250 mg
Apothecon Bristol 7893

℞

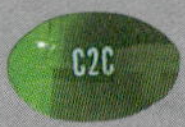

Lanoxicaps 0.2 mg
Glaxo Wellcome C2C

℞

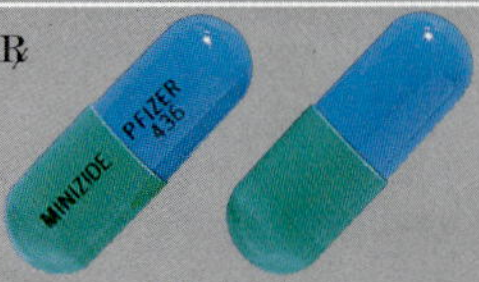

Minizide 5
Pfizer 436

℞

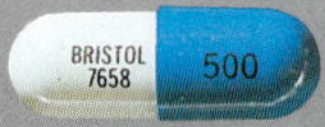

Dynapen 500 mg
Apothecon Bristol 7658

℞

Minipress 5 mg
Pfizer 438

℞

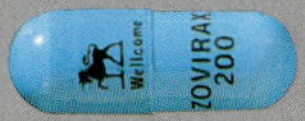

Zovirax 200 mg
Glaxo Wellcome 200

℞

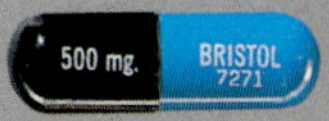

Ultracef 500 mg
Bristol 7271 500

℞

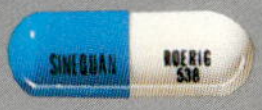

Sinequan 100 mg
Roerig 538

℞

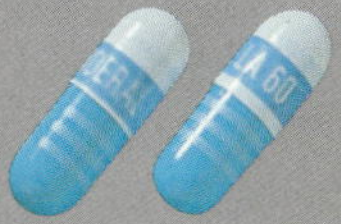

Inderal LA 60 mg
Wyeth-Ayerst 60

℞

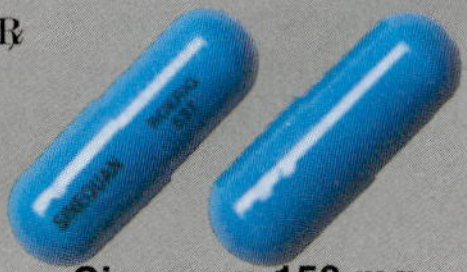

Sinequan 150 mg
Roerig 537

C-II

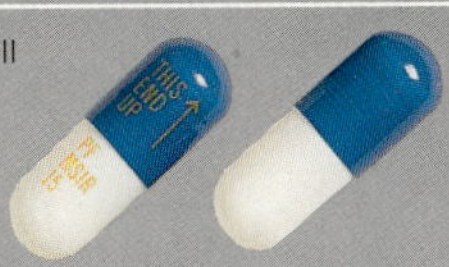

MSIR 15 mg
Purdue Frederick PF 15

℞

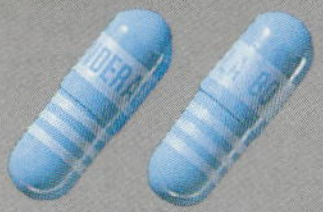

Inderal LA 80 mg
Wyeth-Ayerst 80

℞

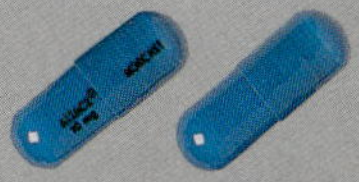

Altace 10 mg
Hoechst Marion Roussel 10

℞

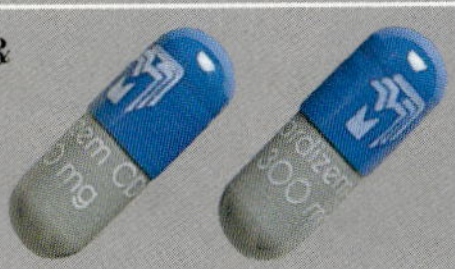

Cardizem CD 300 mg
Hoechst Marion Roussel 300

℞

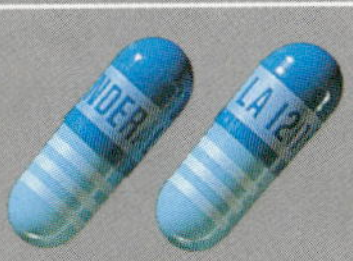

Inderal LA 120 mg
Wyeth-Ayerst 120

℞

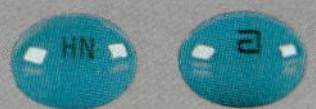

Hytrin 10 mg
Abbott HN

℞

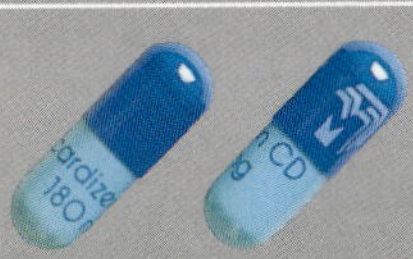

Cardizem CD 180 mg
Hoechst Marion Roussel 180

℞

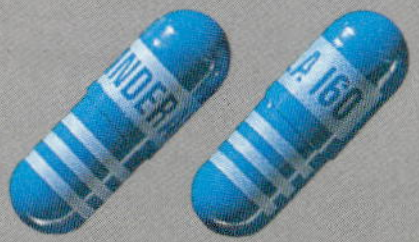

Inderal LA 160 mg
Wyeth-Ayerst 160

C-III

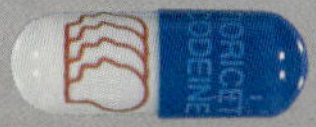

Fioricet w/Codeine
Sandoz

℞

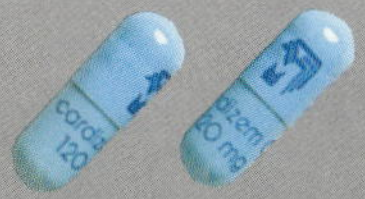

Cardizem CD 120 mg
Hoechst Marion Roussel 120

℞

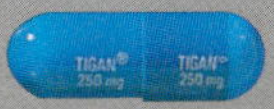

Tigan 250 mg
SmithKline Beecham 250

℞

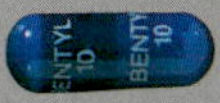

Bentyl 10 mg
Hoechst Marion Roussel 10

℞

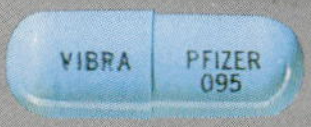

Vibramycin 100 mg
Pfizer 095

℞

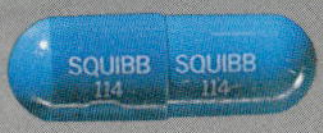

Velosef 500 mg
Apothecon Squibb 114

℞

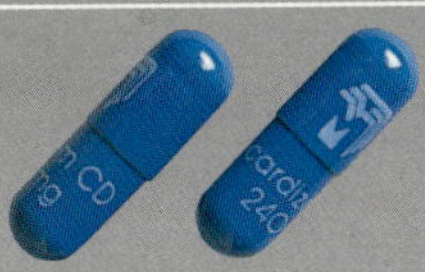

Cardizem CD 240 mg
Hoechst Marion Roussel 240

℞

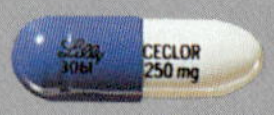

Ceclor 250 mg
Lilly 3061 250

C-IV

Restoril 30 mg
Sandoz 30

℞

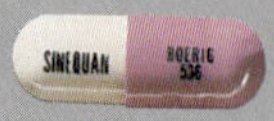

Sinequan 50 mg
Roerig 536

℞

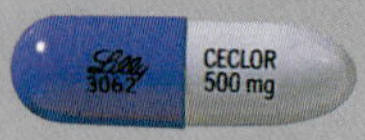

Ceclor 500 mg
Lilly 3062 500

℞

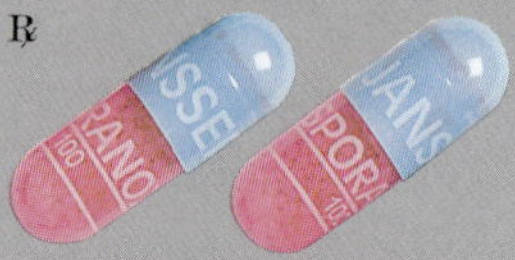

Sporanox 100 mg
Janssen 100

℞

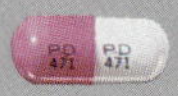

Benadryl 25 mg
Parke-Davis P-D 471

C-II

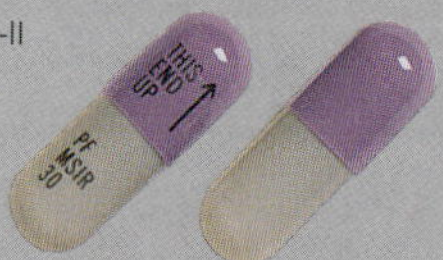

MSIR 30 mg
Purdue Frederick PF 30

℞

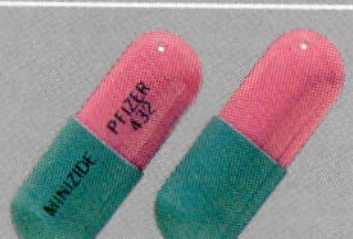

Minizide 2
Pfizer 432

℞

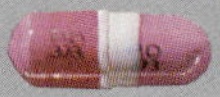

Benadryl 50 mg
Parke-Davis P-D 373

℞

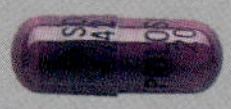

Prilosec 20 mg
Astra Merck MSD 742 20

℞

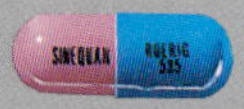

Sinequan 25 mg
Roerig 535

℞

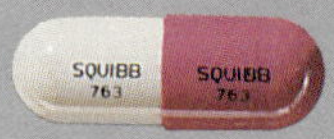

Sumycin 500 mg
Apothecon Squibb 763

℞

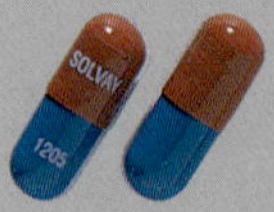

Creon 5
Solvay 1205

℞

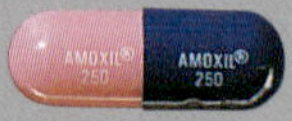

Amoxil 250 mg
SmithKline Beecham 250

℞

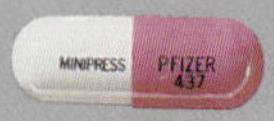

Minipress 2 mg
Pfizer 437

C-II

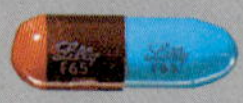

Tuinal 100 mg
Lilly F65

℞

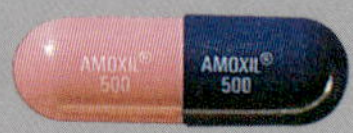

Amoxil 500 mg
SmithKline Beecham 500

C-IV

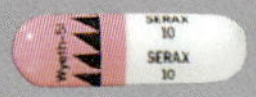

Serax 10 mg
Wyeth-Ayerst 51

℞

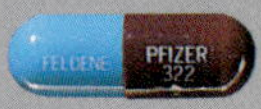

Feldene 10 mg
Pfizer 322

℞

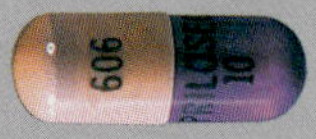

Prilosec 10 mg
Astra Merck 606 10

℞

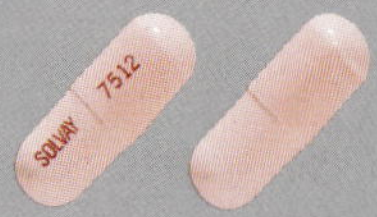

Lithonate 300 mg
Solvay 7512

℞

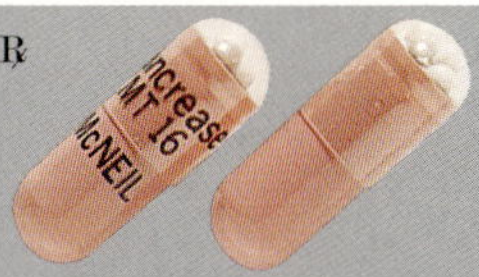

Pancrease MT 16
McNeil MT 16

℞

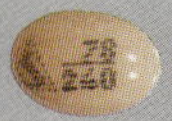

Sandimmune 25 mg
Sandoz 78-240

℞

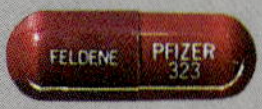

Feldene 20 mg
Pfizer 323

℞

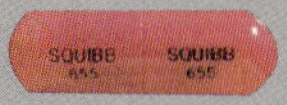

Sumycin 250 mg
Apothecon Squibb 655

℞

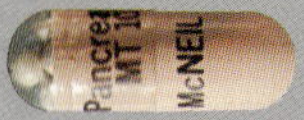

Pancrease MT 10
McNeil MT 10

℞

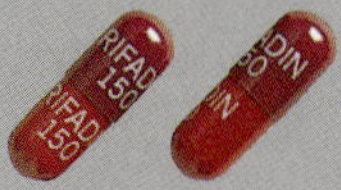

Rifadin 150 mg
Hoechst Marion Roussel 150

℞

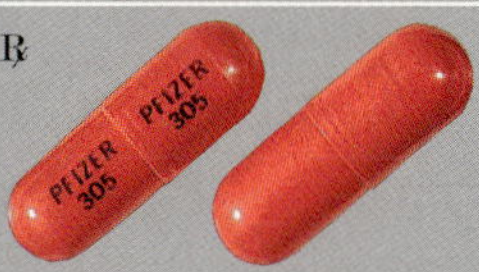

Zithromax 250 mg
Pfizer 305

℞

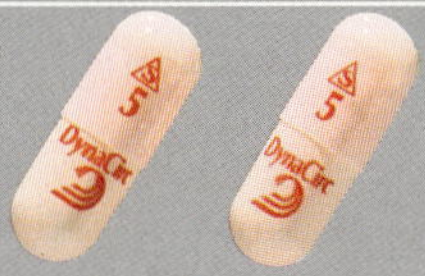

DynaCirc 5 mg
Sandoz 5

℞

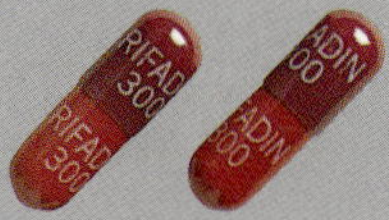

Rifadin 300 mg
Hoechst Marion Roussel 300

℞

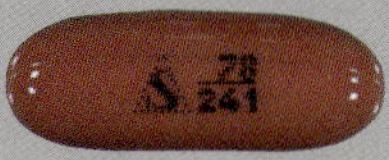

Sandimmune 100 mg
Sandoz 78-241

C-IV

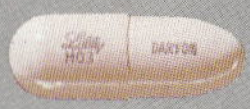

Darvon 65 mg
Lilly H03

℞

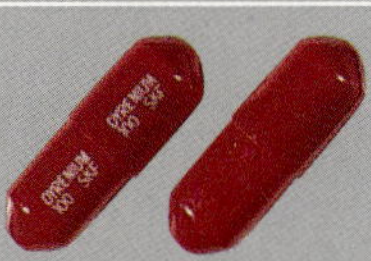

Dyrenium 100 mg
SmithKline Beecham 100 SKF

℞

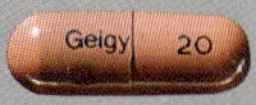

Tofranil-PM 75 mg
Ciba Geneva Geigy 20

℞

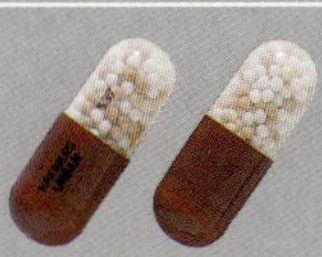

Levsinex Timecaps 0.375 mg
Schwarz Pharma 537

℞

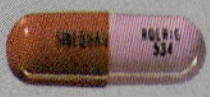

Sinequan 10 mg
Roerig 534

℞

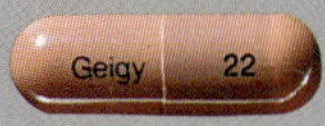

Tofranil-PM 150 mg
Ciba Geneva Geigy 22

℞

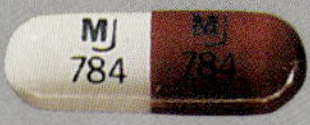

Duricef 500 mg
B-M Squibb MJ 784

℞

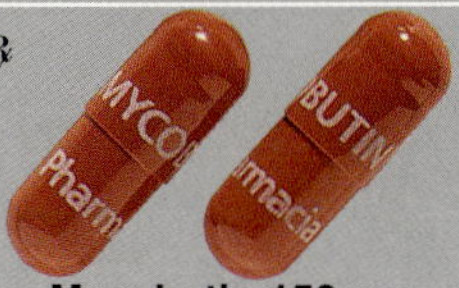

Mycobutin 150 mg
Pharmacia

℞

VePesid 50 mg
BMSOI 3091

C-IV

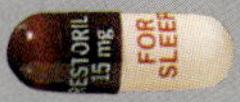

Restoril 15 mg
Sandoz 15

℞

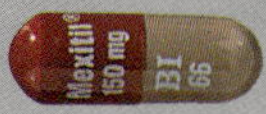

Mexitil 150 mg
Boehringer Ingelheim BI 66

℞

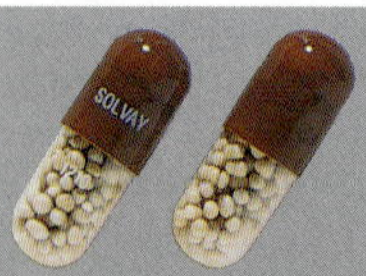

Creon 10
Solvay 1210

C-IV

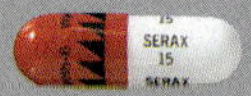

Serax 15 mg
Wyeth-Ayerst 6

℞

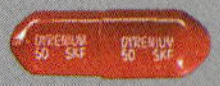

Dyrenium 50 mg
SmithKline Beecham 50 SKF

℞

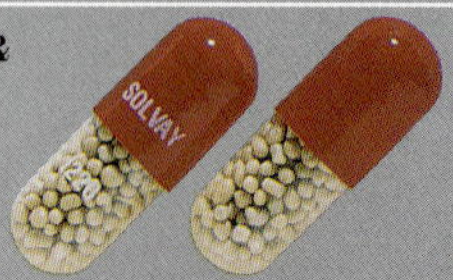

Creon 20
Solvay 1220

℞

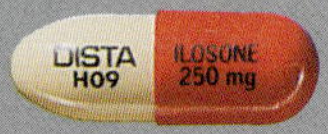

Ilosone 250 mg
Dista H09 250

℞

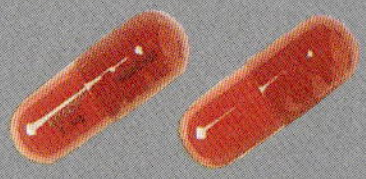

Altace 5 mg
Hoechst Marion Roussel 5

℞

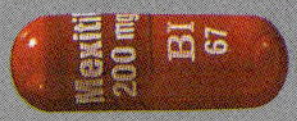

Mexitil 200 mg
Boehringer Ingelheim BI 67

℞

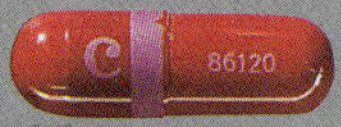

Midrin
Carnrick C 86120

℞

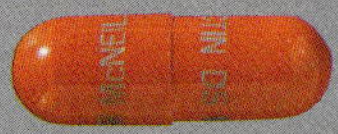

Tolectin DS 400 mg
McNeil DS

℞

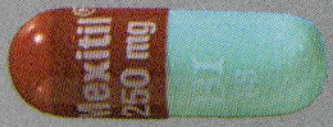

Mexitil 250 mg
Boehringer Ingelheim BI 68

C-II

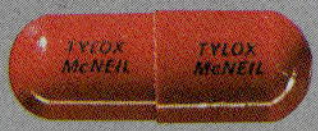

Tylox
McNeil

℞

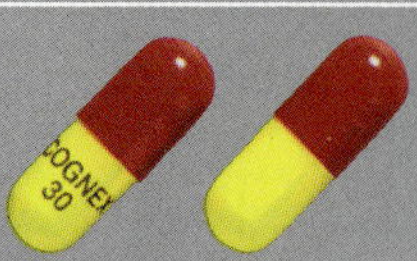

Cognex 30 mg
Parke-Davis 30

℞

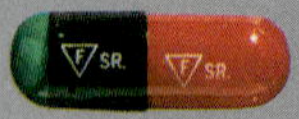

Extendryl SR.
Fleming F SR

℞

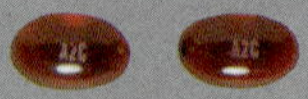

Lanoxicaps 0.05 mg
Glaxo Wellcome A2C

C-IV

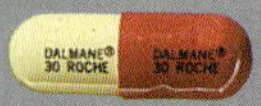

Dalmane 30 mg
Roche 30

℞

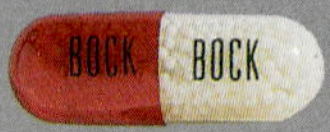

Poly-Histine-D Caps
Bock

℞

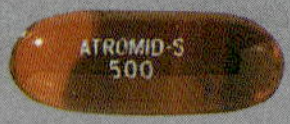

Atromid-S 500 mg
Wyeth-Ayerst 500

℞

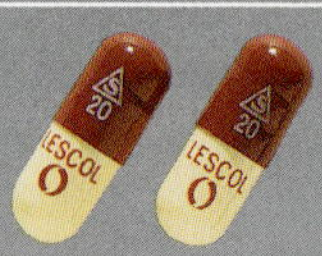

Lescol 20 mg
Sandoz 20

℞

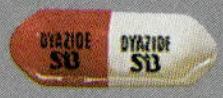

Dyazide
SmithKline Beecham

℞

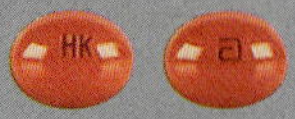

Hytrin 5 mg
Abbott HK

℞

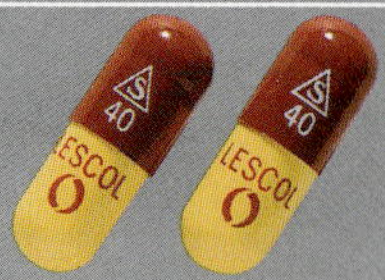

Lescol 40 mg
Sandoz 40

℞
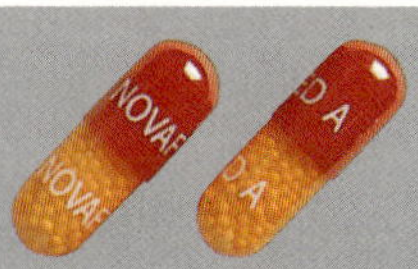

Novafed A
Hoechst Marion Roussel

℞
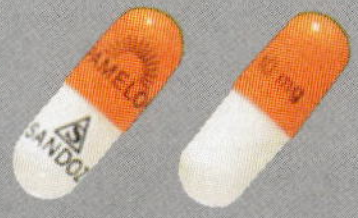

Pamelor 10 mg
Sandoz 10

℞
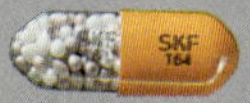

Thorazine Spansule 75 mg
SmithKline Beecham SKF T64

℞
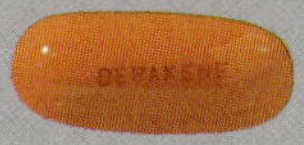
Depakene 250 mg
Abbott

℞
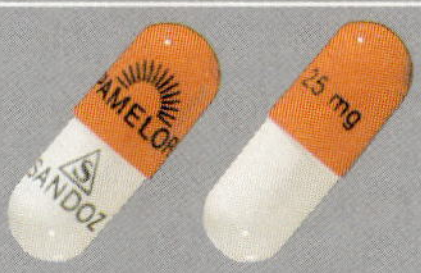

Pamelor 25 mg
Sandoz 25

℞
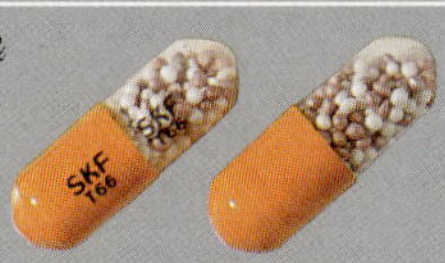

Thorazine Spansule 150 mg
SmithKline Beecham SKF T66

℞
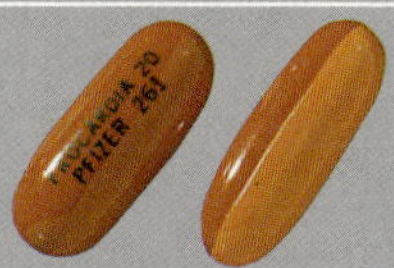

Procardia 20 mg
Pratt Pfizer 20 261

℞
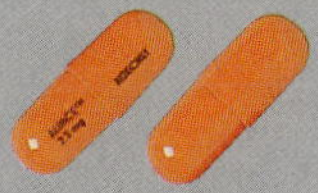
Altace 2.5 mg
Hoechst Marion Roussel 2.5

℞
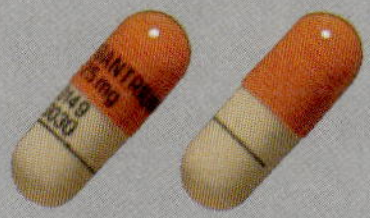
Dantrium 25 mg
Procter & Gamble 0149 0030

℞
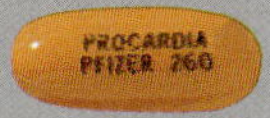

Procardia 10 mg
Pratt Pfizer 260

℞
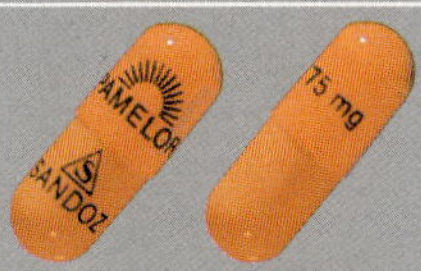

Pamelor 75 mg
Sandoz

℞
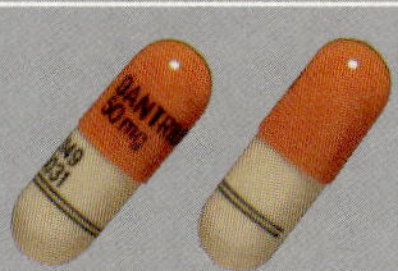
Dantrium 50 mg
Procter & Gamble 0149 0031

℞
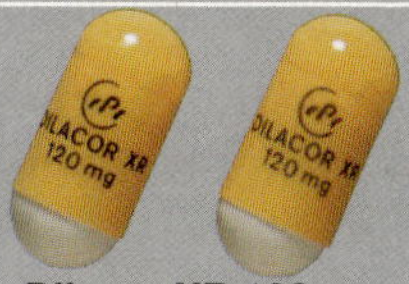

Dilacor XR 120 mg
Rhone-Poulenc Rorer 120

℞
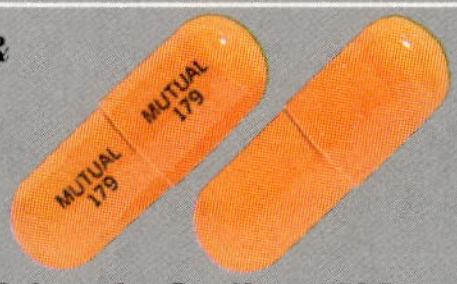

Tolmetin Sodium 400 mg
Mutual 179

℞
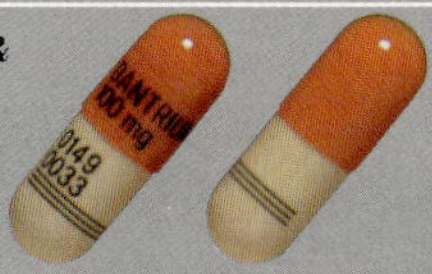

Dantrium 100 mg
Procter & Gamble 0149 0033

℞
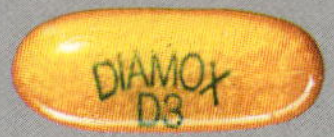

Diamox Sequels 500 mg
Lederle D3

℞
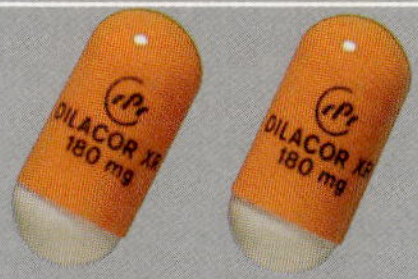

Dilacor XR 180 mg
Rhone-Poulenc Rorer 180

℞
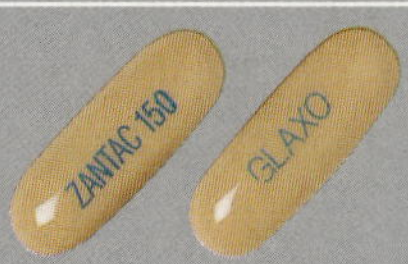

Zantac 150 GELdose 150 mg
Glaxo Wellcome 150

℞
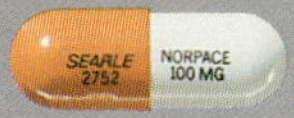

Norpace 100 mg
Searle 2752 100

℞
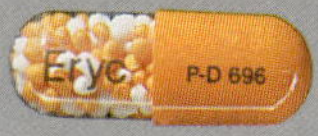

Eryc 250 mg
Parke-Davis P-D 696

℞
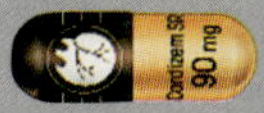

Cardizem SR 90 mg
Hoechst Marion Roussel 90

℞

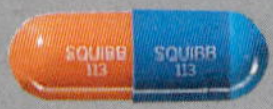

Velosef 250 mg
Apothecon Squibb 113

℞

Sectral 400 mg
Wyeth-Ayerst 4179 400

℞

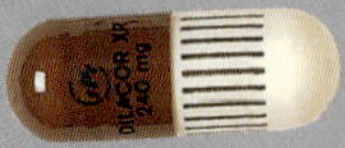

Dilacor XR 240 mg
Rhone-Poulenc Rorer 240

℞

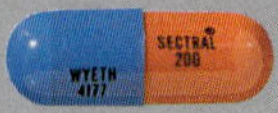

Sectral 200 mg
Wyeth-Ayerst 4177 200

℞

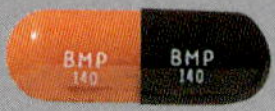

Totacillin 250 mg
SmithKline Beecham BMP 140

℞

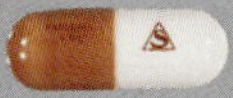

Parlodel 5 mg
Sandoz 5

℞

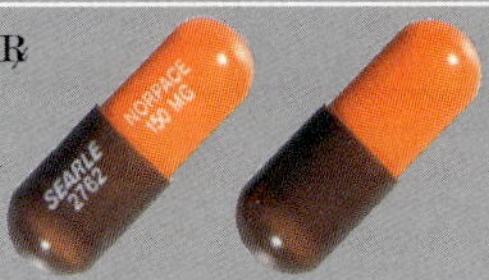

Norpace 150 mg
Searle 2762 150

℞

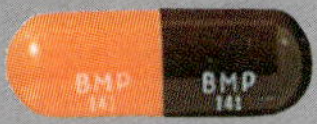

Totacillin 500 mg
SmithKline Beecham BMP 141

℞

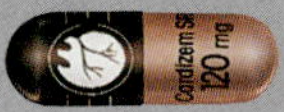

Cardizem SR 120 mg
Hoechst Marion Roussel 120

INDEX

A

Trade names appear in italics. CL indicates color locator page.

B

C

Trade names appear in italics. CL indicates color locator page.

D

H

I

Trade names appear in italics. CL indicates color locator page.

J

K

L

M

N

O

Trade names appear in italics. CL indicates color locator page.

P

Q

R

T

Trade names appear in italics. CL indicates color locator page.

U

V